KEY TO ESSENTIAL TERMINOLOGY

CLIENT ASSESSMENT DATABASE

Provides an overview of the more commonly occurring etiology and coexisting factors associated with a specific medical/surgical diagnosis as well as the signs/symptoms and corresponding diagnostic findings.

NURSING PRIORITIES

Establishes a general ranking of needs/concerns on which the Nursing Diagnoses are ordered in constructing the plan of care. This ranking would be altered according to the individual client situation.

DISCHARGE GOALS

Identifies generalized statements that could be developed into short-term and intermediate goals to be achieved by the client before being "discharged" from nursing care. They may also provide guidance for creating long-term goals for the client to work on after discharge.

NURSING DIAGNOSIS

The general problem/need (diagnosis) is stated without the distinct cause and signs/symptoms, which would be added to create a client diagnostic statement when specific client information is available. For example, when a client displays increased tension, apprehension, quivering voice, and focus on self, the nursing diagnosis of Anxiety might be stated: severe Anxiety, related to unconscious conflict, threat to self-concept as evidenced by statements of increased tension, apprehension; observations of quivering voice, focus on self.

In addition, diagnoses identified within these guides for planning care as actual or risk can be changed or deleted and new diagnoses added, depending entirely on the specific client information.

MAY BE RELATED TO/POSSIBLY EVIDENCED BY

These lists provide the usual/common reasons (etiology) why a particular problem may occur with probable signs/symptoms, which would be used to create the "related to" and "evidenced by" portions of the *client diagnostic statement* when the specific situation is known.

When a risk diagnosis has been identified, signs/symptoms have not yet developed and therefore are not included in the nursing diagnosis statement. However, interventions are provided to prevent progression to an actual problem. The exception to this occurs in the nursing diagnosis risk for Violence, which has possible indicators that reflect the client's risk status.

DESIRED OUTCOMES/EVALUATION CRITERIA—CLIENT WILL

These give direction to client care as they identify what the client or nurse hopes to achieve. They are stated in general terms to permit the practitioner to modify/individualize them by adding time lines and individual client criteria so they become "measurable." For example, "Client will appear relaxed and report anxiety is reduced to a manageable level within 24 hours."

Nursing Outcomes Classification (NOC) labels are also included. The outcome label is selected from a standardized nursing language and serves as a general header for the outcome indicators that follow.

ACTIONS/INTERVENTIONS

NIC (Nursing Interventions Classification) intervention labels are drawn from a standardized nursing language and serve as a general header for the nursing actions that follow.

Nursing actions are divided into independent (those actions that the nurse performs autonomously) and collaborative (those actions that the nurse performs in conjunction with others, such as implementing physician orders) and are ranked in this book from most to least common. When creating the individual plan of care, interventions would normally be ranked to reflect the client's specific needs/situation. In addition, the division of independent/collaborative is arbitrary and is actually dependent on the individual nurse's capabilities and hospital/community standards.

RATIONALE

Although not commonly appearing in client plans of care, rationale has been included here to provide a pathophysiologic basis to assist the nurse in deciding about the relevance of a specific intervention for an individual client situation.

CLINICAL PATHWAY

This abbreviated plan of care or care map is event (task) oriented and provides outcome-based guidelines for goal achievement within a designated length of stay. Several samples have been included to demonstrate alternative planning formats.

NURSING DIAGNOSES ACCEPTED FOR USE AND RESEARCH THROUGH 2006

Activity Intolerance [specify level]
Activity Intolerance, risk for
Adjustment, impaired
Airway Clearance, ineffective
Allergy Response, latex
Allergy response, risk for latex
Anxiety [specify level]
Anxiety, death
Aspiration, risk for
Attachment, risk for impaired parent/infant/child
Autonomic Dysreflexia
Autonomic Dysreflexia, risk for
Body Image, disturbed
Body Temperature, risk for imbalanced
Bowel Incontinence
Breastfeeding, effective
Breastfeeding, ineffective
Breastfeeding, interrupted
Breathing Pattern, ineffective
Cardiac Output, decreased
Caregiver Role Strain
Caregiver Role Strain, risk for
Communication, impaired verbal
Communication, readiness for enhanced
Conflict, decisional (specify)
Conflict, parental role
Confusion, acute
Confusion, chronic
Constipation
Constipation, perceived
Constipation, risk for
Coping, defensive
Coping, ineffective
Coping, readiness for enhanced
Coping, ineffective community
Coping, readiness for enhanced community
Coping, compromised family
Coping, disabled family
Coping, readiness for enhanced family
Death syndrome, risk for sudden infant
Denial, ineffective
Dentition, impaired
Development, risk for delayed
Diarrhea
Disuse Syndrome, risk for
Diversional Activity, deficient
Energy Field disturbed
Environmental Interpretation Syndrome, impaired
Failure to Thrive, adult
Falls, risk for
Family Processes: alcoholism, dysfunctional
Family Processes, interrupted
Family Processes, readiness for enhanced
Fatigue
Fear
Fluid Balance, readiness for enhanced
[Fluid Volume, deficient hyper/hypotonic]
Fluid Volume, deficient [isotonic]
Fluid Volume, excess
Fluid Volume, risk for deficient
Fluid Volume risk for imbalanced
Gas Exchange, impaired
Grieving, anticipatory
Grieving, dysfunctional
Grieving, risk for dysfunctional
Growth & Development, delayed
Growth, risk for disproportionate
Health Maintenance, ineffective
Health-Seeking Behaviors (specify)
Home Maintenance, impaired
Hopelessness
Hyperthermia
Hypothermia
Identity, disturbed personal
Infant Behavior, disorganized
Infant Behavior, readiness for enhanced organized
Infant Behavior, risk for disorganized
Infant Feeding Pattern, ineffective
Infection, risk for
Injury, risk for
Injury, risk for perioperative positioning
Intracranial Adaptive Capacity, decreased
Knowledge, deficient [Learning Need] [specify]
Knowledge [specify], readiness for enhanced
Lifestyle, sedentary
Loneliness, risk for
Memory, impaired
Mobility, impaired bed
Mobility, impaired physical
Mobility, impaired wheelchair
Nausea
Neglect, unilateral
Noncompliance, [Adherence, ineffective] [specify]
Nutrition: less than body requirements, imbalanced
Nutrition: more than body requirements, imbalanced
Nutrition, readiness for enhanced
Nutrition: more than body requirements, risk for imbalanced
Oral Mucous Membrane, impaired
Pain, acute
Pain, chronic
Parenting, impaired
Parenting, readiness for enhanced
Parenting, risk for impaired
Peripheral Neurovascular Dysfunction, risk for
Poisoning, risk for
Post-Trauma Syndrome [specify stage]
Post-Trauma Syndrome, risk for
Powerlessness [specify level]
Powerlessness, risk for
Protection, ineffective
Rape-Trauma Syndrome
Rape-Trauma Syndrome: compound reaction
Rape-Trauma Syndrome: silent reaction
Religiosity, impaired
Religiosity, risk for impaired
Religiosity, readiness for enhanced
Relocation Stress Syndrome
Relocation Stress Syndrome, risk for
Role Performance, ineffective
Self-Care Deficit: bathing/hygiene
Self-Care Deficit: dressing/grooming
Self-Care Deficit: feeding
Self-Care Deficit: toileting
Self-Concept, readiness for enhanced
Self-Esteem, chronic low
Self-Esteem, situational low
Self-Esteem, risk for situational low
Self-Mutilation
Self-Mutilation, risk for
Sensory Perception, disturbed: (specify: visual, auditory, kinesthetic, gustatory, tactile, olfactory)
Sexual Dysfunction
Sexuality Pattern, ineffective
Skin Integrity, impaired
Skin Integrity, risk for impaired
Sleep Deprivation
Sleep, readiness for enhanced
Sleep Pattern, disturbed
Social Interaction, impaired
Social Isolation
Sorrow, chronic
Spiritual Distress
Spiritual Distress, risk for
Spiritual Well-Being, readiness for enhanced
Suffocation, risk for
Suicide, risk for
Surgical Recovery, delayed
Swallowing, impaired
Therapeutic Regimen Management, effective
Therapeutic Regimen Management, ineffective
Therapeutic Regimen Management, ineffective community
Therapeutic Regimen Management, ineffective family
Therapeutic Regimen Management, readiness for enhanced
Thermoregulation, ineffective
Thought Processes, disturbed
Tissue Integrity, impaired
Tissue Perfusion, ineffective (specify type: cerebral, cardiopulmonary, renal, gastrointestinal, peripheral)
Transfer Ability, impaired
Trauma, risk for
Urinary Elimination, impaired
Urinary Elimination, readiness for enhanced
Urinary Incontinence, functional
Urinary Incontinence, reflex
Urinary Incontinence, stress
Urinary Incontinence, total
Urinary Incontinence, urge
Urinary Incontinence, risk for urge
Urinary Retention [acute/chronic]
Ventilation, impaired spontaneous
Ventilatory Weaning Response, dysfunctional
Violence, [actual/] risk for other-directed
Violence, [actual/] risk for self-directed
Walking, impaired
Wandering [specify sporadic or continual]
[ ] author recommendations

NURSING CARE PLANS

GUIDELINES FOR INDIVIDUALIZING CLIENT CARE ACROSS THE LIFE SPAN
EDITION 7

Marilynn E. Doenges, APRN, BC-Retired
Clinical Specialist, Adult Psychiatric/Mental Health Nursing, Retired
Adjunct Faculty
Beth-El College of Nursing and Health Sciences, UCCS
Colorado Springs, Colorado

Mary Frances Moorhouse, RN, MSN, CRRN, LNC
Adjunct Faculty/Clinical Instructor
Pikes Peak Community College
Nurse Consultant/TNT-RN Enterprises
Colorado Springs, Colorado

Alice C. Murr, RN, BSN, LNC
Legal Nurse Consultant
Telephone Triage Nurse
Jackson, Mississippi

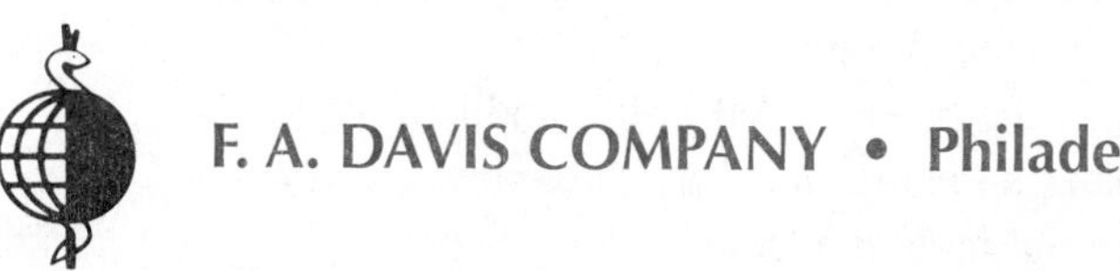

NURSING CARE PLANS, 7th Edition...

The Guideline Approach to Individualized Care Planning

Contains all the elements needed to make individualized patient care choices, while teaching you how to critically analyze each component and create the correct care plan for your patient. More than just a book of Med-Surg care plans—this is an *all-in-one resource* that includes four new care plans, an introduction to Mind Mapping, and a bonus CD-ROM covering all the care plans found in the book (plus 84 only available on the disc) and the top 400 health conditions.

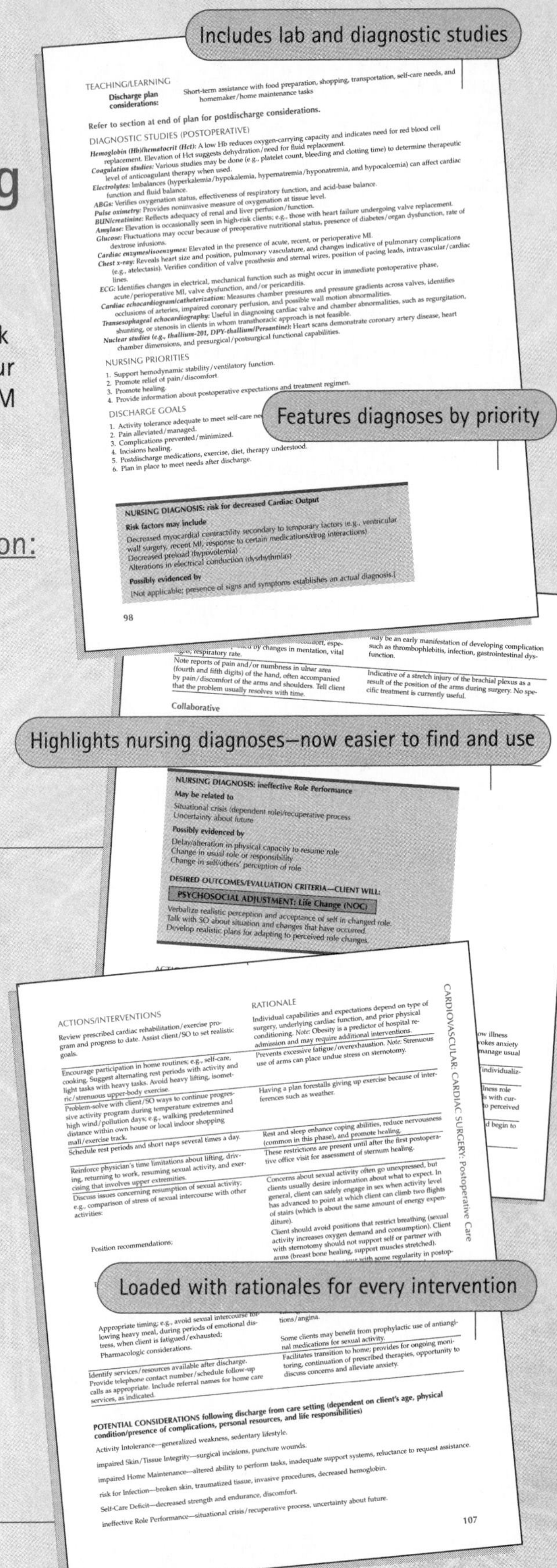

Loaded with care plans, including four new to this edition:

- ⇨ **Obesity Surgery** – Complete coverage of gastric bypass surgery; a procedure becoming more common across the country.
- ⇨ **Fluid and Electrolyte Imbalances** – Clear and definitive care planning covering the role fluid and electrolyte imbalances play in many disorders.
- ⇨ More Life Span coverage – **Extended Care** and **Pediatric** care plans are also included.

Here's just a sample of what you'll find in the pages that follow...

- ⇨ Care plans you can adapt and customize to fit patient needs:
  - CD-ROM includes all 116 care plans from the book plus 84 more—200 care plans!
    - 115 Medical/Surgical care plans
    - 34 Psychiatric care plans
    - 50 Maternal/Newborn care plans
    - Pediatric Considerations
- ⇨ Prioritized nursing diagnoses to help students write measurable goal statements
- ⇨ Focused on the patient, and applies the body system approach to care planning
- ⇨ Guidelines covering total patient needs—physical, cultural, sexual, nutritional, and psychosocial
- ⇨ Updated with the latest NANDA, NIC, and NOC content
- ⇨ New emphasis on complementary therapies
- ⇨ New chapter on mind mapping

Includes a Bonus CD-ROM—a Valuable Package of Resources You Can Use!

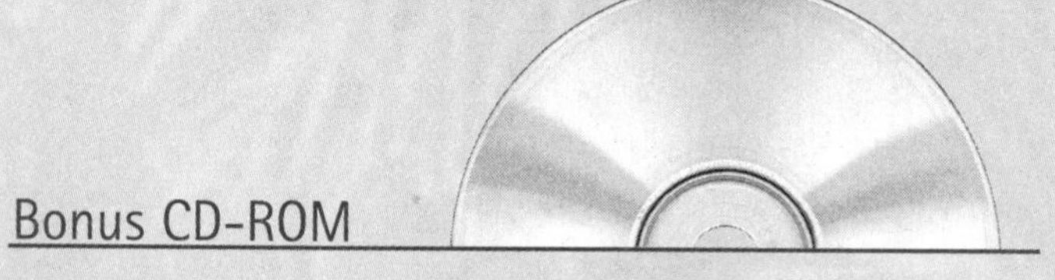

Bonus CD-ROM

You will find **200 Care Plans** with an index of the top **400 Diseases/Disorders** and their associated nursing diagnoses. To help make navigating the CD-ROM even easier, we've provided a complete Table of Contents to the CD in the book. The CD is a robust resource that will save valuable time and help you put all the pieces together quickly and accurately!

Main Menu

Care Plan Content
Select this link to view Medical Surgical, Maternal/NewBorn and Psychological care plans to print and customize.

Diseases/Disorders
Select this link to view 400 Conditions with Associated Nursing Diagnoses.

◂Help▸

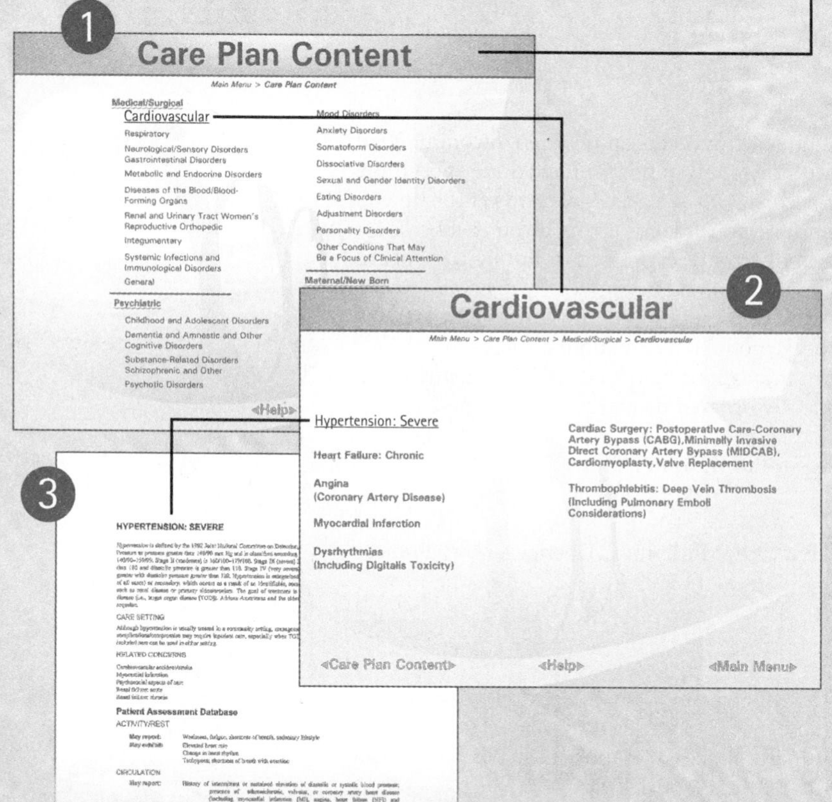

200 Care Plans

The bonus CD-ROM contains 200 care plans that students can adapt and customize to fit their needs. It also includes four NEW care plans covering obesity surgery, fluids and electrolytes, extended care, and pediatric considerations. A complete package including all 116 care plans featured in the book *plus 84 additional found only on the CD-ROM*—that's 200 care plans!

400 Diseases/Disorders

A complete index of 400 Disorders and Health Conditions, with their associated nursing diagnoses, is also included. The menu screen features a user-friendly A to Z listing reflecting all specialty areas, with associated nursing diagnoses, that include "related to" and "evidenced by" statements.

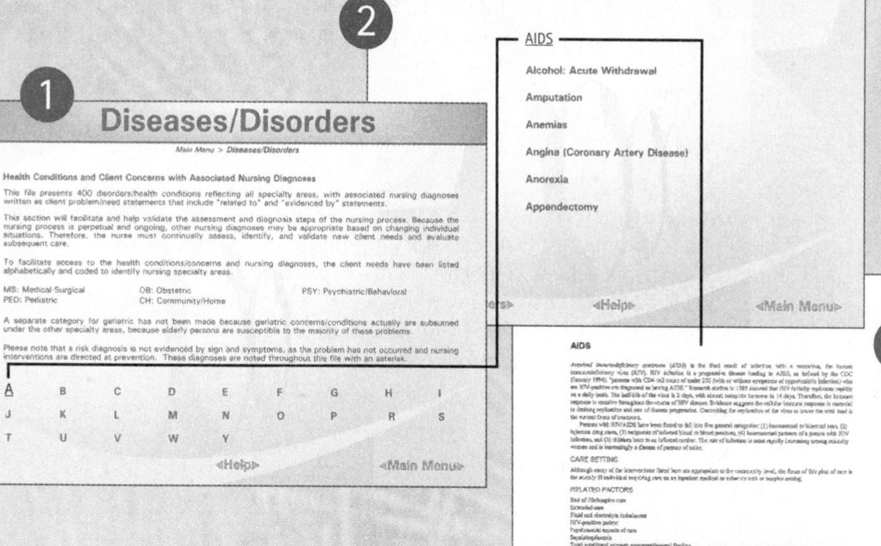

Includes 3+ books in 1, that feature:

- 115 Medical/Surgical care plans
- 34 Psychiatric care plans
- 50 Maternal/Newborn care plans
- Pediatric Considerations

F. A. Davis Company
1915 Arch Street
Philadelphia, PA 19103
www.fadavis.com

Printed in the United States of America

Last digit indicates print number: 10 9 8 7 6 5 4 3

Acquisitions Editor: Joanne P. DaCunha, RN, MSN
Developmental Editor: Alan Sorkowitz
Art and Design Manager: Carolyn O'Brien

Library of Congress Cataloging-in-Publication Data

Doenges, Marilynn E., 1922-
Nursing care plans : guidelines for individualizing client care/Marilynn E. Doenges, Mary Frances Moorhouse, Alice C. Murr.—Ed. 7.
p. ; cm.
Includes bibliographical references and index.
ISBN 10: 0-8036-1294-X ISBN 13: 978-0-8036-1294-5
1. Intensive nursing care—Handbooks, manuals, etc. 2. Nursing care plans—Handbooks, manuals, etc.
[DNLM: 1. Patient Care Planning—Handbooks. 2. Nursing Process—Handbooks. WY 49 D651na 2006] I. Moorhouse, Mary Frances, 1947-II. Geissler-Murr, Alice, 1946-III. Title.
RT49.D64 2006
610.73—dc22

2005036714

DEDICATION

To our spouses, children, parents, and friends, who much of the time have had to manage without us while we work as well as having to cope with our struggles and frustrations.

The Doenges families: the late Dean, whose support and encouragement is sorely missed; Jim; Barbara and Bob Lanza; David, Monita, Matthew, and Tyler; John, Holly, Nicole, and Kelsey; and the Daigle family, Nancy, Jim, Jennifer, Brandon, Anna, Will, and Henry Smith-Daigle, and Jonathan and Kim.

The Moorhouse family: Jan, Paul, Jason, Thenderlyn, Alexa, and Mary.

To Mary and Marilynn, couldn't have done it without you. In loving memory of my parents, who were my biggest promoters in my early days of writing. To my children and grandchildren with love. You have expanded my horizons so wonderfully! Alice

To our FAD family, especially Bob Martone and Bob Butler, whose support is so vital to the completion of a project of this magnitude. And to Alan Sorkowitz, the one who really kept us all together, our go-to-guy when the going got tough. We are fourtunate to have you working with us.

To the nurses we are writing for, who daily face the challenge of caring for the acutely ill client and are looking for a practical way to organize and document this care. We believe that nursing diagnosis and these guides will help.

To NANDA and to the international nurses who are developing and using nursing diagnoses—here we come!

Finally, to the late Mary Lisk Jeffries, who initiated the original project. The memory of our early friendship and struggles remains with us. We miss her and wish she were here to see the growth of the profession and how nursing diagnosis has contributed to the process.

REVIEWERS FOR THE BOOK

JANE V. ARNDT, MS, RN, CWOCN
Nurse Clinician, Enterostomal Therapy
Poudre Valley Hospital
Ft. Collins, Colorado

JENNIFER AVERY
Senior Nursing Student
College of the Sequoias
Visalia, California

BETH HAMSTRA, RN, CNS, RCIS, PHD
Clinical Manager Invasive Cardiology
Memorial Hospital
Colorado Springs, Colorado

SANDRA HARPER, RN, CCRN
Rehabilitation Care Specialist
HealthSouth Rehabilitation Hospital
Colorado Springs, Colorado

CHRISTIE A. HINDS, MSN, APRN-BC
Primary Care Nurse Practitioner
Health Essentials
Chattanooga, Tennesse

SUSAN JANTY, VN, ACRN
SCD/HIV Medical Coordinator
El Paso Department of Heath and Environment
Colorado Springs, Colorado

LAURA RUTH TEIGEN JOHNSON, RN, MNE, CNOR
Perioperative Services Manager
Colorado Springs, Colorado

LENORA KRAFT, RN
Surgical Clinical Manager
Penrose St-Francis Hospital
Colorado Springs, Colorado

SUZANNE LOGAN, MS, RD
Manager, Dietetic Internship
Clinical Manager
Penrose–St. Francis Health Services
Colorado Springs, Colorado

MARY BETH FLYNN-MAKIC, RN, MS, CNS, CCRN
Clinical Nurse Specialist/Educator
University of Colorado Hospital
Senior Instructor
University of Colorado Health Science Center School of Nursing
Denver, Colorado

KIMBERLY TUCKER PFENNIGS, MA, BAN, RN
Pikes Peak Mental Health
Program Manager, Lighthouse Assessment Center
Adult Treatment Units
Colorado Springs, Colorado

GILDA ROLLS-DELLINGER, RN
Staff Nurse, Skin, Wound, and Burn Team
Penrose-St. Francis Health Services
Colorado Springs, Colorado

ROCHELLE SALMORE, MSN, RN, CGRN, CAN, BC
Clincal Manager
Digestive Disease Center
Penrose–St. Francis Health Services
Colorado Springs, Colorado

TRACY STEINBERG, RN, MSN, CNS
Liver Transplant Coordinator
Division of Transplant Surgery
University of Colorado Health Sciences Center
Denver, Colorado

GERI L. TIERNEY, RN, BSN, ONC
Nursing Simulation Lab Coordinator
Pikes Peak Community College
Past-President National Association of Orthopaedic Nurses
Colorado Springs, Colorado

KATHLEEN H. WINDER, RN, BSN
Clinical Manager, Pediatric Specialty Clinic
Memorial Hospital
Colorado Springs, Colorado

ANNE ZOBEC, MS, RN, CS, NP, AOCN
Oncology Nurse Practitioner
The Oncology Clinic, P. C.
Colorado Springs, Colorado

REVIEWERS FOR THE CD-ROM

CYNTHIA ASKVIG, RN, MS
Nursing Faculty
Pikes Peak Community College
Colorado Springs, Colorado

SUSAN JANTY, VN, ACRN
Board Certified in HIV/AIDS Nursing
SCD/HIV Medical Coordinator
El Paso Department of Heath and Evironment
Colorado Springs, Colorado

NOLA LANGE, MS, APRN, BC
Adjunct Psychiatric Instructor
Pikes Peak Community College
Colorado Springs, Colorado

JILL MEIDER, APRN, BC
Adjunct Instructor
Pikes Peak Community College
Colorado Springs, Colorado

SUSAN M. MOBERLY, RNC, BSN, ICCE
Maternal/Newborn Nurse Consultant
ICEA Certified Childbirth Educator
Pikes Peak Choices in Childbirth
Colorado Springs, Colorado

LESLIE MURTAGH, MS, APRN, BC
Board Certified Child and Adolescent
Clinical Nurse Specialist
Casper, Wyoming

ACKNOWLEDGEMENTS

JOE RUSKIN, RPH
Colorado Springs, Colorado

JAMES I. BURNS, BS
Systems Analyst
Disaster Science
Coronado, California

THE LATE NANCY LEA CARTER, RN, MA
Clinical Nurse, Orthopedics
Albuquerque, New Mexico

INTRODUCTION

We are often asked how we came to write the Care Plan books. In the late 1970s we were involved with some publishing efforts that did not come to fruition. In this work we had included care plans, so ensuing discussions revolved around the need for a Care Plan book. We spent a year struggling to write care plans before we realized our major difficulty was the lack of standardized labels for client problems. At that time, we were given a list of nursing diagnoses from the Clearinghouse for Nursing Diagnosis, which became the North American Nursing Diagnosis Association (NANDA), and is now NANDA International. This work answered our need by providing concise titles that could be used in various care plans and followed across the spectrum of client care. We believed these nursing diagnosis labels would both define and focus nursing care.

Because we had long been involved in direct client care in our nursing careers, we knew there was a need for guidelines to assist nurses in planning care. As we began to write, our focus was the nurse in a small rural community who at 2 AM needed the answer to a burning question for her client and had few resources available. We believed the book would give definition and direction to the development and use of individualized nursing care. Thus, in the first edition, the theory of nursing process, diagnosis, and intervention was brought to the clinical setting for implementation by the nurse. We also anticipated that nursing students would appreciate having access to these guidelines as they struggled to learn how to give nursing care. Therefore, we did not consider the book to be an end in itself, but rather a vehicle for the continuing growth and development of the profession. Obviously we struck a chord and met a need because the first edition was an immediate success.

In becoming involved with NANDA, we acknowledged that maintaining a strict adherence to their wording, while adding our own clearly identified recommendations, would help develop this neophyte standardized language and would promote the growth of nursing as a profession. We have continued our involvement with NANDA, promoting the use of the language by practicing nurses in the United States and around the world and encouraging them to participate in updating and refining the diagnoses. The wide use of our books within the student population has supported and fostered the acceptance of both the activity of diagnosing client problems/needs and the use of standardized language.

Nursing instructors initially expressed concern that students would simply copy the plans of care and thus limit their learning. However, as students used the plans to individualize care and to develop practice priorities and client care outcomes, the book met with more acceptance. Instructors began not only to recommend the book, but also to adopt it as an adjunct text. Today, it remains the best-selling nursing care plan book recognized as an important adjunct for student learning.

In writing the second edition, we recognized the need for an assessment tool with a nursing focus instead of a medical focus. Not finding one that met our needs, we constructed our own. To facilitate problem identification, we categorized the nursing diagnosis labels and the information obtained in the client assessment database into a framework entitled "Diagnostic Divisions." Our philosophy is to provide a way in which to gather information and to intervene beneficially, while thinking about the rationale for every action we take and the standardized language that best expresses it. When nurses do this they are defining their practice and are able to identify it with a code and charge for it. By doing this, we promote client protection (quality of care issue), provide for the definition and protection of nursing practice, and the protection of the individual (legal implications). The latter is important because we live in a litigation-minded society and the nurse's license and livelihood are at stake.

One of the most significant achievements in the healthcare field over the past 20 or more years has been the emergence of the nurse as an active coordinator and initiator of client care. Although the transition from physician's helpmate to healthcare professional has been painfully slow and is not yet complete, the importance of the nurse within the system can no longer be denied or ignored. Today's nurse designs nursing care interventions that move the total client toward improved health and maximum independence.

Professional care standards and healthcare providers and consumers will continue to increase the expectations for nurses' performance. Each day brings new challenges in client care and the struggle to understand the human responses to actual and potential health problems. To meet these challenges competently, the nurse must have up-to-date assessment skills and a working knowledge of pathophysiologic concepts concerning the common diseases/conditions presented. We believe that this book is a tool, providing a means of attaining that competency.

In the past, plans of care were viewed principally as learning tools for students and seemed to have little relevance after graduation. However, the need for a written format to communicate and document client care has been recognized in all care settings. In addition, healthcare policy, governmental regulations, and third-party payor requirements have created the need to validate many things, including appropriateness of care provided, staffing patterns, and monetary charges. Thus, although the student's "case studies" were considered to be too cumbersome to be practical in the clinical setting, it has long been recognized that the client plan of care meets certain needs and therefore its appropriate use was validated.

The practicing nurse, as well as the nursing student, can welcome this text as a ready reference in clinical practice. It is designed for use in the acute care, community, and homecare settings. It is organized by systems for easy reference.

Chapter 1 examines current issues and trends and their implications for the nursing profession. An overview of cultural, community, sociologic, and ethical concepts affecting the nurse is included. The importance of the nurse's role in collaboration and coordination with other healthcare professionals is integrated throughout the plans of care.

Chapter 2 reviews the historical use of the nursing process in formulating plans of care and the nurse's role in the delivery of that care. Nursing diagnoses, outcomes, and interventions are discussed to assist the nurse in understanding her or his role in the nursing process. In this book, we have also linked NANDA diagnoses with Nursing Intervention Classification (NIC) and Nursing Outcomes Classification (NOC) language.

Chapter 3 discusses care plan construction and describes the use and adaptation of the guides presented in this book. A nursing-based assessment tool is provided to assist the nurse in identifying appropriate nursing diagnoses. A sample client situation (with individual database and a corresponding plan of care) is included to demonstrate how critical thinking is used to adapt nursing process theory to practice. Finally, a dynamic and creative approach for developing and documenting the planning of care is also included. Mind Mapping is a new technique or learning tool provided to assist you in achieving a holistic view of your client, enhance your critical thinking skills, and facilitate the creative process of planning client care.

Chapters 4 through 15 present plans of care that include information from multiple disciplines to assist the nurse in providing holistic care. Each plan includes a Client Assessment Database (presented in a nursing format) and associated Diagnostic Studies. After the database is collected, Nursing Priorities are sifted from the information to help focus and structure the care. Discharge Goals are created to identify what should be generally accomplished by the time of discharge from the care setting. Next, Desired Client Outcomes are stated in measurable behavioral terms to evaluate both the client's progress and the effectiveness of care provided.

The nursing diagnoses listed in the plans of care are developed by identifying "may be related to" and "possibly evidenced by" factors that provide an explanation of client problems/needs.

Corresponding actions/interventions are designed to promote resolution of the identified client needs. The nurse acting independently or collaboratively within the health team then uses a decision-making model to organize and prioritize nursing interventions. No attempt is made in this book to indicate whether independent or collaborative actions come first because this must be dictated by the individual situation. We do, however, believe that every collaborative action has a component that the nurse must identify and for which nursing has responsibility and accountability.

Rationales for the nursing actions (which are not required in the customary plan of care) are included to assist the nurse in deciding whether the interventions are appropriate for an individual client. Additional information is provided to further assist the nurse in identifying and planning for rehabilitation as the client progresses toward discharge and across all care settings. A bibliography is provided as a reference and to allow further research as desired.

This book is designed for students who will find the plans of care helpful as they learn and develop skills in applying the nursing process and using nursing diagnoses. It will complement their classroom work and support the critical thinking process. The book also provides a ready reference for the practicing nurse as a catalyst for thought in planning, evaluating, and documenting care.

As a final note, this book is not intended to be a procedure manual, and efforts have been made to avoid detailed descriptions of techniques or protocols that might be viewed as individual or regional in nature. Instead the reader is referred to a procedure manual or text covering Standards of Care if detailed direction is desired.

As we always say when we sign a book, "Use and enjoy." MD, MM, and AM

CONTENTS IN BRIEF

A TABLE OF CONTENTS INCLUDING NURSING DIAGNOSES FOLLOWS.

DETAILED CONTENTS

CONTENTS OF THE CD-ROM

1 CHAPTER

Issues and Trends in Medical/Surgical Nursing

THE EVER-CHANGING HEALTHCARE ENVIRONMENT

Understanding trends in client care and dealing with the current issues in nursing require looking at the overall trends in healthcare practice and the ongoing restructuring of healthcare delivery systems within the healthcare industry.

Factors driving the changes in healthcare include the rising cost of care, the ever-increasing numbers of uninsured/underinsured healthcare consumers, and the need for allocation of limited healthcare dollars and resources. In addition, other factors, such as technologic advances, ever-enlarging populations with special needs; changing roles for, and shortages of, healthcare providers; ethical issues associated with living in a technologic age; the potential conflict of the client's or family's wishes and prudent medical care; and liability concerns will continue to affect nursing practice in the future.

Nurses must be aware of these influences and be actively involved in the formulation of policies and legislation affecting practice. As the definers of nursing practice, nurses must set the standards of practice so that quality nursing care is provided with a high degree of client satisfaction and within the constraints of available resources.

HEALTHCARE COSTS AND THE ALLOCATION OF RESOURCES

Healthcare expenditures continue to rise. Both government and private payors of healthcare are pursuing various methods of cost containment. One of the most widespread solutions for cost containment has been the implementation of managed care services, and health maintenance organizations (HMOs) or physician provider organizations (PPOs). In some cases, special incentives are provided for the consumer to promote wellness or manage disease risk factors (e.g., providing health club memberships or smoking cessation programs). There may also be provider incentives such as bonus checks when the cost of care is below projected costs for the program or the individual provider.

Most insurance plans require preauthorization for many services and/or procedures based on established protocols, and encourage early discharge from acute or hospital services, preferring to provide payment for outpatient services, or in some cases, in-home care. Third-party payors are negotiating contracts with healthcare providers, including physicians, provider agencies, and facilities, in order to reduce reimbursement rates or even to capitate fees (providing services for a preset fee regardless of actual cost). This method of payment is based on both the number and specific demographics of the insured population. At the same time, third-party payors continue to pay for extra care associated with medical errors, but seem reluctant to pay for best practices or increase reimbursement in ways that can reduce untoward outcomes.

Public Law 98–21 changed the method of payment for federally subsidized (Medicare) inpatient healthcare services from a cost-based retrospective payment system (payment for services after care was provided) to a prospective payment system based on 467 diagnoses or diagnosis-related groups, referred to as DRGs. Upgrades to this payment system have been made to better reflect the severity of client condition/care needs (known as all-patient-related, or APR-DRGs). However, reimbursement remains below billed costs. Most states are considering or have developed options to similarly curb Medicaid reimbursement.

Finally, although the federal government has recently agreed to provide a measure of funding to states located along the southern U.S. border to reimburse facilities for services provided to undocumented aliens, the high cost of emergent care has required some hospitals to engage in cost-shifting to insurance carriers and cash pay clients, or in some cases, to even close emggergency departments. Adults who lack health insurance coverage are more likely to rate their health status as poor or fair, and are less likely to often rely on emergent care, receive preventive services, cancer screenings, or dental care than adults with insurance, increasing their overall care costs (State Health, 2002).

MANAGED CARE: RESTRUCTURING HEALTHCARE

In recent years, these changes in reimbursement and the practice of managed healthcare delivery have required hospitals to restructure. They adopted methods used in industry (such as reengineering and work redesign) or used methods developed specifically for the healthcare arena. The intent was to implement change aimed at reducing costs without jeopardizing quality or consumer satisfaction.

Restructuring the workforce and the client care system was initially accomplished through mergers and consolidation of services, as well as downsizing professional staff by means of normal attrition, early retirement programs, and layoffs. The responsibility for hands-on care in many settings shifted away from registered nurses (RNs) to other providers such as licensed practical nurses (LPNs) and unlicensed assistive personnel (UAPs).

Many healthcare professionals expressed great concern regarding the effect of downsizing on the quality of care provided, noting the decline in healthcare consumer satisfaction reported on discharge surveys. Furthermore, a 1999 study by the Institute of Medicine conservatively projects that 98,000 people a year die from medical errors. In contrast, other studies (e.g., Blegen et al., 1998; Yang, 2003) have shown that a higher ratio of professional nursing staff improves client outcomes and can lower medication errors and adverse events such as falls, and may even reduce mortality rates. However, facilities have been slow to improve staffing ratios (partly due to nursing shortages in some geographic areas and nursing specialties), resulting in increased stress for staff and higher rates of errors and adverse incidents.

Responding to these concerns, many healthcare providers have formed collaborative practice teams whose goal is to revise the client care delivery system by reducing redundancy of services, eliminating nonproductive activities, and relocating ancillary services such as laboratory and radiography to client care areas. The addition of a pharmacist as an active member of the healthcare team has been shown to reduce preventable drug reactions by 78% (Leape and Berwick, 2005). Employers have implemented cross-training of staff to enhance provider scope of services and qualifications. The reduction in the number of professional nurses providing direct client care has necessitated creative problem solving to find ways to help nurses "work smarter" and safer.

The federal government has directed facilities to expand computer capabilities to reduce errors and untoward outcomes by improving order entry, streamlining documentation, facilitating data retrieval, and developing structured care methodologies. Computerizing physician order entry can reduce prescriptions errors by as much as 81% (Leape and Berwick, 2005). Access to computers, whether by central location, bedside terminal, or hand-held units, allows for the immediate entry and retrieval of client data by care providers. Beepers, pagers, and cordless or cell phones have facilitated communication between the nurse and other healthcare team members and clients, reducing response time for meeting client needs. Documentation time can be reduced through use of detailed flow sheets, charting by exception, standardized and computerized plans of care, and/or developing clinical pathways (care maps).

Clinical pathways support the coordination and evaluation of interdisciplinary care through the identification of specific outcomes (important in today's focus of "outcomes-based" client care) and corresponding activities for a given condition/procedure based on the DRG or the agency expected length of stay (ELOS). Their use provides a mechanism for modifying care to reflect current clinical practice expectations based on clinical innovations and research findings. Clinical pathways may also be useful for timely identification of actual or potential outlyers, thus allowing reallocation of resources to maximize client outcomes while controlling costs. However, although clinical pathways are useful for clients who fall within an expected course of illness, their lack of flexibility to accommodate preexisting multiple diagnoses (e.g., coronary bypass surgery for a client with diabetes mellitus and chronic renal insufficiency) or the development of complications generally precludes their use when greater individualization of care is required. In addition, because pathways generally address a specific episode of care, they may not focus on care over a continuum.

Other structured care methodologies promoting standardization of care processes include the use of algorithms, guidelines, or protocols (standing orders). In the field of medicine, criteria have been developed such as the computer program APACHE (Acute Physiology and Chronic Health Evaluation) to assist providers in choosing appropriate treatment options and to help allocate resources. This program provides data on the likely outcomes of various treatments in specific client populations. Thus, reimbursement could conceivably be tied to a scoring system reflecting the likelihood of survival and corresponding treatment protocols.

The advancement of knowledge continues with the work of the U.S. Department of Health and Human Services' Agency for Healthcare Research and Quality (formerly the Agency for Health Care Policy and Research), whose purpose is to enhance the quality, appropriateness, and effectiveness of healthcare services. Multidisciplinary panels of clinicians (including nurses) created clinical practice and client teaching guidelines addressing specific client care situations. These guidelines are intended not only to assist in the prevention, diagnosis, and management of clinical conditions, but also to provide a resource by which client care can be evaluated, the provider is held accountable, and reimbursement is justified. The agency now serves as a repository for research resources and documents to provide a comprehensive database for the development of evidence-based clinical practice guidelines.

These processes tend to stabilize care practices and system processes and are designed to improve outcomes. By shifting some routine or nondirect care activities from the nurse to another provider, even the client or family, better use may be made of nursing time and efforts. In addition, promoting client self-care (through participation in the planning of care and mutual goal setting as well as the self-administration of some therapies/medications) provides opportunities for the client/family to maximize their control of/contribution to their health status, improve their acute care experience, and demonstrate newly learned skills.

The need to provide services at lower costs has forced providers to seek alternatives to inpatient care. Currently, the emphasis is on outpatient services and affiliations with other provider groups to provide a wider continuum of client care. Healthcare networks have been created, some of which encompass a major hub or tertiary hospital and smaller affiliating hospitals, freestanding emergency clinics and surgical centers, subacute units, rehabilitation centers, long-term care facilities, and home-care agencies. These networks are designed to meet all the client's healthcare needs while keeping all the revenue within the network. However, this practice has the potential of limiting competition, thereby causing the decline of independent healthcare agencies, especially when physicians, pharmacies, and equipment supply companies join one network.

One innovation was the creation of Community Nursing Organization (CNO) demonstration projects that offered direct access to professional nursing care and nursing coordination of all services with community-based care delivery. The Centers for Medicare and Medicaid Services (CMS), formerly the Health Care Financing Administration (HCFA), developed this nursing model to provide Medicare beneficiaries with a specific package of services (including prevention and health promtion) plus case management to promote health and manage acute or chronic illnesses under a capitated payment methodology. At four demonstration sites, all members were seen a minimum of twice a year to evaluate their health and to develop or check on progress of a plan of care. The final report to Congress (Abt Associates, 2003) revealed that although an overwhelming majority of enrollees in the CNOs were satisfied with the care received and believed that the services helped with health needs and problems, the CNOs actually significantly increased the average monthly Medicare spending per client instead of decreasing costs. Further study is required to determine if decreasing the capitated rate can reduce costs without negatively impacting client satisfaction.

Significant changes in client care management are taking place because of implementation of case management, disease-state management, and evidence-based care. Case management services are now provided across all settings from case managers employed by insurers to entrepreneurial individuals engaged in "continuum of care" specialty areas and alternate sites, including outpatient, subacute, and home care.

Healthcare-delivery systems use managed care to keep clients out of acute care hospitals by providing early intervention treatment, and by using less costly services within the network. Whether the case manager is a physician, nurse, or insurance adjuster, all individuals involved in care are responsible for evaluating both the therapeutic benefit and cost effectiveness of the services provided. This need is especially critical for end-of-life care, for which a high percentage of healthcare dollars are spent.

NURSING CARE COSTS

Nurses have always been mainstays of care for people throughout the life span and especially at the end of their lives. They continue to play a vital role in promoting responsible, appropriate, and ethical healthcare.

Today, the nurse's attention is focused on providing nursing care to clients within the guidelines of prospective reimbursement and capitation, scarce dollars, limited time, reduced beds and staff, and restricted numbers of therapy and home-care visits. Quantifying the contribution of nursing to client care requires identification of the level of nursing care necessary for each client and translating that into direct billing of services rendered. In those facilities/agencies already billing for nursing services, the client plan of care is an integral part of the justification of nursing care costs.

The "what" and "how" of the work of nursing have been explained in part in a number of existing publications that help operationalize the work of nursing. NANDA International (formerly The North American Nursing Diagnosis Association) developed a taxonomy in 1989 that began a classification scheme to categorize and classify nursing diagnostic labels, which was subsequently revised in 2000. In 1992, the Iowa Intervention Project: Nursing Interventions Classification (NIC) directed our focus to the content and process of nursing care by identifying and standardizing some of the direct care activities nurses perform. A second group, the Iowa Outcomes Project: Nursing Outcomes Classification (NOC), addresses client outcomes responsive to and associated with nursing interventions.

EARLY DISCHARGE

Clients are discharged from acute care as soon as they are out of danger or their condition is stabilized, but they may still require specialized care. Subacute or transitional units provide routine services (such as monitoring), ongoing therapies, and complex care (such as intravenous therapy, pain and wound management, airway care, and ventilator weaning), rehabilitation services, and postsurgical recovery care.

Shorter hospital stays have also shifted recovery care to the home setting. Families are expected to be more involved in postdischarge care. Although the rate of nosocomial infections may decline, clients could be "abandoned" or recovery delayed or prolonged if the family's personal resources cannot meet the new challenges associated with the recovery process.

AGING POPULATION

Individuals are living longer and often more active lives. As a result they expect access to procedures such as coronary artery bypass, total joint replacements, aggressive cancer care, and other interventions that in the past were not recommended in the presence of advanced age. The increased mean age of clients requiring hospitalization necessitates some changes in the way their healthcare is provided. A general lack of knowledge among healthcare providers regarding special needs of the elderly, along with limited resources to meet these needs and the high incidence of adverse events (such as confusion, falls, and incontinence), can contribute to instances of suboptimal client care. At the least, these factors can cause prolonged facility stays, and increase the number and complexity of treatments, readmissions, and adverse outcomes. To this end, the nursing profession is working to develop models that will improve the care provided to this population (e.g., Nurses Improving Care to the Hospitalized Elderly [NICHE] Project). The provision of primary nurse case managers to follow chronically ill clients across the continuum of care (and other projects such as the CNO) work to ensure that elderly clients are not lost to follow-up and receive ongoing monitoring for timely, cost-effective intervention.

Healthcare decision making has changed dramatically in recent decades, with an explicit acknowledgment of the client's right to determine the course of care. In the nursing profession, there has been a long-standing allegiance to the client's role in decision making, but nurses, especially those in elder care, fear that the interpretation and use of advance directives are creating ethical conflicts regarding the withdrawal or withholding of treatment or care, especially when the client is concerned about being a "burden to others." Living wills and advance directives cannot be expected to anticipate all situations that clients may encounter; however, they can provide information to a proxy (named in a medical durable power of attorney) to help in the decision-making process. Even with advance directives in place, clients have a right to change their minds and redefine their wishes based on changes in their health status/care options.

TECHNOLOGIC ADVANCES

Technology continues to evolve at an astounding rate in both treatment and equipment. The purpose of technology is to improve clinical decision making and symptom management, facilitate early detection/prevention of illness, and enhance self-care and client outcomes. Robots are being used to dispense medications in pharmacies and to assist with surgical procedures such as coronary artery bypass, mitral valve repair, and prostate removal. Clients undergoing minimally invasive surgery report less pain, have less blood loss and scarring, have shorter lengths of stay, and report faster healing.

The use of in-room cameras and computers combined with video conferencing (eICU) to monitor the vital signs and status of multiple clients in intensive care units promotes earlier recognition of changes and timely response by nurses and physicians, improving client outcomes and reducing mortality rates. Biventricular pacing for cardiac resynchronization is available, although underused, for the treatment of clients with classes 3 and 4 heart failure. Brain stimulators are being used to treat movement disorders such as Parkinson's disease, dystonia, and essential tremors. And implantable insulin pumps are reducing or delaying the complications associated with type 1 diabetus mellitus.

In the near future, the expanded use of monoclonal antibodies to carry chemotherapy agents or radionuclides to cancer cells will reduce adverse reactions and possibly the need for acute care. Endotoxin antibodies (immune system molecules that can mediate sepsis) and gene therapies are being developed that can manage or even eliminate hereditary/degenerative diseases, thereby reducing high-cost therapy needs. Equipment developments that allow clients to leave acute care settings more quickly include user-friendly ventilators, smaller implantable ventilator-assist devices, and artificial hearts. The cost of care and the incidence of complications or adverse outcomes have been reduced for many clients with the use of such procedures as noninvasive intracranial pressure monitoring, tube locators to verify placement of catheters or enteral tubes, and bedside monitoring of many laboratory studies (such as electrolytes, blood urea nitrogen, hematocrit, glucose, and coagulation times).

Additionally, point-of-care computer systems are being refined in an effort to cut documentation time, and to track nursing time for the costing of care. Computers providing real-time updating of the client plan of care enable the nurse to process data from monitoring activities and facilitate evaluation of the effectiveness of nursing actions and other therapies.

Telehealth is being used in the community to not only triage the needs of large populations, but also to provide direct client care to underserved areas via long-distance communication lines. Video conferencing, the Internet, and interactive voice-response systems are being used to monitor chronically ill clients in their own homes.

Finally, work is progressing toward the creation of a computerized patient record (CPR) or electronic health record (EHR) that will provide a composite "cradle to grave" record for each individual accessing healthcare in this country. However, many questions and concerns remain about online security and privacy.

We are living in an age of escalating uncertainty and tension. Scientific and technologic advances we so covet are the same advances that strip life of its simplicity. In the future, technologies can and will be created to support and, in some cases, replace dependent and interdependent activities of nursing. As a result of the efficiencies afforded by advances in automation and information management, the focus of nursing practice could shift from primarily task-oriented client interactions. Concrete activities, such as inserting an intravenous line, assessing for respiratory sounds, and providing client teaching, although vital, do not reflect what nurses believe and value as the most important elements of practice. For even in a technologically driven healthcare system, clients will always feel the need to be comforted, listened to, and treated with dignity and respect.

Nurses have long placed emphasis on the psychosocial, spiritual, and physical needs of their clients within the medical regimen. Today, individuals spend billions of dollars annually for therapies (ranging from guided imagery and meditation to homeopathy and acupuncture) not generally provided by their physicians or approved by their Health Maintenance Organizations. As technology changes and more people become knowledgeable partners in healthcare, many direct their therapies (challenging therapeutic plans developed by healthcare providers or withdrawing from established medical care), choosing alternative therapies and modalities. Nurses need to be knowledgeable and open minded regarding complementary/alternative therapies—supporting client choices and learning and evaluating new techniques as appropriate. Although nurses and clients alike are turning to the Internet for medical information and therapeutic options, this resource can be a double-edged sword because data provided may or may not be accurate. Therefore, nurses need to be aware and knowledgeable regarding various sites in order to direct their clients to reputable and valid resources.

FUTURE OF NURSING

Healthcare reform remains the focus of much writing and debate in this new century. Questions still abound about what constitutes healthcare reform. Whether brought about by statute, insurance payors, or healthcare providers, the changes in healthcare delivery are continuing and far reaching. These changes are, and should be, of great concern to nurses.

We, the authors, are nurses who still believe that a nursing perspective is essential if nurses are to position themselves for a role in future healthcare-delivery systems. As Virginia Henderson said, "The beauty of nursing is the combination of the heart, head, and hands" (Buerhaus, 1998). We are opposed to any system that reduces or eliminates the role of nursing. Clients depend on the nurse to advocate for the rights of the client and the quality of care provided.

In general, the public's image of nursing remains positive; however, we can fall short of meeting the public's expectations because people are sometimes unaware of nurses' varied capabilities or their advanced practice potential. Although the public expects nurses to demonstrate technical competence and academic knowledge, it is also now demanding better consumer service; that is, friendliness, attention to the client's personal or special needs, concern for privacy, information about tests and therapies, and inclusion of the family in the information loop. As the number of RNs in acute care facilities declines, and as they are replaced with less knowledgeable client care providers, nurses need to delegate and supervise appropriately, using team members effectively and safely. Nurses, who now have less time for nonclinical activities, are nonetheless spending more time collaborating with a wide variety of healthcare professionals to manage and coordinate care, as well as to communicate data regarding effectiveness of therapies. Nurses are interacting more with families, providing them with the information they need to make treatment decisions that reflect the client's goals and values, and incorporating them into the caregiving process in preparation for the client's discharge.

To ensure that clients are getting what they need without wasting healthcare dollars, nurses must be knowledgeable about costs and reimbursement plans, as well as the relative benefits of treatment options. Downsizing produced the stimulus to nurses to broaden their skill base through cross-training and certification in order to document their expertise in a given area. Staff cutting requires that nurses remain flexible and perhaps trained to work in more than one clinical area. Healthcare systems can no longer employ RNs in roles that do not directly, critically, and clearly contribute to the outcomes of the organization. Today's nurse must be technically competent, skilled at critical thinking and problem solving, able to work with a variety of people, and fiscally responsible.

This is not enough, however, because the outcomes of nursing care are the true measurement of the ability to provide care. Nurses are entering (and even creating) new practice environments in which to use their skills. They are also working to further define nursing practice and the special contribution that nursing will continue to offer because that is how services will be evaluated and reimbursed. If nursing fails to define its contribution, then, as far as the reimburser is concerned, the contribution does not exist.

A recent focus of growth in the profession has been the effort to standardize nursing language to better demonstrate what nursing is and what nurses do. As of this edition, more than 10 versions of standardized nursing languages have been recognized by the American Nurses Association (ANA) and submitted to the National Library of Medicine for inclusion in the Unified Medical Language System Metathesaurus. These nursing languages (e.g., NANDA, NIC/NOC, Omaha System, Clinical Care Classification, the Perioperative Minimum Data Set, and Ozbolt Patient Care Data Set) can enhance the ability of nurses to communicate and document the care they provide, and to charge for these services. This facilitates the recognition of nursing's contribution to client care and promotes the view that nursing is a revenue-generating center.

In the midst of this whirlwind of change, as we experiment with new ways to provide cost-effective care within a specified time frame, it is imperative that we build on the foundation of the profession; that is, nursing is a science as well as an art, and nursing practice is rooted in the scientific process. Whether or not we choose to rename the steps we engage in (assessing clients and determining their needs, choosing actions to meet those needs, and evaluating the effectiveness of those actions), our purpose remains the same—the diagnosis and treatment of human responses to health and illness. It reinforces the importance of critical thinking and reasoning to professional nursing practice as well as the differences between basic and advanced nursing practice. If we allow our nursing focus to be replaced by the medical model, our practice will be subsumed, and much more will be lost than the essence of our profession.

CONCLUSION

Rapid and continuous changes in the healthcare environment have greatly increased the responsibilities facing today's nurse. To fulfill these responsibilities, planning and documentation of care are essential to satisfy client needs and meet legal obligations. Documentation of the impact of nursing on desired client outcomes provides a basis for evaluating continuing care needs, dealing with legal concerns, and determining payment.

Therefore, as nurses work collaboratively with other disciplines to provide client care, we need to continue to identify and document the nursing care needs of clients through the use of the nursing process and nursing diagnosis. Although this journey into change is not optional, nursing does have the opportunity and responsibility to take an active role in shaping that change.

What lies ahead for nursing and planning of client care? Definitely, a tremendously exciting and exacting challenge!

2

CHAPTER

The Nursing Process: Planning Care Using Nursing Diagnoses

Nurses and healthcare consumers agree that nursing care is a key factor in achieving positive outcomes and enhancing client satisfaction. Nursing care is instrumental in all phases of acute care as well as in the maintenance of general well-being (i.e., prevention of illness, rehabilitation, and maximization of health), or where a return to health is not possible, the relief of pain and discomfort and a peaceful death. To this end, the nursing profession has identified a problem-solving process that "combines the most desirable elements of the art of nursing with the most relevant elements of systems theory, using the scientific method" (Shore, 1988).

The original concept of nursing process was introduced in the 1950s as a three-step process of assessment, planning, and evaluation based on the scientific method of observing, measuring, gathering data, and analyzing the findings. Over time, this process became part of the conceptual framework of all nursing curricula and is included in the legal definition of nursing in the nurse practice acts of most states. After years of study, use, and refinement, the three-step process was expanded. The five steps—(1) assessment (systematic collection of data relating to clients and their problems/needs), (2) problem identification (analysis and interpretation of data), (3) planning (prioritizing needs, identifying goals, and choosing solutions), (4) implementation (putting the plan into action), and (5) evaluation (assessing the effectiveness of the plan and changing the plan as indicated by current needs)—are central to nursing actions and the delivery of high-quality, individualized client care in any setting.

When a client enters the healthcare system, the nurse uses the steps of the nursing process to work toward achieving the desired outcomes and goals identified for the client. The effectiveness of the plan of care is evaluated by ascertaining whether or not the desired outcomes and goals have been attained (client's problems/needs have been resolved) or whether problems remain at the time of discharge. If problems are unresolved, plans need to be made for further follow-up including assessment, additional problem/need identification, alteration of desired outcomes and goals, and/or changes of interventions in the next care settings.

Although some nurses view the nursing process as separate, progressive steps; in reality, the elements are interrelated. Together, they form a continuous circle of thought and action throughout the client's contact with the healthcare system. The process combines all the skills of critical thinking and good nursing care because it creates a method of active problem solving that is both dynamic and cyclic. Figure 2–1 visualizes the way this cyclic process works. As we learn more about diagnostic reasoning and critical thinking, some scholars are proposing a new model of describing what nurses do. With the emphasis on outcomes (the most recent revision of the American Nurses Association [ANA] Social Policy Statement [1995] focused on outcomes and deemphasized problem-focused approaches to nursing care) and new research into the nature of thinking and reasoning, the nursing process continues to be redefined (Pesut and Herman, 1999).

The "what" and "how" of the work of nursing have been explained in part in a number of existing publications that help operationalize the work of nursing. The ANA Social Policy Statement (1980) defined nursing as the "diagnosis and treatment of human responses to actual and potential health problems." It represents a framework for understanding nursing's relationship with society and nursing's obligations to those who receive nursing care. In 1991, the ANA *Standards of Clinical Nursing Practice* described the client care process and standards for professional performance, providing impetus and support for the use of nursing diagnosis in the practice setting. The work of NANDA International (formerly North American Nursing Diagnosis Association) has been ongoing for more than 25 years, beginning with efforts to identify client problems/needs for which nurses are accountable. NANDA continues to develop nursing diagnostic labels (Table 2–1), which are now being complemented by the Iowa Intervention Project: Nursing Interventions Classification (NIC) and the Iowa Outcomes Project: Nursing Outcomes Classification (NOC). NIC directs our focus to the content and process of nursing care by identifying and standardizing the care activities nurses perform while NIC describes client outcomes that are responsive to nursing intervention and developing corresponding measurement scales.

The implementation of prospective/capitated payment plans has moved a greater portion of healthcare delivery away from acute care hospitals into the community, with an emphasis on multifaceted free-standing care centers and home health services. Standards of care such as those published by the American Association of Critical-Care Nurses (AACN) and the Joint Commission on Accreditation of

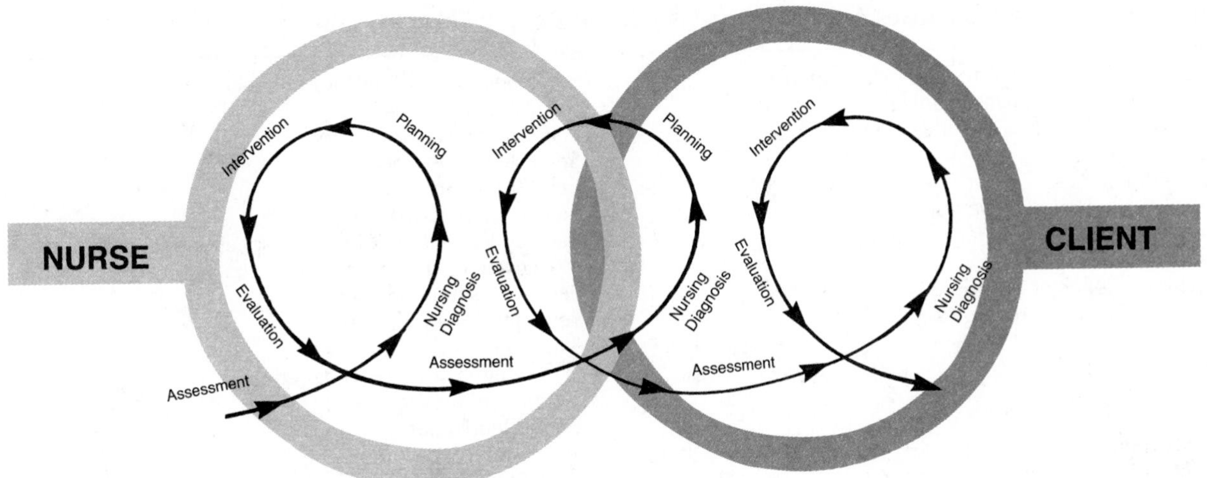

Figure 2–1. Diagram of the nursing process. The steps of the nursing process are interrelated, forming a continuous circle of thought and action that is both dynamic and cyclic.

Table 2–1 Nursing Diagnoses Accepted for Use and Research Through 2006

Activity Intolerance [specify level]
Activity Intolerance, risk for
Adjustment, impaired
Airway Clearance, ineffective
Allergy Response, latex
Allergy Response, risk for latex
Anxiety [specify level]
Anxiety, death
Aspiration, risk for
Attachment, risk for impaired parent/infant/child
Autonomic Dysreflexia
Autonomic Dysreflexia, risk for

Body Image, disturbed
Body Temperature, risk for imbalanced
Bowel Incontinence
Breastfeeding, effective
Breastfeeding, ineffective
Breastfeeding, interrupted
Breathing Pattern, ineffective

Cardiac Output, decreased
Caregiver Role Strain
Caregiver Role Strain, risk for
Communication, impaired verbal
Communication, readiness for enhanced
Conflict, decisional (specify)
Conflict, parental role
Confusion, acute
Confusion, chronic
Constipation
Constipation, perceived
Constipation, risk for
Coping, compromised family
Coping, defensive
Coping, disabled family
Coping, ineffective
Coping, readiness for enhanced
Coping, ineffective community
Coping, readiness for enhanced community
Coping readiness for enhanced family

Death Syndrome, risk for sudden infant
Denial, ineffective
Dentition, impaired
Development, risk for delayed
Diarrhea
Disuse Syndrome, risk for
Diversional Activity, deficient

Energy Field, disturbed
Environmental Interpretation Syndrome, impaired

Failure to Thrive, adult
Falls, risk for
Family Processes: alcoholism, dysfunctional
Family Processes, interrupted
Family Processes, readiness for enhanced
Fatigue
Fear [specify focus]
Fluid Balance, readiness for enhanced
[Fluid Volume, deficient hyper/hypotonic]
Fluid Volume, deficient [isotonic]
Fluid Volume, excess
Fluid Volume, risk for deficient
Fluid Volume, risk for imbalanced

Gas Exchange, impaired
Grieving, anticipatory
Grieving, dysfunctional
Grieving, risk for dysfunctional
Growth, risk for disproportionate
Growth & Development, delayed

Health Maintenance, ineffective
Health-Seeking Behaviors [specify]
Home Maintenance, impaired
Hopelessness
Hyperthermia
Hypothermia

Identity, disturbed personal
Infant Behavior, disorganized

(Continued on the following page)

Table 2–1 Nursing Diagnoses Accepted for Use and Research Through 2006 *(Continued)*

Infant Behavior, readiness for enhanced organized
Infant Behavior, risk for disorganized
Infant Feeding Pattern, ineffective
Infection, risk for
Injury, risk for
Injury, risk for perioperative positioning
Intracranial Adaptive Capacity, decreased

Knowledge, deficient [Learning Need] [specify]
Knowledge [specify], readiness for enhanced

Lifestyle, sedentary
Loneliness, risk for

Memory, impaired
Mobility, impaired bed
Mobility, impaired physical
Mobility, impaired wheelchair

Nausea
Neglect, unilateral
Noncompliance, [ineffective Adherence] [specify]
Nutrition: less than body requirements, imbalanced
Nutrition: more than body requirements, imbalanced
Nutrition: more than body requirements, risk for imbalanced
Nutrition, readiness for enhanced

Oral Mucous Membrane, impaired

Pain, acute
Pain, chronic
Parenting, impaired
Parenting, readiness for enhanced
Parenting, risk for impaired
Peripheral Neurovascular Dysfunction, risk for
Poisoning, risk for
Post-Trauma Syndrome [specify stage]
Post-Trauma Syndrome, risk for
Powerlessness [specify level]
Powerlessness, risk for
Protection, ineffective

Rape-Trauma Syndrome
Rape-Trauma Syndrome: compound reaction
Rape-Trauma Syndrome: silent reaction
Religiosity, impaired
Religiosity, risk for impaired
Religiosity, readiness for enhanced
Relocation Stress Syndrome
Relocation Stress Syndrome, risk for
Role Performance, ineffective

Self-Care Deficit, bathing/hygiene
Self-Care Deficit, dressing/grooming
Self-Care Deficit, feeding
Self-Care Deficit, toileting
Self-Concept, readiness for enhanced
Self-Esteem, chronic low
Self Esteem, situational low
Self Esteem, risk for situational low
Self-Mutilation
Self-Mutilation, risk for
Sensory Perception, disturbed (specify: visual, auditory, kinesthetic, gustatory, tactile, olfactory)
Sexual Dysfunction
Sexuality Pattern, ineffective
Skin Integrity, impaired
Skin Integrity, risk for impaired
Sleep, readiness for enhanced
Sleep Deprivation
Sleep Pattern, disturbed
Social Interaction, impaired
Social Isolation
Sorrow, chronic
Spiritual Distress
Spiritual Distress, risk for
Spiritual Well-Being, readiness for enhanced
Suffocation, risk for
Suicide, risk for
Surgical Recovery, delayed
Swallowing, impaired

Therapeutic Regimen Management, effective
Therapeutic Regimen Management, ineffective
Therapeutic Regimen Management, ineffective community
Therapeutic Regimen Management, ineffective family
Therapeutic Regimen Management, readiness for enhanced
Thermoregulation, ineffective
Thought Processes, disturbed
Tissue Integrity, impaired
Tissue Perfusion, ineffective (specify type: cerebral, cardiopulmonary, renal, gastrointestinal, peripheral)
Transfer Ability, impaired
Trauma, risk for

Urinary Elimination, impaired
Urinary Elimination, readiness for enhanced
Urinary Incontinence, functional
Urinary Incontinence, reflex
Urinary Incontinence, risk for urge
Urinary Incontinence, stress
Urinary Incontinence, total
Urinary Incontinence, urge
Urinary Retention [acute/chronic]

Ventilation, impaired spontaneous
Ventilatory Weaning Response, dysfunctional
Violence, [actual/] risk for other-directed
Violence, [actual/] risk for self-directed

Walking, impaired
Wandering [specify sporadic or continual]

[ ] author recommendations

Used with permission from NANDA International: Definitions and Classification, 2005–2006. NANDA, Philadelphia, 2005.

Healthcare Organizations (JCAHO) emphasize that, even in these environments, nursing must meet standards that further specify the parameters of client assessment and documentation of care.

Changes in the healthcare system continue to occur at an ever-increasing rate, requiring the profession of nursing to define itself in a way that will complement and facilitate the provision of appropriate, cost-effective evidenced-based care to all persons. Nurses need a common framework of communication and documentation so their contribution to healthcare is recognized as being essential and they are remunerated appropriately. At the very least, nursing requires a commonality of words describing practice so it can be captured and is visible in the healthcare databases.

The linkage of nursing diagnoses to specific nursing interventions and client outcomes has led to the development of a number of standardized nursing languages (e.g., Omaha System, Clinical Care Classification [formerly Home Healthcare Classification], Ozbolt Patient Care Data Set, Perioperative Minimum Data Set). The purpose of these languages is to help ensure continuity of appropriate high-quality nursing care for the client regardless of setting. This is accomplished in part through enhanced communication, standardization of the process evaluating the care provided, and facilitation of documentation.

PLANNING CARE

Medicine and nursing as well as other healthcare disciplines are interrelated, and therefore the actions for each discipline have implications for the others. This interrelationship allows for exchange of information and ideas and for development of plans of care that include all data pertinent to the individual client and/or family. In this book, the plan of care contains not only the actions initiated by medical and nursing orders, but also the coordination of care provided by all related healthcare disciplines. The nurse is often the person responsible for coordinating these various activities into a comprehensive functional plan, essential in providing holistic care for the client. Although independent nursing actions are an integral part of this process, collaborative actions are usually present based on the medical regimen or orders from other disciplines participating in the care of the client. We believe that nursing is an essential part of collaborative practice, and, as such, nursing has a responsibility and accountability in every collaborative problem in which the nurse interacts with the client. The educational background and expertise of the nurse, standing protocols, delegation of tasks, the use of care partners, and the area of practice (rural or urban, acute care or community care settings) influence whether an intervention is actually an independent nursing function or requires collaboration.

The well-written plan of care communicates the client's past and present health status and current needs to all members of the healthcare team involved in providing care. It identifies problems solved and those yet to be solved, can inform of approaches that have been successful, and notes patterns of client responses to interventions. In legal terms, the plan of care documents client care in areas of liability, accountability, and quality improvement. It also provides a mechanism to help ensure continuity of care when the client leaves a care setting while still needing services.

COMPONENTS OF THE PLAN OF CARE

The critical element for providing effective planned nursing care is its relevance as identified in client assessments. According to ANA Standards of Clinical Nursing Practice (ANA, 1991), client assessment is required in the following areas: physical, psychologic, sociocultural, spiritual, cognitive, functional abilities, developmental, economic, and lifestyle. These assessments, combined with the results of medical findings and diagnostic studies, are documented in the client database and form the foundation for development of the client's plan of care. For each plan of care presented in this book, a client assessment database is created from information that would likely be obtained from the history, physical examination, and related diagnostic studies. Nursing priorities are then determined and ranked. Priorities are simply stated and represent a general ranking system for the nursing diagnoses in the plan of care. They can be reworded and/or reorganized along with their timelines to create short- and long-term goals. Next, the nursing diagnosis statements, which include possible related factors (etiology) and corresponding signs and symptoms (cues) when appropriate, are presented. Desired client outcomes are then identified and followed by appropriate independent and collaborative interventions with accompanying rationales.

Client Database

In this book, each selected medical condition has an accompanying client database that includes subjective ("may report") and objective ("may exhibit") data that would likely be collected through the history-taking interview, physical assessment, diagnostic studies, and review of prior records. The client database is organized within the 13 categories of the Diagnostic Divisions. A sample medical/surgical assessment tool, definitions of the divisions, and a client situation are included in Chapter 3. As the nurse develops the plan of care, it will also be individualized to the client's situation.

Interviewing

Interviewing the client and/or significant other(s) provides data that the nurse obtains through conversation and observation. This information includes the individual's perceptions; that is, what the client perceives to be a problem and typically what he or she wants to share. Data may be collected during one or more contact periods and should include all relevant information. All participants in the interview process need to know that collected data are used in planning the client's care. Organizing and updating the data assists in the ongoing identification of client care needs and nursing diagnoses.

Physical Assessment

During information gathering, the nurse exercises perceptual and observational skills, assessing the client through the senses of sight, hearing, touch, and smell. The duration and depth of any physical assessment depend on the current condition of the client and the urgency of the situation, but it usually includes inspection, palpation, percussion, and auscultation. In this book, the physical assessment data are presented within the client database as objective data.

Diagnostic Studies

Interpretation of diagnostic test results is integrated with the history and physical findings as part of objective findings. Some tests are used to diagnose disease, whereas others are useful in following the course of a disease or in adjusting therapies. The nurse needs to be aware of significant test results that require reporting to the physician and/or initiation of specific nursing interventions. In many cases, the relationship of the test to the pathological physiology is clear, but in other cases it is not. This is the result of the interrelationship between various organs and body systems.

Nursing Priorities

In this book, nursing priorities are listed in a certain order to facilitate the linking/ranking of selected associated nursing diagnoses that appear in the plan of care guidelines. In any given client situation, nursing priorities are based on the client's specific needs and can vary from minute to minute. A nursing diagnosis that is a priority today may be less of a priority tomorrow, depending on the fluctuating physical and psychosocial condition of the client or the client's changing responses to the existing condition.

An example of nursing priorities for a client diagnosed with severe hypertension would include:

1. Maintain/enhance cardiovascular functioning.
2. Prevent complications.
3. Provide information about disease process, prognosis, and treatment regimen.
4. Support active client control or management of condition.

Discharge Goals

Once the nursing priorities are determined, the next step is to establish goals of treatment. In this book, each medical condition has established discharge goals, which are broadly stated and reflect the desired general status of the client on discharge or transfer to another care setting.

Discharge goals for a client with severe hypertension would include:

1. Blood pressure within acceptable limits for individual.
2. Cardiovascular and systemic complications prevented/minimized.
3. Disease process/prognosis and therapeutic regimen understood.
4. Necessary lifestyle/behavioral changes initiated.

Nursing Diagnosis (Problem/ Need Identification)

Nursing diagnoses are a uniform way of identifying, focusing on, and dealing with specific client needs and responses to actual and high-risk problems. Nursing diagnosis labels (see Table 2–1) provide a format for expressing the problem identification portion of the nursing process. In 1989, NANDA developed a taxonomy or classification scheme to categorize and classify nursing diagnostic labels. (This was replaced by a second taxonomy in 2000.) The NANDA definition of nursing diagnosis approved in 1990 further clarified the second step of the nursing process (i.e., problem identification/diagnosis). The definition of nursing diagnosis developed by NANDA is presented in Box 2–1.

BOX 2–1. NANDA DEFINITION OF NURSING DIAGNOSIS

> Nursing diagnosis is a clinical judgment about individual, family, or community responses to actual and potential health problems/life processes. Nursing diagnoses provide the basis for selection of nursing interventions to achieve outcomes for which the nurse is accountable.

There are several steps involved in the process of problem/need identification. Integrating these steps provides a systematic approach to accurately identifying nursing diagnoses using the process of critical thinking.

1. Collecting a client database (nursing interview, physical assessment, and diagnostic studies) combined with information collected by other healthcare providers
2. Reviewing and analyzing the client data
3. Synthesizing the gathered client data as a whole and then labeling your clinical judgment about the client's responses to these actual or high-risk problems/life processes
4. Comparing and contrasting the relationships of your clinical judgments against related factors and defining characteristics for the selected nursing diagnosis. This step is crucial to choosing and validating the appropriate nursing diagnosis label that will be used to create a specific client diagnostic statement.
5. Combining the nursing diagnosis with the related factors and defining characteristics to create the client diagnostic statement. For example, the diagnostic statement for a paraplegic client with a decubitus ulcer could read: impaired Skin Integrity related to pressure, circulatory impairment, and decreased sensation evidenced by draining wound, sacral area.

The nursing diagnosis is as correct as the present information allows because it is supported by the immediate data collected. It documents the client's situation at the present time and should reflect changes as they occur in the client's condition. Accurate need identification and diagnostic labeling provide the basis for selecting nursing interventions.

The nursing diagnosis may be a physical or a psychosocial response. Physical nursing diagnoses include those that pertain to physical processes, such as circulation (ineffective renal Tissue Perfusion), ventilation (impaired Gas Exchange), and elimination (Constipation). Psychosocial nursing diagnoses include those that pertain to the mind (acute Confusion), emotions (Fear), or lifestyle/relationships (ineffective Role Performance). Unlike medical diagnoses, nursing diagnoses change as the client progresses through various stages of illness/maladaptation to resolution of the problem or to the conclusion of the condition. Each decision the nurse makes is time dependent, and, with additional information gathered at a later point in time, decisions may change. For example, the initial problems/needs for a client undergoing cardiac surgery may be acute Pain, decreased Cardiac Output, ineffective Airway Clearance, and Risk for

Infection. As the client progresses, problems/needs are likely to shift to Activity Intolerance, deficient Knowledge, and ineffective Role Performance.

Diagnostic reasoning is used to ensure the accuracy of the client diagnostic statement. The defining characteristics and related factors associated with the chosen nursing diagnosis are reviewed and compared with the client data. If the diagnosis is not consistent with a majority of the cues or is not supported by relevant cues, additional data may be required or another nursing diagnosis needs to be considered.

Desired Client Outcomes

A desired client outcome is defined as the result of achievable nursing interventions and client responses that is desired by the client and/or caregiver and attainable within a defined time period, given the present situation and resources. These desired outcomes are the measurable steps toward achieving the previously established discharge goals and are used to evaluate the client's response to nursing interventions. (The fifth step of the nursing process, evaluation, is addressed in the sample client situation provided in Chapter 3.) Useful desired client outcomes must:

1. Be specific.
2. Be realistic.
3. Be measurable.
4. Indicate a definite time frame for achievement.
5. Consider client's desires and resources.

Desired client outcomes are created by listing items and/or behaviors that can be observed or heard. They are monitored to determine whether an acceptable outcome has been achieved within a specified time frame. Action verbs and time frames are used; for example, "client will ambulate, using cane, within 48 hours of surgery." The action verbs describe the client's behavior to be evaluated. Time frames are dependent on the client's projected or anticipated length of stay, often determined by diagnosis-related group (DRG) classification and considering the presence of complications or extenuating circumstances (e.g., age, debilitating disease process). The ongoing work of NOC in identifying 330 outcomes now also addresses client groups or aggregates. Although the NOC outcomes are listed in general terms such as Ambulation: Walking, 12 indicators are included for this outcome that can be measured by a five-point Likert-type scale ranging from "dependent, does not participate" to "completely independent." This facilitates tracking clients across care settings and can demonstrate client progress even when outcomes are not met.

When outcomes are properly written, they provide direction for planning and validating the selected nursing interventions. Consider the two following client outcomes: "Client will identify individual nutritional needs within 36 hours" and "...formulate a dietary plan based on identified nutritional needs within 72 hours." Based on the clarity of these outcomes, the nurse can select nursing interventions to ensure that the client's dietary knowledge is assessed, individual needs identified, and nutritional education presented. Often, the client outcomes identified are not unique to nursing because we provide care in a team approach with other disciplines. However, the NOC indicators for outcomes are more sensitive to nursing interventions. Other team members can use the majority of NOC labels and identify different indicators relative to their specialty focus to demonstrate their contribution to client improvement or to track deterioration. In this book, the identified outcomes in each plan of care are organized by using NOC labels (which are boxed to call attention to their introduction in this text).

Planning (Goals and Actions/Interventions)

Nursing interventions are prescriptions for specific behaviors expected from the client and actions to be carried out/facilitated by nurses. These actions/interventions are selected to assist the client in achieving the stated desired client outcomes and discharge goals. The expectation is that the prescribed behavior will benefit the client/family in a predictable way related to the identified problem/need and chosen outcomes. These interventions have the intent of individualizing care by meeting a specific client need and should incorporate identified client strengths when possible.

Nursing interventions should be specific and clearly stated, beginning with an action verb. Qualifiers of how, when, where, time/frequency, and amount provide the content of the planned activity; for example, "Assist as needed with self-care activities each morning," "Record respiratory and pulse rates before, during, and after activity," and "Instruct family in postdischarge care."

The NIC project has identified 514 interventions (both direct and indirect) that are stated in general terms, such as Respiratory Monitoring. Each label has a varied number of activities that may be chosen to accomplish the intervention. The interventions encompass a broad range of nursing practice, with some requiring specialized training/advanced certification. Others may be appropriate for delegation to other care providers (e.g., licensed practical nurses [LPNs], nursing assistants, unlicensed personnel) but still require planning and evaluation by registered nurses. In this text, these NIC labels are boxed to help the user begin to identify how they can be used.

This book divides the nursing interventions/actions into independent (nurse initiated) and collaborative (initiated by/performed in conjunction with other care providers) under the appropriate NIC labels. Examples of these two different professionally initiated actions are:

- Independent: Provide calm, restful surroundings, minimize environmental activity/noise, and limit numbers of visitors and length of stay.
- Collaborative: Administer antianxiety medication as indicated.

RATIONALE

Although rationales do not appear on regular plans of care, they are included in this book to assist the student and practicing nurse in associating the pathophysiologic and/or psychologic principles with the selected nursing intervention. This will help the nurse determine whether an intervention is appropriate for a specific client.

CONCLUSION

This book is intended to facilitate the application of the nursing process and the use of nursing diagnosis in medical/surgical clients. Each plan of care guideline was designed to provide generalized information on the associated medical condition. The guidelines can be modified either by using portions of the information provided or by adding more client care information to the existing guides. The plan of care guidelines were developed according to the NANDA recommendations except in a few examples where the authors believed more clarification and enhancement were required. The ongoing controversy on the validity of the NANDA-approved nursing diagnosis deficient Knowledge is one example where further clarification was added. The term *Learning Need* has been added to the nursing diagnosis label. Also, some diagnoses, such as Anxiety/Fear, have been combined for convenience; the combination indicates that two or more factors may be involved, and the nurse can then choose the most appropriate diagnosis for a specific client. We recognize that not all of the NANDA-approved nursing diagnoses have been used in these plan of care guidelines, but we hope that these guidelines will assist you in determining your clients' needs, outcomes, and nursing interventions.

Next, Chapter 3 will assist you in applying and adapting theory to practice.

3

CHAPTER

Critical Thinking: Adaptation of Theory to Practice

Critical thinking is defined as the "intellectually disciplined process of actively and skillfully conceptualizing, applying, analyzing, synthesizing, and evaluating information gathered from or generated by observation, experience, reflection, reasoning, or communication, as a guide to belief and action" (National Council for Excellence in Critical Thinking, 1992). Critical thinking requires cognitive, psychomotor, and affective skills to use the tools of a comprehensive knowledge base, the nursing process, and established standards of care, as well as nursing research, to analyze data and plan a course of action based on new insights and conclusions. Although critical thinking skills are used in all aspects of nursing practice, they are most evident when assessment data are analyzed to identify relevant information, make decisions about client needs, and develop an individualized plan of care. Therefore, client assessment is the foundation on which identification of individual needs, responses, and problems is based. Nurses of the future will need to manage and interpret data and evaluate nursing activities and interventions. They will also need competencies in case and financial management, healthcare policy and economics, legislative outcomes, and research methods. Additionally, they will need skills of delegation and the ability to think and reason across a diversity of settings in which they will practice (Pesut and Herman, 1999).

To facilitate the steps of assessing and diagnosing in the nursing process and to aid in the critical thinking process, assessment databases have been developed (Figure 3–1) that use a nursing focus instead of the traditional medical approach of review of systems. To achieve this nursing focus, we have grouped the NANDA International (formerly the North American Nursing Diagnosis Association) nursing diagnoses into related categories titled Diagnostic Divisions (Box 3–1), which reflect a blending of theories, primarily Maslow's Hierarchy of Needs and a self-care philosophy. These divisions serve as the framework or outline for collection of data and direct the nurse to the corresponding nursing diagnosis labels.

Because these divisions are based on human responses/needs and are not specific "systems," data may be recorded in more than one area. For this reason, the nurse is encouraged to keep an open mind and to collect as much information as possible before choosing the nursing diagnosis label. The results (synthesis) of the collected data are written concisely (client diagnostic statements) to best reflect the client's situation.

From the specific data recorded in the database, the related/risk factors (etiology) and signs and symptoms can be identified, and an individualized client diagnostic statement can be formulated according to the problem, etiology, and signs/symptoms (PES) format to accurately represent the client's situation. For example, the diagnostic statement may read: ineffective peripheral Tissue Perfusion related to decreased arterial flow, evidenced by decreased pulses, pale/cool feet, thick brittle nails, numbness/tingling of feet when walks 1/4 mile.

Outcomes are identified to facilitate choosing appropriate interventions and to serve as evaluators of both nursing care and client response. In addition to being measurable, outcomes must be achievable and desired by the client. These outcomes also form the framework for documentation.

Interventions are designed to specify the action of the nurse, the client, and/or significant other(s). They are not all-inclusive because such basic nursing actions as "bathe the client" or "notify the physician of changes" have been omitted. It is expected that these actions are included in routine client care. Sometimes controversial issues or treatments are presented for the sake of information and/or because different therapies may be used in different care settings or geographic locations.

Interventions need to promote the client's movement toward health and independence. This requires involvement of the client in his or her own care, including participation in decisions about the care activities and projected outcomes. This promotes client responsibility, negating the idea that healthcare providers control clients' lives.

To assist in visualizing this critical thinking process, a prototype client situation (Figure 3–2) is provided as an example of data collection and construction of a plan of care. As the client assessment database is reviewed, the nurse can identify the related/risk factors and defining characteristics (signs/symptoms) that were used to formulate the client diagnostic statements. The addition of timelines to specific client outcomes and goals reflects the anticipated length of stay and individual client/nurse expectations. Interventions are based on concerns/needs identified by the client and nurse during data collection in addition to physician orders. Although not normally included in a plan of care, rationales are included in this sample for the purpose of explaining or clarifying the choice of interventions. *(Text continues on p. 26)*

ADULT MEDICAL/SURGICAL ASSESSMENT TOOL

General Information

Name: ______________________________

Age: __________ DOB: __________ Gender: __________ Race: __________

Admission Date: __________ Time: __________ From: __________

Source of Information: __________ Reliability (1–4 with 4 being very reliable): __________

Activity/Rest

Subjective (Reports)

Occupation: __________ Usual activities: __________

Leisure time activities/hobbies: __________

Limitations imposed by condition: __________

Sleep: Hours: ______ Naps: ______ Aids: ______

Insomnia: __________ Related to: __________

Rested on awakening: __________

Excessive grogginess: __________

Feelings of boredom/dissatisfaction: __________

Objective (Exhibits)

Observed response to activity:

Cardiovascular: ______ Respiratory: ______

Mental Status (e.g., withdrawn/lethargic): __________

Neuromuscular Assessment:

Muscle mass/tone: ______ Posture: ______

ROM: ______ Strength: ______ Tremors: ______

Deformity: __________

Circulation

Subjective (Reports)

History of: Hypertension: ______ Heart trouble: ______

Rheumatic fever: ______ Ankle/leg edema: ______

Phlebitis: ______ Slow healing: ______

Claudication: ______ Dysreflexia: ______

Bleeding tendencies/episodes: __________

Palpitations: ______ Syncope: ______

Extremities: Numbness: ______Tingling: ______

Cough/hemoptysis: __________

Change in frequency/amount of urine: __________

Objective (Exhibits)

BP: R and L: Lying/sit/stand: __________

Pulse pressure: ______ Auscultatory gap: ______

Pulses (palpation): ______ Carotid: ______

Temporal: ______ Jugular: ______ Radial: ______

Femoral: ______ Popliteal: ______

Posttibial: ______ Dorsalis pedis: ______

Cardiac (palpation): Thrill: ______ Heaves: ______

Heart sounds: Rate: ______ Rhythm: ______

Quality: ______ Friction rub: ______

Murmur: __________

Vascular bruit: __________

Jugular vein distention (JVD): __________

Breath sounds: __________

Extremities: Temperature: ______ Color: ______

Capillary refill: ______ Homans' sign: ______

Varicosities: ______ Nail abnormalities: ______

Edema: __________

Distribution/quality of hair: __________

Trophic skin changes: __________

Color: General: __________

Mucous membranes: ______ Lips: ______

Nailbeds: ______ Conjunctiva: ______

Sclera: __________

Diaphoresis: __________

Figure 3–1. Adult medical-surgical assessment tool. This is a suggested guide and tool for creating a database reflecting a nursing focus. Although the diagnostic divisions are alphabetized here for ease of presentation, they can be prioritized or rearranged in any manner to meet individual needs. In addition, this assessment tool can be adapted to meet the needs of specific client populations.

Ego Integrity

Subjective (Reports)

Stress factors: ______
Ways of handling stress: ______
Financial concerns: ______
Relationship status: ______
Cultural factors/ethnic ties: ______
Religion: ______ Practicing: ______
Lifestyle: ______ Recent changes: ______
Sense of connectedness/harmony with self: ______
Feeling of: Helplessness: ______
Hopelessness: ______ Powerlessness: ______

Objective (Exhibits)

Emotional status (check those that apply):
Calm: ______ Anxious: ______ Angry: ______
Withdrawn/Fearful: ______ Irritable: ______
Restive: ______ Euphoric: ______
Observed physiological response(s): ______
Changes in energy field:
Temperature: ______ Color: ______
Distribution: ______ Movement: ______
Sounds: ______

Elimination

Subjective (Reports)

Usual bowel pattern: ______
Laxative use: ______
Character of stool: ______ Last BM: ______
Constipation: ______ Diarrhea: ______
History of bleeding: ______ Hemorrhoids: ______
Usual voiding pattern: ______
Incontinence/when: ______ Urgency: ______
Frequency: ______ Retention: ______
Character of urine: ______
Pain/burning/difficulty voiding: ______
History of kidney/bladder disease: ______
Diuretic use: ______

Objective (Exhibits)

Abdomen: Tender: ______ Soft/firm: ______
Palpable mass: ______ Size/girth: ______
Bowel sounds: Location/type: ______
Hemorrhoids: ______ Stool guaiac: ______
Bladder palpable: ______
Overflow voiding: ______
CVA tenderness: ______

Food/Fluid

Subjective (Reports)

Usual diet (type): ______ Last meal/intake: ______
Cultural/religious restrictions: ______
Dietary pattern/content: B: ______ L: ______ D: ______
Carbohydrate/protein/fat intake: g/d ______
Number of meals daily: ______
Vitamin/food supplement use: ______
Last meal/intake: ______
Loss of appetite: ______ Nausea/vomiting: ______
Heartburn/indigestion: ______ Related to: ______
Relieved by: ______
Food preferences: ______ Food prohibitions: ______
Allergy/food intolerance: ______

Objective (Exhibits)

Current weight: ______ Height: ______
Body build: ______ Skin turgor: ______
Mucous membranes: Moist/dry: ______
Breath sounds: Crackles: ______
Wheezes: ______
Edema: General: ______ Dependent: ______
Periorbital: ______ Ascites: ______
Jugular vein distention (JVD): ______
Thyroid enlarged: ______
Condition of teeth/gums: ______
Appearance of tongue: ______
Mucous membranes: ______ Halitosis: ______

Figure 3–1. *(Continued)*

Mastication/swallowing problems: ______
Dentures: ______
Usual weight: ______ Changes in weight: ______
Diuretic use: ______

Bowel sounds: ______
Hernia/masses: ______
Urine S/A or Chemstix: ______
Serum glucose (Glucometer): ______

Hygiene

Subjective (Reports)

Activities of daily living: Independent/dependent (level):
Mobility: ______ Feeding: ______ Hygiene: ______
Dressing/grooming: ______ Toileting: ______
Preferred time of personal care/bath: ______
Equipment/prosthetic devices required: ______
Assistance provided by: ______

Objective (Exhibits)

General appearance: ______
Manner of dress: ______
Personal habits: ______
Body odor: ______
Condition of scalp: ______
Presence of vermin: ______

Neurosensory

Subjective (Reports)

Fainting spells/dizziness: ______
Headaches: Location: ______ Frequency: ______
Tingling/numbness/weakness (location): ______
Stroke/brain injury (residual effects): ______
Seizures: ______ Type: ______ Aura: ______
Frequency: ______ Postictal state: ______
How controlled: ______
Eyes: Vision loss: ______ Last exam: ______
Glaucoma: ______ Cataract: ______
Ears: Hearing loss: ______ Last exam: ______
Sense of smell: ______ Epistaxis: ______

Objective (Exhibits)

Mental status (Note duration of change):
Oriented/disoriented: Person: ______
Place: ______ Time: ______ Situation: ______
Check all that apply:
Alert: ______ Drowsy: ______ Lethargic: ______
Stuporous: ______ Comatose: ______
Cooperative: ______ Combative: ______
Delusions: ______ Hallucinations: ______
Affect (describe): ______
Memory: Recent: ______ Remote: ______
Glasses: ______ Contacts: ______ Hearing aids: ______
Pupil: Shape: ______ Size/reaction: R/L: ______
Facial droop: ______ Swallowing: ______
Handgrasp/release, R/L:
Deep tendon reflexes: ______
Posturing: ______ Paralysis: ______

Pain/Discomfort

Subjective (Reports)

Primary focus: ______ Location: ______
Intensity (0–10 with 10 being most severe): ______
Frequency: ______ Quality: ______
Duration: ______ Radiation: ______
Precipitating/aggravating factors: ______
How relieved: ______
Associated symptoms: ______
Effect on activities: ______ Relationships: ______
Additional focus: ______

Objective (Exhibits)

Facial grimacing: ______
Guarding affected area: ______
Emotional response: ______
Narrowed focus: ______
Change in blood pressure: ______ Pulse: ______

Figure 3–1. *(Continued)*

Respiration

Subjective (Reports)

Dyspnea/related to: ______
Cough/sputum: ______
History of bronchitis: ______ Asthma: ______
Emphysema: ______ Tuberculosis: ______
Recurrent pneumonia: ______
Exposure to noxious fumes: ______
Smoker: ______ Pack/day: ______
No. of pack years: ______
Use of respiratory aids: ______ Oxygen: ______

Objective (Exhibits)

Respiratory: Rate: ______ Depth: ______
Symmetry: ______
Use of accessory muscles: ______
Nasal flaring: ______
Fremitus: ______
Breath sounds: ______ Egophony: ______
Cyanosis: ______
Clubbing of fingers: ______
Sputum characteristics: ______
Mentation/restlessness: ______

Safety

Subjective (Reports)

Allergies/sensitivity: ______ Reaction: ______
Exposure to infectious diseases: ______
Previous alteration of immune system: ______
Cause: ______
History of sexually transmitted disease (date/type): ______ Testing: ______
High-risk behaviors: ______
Blood transfusion/number: ______ When: ______
Reaction: ______ Describe: ______
Geographic areas lived in/visited: ______
Seat belt/helmet use: ______
Workplace safety/health issues: ______
History of accidental injuries: ______
Fractures/dislocations: ______
Arthritis/unstable joints: ______
Back problems: ______
Changes in moles: ______ Enlarged nodes: ______
Delayed healing: ______
Cognitive limitations: ______
Impaired vision/hearing: ______
Prosthesis: ______ Ambulatory devices: ______

Objective (Exhibits)

Temperature: ______ Diaphoresis: ______
Skin integrity: Scars: ______ Rashes: ______
Lacerations: ______ Ulcerations: ______
Ecchymosis: ______ Blisters: ______ Burns (degree/percent): ______ Drainage: ______
Mark location of the above on diagram:

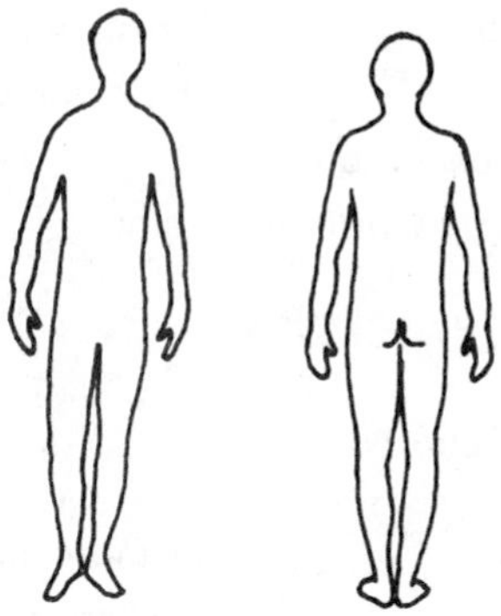

General strength: ______
Muscle tone: ______
Gait: ______ ROM: ______
Paresthesia/paralysis: ______
Results of cultures: ______
Immune system testing: ______
Tuberculosis testing: ______

Figure 3–1. *(Continued)*

Sexuality (Component of Ego Integrity and Social Interaction)

Subjective (Reports)

Sexually active: ________ Use of condoms: __________
Birth control method: ______________________________
Sexual concerns/difficulties: ______________________
Recent change in frequency/interest: _______________

Objective (Exhibits)

Comfort level with subject matter: ________________

Female:

Subjective (Reports)

Age at menarche: ________ Length of cycle: ________
Duration: ________ Number of pads used/d: ______
Last menstrual period: ______ Pregnant now: ______
Bleeding between periods: ______________________
Menopause: ___________ Vaginal lubrication: ________
Vaginal discharge: ______________________________
Surgeries: ______________________________________
Hormonal therapy/calcium use: ___________________
Practices breast self-exam: ______________________
Last mammogram: ________ PAP smear: ________

Objective (Exhibits)

Breast exam: ____________________________________
Genital warts/lesions: ___________________________
Discharge: ______________________________________

Male:

Subjective (Reports)

Penile discharge: ________ Prostate disorder: ________
Circumcised: ___________ Vasectomy: ___________
Practice self-exam: Breast: ________ Testicles: ________
Last proctoscopic/prostate exam: ________________

Objective (Exhibits)

Breast: __________________ Testicles: ______________
Genital warts/lesions: ___________________________
Discharge: ______________________________________

Social Interactions

Subjective (Reports)

Marital status: ________ Years in relationship: ________
Living with: ________ Concerns/stresses: ________
Extended family: ________________________________
Other support person(s): _________________________
Role within family structure: ____________________
Perception of relationships with family members: _____
Ethnic affiliation: ______________________________
Strength of ethnic identity: ______________________
Lives in ethnic community (y/n): _________________
Feelings of: Mistrust: __________ Rejection: ________
Unhappiness: ______ Loneliness/isolation: ________
Problems related to illness/condition: ______________
Problems with communication: ___________________

Objective (Exhibits)

Speech: Clear: ____________ Slurred: ______________
Unintelligible: ____________ Aphasic: ___________
Usual speech pattern/impairment: ________________
Use of speech/communication aids: ______________
Laryngectomy present: _________________________

Verbal/nonverbal communication with family/SO(s): ______________________________
Family interaction (behavioral) pattern:
____

Figure 3–1. *(Continued)*

Teaching/Learning

Subjective (Reports)

Dominant language (specify): ____________
Second language: ____________
Literate: ______ Education level: ______
Learning disabilities: (specify): ____________
Cognitive limitations: ____________
Where born: ______ If immigrant how long in this country: ____________
Health and illness beliefs/practices (e.g., complementary therapies)/customs: ______
Which family member makes healthcare decisions/ is spokesperson: ____________
Presence of Advance Directives/Durable Medical Power of Attorney: ____________
Special healthcare concerns (e.g., impact of religious/cultural practices): ____________
Health goals: ____________
Familial risk factors (indicate relationship):
Diabetes: ______ Thyroid (specify): ______
Tuberculosis: ______ Heart disease: ______
Strokes: ______ High BP: ______ Epilepsy: ______
Kidney disease: ______ Cancer: ______
Mental illness: ______ Other: ______

Prescribed medications:
Drug: ______ Dose: ______
Times (circle last dose): ____________
Take regularly: ______ Purpose: ______
Side effects/problems: ____________
Nonprescription drugs: OTC drugs: ______
Herbal supplements (specify): ______
Street drugs: ______ Tobacco: ______
Smokeless tobacco: ____________
Alcohol (amount/frequency): ____________
Admitting diagnosis per provider: ____________
Reason for admission per client: ____________
History of current complaint: ____________
Client expectations of care: ____________
Previous illnesses and/or hospitalizations/ surgeries: ____________
Evidence of failure to improve: ____________
Last complete physical exam: ____________

Discharge Plan Considerations

DRG projected mean length of stay: ____________
Date information obtained: ____________
Anticipated date of discharge: ____________
Resources available: Persons: ____________
Financial: ______ Community: ______ Support groups: ______ Socialization: ______
Areas that may require alteration/assistance:
Food preparation: ______ Shopping: ______
Transportation: ______ Ambulation: ______
Medication/IV therapy: ____________
Treatments: ______ Wound care: ______
Supplies: ______ Self-care (specify): ______
Homemaker/maintenance (specify): ______

Physical layout of home (specify): ______
Anticipated changes in living situation after discharge: ____________
Living facility other than home (specify):
____
Referrals (date, source, services):
Social Services: ____________
Rehabilitation services: ____________
Dietary: ______ Home care: ______
Resp/O_2: ______ Equipment: ______
Supplies: ____________
Other: ____________

BOX 3–1. NURSING DIAGNOSES ORGANIZED ACCORDING TO DIAGNOSTIC DIVISIONS

After data are collected and areas of concern/need identified, the nurse is directed to the Diagnostic Divisions to review the list of nursing diagnoses that fall within the individual categories. This will assist the nurse in choosing the specific diagnostic label to accurately describe the data. Then, with the addition of etiology or related/risk factors (when known) and signs and symptoms, or cues (defining characteristics), the client diagnostic statement emerges.

Activity/Rest—Ability to engage in necessary/desired activities of life (work and leisure) and to obtain adequate sleep/rest

- Activity Intolerance
- Activity Intolerance, risk for
- Disuse Syndrome, risk for
- Diversional Activity, deficient
- Fatigue
- Lifestyle, sedentary
- Mobility, impaired bed
- Mobility, impaired physical
- Mobility, impaired wheelchair
- Sleep Deprivation
- Sleep Pattern, disturbed
- Sleep, readiness for enhanced
- Transfer Ability, impaired
- Walking, impaired

Circulation—Ability to transport oxygen and nutrients necessary to meet cellular needs

- Autonomic Dysreflexia
- Autonomic Dysreflexia, risk for
- Cardiac Output, decreased
- Intracranial Adaptive Capacity, decreased
- Tissue Perfusion, ineffective (specify type: renal, cerebral, cardiopulmonary, gastrointestinal, peripheral)

Ego Integrity—Ability to develop and use skills and behaviors to integrate and manage life experiences

- Adjustment, impaired
- Anxiety [specify level]
- Anxiety, death
- Body Image, disturbed
- Conflict, decisional (specify)
- Coping, defensive
- Coping, ineffective
- Coping, readiness for enhanced
- Denial, ineffective
- Energy Field, disturbed
- Fear
- Grieving, anticipatory
- Grieving, dysfunctional
- Grieving, risk for dysfunctional
- Hopelessness
- Personal Identity, disturbed
- Post-Trauma Syndrome
- Post-Trauma Syndrome, risk for
- Powerlessness
- Powerlessness, risk for
- Rape-Trauma Syndrome
- Rape-Trauma Syndrome: compound reaction
- Rape-Trauma Syndrome: silent reaction
- Religiosity, readiness for enhanced
- Religiosity, impaired
- Religiosity, risk for impaired
- Relocation Stress Syndrome
- Relocation Stress Syndrome, risk for
- Self-Concept, readiness for enhanced
- Self-Esteem, chronic low
- Self-Esteem, situational low
- Self-Esteem, risk for situational low
- Sorrow, chronic
- Spiritual Distress
- Spiritual Distress, risk for
- Spiritual Well-Being, readiness for enhanced

Elimination—Ability to excrete waste products

- Bowel Incontinence
- Constipation
- Constipation, perceived
- Constipation, risk for
- Diarrhea
- Urinary Elimination, impaired
- Urinary Elimination, readiness for enhanced
- Urinary Incontinence, functional
- Urinary Incontinence, reflex
- Urinary Incontinence, stress
- Urinary Incontinence, total
- Urinary Incontinence, urge
- Urinary Incontinence, risk for urge
- Urinary Retention [acute/chronic]

Food/Fluid—Ability to maintain intake of and utilize nutrients and liquids to meet physiological needs

- Breastfeeding, effective
- Breastfeeding, ineffective
- Breastfeeding, interrupted
- Dentition, impaired
- Failure to Thrive, adult
- [Fluid Volume, deficient hyper/hypotonic]
- Fluid Volume, deficient [isotonic]
- Fluid Volume excess
- Fluid Volume, risk for deficient
- Fluid Volume, risk for imbalanced
- Infant Feeding Pattern, ineffective
- Nausea
- Nutrition, less than body requirements, imbalanced
- Nutrition, more than body requirements, imbalanced
- Nutrition, risk for more than body requirements, imbalanced
- Nutrition, readiness for enhanced
- Oral Mucous Membrane, impaired
- Swallowing, impaired

(Continued on the following page)

Hygiene—Ability to perform activities of daily living
- Self-Care Deficit: bathing/hygiene, dressing/grooming, feeding, toileting

Neurosensory—Ability to perceive, integrate, and respond to internal and external cues
- Confusion, acute
- Confusion, chronic
- Infant Behavior, disorganized
- Infant Behavior, risk for disorganized
- Infant Behavior, readiness for enhanced organized
- Memory, impaired
- Peripheral Neurovascular Dysfunction, risk for
- Sensory Perception, disturbed (specify: visual, auditory, kinesthetic, gustatory, tactile, olfactory)
- Thought Processes, disturbed
- Unilateral Neglect

Pain/Discomfort—Ability to control internal/external environment to maintain comfort
- Pain, acute
- Pain, chronic

Respiration—Ability to provide and use oxygen to meet physiological needs
- Airway Clearance, ineffective
- Aspiration, risk for
- Breathing Pattern, ineffective
- Gas Exchange, impaired
- Ventilation, impaired spontaneous
- Ventilatory Weaning Response, dysfunctional

Safety—Ability to provide safe, growth-promoting environment
- Allergy Response, latex
- Allergy Response, risk for latex
- Body Temperature, risk for imbalanced
- Environmental Interpretation Syndrome, impaired
- Falls, risk for
- Health Maintenance, ineffective
- Home Maintenance, impaired
- Hyperthermia
- Hypothermia
- Infection, risk for
- Injury, risk for
- Injury, risk for perioperative positioning
- Mobility, impaired physical
- Poisoning, risk for
- Protection, ineffective
- Self-Mutilation
- Self-Mutilation, risk for
- Skin Integrity, impaired
- Skin Integrity, risk for impaired
- Suffocation, risk for
- Suicide, risk for
- Surgical Recovery, delayed
- Thermoregulation, ineffective
- Tissue Integrity, impaired
- Trauma, risk for
- Violence, [actual/]risk for other-directed
- Violence, [actual/]risk for self-directed
- Wandering [specify sporadic or continual]

Sexuality [Component of Ego Integrity and Social Interaction]—Ability to meet requirements/characteristics of male/female role
- Sexual Dysfunction
- Sexuality Pattern, ineffective

Social Interaction—Ability to establish and maintain relationships
- Attachment, risk for impaired parent/infant/child
- Caregiver Role Strain
- Caregiver Role Strain, risk for
- Communication, impaired verbal
- Communication, readiness for enhanced
- Coping, ineffective community
- Coping, readiness for enhanced community
- Coping, compromised family
- Coping, disabled family
- Coping, readiness for enhanced family
- Family Processes, interrupted
- Family Processes, alcoholism, dysfunctional
- Loneliness, risk for
- Parental Role Conflict
- Parenting, impaired
- Parenting, risk for impaired
- Parenting, readiness for enhanced
- Role Performance, ineffective
- Social Interaction, impaired
- Social Isolation

Teaching/Learning—Ability to incorporate and use information to achieve healthy lifestyle/optimal wellness
- Development, risk for delayed
- Growth and Development, delayed
- Growth, risk for disproportionate
- Health-Seeking Behaviors (specify)
- Knowledge, deficient (specify)
- Knowledge (specify), readiness for enhanced
- Noncompliance [Adherence, ineffective] [specify]
- Therapeutic Regimen Management, effective
- Therapeutic Regimen Management, ineffective community
- Therapeutic Regimen Management, ineffective family
- Therapeutic Regimen Management, ineffective

Client Situation: Diabetes Mellitus

Mr. R.S., a type 2 diabetic (formerly a non–insulin-dependent diabetic, or NIDDM) for 10 years, presented to his physician's office with a nonhealing ulcer of 3 weeks' duration on his left foot. Screening studies done during the exam revealed blood glucose (BG) of 356/fingerstick and urine Chemstix of 2%. Because of distance from medical provider and lack of local community services, he is admitted to the hospital.

Admitting Physician's Orders

Culture/sensitivity and Gram's stain of foot ulcer
Random blood glucose on admission and fingerstick BG qid
CBC, electrolytes, serum lipid profile, glycosylated Hb in AM
Chest x-ray and ECG in AM
DiaBeta 10 mg, PO, bid
Glucophage 500 mg, PO, daily to start—will increase gradually
Humulin N 10 U SC q AM and hs. Begin insulin instruction for postdischarge self-care, if necessary
Dicloxacillin 500 mg PO, q6h, start after culture obtained
Darvocet-N 100 mg q4h PRN pain
Diet—2400 calories/three meals with two snacks
Up in chair ad lib with feet elevated
Foot cradle for bed
Irrigate lesion L foot with normal saline tid then apply wet to dry sterile dressing
Vital signs qid

Client Assessment Database

Name: R.S. Informant: Client Reliability (scale 1–4): 3, Age: 73 DOB: 5/3/31 Race: White Gender: M
Admission date: 6/28/2004 Time: 7 PM From: Home

ACTIVITY/REST

Reports (Subjective):
Occupation: Farmer
Usual activities/hobbies: Reading, playing cards. "Don't have time to do much. Anyway I'm too tired most of the time to do anything after the chores."
Limitations imposed by illness: "Have to watch what I order if I eat out."
Sleep: Hours: 6–8 hr/night Naps: No Aids: No
Insomnia: "Not unless I drink coffee after supper."
Usually feels rested when awakens at 4:30 AM

Exhibits (Objective):
Observed response to activity: Limps, favors L foot when walking
Mental status: Alert/active
Neuromuscular assessment: Muscle mass/tone: bilaterally equal/firm
Posture: Erect ROM: normal all extremities
Strength: Equal 3 extremities/favors L leg currently

CIRCULATION

Reports (Subjective):
Slow healing: lesion L foot, 3 weeks' duration
Extremities: Numbness/tingling: "My feet feel cold and tingly like sharp pins poking the bottom of my feet when I walk the quarter mile to the mailbox."
Cough/character of sputum: Occasional/white
Change in frequency/amount of urine: Yes, voiding more lately

Exhibits (Objective):
Peripheral pulses: Radials 3+; popliteal, dorsalis, posttibial/pedal, all 1+
BP: R: Lying: 146/90 Sitting: 140/86 Standing: 138/90
L: Lying: 142/88 Sitting: 138/88 Standing: 138/84
Pulse: Apical: 86 Radial: 86 Quality: Strong Rhythm: Regular
Chest auscultation: Few wheezes clear with cough, no murmurs/rubs
JVD: -0-
Extremities: Temperature: Feet cool bilat/legs warm
Color: Skin: Legs pale Capillary refill: Slow both feet (approx 5 sec)

Figure 3–2. Client situation: Diabetes Mellitus.

Homans' sign: -0- Varicosities: Few enlarged superficial veins both calves
Nails: Toenails thickened, yellow, brittle
Distribution and quality of hair: Coarse hair to midcalf, none on ankles/toes
Color: General: Ruddy face/arms Mucous membranes/lips: Pink
Nail beds: Fingers blanch well Conjunctiva and sclera: White

EGO INTEGRITY

Reports (Subjective): Stress factors: "Normal farmer's problems: weather, pests, bankers, and so on."
Ways of handling stress: "I get busy with the chores and talk things over with my livestock; they listen pretty good."
Financial concerns: No supplemental insurance; needs to hire someone to do chores while in hospital
Relationship status: Married—45 years
Cultural factors: Rural/agrarian, Eastern European descent, "American," no ethnic ties
Religion: Protestant/practicing
Lifestyle: Middle class/self-sufficient farmer
Recent changes: -0-
Feelings: "I'm in control of most things, except the weather and this diabetes."
Concerned regarding possible therapy "change from pills to shots"

Exhibits (Objective): Emotional status: Generally calm; appears frustrated at times
Observed physiologic response(s): Occasionally sighs deeply/frowns, fidgeting with coin, shoulders tense, shrugs shoulders/throws up hands

ELIMINATION

Reports (Subjective): Usual bowel pattern: Almost every PM
Last bowel movement: Last night Character of stool: Firm/brown
Bleeding: -0- Hemorrhoids: -0- Constipation: Occasional
Laxative used: Hot prune juice as needed
Urinary: No problems Character of urine: Pale yellow

Exhibits (Objective): Abdomen tender: No Soft/Firm: Soft Palpable mass: -0-
Bowel sounds: Active all 4 quads

FOOD/FLUID

Reports (Subjective): Usual diet (type): 2400 calories (occasionally "cheats" with dessert; "My wife watches it pretty closely.") Number of meals daily: 3/1 snack
Dietary Pattern: Breakfast: Fruit juice, toast, ham, decaf coffee
Lunch: Meat, potatoes, vegetables, fruit, milk
Dinner: Meat sandwich, soup, fruit, decaf coffee
Snack: Milk/crackers at hs. Usual beverage: Skim milk, 2–3 cups decaf coffee. Drinks "a lot of water"—several qt
Last meal/intake: Dinner: Hot roast beef sandwich, vegetable soup, pear with cheese, decaf coffee
Loss of appetite: "Never, but lately I don't feel as hungry as usual."
Nausea/vomiting: -0- Food allergies: None
Heartburn/food intolerance: Cabbage causes gas, coffee after supper causes heartburn
Mastication/swallowing problems: -0- Dentures: Partial upper plate fits OK
Usual weight: 175 lb Recent changes: Has lost about 5 lb this month
Diuretic therapy: No

Exhibits (Objective): Wt: 171 lb Ht: 5 ft 10 in Build: Stocky
Skin turgor: Good/leathery
Appearance of tongue: Midline, pink Mucous membranes: Pink, intact
Condition of teeth/gums: Good; no irritation/bleeding noted
Breath sounds: Few wheezes cleared with cough
Bowel sounds: Active all 4 quads
Urine Chemstix: 2% Fingerstick: 356 (Dr. office) Random BG drawn on admission 450

HYGIENE

Reports (Subjective): Activities of daily living: Independent in all areas
Preferred time of bath: PM

Figure 3–2. *(Continued)*

Exhibits (Objective): General appearance: Clean, shaven, short-cut hair, hands rough and dry, skin on feet dry, cracked, and scaly
Scalp and eyebrows: Scaly white patches
Body odor: -0-

NEUROSENSORY

Reports (Subjective): Headaches: "Occasionally behind my eyes when I worry too much."
Tingling/Numbness: Feet, once or twice a week (as noted)
Eyes: Vision loss, farsighted, "seems a little blurry now." Examination: 2 years ago
Ears: Hearing loss: R: "Some." L: No (has not been tested)
Nose: Epistaxis: -0-. Sense of smell: "No problems"

Exhibits (Objective): Mental status: Alert, oriented to time, place, person, situation
Affect: Concerned Memory: Remote/recent: clear and intact
Speech: Clear, coherent, appropriate
Pupil reaction: PERLA/small Glasses: Reading Hearing aid: No
Handgrip/release: Strong/equal

PAIN/DISCOMFORT

Reports (Subjective): Primary focus: L foot Location: Medial aspect, heel of L foot
Intensity (0–10): 4–5/10 Quality: Dull ache with occasional sharp stabbing sensation
Frequency/duration: "Seems like all the time" Radiation: No
Precipitating factors: Shoes, walking How relieved: ASA, not helping
Additional complaints: Sometimes has back pain following chores/heavy lifting
Relieved by: ASA/liniment rubdown

Exhibits (Objective): Facial grimacing: When lesion border palpated
Guarding affected area: Pulls foot away Narrowed focus: -0-
Emotional response: Tense, irritated

RESPIRATORY

Reports (Subjective): Dyspnea: -0- Cough: Occasional morning cough, white sputum
Emphysema: -0- Bronchitis: -0- Asthma: -0- Tuberculosis: -0-
Smoker: Filters Packs/day: 1/2 Number of pack years: 25
Use of respiratory aids: -0-

Exhibits (Objective): Respiratory rate: 22 Depth: Good Symmetry: Equal, bilateral
Auscultation: Few wheezes, clear with cough
Cyanosis: -0- Clubbing of fingers: -0-
Sputum characteristics: None to observe
Mentation/restlessness: Alert/oriented/fairly relaxed

SAFETY

Reports (Subjective): Allergies: -0- Blood transfusions: -0-
Sexually transmitted disease: -0-
Fractures/dislocations: L clavicle, 1966, fell getting off tractor
Arthritis/unstable joints: "Think I've got some arthritis in my knees."
Back problems: Occasional lower back pain
Vision impaired: Requires glasses for reading
Hearing impaired: Slightly (R), compensates by turning "good ear" toward speaker

Exhibits (Objective): Temperature: 99.4°F (37.4°C) tympanic
Skin integrity: Impaired L foot Scars: R Ing, surgical
Rashes: -0- Bruises: -0- Lacerations: -0- Blisters: -0-
Ulcerations: Medial aspect L heel, 2.5 cm diameter, approximately 3 mm deep, draining small amount cream colored/pink-tinged matter, no odor noted
Strength (general): Equal 3 extremities/favors L leg Muscle tone: Firm
ROM: Good. Gait: Favors L foot Paresthesia/Paralysis: -0-

SEXUALITY: MALE

Reports (Subjective): Sexually active: Yes Use of condoms: No (monogamous)
Recent changes in frequency/interest: "I've been too tired lately."
Penile discharge: -0- Prostate disorder: -0- Vasectomy: -0-
Last proctoscopic examination: 2 years ago Prostate examination: 1 year ago
Practice self-examination: Breast/testicles: No
Problems/complaints: "I don't have any problems, but you'd have to ask my wife if there are any complaints."

Figure 3–2. *(Continued)*

Exhibits (Objective):
Examination: Breast: No masses Testicles: Deferred
Prostate: Deferred

SOCIAL INTERACTIONS

Reports (Subjective):
Marital status: Married, 48 years Living with: Wife
Report of problems: -0-
Extended family: 1 daughter lives in town (30 miles away); 1 daughter married/grandson, living out of state
Other: Several couples; he and wife play cards/socialize 2 or 3 times a month
Role: Works farm alone; husband/father/grandfather
Report of problems related to illness/condition: None until now
Coping behaviors: "My wife and I have always talked things out. You know the eleventh commandment is 'Thou shalt not go to bed angry.'"

Exhibits (Objective):
Speech: Clear, intelligible
Verbal/nonverbal communication with family/SO(s): Speaks quietly with wife, looking her in the eye; relaxed posture
Family interaction patterns: Wife sitting at bedside, relaxed, both reading paper, making occasional comments to each other

TEACHING/LEARNING

Reports (Subjective):
Dominant language: English Second language: -0- Literate: Yes
Education level: 2 years of college
Health and illness beliefs/practices/customs: "I take care of the minor problems and only see the doctor when something's broken."
Advance Directives: in chart
Familial risk factors/relationship:
Diabetes: Maternal uncle Tuberculosis: Brother died age 27
Heart Disease: Father died age 78, heart attack
Strokes: Mother died age 81 High BP: Mother
Prescribed medications:

Drug	*Dose*	*Schedule*	*Last dose*	*Purpose*
DiaBeta	10 mg bid	8 AM/6 PM	6 PM today	Control diabetes

Take medications regularly: Yes
Home urine/glucose monitoring: "Stopped several months ago when I ran out of Tes-Tape. It was always negative anyway."
Nonprescription (OTC) drugs: Occasionally ASA
Use of alcohol (amount/frequency): Socially, occasional beer
Tobacco: Smokes 1/2 pack/day
Admitting diagnosis (physician): Hyperglycemia with nonhealing lesion L foot
Reason for hospitalization (client): "Sore on foot, and the doctor is concerned about my blood sugar and says I'm supposed to learn this fingerstick test now."
History of current complaint: "Three weeks ago, I got a blister on my foot from breaking in my new boots. It got sore so I lanced it, but it isn't getting any better."
Client's expectations of this hospitalization: "Clear up this infection and control my diabetes."
Other relevant illness and/or previous hospitalizations/surgeries: 1969, R inguinal hernia repair
Evidence of failure to improve: Lesion L foot, 3 weeks
Last physical examination: Complete 1 year ago, office follow-up 3 months ago

Discharge Considerations (as of 6/28):
Anticipated discharge: 7/1/04 (3 days)
Resources: Person: Self, wife Financial: "If this doesn't take too long to heal, we got some savings to cover things."
Community supports: Diabetic support group (has not participated)
Anticipated lifestyle changes: Become more involved in management of condition
Assistance needed: May require farm help for several days
Teaching: Learn new medication regimen, glucose monitoring, and wound care; review diet; encourage smoking cessation
Referrals: Supplies: Downtown Pharmacy or AARP
Equipment: Glucometer—AARP
Follow-up: Primary care provider 1 wk after discharge to evaluate wound healing and potential need for additional changes in diabetic regimen

Another way to conceptualize the client's care needs is to create a *Mind Map* (Figure 3–3). This new technique or learning tool has been developed to help visualize the linkages or interconnections between various client symptoms, interventions, or problems as they impact each other. The parts that are great about traditional care plans (problem solving and categorizing) are retained but the linear/columnar nature of the plan is changed to a design that uses the whole brain—a design that brings left-brained, linear problem-solving thinking together with the free-wheeling, interconnected, creative right brain. Joining mind mapping and care planning enables the nurse to create a holistic view of a client, strengthening critical thinking skills, and facilitating the creative process of planning client care.

Mind mapping starts in the center of the page with a representation of the main concept—the client. (This helps keep in mind that the client is the focus of the plan, not the medical diagnosis or condition.) From that central thought, other main ideas that relate to the client radiate out from the center similar to spokes of a wheel (however, they do not have to be added in a balanced manner; it does not have to be a round "wheel"). Different concepts can be grouped together by geometric shapes, color coding, or by placement on the page. Connections and interconnections between groups of ideas are represented by the use of arrows or lines with defining phrases added that explain how the interconnected thoughts relate to one another. In this manner, many different pieces of information *about* the client can be connected directly *to* the client.

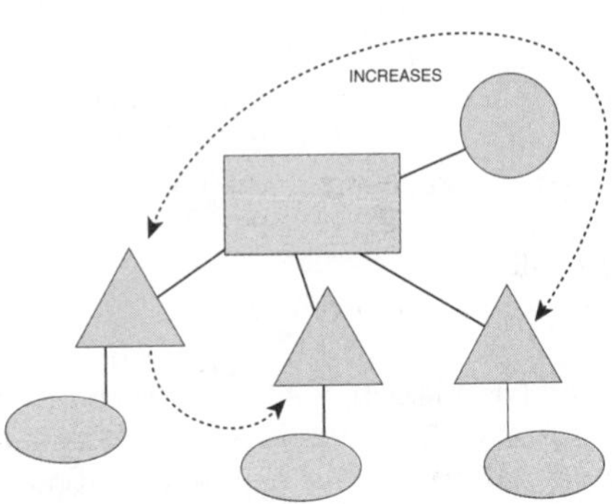

Whichever piece is chosen becomes the first layer of connections—clustered assessment data, nursing diagnoses, or outcomes. For example, a map could start with nursing diagnoses featured as the first "branches," each one being listed separately in some way on the map. Next, the signs and symptoms or data supporting the diagnoses could be added. Or the plan could begin with the client outcomes to be achieved with connections then to nursing diagnoses. When the plan is completed, there should be a nursing diagnosis (supported by subjective and objective assessment data), nursing interventions, desired client outcome(s), and any evaluation data, all connected in a manner that shows there is a relationship between them. It is critical to understand that there is no preset order for the pieces because one cluster is not more or less important than another (or one is not "subsumed" under another). It is important, however, that those pieces within a branch be in the same order in each branch.

Finally, to complete the learning experience, we present samples of the evaluation step based on the client situation.

EVALUATION

As nursing care is provided, ongoing assessment evaluates the client's response to therapy and progress toward accomplishing the desired outcomes. This activity serves as the feedback and control part of the nursing process through which the status of the individual client diagnostic statement is judged to be resolved, continuing, or requiring revision.

This process is visualized in Figure 3–4. Observation of Mr. R.S.'s wound reveals that edges are clean and pink and drainage is scant. Therefore, he is progressing toward achieving wound healing, and this problem will continue to be addressed, although no revision in the treatment plan is required at this time.

DOCUMENTATION

To date, a number of charting formats are being used for documentation. These include block notes, with a single entry covering an entire shift (e.g., 7–3 PM); narrative timed notes (e.g., 8:30 AM, ate all of breakfast); the problem-oriented medical record system (POMR or PORS) using the SOAP/SOAPIER approach; and the use of flow sheets with charting by exception, to name a few. The POMR can provide thorough documentation, but it was designed by physicians for episodic care and requires that the entries be tied to a problem identified from a problem list.

A charting system format created by nurses for documentation of frequent/repetitive care is Focus Charting®. It was designed to encourage looking at the client from a positive rather than a negative (or problem-oriented) perspective by using precise documentation to record the nursing process. Recording of assessment, interventions, and evaluation information in *data, action,* and *response* (DAR) categories facilitates tracking and following what is happening to the client at any given moment. Charting focuses on client and nursing concerns, with the focal point being client status and the associated nursing care. The focus is always stated in a way that reflects the client's concern/need rather than a nursing task or medical diagnosis. Thus, the focus can be a client problem/concern or nursing diagnosis, signs/symptoms of potential importance (e.g., fever, dysrhythmia, edema), a significant event or change in status, or a specific standard of care/hospital policy. An expansion of this format is DATRP—data, action, teaching, response, plan.

A more recent way to evaluate and document the client's progress (response to care) is through the use of clinical pathways. These were originally developed as tools for providing care in case management systems and are now used in many settings. A clinical pathway is a type of abbreviated plan of care that is event oriented (task oriented) and provides outcome-based guidelines for goal achievement within a designated length of stay. The pathway incorporates agency and professional standards of care and may be interdisciplinary, depending on the care setting. As a rule, however, the standardized clinical pathways address a specific diagnosis/condition or procedure (e.g., myocardial infarction, total hip replacement, chemotherapy) and do not provide for inclusion of secondary diagnoses or complications (e.g., asthmatic client in alcohol withdrawal). In short, if the client does not achieve the daily outcomes or goals of care, the variance is identified, and a separate plan of care must be developed to meet the client's individual needs. Therefore, although clinical pathways are becoming more common in the clinical setting, they have limited value (in place of more individualized plans of care) as learning tools for students who are working to practice the nursing process, critical thinking, and a holistic approach to meeting client needs. A sample clinical pathway (Figure 3–5) reflects Mr. R.S.'s primary diagnostic problem: nonhealing lesion, diabetic.

PLAN OF CARE: Mr. R.S.

CLIENT DIAGNOSTIC STATEMENT:

impaired Skin Integrity related to pressure, altered metabolic state, circulatory impairment, and decreased sensation, as evidenced by draining wound L foot.

OUTCOME: Blood Glucose Control (NOC) Indicators:

CLIENT WILL:

Demonstrate correction of metabolic state as evidenced by FBS less than 120 mg/dL within 36 hours (6/30 0700).

OUTCOME: Wound Healing: Secondary Intention (NOC) Indicators:

CLIENT WILL:

Be free of purulent drainage within 48 hours (6/30 1900).
Display signs of healing with wound edges clean/pink within 60 hours (7/1 0700).

ACTIONS/INTERVENTIONS	RATIONALE
Wound Care (NIC)	
Irrigate wound with room-temperature sterile NS tid.	Cleans wound without harming delicate tissues.
Assess wound with each dressing change. Obtain wound tracing on admission and at discharge.	Provides information about effectiveness of therapy, and identifies additional needs.
Apply wet to dry sterile dressing. Use paper tape.	Keeps wound clean/minimizes cross-contamination. Adhesive tape may be abrasive to fragile tissues.
Infection Control (NIC)	
Follow wound precautions.	Use of gloves and proper handling of contaminated dressings reduces likelihood of spread of infection.
Obtain sterile specimen of wound drainage on admission for laboratory analysis.	Culture/sensitivity identifies pathogens and therapy of choice.
Administer dicloxacillin 500 mg PO q6h, starting 10 PM. Observe for signs of hypersensitivity: pruritus, urticaria, rash.	Treatment of infection/prevention of complications. Food interferes with drug absorption, requiring scheduling around meals. Although no prior history of penicillin reaction, it may occur at any time.
Administer antidiabetic medications: 10 U Humulin N insulin SC q AM/hs after fingerstick BG; DiaBeta 10 mg PO bid; Glucophage 500 mg PO daily. Note onset of side effects.	Treats underlying metabolic dysfunction, reducing hyperglycemia and promoting healing. Glucophage lowers serum glucose levels by improving insulin sensitivity, increasing glucose utilization in the muscles. By using in conjunction with DiaBeta, client may be able to discontinue insulin once target dosage is achieved (e.g., 2000 mg/day). Increase of 1 tablet per week is necessary to limit side effects of diarrhea, abdominal cramping, vomiting, possibly leading to dehydration and prerenal azotemia.

(Continued on following page)

CLIENT DIAGNOSTIC STATEMENT:

acute Pain related to physical agent (wound L foot) evidenced by verbal report of pain and guarding behavior.

OUTCOMES: Pain Self-Control (NOC) Indicators:

CLIENT WILL:

Report pain is minimized/relieved within 1 hour of analgesic administration (ongoing).
Report absence or control of pain by discharge (7/1).

OUTCOME: Pain Disruptive Effects (NOC) Indicators:

Ambulate normally, full weight bearing by discharge (7/1).

ACTIONS/INTERVENTIONS	RATIONALE
Pain Management (NIC)	
Determine pain characteristics through client's description.	Establishes baseline for assessing improvement/changes.
Place foot cradle on bed/encourage use of loose-fitting slipper, when up.	Avoids direct pressure to area of injury, which could result in vasoconstriction/increased pain.
Administer Darvocet-N 100 mg PO q4h as needed. Document effectiveness.	Provides relief of persistent pain unrelieved by other measures.

CLIENT DIAGNOSTIC STATEMENT:

ineffective peripheral Tissue Perfusion related to decreased arterial flow as evidenced by decreased pulses, pale/cool feet, thick brittle nails, numbness/tingling of feet "when walks 1/4 mile."

OUTCOMES: Knowledge: Diabetes Management (NOC) Indicators:

CLIENT WILL:

Verbalize understanding of relationship between chronic disease (diabetes mellitus) and circulatory changes within 48 hours (6/30 1900).
Demonstrate awareness of safety factors/proper foot care within 48 hours (6/30 1900).
Maintain adequate level of hydration to maximize perfusion (ongoing), as evidenced by balanced intake/output, moist skin/mucous membranes, capillary refill less than 4 sec (ongoing).

ACTIONS/INTERVENTIONS	RATIONALE
CIRCULATORY CARE: Arterial Insufficiency (NIC)	
Elevate feet when up in chair. Avoid long periods with feet in dependent position.	Minimizes interruption of blood flow, reduces venous pooling.
Assess for signs of dehydration. Monitor intake/output. Encourage oral fluids.	Glycosuria may result in dehydration with consequent reduction of circulating volume and further impairment of peripheral circulation.
Recommend cessation of smoking.	Vascular constriction associated with smoking and diabetes impairs peripheral circulation.

(Continued on following page)

ACTIONS/INTERVENTIONS	RATIONALE
Instruct client to avoid constricting clothing/socks and ill-fitting shoes.	Compromised circulation and decreased pain sensation may precipitate or aggravate tissue breakdown.
Reinforce safety precautions regarding use of heating pads, hot water bottles/soaks.	Heat increases metabolic demands on compromised tissues. Vascular insufficiency alters pain sensation, increasing risk of injury.
Discuss complications of disease that result from vascular changes: ulceration, gangrene, muscle or bony structure changes.	Although proper control of diabetes mellitus may not prevent complications, severity of effects may be minimized. Diabetic foot complications are the leading cause of nontraumatic lower extremity amputations. *Note:* Skin dry, cracked, scaly; feet cool, pain when walking a distance suggest mild to medium vascular disease (autonomic neuropathy) that can limit response to infection, impair wound healing, and increase risk of bony deformities.
Review proper foot care as outlined in teaching plan.	Altered perfusion of lower extremities may led to serious/persistent complications at the cellular level.

CLIENT DIAGNOSTIC STATEMENT:

Learning Need regarding diabetic condition, related to misinterpretation of information and/or lack of recall as evidenced by inaccurate follow-through of instructions regarding home glucose monitoring and foot care and failure to recognize signs/symptoms of hyperglycemia.

OUTCOMES: Knowledge: Diabetes Management (NOC) Indicators:

CLIENT WILL:

Perform procedure of home glucose monitoring correctly within 36 hours (6/30 0700).
Verbalize basic understanding of disease process and treatment within 38 hours (6/30 0900).
Explain reasons for actions within 38 hours (6/30 0900).
Perform insulin administration correctly within 60 hours (7/1 0700).

ACTIONS/INTERVENTIONS	RATIONALE
TEACHING: Disease Process (NIC)	
Determine client's level of knowledge, priorities of learning needs, desire/need for including wife in instruction.	Establishes baseline and direction for teaching/planning. Involvement of wife, if desired, will provide additional resource for recall/understanding and may enhance client's follow-through.
Provide teaching guide, *Understanding Your Diabetes,* 6/28 PM. Show film *Living with Diabetes,* 6/29, 4 PM when wife is visiting. Include in group teaching session 6/30 AM. Review information and obtain feedback from client and wife.	Provides different methods for accessing/reinforcing information, and enhances opportunity for learning/understanding.
Discuss factors related to/altering diabetic control, such as stress, illness, exercise.	Drug therapy/diet may need to be altered in response to both short- and long-term stressors, changes in activity level.
Review signs/symptoms of hyperglycemia (e.g., fatigue, nausea/vomiting, polyuria/polydipsia). Discuss how to prevent and evaluate this situation and when to seek medical care. Have client identify appropriate interventions.	Recognition/understanding of these signs/symptoms and timely intervention will aid client in avoiding recurrences and preventing complications.

(Continued on following page)

ACTIONS/INTERVENTIONS	RATIONALE
Review and provide information about necessity for routine examination of feet and proper foot care (e.g., daily inspection for injuries, pressure areas, corns, calluses; proper nail cutting; daily washing, application of good moisturizing lotion such as Eucerin, Keri, or Nivea bid). Recommend loose-fitting socks, shoes that fit (break new shoes in gradually), and not going barefoot. If foot injury/skin break occurs, wash with soap/dermal cleanser and water, cover with sterile dressing, inspect wound, and change dressing daily; report redness, swelling, or presence of drainage.	Reduces risk of tissue injury, promotes understanding and prevention of stasis ulcer formation and wound healing difficulties.
TEACHING: Prescribed Medication (NIC)	
Instruct regarding prescribed insulin therapy:	May be a temporary treatment of hyperglycemia with infection or may be permanent replacement of oral hypoglycemic agent.
Humulin N insulin, SC.	Intermediate-acting insulin generally lasts 18–28 hr, with peak effect 6–12 hr.
Keep vial in current use at room. temperature (if used within 30 days).	Cold insulin is poorly absorbed.
Store extra vials in refrigerator.	Refrigeration prolongs the drug shelf life by preventing wide fluctuations in temperature.
Roll bottle and invert to mix, or shake gently, avoiding bubbles.	Vigorous shaking may create foam, which can interfere with accurate dose withdrawal and damage the insulin molecule. *Note:* New research suggests that shaking the vial may be more effective in mixing suspension.
Choice of injection sites (e.g., across lower abdomen in Z pattern).	Provides for steady absorption of medication. Site is easily visualized and accessible by client; and Z pattern minimizes tissue damage.
Demonstrate, then observe client in drawing insulin into syringe, reading syringe markings, and administering dose. Assess for accuracy.	May require several instruction sessions and practice before client and wife feel comfortable drawing up and injecting medication.
Instruct in signs/symptoms of insulin reaction/ hypoglycemia: fatigue, nausea, headache, hunger, sweating, irritability, shakiness, anxiety, difficulty concentrating.	Knowing what to watch for and appropriate treatment (such as ½ cup grape juice for immediate response and snack within ½ hr; e.g., 1 slice bread with peanut butter or cheese, fruit and slice of cheese for sustained effect) may prevent or minimize complications.
Review "sick day rules," e.g., call doctor if too sick to eat normally/stay active; take insulin as ordered. Keep record as noted in Sick Day Guide.	Understanding of necessary actions in the event of mild/severe illness promotes competent self-care and reduces risk of hyperglycemia or hypoglycemia.
Instruct client/wife in fingerstick glucose monitoring to be done 4×/day until stable, then bid at rotating times, such as FBS and before dinner; before lunch, and hs. Observe return demonstrations of the procedure.	Fingerstick monitoring provides accurate and timely information regarding diabetic status. Return demonstration verifies correct learning.
Recommend client maintain record/log of fingerstick testing, antidiabetic medication and insulin dosage/site, unusual physiological response, dietary intake. Outline desired goals; e.g., FBS 80–110, premeal 80–120.	Provides accurate record for review by caregivers for assessment of therapy effectiveness/needs.
Schedule consultation with dietitian to restructure meal plan and evaluate food choices.	Calories are unchanged on new orders but have been redistributed to three meals and two snacks. Dietary choices (e.g., increased vitamin C) may enhance healing.
Discuss other healthcare issues, such as smoking habits, self-monitoring for cancer (breasts/testicles), and reporting changes in general well-being.	Encourages client involvement, awareness, and responsibility for own health; promotes wellness. *Note:* Smoking tends to increase client's resistance to insulin.

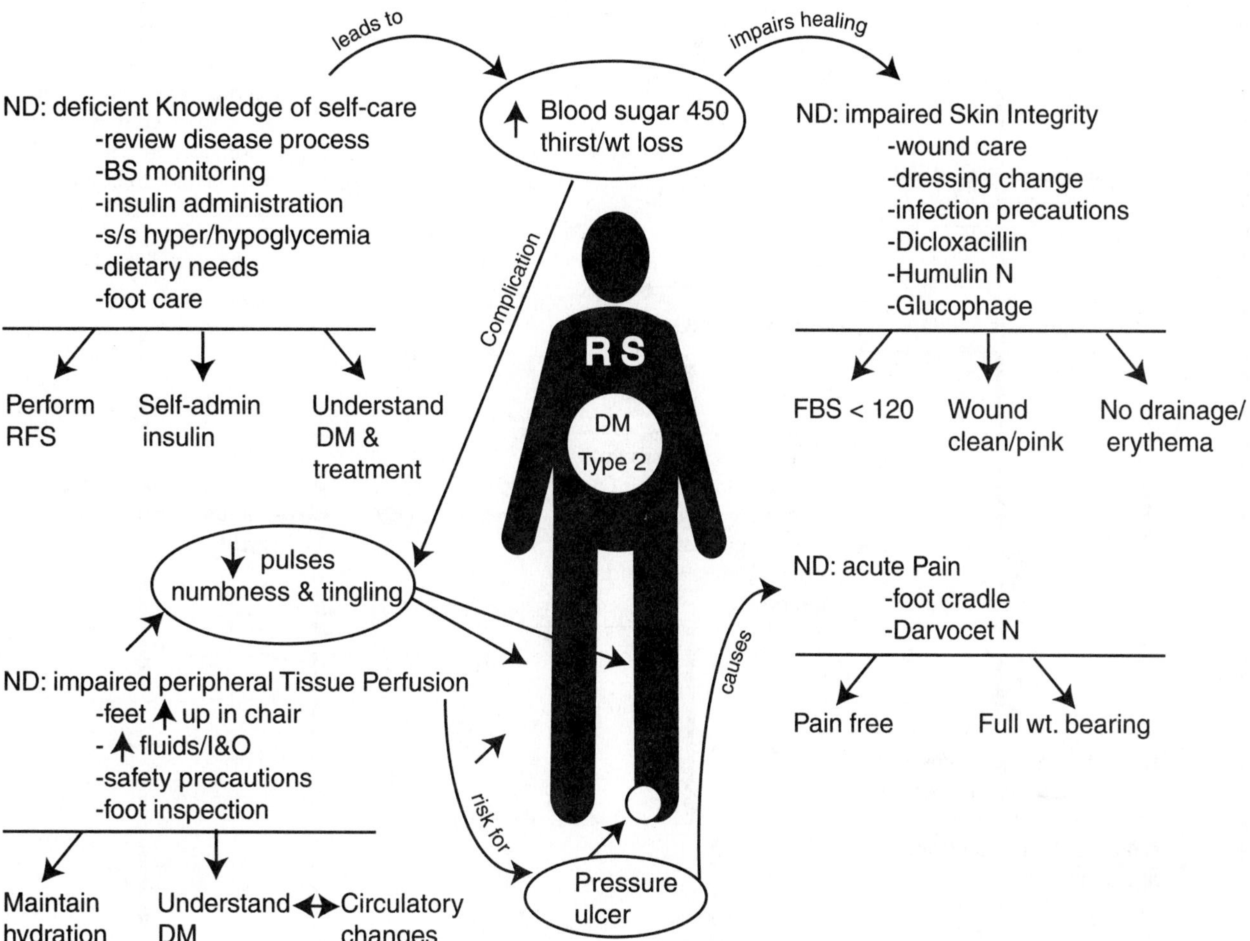

Figure 3–3. Mind map for Mr. R.S.

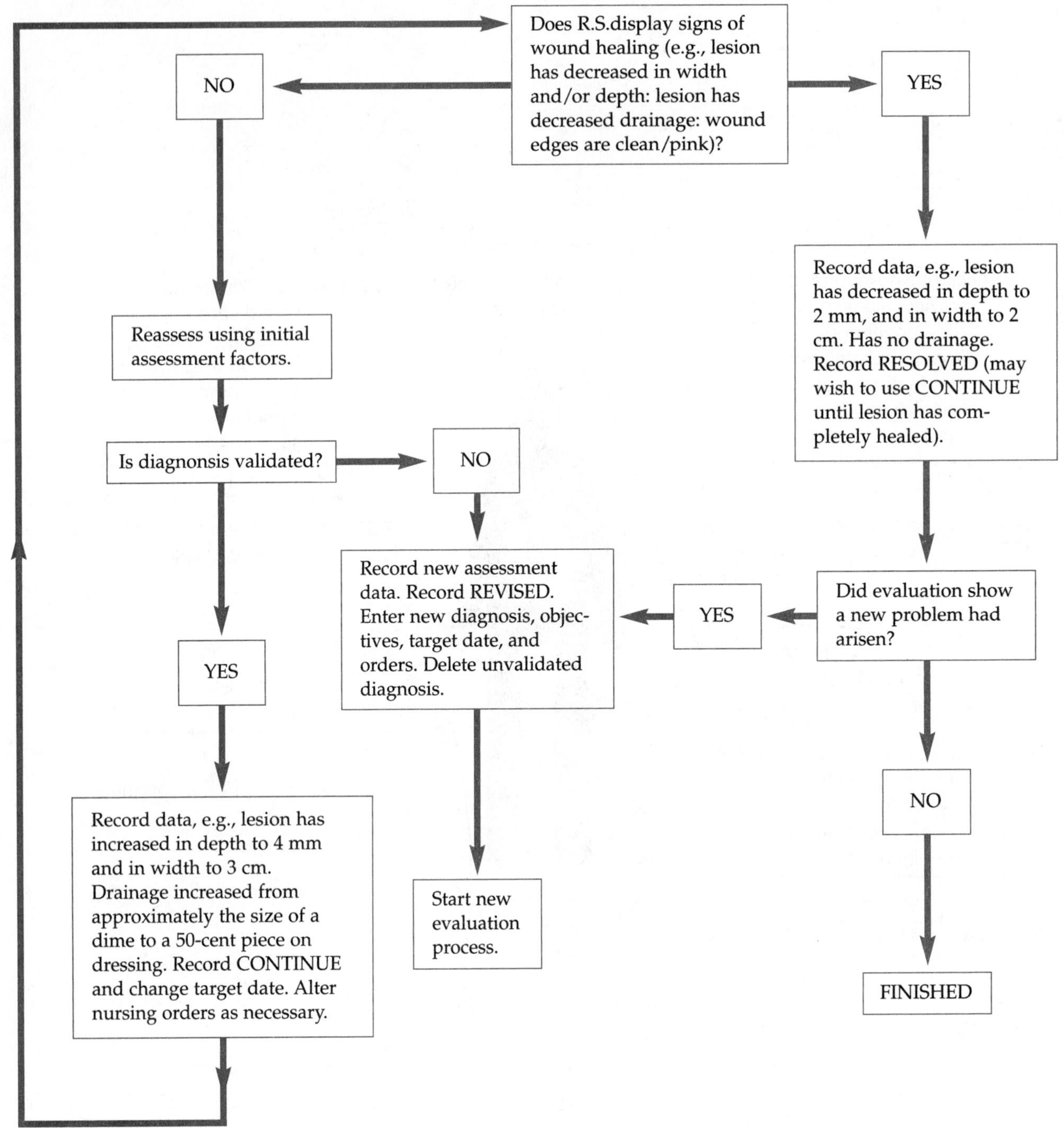

FIGURE 3–4. Outcome-based evaluation of the client's response to therapy. (Adapted from Cox, HC, et al: *Clinical Applications of Nursing Diagnosis,* ed. 3. FA Davis, Philadelphia, 1996.)

CP: Non-healing Lesion—Diabetic. ELOS: 3 Days—Variations from Designated Pathway Should Be Documented in Progress Notes

ND and Categories of Care	Adm Day <u>6/28</u> 7pm	Day 1 <u>6/29</u>	Day 2 <u>6/30</u>	Day 3 <u>7/1</u> Discharge
Impaired skin/tissue integrity	Actions: Goals:	Actions: Goals: Verbalize understanding of condition Display blood glucose WNL (ongoing)	Actions: Goals: Be free of signs of dehydration Wound free of purulent drainage Verbalize understanding of treatment need Perform self-care tasks No. 1 & 3 correctly Explain reasons for actions	Actions: Goals: Wound edges show signs of healing process Perform self-care task: No. 2 correctly Explain reason for actions Plan in place to meet discharge needs
Referrals		Dietician & determine need for: Home care Physical therapy Visiting nurse		
Diagnostic studies	Wound culture/sensitivity Gram's stain Random blood glucose Fingerstick BG hs	CBC, electrolytes Glycosylated Hb Serum lipid profile →Fingerstick BG qid Chest x-ray (if indicated) ECG (if indicated)	 →	 Fingerstick BG bid if stable
Additional assessments	VS qid I&O/level of hydration qd Character of wound tid Level of knowledge and priorities of learning needs Observe for signs of antibiotic hypersensitivity reaction	→ → → Anticipated discharge needs	→ VS each shift → →	→ →D/C →
Medications	Antibiotic: *Dicloxacillin 500 mg PO q6h* Antidiabetic: *Humulin N insulin 0 units SC hs*	Antibiotic: same Antidiabetic: *Humulin N insulin 10 U SC q AM/hs* *DiaBeta 10 mg PO bid* *Glucophage 500 mg PO qd*	Antibiotic: same Antidiabetic: same	Antibiotic: same Antidiabetic: same
Client education	Provide: *Understanding Your Diabetes*	Film *Living with Diabetes* Demonstrate and practice self-care activities: 1. Fingerstick BG 2. Insulin administration 3. Wound care 4. Routine foot care	Group sessions: *Diabetic management*	Practice self-care activities 2: *insulin administration* Review discharge instructions
Additional nursing actions	Up ad lib NS soaks/dressing change tid Goals:	→ →	→ →	→ →

Figure 3–5. Sample clinical pathway.

(Continued on following page)

CP: Non-healing Lesion—Diabetic. ELOS: 3 Days—Variations from Designated Pathway Should Be Documented in Progress Notes *(Continued)*

ND and Categories of Care	Adm Day 6/28 7pm	Day 1 6/29	Day 2 6/30	Day 3 7/1 Discharge
Acute Pain	Actions: State pain relieved or minimized with 1 hr of analgesic administration (ongoing) Verbalize understanding of when to report pain and rating scale used Verbalize understanding of self-care measures No. 1–2 Explain reason for actions	Actions: Goals: Verbalize understanding of self-care measure No. 3 Explain reason for actions	Actions: Goals: Able to participate in usual level: *ambulate full weight bearing*	Actions: Goals: State pain-free/controlled with medication Verbalize understanding of correct medication use
Additional assessments	Characteristics of pain Level of participation activities Individual analgesic needs	→ → →	→ → →	→ → →
Medications Allergies: -0-	Analgesic: Darvocet-N 100 mg PO q4h PRN	Analgesic: same	Analgesic: same	Analgesic: same
Client education	Orient to unit/room Guidelines for self-report of pain and rating scale *0–10* Safety/comfort measures: *1 elevation of feet* *2 proper footwear*	Safety/comfort measures *3 prevention of injury*		Review discharge medication instructions: dosage, route, frequency, side effects
Additional nursing actions	Bed cradle as indicated			

4
CHAPTER

Cardiovascular

HYPERTENSION: SEVERE

Hypertension was previously defined as blood pressure greater than 140/90 mm Hg by the 1992 Joint National Committee on Detection, Evaluation, and Treatment of High Blood Pressure and was classified in stages, according the the degree of severity. In 2003, new guidelines were issued by the National Heart, Lung, and Blood Institute (NHLBI) that include a lower "normal blood pressure," a "prehypertension" level, and a merging of staging categories.

Normal blood pressure is now defined as measurements less than 120/80 mm Hg and prehypertension as 120–139/80–89 mm Hg. Hypertension is defined as pressure greater than 140/90 mm Hg; and is classified according to the degree of severity. Stage I (mild) is 140/90–159/99. Stage II (moderate) is 160/100 or greater. Stage III (severe) is present when systolic pressure is greater than 180 and diastolic pressure is greater than 110. Stage IV (very severe) occurs when systolic pressure is 210 or greater with diastolic pressure greater than 120. Stages II and III hypertension have essentially been combined in the new guidelines, as their treatment is the same.

Hypertension is also categorized according to etiology: as *primary/essential* (approximately 95% of all cases), when it has no identifiable cause; or *secondary,* which occurs as a result of an identifiable, sometimes correctable, pathologic condition (e.g., kidney disorders, use of medications, drugs or other chemicals, adrenal gland tumors, or primary aldosteronism).

Hypertension increases with age and is one of the major risk factors in the development of cardiovascular disease. Current research has demonstrated that the systolic blood pressure is a more important determinant of cardiovascular risk in people over 50 years of age; however, in clients under 50 years old, the diastolic blood pressure is the major predictor.

Blood pressure in the "prehypertension" range responds well to lifestyle changes (e.g., weight management and exercise), and is not usually treated with medications unless other risk factors are present, such as diabetes or heart disease. However, recent studies indicate that persons with prehypertension are at high risk for developing hypertension and death from heart diease and stroke.

The goal of treatment is to prevent the long-term sequelae of the disease (i.e., target organ disease [TOD]). Although the elderly are most prone to this disorder and its sequelae, it is a growing health problem across many cultures, and is demonstrated in youger people in multiple populations.

CARE SETTING

Although hypertension is usually treated in a community setting, management of stages III and IV with symptoms of complications/compromise may require inpatient care, especially when TOD is present. The majority of interventions included here can be used in either setting.

RELATED CONCERNS

Cerebrovascular accident/stroke, page 236
Myocardial infarction, page 72
Psychosocial aspects of care, page 770
Renal failure: acute, page 541
Renal failure: chronic, page 553

Client Assessment Database

ACTIVITY/REST

May report: Weakness, fatigue, shortness of breath
Sedentary lifestyle (major risk factor)

May exhibit: Elevated heart rate
Change in heart rhythm
Tachypnea; shortness of breath with exertion

CIRCULATION

May report: History of intermittent or sustained elevation of diastolic or systolic blood pressure; presence of atherosclerotic, valvular, or coronary artery heart disease (including myocardial infarction [MI], angina, heart failure [HF]) and cerebrovascular disease (reflecting TOD)

Episodes of palpitations, diaphoresis

May exhibit: Elevated blood pressure (BP) (serial elevated measurements are necessary to confirm diagnosis)

Note: Postural hypotension, when present, may be related to drug regimen or reflect dehydration or reduced ventricular function.

Pulse: Bounding carotid, jugular, radial pulsations; pulse disparities (e.g., femoral delay as compared with radial or brachial pulsation); absence of/diminished popliteal, posterior tibial, pedal pulses

Apical pulse: Point of maximal impulse (PMI) possibly displaced and/or forceful

Rate/rhythm: Tachycardia, various dysrhythmias

Heart sounds: Accentuated S_2 at base; S_3 (early HF); S_4 (rigid left ventricle/left ventricular hypertrophy)

Murmurs of valvular stenosis

Vascular bruits audible over carotid, femoral, or epigastrium (artery stenosis); jugular venous distension (JVD) (venous congestion)

Extremities: discoloration of skin, cool temperature (peripheral vasoconstriction); capillary refill possibly slow/delayed (vasoconstriction)

Skin: Pallor, cyanosis, and diaphoresis (congestion, hypoxemia); flushing (pheochromocytoma)

EGO INTEGRITY

May report: History of personality changes, anxiety, depression, euphoria, or chronic anger (may imdicate cerebral impairment)

Multiple stress factors (relationship, financial, job related)

May exhibit: Mood swings, restlessness, irritability, narrowed attention span, outbursts of crying

Emphatic hand gestures, tense facial muscles (particularly around the eyes), quick physical movement, expiratory sighs, accelerated speech pattern

ELIMINATION

May report: Past or present renal insult (e.g., infection/obstruction or past history of kidney disease)

FOOD/FLUID

May report: Food preferences, which include high-salt, high-fat, high-cholesterol foods (e.g., fried foods, cheese, eggs); licorice; high caloric content; low dietary intake of potassium, calcium, and magnesium

Nausea, vomiting

Recent weight changes (gain/loss)

Current/history of diuretic use

May exhibit: Normal weight or obesity

Presence of edema (may be generalized or dependent); venous congestion, JVD

Glycosuria (almost 10% of hypertensive clients are diabetic, reflecting TOD)

NEUROSENSORY

May report: Fainting spells/dizziness

Throbbing, suboccipital headaches (present on awakening and disappearing spontaneously after several hours)

Episodes of numbness and/or weakness on one side of the body; brief periods of confusion or difficulty with speech (transient ischemic attack [TIA]); or history of cerebrovascular accident (CVA)

Visual disturbances (diplopia, blurred vision)

Episodes of epistaxis

May exhibit: Mental status: changes in alertness, orientation, speech pattern/content, affect, thought process, or memory

Motor responses: decreased strength, hand grip, and/or deep tendon reflexes

Optic retinal changes: from mild sclerosis/arterial narrowing to marked retinal and sclerotic changes with edema or papilledema, exudates, hemorrhages, and arterial nicking, dependent on severity/duration of hypertension (TOD)

PAIN/DISCOMFORT

May report: Angina (coronary artery disease/cardiac involvement)
Intermittent pain in legs/claudication (indicative of arteriosclerosis of lower extremity arteries)
Severe occipital headaches as previously noted
Abdominal pain/masses (pheochromocytoma)

RESPIRATION

(Generally associated with advanced cardiopulmonary effects of sustained/severe hypertension)

May report: Dyspnea associated with activity/exertion
Tachypnea, orthopnea, paroxysmal nocturnal dyspnea
Cough with/without sputum production
Smoking history (major risk factor)

May exhibit: Respiratory distress/use of accessory muscles
Adventitious breath sounds (crackles/wheezes)
Pallor or cyanosis

SAFETY

May report/exhibit: Impaired coordination/gait
Transient episodes of numbness, unilateral paresthesias
Light-headedness with position changes

SEXUALITY

May report: Postmenopausal (major risk factor)
Erectile dysfunction (medication related)

TEACHING/LEARNING

May report: Familial risk factors: hypertension, atherosclerosis, heart disease, diabetes mellitus, cerebrovascular/kidney disease
Ethnic/racial risk factors; e.g., more prevalent in African-American and southeast Asian populations
Use of birth control pills or other hormones; drug/alcohol use
Use of herbal supplements to manage blood pressure (e.g. garlic, hawthorn, black cohash, celery seed, coleus, evening primrose)

Discharge plan considerations: Assistance with self-monitoring of blood pressure (BP)
Periodic evaluation of and alterations in medication therapy

Refer to section at end of plan for postdischarge considerations.

DIAGNOSTIC STUDIES

Hemoglobin/hematocrit: Not diagnostic but assesses relationship of cells to fluid volume (viscosity) and may indicate risk factors such as hypercoagulability, anemia.

Blood urea nitrogen (BUN)/creatinine: Provides information about renal perfusion/function.

Glucose: Hyperglycemia (diabetes mellitus is a precipitator of hypertension) may result from elevated catecholamine levels (increases hypertension), and/or use of thiazide diuretics.

Serum potassium: Hypokalemia may indicate the presence of primary aldosteronism (cause) or be a side effect of diuretic therapy.

Serum calcium and magnesium: Imbalances may contribute to hypertension.

Lipid panel (total lipids, high-density lipoprotein [HDL], low-density lipoprotein [LDL], cholesterol, triglycerides, phospholipids [usually done by blood testing, however, a new test called PREVU measuring skin sterol may be used in some facilities]): Elevated level may indicate predisposition for/presence of atheromatous plaquing. *Note:* Diuretics and β-blockers can also raise triglyceride and LDL levels.

Thyroid studies: Hyperthyroidism may lead or contribute to vasoconstriction and hypertension.

Serum/urine aldosterone level: May be done to assess for primary aldosteronism.

Urinalysis: May show blood, protein, or white blood cells; or glucose suggests renal dysfunction and/or presence of diabetes.

Creatinine clearance: May be reduced, reflecting renal damage.

Urine vanillylmandelic acid (VMA) (catecholamine metabolite): Elevation may indicate presence of pheochromocytoma (cause); 24-hour urine VMA may be done for assessment of pheochromocytoma if hypertension is intermittent.

Uric acid: Hyperuricemia has been implicated as a risk factor for the development of hypertension.
Renin: Elevated in renovascular and malignant hypertension, salt-wasting disorders.
Urine steroids: Elevation may indicate hyperadrenalism, pheochromocytoma, pituitary dysfunction, Cushing's syndrome.
Intravenous pyelogram (IVP): May identify cause of secondary hypertension; e.g., renal parenchymal disease, renal/ureteral calculi.
Kidney and renography nuclear scan: Evaluates renal status (TOD).
Excretory urography: May reveal renal atrophy, indicating chronic renal disease.
Chest x-ray: May demonstrate obstructing calcification in valve areas; deposits in and/or notching of aorta; cardiac enlargement.
Computed tomography (CT) scan: Assesses for cerebral tumor, CVA, or encephalopathy or to rule out pheochromocytoma.
Electrocardiogram (ECG): May demonstrate enlarged heart, strain patterns, conduction disturbances. *Note:* Broad, notched P wave is one of the earliest signs of hypertensive heart disease.

NURSING PRIORITIES

1. Maintain/enhance cardiovascular functioning.
2. Prevent complications.
3. Provide information about disease process/prognosis and treatment regimen.
4. Support active client control of condition.

DISCHARGE GOALS

1. BP within acceptable limits for individual.
2. Cardiovascular and systemic complications prevented/minimized.
3. Disease process/prognosis and therapeutic regimen understood.
4. Necessary lifestyle/behavioral changes initiated.
5. Plan in place to meet needs after discharge.

NURSING DIAGNOSIS: risk for decreased Cardiac Output

Risk factors may include

Increased vascular resistance, vasoconstriction
Myocardial ischemia
Ventricular hypertrophy/rigidity

Possibly evidenced by

[Not applicable; presence of signs and symptoms establishes an *actual* diagnosis.]

DESIRED OUTCOMES/EVALUATION CRITERIA—CLIENT WILL:

Circulation Status (NOC)

Participate in activities that reduce BP/cardiac workload.
Maintain BP within individually acceptable range.
Demonstrate stable cardiac rhythm and rate within client's normal range.

ACTIONS/INTERVENTIONS	RATIONALE
Hemodynamic Regulation (NIC)	
Independent	
Monitor BP. Measure in both arms/thighs three times, 3–5 min apart while client is at rest, then sitting, then standing for initial evaluation. Use correct cuff size and accurate technique.	Comparison of pressures provides a more complete picture of vascular involvement/scope of problem. Severe hypertension is classified in the adult as a diastolic pressure elevation to 110 mm Hg; progressive diastolic readings above 120 mm Hg are considered first accelerated, then malignant

ACTIONS/INTERVENTIONS	RATIONALE
	(very severe). Systolic hypertension also is an established risk factor for cerebrovascular disease and ischemic heart disease even when diastolic pressure is not elevated. In younger clients, diastolic with normal systolic readings, elevation of diastolic readings may indicate prehypertension.
Note presence, quality of central and peripheral pulses.	Bounding carotid, jugular, radial, and femoral pulses may be observed/palpated. Pulses in the legs/feet may be diminished, reflecting effects of vasoconstriction (increased systemic vascular resistance [SVR]) and venous congestion.
Auscultate heart tones and breath sounds.	S_4 heart sound is common in severely hypertensive clients because of the presence of atrial hypertrophy (increased atrial volume/pressure). Development of S_3 indicates ventricular hypertrophy and impaired functioning. Presence of crackles, wheezes may indicate pulmonary congestion secondary to developing or chronic heart failure.
Observe skin color, moisture, temperature, and capillary refill time.	Presence of pallor; cool, moist skin; and delayed capillary refill time may be due to peripheral vasoconstriction or reflect cardiac decompensation/decreased output.
Note dependent/general edema.	May indicate heart failure, renal or vascular impairment.
Provide calm, restful surroundings, minimize environmental activity/noise. Limit the number of visitors and length of stay.	Helps reduce sympathetic stimulation; promotes relaxation.
Maintain activity restrictions; e.g., bed rest/chair rest; schedule periods of uninterrupted rest; assist client with self-care activities as needed.	Reduces physical stress and tension that affect blood pressure and the course of hypertension.
Provide comfort measures; e.g., back and neck massage, elevation of head.	Decreases discomfort and may reduce sympathetic stimulation.
Instruct in relaxation techniques, guided imagery, distractions.	Can reduce stressful stimuli, produce calming effect, thereby reducing BP.
Monitor response to medications to control blood pressure.	Response to drug therapy (usually consisting of several drugs, including diuretics, angiotensin-converting enzyme [ACE] inhibitors, angiotensin receptor blockers [ARBs], vascular smooth muscle relaxants, and alpha, beta, and calcium channel blockers) is dependent on both the individual as well as the synergistic effects of the drugs. Because of side effects, drug interactions, and client's motivation for taking antihypertensive medication, it is important to use the smallest number and lowest dosage of medications.

Collaborative

Administer medications as indicated:

Thiazide diuretics; e.g., chlorothiazide (Diuril); hydrochlorothiazide (Esidrix/HydroDIURIL); hydrochlorothiazide with triamterene (Diazide, Maxide) or amiloride (Modiuretic); bendroflumethiazide (Naturetin); indapamide (Lozol), metolazone (Mykrox, Zaroxolyn);	Diuretics are considered first-line medications for uncomplicated stage I or II hypertension and may be used alone or in association with other drugs (such as β-blockers) to reduce BP in clients with relatively normal renal function. These diuretics potentiate the effects of other antihypertensive agents as well by limiting fluid retention, and may reduce the incidence of strokes and heart failure.
Loop diuretics; e.g., furosemide (Lasix), bumetanide (Bumex), torsemide (Demadex);	These drugs produce marked diuresis by inhibiting resorption of sodium and chloride and are effective antihypertensives, especially in clients who are resistant to thiazides or have renal impairment.
Potassium-sparing diuretics; e.g., spironolactone (Aldactone); triamterene (Dyrenium); amiloride (Midamor);	May be given in combination with a thiazide diuretic to minimize potassium loss.

ACTIONS/INTERVENTIONS	RATIONALE
α-adrenergic, β-adrenergic, or centrally acting adrenergic antagonists; e.g., doxazosin (Cardura); propranolol (Inderal); acebutolol (Sectral); metoprolol (Lopressor), labetalol (Normodyne); atenolol (Tenormin); nadolol (Corgard), carvedilol (Coreg); methyldopa (Aldomet); clonidine (Catapres); prazosin (Minipress); terazosin (Hytrin); pindolol (Visken);	β-Blockers may be ordered instead of diuretics for clients with ischemic heart disease; obese clients with cardiogenic hypertension; and clients with concurrent supraventricular arrhythmias, angina, or hypertensive cardiomyopathy. Specific actions of these drugs vary, but they generally reduce BP through the combined effect of decreased total peripheral resistance, reduced cardiac output, inhibited sympathetic activity, and suppression of renin release. *Note:* Clients with diabetes should use Corgard and Visken with caution because they can prolong and mask the hypoglycemic effects of insulin. The elderly may require smaller doses because of the potential for bradycardia and hypotension. African-American clients tend to be less responsive to β-blockers in general and may require increased dosage or use of another drug; e.g., monotherapy with a diuretic.
Calcium channel antagonists; e.g., nifedipine (Adalat, Procardia); verapamil (Calan, Isoptin, Verelan); diltiazem (Cardizem); amlodipine (Norvasc); isradipine (DynaCirc); nicardipine (Cardene);	May be used to treat severe hypertension when a combination of a diuretic and a sympathetic inhibitor does not sufficiently control BP. Vasodilation of healthy cardiac vasculature and increased coronary blood flow are secondary benefits of vasodilator therapy.
Adrenergic neuron blockers: guanadrel (Hylorel); guanethidine (Ismelin); reserpine (Serpalan);	Reduce arterial and venous constriction activity at the sympathetic nerve endings.
Direct-acting oral vasodilators: hydralazine (Apresoline); minoxidil (Loniten);	Action is to relax vascular smooth muscle, thereby reducing vascular resistance.
Direct-acting parenteral vasodilators: diazoxide (Hyperstat), nitroprusside (Nitropress); labetalol (Normodyne);	These are given intravenously for management of hypertensive emergencies.
Angiotensin-converting enzyme (ACE) inhibitors; e.g., captopril (Capoten); enalapril (Vasotec); benazepril (Lotensin); lisinopril (Zestril); fosinopril (Monopril); ramipril (Altace) Angiotensin II blockers; e.g., valsartan (Diovan), guanethidine (Ismelin).	The use of an additional sympathetic inhibitor may be required for its cumulative effect when other measures have failed to control BP or when congestive heart failure (CHF) or diabetes is present.
Implement dietary restrictions (e.g., calories, refined carbohydrates, sodium, fat, and cholesterol) as indicated.	These restrictions can help manage fluid retention and, with associated hypertensive response, decrease myocardial workload.
Prepare for surgery when indicated.	When hypertension is due to pheochromocytoma, removal of the tumor will correct condition.

NURSING DIAGNOSIS: Activity Intolerance

May be related to

Generalized weakness
Imbalance between oxygen supply and demand

Possibly evidenced by

Verbal report of fatigue or weakness
Abnormal heart rate or BP response to activity
Exertional discomfort or dyspnea
Electrocardiogram (ECG) changes reflecting ischemia; dysrhythmias

DESIRED OUTCOMES/EVALUATION CRITERIA—CLIENT WILL:

Endurance (NOC)

Participate in necessary/desired activities.
Report a measurable increase in activity tolerance.
Demonstrate a decrease in physiologic signs of intolerance.

ACTIONS/INTERVENTIONS	RATIONALE
Energy Management (NIC)	
Independent	
Assess the client's response to activity, noting pulse rate more than 20 beats/min faster than resting rate; marked increase in BP during/after activity (systolic pressure increase of 40 mm Hg or diastolic pressure increase of 20 mm Hg); dyspnea or chest pain; excessive fatigue and weakness; diaphoresis; dizziness or syncope.	The stated parameters are helpful in assessing physiologic responses to the stress of activity and, if present, are indicators of overexertion.
Instruct client in energy-conserving techniques; e.g., using chair when showering, sitting to brush teeth or comb hair, carrying out activities at a slower pace.	Energy-saving techniques reduce the energy expenditure, thereby assisting in equalization of oxygen supply and demand.
Encourage progressive activity/self-care when tolerated. Provide assistance as needed.	Gradual activity progression prevents a sudden increase in cardiac workload. Providing assistance only as needed encourages independence in performing activities.

NURSING DIAGNOSIS: acute headache Pain

May be related to

Increased cerebral vascular pressure

Possibly evidenced by

Reports of throbbing pain located in suboccipital region, present on awakening, and disappearing spontaneously after being up and about
Reluctance to move head, rubbing head, avoidance of bright lights and noise, wrinkled brow, clenched fists
Reports of stiffness of neck, dizziness, blurred vision, nausea, and vomiting

DESIRED OUTCOMES/EVALUATION CRITERIA—CLIENT WILL:

Pain Control (NOC)

Report pain/discomfort is relieved/controlled.
Verbalize methods that provide relief.
Follow prescribed pharmacologic regimen.

ACTIONS/INTERVENTIONS	RATIONALE
Pain Management (NIC)	
Independent	
Determine specifics of pain; e.g., location, characteristics, intensity (0–10 scale), onset/duration. Note nonverbal cues.	Facilitates diagnosis of problem and initiation of appropriate therapy. Helpful in evaluating effectiveness of therapy.
Encourage/maintain bedrest during acute phase.	Minimizes stimulation/promotes relaxation.
Provide/recommend nonpharmacologic measures for relief of headache; e.g., cool cloth to forehead; back and neck rubs; quiet, dimly lit room; relaxation techniques (guided imagery, distraction); and diversional activities.	Measures that reduce cerebral vascular pressure and that slow/block sympathetic response are effective in relieving headache and associated complications.
Eliminate/minimize vasoconstricting activities that may aggravate headache; e.g., straining at stool, prolonged coughing, bending over.	Activities that increase vasoconstriction accentuate the headache in the presence of increased cerebral vascular pressure.

ACTIONS/INTERVENTIONS	RATIONALE
Assist client with ambulation as needed.	Dizziness and blurred vision frequently are associated with vascular headache. Client may also experience episodes of postural hypotension, causing weakness when ambulating.
Provide liquids, soft foods, frequent mouth care if nosebleeds occur or nasal packing has been done to stop bleeding.	Promotes general comfort. Nasal packing may interfere with swallowing or require mouth breathing, leading to stagnation of oral secretions and drying of mucous membranes.
Collaborative	
Administer medications as indicated: analgesics	Reduce/control pain and decrease stimulation of the sympathetic nervous system.
Antianxiety agents; e.g., lorazepam (Ativan), alprazolam (Xanax), diazepam (Valium)	May aid in the reduction of tension and discomfort that is intensified by stress.

NURSING DIAGNOSIS: imbalanced Nutrition: More than Body Requirements

May be related to

Excessive intake in relation to metabolic need
Sedentary lifestyle
Cultural preferences

Possibly evidenced by

Weight 10%–20% more than ideal for height and frame
Triceps skinfold more than 15 mm in men and 25 mm in women (maximum for age and sex)
Reported or observed dysfunctional eating patterns

DESIRED OUTCOMES/EVALUATION CRITERIA—CLIENT WILL:

KNOWLEDGE: Treatment Regimen (NOC)

Identify correlation between hypertension and obesity.

NUTRITIONAL STATUS: Nutrient Intake (NOC)

Demonstrate change in eating patterns (e.g., food choices, quantity) to attain desirable body weight with optimal maintenance of health.
Initiate/maintain individually appropriate exercise program.

ACTIONS/INTERVENTIONS	RATIONALE
Weight Reduction Assistance (NIC)	
Independent	
Assess client understanding of direct relationship between hypertension and obesity.	Obesity is an added risk with high blood pressure because of the disproportion between fixed aortic capacity and increased cardiac output associated with increased body mass. Reduction in weight may obviate the need for drug therapy or decrease the amount of medication needed for control of BP. *Note:* Recent research suggests that bringing weight within 15% of ideal weight can result in a drop of 10 mm Hg in both systolic and diastolic BP.

ACTIONS/INTERVENTIONS	RATIONALE
Discuss necessity for decreased caloric intake and limited intake of fats, salt, and sugar as indicated.	Faulty eating habits contribute to atherosclerosis and obesity, which predispose to hypertension and subsequent complications; e.g., stroke, kidney disease, heart failure. Excessive salt intake expands the intravascular fluid volume and may damage kidneys, which can further aggravate hypertension. *Note:* One study showed that sodium reduction reduced the need for medication by 31%. Weight loss lowered the need for medication by 36% and the combination of the two by 53%.
Determine client's desire to lose weight.	Motivation for weight reduction is internal. The individual must want to lose weight, or the program most likely will not succeed.
Review usual daily caloric intake and dietary choices.	Identifies current strengths/weaknesses in dietary program. Aids in determining individual need for adjustment/teaching.
Establish a realistic weight reduction plan with the client; e.g., 1-lb weight loss/wk.	Reducing caloric intake by 500 calories daily theoretically yields a weight loss of 1 lb/wk. Slow reduction in weight is therefore indicative of fat loss with muscle sparing and generally reflects a change in eating habits.
Encourage client to maintain a diary of food intake, including when and where eating takes place and the circumstances and feelings around which the food was eaten.	Provides a database for both the adequacy of nutrients eaten and the emotional conditions of eating. Helps focus attention on factors that client has control over/can change.
Instruct and assist in appropriate food selections, such as a diet rich in fruits, vegetables, and low-fat dairy foods referred to as the DASH (dietary approaches to stop hypertension) diet and avoiding foods high in saturated fat (butter, cheese, eggs, ice cream, meat) and cholesterol (fatty meat, egg yolks, whole dairy products, shrimp, organ meats).	Avoiding foods high in saturated fat and cholesterol is important in preventing progressing atherogenesis. Moderation and use of low-fat products in place of total abstinence from certain food items may prevent sense of deprivation and enhance cooperation with dietary regimen. The DASH diet, in conjunction with exercise, weight loss, and limits on salt intake, may reduce or even eliminate the need for drug therapy.

Collaborative

Refer to dietitian as indicated.	Can provide additional counseling and assistance with meeting individual dietary needs.

NURSING DIAGNOSIS: ineffective Coping

May be related to

Situational/maturational crisis; multiple life changes
Inadequate relaxation; little or no exercise, work overload
Inadequate support systems
Poor nutrition
Unmet expectations; unrealistic perceptions
Inadequate coping methods

Possibly evidenced by

Verbalization of inability to cope or ask for help
Inability to meet role expectations/basic needs or problem-solve
Destructive behavior toward self; overeating, lack of appetite; excessive smoking/drinking, proneness to alcohol abuse
Chronic fatigue/insomnia; muscular tension; frequent head/neck aches; chronic worry, irritability, anxiety, emotional tension, depression

DESIRED OUTCOMES/EVALUATION CRITERIA—CLIENT WILL:

Coping (NOC)

Identify ineffective coping behaviors and consequences.
Verbalize awareness of own coping abilities/strengths.
Identify potential stressful situations and steps to avoid/modify them.
Demonstrate the use of effective coping skills/methods.

ACTIONS/INTERVENTIONS	RATIONALE
Coping Enhancement (NIC)	
Independent	
Assess effectiveness of coping strategies by observing behaviors; e.g., ability to verbalize feelings and concerns, willingness to participate in the treatment plan.	Adaptive mechanisms are necessary to appropriately alter one's lifestyle, deal with the chronicity of hypertension, and integrate prescribed therapies into daily living.
Note reports of sleep disturbances, increasing fatigue, impaired concentration, irritability, decreased tolerance of headache, inability to cope/problem-solve.	Manifestations of maladaptive coping mechanisms may be indicators of repressed anger and have been found to be major determinants of diastolic BP.
Assist client to identify specific stressors and possible strategies for coping with them.	Recognition of stressors is the first step in altering one's response to the stressor.
Include client in planning of care, and encourage maximum participation in treatment plan/interdisciplinary team.	Involvement provides client with an ongoing sense of control, improves coping skills, and can enhance cooperation with therapeutic regimen. Ongoing intensive assessment and management by an interdisciplinary team promotes timely adjustments to therapeutic regimen.
Encourage client to evaluate life priorities/goals. Ask questions such as, "Is what you are doing getting you what you want?"	Focuses client's attention on reality of present situation relative to client's view of what is wanted. Strong work ethic, need for "control," and outward focus may have led to lack of attention to personal needs.
Assist client to identify and begin planning for necessary lifestyle changes. Assist to adjust, rather than abandon, personal/family goals.	Necessary changes should be realistically prioritized so client can avoid being overwhelmed and feeling powerless.

NURSING DIAGNOSIS: deficient Knowledge [Learning Need] regarding condition, treatment plan, self-care, and discharge needs

May be related to

Lack of knowledge/recall
Information misinterpretation
Cognitive limitation
Denial of diagnosis

Possibly evidenced by

Verbalization of the problem
Request for information
Statement of misconception
Inaccurate follow-through of instructions; inadequate performance of procedures
Inappropriate or exaggerated behaviors; e.g., hostile, agitated, apathetic

DESIRED OUTCOMES/EVALUATION CRITERIA—CLIENT WILL:

KNOWLEDGE: Disease Process (NOC)

Verbalize understanding of disease process and treatment regimen.
Identify drug side effects and possible complications that necessitate medical attention.
Maintain BP within individually acceptable parameters.

KNOWLEDGE: Treatment Regimen (NOC)

Describe reasons for therapeutic actions/treatment regimen.

ACTIONS/INTERVENTIONS	RATIONALE
TEACHING: Disease Process (NIC)	
Independent	
Assist client in identifying modifiable risk factors; e.g., obesity; diet high in sodium, saturated fats, and cholesterol; sedentary lifestyle; smoking; alcohol intake (more than 2 oz/day on a regular basis); stressful lifestyle.	These risk factors have been shown to contribute to hypertension and cardiovascular and renal disease.
Problem-solve with client to identify ways in which appropriate lifestyle changes can be made to reduce modifiable risk factors.	Changing "comfortable/usual" behavior patterns can be very difficult and stressful. Support, guidance, and empathy can enhance client's success in accomplishing these tasks.
Discuss importance of eliminating smoking, and assist client in formulating a plan to quit smoking.	Nicotine increases catecholamine discharge, resulting in increased heart rate, BP, vasoconstriction, and myocardial workload, and reduces tissue oxygenation.
Reinforce the importance of adhering to treatment regimen and keeping follow-up appointments.	Lack of engagement in the treatment plan is a common reason for failure of antihypertensive therapy. Therefore, ongoing evaluation for client cooperation is critical to successful treatment. Compliance usually improves when client understands causative factors and consequences of inadequate intervention and health maintenance.
Instruct and demonstrate technique of BP self-monitoring. Evaluate client's hearing, visual acuity, manual dexterity, and coordination.	Monitoring BP at home is reassuring to client because it provides visual/positive reinforcement for efforts in following the medical regimen and promotes early detection of deleterious changes.
Help client develop a simple, convenient schedule for taking medications.	Individualizing medication schedule to fit client's personal habits/needs may facilitate cooperation with long-term regimen.
Explain prescribed medications along with their rationale, dosage, expected and adverse side effects, and idiosyncrasies; e.g.:	Adequate information and understanding that side effects (e.g., mood changes, initial weight gain, dry mouth) are common and often subside with time can enhance cooperation with treatment plan.
Diuretics: Take daily doses (or larger dose) in the early morning;	Scheduling minimizes nighttime urination.
Weigh self on a regular schedule and record;	Primary indicator of effectiveness of diuretic therapy.
Avoid/limit alcohol intake;	The combined vasodilating effect of alcohol and the volume-depleting effect of a diuretic greatly increase the risk of orthostatic hypotension.
Notify physician if unable to tolerate food or fluid;	Dehydration can develop rapidly if intake is poor and client continues to take a diuretic.

ACTIONS/INTERVENTIONS	RATIONALE
Antihypertensives: Take prescribed dose on a regular schedule; avoid skipping, altering, or making up doses; and do not discontinue without notifying the healthcare provider. Review potential side effects and/or drug interactions;	Because clients often cannot feel the difference the medication is making in blood pressure, it is critical that there be understanding about the medication's working and side effects. For example, abruptly discontinuing a drug may cause rebound hypertension leading to severe complications, or medication may need to be altered to reduce adverse effects.
Rise slowly from a lying to standing position, sitting for a few minutes before standing. Sleep with the head slightly elevated.	Measures reduce severity of orthostatic hypotension associated with the use of vasodilators and diuretics.
Suggest frequent position changes, leg exercises when lying down.	Decreases peripheral venous pooling that may be potentiated by vasodilators and prolonged sitting/standing.
Recommend avoiding hot baths, steam rooms, and saunas, especially with concomitant use of alcoholic beverages.	Prevents vasodilation with potential for dangerous side effects of syncope and hypotension.
Instruct client to consult healthcare provider before taking other prescription or over-the-counter (OTC) medications.	Precaution is important in preventing potentially dangerous drug interactions. Any drug that contains a sympathetic nervous stimulant may increase BP or counteract antihypertensive effects.
Instruct client about increasing intake of foods/fluids high in potassium (e.g., oranges, bananas, figs, dates, tomatoes, potatoes, raisins, apricots, Gatorade, and fruit juices) and foods/fluids high in calcium; e.g., low-fat milk, yogurt, or calcium supplements, as indicated.	Diuretics can deplete potassium levels. Dietary replacement is more palatable than drug supplements and may be all that is needed to correct deficit. Some studies show that 400 mg of calcium/day can lower systolic and diastolic BP. Correcting mineral deficiencies can also affect BP.
Review signs/symptoms requiring notification of healthcare provider; e.g., headache present on awakening that does not abate, sudden and continued increase of BP, chest pain/shortness of breath, irregular/increased pulse rate, significant weight gain (2 lb/day or 5 lb/wk) or peripheral/abdominal swelling, visual disturbances, frequent, uncontrollable nosebleeds, depression/emotional lability, severe dizziness or episodes of fainting, muscle weakness/cramping, nausea/vomiting; excessive thirst.	Early detection of developing complications/decreased effectiveness of drug regimen or adverse reactions to it allows for timely intervention.
Explain rationale for prescribed dietary regimen (usually a diet low in sodium, saturated fat, and cholesterol).	Excess saturated fats, cholesterol, sodium, alcohol, and calories have been defined as nutritional risks in hypertension. A diet low in fat and high in polyunsaturated fat reduces BP; possibly through prostaglandin balance in both normotensive and hypertensive people.
Help client identify sources of sodium intake (e.g., table salt, salty snacks, processed meats and cheeses, sauerkraut, sauces, canned soups and vegetables, baking soda, baking powder, monosodium glutamate). Stress the importance of reading ingredient labels of foods and OTC drugs.	Two years on a moderate low-salt diet may be sufficient to control mild hypertension or reduce the amount of medication required.
Encourage foods rich in essential fatty acids (e.g., salmon, cod, mackeral, tuna).	Omega-3 fatty acids in fish tend to relax artery walls, reducing blood pressure. They also make blood thinner and less likely to clot.
Encourage client to establish an individual exercise program incorporating aerobic exercise (walking, swimming) within client's capabilities. Stress the importance of avoiding isometric activity.	Besides helping to lower BP, aerobic activity aids in toning the cardiovascular system. Isometric exercise can increase serum catecholamine levels, further elevating BP.
Demonstrate application of ice pack to the back of the neck and pressure over the distal third of nose, and recommend that client lean the head forward if nosebleed occurs.	Nasal capillaries may rupture as a result of excessive vascular pressure. Cold and pressure constrict capillaries to slow or halt bleeding. Leaning forward reduces the amount of blood that is swallowed.
Provide information regarding community resources, and support client in making lifestyle changes. Initiate referrals as indicated.	Community resources such as the American Heart Association, "coronary clubs," stop smoking clinics, alcohol (drug) rehabilitation, weight loss programs, stress management classes, and counseling services may be helpful in client's efforts to initiate and maintain lifestyle changes.

POTENTIAL CONSIDERATIONS following acute hospitalization (dependent on client's age, physical condition/presence of complications, personal resources, and life responsibilities)

Activity Intolerance—frequently occurs as a result of alterations in cardiac output and side effects of medication.

imbalanced Nutrition: more than body requirements—obesity is often present and a factor in blood pressure control.

ineffective Therapeutic Regimen Management—result of the complexity of the therapeutic regimen, required lifestyle changes, side effects of medication, and frequent feelings of general well-being ("I'm not really sick.").

ineffective Sexuality Pattern—interference in sexual functioning may occur because of activity intolerance and side effects of medication.

readiness for enhanced family Coping—opportunity exists for family members to support client while reducing risk factors for themselves and improving quality of life for family as a whole.

HEART FAILURE: CHRONIC

Heart failure afflicts more than 22 million people worldwide, and in the United States, is the most costly heart-related disease because of its chronicity (Collins, 2003). Failure of the left and/or right chambers of the heart results in insufficient output to meet tissue needs and causes pulmonary and systemic vascular congestion. Remodeling of the myocardium as a structural response to injury is one of the pathophysiologic causes of heart failure (HF). During remodeling the heart changes from an efficient football shape to an inefficient basketball shape, making coordinated contractility difficult. Despite diagnostic and therapeutic advances, HF continues to be associated with high morbidity and mortality. (Agency for Health Care Policy and Research [AHCPR] guidelines [6/94] promote the term *heart failure* [HF] in place of *congestive heart failure* [CHF] because many clients with heart failure do not manifest pulmonary or systemic congestion.) The New York Heart Association Functional Classification System for HF includes classes I– IV. Common causes of HF include ventricular dysfunction, cardiomyopathies, hypertension, coronary artery disease, valvular disease, and dysrhythmias.

CARE SETTING

Although generally managed at the community level, inpatient stay may be required for periodic exacerbation of failure/development of complications.

RELATED CONCERNS

Myocardial infarction, page 72
Hypertension, page 35
Cardiac surgery, page 96
Dysrhythmias, page 85
Psychosocial aspects of care, page 770

Client Assessment Database

ACTIVITY/REST

May report:
Fatigue/exhaustion progressing throughout the day; exercise intolerance
Insomnia
Chest pain/pressure with activity
Dyspnea at rest or with exertion

May exhibit:
Restlessness, mental status changes; e.g., anxiety and lethargy
Vital sign changes with activity

CIRCULATION

May report:
History of hypertension, recent/acute multiple MIs, previous episodes of HF, valvular heart disease, cardiac surgery, endocarditis, systemic lupus erythematosus (SLE), anemia, septic shock
Swelling of feet, legs, abdomen, "belt too tight" (right-sided heart failure)

May exhibit:
BP may be low (pump failure), normal (mild or chronic HF), or high (fluid overload/increased systemic vascular resistance [SVR])
Pulse pressure may be narrow, reflecting reduced stroke volume

Tachycardia (may be left- or right-sided heart failure)
Dysrhythmias; e.g., atrial fibrillation, premature ventricular contractions/tachycardia, heart blocks
Apical pulse: PMI may be diffuse and displaced inferiorly to the left
Heart sounds: S_3 (gallop) is diagnostic of congestive failure; S_4 may occur; S_1 and S_2 may be softened
Systolic and diastolic murmurs may indicate the presence of valvular stenosis or insufficiency, both atrial and ventricular
Pulses: Peripheral pulses diminished; central pulses may be bounding; e.g., visible jugular, carotid, abdominal pulsations; alteration in strength of beat may be noted
Color ashen, pale, dusky, or even cyanotic
Nailbeds pale or cyanotic, with slow capillary refill
Liver may be enlarged/palpable, positive hepatojugular reflex
Breath sounds: Crackles, rhonchi
Edema may be dependent, generalized, or pitting, especially in extremities; JVD may be present

EGO INTEGRITY

May report: Anxiety, apprehension, fear
Stress related to illness/financial concerns (job/cost of medical care)

May exhibit: Various behavioral manifestations; e.g., anxiety, anger, fear, irritability

ELIMINATION

May report: Decreased voiding, dark urine
Night voiding (nocturia)
Diarrhea/constipation

FOOD/FLUID

May report: Loss of appetite/anorexia
Nausea/vomiting
Significant weight gain (may not respond to diuretic use)
Lower extremity swelling
Tight clothing/shoes
Diet high in salt/processed foods, fat, sugar, and caffeine
Use of diuretics

May exhibit: Rapid/continuous weight gain
Abdominal distention (ascites); edema (general, dependent, pitting, brawny)
Abdominal tenderness (ascites, hepatic engorgement)

HYGIENE

May report: Fatigue/weakness, exhaustion during self-care activities

May exhibit: Appearance indicative of neglect of personal care

NEUROSENSORY

May report: Weakness, dizziness, fainting episodes

May exhibit: Lethargy, confusion, disorientation
Behavior changes, irritability

PAIN/DISCOMFORT

May report: Chest pain, chronic or acute angina
Right upper abdominal pain (right-sided heart failure [RHF])
Generalized muscle aches/pains

May exhibit: Nervousness, restlessness
Narrowed focus (withdrawal)
Guarding behavior

RESPIRATION

May report: Dyspnea on exertion, sleeping sitting up or with several pillows
Cough with/without sputum production, dry/hacking—especially when recumbent

History of chronic lung disease
Use of respiratory aids; e.g., oxygen and/or medications

May exhibit: Tachypnea; shallow, labored breathing; use of accessory muscles, nasal flaring
Cough: Dry/hacking/nonproductive or may be gurgling with/without sputum production
Sputum may be blood-tinged, pink/frothy (pulmonary edema)
Breath sounds may be diminished, with bibasilar crackles and wheezes
Mentation may be diminished; lethargy, restlessness present
Color: Pallor or cyanosis

SAFETY

May exhibit: Changes in mentation/confusion
Loss of strength/muscle tone
Skin excoriations, rashes

SOCIAL INTERACTION

May report: Decreased participation in usual social activities

TEACHING/LEARNING

May report: Family history of developing HF at young age (genetic form). Family hisotry of heart disease, hypertension, diabetes (risk factors)
Use/misuse of cardiac medications; e.g., β-blockers, calcium channel blockers
Use of vitamins, herbal supplements (e.g., niacin, coenzyme Q10, garlic, ginkgo, black hellebore, dandelion), or aspirin
Recent/recurrent hospitalizations
Evidence of failure to improve

Discharge plan considerations: Assistance with shopping, transportation, self-care needs, homemaker/maintenance tasks
Alteration in medication use/therapy
Changes in physical layout of home

Refer to section at end of plan for postdischarge considerations.

DIAGNOSTIC STUDIES

ECG: Ventricular or atrial hypertrophy, axis deviation, ischemia, and damage patterns may be present. Dysrhythmias; e.g., tachycardia, atrial fibrillation, conduction delays, especially left bundle branch block, frequent premature ventricular contractions (PVCs), may be present. Persistent ST-T segment abnormalities and decreased QRS amplitude may be present.

Chest x-ray: May show enlarged cardiac shadow, reflecting chamber dilatation/hypertrophy, or changes in blood vessels, reflecting increased pulmonary pressure. Abnormal contour; e.g., bulging of left cardiac border, may suggest ventricular aneurysm.

Sonograms (echocardiogram, Doppler and transesophageal echocardiogram): May reveal enlarged chamber dimensions, alterations in valvular function/structure, the degrees of ventricular dilation and dysfunction.

Heart scans:

Technetium-99m (99mTc) pyrophosphate scaning (also known as hot spot myocardial imaging and infarct avid imaging): Used to detect recent myocardial infaction and its extent.

Multigated acquisition (MUGA): Measures cardiac volume during both systole and diastole, measures ejection fraction, and estimates wall motion.

Exercise or pharmacologic stress myocardial perfusion (e.g., dipyridamole [Persantine] or thallium scan): Evaluates blood flow, determines presence of myocardial ischemia and wall motion abnormalities.

Positron emission tomography (PET) scan: Sensitive test for evaluation of myocardial ischemia/detecting viable myocardium.

Cardiac magnetic resonance imaging (MRI): Helps detect congenital heart disease, valvular heart disease, and vascular disorders such as thoracic aneurysm. It also helps detect cardiac tumors and structural anomalies.

Cardiac catheterization: Abnormal pressures are indicative of and help differentiate right-sided versus left-sided heart failure, as well as valve stenosis or insufficiency. Also assesses patency of coronary arteries. Contrast injected into the ventricles reveals abnormal size and ejection fraction/altered contractility. Transvenous endomyocardial biopsy may be useful in some clients to determine the underlying disorder, such as myocarditis or amylodosis.

BNP (Beta-type natruiretic peptide): Affects cardiac function and vascular tone and renal function. Low levels indicate worsening heart failure.

Liver enzymes: Elevated in liver congestion/failure.

Digoxin and other cardiac drug levels: Monitored to determine therapeutic range and correlate expected response with client response.

Bleeding and clotting times: Determine therapeutic range for anticoagulant therapy and/or identify those at risk for excessive clot formation.

Electrolytes: May be altered because of fluid shifts/decreased renal function and medications (e.g., diuretics, ACE inhibitors).

Arterial blood gases (ABGs): Left ventricular failure is characterized by mild respiratory alkalosis (early) or hypoxemia with an increased P_{CO_2} (late).

BUN/creatinine: Elevated BUN suggests decreased renal perfusion as may occur with HF and/or as a side effect of prescribed medications (e.g., diuretics and ACE inhibitors). Elevation of both BUN and creatinine is indicative of renal failure.

Serum albumin/transferrin: May be decreased as a result of reduced protein intake or reduced protein synthesis in congested liver.

Complete blood count (CBC): May reveal anemia (major contributor/exacerbating factor in HF), polycythemia, or dilutional changes indicating water retention. Levels of white blood cells (WBCs) may be elevated, reflecting recent/acute MI, pericarditis, or other inflammatory or infectious states.

ESR: May be elevated, indicating acute inflammatory reaction (especially if viral infection is cause of HF).

Thyroid studies: Increased thyroid activity suggests thyroid hyperactivity as precipitator of HF. Hypothroydism can also cause or exacerbate HF.

Pulse oximetry: Oxygen saturation may be low, especially when acute HF is imposed on chronic obstructive pulmonary disease (COPD) or chronic HF.

NURSING PRIORITIES

1. Improve myocardial contractility/systemic perfusion.
2. Reduce fluid volume overload.
3. Prevent complications.
4. Provide information about disease/prognosis, therapy needs, and prevention of recurrences.

DISCHARGE GOALS

1. Cardiac output adequate for individual needs.
2. Complications prevented/resolved.
3. Optimum level of activity/functioning attained.
4. Disease process/prognosis and therapeutic regimen understood.
5. Plan in place to meet needs after discharge.

NURSING DIAGNOSIS: decreased Cardiac Output

May be related to

Altered myocardial contractility/inotropic changes
Alterations in rate, rhythm, electrical conduction
Structural changes (e.g., valvular defects, ventricular aneurysm)

Possibly evidenced by

Increased heart rate (tachycardia), dysrhythmias, ECG changes
Changes in BP (hypotension/hypertension)
Extra heart sounds (S_3, S_4)
Decreased urine output
Diminished peripheral pulses
Cool, ashen skin; diaphoresis
Orthopnea, crackles, JVD, liver engorgement, edema
Chest pain

DESIRED OUTCOMES/EVALUATION CRITERIA—CLIENT WILL:

Cardiac Pump Effectiveness (NOC)

Display vital signs within acceptable limits, dysrhythmias absent/controlled, and no symptoms of failure (e.g., hemodynamic parameters within acceptable limits, urinary output adequate).
Report decreased episodes of dyspnea, angina.

Cardiac Disease Self-Management (NOC)

Participate in activities that reduce cardiac workload.

ACTIONS/INTERVENTIONS	RATIONALE
Hemodynamic Regulation (NIC)	
Independent	
Auscultate apical pulse; assess heart rate, rhythm (document dysrhythmia if telemetry available).	Tachycardia is usually present (even at rest) to compensate for decreased ventricular contractility. Premature atrial contractions (PACs), paroxysmal atrial tachycardia (PAT), PVCs, multifocal atrial tachycardia (MAT), and atrial fibrillation (AF) are common dysrhythmias associated with HF, although others may also occur. *Note:* Intractable ventricular dysrhythmias unresponsive to medication suggest ventricular aneurysm.
Note heart sounds.	S_1 and S_2 may be weak because of diminished pumping action. Gallop rhythms are common (S_3 and S_4), produced as blood flows into noncompliant/distended chambers. Murmurs may reflect valvular incompetence/stenosis.
Palpate peripheral pulses.	Decreased cardiac output may be reflected in diminished radial, popliteal, dorsalis pedis, and posttibial pulses. Pulses may be fleeting or irregular to palpation, and pulsus alternans (strong beat alternating with weak beat) may be present.
Monitor BP.	In early, moderate, or chronic HF, BP may be elevated because of increased SVR. In advanced HF, the body may no longer be able to compensate, and profound/irreversible hypotension may occur.
Inspect skin for pallor, cyanosis.	Pallor is indicative of diminished peripheral perfusion secondary to inadequate cardiac output, vasoconstriction, and anemia. Cyanosis may develop in refractory HF. Dependent areas are often blue or mottled as venous congestion increases.
Monitor urine output, noting decreasing output and dark/concentrated urine.	Kidneys respond to reduced cardiac output by retaining water and sodium. Urine output is usually decreased during the day because of fluid shifts into tissues but may be increased at night because fluid returns to circulation when client is recumbent.
Note changes in sensorium; e.g., lethargy, confusion, disorientation, anxiety, and depression.	May indicate inadequate cerebral perfusion secondary to decreased cardiac output.
Encourage rest, semirecumbent in bed or chair. Assist with physical care as indicated.	Physical rest should be maintained during acute or refractory HF to improve efficiency of cardiac contraction and to decrease myocardial oxygen demand/consumption and workload.

ACTIONS/INTERVENTIONS	RATIONALE
Provide quiet environment; explain medical/nursing management; help client avoid stressful situations; listen/respond to expressions of feelings/fears.	Psychologic rest helps reduce emotional stress, which can produce vasoconstriction, elevating BP and increasing heart rate/work.
Provide bedside commode. Have client avoid activities eliciting a vasovagal response; e.g., straining during defecation, holding breath during position changes.	Commode use decreases work of getting to bathroom or struggling to use bedpan. Vasovagal maneuver causes vagal stimulation followed by rebound tachycardia, which further compromises cardiac function/output.
Elevate legs, avoiding pressure under knee. Encourage active/passive exercises. Increase ambulation/activity as tolerated.	Decreases venous stasis, and may reduce incidence of thrombus/embolus formation.
Check for calf tenderness; diminished pedal pulse; swelling, local redness, or pallor of extremity.	Reduced cardiac output, venous pooling/stasis, and enforced bed rest increases risk of thrombophlebitis.
Withhold digitalis preparation as indicated, and notify physician if marked changes occur in cardiac rate or rhythm or signs of digitalis toxicity occur.	Incidence of toxicity is high (20%) because of narrow margin between therapeutic and toxic ranges. Digoxin may have to be discontinued in the presence of toxic drug levels, a slow heart rate, or low potassium level. (Refer to CP: Dysrhythmias; ND: risk for Poisoning: digitalis toxicity.)

Collaborative

Administer supplemental oxygen as indicated.	Increases available oxygen for myocardial uptake to combat effects of hypoxia/ischemia.
Administer medications as indicated:	A variety of medications may be used to increase stroke volume, improve contractility, and reduce congestion.
Diuretics, e.g., furosemide (Lasix), ethacrynic acid (Edecrin), bumetanide (Bumex), spironolactone (Aldactone);	Diuretics, in conjunction with restriction of dietary sodium and fluids, often lead to clinical improvement in clients with stages I and II HF. In general, type and dosage of diuretic depend on cause and degree of HF and state of renal function. Preload reduction is most useful in treating clients with a relatively normal cardiac output accompanied by congestive symptoms. Loop diuretics block chloride reabsorption, thus interfering with the reabsorption of sodium and water.
Vasodilators, e.g., nitrates (Nitro-Dur, Isordil); arteriodilators; e.g., hydralazine (Apresoline); combination drugs; e.g., prazosin (Minipress); nesiritide Natrecor);	Vasodilators are the mainstay of treatment in HF and are used to increase cardiac and renal output, reducing circulating volume (preload and afterload) and decreasing SVR, thereby reducing ventricular workload. *Note:* Nesiritide is used in acutely decompensated CHF and has been used with digoxin, diuretics, and ACE inhibitors. Parenteral vasodilators are reserved for clients with severe HF or those unable to take oral medications.
ACE inhibitors; e.g., benazepril (Lotensin), captopril (Capoten), lisinopril (Prinivil), enalapril (Vasotec), quinapril (Accupril), ramipril (Altace), moexipril (Univasc);	ACE inhibitors represent first-line therapy to control heart failure by decreasing venticular filling pressures and SVR while increasing cardiac output with little or no change in BP and heart rate.
Angiotensin II receptor antagonists, (also known as angiotension receptor blockers [ARBs]); e.g., candesartan (Atacand), losartan (Cozaar), eprosartan (Teveten), ibesartan (Avapro), valsartan (Diovan);	Antihypertensive and cardioprotective effects are attributable to selective blockade of AT_1 (angiotensin II) receptors and angiotensin II synthesis. *Note:* ARBs used in combination with ACE inhibitors and β-blockers are thought to have decreased hospitalizations for HF clients.
Digoxin (Lanoxin);	Increases force of myocardial contraction when diminished contractility is the cause of HF, and slows heart rate by decreasing conduction velocity and prolonging refractory period of the atrioventricular (AV) junction to increase cardiac efficiency/output.

ACTIONS/INTERVENTIONS	RATIONALE
Inotropic agents; e.g., amrinone (Inocor), milrinone (Primacor), vesnarinone (Arkin-Z);	These medications are useful for short-term treatment of HF unresponsive to cardiac glycosides, vasodilators, and diuretics in order to increase myocardial contractility and produce vasodilation. Positive inotropic properties have reduced mortality rates 50% and improved quality of life.
β-adrenergic receptor antagonists; e.g., carvedilol (Coreg), bisoprolol (Zebeta), metoprolol (Lopressor);	Useful in the treatment of HF by blocking the cardiac effects of chronic adrenergic stimulation. Many clients experience improved activity tolerance and ejection fraction.
Aldosterone antagonist; e.g. eplerenone (Inspra);	Approved by the Food and Drug Administration (FDA) in 2003, eplerenone has been shown to improve survival in HF, especially following MI.
Morphine sulfate;	Decreases vascular resistance and venous return, reducing myocardial workload, especially when pulmonary congestion is present. Allays anxiety and breaks the feedback cycle of anxiety to catecholamine release to anxiety.
Antianxiety agents/sedatives;	Promote rest/relaxation, reducing oxygen demand and myocardial workload.
Anticoagulants; e.g., low-dose heparin, warfarin (Coumadin).	May be used prophylactically to prevent thrombus/embolus formation in the presence of risk factors such as venous stasis, enforced bedrest, cardiac dysrhythmias, and history of previous thrombolic episodes.
Administer IV solutions, restricting total amount as indicated. Avoid saline solutions.	Because of existing elevated left ventricular pressure, client may not tolerate increased fluid volume (preload). Clients with HF also excrete less sodium, which causes fluid retention and increases myocardial workload.
Monitor/replace electrolytes.	Fluid shifts and use of diuretics can alter electrolytes (especially potassium and chloride), which affect cardiac rhythm and contractility.
Monitor serial ECG and chest x-ray changes.	ST segment depression and T wave flattening can develop because of increased myocardial oxygen demand, even if no coronary artery disease is present. Chest x-ray may show enlarged heart and changes of pulmonary congestion.
Measure cardiac output and other functional parameters as indicated.	Cardiac index, preload/afterload, contractility, and cardiac work can be measured noninvasively by using thoracic electrical bioimpedance (TEB) technique. Useful in determining effectiveness of therapeutic interventions and response to activity.
Monitor laboratory studies; e.g., BUN, creatinine:	Elevation of BUN/creatinine reflects kidney hypoperfusion/failure.
Liver function studies (AST, LDH);	May be elevated because of liver congestion and indicate need for smaller dosages of medications that are detoxified by the liver.
Prothrombin time (PT)/activated partial thromboplastin time (aPTT) coagulation studies.	Measures changes in coagulation processes or effectiveness of anticoagulant therapy.
Prepare for insertion/maintain pacemaker (or pacemaker/defibrillator), if indicated.	May be necessary to correct bradydysrhythmias unresponsive to drug intervention, which can aggravate congestive failure/produce pulmonary edema. *Note:* Beiventricular pacemaker and cardiac defibirillators are designed to provide resynchronization for the heart by simultaneous electrical activation of both the right and left sides of the heart, thereby creating a more effective and efficient pump.
Prepare for surgery as indicated; e.g., valve replacement, angioplasty, coronary artery bypass grafting (CABG);	Heart failure due to ventricular aneurysm or valvular dysfunction may require aneurysmectomy or valve replacement to improve myocardial contractility/ function. Revascularization of cardiac muscle by CABG may be done to improve cardiac function.

ACTIONS/INTERVENTIONS	RATIONALE
Cardiomyoplasty;	Cardiomyoplasty, an experimental procedure in which the latissimus dorsi muscle is wrapped around the heart and electrically stimulated to contract with each heartbeat, may be done to augment ventricular function while the client is awaiting cardiac transplantation or when transplantation is not an option.
Transmyocardial revascularization.	Other new surgical techniques include transmyocardial revascularization (percutaneous [PTMR]) using CO_2 laser technology, in which a laser is used to create multiple 1-mm diameter channels in viable but underperfused cardiac muscle.
Assist with/maintain mechanical circulatory support system, such as IABP or LVAD, when indicated.	An intra-aortic balloon pump (IABP) may be inserted as a temporary support to the failing heart in the critically ill client with potentially reversible HF. A battery-powered left-ventricular assist device (LVAD) may also be used positioned between the cardiac apex and the descending thoracic or abdominal aorta. This device receives blood from the left ventricle (LV) and ejects it into the systemic circulation, often allowing client to resume a nearly normal lifestyle while awaiting heart transplantation, or in some instances, allows the heart to recover and regain its function.. With end-stage HF, cardiac transplantation may be indicated.

NURSING DIAGNOSIS: Activity Intolerance

May be related to

Imbalance between oxygen supply/demand
Generalized weakness
Prolonged bedrest/immobility

Possibly evidenced by

Weakness, fatigue
Changes in vital signs, presence of dysrhythmias
Dyspnea
Pallor, diaphoresis

DESIRED OUTCOMES/EVALUATION CRITERIA—CLIENT WILL:

Endurance (NOC)

Participate in desired activities; meet own self-care needs.
Achieve measurable increase in activity tolerance, evidenced by reduced fatigue and weakness and by vital signs within acceptable limits during activity.

ACTIONS/INTERVENTIONS	RATIONALE
Energy Management (NIC)	
Independent	
Check vital signs before and immediately after activity, especially if client is receiving vasodilators, diuretics, or β-blockers.	Orthostatic hypotension can occur with activity because of medication effect (vasodilation), fluid shifts (diuresis), or compromised cardiac pumping function.

ACTIONS/INTERVENTIONS	RATIONALE
Document cardiopulmonary response to activity. Note tachycardia, dysrhythmias, dyspnea, diaphoresis, pallor.	Compromised myocardium/inability to increase stroke volume during activity may cause an immediate increase in heart rate and oxygen demands, thereby aggravating weakness and fatigue.
Assess for other precipitators/causes of fatigue; e.g., treatments, pain, medications.	Fatigue is a side effect of some medications (e.g., β-blockers, tranquilizers, and sedatives). Pain and stressful regimens also extract energy and produce fatigue.
Evaluate accelerating activity intolerance.	May denote increasing cardiac decompensation rather than overactivity.
Provide assistance with self-care activities as indicated. Intersperse activity periods with rest periods.	Meets client's personal care needs without undue myocardial stress/excessive oxygen demand.

Collaborative

Implement graded cardiac rehabilitation/activity program.	Strengthens and improves cardiac function under stress if cardiac dysfunction is not irreversible. Gradual increase in activity avoids excessive myocardial workload and oxygen consumption.

NURSING DIAGNOSIS: excess Fluid Volume

May be related to

Reduced glomerular filtration rate (decreased cardiac output)/increased antidiuretic hormone (ADH) production, and sodium/water retention

Possibly evidenced by

Orthopnea, S_3 heart sound
Oliguria, edema, JVD, positive hepatojugular reflex
Weight gain
Hypertension
Respiratory distress, abnormal breath sounds

DESIRED OUTCOMES/EVALUATION CRITERIA—CLIENT WILL:

Fluid Balance (NOC)

Demonstrate stabilized fluid volume with balanced intake and output, breath sounds clear/clearing, vital signs within acceptable range, stable weight, and absence of edema.
Verbalize understanding of individual dietary/fluid restrictions.

ACTIONS/INTERVENTIONS — RATIONALE

Fluid Management (NIC)

Independent

Monitor urine output, noting amount and color, as well as time of day when diuresis occurs.	Urine output may be scanty and concentrated (especially during the day) because of reduced renal perfusion. Recumbency favors diuresis; therefore, urine output may be increased at night/during bedrest.
Monitor/calculate 24-hour intake and output (I&O) balance.	Diuretic therapy may result in sudden/excessive fluid loss (circulating hypovolemia), even though edema/ascites remains.

ACTIONS/INTERVENTIONS	RATIONALE
Maintain chair or bed rest in semi-Fowler's position during acute phase.	Recumbency increases glomerular filtration and decreases production of ADH, thereby enhancing diuresis.
Establish fluid intake schedule if fluids are medically restricted, incorporating beverage preferences when possible. Give frequent mouth care/ice chips as part of fluid allotment.	Involving client in therapy regimen may enhance sense of control and cooperation with restrictions.
Weigh daily.	Documents changes in/resolution of edema in response to therapy. A gain of 5 lb represents approximately 2 L of fluid. Conversely, diuretics can result in rapid/excessive fluid shifts and weight loss.
Assess for distended neck and peripheral vessels. Inspect dependent body areas for edema with/without pitting; note presence of generalized body edema (anasarca).	Excessive fluid retention may be manifested by venous engorgement and edema formation. Peripheral edema begins in feet/ankles (or dependent areas) and ascends as failure worsens. Pitting edema is generally obvious only after retention of at least 10 lb of fluid. Increased vascular congestion (associated with RHF) eventually results in systemic tissue edema.
Change position frequently. Elevate feet when sitting. Inspect skin surface, keep dry, and provide padding as indicated. (Refer to ND: risk for impaired Skin Integrity.)	Edema formation, slowed circulation, altered nutritional intake, and prolonged immobility/bedrest are cumulative stressors that affect skin integrity and require close supervision/preventive interventions.
Auscultate breath sounds, noting decreased and/or adventitious sounds; e.g., crackles, wheezes. Note presence of increased dyspnea, tachypnea, orthopnea, paroxysmal nocturnal dyspnea, persistent cough.	Excess fluid volume often leads to pulmonary congestion. Symptoms of pulmonary edema may reflect acute left-sided HF. RHF's respiratory symptoms (dyspnea, cough, orthopnea) may have slower onset but are more difficult to reverse.
Investigate reports of sudden extreme dyspnea/air hunger, need to sit straight up, sensation of suffocation, feelings of panic or impending doom.	May indicate development of complications (pulmonary edema/embolus) and differs from orthopnea paroxysmal nocturnal dyspnea in that it develops much more rapidly and requires immediate intervention.
Monitor BP and central venous pressure (CVP) (if available).	Hypertension and elevated CVP suggest fluid volume excess and may reflect developing/increasing pulmonary congestion, HF.
Assess bowel sounds. Note complaints of anorexia, nausea, abdominal distention, constipation.	Visceral congestion (occurring in progressive HF) can alter gastric/intestinal function.
Provide small, frequent, easily digestible meals.	Reduced gastric motility can adversely affect digestion and absorption. Small, frequent meals may enhance digestion/prevent abdominal discomfort.
Measure abdominal girth, as indicated.	In progressive RHF, fluid may shift into the peritoneal space, causing increasing abdominal girth (ascites).
Encourage verbalization of feelings regarding limitations.	Expression of feelings/concerns may decrease stress/anxiety, which is an energy drain that can contribute to feelings of fatigue.
Palpate abdomen. Note reports of right upper quadrant pain/tenderness.	Advancing HF leads to venous congestion, resulting in abdominal distention, liver engorgement (hepatomegaly), and pain. This can alter liver function and impair/prolong drug metabolism.
Note increased lethargy, hypotension, muscle cramping.	Signs of potassium and sodium deficits that may occur because of fluid shifts and diuretic therapy.

Collaborative

Fluid/Electrolyte Management (NIC)

Administer medications as indicated:	
Diuretics; e.g., furosemide (Lasix), bumetanide (Bumex);	Increases rate of urine flow and may inhibit reabsorption of sodium/chloride in the renal tubules.

ACTIONS/INTERVENTIONS	RATIONALE
Thiazides with potassium-sparing agents; e.g., spironolactone (Aldactone);	Promotes diuresis without excessive potassium losses.
Potassium supplements; e.g., K-Dur.	Replaces potassium that is lost as a common side effect of diuretic therapy, which can adversely affect cardiac function.
Maintain fluid/sodium restrictions as indicated.	Reduce total body water/prevents fluid reaccumulation.
Consult with dietitian.	May be necessary to provide diet acceptable to client that meets caloric needs within sodium restriction.
Monitor chest x-ray.	Reveals changes indicative of increase/resolution of pulmonary congestion.
Assist with rotating tourniquets/phlebotomy, dialysis, or ultrafiltration as indicated.	Although not frequently used, mechanical fluid removal rapidly reduces circulating volume, especially in pulmonary edema refractory to other therapies.

NURSING DIAGNOSIS: risk for impaired Gas Exchange

Risk factors may include

Alveolar-capillary membrane changes; e.g., fluid collection/shifts into interstitial space/alveoli

Possibly evidenced by

[Not applicable; presence of signs and symptoms establishes an *actual* diagnosis.]

DESIRED OUTCOMES/EVALUATION CRITERIA—CLIENT WILL:

RESPIRATORY STATUS: Gas Exchange (NOC)

Demonstrate adequate ventilation and oxygenation of tissues by ABGs/oximetry within client's normal ranges and free of symptoms of respiratory distress.
Participate in treatment regimen within level of ability/situation.

ACTIONS/INTERVENTIONS	RATIONALE
Airway Management (NIC)	
Independent	
Auscultate breath sounds, noting crackles, wheezes.	Reveals presence of pulmonary congestion/collection of secretions, indicating need for further intervention.
Instruct client in effective coughing, deep breathing.	Clears airways and facilitates oxygen delivery.
Encourage frequent position changes.	Helps prevent atelectasis and pneumonia.
Maintain chair/bedrest with head of bed elevated 20–30 degrees, semi-Fowler's position. Support arms with pillows.	Reduces oxygen consumption/demands and promotes maximal lung inflation.
Collaborative	
Monitor/graph serial ABGs, pulse oximetry.	Hypoxemia can be severe during pulmonary edema. Compensatory changes are usually present in chronic HF. *Note:* In clients with abnormal cardiac index, research suggests pulse oximeter measurements may exceed actual oxygen saturation by up to 7%.

ACTIONS/INTERVENTIONS	RATIONALE
Administer supplemental oxygen as indicated.	Increases alveolar oxygen concentration, which may correct/reduce tissue hypoxemia.
Administer medications as indicated:	
Diuretics; e.g., furosemide (Lasix);	Reduces alveolar congestion, enhancing gas exchange.
Bronchodilators; e.g., aminophylline.	Increase oxygen delivery by dilating small airways, and exerts mild diuretic effect to aid in reducing pulmonary congestion.

NURSING DIAGNOSIS: risk for impaired Skin Integrity

Risk factors may include

Prolonged bedrest
Edema, decreased tissue perfusion

Possibly evidenced by

[Not applicable; presence of signs and symptoms establishes an *actual* diagnosis.]

DESIRED OUTCOMES/EVALUATION CRITERIA—CLIENT WILL:

TISSUE PERFUSION: Peripheral (NOC)

Maintain skin integrity.
Demonstrate behaviors/techniques to prevent skin breakdown.

ACTIONS/INTERVENTIONS	RATIONALE
Pressure Management (NIC)	
Independent	
Inspect skin, noting skeletal prominences, presence of edema, areas of altered circulation/pigmentation, or obesity/emaciation.	Skin is at risk because of impaired peripheral circulation, physical immobility, and alterations in nutritional status.
Provide gentle massage around reddened or blanched areas.	Improves blood flow, minimizing tissue hypoxia. *Note:* Direct massage of compromised area may cause tissue injury.
Encourage frequent position changes in bed/chair, assist with active/passive range of motion (ROM) exercises.	Reduces pressure on tissues, improving circulation and reducing time any one area is deprived of full blood flow.
Provide frequent skin care; minimize contact with moisture/excretions.	Excessive dryness or moisture damages skin and hastens breakdown.
Check fit of shoes/slippers and change as needed.	Dependent edema may cause shoes to fit poorly, increasing risk of pressure and skin breakdown on feet.
Avoid intramuscular route for medication administration.	Interstitial edema and impaired circulation impede drug absorption and predispose to tissue breakdown/development of infection.
Collaborative	
Provide alternating pressure/egg-crate mattress, sheepskin elbow/heel protectors.	Reduces pressure to skin, may improve circulation.

NURSING DIAGNOSIS: deficient Knowledge (Learning Need] regarding condition, treatment regimen, self-care, and discharge needs

May be related to

Lack of understanding/misconceptions about interrelatedness of cardiac function/disease/failure

Possibly evidenced by

Questions
Statements of concern/misconceptions
Recurrent, preventable episodes of HF

DESIRED OUTCOMES/EVALUATION CRITERIA—CLIENT WILL:

KNOWLEDGE: Cardiac Disease Management (NOC)

Identify relationship of ongoing therapies (treatment program) to reduction of recurrent episodes and prevention of complications.
List signs/symptoms that require immediate intervention.
Identify own stress/risk factors and some techniques for handling.
Initiate necessary lifestyle/behavioral changes.

ACTIONS/INTERVENTIONS	RATIONALE
TEACHING: Disease Process (NIC)	
Independent	
Discuss normal heart function. Include information regarding client's variance from normal function. Explain difference between heart attack and HF.	Knowledge of disease process and expectations can facilitate adherence to prescribed treatment regimen.
Reinforce treatment rationale. Include significant other (SO)/family members in teaching as appropriate, especially for complicated regimens such as management of technology (e.g., implantable cardioverter defibrillator [ICD], left vetricular assist device [LVAD]), or dobutamine infusion home therapy when client does not respond to customary combination therapy or cannot be weaned from dobutamine, or those awaiting heart transplant.	Client may believe it is acceptable to alter postdischarge regimen when feeling well and symptom-free or when feeling below par, which can increase the risk of exacerbation of symptoms. Understanding of regimen, medications, tehcnology , and restrictions may augment cooperation with control of symptoms. Home IV therapy requires a significant commitment by caregivers to operate/troubleshoot infusion pump, change dressing for peripherally inserted central catheter (PICC) line, and monitor I&O and signs/symptoms of HF.
Encourage developing a regular home exercise program, and provide guidelines for sexual activity.	Promotes maintenance of muscle tone and organ function for overall sense of well-being. Changing sexual habits (e.g., sex in morning when well rested, client on top, inclusion of other physical expressions of affection) may be difficult but provides opportunity for continuing satisfying sexual relationship.
Discuss importance of being as active as possible without becoming exhausted and need for rest between activities.	Excessive physical activity or overexertion can further weaken the heart, exacerbating failure, and necessitates adjustment of exercise program.
Discuss importance of sodium limitation. Provide list of sodium content of common foods that are to be avoided/limited. Encourage reading of labels on food and drug packages.	Dietary intake of sodium of more than 3 g/day can offset effect of diuretic. Most common source of sodium is table salt and obviously salty foods, although canned soups/vegetables, luncheon meats, and dairy products also may contain high levels of sodium.

ACTIONS/INTERVENTIONS	RATIONALE
Refer to dietitian for counseling specific to individual needs/dietary customs.	Identifies dietary needs, especially in presence of obesity (major risk factor for developing HF), diabetes, or presence of nausea/vomiting and resulting wasting syndrome (cardiac cachexia). Eating six small meals and using liquid dietary supplements and vitamin supplements can limit inappropriate weight loss.
Review medications, purpose, and side effects. Provide both oral and written instructions.	Understanding therapeutic needs and importance of prompt reporting of side effects can prevent occurrence of drug-related complications. Anxiety may block comprehension of input or details, and client/SO may refer to written material at later date to refresh memory.
Recommend taking diuretic early in morning.	Provides adequate time for drug effect before bedtime to prevent/limit interruption of sleep.
Instruct and receive return demonstration of ability to take and record daily pulse and blood pressure and when to notify healthcare provider; e.g., parameters above/below preset rate, changes in rhythm/regularity.	Promotes self-monitoring of condition/drug effect. Early detection of changes allows for timely intervention and may prevent complications, such as digitalis toxicity.
Explain and discuss client's role in control of risk factors (e.g., smoking) and precipitating or aggravating factors (e.g., high-salt diet, inactivity/overexertion, exposure to extremes in temperature).	Adds to body of knowledge, and permits client to make informed decisions regarding control of condition and prevention of recurrence/complications. Smoking potentiates vasoconstriction; sodium intake promotes water retention/edema formation; improper balance between activity and rest and exposure to temperature extremes may result in exhaustion/increased myocardial workload and increased risk of respiratory infections. Alcohol can depress cardiac contractility. Limitation of alcohol use to social occasions or maximum of one drink/day may be tolerated unless cardiomyopathy is alcohol induced (requiring complete abstinence).
Review signs/symptoms that require immediate medical attention; e.g., rapid/significant weight gain, edema, shortness of breath, increased fatigue, cough, hemoptysis, fever.	Self-monitoring increases client responsibility in health maintenance and aids in prevention of complications; e.g., pulmonary edema, pneumonia. Weight gain of more than 3 lb in a week requires medical evaluation/adjustment of diuretic therapy. *Note:* Client should weigh self daily in morning without clothing, after voiding and before eating.
Provide opportunities for client/SO to ask questions, discuss concerns, and make necessary lifestyle changes.	Chronicity and recurrent/debilitating nature of HF often exhausts coping abilities and supportive capacity of both client and SO, leading to depression.
Discuss general health risks (such as infection), recommending avoidance of crowds and individuals with respiratory infections, obtaining yearly influenza immunization and one-time pneumonia immunization.	This population is at increased risk for infection because of circulatory compromise.
Stress importance of reporting signs/symptoms of digitalis toxicity; e.g., development of gastrointestinal (GI) and visual disturbances, changes in pulse rate/rhythm, worsening of heart failure.	Early recognition of developing complications and involvement of healthcare provider may prevent toxicity/hospitalization.
Identify community resources/support groups and visiting home health nurse as indicated.	May need additional assistance with self-monitoring/home management, especially when HF is progressive.
Discuss importance of advance directives and of communicating plan/wishes to family and primary care providers.	Up to 50% of all deaths from heart failure are sudden, with many occurring at home, possibly without significant worsening of symptoms. If client chooses to refuse life-support measures, an alternative contact person (rather than 911) needs to be designated, should cardiac arrest occur.

POTENTIAL CONSIDERATIONS following discharge from care setting (dependent on client's age, physical condition/presence of complications, personal resources, and life responsibilities)

Activity Intolerance—poor cardiac reserve, side effects of medication, generalized weakness.

excess or deficient Fluid Volume—changes in glomerular filtration rate, diuretic use, individual fluid/salt intake.

impaired Skin Integrity—decreased activity level, prolonged sitting, presence of edema, altered circulation.

ineffective Therapeutic Regimen Management—complexity of regimen, economic limitations.

impaired Home Maintenance—chronic/debilitating condition, insufficient finances, inadequate support systems.

Self-Care Deficit—decreased strength/endurance, depression.

CP 4–1 Sample CP: Heart Failure, Hospital. ELOS 4 Days Cardiology or Medical Unit

ND and Categories of Care	Day 1 ____	Day 2 ____	Day 3 ____	Day 4 ____
Decreased cardiac output R/T decreased myocardial contractility, altered electrical conduction, structural changes	Goals Participate in actions to reduce cardiac workload	Display VS within acceptable limits; dysrhythmias controlled; pulse oximetry within acceptable range Meet own self-care needs with assistance as necessary	→ Dysrhythmias controlled or absent Free of signs of respiratory distress Demonstrate measureable increase in activity tolerance	→ → →
Fluid volume excess R/T compromised regulatory mechanism	Verbalize understanding of fluid/food restrictions	Verbalize understanding of general condition and health-care needs Breathing sounds clearing Urinary output adequate Weight loss (reflecting fluid loss)	Plan for lifestyle/behavior changes Breath sounds clear Balanced I&O Edema resolving	Plan in place to meet postdischarge needs Weight stable (continued loss if edema present)
Referrals	Cardiology Dietician	Cardiac Rehab Occupational Therapist (for ADLs) Social Services Home Care	Community Resources	
Diagnostic studies	ECG Echo-Doppler CXR ABGs/pulse oximetry Cardiac enzymes BUN/Cr CBC/electrolytes, MG++ PT/aPTT Liver function studies Serum glucose Albumin Uric acid Digoxin level (as indicated) UA	Echo-Doppler (if not done day 1) or MUGA Cardiac enzymes (if ↑) BUN/Cr Electrolytes PT/aPTT (if taking anticoagulants)	CXR BUN/Cr Electrolytes PT/aPTT (as indicated) Repeat digoxin level (if indicated)	

(Continued on following page)

ND and Categories of Care	Day 1 ____	Day 2 ____	Day 3 ____	Day 4 ____
Additional assessments	Apical pulse, heart/breath sounds q8h	→	→ bid	→
	Cardiac rhythm (telemetry) q4h	→	→ D/C	
	BP, P, R q2h until stable, q4h	→q8h	→	→
	Temp q8h	→	→	→
	I&O q8h	→	→	→D/C
	Weight qAM	→	→	→
	Peripheral edema q8h	→	→bid	→ qd
	Peripheral pulses q8h	→	→bid	→D/C
	Sensorium q8h	→	→bid	→D/C
	DVT check qd	→	→	→
	Response to activity	→	→	→
	Response to therapeutic interventions	→	→	→
Medication Allergies:	IV diuretic	→PO	→	→
	ACE inhibitor	→	→	→
	Digoxin	→	→	→
	PO/cutaneous nitrates	→	→	→
	Morphine sulfate	→	→D/C	
	Daytime/hs sedation	→	→	→D/C
	PO/low-dose anticoagulant	→	→PO or D/C	→
	IV/PO potassium	→	→D/C	
	Stool softener/laxative	→	→	→
Client education	Orient to unit/room	Cardiac education per protocol	Signs/symptoms to report to health-care provider	Provide written instructions for homecare
	Review advance directives	Review medications: Dose, times, route, purpose, side effects	Plan for homecare needs	Schedule for follow-up appointments
	Discuss expected outcomes, diagnostic tests/results	Progressive activity program		
	Fluid/nutritional restrictions/needs	Skin care		
Additional nursing actions	Bed/chair rest	→BPR/Ambulate as tolerated, cardiac program	→Up ad lib/graded program	→
	Assist with physical care	→	→	→
	Egg-crate mattress	→	→	→(send home)
	Dysrhythmia/angina care per protocol	→	→	→
	Supplemental O_2	→	→D/C	→
	Cardiac diet	→	→	

ANGINA (CORONARY ARTERY DISEASE/ACUTE CORONARY SYNDROME)

The classic symptom of coronary artery disease (CAD) is angina—pain caused by loss of oxygen and nutrients to the myocardial tissue because of inadequate coronary blood flow. In most, but not all, clients presenting with angina, CAD symptoms are caused by significant atherosclerosis. Unstable angina is sometimes grouped with myocardial infarction (MI) under the diagnosis of acute coronary syndrome. Angina has three major forms: (1) stable— precipitated by effort, of short duration, and easily relieved, (2) unstable—longer lasting, more severe, may not be relieved by rest/nitroglycerin; may also be new onset of pain with exertion or recent acceleration in severity of pain, and (3) variant—chest pain at rest with ECG changes due to coronary artery spasm. The AHCPR guidelines of May 1994 state that unstable angina is a transitory syndrome that causes significant disability and death in the United States.

CARE SETTING

Clients judged to be at intermediate or high likelihood of significant CAD are often hospitalized for further evaluation and therapeutic intervention. Classification of angina (provided by Canadian Cardiovascular Society Classification [CCSC]) aids in determining the risk of adverse outcomes for clients with unstable angina and, therefore, level of treatment needs. Class III angina is identified as occurring if the client walks less than two blocks and normal activity is markedly limited, and class IV angina occurs at rest or with minimal activity and level of activity is severely limited. These two classes may require inpatient evaluation/therapeutic adjustments.

RELATED CONCERNS

Cardiac surgery: postoperative care, page 96
Dysrhythmias, page 85
Heart failure: chronic, page 47
Myocardial infarction, page 72
Psychosocial aspects of care, page 770

Client Assessment Database

ACTIVITY/REST

May report:
- Sedentary lifestyle, weakness
- Fatigue, feeling incapacitated after exercise
- Chest pain with exertion or at rest
- Awakened by chest pain

May exhibit:
- Exertional dyspnea

CIRCULATION

May report:
- History of heart disease, hypertension, obesity in self/family

May exhibit:
- Tachycardia, dysrhythmias
- Blood pressure normal, elevated, or decreased
- Heart sounds: May be normal; late S_4 or transient late systolic murmur (papillary muscle dysfunction) may be evident during pain
- Moist, cool, pale skin/mucous membranes in presence of vasoconstriction

EGO INTEGRITY

May report:
- Stressors of work, family, others

May exhibit:
- Apprehension, uneasiness

FOOD/FLUID

May report:
- Nausea, "heartburn"/epigastric distress with eating
- Diet high in cholesterol/fats, salt, caffeine, liquor

May exhibit:
- Belching, gastric distention

PAIN/DISCOMFORT

May report:

Note: Reports of pain location and severity differ between men and women.

- Substernal or anterior chest pain that may radiate to jaw, neck, shoulders, and upper extremities (to left side more than right). Women may report pain between shoulder blades, back pain.
- Quality: Varies from transient/mild to moderate, heavy pressure, tightness, squeezing, burning. Women may report dull aching pain.
- Duration: Usually less than 15 min, rarely more than 30 min (average 3 min)
- Precipitating factors: Physical exertion or great emotion, such as anger or sexual arousal; exercise in weather extremes; or may be unpredictable and/or occur during rest or sleep in unstable angina
- Relieving factors: Pain may be responsive to particular relief mechanisms (e.g., rest, antianginal medications [women may not respond to these]).
- New or ongoing chest pain that has changed in frequency, duration, character, or predictability (i.e., unstable, variant, Prinzmetal's)

May exhibit:
- Facial grimacing, placing fist over midsternum, rubbing left arm, muscle tension, restlessness
- Autonomic responses; e.g., tachycardia, blood pressure changes

RESPIRATION

May report: Dyspnea worse with exertion
History of smoking

May exhibit: Respirations: Increased rate/rhythm and alteration in depth

TEACHING/LEARNING

May report: Family history or risk factors of CAD, obesity, sedentary lifestyle, hypertension, stroke, diabetes, cigarette smoking, hyperlipidemia
Use/misuse of cardiac, hypertensive, or OTC drugs. History of hormone replacement therapy in post-menopausal women
Use of vitamins/herbal supplements; e.g., niacin, coenxyme Q10, ginger, bilberry, comfrey, garlic, L-carnitine
Regular alcohol use, illicit drug use; e.g., cocaine, amphetamines

Discharge plan considerations: Alteration in medication use/therapy
Assistance with homemaker/maintenance tasks
Changes in physical layout of home

Refer to section at end of plan for postdischarge considerations.

DIAGNOSTIC STUDIES

ECG: Often normal when client at rest or when pain-free; depression of the ST segment or T wave inversion signifies ischemia. Dysrhythmias and heart block may also be present. Significant Q waves are consistent with a prior MI.

24-hour ECG monitoring (Holter): Done to see whether pain episodes correlate with or change during exercise or activity. ST depression without pain is highly indicative of ischemia.

Exercise or pharmacologic stress electrocardiography: Provides more diagnostic information, such as duration and level of activity attained before onset of angina. A markedly positive test is indicative of severe CAD. *Note:* Studies have shown stress echo studies to be more accurate in some groups than exercise stress testing alone.

Cardiac enzymes (troponin I and cardiac troponin T, CPK, CK and CK-MB; LDH and isoenzymes LD_1, LD_2): Usually within normal limits (WNL); elevation indicates myocardial damage.

Chest x-ray: Usually normal; however, infiltrates may be present, reflecting cardiac decompensation or pulmonary complications.

PCO_2, potassium, and myocardial lactate: May be elevated during anginal attack (all play a role in myocardial ischemia and may perpetuate it).

Serum lipids (total lipids, lipoprotein electrophoresis, and isoenzymes cholesterols [HDL, LDL, VLDL]; triglycerides; phospholipids): May be elevated (CAD risk factor).

Echocardiogram: Motion-mode (M-mode) or two-dimensional (2-D or cross-sectional) echocardiography helps diagnose cardiomyopathy, HF, pericarditis, and abnormal valvular action that might be cause of chest pain.

Nuclear imaging studies (rest or stress scan): *Thallium-201:* Ischemic regions appear as areas of decreased thallium uptake. *MUGA:* Evaluates specific and general ventricle performance, regional wall motion, and ejection fraction.

Calcium scoring (also called coronary artery calcium scoring): Ultrafast CT scan that measures the amount of calcium in the coronary arteries. Elevated calcium scoring in client with other risk factors (e.g., family history, hypertension, diabetes, hypercholesterolemia) is an indication of some level of coronary artery disease (CAD).

Cardiac catheterization with angiography: Definitive test for CAD in clients with known ischemic disease with angina or incapacitating chest pain, in clients with cholesterolemia and familial heart disease who are experiencing chest pain, and in clients with abnormal resting ECGs. Abnormal results are present in valvular disease, altered contractility, ventricular failure, and circulatory abnormalities. *Note:* Ten percent of clients with unstable angina have normal-appearing coronary arteries.

NURSING PRIORITIES

1. Relieve/control pain.
2. Prevent/minimize development of myocardial complications.
3. Provide information about disease process/prognosis and treatment.
4. Support client/SO in initiating necessary lifestyle/behavioral changes.

DISCHARGE GOALS

1. Achieves desired activity level; meets self-care needs with minimal or no pain.
2. Free of complications.
3. Disease process/prognosis and therapeutic regimen understood.
4. Participating in treatment program, behavioral changes.
5. Plan in place to meet needs after discharge.

NURSING DIAGNOSIS: acute Pain

May be related to

Decreased myocardial blood flow
Increased cardiac workload/oxygen consumption

Possibly evidenced by

Reports of pain varying in frequency, duration, and intensity (especially as condition worsens)
Narrowed focus
Distraction behaviors (moaning, crying, pacing, restlessness)
Autonomic responses; e.g., diaphoresis, blood pressure and pulse rate changes, pupillary dilation, increased/decreased respiratory rate

DESIRED OUTCOMES/EVALUATION CRITERIA—CLIENT WILL:

Pain Level (NOC)

Report anginal episodes decreased in frequency, duration, and severity.
Demonstrate relief of pain as evidenced by stable vital signs, absence of muscle tension and restlessness.

ACTIONS/INTERVENTIONS	RATIONALE
Pain Management (NIC)	
Independent	
Instruct client to notify nurse immediately when chest pain occurs.	Pain and decreased cardiac output may stimulate the sympathetic nervous system to release excessive amounts of norepinephrine, which increases platelet aggregation and release of thromboxane A_2. This potent vasoconstrictor causes coronary artery spasm, which can precipitate, complicate, and/or prolong an anginal attack. Unbearable pain may cause vasovagal response, decreasing BP and heart rate.
Assess and document client response/effects of medication.	Provides information about disease progression. Aids in evaluating effectiveness of interventions, and may indicate need for change in therapeutic regimen.
Identify precipitating event, if any; frequency, duration, intensity, and location of pain.	Helps differentiate this chest pain, and aids in evaluating possible progression to unstable angina. (Stable angina usually lasts 3–15 minutes and is often relieved by rest and sublingual nitroglycerin [NTG]; unstable angina is more intense, occurs unpredictably, may last longer, and is not usually relieved by NTG/rest.)
Observe for associated symptoms; e.g., dyspnea, nausea/vomiting, dizziness, palpitations, desire to micturate.	Decreased cardiac output (which may occur during ischemic myocardial episode) stimulates sympathetic/parasympathetic nervous system, causing a variety of vague sensations that client may not identify as related to anginal episode.
Evaluate reports of pain in jaw, neck, shoulder, arm, or hand (typically on left side).	Cardiac pain may radiate; e.g., pain is often referred to more superficial sites served by the same spinal cord nerve level.
Place client at complete rest during anginal episodes.	Reduces myocardial oxygen demand to minimize risk of tissue injury/necrosis.

ACTIONS/INTERVENTIONS	RATIONALE
Elevate head of bed if client is short of breath.	Facilitates gas exchange to decrease hypoxia and resultant shortness of breath.
Monitor heart rate/rhythm.	Clients with unstable angina have an increased risk of acute life-threatening dysrhythmias, which occur in response to ischemic changes and/or stress.
Monitor vital signs every 5 min during initial anginal attack.	Blood pressure may initially rise because of sympathetic stimulation, then fall if cardiac output is compromised. Tachycardia also develops in response to sympathetic stimulation and may be sustained as a compensatory response if cardiac output falls.
Stay with client who is experiencing pain or appears anxious.	Anxiety releases catecholamines, which increase myocardial workload and can escalate/prolong ischemic pain. Presence of nurse can reduce feelings of fear and helplessness.
Maintain quiet, comfortable environment; restrict visitors as necessary.	Mental/emotional stress increases myocardial workload.
Provide light meals. Have client rest for 1 hour after meals.	Decreases myocardial workload associated with work of digestion, reducing risk of anginal attack.

Collaborative

ACTIONS/INTERVENTIONS	RATIONALE
Provide supplemental oxygen as indicated.	Increases oxygen available for myocardial uptake/reversal of ischemia.
Administer antianginal medication(s) promptly as indicated:	
Nitroglycerin: sublingual (Nitrostat), extended release tablets/capsules (Imdur, Isobid, Isordil, Nitrong, Nitrocot); chewable tablets (Isordil, Sorbitrate), metered-dose spray (Nitrolingual); transdermal patch (Nitro-Dur, Nitrodisc); transdermal ointment (Nitro-Dur, Transderm-Nitro);	Nitroglycerin has been the standard for treating and preventing anginal pain for more than 100 years. Today, it is available in many forms and is still the cornerstone of antianginal therapy. Rapid vasodilator effect lasts 10–30 minutes and can be used prophylactically to prevent, as well as abort, anginal attacks. Long-acting preparations are used to prevent recurrences by reducing coronary vasospasms and reducing cardiac workload. May cause headache, dizziness, light-headedness—symptoms that usually pass quickly. If headache is intolerable, alteration of dose or discontinuation of drug may be necessary. *Note:* Isordil may be more effective for clients with variant form of angina.
β-blockers; e.g., acebutolol (Sectral), atenolol (Tenormin), nadolol (Corgard), metroprolol (Lopressor), propranolol (Inderal);	Reduce angina by reducing the heart's workload. (Refer to ND: risk for decreased Cardiac Output, following, p. 67.) *Note:* Often, these drugs alone are sufficient to relieve angina in less severe conditions.
Calcium channel blockers; e.g., bepridil (Vascor), amlodipine (Norvasc), nifedipine (Procardia), felodipine (Plendil), isradipine (DynaCirc), diltiazem (Cardizem);	Produce relaxation of coronary vascular smooth muscle; dilate coronary arteries; decrease peripheral vascular resistance.
Analgesics; e.g., acetaminophen (Tylenol);	Usually sufficient analgesia for relief of headache caused by dilation of cerebral vessels in response to nitrates.
Morphine sulfate (MS).	Potent narcotic analgesic may be used in acute onset because of its several beneficial effects; e.g., causes peripheral vasodilation and reduces myocardial workload, has a sedative effect to produce relaxation, interrupts the flow of vasoconstricting catecholamines and thereby effectively relieves severe chest pain. MS is given IV for rapid action and because decreased cardiac output compromises peripheral tissue absorption.
Monitor serial ECG changes.	Ischemia during anginal attack may cause transient ST segment depression or elevation and T wave inversion. Serial tracings verify ischemic changes, which may disappear when client is pain-free. They also provide a baseline against which to compare later pattern changes.

NURSING DIAGNOSIS: risk for decreased Cardiac Output

Risk factors may include

Inotropic changes (transient/prolonged myocardial ischemia, effects of medications)
Alterations in rate/rhythm and electrical conduction

Possibly evidenced by

[Not applicable; presence of signs and symptoms establishes an *actual* diagnosis.]

DESIRED OUTCOMES/EVALUATION CRITERIA—CLIENT WILL:

Cardiac Pump Effectiveness (NOC)

Demonstrate increased activity tolerance.
Report/display decreased episodes of dyspnea, angina, and dysrhythmias.
Participate in behaviors/activities that reduce the workload of the heart.

ACTIONS/INTERVENTIONS	RATIONALE
Hemolytic Regulation (NIC)	
Independent	
Maintain bed/chair rest in position of comfort during acute episodes.	Decreases oxygen consumption/demand, reducing myocardial workload and risk of decompensation.
Monitor vital signs (e.g., heart rate, BP) and cardiac rhythm.	Tachycardia may be present because of pain, anxiety, hypoxemia, and reduced cardiac output. Changes may also occur in BP (hypertension or hypotension) because of cardiac response. ECG changes reflecting ischemia/dysrhythmias indicate need for additional evaluation and therapeutic intervention.
Auscultate breath sounds and heart sounds. Listen for murmurs.	S_3, S_4, or crackles can occur with cardiac decompensation or some medications (especially β-blockers). Development of murmurs may reveal a valvular cause for chest pain (e.g., aortic stenosis, mitral stenosis) or papillary muscle rupture.
Provide for adequate rest periods. Assist with/perform self-care activities, as indicated.	Conserves energy, reduces cardiac workload.
Stress importance of avoiding straining/ bearing down, especially during defecation.	Valsalva maneuver causes vagal stimulation, reducing heart rate (bradycardia), which may be followed by rebound tachycardia, both of which may impair cardiac output.
Encourage immediate reporting of pain for prompt administration of medications as indicated.	Timely interventions can reduce oxygen consumption and myocardial workload and may prevent/minimize cardiac complications.
Monitor for and document effects of/adverse response to medications, noting BP, heart rate, and rhythm (especially when giving combination of calcium antagonists, β-blockers, and nitrates).	Desired effect is to decrease myocardial oxygen demand by decreasing ventricular stress. Drugs with negative inotropic properties can decrease perfusion to an already ischemic myocardium. Combination of nitrates and β-blockers may have cumulative effect on cardiac output.
Assess for signs and symptoms of heart failure.	Angina is only a symptom of underlying pathology causing myocardial ischemia. Disease may compromise cardiac function to point of decompensation.
Evaluate mental status, noting development of confusion, disorientation.	Reduced perfusion of the brain can produce observable changes in sensorium.
Note skin color and presence/quality of pulses.	Peripheral circulation is reduced when cardiac output falls, giving the skin a pale or gray color (depending on level of hypoxia) and diminishing the strength of peripheral pulses.

ACTIONS/INTERVENTIONS	RATIONALE
Collaborative	
Administer supplemental oxygen as needed.	Increases oxygen available for myocardial uptake to improve contractility, reduce ischemia, and reduce lactic acid levels.
Monitor pulse oximetry or ABGs as indicated.	Determines adequacy of respiratory function and/or O_2 therapy.
Measure cardiac output and other functional parameters as indicated.	Cardiac index, preload/afterload, contractility, and cardiac work can be measured noninvasively through various means, including thoracic electrical bioimpedance (TEB) technique. Useful in evaluating response to therapeutic interventions and identifying need for more aggressive/emergency care. *Note:* Evaluation of changes in heart rate, BP, and cardiac output requires consideration of client's circadian hemodynamic variability (e.g., these measurements are normally expected to be lower at night in clients who are active during the day).
Administer medications as indicated:	
Calcium channel blockers; e.g., diltiazem (Cardizem), nifedipine (Procardia), verapamil (Calan), bepridil (Vascor), amlodipine (Norvasc), felodipine (Plendil), isradipine (DynaCirc);	Although differing in mode of action, calcium channel blockers play a major role in preventing and terminating ischemia induced by coronary artery spasm and in reducing vascular resistance, thereby decreasing BP and cardiac workload.
β-Blockers; e.g., atenolol (Tenormin), nadolol (Corgard), propranolol (Inderal), esmolol (Brevibloc);	These medications decrease cardiac workload by reducing heart rate and systolic BP. *Note:* Overdosage produces cardiac decompensation.
Acetylsalicylic acid (ASA), other antiplatelet agents; e.g., clopidogrel (Plavix), ticlopidine (Ticlid), tirofiban (Aggrastat), eptifibatide (Integrilin);	Useful in unstable angina, ASA diminishes platelet aggregation/clot formation. For clients with major GI intolerance, alternative drugs may be indicated. Newer IV and oral antiplatelet medications (especially Plavix) are frequently being used IV in conjunction with angioplasty and stenting for relief of angina.
IV heparin.	Bolus, followed by continuous infusion, is recommended to help reduce risk of subsequent MI by reducing the thrombotic complications of plaque rupture for clients diagnosed with intermediate or high-risk unstable angina. *Note:* Use of low-molecular-weight heparin is increasing because of its more efficacious and predictable effect with fewer adverse effects (e.g., less risk of bleeding) and longer half-life. It also does not require anticoagulation monitoring.
Monitor laboratory studies; e.g., PTT, aPTT.	Evaluates anticoagulation therapy needs/effectiveness.
Discuss purpose and prepare for stress testing and cardiac catheterization when indicated.	Stress testing provides information about the health/strength of the ventricles.
Prepare for surgical interventions (e.g., angioplasty with/without intracoronary stent placement, valve replacement, CABG) if indicated.	Angioplasty (also called percutaneous transluminal coronary angioplasty [PTCA]) increases coronary blood flow by compression of atheromatous lesions and dilation of the vessel lumen in an occluded coronary artery. Intracoronary stents may be placed at the time of PTCA to provide structural support within the coronary artery and improve the odds of long-term patency. This procedure is preferred over the more invasive CABG surgery. Drug-eluting (drug-coated) stents my be considered for clients at high risk for thrombosis, acute closure, and for diabetics. Several different drugs are available to help decrease restenosis after stenting or angioplasty. Stent placement may also be effective for the variant form of angina where periodic vasospasms impair arterial flow. *Note:* A recent innovation

ACTIONS/INTERVENTIONS	RATIONALE
	in thrombolytic therapy associated with angioplasty and stenting is the Anjiojet (a device approved for removing blood clots from coronary arteries), which can reduce risk of heart attack or death. CABG is the recommended treatment when testing confirms myocardial ischemia as a result of left main coronary artery disease or symptomatic three-vessel disease, especially in those with left ventricular dysfunction.
Prepare for transfer to critical care unit if condition warrants.	Profound/prolonged chest pain with decreased cardiac output reflects development of complications requiring more intense/emergency interventions.

NURSING DIAGNOSIS: Anxiety [specify level]

May be related to

Situational crises
Threat to self-concept (altered image/abilities)
Underlying pathophysiologic response
Threat to or change in health status (disease course that can lead to further compromise, debility, even death)
Negative self-talk

Possibly evidenced by

Expressed concern regarding changes in life events
Increased tension/helplessness
Apprehension, uncertainty, restlessness
Association of diagnosis with loss of healthy body image, loss of place/influence
View of self as noncontributing member of family/society
Fear of death as an imminent reality

DESIRED OUTCOMES/EVALUATION CRITERIA—CLIENT WILL:

Anxiety Self-Control (NOC)

Verbalize awareness of feelings of anxiety and healthy ways to deal with them.
Report anxiety is reduced to a manageable level.
Express concerns about effect of disease on lifestyle, position within family and society.
Demonstrate effective coping strategies/problem-solving skills.

ACTIONS/INTERVENTIONS — RATIONALE

Anxiety Reduction (NIC)

Independent

ACTIONS/INTERVENTIONS	RATIONALE
Explain purpose of tests and procedures; e.g., stress testing.	Reduces anxiety attributable to fear of unknown diagnosis and prognosis.
Promote expression of feelings and fears; e.g., denial, depression, and anger. Let client/SO know these are normal reactions. Note statements of concern, such as, "Heart attack is inevitable."	Unexpressed feelings may create internal turmoil and affect self-image. Verbalization of concerns reduces tension, verifies level of coping, and facilitates dealing with feelings. Presence of negative self-talk can increase level of anxiety and may contribute to exacerbation of anginal attacks.

ACTIONS/INTERVENTIONS	RATIONALE
Encourage family and friends to treat client as before.	Reassures client that role in the family and business has not been altered.
Tell client the medical regimen has been designed to reduce/limit future attacks and increase cardiac stability.	Encourages client to test symptom control (e.g., no angina with certain levels of activity), to increase confidence in medical program, and to integrate abilities into perceptions of self. (Refer to CP: Psychosocial Aspects of Care, ND: Anxiety [specify level]/Fear, p. 770, for additional considerations.)
Collaborative	
Administer sedatives, tranquilizers, as indicated.	May be desired to help client relax until physically able to reestablish adequate coping strategies.

NURSING DIAGNOSIS: deficient Knowledge [Learning Need] regarding condition, treatment needs, self-care, and discharge needs

May be related to

Lack of exposure
Inaccurate/misinterpretation of information
Unfamiliarity with information resources

Possibly evidenced by

Questions; statement of concerns
Request for information
Inaccurate follow-through of instructions

DESIRED OUTCOMES/EVALUATION CRITERIA—CLIENT WILL:

Participate in learning process.
Assume responsibility for own learning, looking for information and asking questions.

KNOWLEDGE: Cardiac Disease Management (NOC)

Verbalize understanding of condition/disease process and potential complications.
Verbalize understanding of /participate in therapeutic regimen.
Initiate necessary lifestyle changes.

ACTIONS/INTERVENTIONS	RATIONALE
TEACHING: Disease Process (NIC)	
Independent	
Discuss pathophysiology of condition. Stress need for preventing and managing anginal attacks.	Clients with angina need to learn why it occurs and what they can do to control it. This is the focus of therapeutic management to reduce likelihood of MI and promote healthy heart lifestyle.

ACTIONS/INTERVENTIONS	RATIONALE
Review significance of cholesterol levels and differentiate between LDL and HDL factors. Emphasize importance of periodic laboratory measurements, and use of cholesterol-lowering drugs.	Although the American Heart Association recommended LDL is ±130mg/dL, clients with two or more risk factors (e.g., smoking, hypertension, diabetes mellitus, positive family history) should keep LDL ±100 mg/dL, and those with diagnosis of CAD need to keep LDL below 100 mg/dL. HDL below 35–45 is considered a risk factor; a level above 60 mg/dL is considered an advantage. *Note:* The National Choleterol Education Program Guidelines now state that all adult high-risk clients with LDL ≥ 100mg/dL should be treated with drug therapy.
Encourage avoidance of factors/situations that may precipitate anginal episode; e.g., emotional stress, extensive or intense physical exertion, ingestion of large/heavy meal, especially at bedtime, exposure to extremes in environmental temperature.	May reduce incidence/severity of ischemic episodes. Helps client manage symptoms.
Assist client/SO to identify sources of physical and emotional stress and discuss ways that they can be avoided.	This is a crucial step in limiting/preventing anginal attacks.
Review importance of cessation of smoking, weight control, dietary changes, and exercise.	Knowledge of the significance of risk factors provides client with opportunity to make needed changes. Clients with high cholesterol who do not respond to 6-month program of low-fat diet and regular exercise will require medication.
Encourage client to follow prescribed reconditioning program; caution to avoid exhaustion.	Fear of triggering attacks may cause client to avoid participation in activity that has been prescribed to enhance recovery (increase myocardial strength and form collateral circulation). Cardiac rehab programs provide a phased approach to increaasing client's activity and exercise tolerance.
Discuss impact of condition on desired lifestyle and activities, including work, driving, sexual activity, and hobbies. Provide information, privacy, or consultation, as indicated.	Client may be reluctant to resume/continue usual activities because of fear of anginal attack or death. Client should take nitroglycerin prophylactically before any activity that is known to precipitate angina.
Demonstrate how/encourage client to monitor own pulse and BP during/after activities, when appropriate, and to schedule/simplify activities, avoid strain, and take rest periods.	Allows client to identify those activities that can be modified to avoid cardiac stress and stay below the anginal threshold.
Discuss steps to take when anginal attacks occur; e.g., cessation of activity, keeping "rescue" NTG on hand, administration of prn medication, use of relaxation techniques.	Being prepared for an event takes away the fear that client will not know what to do if attack occurs.
Review prescribed medications for control/prevention of anginal attacks as previously presented:	Angina is a complicated condition that often requires the use of many drugs given to decrease myocardial workload, improve coronary circulation, and control the occurrence of attacks.
ASA and other antiplatelet agents;	May be given prophylactically on a daily basis to decrease platelet aggregation and improve coronary circulation. May prolong survival rate of clients with unstable angina.
Lipid-lowering agents: bile acid sequestrants; e.g., cholestyramine (Questran), colestipol (Colestid); nicotinic acid (Niacin); fibrates; e.g. fenofibrate (Tricor), gemfibrozil (Lopid); and HMG-CoA reductase inhibitors; e.g., lovastatin (Lipitor), fluvastatin (Lescol) pravastatin (Pravachol), simvastatin (Zocor).	These drugs are considered first-line agents for lowering serum cholesterol levels. *Note:* Questran/Colestid may inhibit absorption of fat-soluble vitamins and some drugs such as Coumadin, Lanoxin, and Inderal. The HMG-CoA reductase inhibitors may cause photosensitivity. Most lipid-lowering agents are inhibited by grapefruit juice.
Stress importance of checking with physician before taking OTC drugs.	OTC drugs may potentiate or negate effects of prescribed medications.
Discuss use of herbals (e.g., gensing, garlic, ginkgo, hawthorn, bromelain) as indicated.	Some herbals (e.g., ginkgo, gensing, bromelain) can impact bleeding/clotting, especially when added to medications such as Plavix or Coumadin (increases bleeding). Others (e.g., hawthorn) can increase the effects of certain heart medications.

ACTIONS/INTERVENTIONS	RATIONALE
Review symptoms to be reported to physician; e.g., increase in frequency/duration of attacks, changes in response to medications.	Knowledge of expectations can avoid undue concern for insignificant reasons or delay in treatment of important symptoms.
Discuss importance of follow-up appointments.	Angina is a symptom of progressive coronary artery disease that should be monitored and may require occasional adjustment of treatment regimen.

POTENTIAL CONSIDERATIONS following discharge from care setting (dependent on client's age, physical condition/presence of complications, personal resources, and life responsibilities)

acute Pain—episodes of decreased myocardial blood flow/ischemia

Activity Intolerance—imbalance between oxygen supply/demand, sedentary/stressful lifestyle

ineffective Denial—learned response patterns (e.g., avoidance), cultural factors, personal and family value systems

interrupted Family Processes—situational transition and crisis

impaired Home Maintenance—altered ability to perform tasks, inadequate support systems, reluctance to request assistance

MYOCARDIAL INFARCTION

Myocardial infarction (MI) is caused by marked reduction/loss of blood flow through one or more of the coronary arteries, resulting in cardiac muscle ischemia and necrosis.

CARE SETTING

Inpatient acute hospital, step-down, or medical unit.

RELATED CONCERNS

Angina, page 62
Dysrhythmias, page 85
Heart failure: chronic, page 47
Psychosocial aspects of care, page 770
Thrombophlebitis: deep vein thrombosis, page 108

Client Assessment Database

ACTIVITY/REST

May report: Weakness, fatigue, loss of sleep
Sedentary lifestyle, sporadic exercise schedule

May exhibit: Tachycardia, dyspnea with rest/activity

CIRCULATION

May report: History of previous MI, CAD, HF, hypertension, diabetes mellitus

May exhibit: BP may be normal, increased, or decreased; postural changes may be noted from lying to sitting/standing
Pulse may be normal, full/bounding, or have a weak/thready quality with delayed capillary refill; irregularities (dysrhythmias) may be present
Heart sounds S_3/S_4 may reflect a pathologic condition (e.g., cardiac failure, decreased ventricular contractility or compliance)
Murmurs may reflect valvular insufficiency or papillary muscle dysfunction
Friction rub (suggests pericarditis)
Heart rate regular or irregular; tachycardia/bradycardia may be present
Edema: Jugular vein distention, peripheral/dependent edema, generalized edema
Color: Pallor or cyanosis/mottling of skin, nail beds, mucous membranes, and lips may be noted

EGO INTEGRITY

May report: Denial of significance of symptoms/presence of condition
Fear of dying, feelings of impending doom
Anger at inconvenience of illness/"unnecessary" hospitalization
Worry about family, employment, finances

May exhibit: Denial, withdrawal, anxiety, lack of eye contact
Irritability, anger, combative behavior
Focus on self/pain

ELIMINATION

May exhibit: Normal or decreased bowel sounds

FOOD/FLUID

May report: Nausea, loss of appetite, belching, indigestion/heartburn

May exhibit: Poor skin turgor; dry or diaphoretic skin
Vomiting

HYGIENE

May report/exhibit: Difficulty in performing self-care tasks

NEUROSENSORY

May report: Dizziness, fainting spells in or out of bed (upright or at rest)

May exhibit: Changes in mentation
Weakness

PAIN/DISCOMFORT

May report: **Note: Reports of location and intensity of pain differ between men and women.**
Sudden onset of chest pain unrelieved by rest or nitroglycerin (although most pain is deep and visceral, 20% of MIs are painless)
Location: Typically, anterior chest (substernal, precordium); may radiate to arms, jaw, face; may have atypical location such as epigastrium/abdomen, elbow, jaw, back, neck, between shoulder blades, severe sore throat. Women may report pain between shoulder blades, back pain, tiredness, throat fullness
Quality: Crushing, constricting, vise-like, squeezing, heavy, steady. Women may report dull aching pain
Intensity: Usually 10 on a scale of 0–10 or "worst pain ever experienced." *Note:* Pain is sometimes absent in women, postoperative clients, those with prior stroke or heart failure, diabetes mellitus or hypertension, or the elderly. Studies indicate that up to one-third of persons experiencing MI do not have typical chest pain.
Precipitating factor: May/may not be associated with activity

May exhibit: Facial grimacing, changes in body posture, may place clenched fist on midsternum when describing pain
Crying, groaning, squirming, stretching
Withdrawal, lack of eye contact
Autonomic responses: Changes in heart rate/rhythm, BP, respirations, skin color/moisture, level of consciousness

RESPIRATION

May report: Dyspnea with/without exertion, nocturnal dyspnea
Cough with/without sputum production
History of smoking, chronic respiratory disease

May exhibit: Increased respiratory rate, shallow/labored breathing
Pallor or cyanosis
Breath sounds clear or crackles/wheezes
Sputum clear, possibly pink-tinged

SOCIAL INTERACTION

May report: Recent stress; e.g., work, family
Difficulty coping with recent/current stressors; e.g., money, work, family problems made worse by this illness/hospitalization

May exhibit: Difficulty resting quietly, overemotional responses (intense anger, fear)
Withdrawal from family

TEACHING/LEARNING

May report: Family history of heart disease/MI, diabetes, stroke, hypertension, peripheral vascular disease
Use of tobacco
Use/misuse cardiac medications, OTC preparations
Use of vitamins/herbal supplements (e.g., vitamin E, gensing, garlic, ginkgo, hawthorn, bromelain)

Discharge plan considerations: May require assistance with food preparation, shopping, transportation, homemaking/maintenance tasks; physical layout of home

Refer to section at end of plan for postdischarge considerations.

DIAGNOSTIC STUDIES

ECG: ST elevation signifying ischemia; peaked upright or inverted T wave indicating injury; development of Q waves signifying prolonged ischemia or necrosis.

Blood tests:

Cardiac enzymes and isoenzymes: CPK-MB (isoenzyme in cardiac muscle): Elevates within 4–8 hours, peaks in 12–20 hours, returns to normal in 48–72 hours.

Troponins: Troponin I (cTnI) and troponin T (cTnT): Levels are elevated at 4–6 hours, peak at 14–18 hours, and return to baseline over 6–7 days. These enzymes have increased specificity for necrosis and are therefore useful in diagnosing postoperative MI when MB-CPK may be elevated related to skeletal trauma.

Myoglobin: A heme protein of small molecular weight that is more rapidly released from damaged muscle tissue with elevation within 2 hr after an acute MI, and peak levels occurring in 3–15 hours.

Electrolytes: Imbalances of sodium and potassium can alter conduction and compromise contractility.

WBC: Leukocytosis (10,000–20,000) usually appears on the second day after MI due to the inflammatory process.

Chemistry profiles: May be abnormal depending on acute/chronic abnormal organ function/perfusion.

ABGs/pulse oximetry: May indicate hypoxia or acute/chronic lung disease processes.

Lipids (total lipids, HDL, LDL, VLDL, total cholesterol, triglycerides, and phospholipids): Elevations may reflect arteriosclerosis as a cause for coronary narrowing or spasm.

Coronary angiography: In hospitals with catheterization lab facilities, coronary angiography has become the gold standard for the assessment and treatment of myocardial infarction. Visualizes narrowing/occlusion of coronary arteries and is usually done in conjunction with measurements of chamber pressures and assessment of left ventricular function (ejection fraction). Procedure is not usually done in acute phase of MI unless angioplasty with/without stenting, or emergency heart surgery is imminent.

Chest x-ray: May be normal or show an enlarged cardiac shadow suggestive of HF or ventricular aneurysm.

Two-dimensional echocardiogram: May be done to determine dimensions of chambers, septal/ventricular wall motion, ejection fraction (blood flow), and valve configuration/function.

Nuclear imaging studies:

Persantine or thallium: Evaluates myocardial blood flow and status of myocardial cells; e.g., location/extent of acute/previous MI.

Cardiac blood imaging/MUGA: Evaluates specific and general ventricular performance, regional wall motion, and ejection fraction.

Technetium: Accumulates in ischemic cells, outlining necrotic area(s).

Digital subtraction angiography (DSA): Technique used to visualize status of arterial bypass grafts and to detect peripheral artery disease.

MRI: Allows visualization of blood flow, cardiac chambers/intraventricular septum, valves, vascular lesions, plaque formations, areas of necrosis/infarction, and blood clots.

Exercise stress test: Determines cardiovascular response to activity (often done in conjunction with thallium imaging in the recovery phase).

NURSING PRIORITIES

1. Relieve pain, anxiety.
2. Reduce myocardial workload.
3. Prevent/detect and assist in treatment of life-threatening dysrhythmias or complications.
4. Promote cardiac health, self-care.

DISCHARGE GOALS

1. Chest pain absent/controlled.
2. Heart rate/rhythm sufficient to sustain adequate cardiac output/tissue perfusion.
3. Achievement of activity level sufficient for basic self-care.
4. Anxiety reduced/managed.
5. Disease process, treatment plan, and prognosis understood.
6. Plan in place to meet needs after discharge.

NURSING DIAGNOSIS: acute Pain

May be related to

Tissue ischemia (coronary artery occlusion)

Possibly evidenced by

Reports of chest pain with/without radiation
Facial grimacing
Restlessness, changes in level of consciousness
Changes in pulse, BP

DESIRED OUTCOMES/EVALUATION CRITERIA—CLIENT WILL:

Pain Level (NOC)

Verbalize relief/control of chest pain within appropriate time frame for administered medications.
Display reduced tension, relaxed manner, ease of movement.

Pain Control (NOC)

Demonstrate use of relaxation techniques.

ACTIONS/INTERVENTIONS	RATIONALE
Pain Management (NIC)	
Independent	
Monitor/document characteristics of pain, noting verbal reports, nonverbal cues (e.g., moaning, crying, restlessness, diaphoresis, clutching chest, rapid breathing), and hemodynamic response (BP/heart rate changes).	Variation of appearance and behavior of clients in pain may present a challenge in assessment (e.g., men and women consistently present differently; or an individual may present differently from one episode to another). However, most clients with an acute MI appear ill, distracted, and focused on pain. Verbal history and deeper investigation of precipitating factors should be postponed until pain is relieved. Respirations may be increased as a result of pain and associated anxiety; release of stress-induced catecholamines increases heart rate and BP.
Obtain full description of pain from client including location, intensity (0–10), duration, characteristics (dull/crushing), and radiation. Assist client to quantify pain by comparing it to other experiences.	Pain is a subjective experience and must be described by client. Provides baseline for comparison to aid in determining effectiveness of therapy, resolution/progression of problem.
Review history of previous angina, anginal equivalent, or MI pain. Discuss family history if pertinent.	May differentiate current pain from preexisting patterns, as well as identify complications such as extension of infarction, pulmonary embolus, or pericarditis.

ACTIONS/INTERVENTIONS	RATIONALE
Instruct client to report pain immediately.	Delay in reporting pain hinders pain relief/may necessitate increased dosage of medication to achieve relief. In addition, severe pain may induce shock by stimulating the sympathetic nervous system, thereby creating further damage and interfering with diagnostics and relief of pain.
Provide quiet environment, calm activities, and comfort measures (e.g., dry/wrinkle-free linens, backrub). Approach client calmly and confidently.	Decreases external stimuli, which may aggravate anxiety and cardiac strain, limit coping abilities and adjustment to current situation.
Assist/instruct in relaxation techniques; e.g., deep/slow breathing, distraction behaviors, visualization, guided imagery.	Helpful in decreasing perception of/response to pain. Provides a sense of having some control over the situation, increase in positive attitude.
Check vital signs before and after administration of narcotic medication.	Hypotension/respiratory depression can occur as a result of narcotic administration. These problems may increase myocardial damage in presence of ventricular insufficiency.

Collaborative

Administer supplemental oxygen by means of nasal cannula or face mask, as indicated.	Increases amount of oxygen available for myocardial uptake and thereby may relieve discomfort associated with tissue ischemia.
Administer medications as indicated:	
Aspirin (ASA);	Aspirin is the mainline medication to be given first to all acute MI clients. ASA possesses anti-inflammatory, analgesic, and anitplatelet qualities that assist in the stabilization of plaque while decreasing clotting potential.
Antianginals; e.g., nitroglycerin (Nitro-Bid, Nitrostat, Nitro-Dur), isosorbide dinitrate (Isordil), mononitrate (Imdur);	Nitrates are useful for pain control by coronary vasodilating effects, which increase coronary blood flow and myocardial perfusion. Peripheral vasodilation effects reduce the volume of blood returning to the heart (preload), thereby decreasing myocardial workload and oxygen demand.
β-Blockers; e.g., atenolol (Tenormin), pindolol (Visken), propranolol (Inderal), nadolol (Corgard), metoprolol (Lopressor);	Important second-line agents for pain control through effect of blocking sympathetic stimulation, thereby reducing heart rate, systolic BP, and myocardial oxygen demand. May be given alone or with nitrates. *Note:* β-blockers may be contraindicated if myocardial contractility is severely impaired because negative inotropic properties can further reduce contractility.
Analgesics; e.g., morphine sulfate.	Although intravenous (IV) morphine is the usual drug of choice, other injectable narcotics may be used in acute-phase/recurrent chest pain unrelieved by nitroglycerin to reduce severe pain, provide sedation, and decrease myocardial workload. IM injections should be avoided, if possible, because they can alter the CPK diagnostic indicator and are not well absorbed in underperfused tissue.

NURSING DIAGNOSIS: Activity Intolerance

May be related to

Imbalance between myocardial oxygen supply and demand
Presence of ischemia/necrotic myocardial tissues
Cardiac depressant effects of certain drugs (beta-blockers, antidysrhythmics)

Possibly evidenced by

Alterations in heart rate and BP with activity
Development of dysrhythmias

Changes in skin color/moisture
Exertional angina
Generalized weakness

DESIRED OUTCOMES/EVALUATION CRITERIA—CLIENT WILL:

Activity Tolerance (NOC)

Demonstrate measurable/progressive increase in tolerance for activity with heart rate/rhythm and BP within client's normal limits and skin warm, pink, dry.
Report absence of angina with activity.

ACTIONS/INTERVENTIONS	RATIONALE
Energy Management (NIC)	
Independent	
Record/document heart rate and rhythm and BP changes before, during, and after activity as indicated. Correlate with reports of chest pain/shortness of breath. (Refer to ND: risk for decreased Cardiac Output.)	Trends determine client's response to activity and may indicate myocardial oxygen deprivation that may require decrease in activity level/return to bedrest, changes in medication regimen, or use of supplemental oxygen.
Encourage rest (bed/chair) initially. Thereafter, limit activity on basis of pain/ adverse cardiac response. Provide nonstress diversional activities.	Reduces myocardial workload/oxygen consumption, reducing risk of complications (e.g., extension of MI). *Note:* American Heart Association/American College of Cardiology guidelines (1996) suggest that clients with cardiac conditions should not be kept in bed longer than 24 hours. Clients with uncomplicated MI are encouraged to engage in mild activity out of bed, including short walks 12 hours after incident.
Instruct client to avoid increasing abdominal pressure; e.g., straining during defecation.	Activities that require holding the breath and bearing down (Valsalva's maneuver) can result in bradycardia (temporarily reduced cardiac output) and rebound tachycardia with elevated BP.
Explain pattern of graded increase of activity level; e.g., getting up to commode or sitting in chair, progressive ambulation, and resting after meals.	Progressive activity provides a controlled demand on the heart, increasing strength and preventing overexertion.
Review signs/symptoms reflecting intolerance of present activity level or requiring notification of nurse/physician.	Palpitations, pulse irregularities, development of chest pain, or dyspnea may indicate need for changes in exercise regimen or medication.
Collaborative	
Refer to cardiac rehabilitation program.	Provides continued support/additional supervision and participation in recovery and wellness process.

NURSING DIAGNOSIS: Anxiety [specify level]/Fear

May be related to

Threat to or change in health and socioeconomic status
Threat of loss/death
Unconscious conflict about essential values, beliefs, and goals of life
Interpersonal transmission/contagion

Possibly evidenced by

Fearful attitude
Apprehension, increased tension, restlessness, facial tension
Uncertainty, feelings of inadequacy
Somatic complaints/sympathetic stimulation
Focus on self, expressions of concern about current and future events
Fight (e.g., belligerent attitude) or flight behavior

DESIRED OUTCOMES/EVALUATION CRITERIA—CLIENT WILL:

Anxiety Self-Control/Fear Self-Control (NOC)

Recognize feelings.
Identify causes, contributing factors.
Verbalize reduction of anxiety or fear.
Demonstrate positive problem-solving skills.
Identify/use resources appropriately.

ACTIONS/INTERVENTIONS	RATIONALE
Anxiety Reduction (NIC)	
Independent	
Identify and acknowledge client's perception of threat/situation. Encourage expressions of, and do not deny feelings of, anger, grief, sadness, fear.	Coping with the pain and emotional trauma of an MI is difficult. Client may fear death and/or be anxious about immediate environment. Ongoing anxiety (related to concerns about impact of heart attack on future lifestyle, matters left unattended/unresolved, and effects of illness on family) may be present in varying degrees for some time and may be manifested by symptoms of depression.
Note presence of hostility, withdrawal, and/or denial (inappropriate affect or refusal to comply with medical regimen).	Research into survival rates between type A and type B individuals and the impact of denial has been ambiguous; however, studies show some correlation between degree/expression of anger or hostility and an increased risk for MI.
Maintain confident manner (without false reassurance).	Client and SO can be affected by the anxiety/uneasiness displayed by health team members. Honest explanations can alleviate anxiety.
Observe for verbal/nonverbal signs of anxiety, and stay with client. Intervene if client displays destructive behavior.	Client may not express concern directly, but words/actions may convey sense of agitation, aggression, and hostility. Intervention can help client regain control of own behavior.
Accept but do not reinforce use of denial. Avoid confrontations.	Denial can be beneficial in decreasing anxiety but can postpone dealing with the reality of the current situation. Confrontation can promote anger and increase use of denial, reducing cooperation and possibly impeding recovery.
Orient client/SO to routine procedures and expected activities. Promote participation when possible.	Predictability and information can decrease anxiety for client.
Answer all questions factually. Provide consistent information; repeat as indicated.	Accurate information about the situation reduces fear, strengthens nurse-client relationship, and assists client/SO to deal realistically with situation. Attention span may be short, and repetition of information helps with retention.
Encourage client/SO to communicate with one another, sharing questions and concerns.	Sharing information elicits support/comfort and can relieve tension of unexpressed worries.

ACTIONS/INTERVENTIONS	RATIONALE
Provide privacy for client and SO.	Allows needed time for personal expression of feelings; may enhance mutual support and promote more adaptive behaviors.
Provide rest periods/uninterrupted sleep time, quiet surroundings, with client controlling type, amount of external stimuli.	Conserves energy and enhances coping abilities.
Support normality of grieving process, including time necessary for resolution.	Can provide reassurance that feelings are normal response to situation/perceived changes.
Encourage independence, self-care, and decision making within accepted treatment plan.	Increased independence from staff promotes self-confidence and reduces feelings of abandonment that can accompany transfer from coronary unit/discharge from hospital.
Encourage discussion about postdischarge expectations.	Helps client/SO identify realistic goals, thereby reducing risk of discouragement in face of the reality of limitations of condition/pace of recuperation.
Collaborative	
Administer antianxiety/hypnotics as indicated; e.g., alprazolam (Xanax), diazepam (Valium), lorazepam (Ativan), flurazepam (Dalmane).	Promotes relaxation/rest and reduces feelings of anxiety.

NURSING DIAGNOSIS: risk for decreased Cardiac Output

Risk factors may include

Changes in rate, rhythm, electrical conduction
Reduced preload/increased SVR
Infarcted/dyskinetic muscle, structural defects; e.g., ventricular aneurysm, septal defects

Possibly evidenced by

[Not applicable; presence of signs and symptoms establishes *actual* diagnosis.]

DESIRED OUTCOMES/EVALUATION CRITERIA—CLIENT WILL:

Cardiac Pump Effectiveness (NOC)

Maintain hemodynamic stability; e.g., BP, cardiac output within normal range, adequate urinary output, decreased frequency/absence of dysrhythmias.
Report decreased episodes of dyspnea, angina.
Demonstrate an increase in activity tolerance.

ACTIONS/INTERVENTIONS	RATIONALE
CARDIAC CARE: Acute (NIC)	
Independent	
Auscultate BP. Compare both arms and obtain lying, sitting, and standing pressures when able.	Hypotension may occur related to ventricular dysfunction, hypoperfusion of the myocardium, and vagal stimulation. However, hypertension is also a common phenomenon, possibly related to pain, anxiety, catecholamine release, and/or preexisting vascular problems. Orthostatic (postural) hypotension may be associated with complications of infarct; e.g., HF.

ACTIONS/INTERVENTIONS	RATIONALE
Evaluate quality and equality of pulses, as indicated.	Decreased cardiac output results in diminished weak/thready pulses. Irregularities suggest dysrhythmias, which may require further evaluation/monitoring.
Auscultate heart sounds:	
Note development of S_3, S_4;	S_3 is usually associated with HF, but it may also be noted with the mitral insufficiency (regurgitation) and left ventricular overload that can accompany severe infarction. S_4 may be associated with myocardial ischemia, ventricular stiffening, and pulmonary or systemic hypertension.
Presence of murmurs/rubs.	Indicates disturbances of normal blood flow within the heart; e.g., incompetent valve, septal defect, or vibration of papillary muscle/chordae tendineae (complication of MI). Presence of rub with an infarction is also associated with inflammation; e.g., pericardial effusion and pericarditis.
Auscultate breath sounds.	Crackles reflecting pulmonary congestion may develop because of depressed myocardial function.
Monitor heart rate and rhythm. Document dysrhythmias via telemetry.	Heart rate and rhythm respond to medication, activity, and developing complications. Dysrhythmias (especially premature ventricular contractions or progressive heart blocks) can compromise cardiac function or increase ischemic damage. Acute or chronic atrial flutter/fibrillation may be seen with coronary artery or valvular involvement and may or may not be pathologic.
Note response to activity and promote rest appropriately. (Refer to ND: Activity Intolerance.)	Overexertion increases oxygen consumption/demand and can compromise myocardial function.
Provide small/easily digested meals. Limit caffeine intake; e.g., coffee, chocolate, cola as indicated.	Large meals may increase myocardial workload and cause vagal stimulation, resulting in bradycardia/ectopic beats. Caffeine is a direct cardiac stimulant that can increase heart rate but may not be a problem for everyone (e.g., some clients with regular daily caffeine intake).
Have emergency equipment/medications available.	Sudden coronary occlusion, lethal dysrhythmias, extension of infarct, and unrelenting pain are situations that may precipitate cardiac arrest, requiring immediate life-saving therapies/transfer to critical/coronary care unit (CCU).

Collaborative

Administer supplemental oxygen, as indicated.	Increases amount of oxygen available for myocardial uptake, reducing ischemia and resultant cellular irritation/dysrhythmias.
Measure cardiac output and other functional parameters as appropriate.	Cardiac index, preload/afterload, contractility, and cardiac work can be measured noninvasively with thoracic electrical bioimpedance (TEB) technique. Useful in evaluating response to therapeutic interventions and identifying need for more aggressive/emergency care.
Maintain IV/Hep-Lock access as indicated.	Patent line is important for administration of emergency drugs in presence of persistent lethal dysrhythmias or chest pain.
Review serial ECGs.	Provides information regarding progression/resolution of infarction, status of ventricular function, electrolyte balance, and effects of drug therapies.
Review chest x-ray.	May reflect pulmonary edema related to ventricular dysfunction.
Monitor laboratory data; e.g., cardiac enzymes, ABGs, electrolytes.	Enzymes monitor resolution/extension of infarction. Presence of hypoxia indicates need for supplemental oxygen. Electrolyte imbalance; e.g., hypokalemia/hyperkalemia, adversely affects cardiac rhythm/contractility.

ACTIONS/INTERVENTIONS	RATIONALE
Administer antidysrhythmic drugs as indicated. (Refer to CP: Dysrhythmias.)	Dysrhythmias are usually treated symptomatically. Early inclusion of ACE inhibitor therapy (especially in presence of large anterior MI, ventricular aneurysm, or HF) enhances ventricular output, increases survival, and may slow progression of HF. *Note:* Use of routine lidocaine is no longer recommended.
Assist with insertion/maintain pacemaker/automatic internal cardiac defibrillator (AICD) when used.	Pacing may be a temporary support measure during acute phase or may be needed permanently if infarction severely damages conduction system, impairing systolic function. Use of AICD is currently advocated in client who has had ventricular fibrillation or tachycardia resulting in arrest. Strong supporting data document the benefits of ICDs for the primary prevention of sudden cardiac death.

NURSING DIAGNOSIS: ineffective Tissue Perfusion

Risk factors may include

Reduction/interruption of blood flow; e.g., vasoconstriction, hypovolemia/shunting, and thromboembolic formation

Possibly evidenced by

[Not applicable; presence of signs and symptoms establishes an *actual* diagnosis.]

DESIRED OUTCOMES/EVALUATION CRITERIA—CLIENT WILL:

Cardiac Pump Effectiveness (NOC)

Demonstrate adequate perfusion as individually appropriate; e.g., skin warm and dry, peripheral pulses present/strong, vital signs within client's normal range, client alert/oriented, balanced I&O, absence of edema, free of pain/discomfort.

ACTIONS/INTERVENTIONS	RATIONALE
Hemodynamic Regulation (NIC)	
Independent	
Investigate sudden changes or continued alterations in mentation; e.g., anxiety, confusion, lethargy, stupor.	Cerebral perfusion is directly related to cardiac output and is also influenced by electrolyte/acid-base variations, hypoxia, and systemic emboli.
Inspect for pallor, cyanosis, mottling, cool/clammy skin. Note strength of peripheral pulse.	Systemic vasoconstriction resulting from diminished cardiac output may be evidenced by decreased skin perfusion and diminished pulses. (Refer to ND: risk for decreased Cardiac Output, p. 38.)
Monitor respirations, note work of breathing.	Cardiac pump failure and/or ischemic pain may precipitate respiratory distress; however, sudden/continued dyspnea may indicate thromboembolic pulmonary complications.
Monitor intake, note changes in urine output. Record urine specific gravity as indicated.	Decreased intake/persistent nausea may result in reduced circulating volume, which negatively affects perfusion and organ function. Specific gravity measurements reflect hydration status and renal function.

ACTIONS/INTERVENTIONS	RATIONALE
Assess GI function, noting anorexia, decreased/absent bowel sounds, nausea/vomiting, abdominal distention, constipation.	Reduced blood flow to mesentery can produce GI dysfunction; e.g., loss of peristalsis. Problems may be potentiated/aggravated by use of analgesics, decreased activity, and dietary changes.

CIRCULATORY CARE: Venous Insufficiency (NIC)

Encourage active/passive leg exercises, avoidance of isometric exercises.	Enhances venous return, reduces venous stasis, and decreases risk of thrombophlebitis; however, isometric exercises can adversely affect cardiac output by increasing myocardial work and oxygen consumption.
Assess for pain in lower extremity/Homans' sign, erythema, edema.	Indicators of deep vein thrombosis (DVT), although calf pain is not always present.
Instruct client in application/periodic removal of antiembolic hose when used.	Limits venous stasis, improves venous return, and reduces risk of thrombophlebitis in client who is limited in activity.

Collaborative

Monitor laboratory data; e.g., ABGs, BUN, creatinine, electrolytes, coagulation studies (PT, aPTT, clotting times).	Indicators of organ perfusion/function. Abnormalities in coagulation may occur as a result of therapeutic measures (e.g., heparin/Coumadin use and some cardiac drugs).
Administer medications as indicated:	
Antiplatelet agents; e.g., aspirin, abciximab (ReoPro), clopidogrel (Plavix); eptifibatide (Integrilin);	Reduces mortality in MI clients, and is taken daily. Aspirin also reduces coronary reocclusion after percutaneous transluminal coronary angioplasty (PTCA). IV antiplatelet drugs (e.g., ReoPro, Integrilin) are used as adjuncts to PTCA to decrease complication of platelet clumping within stent when placed.
Anticoagulants; e.g., heparin/enoxaparin (Lovenox);	Low-dose heparin is given during PTCA and may be given prophylactically in high-risk clients (e.g., atrial fibrillation, obesity, ventricular aneurysm, or history of thrombophlebitis) to reduce risk of thrombophlebitis or mural thrombus formation.
Cimetidine (Tagamet), ranitidine (Zantac), antacids.	May occasionally be used to reduce or neutralize gastric acid, preventing discomfort and gastric irritation, especially in presence of reduced mucosal circulation.
Assist with reperfusion therapy:	
Administer thrombolytic agents; e.g., alteplase (Activase, rt-PA), reteplase (Retavase), streptokinase (Streptase), anistreplase (Eminase), urokinase, (Abbokinase).	Thrombolytic therapy is the treatment of choice if angioplasty is not immediately (within 90 minutes) available. The goal is to restore pefusion to the myocardium.
Prepare for procedures; e.g., balloon coronary angioplasty (PTCA), with/without intracoronary stents.	Angioplasty is used to open blocked coronary arteries, and immediately restore myocardial perfusion. The mechanism includes a combination of vessel stretching and plaque compression and/or removal of thrombotic material. Intracoronary stents may be placed at the time of PTCA to provide structural support within the coronary artery. Drug-eluting (drug-coated) stents may be used to decrease risk of restenosis/improve long-term patency.
Transfer to critical care or step-down unit.	Depending on client's condition/heart damage, other chronic health conditions, telemetry or more intensive monitoring and aggressive interventions may be necessary to promote optimum outcome.

NURSING DIAGNOSIS: risk for excess Fluid Volume

Risk factors may include

Decreased organ perfusion (renal)
Increased sodium/water retention
Increased hydrostatic pressure or decreased plasma proteins (sequestering of fluid in interstitial space/tissues)

Possibly evidenced by

[Not applicable; presence of signs and symptoms establishes an *actual* diagnosis.]

DESIRED OUTCOMES/EVALUATION CRITERIA—CLIENT WILL:

Fluid Balance (NOC)

Maintain fluid balance as evidenced by BP within client's normal limits.
Be free of peripheral/venous distention and dependent edema, with lungs clear and weight stable.

ACTIONS/INTERVENTIONS	RATIONALE
Fluid Management (NIC)	
Independent	
Auscultate breath sounds for presence of crackles.	May indicate pulmonary edema secondary to cardiac decompensation.
Note JVD, development of dependent edema.	Suggests developing congestive failure/fluid volume excess.
Measure I&O, noting decrease in output, concentrated appearance. Calculate fluid balance.	Decreased cardiac output results in impaired kidney perfusion, sodium/water retention, and reduced urine output.
Weigh daily.	Sudden changes in weight reflect alterations in fluid balance.
Maintain total fluid intake at 2000 mL/24 hour within cardiovascular tolerance.	Meets normal adult body fluid requirements, but may require alteration/restriction in presence of cardiac decompensation.
Collaborative	
Provide low-sodium, low caffeine diet/beverages.	Sodium enhances fluid retention and should therefore be restricted during active MI phase and/or if heart failure is present. Caffeine may cause vasospasm.
Administer diuretics; e.g., furosemide (Lasix), spironolactone with hydrochlorothiazide (Aldactazide), hydralazine (Apresoline).	May be necessary to correct fluid overload. Drug choice is usually dependent on acute/chronic nature of symptoms.
Monitor potassium as indicated.	Hypokalemia can limit effectiveness of therapy and can occur with use of potassium-depleting diuretics.

NURSING DIAGNOSIS: deficient Knowledge [Learning Need] regarding cause/treatment of condition, self-care, and discharge needs

May be related to

Lack of information/misunderstanding of medical condition/therapy needs
Unfamiliarity with information resources
Lack of recall

Possibly evidenced by

Questions; statement of misconception
Failure to improve on previous regimen
Development of preventable complications

DESIRED OUTCOMES/EVALUATION CRITERIA—CLIENT WILL:

KNOWLEDGE: Cardiac Disease Management (NOC)

Verbalize understanding of condition, potential complications, individual risk factors, and function of pacemaker (if used).
Relate signs of pacemaker failure.
Verbalize understanding of therapeutic regimen.
List desired action and possible adverse side effects of medications.

Cardiac Disease Self-Management (NOC)

Correctly perform necessary procedures and explain reasons for actions.

ACTIONS/INTERVENTIONS	RATIONALE
TEACHING: Individual (NIC)	
Independent	
Assess client/SO level of knowledge and ability/desire to learn.	Necessary for creation of individual instruction plan. Reinforces expectation that this will be a "learning experience." Verbalization identifies misunderstandings and allows for clarification.
Be alert to signs of avoidance; e.g., changing subject away from information being presented or extremes of behavior (withdrawal/euphoria).	Natural defense mechanisms, such as anger or denial of significance of situation, can block learning, affecting client's response and ability to assimilate information. Changing to a less formal/structured style may be more effective until client/SO is ready to accept/deal with current situation.
Present information in varied learning formats; e.g., programmed books, audiovisual tapes, question-and-answer sessions, group activities.	Using multiple learning methods enhances retention of material.
CARDIAC CARE: Rehabilitation (NIC)	
Reinforce explanations of risk factors, dietary/activity restrictions, medications, and symptoms requiring immediate medical attention.	Provides opportunity for client to retain information and to assume control/participate in rehabilitation program.
Discuss use of herbals (e.g., gensing, garlic, ginkgo, hawthorn, bromelain) as indicated.	Use of supplements/herbal remedies can result in alterations in blood clotting, especially when anticoagulant therapy; e.g., Plavix or ASA, is prescribed. Other herbals (e.g., hawthorn) can increase the effect of certain cardiac medications.
Encourage identification/reduction of individual risk factors; e.g., smoking/alcohol consumption, obesity.	These behaviors/chemicals have direct adverse effects on cardiovascular function and may impede recovery, increase risk for complications.
Warn against isometric activity, Valsalva's maneuver, and activities requiring arms positioned above head.	These activities greatly increase cardiac workload and myocardial oxygen consumption and may adversely affect myocardial contractility/output.

ACTIONS/INTERVENTIONS	RATIONALE
Review programmed increases in levels of activity. Educate client regarding gradual resumption of activities; e.g., walking, work, recreational and sexual activity. Provide guidelines for gradually increasing activity and instruction regarding target heart rate and pulse taking, as appropriate.	Gradual increase in activity increases strength and prevents overexertion, may enhance collateral circulation, and promotes return to normal lifestyle. *Note:* Sexual activity can be safely resumed once client can accomplish activity equivalent to climbing two flights of stairs without adverse cardiac effects.
Identify alternative activities for "bad weather" days, such as measured walking in house or shopping mall.	Provides for continuing daily activity program.
Review signs/symptoms requiring reduction in activity and notification of healthcare provider. Differentiate between increased heart rate that normally occurs during various activities and worsening signs of cardiac stress (e.g., chest pain, dyspnea, palpitations, increased heart rate lasting more than 15 min after cessation of activity, excessive fatigue the following day).	Pulse elevations beyond established limits, development of chest pain, or dyspnea may require changes in exercise and medication regimen.
Stress importance of follow-up care, and identify community resources/support groups; e.g., cardiac rehabilitation programs, "coronary clubs," smoking cessation clinics.	Reinforces that this is an ongoing/continuing health problem for which support/assistance is available after discharge. *Note:* After discharge, client can encounter limitations in physical functioning and often incur difficulty with emotional, social, and role functioning requiring ongoing support.
Emphasize importance of contacting physician if chest pain, change in anginal pattern, or other symptoms recur.	Timely evaluation/intervention may prevent complications.
Stress importance of reporting development of fever in association with diffuse/atypical chest pain (pleural, pericardial) and joint pain.	Post-MI complication of pericardial inflammation (Dressler's syndrome) requires further medical evaluation and intervention.
Encourage client/SO to share concerns/feelings. Discuss signs of pathologic depression versus transient feelings frequently associated with major life events. Recommend seeking professional help if depressed feelings persist.	Depressed clients have a greater risk of dying 6–18 months following a heart attack. Timely intervention may be beneficial. *Note:* Selective serotonin reuptake inhibitors (SSRIs), e.g., paroxetine (Paxil), have been found to be as effective as tricyclic antidepressants but with significantly fewer adverse cardiac complications.

POTENTIAL CONSIDERATIONS following discharge from care setting (dependent on client's age, physical condition/presence of complications, personal resources, and life responsibilities)

Activity Intolerance —imbalance between myocardial oxygen supply/demand.

anticipatory Grieving—perceived loss of general well-being, required changes in lifestyle, confronting mortality.

decisional Conflict (treatment)—multiple/divergent sources of information, perceived threat to value system, support system deficit.

interrupted Family Processes—situational transition and crisis.

impaired Home Management—altered ability to perform tasks, inadequate support systems, reluctance to request assistance.

DYSRHYTHMIAS (INCLUDING DIGITALIS TOXICITY)

A cardiac dysrhythmia is any disturbance in the normal rhythm of the electrical excitation of the heart. It can be the result of a primary cardiac disorder, a response to a systemic condition, or the result of electrolyte imbalance or drug toxicity. Dysrhythmias vary in severity and in their effects on cardiac function, which are partially influenced by the site of origin (ventricular or supraventricular).

CARE SETTINGS

Generally, minor dysrhythmias are monitored and treated in the community setting; however, potential life-threatening situations (including heart rates above 150 beats/min) may require a short inpatient stay.

RELATED CONCERNS

Angina, page 62
Heart failure: chronic, page 47
Myocardial infarction, page 72
Psychosocial aspects of care, page 770

Client Assessment Database

ACTIVITY/REST

May report: Generalized weakness and exertional fatigue
May exhibit: Changes in heart rate/BP with activity/exercise

CIRCULATION

May report: History of previous/acute MI (90%–95% experience dysrhythmias), cardiac surgery, cardiomyopathy, rheumatic/HF, valvular heart disease, long-standing hypertension, use of pacemaker

Pulse: Fast, slow, or irregular; palpitations, skipped beats

May exhibit: BP changes (hypertension or hypotension) during episodes of dysrhythmia

Pulses may be irregular; e.g., skipped beats; pulsus alternans (regular strong beat/weak beat); bigeminal pulse (irregular strong beat/weak beat)

Pulse deficit (difference between apical pulse and radial pulse)

Heart sounds: irregular rhythm, extra sounds, dropped beats

Skin color and moisture changes; e.g., pallor, cyanosis, diaphoresis (heart failure, shock)

Edema dependent, generalized, JVD (in presence of heart failure)

Urine output decreased if cardiac output is severely diminished

EGO INTEGRITY

May report: Feeling nervous (certain tachydysrhythmias), sense of impending doom

Stressors related to current medical problems

May exhibit: Anxiety, fear, withdrawal, anger, irritability, crying

FOOD/FLUID

May report: Loss of appetite, anorexia

Food intolerance (with certain medications)

Nausea/vomiting

Changes in weight

May exhibit: Weight gain or loss

Edema

Changes in skin moisture/turgor

Respiratory crackles

NEUROSENSORY

May report: Dizzy spells, fainting, headaches
May exhibit: Mental status/sensorium changes; e.g., disorientation, confusion, loss of memory; changes in usual speech pattern/consciousness, stupor, coma

Behavioral changes; e.g., combativeness, lethargy, hallucinations

Pupil changes (equality and reaction to light)

Loss of deep tendon reflexes with life-threatening dysrhythmias (ventricular tachycardia, severe bradycardia)

PAIN/DISCOMFORT

May report: Chest pain, mild to severe, which may or may not be relieved by antianginal medication
May exhibit: Distraction behaviors; e.g., restlessness

RESPIRATION

May report: Chronic lung disease
History of or current tobacco use
Shortness of breath
Coughing (with/without sputum production)

May exhibit: Changes in respiratory rate/depth during dysrhythmia episode
Breath sounds: Adventitious sounds (crackles, rhonchi, wheezing) may be present, indicating respiratory complications, such as left-sided heart failure (pulmonary edema) or pulmonary thromboembolic phenomena
Hemoptysis

SAFETY

May exhibit: Fever
Skin: Rashes (medication reaction)
Loss of muscle tone/strength

TEACHING/LEARNING

May report: Familial risk factors; e.g., heart disease, stroke
Use/misuse of prescribed medications, such as heart medications (e.g., digitalis), anticoagulants (e.g., warfarin [Coumadin]), benzodiazepines (e.g., diazepam [Valium]), tricyclic antidepressants (e.g., amitriptyline [Elavil]), or antipsychotic agents (e.g., fluphenazine [Prolixin], chlorpromazine [Thorazine]), or OTC medications (e.g., cough syrup and analgesics containing ASA)
Use of vitamins/herbal supplements for heart rhythm (e.g., belladonna, camphor, dong quai, gensing, goldenseal)
Stimulant abuse, including caffeine/nicotine; street drugs (e.g., cocaine derivitives, methamphetamines, ecstasy, inhalants
Lack of understanding about disease process/therapeutic regimen
Evidence of failure to improve; e.g., recurrent/intractable dysrhythmias that are life-threatening

Discharge plan considerations: Alteration of medication use/therapy

Refer to section at end of plan for postdischarge considerations.

DIAGNOSTIC STUDIES

ECG: Reveals type/source of dysrhythmia and effects of electrolyte imbalances and cardiac medications. Demonstrates patterns of ischemic injury and conduction aberrance. *Note:* Exercise ECG can reveal dysrhythmias occurring only when client is not at rest (can be diagnostic for cardiac cause of syncope).

Extended or event monitoring (e.g., Holter monitor): Extended ECG tracing (24 hours to weeks) may be desired to determine which dysrhythmias may be causing specific symptoms when client is active (home/work) or at rest. May also be used to evaluate pacemaker function, antidysrhythmic drug effect, or effectiveness of cardiac rehabilitation.

Signal-averaged ECG (SAE): May be used to screen high-risk clients (especially post-MI or unexplained syncope) for ventricular dysrhythmias, presence of delayed conduction, and late potentials (as occurs with sustained ventricular tachycardia).

Chest x-ray: May show enlarged cardiac shadow due to ventricular or valvular dysfunction.

Myocardial imaging scans: May demonstrate ischemic/damaged myocardial areas that could impede normal conduction or impair wall motion and pumping capabilities.

Electrophysiologic (EP) studies: Provides cardiac mapping of entire conduction system to evaluate normal and abnormal pathways of electrical conduction. Used to diagnose dysrhythmias and evaluate effectiveness of medication or pacemaker therapies.

Electrolytes: Elevated or decreased levels of potassium, calcium, and magnesium can cause dysrhythmias.

Drug screen: May reveal toxicity of cardiac drugs, presence of street drugs, or suggest interaction of drugs; e.g., digitalis and quinidine.

Thyroid studies: Elevated or depressed serum thyroid levels can cause/aggravate dysrhythmias.

ESR: Elevation may indicate acute/active inflammatory process, e.g., endocarditis, as a precipitating factor for dysrhythmias.

ABGs/pulse oximetry: Hypoxemia can cause/exacerbate dysrhythmias.

NURSING PRIORITIES

1. Prevent/treat life-threatening dysrhythmias.
2. Support client/SO in dealing with anxiety/fear of potentially life-threatening situation.
3. Assist in identification of cause/precipitating factors.
4. Review information regarding condition/prognosis/treatment regimen.

DISCHARGE GOALS

1. Free of life-threatening dysrhythmias and complications of impaired cardiac output/tissue perfusion.
2. Anxiety reduced/managed.
3. Disease process, therapy needs, and prevention of complications understood.
4. Plan in place to meet needs after discharge.

NURSING DIAGNOSIS: risk for decreased Cardiac Output

Risk factors may include

Altered electrical conduction
Reduced myocardial contractility

Possibly evidenced by

[Not applicable; presence of signs and symptoms establishes an *actual* diagnosis.]

DESIRED OUTCOMES/EVALUATION CRITERIA—CLIENT WILL:

Cardiac Pump Effectiveness (NOC)

Maintain/achieve adequate cardiac output as evidenced by BP/pulse within normal range, adequate urinary output, palpable pulses of equal quality, usual level of mentation.
Display reduced frequency/absence of dysrhythmia(s).
Participate in activities that reduce myocardial workload.

ACTIONS/INTERVENTIONS	RATIONALE
Dysrhythmia Management (NIC)	
Independent	
Palpate pulses (radial, carotid, femoral, dorsalis pedis), noting rate, regularity, amplitude (full/thready), and symmetry. Document presence of pulsus alternans, bigeminal pulse, or pulse deficit.	Differences in equality, rate, and regularity of pulses are indicative of the effect of altered cardiac output on systemic/peripheral circulation.
Auscultate heart sounds, noting rate, rhythm, presence of extra heartbeats, dropped beats.	Specific dysrhythmias are more clearly detected audibly than by palpation. Hearing extra heartbeats or dropped beats helps identify dysrhythmias in the unmonitored client.
Monitor vital signs. Assess adequacy of cardiac output/tissue perfusion, noting significant variations in BP/pulse rate equality, respirations, changes in skin color/temperature, level of consciousness/sensorium, and urine output during episodes of dysrhythmias.	Although not all dysrhythmias are life-threatening, immediate treatment may be required to terminate dysrhythmia in the presence of alterations in cardiac output and tissue perfusion.
Determine type of dysrhythmia and document with rhythm strip (if cardiac/telemetry monitoring is available):	Useful in determining need for/type of intervention required.

ACTIONS/INTERVENTIONS	RATIONALE
Sinus tachycardia;	Tachycardia can occur in response to stress, pain, fever, infection, coronary artery blockage, valvular dysfunction, hypovolemia, hypoxia, or as a result of decreased vagal tone or of increased sympathetic nervous system activity associated with the release of catecholamines. Although it generally does not require treatment, persistent tachycardia may worsen underlying pathology in clients with ischemic heart disease because of shortened diastolic filling time and increased oxygen demands. These clients may require medications.
Sinus bradycardia;	Bradycardia is common in clients with acute MI (especially anterior and inferior) and is the result of excessive parasympathetic activity, blocks in conduction to the SA or AV nodes, or loss of automaticity of the heart muscle. Clients with severe heart disease may not be able to compensate for a slow rate by increasing stroke volume. Therefore, decreased cardiac output, HF, and potentially lethal ventricular dysrhythmias may occur.
Atrial dysrhythmias; e.g., PACs, atrial flutter, atrial fibrillation (AF), atrial supraventricular tachycardias) (i.e., PAT, MAT, SVT);	PACs can occur as a response to ischemia and are normally harmless but can precede or precipitate atrial fibrillation. Acute and chronic atrial flutter and/or fibrillation (the most common dysrhythmia) can occur with coronary artery or valvular disease and may or may not be pathological. Rapid atrial flutter/fibrillation reduces cardiac output as a result of incomplete ventricular filling (shortened cardiac cycle) and increased oxygen demand.
Ventricular dysrhythmias; e.g., premature ventricular contractions/ventricular premature beats (PVCs/VPBs), ventricular tachycardia (VT), ventricular flutter/fibrillation (VF);	PVCs or VPBs reflect cardiac irritability and are commonly associated with MI, digitalis toxicity, coronary vasospasm, and misplaced temporary pacemaker leads. Frequent, multiple, or multifocal PVCs result in diminished cardiac output and may lead to potentially lethal dysrhythmias; e.g., VT or sudden death/cardiac arrest from ventricular flutter/fibrillation. *Note:* Intractable ventricular dysrhythmias unresponsive to medication may reflect ventricular aneurysm. Polymorphic VT (torsades de pointes) is recognized by inconsistent shape of QRS complexes and is often drug related; e.g., procainamide (Pronestyl), quinidine (Quinaglute), disopyramide (Norpace), and sotalol (Betapace).
Heart blocks.	Reflect altered transmission of impulses through normal conduction channels (slowed, altered) and may be the result of MI, coronary artery disease with reduced blood supply to sinoatrial (SA) or atrioventricular (AV) nodes, drug toxicity, and sometimes cardiac surgery. Progressing heart block is associated with slowed ventricular rates, decreased cardiac output, and potentially lethal ventricular dysrhythmias or cardiac standstill.
Provide calm/quiet environment. Review reasons for limitation of activities during acute phase.	Reduces stimulation and release of stress-related catecholamines, which can cause/aggravate dysrhythmias and vasoconstriction, increasing myocardial workload.
Demonstrate/encourage use of stress management behaviors; e.g., relaxation techniques, guided imagery, slow/deep breathing.	Promotes client participation in exerting some sense of control in a stressful situation.
Investigate reports of chest pain, documenting location, duration, intensity (0–10 scale), and relieving/aggravating factors. Note nonverbal pain cues; e.g., facial grimacing, crying, changes in BP/heart rate.	Reasons for chest pain are variable and depend on underlying cause. However, chest pain may indicate ischemia due to altered electrical conduction, decreased myocardial perfusion, or increased oxygen need (e.g., impending/evolving MI).

ACTIONS/INTERVENTIONS	RATIONALE
Be prepared to initiate cardiopulmonary resuscitation (CPR) as indicated.	Development of life-threatening dysrhythmias requires prompt intervention to prevent ischemic damage/death.

Collaborative

ACTIONS/INTERVENTIONS	RATIONALE
Monitor laboratory studies:	
Electrolytes;	Imbalance of electrolytes, such as potassium, magnesium, and calcium, adversely affects cardiac rhythm and contractility.
Medication/drug levels.	Reveal therapeutic/toxic level of prescription medications or street drugs that may affect/contribute to presence of dysrhythmias.
Administer supplemental oxygen as indicated.	Increases amount of oxygen available for myocardial uptake, reducing irritability caused by hypoxia.
Prepare for/assist with diagnostic/treatment procedures (e.g., electrophysiology studies, radiofrequency ablation [RFA]; cryo-ablation [CA]).	Treatment for several tachycardia dysrhythmias (e.g., SVT, atrial flutter, WPW [Wolf-Parkinson-White], atrial fibrillation, VT) is often carried out as first-line treatment via heart catheterization/angiographic procedures. After rhythm is confirmed with electrophysiologic study, the client will then often have either an RFA or CA to terminate or disrupt the dysfunctional pattern. Medications may be trialed first or added after ablation for increased treatment success.
Administer medications as indicated:	
Potassium;	Dysrhythmias are generally treated symptomatically.
Antidysrhythmics, such as:	Correction of hypokalemia may be sufficient to terminate some ventricular dysrhythmias. *Note:* Potassium imbalance is the number one cause of atrial fibrillation.
Class I drugs: e.g.,	Class I drugs depress depolarization and alter repolarization, stabilizing the cell. These drugs are divided into groups a, b, and c based on their unique effects.
Class Ia; e.g., disopyramide (Norpace), procainamide (Pronestyl, Procan SR), quinidine (Quinaglute, Cardioquin);	These drugs increase action potential, duration, and effective refractory period and decrease membrane responsiveness, prolonging both QRS complex and QT interval. Useful for treatment of atrial and ventricular premature beats, repetitive dysrhythmias (e.g., atrial tachycardias and atrial flutter/fibrillation). *Note:* Myocardial depressant effects may be potentiated when class Ia drugs are used in conjunction with any drugs possessing similar properties.
Class Ib; e.g., lidocaine (Xylocaine), phenytoin (Dilantin), tocainide (Tonocard), mexiletine (Mexitil), moricizine (Ethmozine);	These drugs shorten the duration of the refractory period (QT interval), and their action depends on the tissue affected and the level of extracellular potassium. Drugs of choice for ventricular dysrhythmias, they are also effective for automatic and re-entrant dysrhythmias and digitalis-induced dysrhythmias. *Note:* These drugs may aggravate myocardial depression.
Class Ic; e.g., flecainide (Tambocor), propafenone (Rhythmol), encainide (Enkaid);	These drugs slow conduction by depressing SA node automaticity and decreasing conduction velocity through the atria, ventricles, and Purkinje's fibers. The result is prolongation of the PR interval and lengthening of the QRS complex. They suppress and prevent all types of ventricular dysrhythmias. *Note:* Flecainide increases risk of drug-induced dysrhythmias post MI. Propafenone can worsen or cause new dysrhythmias, a tendency called the "pro-arrhythmic effect." Encainide is available only for clients who demonstrated a good result before the drug was removed from the market.

ACTIONS/INTERVENTIONS	RATIONALE
Class II drugs; e.g., atenolol (Tenormin), propranolol (Inderal), nadolol (Corgard), acebutolol (Sectral), esmolol (Brevibloc), sotalol (Betapace); bisoprolol (Zebeta);	β-adrenergic blockers have antiadrenergic properties and decrease automaticity. Therefore, they are useful in the treatment of dysrhythmias caused by SA and AV node dysfunction (e.g., SVTs, atrial flutter or fibrillation). *Note:* These drugs may exacerbate bradycardia and cause myocardial depression, especially when combined with drugs that have similar properties.
Class III drugs; e.g., bretylium tosylate (Bretylol), amiodarone (Cordarone), sotalol (Betapace), ibutilide (Corvert);	These drugs prolong the refractory period and action potential duration, consequently prolonging the QT interval. They are used to terminate ventricular fibrillation and other life-threatening ventricular dysrhythmias/sustained ventricular tachyarrhythmias, especially when lidocaine/procainamide are not effective. *Note:* Sotalol is a nonselective β-blocker with characteristics of both class II and class III.
Class IV drugs; e.g., verapamil (Calan), nifedipine (Procardia), diltiazem (Cardizem);	Calcium antagonists (also called calcium channel blockers) slow conduction time through the AV node (prolonging PR interval) to decrease ventricular response in SVTs, atrial flutter/fibrillation. Calan and Cardizem may be used for bedside conversion of acute atrial fibrillation.
Class V drugs; e.g., atropine sulfate, isoproterenol (Isuprel), cardiac glycosides: digoxin (Lanoxin);	Miscellaneous drugs useful in treating bradycardia by increasing SA and AV conduction and enhancing automaticity. Cardiac glycosides may be used alone or in combination with other antidysrhythmic drugs to reduce ventricular rate in presence of uncontrolled/poorly tolerated atrial tachycardias or flutter/fibrillation.
Adenosine (Adenocard).	First-line treatment for paroxysmal supraventricular tachycardia (PVST). Slows conduction and interrupts reentry pathways in AV node. *Note:* Contraindicated in clients with second- or third-degree heart block or those with sick sinus syndrome who do not have a functioning pacemaker.
Prepare for/assist with elective cardioversion.	May be used in atrial fibrillation (after trials of first-line drugs [e.g., atenolol, metoprolol, diltiazem, verapamil] have failed to control heart rate), or certain unstable dysrhythmias to restore normal heart rate/relieve symptoms of heart failure.
Assist with insertion/maintain pacemaker (e.g., external/temporary or internal/permanent) function.	Temporary pacing may be necessary to accelerate impulse formation in bradydysrhythmias, synchronize electrical impulsivity, or override tachydysrhythmias and ectopic activity, to maintain cardiovascular function until spontaneous pacing is restored or permanent pacing is initiated. These devices may include atrial and/or ventricular pacemakers and may provide single chamber or dual chamber pacing. The placment of implantable cardioverter defibrillators (ICDs) is on the rise.
Insert/maintain IV access.	Patent access line may be required for administration of emergency drugs.
Prepare for surgery (e.g., aneurysmectomy, CABG, Maze) as indicated.	Differential diagnosis of underlying cause may be required to formulate appropriate treatment plan. Resection of ventricular aneurysm may be required to correct intractable ventricular dysrhythmias unresponsive to medical therapy. Surgery, e.g., CABG, may be indicated to enhance circulation to myocardium and conduction system. *Note:* A Maze procedure is an open- heart surgical procedure sometimes used to treat refractive atrial fibrillation by surgically redirecting electrical conduction pathways.

ACTIONS/INTERVENTIONS	RATIONALE
Prepare for implantation of cardioverter/defibrillator (ICD) when indicated.	This device may be surgically implanted in those clients with recurrent, life-threatening ventricular dysrhythmias unresponsive to tailored drug therapy. The latest generation of devices can provide multilevel ("tiered") therapy; that is, antitachycardia and antibradycardia pacing, cardioversion, or defibrillation depending on how each device is programmed.

NURSING DIAGNOSIS: risk for Poisoning [digitalis toxicity]

Risk factors may include

Limited range of therapeutic effectiveness, lack of education/proper precautions, reduced vision/cognitive limitations

Possibly evidenced by

[Not applicable; presence of signs and symptoms establishes an *actual* diagnosis.]

DESIRED OUTCOMES/EVALUATION CRITERIA—CLIENT WILL:

KNOWLEDGE: Medication (NOC)

Verbalize understanding of individual prescription, how it interacts with other drugs/substances, and importance of maintaining prescribed regimen.
Recognize signs of digitalis overdose and developing heart failure, and what to report to physician.

Cardiac Pump Effectiveness (NOC)

Be free of signs of toxicity; display serum drug level within individually acceptable range.

ACTIONS/INTERVENTIONS	RATIONALE
Medication Management (NIC)	
Independent	
Explain client's specific type of digitalis preparation and its specific therapeutic use.	Reduces confusion due to digitalis preparations varying in name (although they may be similar), dosage strength, and onset and duration of action. Up to 15% of all clients receiving digitalis develop toxicity at some time during the course of therapy because of its narrow therapeutic range.
Instruct client not to change dose for any reason, not to omit dose (unless instructed to, depending on pulse rate), not to increase dose or take extra doses, and to contact physician if more than one dose is omitted.	Alterations in drug regimen can reduce therapeutic effects, result in toxicity, and cause complications.
Advise client that digitalis may interact with many other drugs (e.g., barbiturates, neomycin, cholestyramine, quinidine, and antacids) and that physician should be informed that digitalis is taken whenever new medications are prescribed. Advise client not to use OTC drugs (e.g., laxatives, antidiarrheals, antacids, cold remedies, diuretics, herbals) without first checking with the pharmacist or healthcare provider.	Knowledge may help prevent dangerous drug interactions.

ACTIONS/INTERVENTIONS	RATIONALE
Review importance of dietary and supplemental intake of potassium, calcium, and magnesium.	Maintaining electrolytes at normal ranges may prevent or limit development of toxicity and correct many associated dysrhythmias.
Provide information and have the client/SO verbalize understanding of toxic signs/symptoms to report to the healthcare provider.	Nausea, vomiting, diarrhea, unusual drowsiness, confusion, very slow or very fast irregular pulse, thumping in chest, double/blurred vision, yellow/green tint or halos around objects, flickering color forms or dots, altered color perception, and worsening heart failure (e.g., dependent/generalized edema, dyspnea, decreased amount/frequency of voiding) indicate need for prompt evaluation/intervention. Mild symptoms of toxicity may be managed with a brief drug holiday. *Note:* In severe/refractory heart failure, altered cardiac binding of digitalis may result in toxicity even with previously appropriate drug doses.
Discuss necessity of periodic laboratory evaluations as indicated:	
Serum digoxin (Lanoxin) or digitoxin (Crystodigin) level;	Digitalis has a narrow therapeutic serum range, with toxicity occurring at levels that are dependent on individual response. Laboratory levels are evaluated in conjunction with clinical manifestations and ECG to determine individual therapeutic levels/resolution of toxicity.
Electrolytes, BUN, creatinine, liver function studies.	Abnormal levels of potassium, calcium, or magnesium increase the heart's sensitivity to digitalis. Impaired kidney function can cause digoxin (mainly excreted by the kidney) to accumulate to toxic levels. Digitoxin levels (mainly excreted by the bowel) are affected by impaired liver function.

Collaborative

ACTIONS/INTERVENTIONS	RATIONALE
Administer medications as appropriate: Other antidysrhythmia medications; e.g., lidocaine (Xylocaine), propranolol (Inderal), and procainamide (Pronestyl).	May be necessary to maintain/improve cardiac output in presence of excess effect of digitalis.
Digoxin immune Fab (Digibind).	A digoxin/digitoxin antagonist that increases drug excretion by the kidneys in acute or severe toxicity when standard therapies are unsuccessful.
Prepare client for transfer to CCU as indicated (e.g., dangerous dysrhythmias, exacerbation of heart failure).	In the presence of digitalis toxicity, clients frequently require intensive monitoring until therapeutic levels have been restored. Because all digitalis preparations have long serum half-lives, stabilization can take several days.

NURSING DIAGNOSIS: deficient Knowledge [Learning Need] regarding cause, treatment, self-care, and discharge needs

May be related to

Lack of information/misunderstanding of medical condition/therapy needs
Unfamiliarity with information resources
Lack of recall

Possibly evidenced by

Questions, statement of misconception
Failure to improve on previous regimen
Development of preventable complications

DESIRED OUTCOMES/EVALUATION CRITERIA—CLIENT WILL:

KNOWLEDGE: Disease Process (NOC)

Verbalize understanding of condition, prognosis, and function of pacemaker (if used).
Relate signs of pacemaker failure.

KNOWLEDGE: Treatment Regimen (NOC)

Verbalize understanding of therapeutic regimen.
List desired action and possible adverse side effects of medications.
Correctly perform necessary procedures and explain reasons for actions.

ACTIONS/INTERVENTIONS	RATIONALE
TEACHING: Individual (NIC)	
Independent	
Assess client/SO level of knowledge and ability/desire to learn.	Necessary for creation of individual instruction plan. Reinforces expectation that this will be a "learning experience." Verbalization identifies misunderstandings and allows for clarification.
Be alert to signs of avoidance; e.g., changing subject away from information being presented or extremes of behavior (withdrawal/euphoria).	Natural defense mechanisms, such as anger or denial of significance of situation, can block learning, affecting client's response and ability to assimilate information. Changing to a less formal/structured style may be more effective until client/SO is ready to accept/deal with current situation.
Present information in varied learning formats; e.g., programmed books, audiovisual tapes, question-and-answer sessions, group activities.	Multiple learning methods may enhance retention of material.
Provide information in written form for client/SO to take home.	Follow-up reminders may enhance client's understanding and cooperation with the desired regimen. Written instructions are a helpful resource when client is not in direct contact with healthcare team.
TEACHING: Disease Process (NIC)	
Reinforce explanations of risk factors, dietary/activity restrictions, medications, and symptoms requiring immediate medical attention.	Provides opportunity for client to retain information and to assume control/participate in rehabilitation program.
Encourage identification/reduction of individual risk factors; e.g., smoking and alcohol consumption, obesity.	These behaviors/chemicals have direct adverse effect on cardiovascular function and may impede recovery and increase risk for complications.
Review normal cardiac function/electrical conduction.	Provides a knowledge base to understand individual variations and reasons for therapeutic interventions.
Explain/reinforce specific dysrhythmia problem and therapeutic measures to client/SO.	Ongoing/updated information (e.g., whether the problem is resolving or may require long-term control measures) can decrease anxiety associated with the unknown and prepare client/SO to make necessary lifestyle adaptations. Educating the SO may be especially important if client is elderly, visually or hearing impaired, or unable or even unwilling to learn/follow instructions. Repeated explanations may be needed because anxiety and/or bulk of new information can block/limit learning.

ACTIONS/INTERVENTIONS	RATIONALE
Identify adverse effects/complications of specific dysrhythmias; e.g., fatigue, dependent edema, progressive changes in mentation, vertigo.	Dysrhythmias may decrease cardiac output, manifested by symptoms of developing cardiac failure/altered cerebral perfusion. Tachydysrhythmias may also be accompanied by debilitating anxiety/feelings of impending doom.
Instruct and document teaching regarding medications. Include why the drug is needed (desired action), how and when to take the drug, what to do if a dose is forgotten (dosage and usage information), and expected side effects or possible adverse reactions/interactions with other prescribed/OTC drugs or substances (alcohol, tobacco, herbal remedies), as well as what and when to report to the healthcare provider.	Information necessary for client to make informed choices and to manage medication regimen. *Note:* Use of herbal remedies in conjunction with drug regimen may result in adverse effects (e.g., cardiac stimulation, impaired clotting), necessitating evaluation of product for safe use.
Encourage development of regular exercise routine, avoiding overexertion. Identify signs/symptoms requiring immediate cessation of activities; e.g., dizziness, lightheadedness, dyspnea, chest pain.	When dysrhythmias are properly managed, normal activity should not be affected. Exercise program is useful in improving overall cardiovascular well-being.
Review individual dietary needs/restrictions; e.g., potassium, caffeine.	Depending on specific problem, client may need to increase dietary potassium, such as when potassium-depleting diuretics are used. Caffeine may be limited to prevent cardiac excitation.
Demonstrate proper pulse-taking technique. Recommend weekly checking of pulse for 1 full minute or daily recording of pulse before medication and during exercise as appropriate. Identify situations requiring immediate medical intervention; e.g., dizziness or irregular heartbeat, fainting, chest pain.	Continued self-observation/monitoring provides for timely intervention to avoid complications. Medication regimen may be altered or further evaluation may be required when heart rate varies from desired rate or pacemaker's preset rate.
Review safety precautions, techniques to evaluate/maintain pacemaker or ICD function, and symptoms requiring medical intervention; e.g., report pulse rate below set limit for demand pacing or less than low-limit rate for rate-adaptive pacers, prolonged hiccups.	Promotes self-care, provides for timely interventions to prevent serious complications. Instructions/concerns depend on function and type of device, as well as client's condition and presence/absence of family or caregivers.
Recommend wearing medical alert bracelet or necklace and carrying pacemaker ID card.	Allows for appropriate evaluation and timely intervention, especially if client is unable to respond in an emergency situation.
Discuss monitoring and environmental safety concerns in presence of pacemaker/implantable defibrillator, e.g., microwave ovens and other electrical appliances (including electrical blankets, razors, radio/TV), can be safely operated if they are properly grounded and in good repair; there is no problem with metal detectors, although pacemaker may trigger sensitive detectors; although cordless phones are safe, cellular phones held directly over pacemaker may cause interference, so it is recommended that client not carry phone in shirt pocket when phone is on; high-voltage areas, magnetic fields, and radiation can interfere with optimal pacemaker function, so client should avoid high-tension electric wires, arc welding, and large industrial magnets, such as demolition sites and MRIs.	Aids in clarifying misconceptions and fears, and encourages client to be proactive in avoiding potentially harmful situations.

POTENTIAL CONSIDERATIONS following discharge from care setting (dependent on client's age, physical condition/presence of complications, personal resources, and life responsibilities)

Activity Intolerance—imbalance between oxygen supply/demand.

ineffective Therapeutic Regimen Management—complexity of therapeutic regimen, decisional conflicts, economic difficulties, inadequate number/types of cues to action.

CARDIAC SURGERY: POSTOPERATIVE CARE—CORONARY ARTERY BYPASS GRAFT (CABG), MINIMALLY INVASIVE DIRECT CORONARY ARTERY BYPASS (MIDCAB), CARDIOMYOPLASTY, VALVE REPLACEMENT

The goal of surgical treatment for heart disease is to maximize cardiac output. This can be accomplished by improving blood flow and myocardial muscle function through procedures such as the traditional coronary artery bypass grafting (CABG) and/or open-heart valve replacement, which requires the use of heart–lung machine during surgery. Less invasive procedures are also being tried such as the minimally invasive direct coronary bypass (MIDCAB) and the off-pump coronary revascularization with endoscopic saphenous vein harvesting (OCPRES). Variants of the MIDCAB include percutaneous transmyocardial revascularization (PTMR) and/or port access, keyhole surgery (also called buttonhole surgery or laparoscopic bypass) requiring four laparoscopic incisions on the chest and leg and permitting operation on a beating heart without the need for heart–lung machine.

Of the three types of cardiac surgery—(1) reparative (e.g., closure of atrial or ventricular septal defect, repair of mitral stenosis), (2) reconstructive (e.g., CABG, reconstruction of an incompetent valve), and (3) substitutional (e.g., valve replacement, cardiac transplant)—reparative surgeries are more likely to produce cure or prolonged improvement.

CARE SETTING

Inpatient acute hospital on a surgical or post-ICU step-down unit.

RELATED CONCERNS

Angina, page 62
Heart failure: chronic, page 47
Dysrhythmias, page 85
Myocardial infarction, page 72
Pneumothorax/hemothorax, page 150
Psychosocial aspects of care, page 770
Surgical intervention, page 788
Transplantation (postoperative and lifelong), page 761

Client Assessment Database

The preoperative data presented here depend on the specific disease process and underlying cardiac condition/reserve.

ACTIVITY/REST

May report:
History of exercise intolerance
Generalized weakness, fatigue
Inability to perform expected/usual life activities
Insomnia/sleep disturbance

May exhibit:
Abnormal heart rate, BP changes with activity
Exertional discomfort or dyspnea
ECG changes/dysrhythmias

CIRCULATION

May report:
History of recent/acute MI, three (or more) vessel coronary artery disease, valvular heart disease, hypertension

May exhibit:
Variations in BP, heart rate/rhythm
Abnormal heart sounds: S_3/S_4, murmurs
Pallor/cyanosis of skin or mucous membranes
Cool/cold, clammy skin
Edema, JVD
Diminished peripheral pulses
Abnormal breath sounds: crackles
Restlessness/other changes in mentation or sensorium (severe cardiac decompensation)

EGO INTEGRITY

May report:
Feeling frightened/apprehensive, helpless
Distress over current events (anger/fear)
Fear of death/eventual outcome of surgery, possible complications
Fear about changes in lifestyle/role functioning

May exhibit:	Apprehension, restlessness Facial/general tension; withdrawal/lack of eye contact Focus on self; hostility, anger; crying Changes in heart rate, BP, breathing patterns

FOOD/FLUID

May report:	Change in weight Loss of appetite Abdominal pain, nausea/vomiting Change in urine frequency/amount
May exhibit:	Weight gain/loss Dry skin, poor skin turgor Postural hypotension Diminished/absent bowel sounds Edema (generalized, dependent, pitting)

NEUROSENSORY

May report:	Fainting spells, vertigo
May exhibit:	Changes in orientation or usual response to stimuli Restlessness; irritability, exaggerated emotional responses; apathy

PAIN/DISCOMFORT

May report:	Chest pain, angina

RESPIRATION

May report:	Shortness of breath
May exhibit:	Crackles Productive cough

SAFETY

May report:	Infectious episode with valvular involvement or myopathy

TEACHING/LEARNING

May report:	Familial risk factors of diabetes, heart disease, hypertension, strokes Use of various cardiovascular drugs Failure to improve

Postoperative Assessment

PAIN/DISCOMFORT

May report:	Incisional discomfort Pain/paresthesia of shoulders, arms, hands, legs
May exhibit:	Guarding Facial mask of pain; grimacing Distraction behaviors; moaning; restlessness Changes in BP/pulse/respiratory rate

RESPIRATION

May report:	Inability to cough or take a deep breath
May exhibit:	Decreased chest expansion Splinting/muscle guarding Dyspnea (normal response to thoracotomy) Areas of diminished or absent breath sounds (atelectasis) Anxiety Changes in ABGs/pulse oximetry

SAFETY

May exhibit:	Oozing/bleeding from chest or donor site incisions

TEACHING/LEARNING

Discharge plan considerations: Short-term assistance with food preparation, shopping, transportation, self-care needs, and homemaker/home maintenance tasks

Refer to section at end of plan for postdischarge considerations.

DIAGNOSTIC STUDIES (POSTOPERATIVE)

Hemoglobin (Hb)/hematocrit (Hct): A low Hb reduces oxygen-carrying capacity and indicates need for red blood cell replacement. Elevation of Hct suggests dehydration/need for fluid replacement.

Coagulation studies: Various studies may be done (e.g., platelet count, bleeding and clotting time) to determine therapeutic level of anticoagulant therapy when used.

Electrolytes: Imbalances (hyperkalemia/hypokalemia, hypernatremia/hyponatremia, and hypocalcemia) can affect cardiac function and fluid balance.

ABGs: Verifies oxygenation status, effectiveness of respiratory function, and acid-base balance.

Pulse oximetry: Provides noninvasive measure of oxygenation at tissue level.

BUN/creatinine: Reflects adequacy of renal and liver perfusion/function.

Amylase: Elevation is occasionally seen in high-risk clients; e.g., those with heart failure undergoing valve replacement.

Glucose: Fluctuations may occur because of preoperative nutritional status, presence of diabetes/organ dysfunction, rate of dextrose infusions.

Cardiac enzymes/isoenzymes: Elevated in the presence of acute, recent, or perioperative MI.

Chest x-ray: Reveals heart size and position, pulmonary vasculature, and changes indicative of pulmonary complications (e.g., atelectasis). Verifies condition of valve prosthesis and sternal wires, position of pacing leads, intravascular/cardiac lines.

ECG: Identifies changes in electrical, mechanical function such as might occur in immediate postoperative phase, acute/perioperative MI, valve dysfunction, and/or pericarditis.

Cardiac echocardiogram/catheterization: Measures chamber pressures and pressure gradients across valves, identifies occlusions of arteries, impaired coronary perfusion, and possible wall motion abnormalities.

Transesophageal echocardiography: Useful in diagnosing cardiac valve and chamber abnormalities, such as regurgitation, shunting, or stenosis in clients in whom transthoracic approach is not feasible.

Nuclear studies (e.g., thallium-201, DPY-thallium/Persantine): Heart scans demonstrate coronary artery disease, heart chamber dimensions, and presurgical/postsurgical functional capabilities.

NURSING PRIORITIES

1. Support hemodynamic stability/ventilatory function.
2. Promote relief of pain/discomfort.
3. Promote healing.
4. Provide information about postoperative expectations and treatment regimen.

DISCHARGE GOALS

1. Activity tolerance adequate to meet self-care needs.
2. Pain alleviated/managed.
3. Complications prevented/minimized.
4. Incisions healing.
5. Postdischarge medications, exercise, diet, therapy understood.
6. Plan in place to meet needs after discharge.

NURSING DIAGNOSIS: risk for decreased Cardiac Output

Risk factors may include

Decreased myocardial contractility secondary to temporary factors (e.g., ventricular wall surgery, recent MI, response to certain medications/drug interactions)
Decreased preload (hypovolemia)
Alterations in electrical conduction (dysrhythmias)

Possibly evidenced by

[Not applicable; presence of signs and symptoms establishes an *actual* diagnosis.]

DESIRED OUTCOMES/EVALUATION CRITERIA—CLIENT WILL:

TISSUE PERFUSION: Cardiac (NOC)

Report/display decreased episodes of angina and dysrhythmias.
Demonstrate an increase in activity tolerance.
Participate in activities that maximize/enhance cardiac function.

ACTIONS/INTERVENTIONS	RATIONALE
Hemodynamic Regulation (NIC)	
Independent	
Monitor/document trends in heart rate and BP, especially noting hypertension. Be aware of specific systolic/diastolic limits defined for client.	Tachycardia is a common response to discomfort and anxiety, inadequate blood/fluid replacement, and the stress of surgery. However, sustained tachycardia increases cardiac workload and can decrease effective cardiac output. Hypertension can occur (fluid excess or preexisting condition), placing stress on suture lines of new grafts and changing blood flow/pressure within heart chambers and across valves, with increased risk for various complications. Hypotension may result from fluid deficit, dysrhythmias, heart failure/shock.
Monitor/document cardiac dysrhythmias. Observe client response to dysrhythmias; e.g., drop in BP.	Life-threatening dysrhythmias can occur because of electrolyte imbalance, myocardial ischemia, or alterations in the heart's electrical conduction. Atrial fibrillation or atrial flutter are the most common dysrhythmias occurring around the second or third day post-CABG (older clients or presence of right coronary artery disease increases risk). Decreased cardiac output and hemodynamic compromise that occur with dysrhythmias require prompt intervention. *Note:* This is the most frequently occurring postoperative complication, often prolonging hospital stay.
Observe for changes in usual mental status/orientation/body movement or reflexes; e.g., onset of confusion, disorientation, restlessness, reduced response to stimuli, stupor.	May indicate decreased cerebral blood flow or oxygenation as a result of diminished cardiac output (sustained or severe dysrhythmias, low BP, heart failure, or thromboembolic phenomena).
Record skin temperature/color and quality/equality of peripheral pulses.	Warm, pink skin and strong, equal pulses are general indicators of adequate cardiac output.
Measure/document I&O and fluid balance.	Useful in determining fluid needs or identifying fluid excesses, which can compromise cardiac output/oxygen consumption.
Schedule uninterrupted rest/sleep periods. Assist with self-care activities as needed.	Prevents fatigue/overexhaustion and excessive cardiovascular stress.
Monitor graded activity program. Note client response, vital signs before/during/after activity, development of dysrhythmias.	Regular exercise stimulates circulation/cardiovascular tone and promotes feeling of well-being. Progression of activity depends on cardiac tolerance.
Evaluate presence/degree of anxiety/emotional duress. Encourage the use of relaxation techniques; e.g., deep breathing, diversional activities.	Excessive/escalating emotional reactions can affect vital signs and SVR, eventually affecting cardiac function.
Inspect for JVD, peripheral or dependent edema, congestion in lungs, shortness of breath, change in mental status.	May be indicative of heart failure (acute or chronic).
Investigate reports of angina/severe chest pain accompanied by restlessness, diaphoresis, ECG changes.	Although not a common complication of CABG, perioperative or postoperative MI can occur.

ACTIONS/INTERVENTIONS	RATIONALE
Investigate/report profound hypotension (unresponsive to fluid challenge), tachycardia, distant heart sounds, stupor/coma.	Development of cardiac tamponade can rapidly progress to cardiac arrest because of the heart's inability to fill adequately for effective cardiac output. *Note:* This is a relatively rare, life-threatening complication that usually occurs in the immediate postoperative period but can occur later in the recovery phase.

Collaborative

Review serial ECGs.	Most frequently done to follow the progress in normalization of electrical conduction patterns/ventricular function after surgery or to identify complications; e.g., perioperative MI.
Measure cardiac output and other functional parameters as indicated.	Useful in evaluating response to therapeutic interventions and identifying need for more aggressive/emergency care. *Note:* Cardiac index, preload/afterload, contractility, and cardiac work can be measured noninvasively by using thoracic electrical bioimpedance (TEB) technique.
Administer IV fluids/blood transfusions as needed.	IV fluids may be discontinued before discharge from the intensive care unit (ICU), or one line (central/peripheral) may remain in place for fluid replacement and/or emergency cardiac medications. Red blood cell (RBC) replacement may be indicated on occasion to restore/maintain adequate circulating volume and enhance oxygen-carrying capacity.
Administer supplemental oxygen as appropriate.	Promotes maximal oxygenation, which can reduce cardiac workload and aid in resolving myocardial ischemia and dysrhythmias.
Administer electrolytes and medications as indicated; e.g., electrolyte solutions/potassium, antidysrhythmics, beta-blockers, digitalis, diuretics, anticoagulants.	Client needs are variable, depending on type of surgery, client's response to surgical intervention, and preexisting conditions (e.g., general health, age, type of heart disease). Electrolytes, antidysrhythmics, and other heart medications may be required on a short-term or long-term basis to maximize cardiac contractility/output.
Maintain surgically placed pacing wires (atrial/ventricular) and initiate pacing if indicated.	May be required to support cardiac output in presence of conduction disturbances (severe dysrhythmias) that compromise cardiac function.

NURSING DIAGNOSIS: acute Pain/[Discomfort]

May be related to

Sternotomy (mediastinal incision) and/or donor site (leg/arm incision)
Myocardial ischemia (acute MI, angina)
Tissue inflammation/edema formation
Intraoperative nerve trauma

Possibly evidenced by

Reports of incisional discomfort/pain; paresthesia; pain in hand, arm, shoulder
Anxiety, restlessness, irritability
Distraction behaviors
Increased heart rate

DESIRED OUTCOMES/EVALUATION CRITERIA—CLIENT WILL:

Pain Level (NOC)

Verbalize relief/absence of pain.
Demonstrate relaxed body posture, ability to rest/sleep appropriately.

Pain Control (NOC)

Differentiate surgical discomfort from angina/preoperative heart pain.

ACTIONS/INTERVENTIONS	RATIONALE
Pain Management (NIC)	
Independent	
Note type/location of incision(s).	Newer procedures (MIDCAB) may require only a "mini" chest incision, with minimal pain.
Encourage client to report type, location, and intensity of pain, rating on a scale of 0–10. Note associated symptoms. Ascertain how this compares with preoperative chest pain.	Pain is perceived, manifested, and tolerated individually. It is important for client to differentiate incisional pain from other types of chest pain, such as angina or discomfort from chest tubes. Many CABG clients do not experience severe discomfort in chest incision and may complain more often of donor site incision discomfort. Severe pain in either area should be investigated further for possible complications. *Note:* There is up to a 24% rate of complications when vessel donor site is a lower extremity.
Observe for anxiety, irritability, crying, restlessness, sleep disturbances.	These nonverbal cues may indicate the presence/degree of pain being experienced.
Monitor vital signs.	Heart rate usually increases with pain, although a bradycardiac response can occur in a severely diseased heart. BP may be elevated slightly with incisional discomfort but may be decreased or unstable if chest pain is severe and/or myocardial damage is occurring.
Identify/promote position of comfort, using adjuncts as necessary.	Pillows/blanket rolls are useful in supporting extremities, maintaining body alignment, and splinting incisions to reduce muscle tension/promote comfort.
Suggest use of saltwater gargle, throat lozenges, or spray.	Helps relieve discomfort in throat associated with endotracheal tube.
Provide comfort measures (e.g., back rubs, position changes), assist with self-care activities, and encourage diversional activities as indicated.	May promote relaxation/redirect attention and reduce analgesic dosage needs/frequency.
Schedule care activities to balance with adequate periods of sleep/rest.	Rest and sleep are vital for cardiac healing (balance between oxygen demand and consumption) and can enhance coping with stress and discomfort.
Identify/encourage use of behaviors such as guided imagery, distractions, visualizations, deep breathing.	Relaxation techniques aid in management of stress, promote sense of well-being, may reduce analgesic needs, and promote healing.
Tell client that it is acceptable, even preferable, to request analgesics as soon as discomfort becomes noticeable.	Presence of pain causes muscle tension, which can impair circulation, slow healing process, and intensify pain.
Medicate before procedures/activities as indicated.	Client comfort and cooperation in respiratory treatments, ambulation, and procedures (e.g., removal of chest tubes, pacemaker wires, and sutures) are facilitated by maximum analgesic blood level.

ACTIONS/INTERVENTIONS	RATIONALE
Investigate reports of pain in unusual areas (e.g., calf of leg, abdomen) or vague complaints of discomfort, especially when accompanied by changes in mentation, vital signs, respiratory rate.	May be an early manifestation of developing complication such as thrombophlebitis, infection, gastrointestinal dysfunction.
Note reports of pain and/or numbness in ulnar area (fourth and fifth digits) of the hand, often accompanied by pain/discomfort of the arms and shoulders. Tell client that the problem usually resolves with time.	Indicative of a stretch injury of the brachial plexus as a result of the position of the arms during surgery. No specific treatment is currently useful.

Collaborative

Administer medications as indicated, e.g., propoxyphene and acetaminophen (Darvocet-N), acetaminophen and oxycodone (Tylox), and/or ketorolac (Toradol).	Usually provides for adequate control of pain and inflammation, and reduces muscle tension, which improves client comfort and promotes healing.

NURSING DIAGNOSIS: ineffective Role Performance

May be related to

Situational crisis (dependent role)/recuperative process
Uncertainty about future

Possibly evidenced by

Delay/alteration in physical capacity to resume role
Change in usual role or responsibility
Change in self/others' perception of role

DESIRED OUTCOMES/EVALUATION CRITERIA—CLIENT WILL:

PSYCHOSOCIAL ADJUSTMENT: Life Change (NOC)

Verbalize realistic perception and acceptance of self in changed role.
Talk with SO about situation and changes that have occurred.
Develop realistic plans for adapting to perceived role changes.

ACTIONS/INTERVENTIONS | RATIONALE

Role Enhancement (NIC)

Independent

Assess client role in family constellation. Identify concerns about role dysfunction/interruption; e.g., recuperation, health-illness transitions.	Helps to know client's responsibilities and how illness affects this role. Dependent role of client provokes anxiety and concern about how client will be able to manage usual role responsibilities.
Assess level of anxiety, client's perception of degree of threat to self/life.	Information provides baseline for identifying/individualizing plan of care.
Note cultural factors affecting role changes.	Cultural expectations regarding male/female illness role can determine how client/SO reacts to and deals with current situation and may affect future adaptation to perceived changes.
Maintain positive attitude toward client, providing opportunities for client to exercise control as much as possible.	Helps client accept changes that are occurring and begin to realize that control over self/situation is possible.

ACTIONS/INTERVENTIONS	RATIONALE
Assist client/SO to develop strategies for dealing with changes; e.g., shift responsibilities to other family members/friends or neighbors, acquire temporary assistance (homemaker/yardwork), investigate avenues for financial assistance.	Planning for changes that may occur/be required promotes sense of control and accomplishment without loss of self-esteem.
Acknowledge reality of grieving process related to change in usual role (even if only temporary) and help client deal realistically with feelings of anger and sadness.	Cardiac surgery constitutes a dramatic point in client's life, which will never be the same again. These feelings need to be recognized and dealt with by client/family to move forward. *Note:* Because of shorter hospitalization times and fact that client often feels better quickly after revascularization procedures, the client and SO may have the sense that client is cured and no further cardiac problems are anticipated. While this attitude may keep client from becoming a "cardiac cripple," it causes difficulty in dealing realistically with limitations.

NURSING DIAGNOSIS: risk for ineffective Breathing Pattern

Risk factors may include

Inadequate ventilation (pain/muscular weakness)
Diminished oxygen-carrying capacity (blood loss)
Decreased lung expansion (atelectasis or pneumothorax/hemothorax)

Possibly evidenced by

[Not applicable; presence of signs and symptoms establishes an *actual* diagnosis.]

DESIRED OUTCOMES/EVALUATION CRITERIA—CLIENT WILL:

RESPIRATORY STATUS: Ventilation (NOC)

Maintain a normal/effective respiratory pattern free of cyanosis and other signs/symptoms of hypoxia with breath sounds equal bilaterally, lung fields clearing.
Display complete reexpansion of lungs with absence of pneumothorax/hemothorax.

ACTIONS/INTERVENTIONS	RATIONALE
Respiratory Monitoring (NIC)	
Independent	
Evaluate respiratory rate and depth. Note respiratory effort; e.g., presence of dyspnea, use of accessory muscles, nasal flaring.	Client responses are variable. Rate and effort may be increased by pain, fear, fever, diminished circulating volume (blood or fluid loss), accumulation of secretions, hypoxia, or gastric distention. Respiratory suppression (decreased rate) can occur from excessive use of narcotic analgesics. Early recognition and treatment of abnormal ventilation may prevent complications.
Auscultate breath sounds. Note areas of diminished/absent breath sounds and presence of adventitious sounds; e.g., crackles or rhonchi.	Breath sounds are often diminished in lung bases for a period of time after surgery because of normally occurring atelectasis. Loss of active breath sounds in an area of previous ventilation may reflect collapse of the lung segment, especially if chest tubes have recently been removed. Crackles or rhonchi may be indicative of fluid accumulation (interstitial edema, pulmonary edema, or infection) or partial airway obstruction (pooling of secretions).

ACTIONS/INTERVENTIONS	RATIONALE
Observe chest excursion. Investigate decreased expansion or lack of symmetry in chest movement.	Air or fluid in the pleural space prevents complete expansion (usually on one side) and requires further assessment of ventilation status.
Observe character of cough and sputum production.	Frequent coughing may simply be throat irritation from operative endotracheal tube (ET) placement or can reflect pulmonary congestion. Purulent sputum suggests onset of pulmonary infection.
Inspect skin and mucous membranes for cyanosis.	Cyanosis of lips, nail beds, or earlobes or general duskiness may indicate a hypoxic condition due to heart failure or pulmonary complications. General pallor (commonly present in immediate postoperative period) may indicate anemia from blood loss/insufficient blood replacement or RBC destruction from cardiopulmonary bypass pump.
Elevate head of bed, place in upright or semi-Fowler's position. Assist with early ambulation/increased time out of bed.	Stimulates respiratory function/lung expansion. Effective in preventing and resolving pulmonary congestion.
Encourage client participation/responsibility for deep-breathing exercises, use of adjuncts, and coughing, as indicated.	Aids in reexpansion/maintaining patency of small airways, especially after removal of chest tubes. Coughing is not necessary unless wheezes/rhonchi are present, indicating retention of secretions.
Reinforce splinting of chest with pillows during deep breathing/coughing.	Reduces incisional tension, promotes maximal lung expansion, and may enhance effectiveness of cough effort.
Explain that coughing/respiratory treatments will not loosen/damage grafts or reopen chest incision.	Provides reassurance that injury will not occur and may enhance cooperation with therapeutic regimen.
Encourage maximal fluid intake within cardiac reserves.	Adequate hydration helps liquefy secretions, facilitating expectoration.
Medicate with analgesic before respiratory treatments, as indicated.	Allows for easier chest movement and reduces discomfort related to incisional pain, facilitating client cooperation with/effectiveness of respiratory treatments.
Record response to deep-breathing exercises or other respiratory treatment, noting breath sounds (before/after treatment), cough/sputum production.	Documents effectiveness of therapy or need for more aggressive interventions.
Investigate/report respiratory distress, diminished or absent breath sounds, tachycardia, severe agitation, drop in BP.	Although not a common complication, hemothorax/pneumothorax may occur following removal of the chest tubes and requires prompt intervention to maintain respiratory function.

Collaborative

Review chest x-ray reports and laboratory studies (ABGs, Hb) as indicated.	Monitors effectiveness of respiratory therapy and/or documents developing complications. A blood transfusion may be needed if blood loss is the reason for respiratory hypoxemia.
Instruct in/assist with use of incentive spirometer.	Used to maximize lung inflation, reduce atelectasis, and prevent pulmonary complications.
Administer supplemental oxygen by cannula or mask, as indicated.	Enhances oxygen delivery to the lungs for circulatory uptake, especially in presence of reduced/altered ventilation.
Assist with reinsertion of chest tubes or thoracentesis if indicated.	Reexpands lung by removal of accumulated blood/air and restoration of negative pleural pressure.

NURSING DIAGNOSIS: impaired Skin Integrity

May be related to

Surgical incisions, puncture wounds

Possibly evidenced by

Disruption of skin surface

DESIRED OUTCOMES/EVALUATION CRITERIA—CLIENT WILL:

WOUND HEALING: Primary Intention (NOC)

Demonstrate behaviors/techniques to promote healing, prevent complications.
Display timely wound healing.

ACTIONS/INTERVENTIONS	RATIONALE
Incision Site Care (NIC)	
Independent	
Inspect all incisions. Evaluate healing progress. Review expectations for healing with client.	Healing begins immediately, but complete healing takes time. Chest incision heals first (minimal muscle tissue), but donor site incision (when saphenous vein is used) requires more time (more muscle tissue, longer incision, slower circulation). As healing progresses, the incision lines may appear dry, with crusty scabs. Underlying tissue may look bruised and feel tense, warm, and lumpy (resolving hematoma).
Suggest wearing soft cotton shirts and loose-fitting clothing, leaving incisions open to air as much as possible, covering/padding portion of incisions as necessary.	Reduces suture line irritation and pressure from clothing. Leaving incisions open to air promotes healing process and may reduce risk of infection.
Have client shower in warm water, washing incisions gently. Instruct client to avoid tub baths until approved by physician.	Keeps incision clean, promotes circulation/healing. *Note:* "Climbing" out of tub requires use of arms and pectoral muscles, which can put undue stress on sternotomy.
Encourage ankle exercises and elevation of legs when sitting in chair.	Promotes circulation, reduces edema to improve tissue healing.
Review normal signs of healing; e.g., itching along wound line, bruising, slight redness, scabbing. Instruct to watch for/report to physician places in incision that do not heal; reopening of healed incision; any drainage (bloody or purulent); localized area that is swollen with redness, feels increasingly painful, and is hot to touch; temperature greater than 101.5°F (38.6°C) for longer than 24 hours.	Helps client understand expected progression of healing and recognize signs of complications/nonhealing requiring further evaluation/intervention. *Note:* Incisional problems rank second behind chest pain as cause of readmission after CABG. Leg wound complications most often occur on or about the 10th postoperative day.
Promote adequate nutritional and fluid intake.	Helps maintain good circulating volume for tissue perfusion and meets cellular energy requirements to facilitate tissue regeneration/healing process.
Collaborative	
Obtain specimen of wound drainage as indicated.	If infection occurs, local and systemic treatments may be required; e.g., peroxide/saline/Betadine soaks, antibiotic therapy.

NURSING DIAGNOSIS: deficient Knowledge [Learning Need] regarding condition, postoperative care, self-care, and discharge needs

May be related to

Lack of exposure/recall
Information misinterpretation

Possibly evidenced by

Questions/requests for information
Verbalization of problem, statement of misconception
Inaccurate follow-through of instructions

DESIRED OUTCOMES/EVALUATION CRITERIA—CLIENT WILL:

Cardiac Disease Self-Management (NOC)

Participate in learning process.
Assume responsibility for own learning.
Begin to look for information/ask questions.

KNOWLEDGE: Treatment Regimen (NOC)

Verbalize understanding of condition, prognosis, and potential complications.
Describe reasons for therapeutic actions.

ACTIONS/INTERVENTIONS	RATIONALE
TEACHING: Disease Process (NIC)	
Independent	
Reinforce surgeon's explanation of particular surgical procedure, providing diagram as appropriate.	Provides individually specific information, creating knowledge base for subsequent learning regarding home management.
Incorporate this information into discussion about short- and long-term recovery expectations.	Length of rehabilitation and prognosis are dependent on type of surgical procedure, preoperative physical condition, and duration/severity of complications. *Note:* Encephalopathy resulting in memory loss, psychosis, and cognitive impairment is reported in up to 30% of clients following the use of cardiopulmonary bypass pump. Symptoms may persist for 6–7 months.
CARDIAC CARE: Rehabilitation (NIC)	
Reinforce continuation of breathing exercises, incentive spirometry, and coughing with splinting incision.	Promotes alveolar ventilation, reducing risk of lung congestion.
Discuss routine/prophylactic medications and OTC drug use. Stress importance of checking with physician before taking any drugs.	Dependent on type of valve replacement (i.e., synthetic) and presence of atrial fibrillation, anticoagulant therapy may be indicated. Also, antibiotic agent may be required for life, when dental care is provided. Potential for drug interactions must be considered before adding therapeutic agents to regimen. *Note:* Using herbal products (e.g., *Ginkgo biloba*, garlic, vitamins) can alter coagulation and have an adverse effect when taken with anticoagulants.

ACTIONS/INTERVENTIONS	RATIONALE
Review prescribed cardiac rehabilitation/exercise program and progress to date. Assist client/SO to set realistic goals.	Individual capabilities and expectations depend on type of surgery, underlying cardiac function, and prior physical conditioning. *Note:* Obesity is a predictor of hospital readmission and may require additional interventions.
Encourage participation in home routines; e.g., self-care, cooking. Suggest alternating rest periods with activity and light tasks with heavy tasks. Avoid heavy lifting, isometric/strenuous upper-body exercise.	Prevents excessive fatigue/overexhaustion. *Note:* Strenuous use of arms can place undue stress on sternotomy.
Problem-solve with client/SO ways to continue progressive activity program during temperature extremes and high wind/pollution days; e.g., walking predetermined distance within own house or local indoor shopping mall/exercise track.	Having a plan forestalls giving up exercise because of interferences such as weather.
Schedule rest periods and short naps several times a day.	Rest and sleep enhance coping abilities, reduce nervousness (common in this phase), and promote healing.
Reinforce physician's time limitations about lifting, driving, returning to work, resuming sexual activity, and exercising that involves upper extremities.	These restrictions are present until after the first postoperative office visit for assessment of sternum healing.
Discuss issues concerning resumption of sexual activity; e.g., comparison of stress of sexual intercourse with other activities:	Concerns about sexual activity often go unexpressed, but clients usually desire information about what to expect. In general, client can safely engage in sex when activity level has advanced to point at which client can climb two flights of stairs (which is about the same amount of energy expenditure).
Position recommendations;	Client should avoid positions that restrict breathing (sexual activity increases oxygen demand and consumption). Client with sternotomy should not support self or partner with arms (breast bone healing, support muscles stretched).
Expectations of sexual performance;	Impotence appears to occur with some regularity in postoperative cardiac surgery clients. Although etiology is unknown, condition usually resolves in time without specific intervention. If situation persists, may require further evaluation.
Appropriate timing; e.g., avoid sexual intercourse following heavy meal, during periods of emotional distress, when client is fatigued/exhausted;	Timing of activity may reduce occurrence of complications/angina.
Pharmacologic considerations.	Some clients may benefit from prophylactic use of antianginal medications for sexual activity.
Identify services/resources available after discharge. Provide telephone contact number/schedule follow-up calls as appropriate. Include referral names for home care services, as indicated.	Facilitates transition to home; provides for ongoing monitoring, continuation of prescribed therapies, opportunity to discuss concerns and alleviate anxiety.

POTENTIAL CONSIDERATIONS following discharge from care setting (dependent on client's age, physical condition/presence of complications, personal resources, and life responsibilities)

Activity Intolerance—generalized weakness, sedentary lifestyle.

impaired Skin/Tissue Integrity—surgical incisions, puncture wounds.

impaired Home Maintenance—altered ability to perform tasks, inadequate support systems, reluctance to request assistance.

risk for Infection—broken skin, traumatized tissue, invasive procedures, decreased hemoglobin.

Self-Care Deficit—decreased strength and endurance, discomfort.

ineffective Role Performance—situational crisis/recuperative process, uncertainty about future.

THROMBOPHLEBITIS: DEEP VEIN THROMBOSIS (INCLUDING PULMONARY EMBOLI CONSIDERATIONS)

Thrombophlebitis is a condition in which a clot forms in a vein, associated with inflammation/trauma of the vein wall or a partial obstruction of the vein. Clot formation is related to (1) stasis of blood flow, (2) abnormalities in the vessel walls, and (3) alterations in the clotting mechanism (Virchow's triad). Young women (oral estrogen use or pregnancy-related), persons undergoing orthopedic (especially hip and knee) surgery, persons with cancer, and the elderly are at greatest risk. Other predisposing factors include spinal cord injury, immobilization for any cause, heart attack, heart failure, stroke, obesity, inflammatory bowel disease, systemic lupus erythematosus, and central venous catheter use.

Thrombophlebitis can affect superficial or deep veins. Although both conditions can cause symptoms, deep vein thrombosis (DVT) is more serious in terms of potential complications, including pulmonary embolism (can contribute to more than 60,000 deaths annually [Crowther, 2004]), postphlebotic syndrome, chronic venous insufficiency, and vein valve destruction. *Note:* Approximately 50% of clients with DVT are asymptomatic. If the DVT is proximal (extending to the popliteal, femoral, or iliofemoral vessels), the clot is more likely to break away from the vessel and cause pulmonary embolism (PE).

CARE SETTINGS

Primarily treated at the community level, with short inpatient stay generally indicated in the presence of embolization.

RELATED CONCERNS

Surgical intervention, page 788
Ventilatory assistance (mechanical), page 170
Fractures, page 642
Psychosocial aspects of care, page 770

Client Assessment Database

ACTIVITY/REST

May report: Occupation that requires sitting or standing for long periods of time
Prolonged immobility (e.g., fractured hip/orthopedic trauma, long hospitalization/bedrest, prolonged sitting or travel without adequate exercise, complicated pregnancy); spinal cord injury/paralysis; progressive debilitating condition
Pain with activity/prolonged standing
Fatigue/weakness of affected extremity, general malaise

May exhibit: Generalized or extremity weakness

CIRCULATION

May report: History of previous peripheral vascular disease, venous thrombosis, varicose veins
Presence of other predisposing factors; e.g., hypertension (pregnancy-induced), diabetes mellitus, MI/valvular heart disease, thrombotic cerebrovascular accident, blood dyscrasias

May exhibit: Tachycardia
Peripheral pulse may be diminished in the affected extremity (DVT)
Varicosities and/or hardened, bumpy/knotty vein (thrombus)
Skin color/temperature in affected extremity (calf/thigh): pale, cool, edematous (DVT); pinkish red, warm along the course of the vein (superficial)
Positive Homans' sign (absence does not rule out DVT because less than 30% of clients have a positive sign)

FOOD/FLUID

May exhibit: Poor skin turgor, dry mucous membranes (dehydration predisposes to hypercoagulability)
Obesity (predisposes to stasis and pelvic vein pressure)
Edema of affected extremity (present with thrombus in small veins or major venous trunks)

PAIN/DISCOMFORT

May report: Throbbing, tenderness, aching pain aggravated by standing or movement of affected extremity, groin tenderness

May exhibit: Guarding of affected extremity

SAFETY

May report: History of direct or indirect injury to extremity or vein (e.g., major trauma/fractures, orthopedic/pelvic surgery, surgical procedures longer than 2 hours, surgical client age >40 years with other risk factors, urologic surgery, pregnancy, prolonged labor with fetal head pressure on pelvic veins, heart failure, venous cannulation or catheterization/intravenous therapy)

Presence of malignancy (particularly neoplasms of the pancreas, lung, GI system, prostate), sepsis

May exhibit: Fever, chills

TEACHING/LEARNING

May report: Use of oral contraceptives/estrogens, recent anticoagulant therapy (predisposes to hypercoagulability)
Use of vitamins/herbal supplements (e.g., vitamin B6, vitamin E, niacin, magnesium, L-carnitine, bromelain) for heart or blood pressure health
Recurrence/lack of resolution of previous thrombophlebotic episode

Discharge plan considerations: Temporary assistance with shopping, transportation, and homemaker/maintenance tasks
Properly fitted antiembolic hose

DIAGNOSTIC STUDIES

CBC: Hemoconcentration (elevated hematocrit [Hct]) potentiates risk of thrombus formation.

Coagulation profile: Deficits in coagulation modulators (e.g., antithrombin III, protein S or protein C) can predispose client to thrombus formation. Prothrombin time (PT) and the internatonal normalized ratio (INR), plasma thrombin time (PTT), are coagulation tests primarily used to monitor effects of anticoagulaton therapies.

Antithrombin: Useful in determining cause of impaired coagulation/hypercoagulation and in the management of venous thrombotic disease. Elevated in DVT.

D-Dimer Assay: Elevates in presence of DVT due to increased fibrinolysis triggered during thrombogenesis. (May be done to help exclude DVT.)

Noninvasive vascular studies (Doppler ultrasound, compression ultrasonography, impedance plethysmography, and duplex venous scanning): Changes in blood flow and volume identify venous occlusion, vascular damage, and vascular insufficiency. Duplex venous ultrasonography appears to be most accurate noninvasive method for diagnosing multiple proximal DVT (iliac, femoral, popliteal) but is less reliable in detecting isolated calf vein thrombi.

Trendelenburg test: May demonstrate vessel valve incompetence.

Venography: Radiographically confirms diagnosis through changes in blood flow and/or size of channels. *Note:* Although considered the diagnostic gold standard, this study carries a risk of inducing DVT and therefore is reserved for clients with negative or difficult to interpret noninvasive studies in the presence of high clinical suspicion.

MRI: May be done for diagnosis of both proximal and distal DVT, and is believed to be superior to other diagnositic tests for detection of pelvic DVT.

NURSING PRIORITIES

1. Maintain/enhance tissue perfusion, facilitate resolution of thrombus.
2. Promote optimal comfort.
3. Prevent complications.
4. Provide information about disease process/prognosis and treatment regimen.

DISCHARGE GOALS

1. Tissue perfusion improved in affected limb.
2. Pain/discomfort relieved.
3. Complications prevented/resolved.
4. Disease process/prognosis and therapeutic needs understood.
5. Plan in place to meet needs after discharge.

NURSING DIAGNOSIS: ineffective peripheral Tissue Perfusion

May be related to

Decreased blood flow/venous stasis (partial or complete venous obstruction)

Possibly evidenced by

Tissue edema, pain
Diminished peripheral pulses, slow/diminished capillary refill
Skin color changes (pallor, erythema)

DESIRED OUTCOMES/EVALUATION CRITERIA—CLIENT WILL:

TISSUE PERFUSION: Peripheral (NOC)

Demonstrate improved perfusion as evidenced by peripheral pulses present/equal, skin color and temperature normal, absence of edema.
Engage in behaviors/actions to enhance tissue perfusion.
Display increasing tolerance to activity.

ACTIONS/INTERVENTIONS	RATIONALE
EMBOLUS CARE: Peripheral (NIC)	
Independent	
Evaluate circulatory and neurologic studies of involved extremity—both sensory and motor. Inspect for skin color and temperature changes, as well as edema (from groin to foot). Note symmetry of calves; measure and record calf circumference. Report proximal progression of inflammatory process, traveling pain.	Symptoms help distinguish between thrombophlebitis and DVT. Redness, heat, tenderness, and localized edema are characteristic of superficial involvement. *Note*: Unilateral edema is one of the most reliable physical findings in DVT. Calf vein involvement is associated with absence of edema; femoral vein involvement is associated with mild to moderate edema; iliofemoral vein thrombosis is characterized by severe edema.
Examine extremity for obviously prominent veins. Palpate gently for local tissue tension, stretched skin, knots/bumps along course of vein.	Distention of superficial veins can occur in DVT because of backflow through communicating veins. Thrombophlebitis in superficial veins may be visible or palpable.
Assess capillary refill and check for Homans' sign.	Diminished capillary refill usually present in DVT. Positive Homans' sign (deep calf pain in affected leg upon dorsiflexion of foot) is a classic but unreliable sign because many clients with DVT do not have a positive Homans' sign.
Promote early ambulation.	Short frequent walks are determined to be better for extremeties and prevention of pulmonary complications than one long walk. If client is confined to bed, ensure range-of-motion exercises.
Elevate legs when in bed or chair, as indicated.	Reduces tissue swelling and rapidly empties superficial and tibial veins, preventing overdistention and thereby increasing venous return. *Note:* Some physicians believe that elevation may potentiate release of thrombus, thus increasing risk of embolization and decreasing circulation to the most distal portion of the extremity.
Initiate active or passive exercises while in bed (e.g., flex/extend/rotate foot periodically). Assist with gradual resumption of ambulation (e.g., walking 10 min/hr) as soon as client is permitted out of bed.	These measures are designed to increase venous return from lower extremities and reduce venous stasis, as well as improve general muscle tone/strength. They also promote normal organ function and enhance general well-being.
Caution client to avoid crossing legs or hyperflexion at knee (seated position with legs dangling, or lying in jackknife position).	Physical restriction of circulation impairs blood flow and increases venous stasis in pelvic, popliteal, and leg vessels, thus increasing swelling and discomfort.
Instruct client to avoid rubbing/massaging the affected extremity.	This activity potentiates risk of fragmenting/dislodging thrombus, causing embolization, and increasing risk of complications.
Encourage deep-breathing exercises.	Increases negative pressure in thorax, which assists in emptying large veins.
Increase fluid intake to at least 2000 mL/day, within cardiac tolerance.	Dehydration increases blood viscosity and venous stasis, predisposing to thrombus formation.

ACTIONS/INTERVENTIONS	RATIONALE
Collaborative	
Apply warm, moist compresses or heat cradle to affected extremity if indicated.	May be prescribed to promote vasodilation and venous return and resolution of local edema. *Note:* May be contraindicated in presence of arterial insufficiency, in which heat can increase cellular oxygen consumption/nutritional needs, furthering imbalance between supply and demand.
Administer anticoagulants, e.g.:	
heparin sodium, or low-molecular-weight heparin (LMWH) preparations, such as enorxaparin (Lovenox), dalteparin (Fragmin), tinzaparin (Innohep) via continuous or intermittent IV, intermittent subcutaneous (SC) injections, followed by oral coumarin derivatives, e.g., warfarin (Coumadin) or dicumarol (Sintrom);	Heparin may be used initially because of its prompt, predictable, antagonistic action on thrombin as it is formed and also because it removes activated coagulation factors XII, XI, IX, and X (intrinsic pathway), preventing further clot formation. LMWH is the anticogulant of choice after major orthopedic sugery and major trauma due to a lower risk of bleeding, more predictable dose response and longer half-life than heparin. Coumadin has a potent depressant effect on liver formation of prothrombin from vitamin K and impairs formation of factors VII, IX, and X (extrinsic pathway). Coumadin is generally used for long-term/post-discharge therapy to keep international normalized ratio (INR) at 2–3.
Thrombolytic agents; e.g., streptokinase, urokinase.	May be used in hemodynamically unstable client with PE or massive DVT to reduce risk of developing PE, or the presence of valvular damage and/or chronic venous insufficiency. Heparin is usually begun several hours after the completion of thrombolytic therapy. *Note:* Catheter-directed fibrinolysis may be used to infuse a fibrinolytic agent directly into a thrombus, in order to reduce the risks associated with systemic fibrinolytic therapy.
Monitor laboratory studies as indicated:	
PT, PTT, aPTT;	Monitors anticoagulant therapy and presence of risk factors; e.g., hemoconcentration and dehydration, which potentiate clot formation. *Note:* Lovenox does not require serial monitoring because PT and aPTT are not affected.
Platelet count, platelet function/aggregation test, antiheparin antibody assay.	On occasion, platelet count may decrease as a result of an immune reaction leading to platelet aggregation or the formation of "white clots." If bacteremia/DIC (disseminated intravascular coagulation) have been ruled out, condition may be the result of heparin-induced thrombocytopenia and thrombosis (HITT), requiring a change to Coumadin or other agents.
Apply/regulate graduated compression stockings, intermittent pneumatic compression if indicated.	Sequential compression devices may be used to improve blood flow velocity and empty vessels by providing artificial muscle-pumping action.
Apply elastic support hose following acute phase. Take care to avoid tourniquet effect.	Properly fitted support hose are useful (once ambulation has begun) to minimize or delay development of postphlebotic syndrome. They must exert a sustained, evenly distributed pressure over entire surface of calves and thighs to reduce the caliber of superficial veins and increase blood flow to deep veins.
Prepare for surgical intervention when indicated.	Thrombectomy (excision of thrombus) is occasionally necessary if inflammation extends proximally or circulation is severely restricted. Multiple/recurrent thrombotic episodes unresponsive to medical treatment (or when anticoagulant therapy is contraindicated) may require insertion of a vena caval screen/umbrella.

NURSING DIAGNOSIS: acute Pain/[Discomfort]

May be related to

Diminished arterial circulation and oxygenation of tissues with production/accumulation of lactic acid in tissues
Inflammatory process

Possibly evidenced by

Reports of pain, tenderness, aching/burning
Guarding of affected limb
Restlessness, distraction behaviors

DESIRED OUTCOMES/EVALUATION CRITERIA—CLIENT WILL:

Pain Control (NOC)

Report that pain/discomfort is alleviated or controlled.
Verbalize methods that provide relief.
Display relaxed manner; be able to sleep/rest and engage in desired activity.

ACTIONS/INTERVENTIONS	RATIONALE
Pain Management (NIC)	
Independent	
Assess degree and characteristics of discomfort/pain. Note guarding of extremity. Palpate leg with caution.	Degree of pain is directly related to extent of circulatory deficit, inflammatory process, degree of tissue ischemia, and extent of edema associated with thrombus development. Changes in characteristics of pain may indicate progression of problem/development of complications.
Maintain bedrest during acute phase.	Reduces discomfort associated with muscle contraction and movement.
Elevate affected extremity.	Encourages venous return to facilitate circulation, reducing stasis/edema formation.
Provide foot cradle.	Cradle keeps pressure of bedclothes off the affected leg, thereby reducing pressure discomfort.
Encourage client to change position frequently.	Decreases/prevents muscle fatigue, helps minimize muscle spasm, maximizes circulation to tissues.
Monitor vital signs, noting elevated temperature.	Elevations in heart rate may indicate increased pain/discomfort or occur in response to fever and inflammatory process. Fever can also increase client's discomfort.
Investigate reports of sudden and/or sharp chest pain, accompanied by dyspnea, tachycardia, and apprehension, or development of a new pain with signs of another site of vascular involvement.	These signs/symptoms suggest the presence of pulmonary emboli as a complication of DVT or peripheral arterial occlusion associated with heparin-induced thrombocytopenia and thrombosis (HITT). Both conditions require prompt medical evaluation and treatment.
Collaborative	
Administer medications, as indicated:	
Analgesics (narcotic/nonnarcotic);	Relieves pain and decreases muscle tension.
Antipyretic; e.g., acetaminophen (Tylenol).	Reduces fever and inflammation. *Note:* Risk of bleeding may be increased by concurrent use of drugs that affect platelet function; e.g., ASA and nonsteroidal anti-inflammatory drugs (NSAIDs).

ACTIONS/INTERVENTIONS	RATIONALE
Apply moist heat to extremity if indicated.	Causes vasodilation, which increases circulation, relaxes muscles, and may stimulate release of natural endorphins.

NURSING DIAGNOSIS: impaired Gas Exchange (in presence of pulmonary embolus)

May be related to

Altered blood flow to alveoli or to major portions of the lung
Alveolar–capillary membrane changes (atelectasis, airway/alveolar collapse, pulmonary edema/effusion, excessive secretions/active bleeding)

Possibly evidenced by

Profound dyspnea, restlessness, apprehension, somnolence, cyanosis
Changes in ABGs/pulse oximetry; e.g., hypoxemia and hypercapnia

DESIRED OUTCOMES/EVALUATION CRITERIA—CLIENT WILL:

RESPIRATORY STATUS: Gas Exchange (NOC)

Demonstrate adequate ventilation/oxygenation by ABGs within client's normal range.
Report/display resolution or absence of symptoms of respiratory distress.

ACTIONS/INTERVENTIONS	RATIONALE
EMBOLUS CARE: Pulmonary (NIC)	
Independent	
Note respiratory rate and depth, work of breathing (use of accessory muscles/nasal flaring, pursed-lip breathing).	Tachypnea and dyspnea accompany pulmonary obstruction. Dyspnea ("air hunger") and increased work of breathing may be first or only sign of subacute pulmonary embolus (PE). Severe respiratory distress/failure accompanies moderate to severe loss of functional lung units.
Auscultate lungs for areas of decreased/absent breath sounds and the presence of adventitious sounds; e.g., crackles.	Nonventilated areas may be identified by absence of breath sounds. Crackles occur in fluid-filled tissues/airways or may reflect cardiac decompensation.
Observe for generalized duskiness and cyanosis in "warm tissues" such as earlobes, lips, tongue, and buccal membranes.	Indicative of systemic hypoxemia.
Monitor vital signs. Note changes in cardiac rhythm.	Tachycardia, tachypnea, and changes in BP are associated with advancing hypoxemia and acidosis. Rhythm alterations and extra heart sounds may reflect increased cardiac workload related to worsening ventilation imbalance.
Assess level of consciousness/mentation changes.	Systemic hypoxemia may be demonstrated initially by restlessness and irritability, then by progressively decreased mentation.
Assess activity tolerance; e.g., reports of weakness/fatigue, vital sign changes, increased dyspnea during exertion. Encourage rest periods, and limit activities to client tolerance.	These parameters assist in determining client response to resumed activities and ability to participate in self-care.

ACTIONS/INTERVENTIONS	RATIONALE
Airway Management (NIC)	
Institute measures to restore/maintain patent airways; e.g., coughing, suctioning.	Plugged/collapsed airways reduce number of functional alveoli, negatively affecting gas exchange.
Elevate head of bed as client requires/tolerates.	Promotes maximal chest expansion, making it easier to breathe and enhancing physiologic/psychologic comfort.
Assist with frequent changes of position, and get client out of bed/ambulate as tolerated.	Turning and ambulation enhance aeration of different lung segments, thereby improving oxygen diffusion.
Assist client to deal with fear/anxiety that may be present:	Feelings of fear and severe anxiety are associated with inability to breathe and may actually increase oxygen consumption/demand.
Encourage expression of feelings, inform client/SOs of normalcy of anxious feelings, sense of impending doom;	Understanding basis of feelings may help client regain some sense of control over emotions.
Provide brief explanations of what is happening and expected effects of interventions;	Allays anxiety related to unknown and may help reduce fears concerning personal safety.
Monitor frequently, arrange for individual (volunteer, family, others) to stay with client as indicated.	Provides assurance that changes in condition will be noted and that assistance is readily available.
EMBOLUS CARE: Pulmonary (NIC)	
Collaborative	
Prepare for lung scan.	May reveal pattern of abnormal perfusion in areas of ventilation (ventilation/perfusion mismatch), confirming diagnosis of pulmonary embolus (PE) and degree of obstruction. Absence of both ventilation and perfusion reflects alveolar congestion/airway obstruction.
Monitor serial ABGs/pulse oximetry.	Hypoxemia is present in varying degrees, depending on the amount of airway obstruction, usual cardiopulmonary function, and presence/degree of shock. Respiratory alkalosis and metabolic acidosis may also be present.
Airway Management (NIC)	
Administer supplemental oxygen by appropriate method.	Maximizes available oxygen for gas exchange, reducing work of breathing. *Note:* If obstruction is large or hypoxemia does not respond to supplemental oxygenation, it may be necessary to move client to critical care area for intubation and mechanical ventilation.
Administer fluids (IV/PO) as indicated.	Increased fluids may be given to reduce hyperviscosity of blood (potentiates thrombus formation) or to support circulating volume/tissue perfusion.
Administer medications as indicated:	
Thrombolytic agents; e.g., alteplase (Activase, t-PA); anistreplase (APSAC, Eminase); reteplase (Retavase), streptokinase (Kabbikinase, streptase); tenecteplase (TNKase); urokinase (Abbokinase);	Indicated in massive pulmonary obstruction when client is seriously hemodynamically threatened. *Note:* These clients will probably be initially cared for in/transferred to the critical care setting.
Morphine sulfate, antianxiety agents.	May be necessary initially to control pain/anxiety and improve work of breathing, maximizing gas exchange.
Provide supplemental humidification; e.g., ultrasonic nebulizers.	Delivers moisture to mucous membranes and helps liquefy secretions to facilitate airway clearance.
Assist with chest physiotherapy (e.g., postural drainage and percussion of nonaffected area, blow bottles/incentive spirometer).	Facilitates deeper respiratory effort and promotes drainage of secretions from lung segments into bronchi, where they may more readily be removed by coughing/suctioning.
Prepare for/assist with bronchoscopy.	May be done to remove blood clots and clear airways.

ACTIONS/INTERVENTIONS	RATIONALE
Prepare for surgical intervention if indicated.	Vena caval ligation or insertion of an intracaval umbrella may be useful for clients who experience recurrent emboli despite adequate anticoagulation, when anticoagulation is contraindicated, or when septic emboli arising from below the renal veins do not respond to treatment. Additionally, pulmonary embolectomy may be considered in life-threatening situations.

NURSING DIAGNOSIS: deficient Knowledge [Learning Need] regarding condition, treatment program, self-care, and discharge needs

May be related to

Lack of exposure or recall
Misinterpretation of information
Unfamiliarity with information resources

Possibly evidenced by

Request for information, statement of misconception
Inaccurate follow-through of instructions
Development of preventable complications

DESIRED OUTCOMES/EVALUATION CRITERIA—CLIENT WILL:

KNOWLEDGE: Disease Process (NOC)

Verbalize understanding of disease process, treatment regimen, and limitations.
Participate in learning process.
Identify signs/symptoms requiring medical evaluation.

KNOWLEDGE: Treatment Regimen (NOC)

Correctly perform therapeutic actions and explain reasons for actions.

ACTIONS/INTERVENTIONS	RATIONALE
TEACHING: Disease Process (NIC)	
Independent	
Review pathophysiology of condition and signs/symptoms of possible complications; e.g., pulmonary emboli, chronic venous insufficiency, venous stasis ulcers (postphlebitic syndrome).	Provides a knowledge base from which client can make informed choices and understand/identify healthcare needs. Up to 33% experience a recurrence of DVT. *Note:* Genetic blood testing may help identify inherited thrombotic disorders. Screening tests should be done when venous thrombosis occurs in those aged 45 years or younger; when a thrombus occurs at an unusal location such as in GI tract, brain, or arm; and when there is an immediate family history of DVT.
Explain purpose of activity restrictions and need for balance between activity/rest.	Rest reduces oxygen and nutrient needs of compromised tissues and decreases risk of fragmentation of thrombosis. Balancing rest with activity prevents exhaustion and further impairment of cellular perfusion.

ACTIONS/INTERVENTIONS	RATIONALE
Establish appropriate exercise/activity program.	Aids in developing collateral circulation, enhances venous return, and prevents recurrence.
Problem-solve solutions to predisposing factors that may be present; e.g., employment that requires prolonged standing/sitting, wearing restrictive clothing (girdles/garters), use of oral contraceptives, obesity, prolonged bed rest/immobility, dehydration.	Actively involves client in identifying and initiating lifestyle/behavior changes to promote health and prevent recurrence of condition/development of complications.
Recommend sitting with feet touching the floor, avoiding crossing of legs.	Prevents excess pressure on the popliteal space.
Review purpose and demonstrate correct application/removal of antiembolic hose.	Understanding may enhance cooperation with prescribed therapy and prevent improper/ineffective use.
Instruct in meticulous skin care of lower extremities; e.g., prevent/promptly treat breaks in skin and report development of lesions/ulcers or changes in skin color.	Chronic venous congestion/postphlebitic syndrome may develop (especially in presence of severe vascular involvement and/or recurrent episodes), potentiating risk of stasis ulcers/infection.

TEACHING: Prescribed Medication (NIC)

Discuss purpose, dosage of anticoagulant. Emphasize importance of taking drug as prescribed.	Promotes client safety by reducing risk of inadequate therapeutic response/deleterious side effects.
Identify safety precautions; e.g., use of soft toothbrush, electric razor for shaving, gloves for gardening, avoiding sharp objects (including toothpicks), walking barefoot, engaging in rough sports/activities, or forceful blowing of nose.	Reduces the risk of traumatic injury, which potentiates bleeding/clot formation.
Review client's usual medications and foods when on oral anticoagulants, stress need to read ingredient labels of OTC drugs and herbal supplements, and discuss use with healthcare provider prior to starting new medications.	Warfarin (Coumadin) interacts with many foods and drugs, either increasing or decreasing the anticoaglant effect. Salicylates and excess alcohol decrease prothrombin activity, whereas vitamin K (multivitamins, bananas, leafy green vegetables) increases prothrombin activity, and can cause a higher or lower INR, possibly outside of the therapeutic range. Barbiturates increase metabolism of coumarin drugs; antibiotics alter intestinal flora and may interfere with vitamin K synthesis.
Identify untoward anticoagulant effects requiring medical attention; e.g., bleeding from mucous membranes (nose, gums), continued oozing from cuts/punctures, severe bruising after minimal trauma, development of petechiae.	Early detection of deleterious effects of therapy (prolongation of clotting time) allows for timely intervention and may prevent serious complications. *Note:* Even regular use of acetaminophen may prolong clotting times. In addition, use of herbal products, such as *Ginkgo biloba*, garlic, vitamin E, also impairs clotting and should be avoided during anticoagulant therapy.
Stress importance of medical follow-up/laboratory testing.	Understanding that close supervision of anticoagulant therapy is necessary (therapeutic dosage range is narrow and complications may be deadly) promotes client participation.
Encourage wearing of medical identification bracelet/ tag, as indicated.	Alerts emergency healthcare providers to history of thrombotic problems and/or current use of/or need for anticoagulants (e.g., prophylactic before and after any procedure or event with an increased risk of venous thromboembolism.

POTENTIAL CONSIDERATIONS following discharge from care setting (dependent on client's age, physical condition/presence of complications, personal resources, and life responsibilities)

ineffective Therapeutic Regimen Management—perceived seriousness of condition, susceptibility to recurrence, benefit of therapy.

5

CHAPTER

Respiratory

CHRONIC OBSTRUCTIVE PULMONARY DISEASE (COPD) AND ASTHMA

All respiratory diseases characterized by chronic obstruction to airflow fall under the broad classification of COPD, also known as chronic airflow limitations (CAL). COPD is a condition of chronic dyspnea with expiratory airflow limitation that does not significantly fluctuate. Within that broad category, the primary cause of the obstruction may vary; examples include airway inflammation, mucous plugging, narrowed airway lumina, or airway destruction. The term *COPD* includes chronic bronchitis and emphysema. Although asthma also involves airway inflammation and periodic narrowing of the airway lumina (hyperreactivity), the condition is the result of individual response to a wide variety of stimuli/triggers and is therefore episodic in nature with fluctuations/exacerbations of symptoms. Because client response and therapy needs can be similar, asthma has been included in this plan of care.

Asthma: Sometimes called chronic reactive airway disease, asthma is a chronic inflammatory disorder characterized by episodic exacerbations of reversible inflammation and constriction of bronchial smooth muscle, hypersecretion of mucus, and edema. Precipitating factors include allergens (e.g., foods, animals, latex, plants, molds), emotional upheaval, air pollution, cold weather, exercise, chemicals, medications, and viral infections. The prevalence of asthma is rising, accounting for the sixth most common chronic disease in the United States.

Chronic bronchitis: Widespread inflammation of airways with narrowing or blocking of airways, increased production of mucous/sputum (productive cough), and marked cyanosis.

Emphysema: Most severe form of COPD characterized by recurrent inflammation that damages and eventually destroys alveolar walls to create large blebs or bullae (air spaces) and collapsed bronchioles on expiration (air-trapping). Clinically, emphysema typically presents with nonproductive or minimally productive cough and progressive dyspnea.

Note: Chronic bronchitis and emphysema coexist in many clients and are most commonly seen in hospitalized COPD clients when acute exacerbations occur. Chronic bronchitis and emphysema are usually irreversible, although some effects can be mediated.

CARE SETTING

Primarily community level; however, severe exacerbations may necessitate emergency and/or inpatient hospital stay.

RELATED CONCERNS

Heart failure: chronic, page 47
Pneumonia, page 128
Psychosocial aspects of care, page 770
Ventilatory assistance (mechanical), page 170
Surgical intervention, page 788

Client Assessment Database

ACTIVITY/REST

May report:
Fatigue, exhaustion, malaise
Inability to perform basic activities of daily living (ADLs) because of breathlessness
Inability to sleep, need to sleep sitting up
Dyspnea at rest or in response to activity or exercise

May exhibit:
Fatigue
Restlessness, insomnia
General debilitation/loss of muscle mass

CIRCULATION

May report: Swelling of lower extremities

May exhibit: Elevated blood pressure (BP)
Elevated heart rate/severe tachycardia, dysrhythmias
Distended neck veins (advanced disease)
Dependent edema, may not be related to heart disease
Faint heart sounds (due to increased anteroposterior [AP] chest diameter)
Skin color/mucous membranes may be pale or bluish/cyanotic, clubbing of nails and peripheral cyanosis, pallor (can indicate anemia)

EGO INTEGRITY

May report: Increased stress factors
Changes in lifestyle
Feelings of hopelessness, loss of interest in life

May exhibit: Anxious, fearful, irritable behavior, emotional distress
Apathy, change in alertness, dull affect, withdrawal

FOOD/FLUID

May report: Nausea (side effect of medication/mucus production)
Poor appetite/anorexia (emphysema)
Inability to eat because of respiratory distress
Persistent weight loss, decreased muscle mass/subcutaneous fat (emphysema) or weight gain may reflect edema (bronchitis, prednisone use)

May exhibit: Poor skin turgor
Dependent edema
Diaphoresis
Abdominal palpation may reveal hepatomegaly (bronchitis)

HYGIENE

May report: Decreased ability/increased need for assistance with ADLs

May exhibit: Poor hygiene

RESPIRATION

May report: Variable levels of dyspnea, such as insidious and progressive onset (predominant symptom in emphysema), especially on exertion; seasonal or episodic occurrence of breathlessness (asthma); sensation of chest tightness, inability to breathe (asthma); chronic "air hunger"
Persistent cough with sputum production (gray, white, or yellow), which may be copious (chronic bronchitis); intermittent cough episodes, usually nonproductive in early stages, although they may become productive (emphysema); paroxysms of cough (asthma)
History of recurrent pneumonia, long-term exposure to chemical pollution/respiratory irritants (e.g., cigarette smoke), or occupational dust/fumes (e.g., cotton, hemp, asbestos, coal dust, sawdust)
Familial and hereditary factors; i.e., deficiency of α_1-antitrypsin (emphysema)
Use of oxygen at night or continuously

May exhibit: Respirations: Usually rapid, may be shallow; prolonged expiratory phase with grunting, pursed-lip breathing (emphysema)
Assumption of three-point ("tripod") position for breathing (especially with acute exacerbation of chronic bronchitis)
Use of accessory muscles for respiration; e.g., elevated shoulder girdle, retraction of supraclavicular fossae, flaring of nares
Chest may appear hyperinflated with increased AP diameter (barrel-shaped), minimal diaphragmatic movement
Breath sounds may be faint with expiratory wheezes (emphysema); scattered, fine, or coarse moist crackles (bronchitis); rhonchi, wheezing throughout lung fields on expiration, and possibly during inspiration, progressing to diminished or absent breath sounds (asthma)
Percussion may reveal hyperresonance over lung fields (e.g., air-trapping with emphysema) or dullness over lung fields (e.g., consolidation, fluid, mucus)
Difficulty speaking sentences of more than four or five words at one time, loss of voice

Color: Pallor with cyanosis of lips, nail beds; overall duskiness; ruddy color (chronic bronchitis, "blue bloaters"); normal skin color despite abnormal gas exchange and rapid respiratory rate (moderate emphysema, known as "pink puffers")
Clubbing of fingernails (not characteristic of emphysema and if present should alert clinician to another condition; e.g., pulmonary fibrosis, cystic fibrosis, lung cancer, or asbestosis)

SAFETY

May report: History of allergic reactions or sensitivity to substances/environmental factors
Recent/recurrent infections
Flushing/perspiration (asthma)

SEXUALITY

May report: Decreased libido

SOCIAL INTERACTION

May report: Dependent relationship(s)
Insufficient support from/to partner/significant other (SO), lack of support systems
Prolonged disease or disability progression

May exhibit: Inability to converse/maintain voice because of respiratory distress
Limited physical mobility
Neglectful relationships with other family members
Inability to perform/inattention to employment responsibilities, absenteeism/confirmed disability

TEACHING/LEARNING

May report: Use/misuse of respiratory drugs
Use of herbal supplements (e.g., astragalus, coleus, echinacea, elderberry, elencampe, ephedra, garlic, ginkgo, horehound, licorice, marshmallow, mullein, onion, tumeric, goldenseal, Oregon graperoot, wild cherry bark, peppermint, hyssop)
Smoking/difficulty stopping smoking, chronic exposure to second-hand smoke, smoking substances other than tobacco
Regular use of alcohol
Failure to improve over long period of time

Discharge plan considerations: Episodic or long-term assistance with shopping, transportation, self-care needs, homemaker/home maintenance tasks
Changes in medication/therapeutic treatments, use of supplemental oxygen, ventilator support; end-of-life issues

Refer to section at end of plan for postdischarge considerations.

DIAGNOSTIC STUDIES

Chest x-ray: May reveal hyperinflation of lungs with increased anterior-posterior (AP) diameter, flattened diaphragm, increased retrosternal air space, decreased vascular markings/bullae (emphysema), increased bronchovascular markings (bronchitis), normal findings during periods of remission (asthma).

Pulmonary function tests: Spirometry is an established method of measuring lung function, recommended for diagnosis and management of persons with COPD, those at risk of COPD, and follow-up of persons with documented COPD to determine cause of dyspnea, whether functional abnormality is obstructive or restrictive, to estimate degree of dysfunction and to evaluate effects of therapy; e.g., bronchodilators. Exercise pulmonary function studies may also be done to evaluate activity tolerance in those with known pulmonary impairment/progression of disease.

Tidal volume (V_T): Decreased V_T may indicate restrictive disease.

Minute volume (MV): Decreased MV may indicate pulmonary edema; increased MV can occur with acidosis, increased CO_2, decreased PaO_2, and low compliance states.

Forced expiratory volume over 1 second (FEV_1): Reduced FEV_1 not only is the standard way of assessing the clinical course and degree of reversibility in response to therapy but also is an important predictor of prognosis. Measurements done pre- and postbronchodilator help to distinguish obstructive disease (COPD) from restrictive disease (asthma).

Total lung capacity (TLC), functional residual capacity (FRC), and residual volume (RV): May be increased, indicating air-trapping. In obstructive lung disease, the RV will make up the greater portion of the TLC.

Thoracic gas volume (TCV): Increased TCV indicates air-trapping such as might occur with COPD. Body plethysmography may be used to measure pressure and flow or volume changes (e.g., TCV, airway resistance, and conductance).

Maximal voluntary ventilation (MVV), also known as maximum breathing capacity: Decreased in obstructive disease and normal or decreased in restrictive disease.

DLCO: Assesses diffusion in lungs. Carbon monoxide is used to measure gas diffusion across the alveocapillary membrane. Because carbon monoxide combines with hemoglobin 200 times more easily than oxygen, it easily affects the alveoli and small airways where gas exchange occurs. Emphysema is the only obstructive disease that causes diffusion dysfunction.

Arterial blood gases (ABGs): Determines degree and severity of disease process, e.g., most often Pao_2 is decreased, and $Paco_2$ is normal or increased in chronic bronchitis and emphysema, but is often decreased in asthma; pH normal or acidotic, mild respiratory alkalosis secondary to hyperventilation (moderate emphysema or asthma).

Pulse Oximetry: A continuous noninvasive study of arterial blood oxygen diffusion and saturation using a clip or probe attached to a sensor site (usually fingertip or earlobe). The percentage expressed is the ratio of oxygen to hemoglobin. Abnormally low levels (<88%) indicate impaired gas exchange and impending respiratory failure.

Peak Expiratory Flow (PEF or PEFR): Noninvasive meter used by client to monitor disease status by assessing speed at which air is forced out of lungs after deep inhalation.

Bronchogram: Can show cylindrical dilation of bronchi on inspiration, bronchial collapse on forced expiration (emphysema), enlarged mucous ducts (bronchitis).

Lung scan: Perfusion scanning can confirm vascular obstruction such as pulmonary or septic emboli. Ventilation studies may be done to differentiate between the various pulmonary diseases, such as PE, atelectasis, obstruction, tumors and COPD. COPD is characterized by a mismatch of perfusion and ventilation (i.e., areas of abnormal ventilation in area of perfusion defect).

Complete blood count (CBC) and differential: Increased hemoglobin (advanced emphysema), increased eosinophils (asthma). WBCs can be elevated in severe respiratory infection.

Blood chemistry: α_1-Antitrypsin is measured to verify deficiency and diagnosis of primary emphysema.

Sputum culture: Determines presence of infection, identifies pathogen.

Cytologic examination: Rules out underlying malignancy or allergic disorder.

Electrocardiogram (ECG): Right axis deviation, peaked P waves (severe asthma); atrial dysrhythmias (bronchitis), tall, peaked P waves in leads II, III, AVF (bronchitis, emphysema); vertical QRS axis (emphysema).

Exercise ECG, Stress test: May be done for evaluation of hypoxemia and/or desaturation in the presence of dyspnea, known pulmonary disease, abnormal diagnostic tests (e.g., diffusing capacity). Helps in assessing degree of pulmonary dysfunction, evaluating effectiveness of bronchodilator therapy, planning/evaluating exercise program.

NURSING PRIORITIES

1. Maintain airway patency.
2. Assist with measures to facilitate gas exchange.
3. Enhance nutritional intake.
4. Prevent complications, slow progression of condition.
5. Provide information about disease process/prognosis and treatment regimen.

DISCHARGE GOALS

1. Ventilation/oxygenation adequate to meet self-care needs.
2. Nutritional intake meeting caloric needs.
3. Infection treated/prevented.
4. Disease process/prognosis and therapeutic regimen understood.
5. Plan in place to meet needs after discharge.

NURSING DIAGNOSIS: ineffective Airway Clearance

May be related to

Bronchospasm
Increased production of secretions, retained secretions, thick, viscous secretions
Decreased energy/fatigue

Possibly evidenced by

Statement of difficulty breathing
Changes in depth/rate of respirations, use of accessory muscles
Abnormal breath sounds; e.g., wheezes, rhonchi, crackles
Cough (persistent), with/without sputum production

DESIRED OUTCOMES/EVALUATION CRITERIA—CLIENT WILL:

RESPIRATORY STATUS: Airway Patency (NOC)

Maintain patent airway with breath sounds clear/clearing.
Demonstrate behaviors to improve airway clearance; e.g., cough effectively and expectorate secretions.

ACTIONS/INTERVENTIONS	RATIONALE
Airway Management (NIC)	
Independent	
Auscultate breath sounds. Note adventitious breath sounds; e.g., wheezes, crackles, rhonchi.	Some degree of bronchospasm is present with obstructions in airway and may/may not be manifested in adventitious breath sounds; e.g., scattered, moist crackles (bronchitis); faint sounds, with expiratory wheezes (emphysema); or absent breath sounds (severe asthma).
Assess/monitor respiratory rate. Note inspiratory/expiratory ratio.	Tachypnea is usually present to some degree and may be pronounced on admission or during stress/concurrent acute infectious process. Respirations may be shallow and rapid, with prolonged expiration in comparison to inspiration.
Note presence/degree of dyspnea; e.g., reports of "air hunger," restlessness, anxiety, respiratory distress, use of accessory muscles. Use 0–10 scale or American Thoracic Society's "Grade of Breathlessness Scale" to rate breathing difficulty. Ascertain precipitating factors when possible. Differentiate acute episode from exacerbation of chronic dyspnea.	Respiratory dysfunction is variable depending on the underlying process; e.g., infection, allergic reaction, and the stage of chronicity in a client with established COPD. *Note:* Using a 0–10 scale to rate dyspnea aids in quantifying and tracking changes in respiratory distress. Rapid onset of acute dyspnea may reflect pulmonary embolus.
Assist client to assume position of comfort; e.g., elevate head of bed, have client lean on overbed table or sit on edge of bed.	Elevation of the head of the bed facilitates respiratory function by use of gravity; however, client in severe distress will seek the position that most eases breathing. Supporting arms/legs with table, pillows, and so on helps reduce muscle fatigue and can aid chest expansion.
Keep environmental pollution to a minimum (e.g., dust, smoke, and feather pillows), according to individual situation.	Precipitators of allergic type of respiratory reactions that can trigger/exacerbate onset of acute episode.
Encourage/assist with abdominal or pursed-lip breathing exercises.	Provides client with some means to cope with/control dyspnea and reduce air-trapping.
Observe characteristics of cough; e.g., persistent, hacking, moist. Assist with measures to improve effectiveness of cough effort.	Cough can be persistent but ineffective, especially if client is elderly, acutely ill, or debilitated. Coughing is most effective in an upright or in a head-down position after chest percussion.
Increase fluid intake to 3000 mL/day within cardiac tolerance. Provide warm/tepid liquids. Recommend intake of fluids between instead of during meals.	Hydration helps decrease the viscosity of secretions, facilitating expectoration. Using warm liquids may decrease bronchospasm. Fluids during meals can increase gastric distention and pressure on the diaphragm.
Collaborative	
Administer medications as indicated:	
β-Agonists: epinephrine (Adrenalin, AsthmaNefrin, Primatene, Sus-Phrine); albuterol (Proventil, Velmax, Ventolin, AccuNeb, Airet); formoterol (Foradil); levalbuterol (Xopenex); metaproterenol (Alupent): pirbuterol (Maxair): salmeterol, terbutaline (Brethine); salmeterol (Serevent);	Inhaled β_2-adrenergic agonists are first-line therapies for rapid symptomatic improvement of bronchoconstriction. These medications relax smooth muscles and reduce local congestion, reducing airway spasm, wheezing, and mucus production. Medications may be oral, injected, or inhaled. Inhalation by metered-dose inhaler (MDI) with a spacer is recommended, but medications may be nebulized in the event client has severe coughing or is too dyspneic to retain a puff effectively.

ACTIONS/INTERVENTIONS	RATIONALE
Bronchodilators; e.g., anticholinergic agents: ipratropium (Atrovent);	Inhaled anticholinergic agents are now considered the first-line drugs for clients with stable COPD because studies indicate they have a longer duration of action with less toxicity potential, whereas still providing the effective relief of the β-agonists. Some of these medications are available in combinations; e.g., Albuterol and Atrovent are available as Combivent.
Leukotriene antagonists: montelukast (Singulair); zafirlukast (Accolate); zileuton (Zyflo);	Reduce leukotriene activity to limit inflammatory response. In mild to moderate asthma, reduces need for inhaled β_2-agonists and systemic corticosteroids. Not effective in acute exacerbations because there is no bronchodilator effect. *Note:* This drug class is not recommended for clients with COPD because of insufficient testing.
Anti-inflammatories: oral, IV, and inhaled steroids; e.g., prednisone (Cordrol, Deltasone, Pred-Pak, Liquid Pred), methylprednisolone (Medrol), dexamethasone (Decadron), beclomethasone (Beclovent, Vanceril), budesonide (Pulmacort), fluticasone (Flovent), triamcinolone (Azmacort);	Decrease local airway inflammation and edema by inhibiting effects of histamine and other mediators, to reduce severity and frequency of airway spasm, respiratory inflammation, and dyspnea. Studies have shown benefits of systemic steroids in the management of COPD exacerbations. Inhaled steroids may serve as a systemic steroid-sparing agent.
Antimicrobials;	Various antimicrobials may be indicated for control of bacterial exacerbations of COPD; e.g., pneumonia. Refer to CP, Pneumonia, page 128.)
Methylxanthine derivatives; e.g., aminophylline, oxtriphylline (Choledyl), theophylline (Bronkodyl, Theo-Dur, Elixophyllin, Slo-Bid, Slo-Phyllin);	Decrease mucosal edema and smooth muscle spasm (bronchospasm) by indirectly increasing cyclic adenosine monophosphate (AMP). May also reduce muscle fatigue/respiratory failure by increasing diaphragmatic contractility. Use of theophylline may be of little or no benefit in the presence of adequate β-agonist regimen; however, it may sustain bronchodilation because effect of β-agonist diminishes between doses. *Note:* Theophylline products are used with less frequency now and are shied away from in older clients because of their potentially adverse cardiovascular effects.
Analgesics, cough suppressants, or antitussives; e.g., codeine, dextromethorphan products (Benylin DM, Comtrex, Novahistine);	Persistent, exhausting cough may need to be suppressed to conserve energy and permit client to rest. *Note:* Regular use of antitussives is not recommended in COPD since cough can have a significant protective effect.
Artificial surfactant; e.g., colfosceril palmitate (Exosurf).	Research suggests aerosol administration may enhance expectoration of sputum, improve pulmonary function, and reduce lung volumes (air trapping).
Provide supplemental humidification; e.g., ultrasonic nebulizer, aerosol room humidifier.	Humidity helps reduce viscosity of secretions, facilitating expectoration, and may reduce/prevent formation of thick mucous plugs in bronchioles.
Assist with respiratory treatments; e.g., spirometry, chest physiotherapy.	Breathing exercises help enhance diffusion; aerosol/nebulizer medications can reduce bronchospasm and stimulate expectoration. Postural drainage and percussion enhance removal of excessive/sticky secretions and improve ventilation of bottom lung segments. *Note:* Chest physiotherapy may aggravate bronchospasm in asthmatics.
Monitor/graph serial ABGs, pulse oximetry, chest x-ray.	Establishes baseline for monitoring progression/regression of disease process and complications. *Note:* Pulse oximetry readings detect changes in saturation as they are happening, helping to identify trends possibly before client is symptomatic. However, studies have shown that the accuracy of pulse oximetry may be questioned if client has severe peripheral vasoconstriction.

NURSING DIAGNOSIS: impaired Gas Exchange

May be related to

Altered oxygen supply (obstruction of airways by secretions, bronchospasm, air trapping)
Alveoli destruction

Possibly evidenced by

Dyspnea
Confusion, restlessness
Inability to move secretions
Abnormal ABG values (hypoxia and hypercapnia)
Changes in vital signs
Reduced tolerance for activity

DESIRED OUTCOMES/EVALUATION CRITERIA—CLIENT WILL:

RESPIRATORY STATUS: Gas Exchange (NOC)

Demonstrate improved ventilation and adequate oxygenation of tissues by ABGs within client's normal range and be free of symptoms of respiratory distress.
Participate in treatment regimen within level of ability/situation.

ACTIONS/INTERVENTIONS RATIONALE

Acid/Base Management (NIC)

Independent

ACTIONS/INTERVENTIONS	RATIONALE
Assess respiratory rate, depth. Note use of accessory muscles, pursed-lip breathing, and inability to speak/converse.	Useful in evaluating the degree of respiratory distress and/or chronicity of the disease process.
Elevate head of bed, assist client to assume position to ease work of breathing. Include periods of time in prone position as tolerated. Encourage deep-slow or pursed-lip breathing as individually needed/tolerated.	Oxygen delivery may be improved by upright position and breathing exercises to decrease airway collapse, dyspnea, and work of breathing. *Note:* Recent research supports use of prone position to increase PaO_2.
Assess/routinely monitor skin and mucous membrane color.	Cyanosis may be peripheral (noted in nail beds) or central (noted around lips or earlobes). Duskiness and central cyanosis indicate advanced hypoxemia.
Encourage expectoration of sputum; suction when indicated.	Thick, tenacious, copious secretions are a major source of impaired gas exchange in small airways. Deep suctioning may be required when cough is ineffective for expectoration of secretions.
Auscultate breath sounds, noting areas of decreased airflow and/or adventitious sounds.	Breath sounds may be faint because of decreased airflow or areas of consolidation. Presence of wheezes may indicate bronchospasm/retained secretions. Scattered moist crackles may indicate interstitial fluid/cardiac decompensation.
Palpate for fremitus.	Decrease of vibratory tremors suggests fluid collection or air trapping.
Monitor level of consciousness/mental status. Investigate changes.	Restlessness and anxiety are common manifestations of hypoxia. Worsening ABGs accompanied by confusion/somnolence are indicative of cerebral dysfunction due to hypoxemia.

ACTIONS/INTERVENTIONS	RATIONALE
Evaluate level of activity tolerance. Provide calm, quiet environment. Limit client's activity or encourage bed/chair rest during acute phase. Have client resume activity gradually and increase as individually tolerated.	During severe/acute/refractory respiratory distress, client may be totally unable to perform basic self-care activities because of hypoxemia and dyspnea. Rest interspersed with care activities remains an important part of treatment regimen. An exercise program is aimed at improving aerobic capacity and functional performance, increasing endurance and strength without causing severe dyspnea and can enhance sense of well-being.
Evaluate sleep patterns, note reports of difficulties and whether client feels well rested. Provide quiet environment, group care/monitoring activities to allow periods of uninterrupted sleep. Limit stimulants; e.g., caffeine. Encourage position of comfort.	Multiple external stimuli and presence of dyspnea and/or hypoxemia may prevent relaxation and inhibit sleep.
Monitor vital signs and cardiac rhythm.	Tachycardia, dysrhythmias, and changes in blood pressure (BP) can reflect effect of systemic hypoxemia on cardiac function.

Collaborative

Monitor/graph serial ABGs and pulse oximetry.	$Paco_2$ usually elevated (bronchitis, emphysema), and Pao_2 is generally decreased, so that hypoxia is present in a greater or lesser degree. *Note:* A "normal" or increased $Paco_2$ signals impending respiratory failure for asthmatics.
Administer supplemental oxygen judiciously, using appropriate delivery method (e.g., cannula, mask, mechanical ventilator) and titrate as indicated by ABG results and client tolerance.	Used to correct/prevent worsening of hypoxemia, improve survival, and quality of life. Supplemental oxygen can be provided during exacerbations only, or as a long-term therapy.
Administer antianxiety, sedative, or narcotic agents (e.g., morphine) with caution.	May be used to reduce dyspnea by controlling anxiety and restlessness, which increases oxygen consumption/demand, exacerbating dyspnea. Must be monitored closely because depressive effect may lead to respiratory failure.
Assist with noninvasive (or nasal intermittent) positive-pressure ventilation (NIPPV) or intubation, institution/maintenance of mechanical ventilation; transfer to critical care area depending on client directives.	Development of/impending respiratory failure requires prompt life-saving measures. *Note:* NIPPV provides ventilatory support by means of positive pressure typically through a nasal mask. It may be useful in the home setting as well to treat chronic respiratory failure or limit acute exacerbations in clients who are able to maintain spontaneous respiratory effort.
Prepare for additional referrals/interventions; e.g., pulmonary specialist, pulmonary rehabilitation program, surgical intervention, as appropriate.	May be indicated to confirm diagnosis and optimize appropriate treatment. A multidisciplinary approach including education and exercise training may be helpful in improving client function and quality of life. Screened candidates (those with severe dyspnea/end-stage emphysema with FEV_1 (forced expiratory volume in 1 second) less than 35% of the predicted value despite maximal medical therapy, with the ability to complete preoperative pulmonary rehabilitation programs) may benefit from lung volume reduction surgery (LVRS) in which hyperinflated giant bullae/cysts are removed; e.g., those occupying at least one-third of the involved lobe, or areas of lung tissue with small cystic disease. In the absence of fibrosis, this procedure removes ineffective lung tissue, allowing for better lung expansion and elastic recoil, enhanced blood flow to healthy tissues (correction of ventilation-perfusion mismatch), improved respiratory muscle efficiency, and increased venous return to the right ventricle.

NURSING DIAGNOSIS: imbalanced Nutrition: less than body requirements

May be related to

Dyspnea, sputum production
Medication side effects; anorexia, nausea/vomiting
Fatigue

Possibly evidenced by

Weight loss, loss of muscle mass, poor muscle tone
Reported altered taste sensation, aversion to eating, lack of interest in food

DESIRED OUTCOMES/EVALUATION CRITERIA—CLIENT WILL:

Nutritional Status (NOC)

Display progressive weight gain toward goal as appropriate.
Demonstrate behaviors/lifestyle changes to regain and/or maintain appropriate weight.

ACTIONS/INTERVENTIONS	RATIONALE
Nutrition Therapy (NIC)	
Independent	
Assess dietary habits, recent food intake. Note degree of difficulty with eating. Evaluate weight and body size (mass).	Client in acute respiratory distress is often anorectic because of dyspnea, sputum production, and medication effects. In addition, many COPD clients habitually eat poorly even though respiratory insufficiency creates a hypermetabolic state with increased caloric needs. As a result, client often is admitted with some degree of malnutrition. People who have emphysema are often thin with wasted musculature.
Auscultate bowel sounds.	Diminished/hypoactive bowel sounds may reflect decreased gastric motility and constipation (common complication) related to limited fluid intake, poor food choices, decreased activity, and hypoxemia.
Give frequent oral care, remove expectorated secretions promptly, provide specific container for disposal of secretions and tissues.	Noxious tastes, smells, and sights are prime deterrents to appetite and can produce nausea and vomiting with increased respiratory difficulty.
Encourage a rest period of 1 hr before and after meals. Provide frequent small feedings.	Helps reduce fatigue during mealtime, and provides opportunity to increase total caloric intake.
Avoid gas-producing foods and carbonated beverages.	Can produce abdominal distention, which hampers abdominal breathing and diaphragmatic movement and can increase dyspnea.
Avoid very hot or very cold foods.	Extremes in temperature can precipitate/aggravate coughing spasms.
Weigh as indicated.	Useful in determining caloric needs, setting weight goal, and evaluating adequacy of nutritional plan. *Note:* Weight loss may continue initially despite adequate intake, as edema is resolving.
Collaborative	
Consult dietitian/nutritional support team to provide easily digested, nutritionally balanced meals by appropriate means; e.g., oral, supplemental/tube feedings, parenteral nutrition. (Refer to CP: Total Nutritional Support: Parenteral/Enteral Feeding.)	Method of feeding and caloric requirements are based on individual situation/needs to provide maximal nutrients with minimal client effort/energy expenditure.

ACTIONS/INTERVENTIONS	RATIONALE
Review laboratory studies; e.g., serum albumin/prealbumin, transferrin, amino acid profile, iron, nitrogen balance studies, glucose, liver function studies, electrolytes.	Evaluates/treats deficits and monitors effectiveness of nutritional therapy.
Administer supplemental oxygen during meals as indicated.	Decreases dyspnea and increases energy for eating, enhancing intake.

NURSING DIAGNOSIS: deficient Knowledge [Learning Need] regarding condition, treatment, self-care, and discharge needs

May be related to

Lack of information/unfamiliarity with information resources
Information misinterpretation
Lack of recall/cognitive limitation

Possibly evidenced by

Request for information
Statement of concerns/misconception
Inaccurate follow-through of instructions
Development of preventable complications

DESIRED OUTCOMES/EVALUATION CRITERIA—CLIENT WILL:

KNOWLEDGE: Illness Care (NOC)

Verbalize understanding of condition/disease process and treatment.
Identify relationship of current signs/symptoms to the disease process and correlate these with causative factors.
Initiate necessary lifestyle changes and participate in treatment regimen.

ACTIONS/INTERVENTIONS	RATIONALE
TEACHING: Disease Process (NIC)	
Independent	
Explain/reinforce explanations of individual disease process, including factors that lead to exacerbation episodes. Encourage client/significant other (SO) to ask questions.	Understanding decreases anxiety and can lead to improved participation in treatment plan.
Discuss self-management plan:	
Avoidance of triggers, and education regarding zones as appropriate;	Avoiding triggers (e.g., known allergens, environmental temperature extremes, chemical products and fumes) is important in the self-management of asthma and in the prevention of acute exacerbations. Zones may be divided into green (peak expiratory flow rate [PEFR] 80%–100% and no breathing difficulty), yellow (PEFR 50%–80% of baseline and some difficulty breathing with wheezing and coughing), and red (PEFR<50% baseline and does not respond to inhaled bronchodilators).
Review breathing exercises, coughing effectively, and general conditioning exercises;	Pursed-lip and abdominal/diaphragmatic breathing exercises strengthen muscles of respiration, help minimize collapse of small airways, and provide the individual with means to control dyspnea. General paced conditioning exercises (carried out regularly and perhaps timed with activity soon after taking medication or breathing treatments) can increase activity tolerance, muscle strength, and sense of well-being/quality of life.

ACTIONS/INTERVENTIONS	RATIONALE
Regular oral care/dental hygiene;	Decreases bacterial growth in the mouth, which can lead to pulmonary infections.
Importance of avoiding people with active respiratory infections. Stress need for routine influenza/pneumococcal vaccinations;	Decreases exposure to and incidence of acquired acute upper respiratory diseases (URIs).
Identify individual environmental factors that may trigger or aggravate condition; e.g., excessively dry air, wind, environmental temperature extremes, pollen, tobacco smoke, aerosol sprays, air pollution. Encourage client/SO to explore ways to control these factors in and around the home and work setting.	These can induce/aggravate bronchial irritation, leading to increased secretion production and airway blockage.
Review the harmful effects of smoking, and strongly advise cessation of smoking by client and/or SO. Provide information regarding smoking cessation recourses (e.g., QUITLINES, support groups, nicotine substitutes).	Cessation of smoking may slow/halt progression of COPD. Even when client wants to stop smoking, support groups and medical monitoring may be needed. *Note:* Research studies suggest that "side-stream" or "second-hand" smoke can be as detrimental as actually smoking.
Provide information about benefits of regular exercise while addressing individual activity limitations.	Having this knowledge can enable client/SO to make informed choices/decisions to reduce client's dyspnea, maximize functional level, perform most desired activities, and prevent complications. This may include alternating activities with rest periods to prevent fatigue, learning ways to conserve energy during activities (e.g., pulling instead of pushing, sitting instead of standing while performing tasks; use of pursed-lip breathing, side-lying position, and possible need for supplemental oxygen during sexual activity).
Discuss importance of regular medical follow-up care, when to notify healthcare professional of changes in condition, and periodic spirometry testing, chest x-rays, sputum cultures.	Monitoring disease process allows for alterations in therapeutic regimen to meet changing needs and may help prevent complications.
Review oxygen requirements/dosage for client who is discharged on supplemental oxygen. Discuss safe use of oxygen and refer to supplier as indicated.	Reduces risk of misuse (too little/too much) and resultant complications. Promotes environmental/physical safety.
Instruct client/SO in use of NIPPV as appropriate. Problem solve possible side effects and identify adverse signs/symptoms; e.g., increased dyspnea, fatigue, daytime drowsiness, or headaches on awakening.	NIPPV may be used at night/periodically during day to decrease CO_2 level, improve quality of sleep, and enhance functional level during the day. Signs of increasing CO_2 level indicate need for more aggressive therapy.
Instruct asthmatic client in use of peak flow meter as appropriate.	Peak flow level can drop before client exhibits any signs/symptoms of asthma during the "first time" after exposure to a trigger. Regular use of the peak flow meter may reduce the severity of the attack because of earlier intervention.
Provide information/encourage participation in support groups; e.g., American Lung Association, public health department.	These clients and their SOs may experience anxiety, depression, and other reactions as they deal with a chronic disease that has an impact on their desired lifestyle. Support groups and/or home visits may be desired or needed to provide assistance, emotional support, and respite care.
Refer for evaluation of home care if indicated. Provide a detailed plan of care and baseline physical assessment to home care nurse as needed on discharge from acute care.	Provides for continuity of care. May help reduce frequency of rehospitalization.
Assist client/SO in making arrangements for access to emergency assistance (e.g., buddy system for getting help quickly, special phone numbers, "panic button").	Client with chronic respiratory condition should have access to prompt assistance when needed. This is both necessary and psychologically comforting for self-management.
Facilitate discussion about healthcare directives, end-of-life wishes as indicated.	Although many clients have an interest in discussing living wills, their wishes may be unspoken. In client with severe pulmonary disease, it is helpful to discuss specific treatment preferences (e.g., aggressive treatment, home care only, hospitalization for comfort care, full life support). It is useful also to discuss the goals of care (e.g., functional independence or continuation of life support in an extended care nursing facility).

ACTIONS/INTERVENTIONS	RATIONALE
TEACHING: Disease Process (NIC)	
Discuss respiratory medications, side effects, drug interactions, adverse reactions.	Frequently these clients are simultaneously on several respiratory drugs that have similar side effects and potential drug interactions. It is important that client understand the difference between nuisance side effects (medication continued) and untoward or adverse side effects (medication possibly discontinued/dosage changed).
Demonstrate correct technique for using a MDI, such as how to hold it, pausing 2–5 min between puffs, cleaning the inhaler.	Proper administration of drug enhances delivery and effectiveness.
Devise system for recording prescribed intermittent drug/inhaler usage.	Reduces risk of improper use/overdosage of prn medications, especially during acute exacerbations, when cognition may be impaired.
Discuss use of herbals, especially when client is on multiple respiratory medications.	Many interactions can occur between herbals and medications used to treat respiratory disorders. Although most herbals do not have dangerous side effects, effects can be dangerous or lethal if combined with other substances or when taken in larger doses (e.g., ephedra should be used only in very small doses and for a short time; ecchinacea can only alter the actions of a variety of drugs, and is not recommended for persons with HIV infection, multiple sclerosis (MS), and other autoimmune disorders).
Recommend avoidance of sedative antianxiety agents unless specifically prescribed/approved by physician treating respiratory condition.	Although client may be nervous and feel the need for sedatives, these can depress respiratory drive and protective cough mechanisms. *Note:* These drugs may be used prophylactically when client is unable to avoid situations known to increase stress/trigger respiratory response.

POTENTIAL CONSIDERATIONS following acute hospitalization (dependent on client's age, physical condition/presence of complications, personal resources, and life responsibilities)

Self-Care Deficit, specify—intolerance to activity, decreased strength/endurance, depression, severe anxiety.

ineffective Home Maintenance—intolerance to activity, inadequate support system, insufficient finances, unfamiliarity with neighborhood resources.

risk for Infection—decreased ciliary action, stasis of secretions, tissue destruction, increased environmental exposure, chronic disease process, malnutrition.

PNEUMONIA

Pneumonia is an inflammation of the lung parenchyma associated with alveolar edema and congestion that impair gas exchange. *Primary pneumonia* is caused by the client's inhaling or aspirating a pathogen. *Secondary pneumonia* ensues from lung damage caused by the spread of bacteria from an infection elsewhere in the body. Likely causes include various infectious agents (bacterial, viral, or fungal), chemical irritants (including gastric reflux/aspiration, smoke inhalation), and radiation therapy.

Pneumonia may be community acquired (including during the first 2 days of hospitalization) or nosocomial (hospital acquired occurring 48 hours or longer after admission). *Viral pneumonia* accounts for approximately half of all cases of community-acquired pneumonia with common causative organisms including respiratory syncytial virus (RSV) and influenza. *Bacterial pneumonias* are divided into typical and atypical types. Gram-positive *Streptococcus pneumoniae, Haemophilus,* and *Staphylococcus* are the most common bacterial causes. The most common causes of *fungal pneumonia* are *Histoplasma capsulatum,* and *Coccidioides immitis. Pneumocystis carinii and* cytomegalovirus often occur in immunocompromised persons. Nosocomial pneumonias are often caused by different pathogens, including *Staphylococcus aureus* and *Klebsiella.* Other atypical pneumonias can be caused by *Mycoplasma, Mycobacterium tuberculosis, Coxiella burnetii, Chlamydia, Legionella,* and others.

Severe pneumonia is life threatening, (sixth leading cause of death in the United States), especially for the elderly, for very young children, and for persons with asthma, cystic fibrosis, or other chronic respiratory conditions; smokers; immunocompromised persons; and those with heart disease or poorly controlled diabetes.

This plan of care deals primarily with typical bacterial pneumonias.

CARE SETTING

Most clients are treated as outpatients in community settings; however, persons at higher risk (e.g., age >65, persons with other chronic conditions such as COPD, diabetes, cancer, congestive heart failure) are treated in the hospital, as are those already hospitalized for other reasons and have developed nosocomial pneumonia.

RELATED CONCERNS

Acquired immunodeficiency syndrome (AIDS), page 726
Chronic obstructive pulmonary disease (COPD) and asthma, page 117
Psychosocial aspects of care, page 770
Sepsis/septicemia, page 701
Surgical intervention, page 788

Client Assessment Database

ACTIVITY/REST

May report:
Fatigue, weakness
Insomnia

May exhibit:
Prolonged immobility/bedrest
Lethargy
Decreased tolerance to activity

CIRCULATION

May report:
History of recent/chronic heart failure (HF)

May exhibit:
Tachycardia
Flushed appearance, pallor, central cyanosis

EGO INTEGRITY

May report:
Multiple stressors, financial concerns

FOOD/FLUID

May report:
Loss of appetite, nausea/vomiting
May be receiving intestinal/gastric feedings

May exhibit:
Distended abdomen
Hyperactive bowel sounds
Dry skin with poor turgor
Cachectic appearance (malnutrition)

NEUROSENSORY

May report:
Frontal headache (influenza)

May exhibit:
Changes in mentation (confusion, somnolence) or behavior (irritability, restlessness, lethargy)

PAIN/DISCOMFORT

May report:
Headache
Chest pain (pleuritic) aggravated by cough, substernal chest pain (influenza)
Myalgia, arthralgia, abdominal pain

May exhibit:
Splinting/guarding over affected area (client commonly lies on affected side to restrict movement)

RESPIRATION

May report:
History of recurrent/chronic URIs, tuberculosis, COPD, cigarette smoking
Progressive dyspnea
Cough: Dry hacking (initially) progressing to productive cough

May exhibit:
Presence of tracheostomy/endotracheal (ET) tube
Tachypnea, shallow grunting respirations, use of accessory muscles, nasal flaring
Sputum: Scanty or copious; pink, rusty, or purulent (green, yellow, or white)
Percussion: Dull over consolidated areas
Fremitus: Tactile and vocal, gradually increases with consolidation
Pleural friction rub
Breath sounds: Diminished or absent over involved area or bronchial breath sounds over area(s) of consolidation, coarse inspiratory crackles
Color: Pallor or cyanosis of lips/nail beds

SAFETY

May report:

Recurrent chills

History of altered immune system (i.e., systemic lupus erythematosus [SLE], AIDS, active malignancies, neurologic disease, heart failure, diabetes, steroid or chemotherapy use), institutionalization, general debilitation

Fever (e.g., 102°F–104°F/39°C–40°C)

May exhibit:

Diaphoresis

Shaking

Rash may be noted in cases of rubeola or varicella

TEACHING/LEARNING

May report:

History of recent surgery, chronic alcohol use, intravenous (IV) drug therapy or abuse, immunosuppressive therapy

Use of herbal supplements (e.g., garlic, ginkgo, licorice, onion, tumeric, horehound, marshmallow, mullein, wild cherry bark, astragalus, echinacea, elderberry, goldenseal, Oregon graperoot)

Discharge plan considerations:

Assistance with self-care, homemaker tasks

Oxygen may be needed, especially if recovery is prolonged or other predisposing condition exists

Refer to section at end of plan for postdischarge considerations.

DIAGNOSTIC STUDIES

Chest x-ray: Identifies structural distribution (e.g., lobar, bronchial), may also reveal multiple abscesses/infiltrates, empyema (staphylococcus); scattered or localized infiltration (bacterial); or diffuse/extensive nodular infiltrates (more often viral). In *Mycoplasma* pneumonia, chest x-ray may be clear.

Fiberoptic bronchoscopy: May be both diagnostic (qualitative cultures) and therapeutic (reexpansion of lung segment).

ABGs/pulse oximetry: Abnormalities may be present, depending on extent of lung involvement and underlying lung disease. Pulse oximetry <90% indicates significant hypoxia.

Gram stain/cultures: Sputum collection; needle aspiration of empyema, pleural, and transtracheal or transthoracic fluids; lung biopsies and blood cultures may be done to recover causative organism. More than one type of organism may be present; common bacteria include *Diplococcus pneumoniae, Staphylococcus aureus,* α-hemolytic streptococcus, *Haemophilus influenzae,* and cytomegalovirus (CMV). *Note:* Sputum cultures may not identify all offending organisms. Blood cultures may show transient bacteremia.

CBC: Leukocytosis with a left shift is usually present in bacterial pneumonia, although a low white blood cell (WBC) count may be present in viral infection, immunosuppressed conditions such as AIDS, and overwhelming bacterial pneumonia.

Erythrocyte sedimentation rate (ESR): Elevated.

Serologic studies, e.g., viral or Legionella titers, cold agglutinins: Assist in differential diagnosis of specific organism.

Pulmonary function studies: Volumes may be decreased (congestion and alveolar collapse); airway pressure may be increased and compliance decreased. Shunting is present (hypoxemia).

Electrolytes: Sodium and chloride levels may be low.

Bilirubin: May be increased.

Percutaneous aspiration/open biopsy of lung tissues: May reveal typical intranuclear and cytoplasmic inclusions (CMV), characteristic giant cells (rubeola).

NURSING PRIORITIES

1. Maintain/improve respiratory function.
2. Prevent complications.
3. Support recuperative process.
4. Provide information about disease process/prognosis and treatment.

DISCHARGE GOALS

1. Ventilation and oxygenation adequate for individual needs.
2. Complications prevented/minimized.
3. Disease process/prognosis and therapeutic regimen understood.
4. Lifestyle changes identified/initiated to prevent recurrence.
5. Plan in place to meet needs after discharge.

NURSING DIAGNOSIS: ineffective Airway Clearance

May be related to

Tracheal bronchial inflammation, edema formation, increased sputum production
Pleuritic pain
Decreased energy, fatigue

Possibly evidenced by

Changes in rate, depth of respirations
Abnormal breath sounds, use of accessory muscles
Dyspnea, cyanosis
Cough, effective or ineffective; with/without sputum production

DESIRED OUTCOMES/EVALUATION CRITERIA—CLIENT WILL:

RESPIRATORY STATUS: Airway Patency (NOC)

Identify/demonstrate behaviors to achieve airway clearance.
Display patent airway with breath sounds clearing; absence of dyspnea, cyanosis.

ACTIONS/INTERVENTIONS	RATIONALE
Airway Management (NIC)	
Independent	
Assess rate/depth of respirations and chest movement. Monitor for signs of respiratory failure (e.g., cyanosis and severe tachypnea).	Tachypnea, shallow respirations, and asymmetric chest movement are frequently present because of discomfort of moving chest wall and/or fluid in lung. When pneumonia is severe, the client may require endotracheal intubation and mechanical ventilation to keep airways clear.
Auscultate lung fields, noting areas of decreased/absent airflow and adventitious breath sounds; e.g., crackles, wheezes.	Decreased airflow occurs in areas consolidated with fluid. Bronchial breath sounds (normal over bronchus) can also occur in consolidated areas. Crackles, rhonchi, and wheezes are heard on inspiration and/or expiration in response to fluid accumulation, thick secretions, and airway spasm/obstruction.
Elevate head of bed, change position frequently.	Keeping the head elevated lowers diaphragm, promoting chest expansion, aeration of lung segments, and mobilization and expectoration of secretions to keep the airway clear.
Assist client with frequent deep-breathing exercises. Demonstrate/help client learn to perform activity; e.g., splinting chest and effective coughing while in upright position.	Deep breathing facilitates maximum expansion of the lungs/smaller airways. Coughing is a natural self-cleaning mechanism, assisting the cilia to maintain patent airways. Splinting reduces chest discomfort, and an upright position favors deeper, more forceful cough effort. *Note:* Cough associated with pneumonias may last days to weeks or even months.
Suction as indicated (e.g., frequent or sustained cough, adventitious breath sounds, desaturation related to airway secretions).	Stimulates cough or mechanically clears airway in client who is unable to do so because of ineffective cough or decreased level of consciousness.
Force fluids to at least 3000 mL/day (unless contraindicated, as in heart failure). Offer warm, rather than cold, fluids.	Fluids (especially warm liquids) aid in mobilization and expectoration of secretions.

ACTIONS/INTERVENTIONS	RATIONALE
Collaborative	
Assist with/monitor effects of nebulizer treatments and other respiratory physiotherapy; e.g., incentive spirometer, IPPB, percussion, postural drainage. Perform treatments between meals and limit fluids when appropriate.	Facilitates liquefaction and removal of secretions. Postural drainage may not be effective in interstitial pneumonias or those causing alveolar exudate/destruction. Coordination of treatments/schedules and oral intake reduces likelihood of vomiting with coughing and expectorations.
Administer medications as indicated: mucolytics, expectorants, bronchodilators, analgesics.	Aids in reduction of bronchospasm and mobilization of secretions. Analgesics are given to improve cough effort by reducing discomfort, but should be used cautiously because they can decrease cough effort/depress respirations.
Provide supplemental fluids; e.g., IV, humidified oxygen, and room humidification.	Fluids are required to replace losses (including insensible) and aid in mobilization of secretions. *Note:* Some studies indicate that room humidification has been found to provide minimal benefit and is thought to increase the risk of transmitting infection.
Monitor serial chest x-rays, ABGs, pulse oximetry readings. (Refer to ND: impaired Gas Exchange, following.)	Follows progress and effects of disease process/therapeutic regimen, and facilitates necessary alterations in therapy.

NURSING DIAGNOSIS: impaired Gas Exchange

May be related to

Alveolar-capillary membrane changes (inflammatory effects)
Altered oxygen-carrying capacity of blood/release at cellular level (fever, shifting oxyhemoglobin curve)
Altered delivery of oxygen (hypoventilation)

Possibly evidenced by

Dyspnea, cyanosis
Tachycardia
Restlessness/changes in mentation
Hypoxia

DESIRED OUTCOMES/EVALUATION CRITERIA—CLIENT WILL:

RESPIRATORY STATUS: Gas Exchange (NOC)

Demonstrate improved ventilation and oxygenation of tissues by ABGs within client's acceptable range and absence of symptoms of respiratory distress.
Participate in actions to maximize oxygenation.

ACTIONS/INTERVENTIONS	RATIONALE
Respiratory Monitoring (NIC)	
Independent	
Assess respiratory rate, depth, and ease.	Manifestations of respiratory distress are dependent on/indicative of the degree of lung involvement and underlying general health status.
Observe color of skin, mucous membranes, and nail beds, noting presence of peripheral cyanosis (nail beds) or central cyanosis (circumoral).	Cyanosis of nail beds may represent vasoconstriction or the body's response to fever/chills; however, cyanosis of earlobes, mucous membranes, and skin around the mouth ("warm membranes") is indicative of systemic hypoxemia.

ACTIONS/INTERVENTIONS	RATIONALE
Assess mental status.	Restlessness, irritation, confusion, and somnolence may reflect hypoxemia/decreased cerebral oxygenation.
Monitor heart rate/rhythm.	Tachycardia is usually present as a result of fever/dehydration but may represent a response to hypoxemia.
Monitor body temperature, as indicated. Assist with comfort measures to reduce fever and chills; e.g., addition/removal of bedcovers, comfortable room temperature, and tepid or cool water sponge bath.	High fever (common in bacterial pneumonia and influenza) greatly increases metabolic demands and oxygen consumption and alters cellular oxygenation.
Maintain bedrest. Encourage use of relaxation techniques and diversional activities.	Prevents overexhaustion and reduces oxygen consumption/demands to facilitate resolution of infection.
Elevate head and encourage frequent position changes, deep breathing, and effective coughing.	These measures promote maximal inspiration, enhance expectoration of secretions to improve ventilation. (Refer to ND: ineffective Airway Clearance.)
Assess level of anxiety. Encourage verbalization of concerns/feelings. Answer questions honestly. Visit frequently, arrange for SO/visitors to stay with client as indicated.	Anxiety is a manifestation of psychologic concerns and physiologic responses to hypoxia. Providing reassurance and enhancing sense of security can reduce the psychologic component, thereby decreasing oxygen demand and adverse physiologic responses.
Observe for deterioration in condition, noting hypotension, copious amounts of pink/bloody sputum, pallor, cyanosis, change in level of consciousness, severe dyspnea, restlessness.	Shock and pulmonary edema are the most common causes of death in pneumonia and require immediate medical intervention.

Collaborative

Monitor ABGs, pulse oximetry.	Identifies problems (e.g., respiratory failure), follows progress of disease process or improvement; and facilitates alterations in pulmonary therapy.

Oxygen Therapy (NIC)

Administer oxygen therapy by appropriate means; e.g., nasal prongs, mask, Venturi mask.	The purpose of oxygen therapy is to maintain PaO_2 above 60 mm Hg (or greater than 90% O_2 saturation). Oxygen is administered by the method that provides appropriate delivery within the client's tolerance.
Prepare for/transfer to critical care setting if indicated.	Intubation and mechanical ventilation may be required in the event of severe respiratory insufficiency. (Refer to CP: Ventilatory Assistance (Mechanical.)

NURSING DIAGNOSIS: risk for Infection [spread]

Risk factors may include

Inadequate primary defenses (decreased ciliary action, stasis of respiratory secretions)
Inadequate secondary defenses (presence of existing infection, immunosuppression), chronic disease, malnutrition

Possibly evidenced by

[Not applicable; presence of signs and symptoms establishes an *actual* diagnosis.]

DESIRED OUTCOMES/EVALUATION CRITERIA—CLIENT WILL:

Infection Status (NOC)

Achieve timely resolution of current infection without complications.

KNOWLEDGE: Infection Control (NOC)

Identify interventions to prevent/reduce risk/spread of/secondary infection.

ACTIONS/INTERVENTIONS	RATIONALE
Infection Control (NIC)	
Independent	
Monitor vital signs closely, especially during initiation of therapy.	During this period of time, potentially fatal complications (hypotension/shock) may develop.
Instruct client concerning the disposition of secretions (e.g., raising and expectorating versus swallowing) and reporting changes in color, amount, and odor of secretions.	Although client may find expectoration offensive and attempt to limit or avoid it, it is essential that sputum be disposed of in a safe manner. Changes in characteristics of sputum reflect resolution of pneumonia or development of secondary infection.
Demonstrate/encourage good hand washing technique.	Effective means of reducing spread or acquisition of infection.
Change position frequently and provide good pulmonary toilet.	Promotes expectoration, clearing of infection.
Limit visitors as indicated.	Reduces likelihood of exposure to other infectious pathogens.
Institute isolation precautions as individually appropriate.	Dependent on type of infection, response to antibiotics, client's general health, and development of complications, isolation techniques may be desired to prevent spread/protect client from other infectious processes.
Encourage adequate rest balanced with moderate activity. Promote adequate nutritional intake.	Facilitates healing process and enhances natural resistance.
Monitor effectiveness of antimicrobial therapy.	Signs of improvement in condition should occur within 24–48 hr.
Investigate sudden changes/deterioration in condition, such as increasing chest pain, extra heart sounds, altered sensorium, recurring fever, changes in sputum characteristics.	Delayed recovery or increase in severity of symptoms suggests resistance to antibiotics or secondary infection. Complications affecting any/all organ systems include lung abscess/empyema, bacteremia, pericarditis/endocarditis, meningitis/encephalitis, and superinfections.
Collaborative	
Administer antimicrobials as indicated by results of sputum/blood cultures, e.g., macrolides (azithromycin [Zithromax], clarithromycin [Biaxin], erythromycin [E-Mycin]); penicillin combinations (e.g., amoxicillin and clavulanate [Augmentin]); tetracyclines (e.g., doxycycline [Doryx, Vibramycin, Achromycin]); fluoroquinolones (e.g., moxifloxacin[Avelox], levofloxacin [Levaquin], ciprofloxin [Cipro]); cephalosporins, (e.g., cephazolin [Ancef], cephalexin{Keflex}; cefuroxime [Ceftin, Zinacef]).	These drugs are used to combat most of the microbial pneumonias. Combinations of drugs can be used when the pneumonia is a result of mixed organisms.
Prepare for/assist with diagnostic studies as indicated.	Fiberoptic bronchoscopy (FOB) may be done in clients who do not respond in a reasonable amount of time to antimicrobial therapy to clarify diagnosis and therapeutic needs.

NURSING DIAGNOSIS: Activity Intolerance

May be related to

Imbalance between oxygen supply and demand
General weakness
Exhaustion associated with interruption in usual sleep pattern because of discomfort, excessive coughing, and dyspnea

Possibly evidenced by

Verbal reports of weakness, fatigue, exhaustion
Exertional dyspnea, tachypnea
Tachycardia in response to activity
Development/worsening of pallor/cyanosis

DESIRED OUTCOMES/EVALUATION CRITERIA—CLIENT WILL:

Activity Tolerance (NOC)

Report/demonstrate a measurable increase in tolerance to activity with absence of dyspnea and excessive fatigue, and vital signs within client's acceptable range.

ACTIONS/INTERVENTIONS	RATIONALE
Energy Management (NIC)	
Independent	
Evaluate client's response to activity. Note reports of dyspnea, increased weakness/fatigue, and changes in vital signs during and after activities.	Establishes client's capabilities/needs and facilitates choice of interventions.
Provide a quiet environment and limit visitors during acute phase as indicated. Encourage use of stress management and diversional activities as appropriate.	Reduces stress and excess stimulation, promoting rest.
Explain importance of rest in treatment plan and necessity for balancing activities with rest.	Bedrest is maintained during acute phase to decrease metabolic demands, thus conserving energy for healing. Activity restrictions thereafter are determined by individual client response to activity and resolution of respiratory insufficiency.
Assist client to assume comfortable position for rest/sleep.	Client may be comfortable with head of bed elevated, sleeping in a chair, or leaning forward on overbed table with pillow support.
Assist with self-care activities as necessary. Provide for progressive increase in activities during recovery phase.	Minimizes exhaustion and helps balance oxygen supply and demand.

NURSING DIAGNOSIS: acute Pain

May be related to

Inflammation of lung parenchyma
Cellular reactions to circulating toxins
Persistent coughing

Possibly evidenced by

Reports of pleuritic chest pain, headache, muscle/joint pain
Guarding of affected area
Distraction behaviors, restlessness

DESIRED OUTCOMES/EVALUATION CRITERIA—CLIENT WILL:

PAIN: Disruptive Effects (NOC)

Verbalize relief/control of pain.
Demonstrate relaxed manner, resting/sleeping and engaging in activity appropriately.

ACTIONS/INTERVENTIONS	RATIONALE
Pain Management (NIC)	
Independent	
Determine pain characteristics; e.g., sharp, constant, stabbing. Investigate changes in character/location/intensity of pain.	Chest pain, usually present to some degree with pneumonia, may also herald the onset of complications of pneumonia, such as pericarditis and endocarditis.
Monitor vital signs.	Changes in heart rate or BP may indicate that client is experiencing pain, especially when other reasons for changes in vital signs have been ruled out.
Provide comfort measures; e.g., back rubs, change of position, quiet music or conversation. Encourage use of relaxation/breathing exercises.	Nonanalgesic measures administered with a gentle touch can lessen discomfort and augment therapeutic effects of analgesics. Client involvement in pain control measures promotes independence and enhances sense of well-being.
Offer frequent oral hygiene.	Mouth breathing and oxygen therapy can irritate and dry out mucous membranes, potentiating general discomfort.
Instruct and assist client in chest splinting techniques during coughing episodes. (Refer to ND: ineffective Airway Clearance.)	Aids in control of chest discomfort while enhancing effectiveness of cough effort.
Collaborative	
Administer analgesics and antitussives as indicated.	These medications may be used to suppress nonproductive/paroxysmal cough or reduce excess mucus, thereby enhancing general comfort/rest.

NURSING DIAGNOSIS: risk for imbalanced Nutrition: less than body requirements

Risk factors may include

Increased metabolic needs secondary to fever and infectious process
Anorexia associated with bacterial toxins, the odor and taste of sputum, and certain aerosol treatments
Abdominal distention/gas associated with swallowing air during dyspneic episodes

Possibly evidenced by

[Not applicable; presence of signs and symptoms establishes an *actual* diagnosis.]

DESIRED OUTCOMES/EVALUATION CRITERIA—CLIENT WILL:

Nutritional Status (NOC)

Demonstrate increased appetite.
Maintain/regain desired body weight.

ACTIONS/INTERVENTIONS	RATIONALE
Nutrition Therapy (NIC)	
Independent	
Identify factors that are contributing to nausea/vomiting; e.g., copious sputum, aerosol treatments, severe dyspnea, pain.	Choice of interventions depends on the underlying cause of the problem.
Provide covered container for sputum and replace at frequent intervals. Assist with/encourage oral hygiene after emesis, after aerosol and postural drainage treatments, and before meals.	Eliminates noxious sights, tastes, smells from the client's environment and can reduce nausea.
Schedule respiratory treatments at least 1 hr before meals.	Reduces effects of nausea associated with these treatments.
Auscultate for bowel sounds. Observe/palpate for abdominal distention.	Bowel sounds may be diminished/absent if the infectious process is severe/prolonged. Abdominal distention may occur as a result of air swallowing or reflect the influence of bacterial toxins on the gastrointestinal (GI) tract.
Provide small, frequent meals, including dry foods (toast, crackers) and/or foods that are appealing to client.	These measures may enhance intake even though appetite may be slow to return.
Evaluate general nutritional state, obtain baseline weight.	Presence of chronic conditions (e.g., COPD or alcoholism) or financial limitations can contribute to malnutrition, lowered resistance to infection, and/or delayed response to therapy.

NURSING DIAGNOSIS: risk for deficient Fluid Volume

Risk factors may include

Excessive fluid loss (fever, profuse diaphoresis, mouth breathing/hyperventilation, vomiting)
Decreased oral intake

Possibly evidenced by

[Not applicable; presence of signs and symptoms establishes an *actual* diagnosis.]

DESIRED OUTCOMES/EVALUATION CRITERIA—CLIENT WILL:

Demonstrate fluid balance evidenced by individually appropriate parameters; e.g., moist mucous membranes, good skin turgor, prompt capillary refill, stable vital signs.

ACTIONS/INTERVENTIONS	RATIONALE
Fluid Management (NIC)	
Independent	
Assess vital sign changes; e.g., increased temperature/prolonged fever, tachycardia, orthostatic hypotension.	Elevated temperature/prolonged fever increases metabolic rate and fluid loss through evaporation. Orthostatic BP changes and increasing tachycardia may indicate systemic fluid deficit.
Assess skin turgor, moisture of mucous membranes (lips, tongue).	Indirect indicators of adequacy of fluid volume, although oral mucous membranes may be dry because of mouth breathing and supplemental oxygen.
Note reports of nausea/vomiting.	Presence of these symptoms reduces oral intake.
Monitor intake and output (I&O), noting color, character of urine. Calculate fluid balance. Be aware of insensible losses. Weigh as indicated.	Provides information about adequacy of fluid volume and replacement needs.
Force fluids to at least 3000 mL/day or as individually appropriate.	Meets basic fluid needs, reducing risk of dehydration.
Collaborative	
Administer medications as indicated; e.g., antipyretics, antiemetics.	Useful in reducing fluid losses.
Provide supplemental IV fluids as necessary.	In the presence of reduced intake/excessive loss, use of parenteral route may correct/prevent deficiency.

NURSING DIAGNOSIS: deficient Knowledge [Learning Need] regarding condition, treatment, self-care, and discharge needs

May be related to

Lack of exposure
Misinterpretation of information
Altered recall

Possibly evidenced by

Requests for information; statement of misconception
Failure to improve/recurrence

DESIRED OUTCOMES/EVALUATION CRITERIA—CLIENT WILL:

KNOWLEDGE: Illness Care (NOC)

Verbalize understanding of condition, disease process, and prognosis.
Verbalize understanding of therapeutic regimen.
Initiate necessary lifestyle changes.
Participate in treatment program.

ACTIONS/INTERVENTIONS	RATIONALE
TEACHING: Disease Process (NIC)	
Independent	
Review normal lung function, pathology of condition.	Promotes understanding of current situation and importance of cooperating with treatment regimen.
Discuss debilitating aspects of disease, length of convalescence, and recovery expectations. Identify self-care and homemaker needs/resources.	Information can enhance coping and help reduce anxiety and excessive concern. Respiratory symptoms may be slow to resolve, and fatigue and weakness can persist for an extended period. These factors may be associated with depression and the need for various forms of support and assistance.
Provide information in written and verbal form.	Fatigue and depression can affect ability to assimilate information/follow medical regimen.
Stress importance of continuing effective coughing/deep-breathing exercises.	During initial 6–8 weeks after discharge, client is at greatest risk for recurrence of pneumonia.
Emphasize necessity for continuing antibiotic therapy for prescribed period.	Early discontinuation of antibiotics may result in failure to completely resolve infectious process.
Review importance of cessation of smoking.	Smoking destroys tracheobronchial ciliary action, irritates bronchial mucosa, and inhibits alveolar macrophages, compromising body's natural defense against infection.
Outline steps to enhance general health and well-being; e.g., balanced rest and activity, well-rounded diet, program of aerobic exercise or strength training (particularly elderly individuals), avoidance of crowds during cold/flu season and persons with URIs.	Increases natural defenses/immunity, limits exposure to pathogens. Recent research suggests elders with moderate physical limitations can significantly improve immunologic defenses through exercise that increases levels of salivary IgA (immunoglobulin that aids in blocking infectious agents entering through mucous membranes).
Stress importance of continuing medical follow-up and obtaining vaccinations/immunizations as appropriate.	May prevent recurrence of pneumonia and/or related complications.
Identify signs/symptoms requiring notification of healthcare provider; e.g., increasing dyspnea, chest pain, prolonged fatigue, weight loss, fever/chills, persistence of productive cough, changes in mentation.	Prompt evaluation and timely intervention may prevent/minimize complications.

POTENTIAL CONSIDERATIONS following acute hospitalization (dependent on client's age, physical condition/presence of complications, personal resources, and life responsibilities)

Fatigue—increased energy requirements to perform ADLs, discomfort, effects of antimicrobial therapy.

risk for Infection—inadequate secondary response (e.g., leukopenia, suppressed inflammatory response), chronic disease, malnutrition, current use of antibiotics.

ineffective Therapeutic Regimen Management—complexity of therapeutic regimen, economic difficulties, perceived seriousness/susceptibility.

CP 5–1 Sample CP: Bacterial Pneumonia, Hospital. ELOS: 5 Days Medical Unit

ND and Categories of Care	Day 1 ____	Day 2 ____	Day 3 ____	Day 4 ____	Day 5 ____
Impaired gas exchange R/T alveolar congestion, inflammation, hypoventilation	Goals Participate in activities to maximize oxygenation and airway clearance	Demonstrate improving ventilation and oxygenation by lessening symptoms of respiratory distress, ABGs approaching acceptable levels	Verbalize understanding of general healthcare needs	Initiate activities accepting responsibility for therapeutic regimen within level of ability Plan in place to meet postdischarge needs	Demonstrate ABGs within client's acceptable range and absence of respiratory distress
Referrals	Pulmonary specialist		Home care Home O_2/Resp. Therapist		
Diagnostic Studies	CXR				
	ABGs CBC, electrolytes	→ Repeat if pulse ox <87%	Repeat if WBC count elevated, febrile, or ABGs not WNL Hb/Hct		
	Sputum C&S/Gram stain				
	Blood culture				
	Pulse oximetry q4h	→ D/C if 92%			
Additional assessments	Respiratory rate, rhythm, depth; use of accessory muscles; color of skin/mucous membranes q4h	→	→ q8h	→	→
	Breath sounds q4h	→	→ q8h	→	→
	Cough/sputum characteristics	→	→	→	→
	Vital signs q4h	→	→ q8h	→	→
	I&O q8h	→	→	→	→
	Weight qd	→	→	→	→
Medications Allergies:	IV antibiotics	→	→ PO	→	→
	Bronchodilator via MDI or nebulizer	→ MDI	→	→	→
	Mucolytic	→	→	→	→
	Antitussives—prn	→	→	→	→
	Acetaminophen if temperature above 101°F	→	→ D/C		
	Analgesics—prn	→ D/C			
Client education	Orient to unit/room Review advance directives Diagnostic tests/results Pulmonary hygiene: T, C, DB, splinting techniques	Adaptive breathing techniques as indicated Pacing of activities Smoking cessation Fluid/nutritional needs, balancing activity/rest	Individual risk factors, prevention of recurrence, vaccinations/immunizations Signs/symptoms to report to healthcare provider	Medications postdischarge: dose, time, route, purpose, side effects Proper use and care of home care equipment (e.g., O_2, concentrator, nebulizer)	Provide written instructions Schedule for follow-up appointments
Additional nursing actions	Position for maximal respiratory effort	→ per self	→	→	→
	Assist with physical care	→	→ as necessary	→ per self	→
	Incentive spirometry q4h	→	→ per self WA	→	→
	Supplemental O_2	→	→	→ D/C	
	Oral care—prn	→per self	→	→	
	Suction as indicated	→	→	→ D/C	
	Screen visitors/staff for URI	→	→	→ D/C	
	Encourage fluid to 2500 mL/day as tolerated	→	→	→ per self	→

LUNG CANCER (POSTOPERATIVE CARE)

Lung cancer is the leading cause of cancer death in the United States. It usually develops within the wall or epithelium of the bronchial tree and is divided into two major categories—small cell lung cancers (SCLC) and non–small cell lung cancers (NSCLC), which include adenocarcinoma, squamous cell, and large cell carcinomas. Prognosis is generally poor, varying with the type of cancer and extent of involvement at the time of diagnosis. Survival rates are better with NSCLC, especially if treated in early stages. Although NSCLC tumors are frequently associated with metastases, they are generally slow growing. SCLC is more aggressive and fast growing. Surgery is seldom an option in SCLC.

Treatment options can include combinations of surgery, radiation, and chemotherapy. Surgery is the primary treatment for NSCLC stage I and stage II tumors. Selected stage III carcinomas may be operable if the tumor is resectable. Surgical procedures for operable tumors of the lung include:

1. Pneumonectomy (removal of an entire lung); performed for lesions originating in the mainstem bronchus or lobar bronchus.
2. Lobectomy (removal of one lobe); preferred for peripheral carcinoma localized in a lobe.
3. Wedge or segmental resection; performed for lesions that are small and well contained within one segment.
4. Endoscopic laser resection may be done on peripheral tumors to reduce the necessity of cutting through ribs.

CARE SETTING

Inpatient surgical and possibly subacute units.

RELATED CONCERNS

Cancer, page 857
Pneumothorax/hemothorax, page 150
Psychosocial aspects of care, page 770
Radical neck surgery: laryngectomy (postoperative care), page 157
Surgical intervention, page 788

Client Assessment Database (Preoperative)

Findings depend on type, duration of cancer, and extent of metastasis.

ACTIVITY/REST

May report: Fatigue, inability to maintain usual routine, dyspnea with activity

May exhibit: Lassitude (usually in advanced stage)

CIRCULATION

May exhibit: Jugular venous distention (JVD) (with vena caval obstruction)
Heart sounds: Pericardial rub (indicating effusion)
Tachycardia/dysrhythmias
Clubbing of fingers

EGO INTEGRITY

May report: Frightened feelings, fear of outcome of surgery
Denial of severity of condition/potential for malignancy

May exhibit: Restlessness, insomnia, repetitive questioning

ELIMINATION

May report: Intermittent diarrhea (hormonal imbalance, SCLC)
Increased frequency/amount of urine (hormonal imbalance, epidermoid tumor)

FOOD/FLUID

May report: Weight loss, poor appetite, decreased food intake
Difficulty swallowing
Thirst/increased fluid intake

May exhibit: Thin, emaciated, or wasted appearance (late stages)
Edema of face/neck, chest, back (vena caval obstruction); facial/periorbital edema (hormonal imbalance, SCLC)
Glucose in urine (hormonal imbalance, epidermoid tumor)

PAIN/DISCOMFORT

May report: Chest pain (not usually present in early stages and not always present in advanced stages), which may/may not be affected by position change

Shoulder/arm pain (particularly with large cell carcinoma or adenocarcinoma)

Bone/joint pain: Cartilage erosion secondary to increased growth hormones (large cell carcinoma or adenocarcinoma)

Intermittent abdominal pain

May exhibit: Distraction behaviors (restlessness, withdrawal)

Guarding/protective actions

RESPIRATION

May report: Mild cough or change in usual cough pattern and/or sputum production

Shortness of breath

Occupational exposure to pollutants, industrial dusts (e.g., asbestos, iron oxides, coal dust), radioactive material

Hoarseness/change in voice (vocal cord paralysis)

History of smoking

May exhibit: Dyspnea, aggravated by exertion

Increased tactile fremitus (indicating consolidation)

Brief crackles/wheezes on inspiration or expiration (impaired airflow)

Persistent crackles/wheezes; tracheal shift (space-occupying lesion)

Hemoptysis

SAFETY

May exhibit: Fever may be present (large cell carcinoma or adenocarcinoma)

Bruising, discoloration of skin (hormonal imbalance, SCLC)

SEXUALITY

May exhibit: Gynecomastia (neoplastic hormonal changes, large cell carcinoma)

Amenorrhea/impotence (hormonal imbalance, SCLC)

TEACHING/LEARNING

May report: Familial risk factors: Cancer (especially lung), tuberculosis

Failure to improve

Use of vitamins/herbal supplements (e.g., vitamins A, C, E, riboflavin, folic acid, ashwganda, birch, yellow doc, milk thistletumeric, ginger, red clover, echinacea, astragalus, reishi and shiitake mushrooms, zedoary)

Discharge plan considerations: Assistance with transportation, medications, treatments, self-care, homemaker/maintenance tasks.

Refer to section at end of plan for postdischarge considerations.

DIAGNOSTIC STUDIES

Chest x-ray (PA [posteroanterior] and lateral): Lung cancer is usually discovered on chest x-ray. Size and location of mass can be determined. Peripheral nodules, hilar and mediastinal changes can suggest lymphadenopathy. Pleural effusions and endobronchial obstruction may be seen.

Chest computed tomography (CT): Used to confirm abnormalities seen on chest x-ray, to detect early (<1 cm) lesions not visible on chest x-ray, and to assess spread to the mediastinum. Outlines shape, size, and location of lesion. May reveal erosion of ribs or vertebrae.

Abdominal CT: Detects abnormalities below the diaphragm, especially metastases to the liver and adrenal glands, which are often asymptomatic.

Positron emission tomography (PET): Based on the uptake of radioactive glucose in metabolically active cells, it is used to determine differences in the metabolism of normal and neoplastic cells. Identifies occult metastatic disease in the mediastinum and distant sites. More sensitive and specific than CT scans.

Magnetic resonance imaging (MRI) scan: May be used in combination with, or instead of, CT scans to determine tumor size/location and for staging.
Fiberoptic bronchoscopy: Allows for direct visualization, regional washings, and cytologic brushing of lesions (large percentage of bronchogenic carcinomas may be visualized).
Cytologic examinations (sputum, pleural, or lymph node): Performed to assess presence/stage of carcinoma, and may identify tumors of the bronchial wall.
Needle or tissue biopsy: May be performed on scalene nodes, hilar lymph nodes, or pleura to establish diagnosis.
Mediastinoscopy: May be performed to evaluate medialstinal and hilar lymph nodes (especially for nodes larger than 1 cm), to confirm diagnosis, and to aid in determining if client is good candidate for surgical intervention.
Video-assisted thoracoscopy (VATS): Common thoracic surgical procedure that allows more complete staging for lung cancer while reducing surgical trauma and postoperative pain associated with thoracotomy. Allows assessment of suspicious adenopathy in areas inaccessible to conventional mediastinoscopy.
Pulmonary function studies and ABGs: Assess lung capacity to meet postoperative ventilatory needs.
Skin tests, absolute lymphocyte counts: May be done to evaluate for immunocompetence (common in lung cancers).
Bone scan: Evaluate presence of bone metastases in client with bone pain, chest pain, or an elevated calcium or alkaline phosphatase level.
CT or MRI scan of brain: Performed when central nervous system signs or symptoms suggest brain metastases.

NURSING PRIORITIES

1. Maintain/improve respiratory function.
2. Control/alleviate pain.
3. Support efforts to cope with diagnosis/situation.
4. Provide information about disease process/prognosis and therapeutic regimen.

DISCHARGE GOALS

1. Oxygenation/ventilation adequate to meet individual activity needs.
2. Pain controlled.
3. Anxiety/fear decreased to manageable level.
4. Free of preventable complications.
5. Disease process/prognosis and planned therapies understood.
6. Plan in place to meet needs after discharge.

NURSING DIAGNOSIS: impaired Gas Exchange

May be related to

Removal of lung tissue
Altered oxygen supply (hypoventilation)
Decreased oxygen-carrying capacity of blood (blood loss)

Possibly evidenced by

Dyspnea
Restlessness/changes in mentation
Hypoxemia and hypercapnia
Cyanosis

DESIRED OUTCOMES/EVALUATION CRITERIA—CLIENT WILL:

RESPIRATORY STATUS: Gas Exchange (NOC)

Demonstrate improved ventilation and adequate oxygenation of tissues by ABGs within client's normal range.
Be free of symptoms of respiratory distress.

ACTIONS/INTERVENTIONS	RATIONALE
Respiratory Management (NIC)	
Independent	
Note respiratory rate, depth, and ease of respirations. Observe for use of accessory muscles, pursed-lip breathing, changes in skin/mucous membrane color; e.g., pallor, cyanosis.	Respirations may be increased as a result of pain or as an initial compensatory mechanism to accommodate for loss of lung tissue. However, increased work of breathing and cyanosis may indicate increasing oxygen consumption and energy expenditures and/or reduced respiratory reserve; e.g., elderly client or extensive COPD.
Auscultate lungs for air movement and abnormal breath sounds.	Consolidation and lack of air movement on operative side are normal in the pneumonectomy client; however, the lobectomy client should demonstrate normal airflow in remaining lobes.
Investigate restlessness and changes in mentation/level of consciousness.	May indicate increased hypoxia or complications such as mediastinal shift in pneumonectomy client when accompanied by tachypnea, tachycardia, and tracheal deviation.
Assess client response to activity. Encourage rest periods/limit activities to client tolerance.	Increased oxygen consumption/demand and stress of surgery can result in increased dyspnea and changes in vital signs with activity; however, early mobilization is desired to help prevent pulmonary complications and to obtain and maintain respiratory and circulatory efficiency. Adequate rest balanced with activity can prevent respiratory compromise.
Note development of fever.	Fever within the first 24 hr after surgery is frequently due to atelectasis. Temperature elevation within the 5th to 10th postoperative day usually indicates an infection; e.g., wound or systemic.
Airway Management (NIC)	
Maintain patent airway by positioning, suctioning, use of airway adjuncts.	Airway obstruction impedes ventilation, impairing gas exchange. (Refer to ND: ineffective Airway Clearance.)
Reposition frequently, placing client in sitting and supine to side positions.	Maximizes lung expansion and drainage of secretions.
Avoid positioning client with a pneumonectomy on the operative side; instead, favor the "good lung down" position.	Research shows that positioning clients following lung surgery with their "good lung down" maximizes oxygenation by using gravity to enhance blood flow to the healthy lung, thus creating the best possible match between ventilation and perfusion.
Encourage/assist with deep-breathing exercises and pursed-lip breathing as appropriate.	Promotes maximal ventilation and oxygenation and reduces/prevents atelectasis.
TUBE CARE: Chest (NIC)	
Maintain patency of chest drainage system following lobectomy, segmental/wedge resection procedures.	Drains fluid from pleural cavity to promote reexpansion of remaining lung segments.
Note changes in amount/type of chest tube drainage.	Bloody drainage should decrease in amount and change to a more serous composition as recovery progresses. A sudden increase in amount of bloody drainage or return to frank bleeding suggests thoracic bleeding/hemothorax; sudden cessation suggests blockage of tube, requiring further evaluation and intervention.
Observe presence/degree of bubbling in water-seal chamber.	Air leaks immediately postoperatively are not uncommon, especially following lobectomy or segmental resection; however, this should diminish as healing progresses. Prolonged or new leaks require evaluation to identify problems in client versus the drainage system.

ACTIONS/INTERVENTIONS	RATIONALE
Airway Management (NIC)	
Collaborative	
Administer supplemental oxygen via nasal cannula, partial rebreathing mask, or high-humidity face mask, as indicated.	Maximizes available oxygen, especially while ventilation is reduced because of anesthetic, depression, or pain, and during period of compensatory physiologic shift of circulation to remaining functional alveolar units.
Assist with/encourage use of incentive spirometer.	Prevents/reduces atelectasis and promotes reexpansion of small airways.
Monitor/graph ABGs, pulse oximetry readings. Note hemoglobin (Hb) levels.	Decreasing PaO_2 or increasing $PaCO_2$ may indicate need for ventilatory support. Significant blood loss can result in decreased oxygen-carrying capacity, reducing PaO_2.

NURSING DIAGNOSIS: ineffective Airway Clearance

May be related to

Increased amount/viscosity of secretions
Restricted chest movement/pain
Fatigue/weakness

Possibly evidenced by

Changes in rate/depth of respiration
Abnormal breath sounds
Ineffective cough
Dyspnea

DESIRED OUTCOMES/EVALUATION CRITERIA—CLIENT WILL:

RESPIRATORY STATUS: Airway Patency (NOC)

Demonstrate patent airway, with fluid secretions easily expectorated, clear breath sounds, and noiseless respirations.

ACTIONS/INTERVENTIONS	RATIONALE
Airway Management (NIC)	
Independent	
Auscultate chest for character of breath sounds and presence of secretions.	Noisy respirations, rhonchi, and wheezes are indicative of retained secretions and/or airway obstruction.
Assist client with/instruct in effective deep breathing and coughing with upright position (sitting) and splinting of incision.	Upright position favors maximal lung expansion, and splinting improves force of cough effort to mobilize and remove secretions. Splinting may be done by nurse (placing hands anteriorly and posteriorly over chest wall) and by client (with pillows) as strength improves.
Observe amount and character of sputum/aspirated secretions. Investigate changes as indicated.	Increased amounts of colorless (or blood-streaked)/watery secretions are normal initially and should decrease as recovery progresses. Presence of thick/tenacious, bloody, or purulent sputum suggests development of secondary problems (e.g., dehydration, pulmonary edema, local hemorrhage, or infection) that require correction/treatment.

ACTIONS/INTERVENTIONS	RATIONALE
Suction if cough is weak or breath sounds not cleared by cough effort. Avoid deep endotracheal/nasotracheal suctioning in pneumonectomy client if possible.	"Routine" suctioning increases risk of hypoxemia and mucosal damage. Deep tracheal suctioning is generally contraindicated following pneumonectomy to reduce the risk of rupture of the bronchial stump suture line. If suctioning is unavoidable, it should be done gently and only to induce effective coughing.
Encourage oral fluid intake (at least 2500 mL/day) within cardiac tolerance.	Adequate hydration aids in keeping secretions loose/enhances expectoration.
Assess for pain/discomfort and medicate on a routine basis and before breathing exercises.	Encourages client to move, cough more effectively, and breathe more deeply to prevent respiratory insufficiency.

Collaborative

Provide/assist with incentive spirometer; postural drainage/percussion as indicated.	Improves lung expansion/ventilation and facilitates removal of secretions. *Note:* Postural drainage may be contraindicated in some clients, and in any event must be performed cautiously to prevent respiratory embarrassment and incisional discomfort.
Use humidified oxygen/ultrasonic nebulizer. Provide additional fluids via IV as indicated.	Providing maximal hydration helps loosen/liquefy secretions to promote expectoration. Impaired oral intake necessitates IV supplementation to maintain hydration.
Administer bronchodilators, expectorants, and/or analgesics as indicated.	Relieves bronchospasm to improve airflow. Expectorants increase mucus production and liquefy and reduce viscosity of secretions, facilitating removal. Alleviation of chest discomfort promotes cooperation with breathing exercises and enhances effectiveness of respiratory therapies.

NURSING DIAGNOSIS: acute Pain

May be related to

Surgical incision, tissue trauma, and disruption of intercostal nerves
Presence of chest tube(s)
Cancer invasion of pleura, chest wall

Possibly evidenced by

Verbal reports of discomfort
Guarding of affected area
Distraction behaviors; e.g., restlessness
Narrowed focus (withdrawal)
Changes in BP, heart/respiratory rate

DESIRED OUTCOMES/EVALUATION CRITERIA—CLIENT WILL:

Pain Level (NOC)

Report pain relieved/controlled.
Appear relaxed and sleep/rest appropriately.
Participate in desired/needed activities.

ACTIONS/INTERVENTIONS	RATIONALE
Pain Management (NIC)	
Independent	
Ask client about pain. Determine pain location and characteristics; e.g., continuous, aching, stabbing, burning. Have client rate intensity on a 0–10 scale.	Helpful in evaluating cancer-related pain symptoms, which may involve viscera, nerve, or bone tissue. Use of rating scale aids client in assessing level of pain and provides tool for evaluating effectiveness of analgesics, enhancing client control of pain.
Assess client's verbal and nonverbal pain cues.	Discrepancy between verbal/nonverbal cues may provide clues to degree of pain, need for/effectiveness of interventions.
Note possible pathophysiologic and psychologic causes of pain.	Fear, distress, anxiety, and grief over confirmed diagnosis of cancer can impair ability to cope. In addition, a posterolateral incision is more uncomfortable for client than an anterolateral incision. The presence of chest tubes can greatly increase discomfort.
Evaluate effectiveness of pain control. Encourage sufficient medication to manage pain; change medication or time span as appropriate.	Pain perception and pain relief are subjective, thus pain management is best left to client's discretion. If client is unable to provide input, the nurse should observe physiological and nonverbal signs of pain and administer medications on a regular basis.
Encourage verbalization of feelings about the pain.	Fears/concerns can increase muscle tension and lower threshold of pain perception. (Refer to ND: Fear/Anxiety [specify level], following.)
Provide comfort measures; e.g., frequent changes of position, back rubs, support with pillows. Encourage use of relaxation techniques; e.g., visualization, guided imagery, and appropriate diversional activities.	Promotes relaxation and redirects attention. Relieves discomfort and augments therapeutic effects of analgesia.
Schedule rest periods, provide quiet environment.	Decreases fatigue and conserves energy, enhancing coping abilities.
Assist with self-care activities, breathing/arm exercises, and ambulation.	Prevents undue fatigue and incisional strain. Encouragement and physical assistance/support may be needed for some time before client is able or confident enough to perform these activities because of pain or fear of pain.
Collaborative	
Assist with client-controlled analgesia (PCA) or analgesia through epidural catheter. Administer intermittent analgesics routinely as indicated, especially 45–60 min before respiratory treatments, deep-breathing/coughing exercises.	Maintaining a constant drug level avoids cyclic periods of pain, aids in muscle healing, and improves respiratory function and emotional comfort/coping.

NURSING DIAGNOSIS: Fear/Anxiety [specify level]

May be related to

Situational crises
Threat to/change in health status
Perceived threat of death

Possibly evidenced by

Withdrawal
Apprehension

Anger
Increased pain, sympathetic stimulation
Expressions of denial, shock, guilt, insomnia

DESIRED OUTCOMES/EVALUATION CRITERIA—CLIENT WILL:

Fear Self-Control/Anxiety Self-Control (NOC)

Acknowledge and discuss fears/concerns.
Demonstrate appropriate range of feelings and appear relaxed/resting appropriately.
Verbalize accurate knowledge of situation.
Report beginning use of individually appropriate coping strategies.

ACTIONS/INTERVENTIONS	RATIONALE
Anxiety Reduction (NIC)	
Independent	
Evaluate client/SO level of understanding of diagnosis.	Client and SO are hearing and assimilating new information that includes changes in self-image and lifestyle. Understanding perceptions of those involved sets the tone for individualizing care and provides information necessary for choosing appropriate interventions.
Acknowledge reality of client's fears/concerns and encourage expression of feelings.	Support may enable client to begin exploring/dealing with the reality of cancer and its treatment. Client may need time to identify feelings and even more time to begin to express them.
Provide opportunity for questions and answer them honestly. Be sure that client and care providers have the same understanding of terms used.	Establishes trust and reduces misperceptions/misinterpretation of information.
Accept, but do not reinforce, client's denial of the situation.	When extreme denial or anxiety is interfering with progress of recovery, the issues facing client need to be explained and resolutions explored.
Note comments/behaviors indicative of beginning acceptance and/or use of effective strategies to deal with situation.	Fear/anxiety will diminish as client begins to accept/deal positively with reality. Indicator of client's readiness to accept responsibility for participation in recovery and to "resume life."
Involve client/SO in care planning. Provide time to prepare for events/treatments.	May help restore some feeling of control/independence to client who feels powerless in dealing with diagnosis and treatment.
Provide for client's physical comfort.	It is difficult to deal with emotional issues when experiencing extreme/persistent physical discomfort.

NURSING DIAGNOSIS: deficient Knowledge [Learning Need] regarding condition, treatment, prognosis, self-care, and discharge needs

May be related to

Lack of exposure, unfamiliarity with information/resources
Information misinterpretation
Lack of recall

Possibly evidenced by

Statements of concern; request for information
Inadequate follow-through of instruction
Inappropriate or exaggerated behaviors; e.g., hysterical, hostile, agitated, apathetic

DESIRED OUTCOMES/EVALUATION CRITERIA—CLIENT WILL:

KNOWLEDGE: Disease Process (NOC)

Verbalize understanding of ramifications of diagnosis, prognosis, possible complications.
Participate in learning process.

KNOWLEDGE: Treatment Regimen (NOC)

Verbalize understanding of therapeutic regimen.
Correctly perform necessary procedures and explain reasons for the actions.
Initiate necessary lifestyle changes.

ACTIONS/INTERVENTIONS	RATIONALE
TEACHING: Disease Process (NIC)	
Independent	
Discuss diagnosis, current/planned therapies, and expected outcomes.	Provides individually specific information, creating knowledge base for subsequent learning regarding home management. Radiation or chemotherapy may follow surgical intervention, and information is essential to enable the client/SO to make informed decisions.
Reinforce surgeon's explanation of particular surgical procedure, providing diagram as appropriate. Incorporate this information into discussion about short-/long-term recovery expectations.	Length of rehabilitation and prognosis depend on type of surgical procedure, preoperative physical condition, and duration/degree of complications.
Discuss necessity of planning for follow-up care before discharge.	Follow-up assessment of respiratory status and general health is imperative to assure optimal recovery. Also provides opportunity to readdress concerns/questions at a less stressful time.
Identify signs/symptoms requiring medical evaluations; e.g., changes in appearance of incision, development of respiratory difficulty, fever, increased chest pain, changes in appearance of sputum.	Early detection and timely intervention may prevent/minimize complications.
Help client determine activity tolerance and set goals.	Weakness and fatigue should decrease as lung(s) heals and respiratory function improves during recovery period, especially if cancer was completely removed. If cancer is advanced, it is emotionally helpful for client to be able to set realistic activity goals to achieve optimal independence.
Evaluate availability/adequacy of support system(s) and necessity for assistance in self-care/home management.	General weakness and activity limitations may reduce individual's ability to meet own needs.
Recommend alternating rest periods with activity and light tasks with heavy tasks. Stress avoidance of heavy lifting, isometric/strenuous upper body exercise. Reinforce physician's time limitations about lifting.	Generalized weakness and fatigue are usual in the early recovery period but should diminish as respiratory function improves and healing progresses. Rest and sleep enhance coping abilities, reduce nervousness (common in this phase), and promote healing. *Note:* Strenuous use of arms can place undue stress on incision because chest muscles may be weaker than normal for 3–6 months following surgery.
Recommend stopping any activity that causes undue fatigue or increased shortness of breath.	Exhaustion aggravates respiratory insufficiency.
Encourage inspection of incisions. Review expectations for healing with client.	Healing begins immediately, but complete healing takes time. As healing progresses, incision lines may appear dry with crusty scabs. Underlying tissue may look bruised and feel tense, warm, and lumpy (resolving hematoma).

ACTIONS/INTERVENTIONS	RATIONALE
Instruct client/SO to watch for/report places in incision that do not heal or reopening of healed incision, any drainage (bloody or purulent), localized area of swelling with redness or increased pain that is hot to touch.	Signs/symptoms indicating failure to heal, development of complications requiring further medical evaluation/intervention.
Suggest wearing soft cotton shirts and loose-fitting clothing, cover/pad portion of incision as indicated, leave incision open to air as much as possible.	Reduces suture line irritation and pressure from clothing. Leaving incisions open to air promotes healing process and may reduce risk of infection.
Shower in warm water, washing incision gently. Avoid tub baths until approved by physician.	Keeps incision clean, promotes circulation/healing. *Note:* "Climbing" out of tub requires use of arms and pectoral muscles, which can put undue stress on incision.
Support incision with Steri-Strips as needed when sutures/staples are removed.	Aids in maintaining approximation of wound edges to promote healing.
Instruct/provide rationale for arm/shoulder exercises. Have client/SO demonstrate exercises. Encourage following graded increase in number/intensity of routine repetitions.	Simple arm circles and lifting arms over the head or out to the affected side are initiated on the first or second postoperative day to restore normal range of motion (ROM) of shoulder and to prevent ankylosis of the affected shoulder.
Stress importance of avoiding exposure to smoke, air pollution, and contact with individuals with URIs.	Protects lung(s) from irritation and reduces risk of infection.
Review nutritional/fluid needs. Suggest increasing protein and use of high-calorie snacks as appropriate.	Meeting cellular energy requirements and maintaining good circulating volume for tissue perfusion facilitate tissue regeneration/healing process.
Identify individually appropriate community resources; e.g., American Cancer Society, visiting nurse, social services, home care.	Agencies such as these offer a broad range of services that can be tailored to provide support and meet individual needs.

POTENTIAL CONSIDERATIONS following hospitalization (dependent on client's age, physical condition/presence of complications, personal resources, and life responsibilities)

ineffective Airway Clearance—increased amount/viscosity of secretions, restricted chest movement/pain, fatigue/weakness.

acute Pain—surgical incision, tissue trauma, disruption of intercostal nerves, presence of distress/anxiety.

Self-Care Deficit—decreased strength/endurance, presence of pain, intolerance to activity, depression, presence of therapeutic devices; e.g., IV lines.

Refer to CP, Cancer for other considerations, p. 857

PNEUMOTHORAX/HEMOTHORAX

Pneumothorax is defined as the presence of air or gas in the pleural cavity. It can be spontaneous, traumatic, or iatrogenic, and typically involves one lobe of the lung on one side of the chest. However, it can involve more than one lobe and/or occur on both sides of the chest. When accompanied by/or caused by bleeding, the condition is called *hemothorax.*

Primary spontaneous pneumothorax is the result of rupture of pleural blebs and typically occurs in young people without parenchymal lung disease. *Secondary spontaneous pneumothorax* occurs in the presence of lung disease, primarily emphysema, but can also occur with TB, sarcoidosis, cystic fibrosis, malignancy, and pulmonary fibrosis. *Iatrogenic pneumothorax* is a complication of medical or surgical procedures (e.g., therapeutic thoracentesis, tracheostomy, pleural biopsy, central venous catheter insertion, positive pressure mechanical ventilation, inadvertent intubation of right mainstem bronchus). *Traumatic pneumothorax* occurs more frequently than the spontaneous or iatrogenic type and is the focus of this care plan.

The most common cause of pneumothorax/hemothorax is open or closed chest trauma related to blunt or penetrating injuries. The lung collapses partially or completely because of air (pneumothorax), blood (hemothorax), or other fluid (pleural effusion) collecting in the pleural space. The intrathoracic pressure changes induced by increased pleural space volumes reduce lung capacity, causing respiratory distress and gas exchange problems and producing tension on mediastinal structures that can impede cardiac and systemic circulation. Complications include hypoxemia, respiratory failure, and cardiac arrest.

CARE SETTING

Inpatient medical or surgical unit.

RELATED CONCERNS

Cardiac surgery: postoperative care, page 96
Chronic obstructive pulmonary disease (COPD) and asthma, page 117
Psychosocial aspects of care, page 770
Pulmonary tuberculosis (TB), page 184
Ventilatory assistance (mechanical), page 170

Client Assessment Database

Findings vary depending on the amount of air and/or fluid accumulation, rate of accumulation, and underlying lung function.

ACTIVITY/REST

May report: Dyspnea with activity or even at rest

CIRCULATION

May exhibit:
Tachycardia; irregular rate/dysrhythmias
S_3 or S_4/gallop heart rhythm (heart failure secondary to effusion)
Apical pulse reveals point of maximal impulse (PMI) displaced in presence of mediastinal shift (with tension pneumothorax)
Hamman's sign (crunching sound correlating with heartbeat, reflecting air in mediastinum)
BP: Hypertension/hypotension
Jugular venous distention (JVD), especially with tension pneumothorax

EGO INTEGRITY

May exhibit: Apprehension, irritability

PAIN/DISCOMFORT

May report (depending on the size/area involved):
Unilateral chest pain, aggravated by breathing, coughing, and movement
Sudden onset of symptoms while coughing or straining (spontaneous pneumothorax)
Sharp, stabbing pain aggravated by deep breathing, possibly radiating to neck, shoulders, abdomen (pleural effusion)

May exhibit:
Guarding affected area
Distraction behaviors
Facial grimacing

RESPIRATION

May report:
Difficulty breathing, "air hunger"
Coughing (may be presenting symptom)
History of recent chest surgery/trauma; chronic lung disease, lung inflammation/infection (empyema/effusion); diffuse interstitial disease (sarcoidosis); malignancies (e.g., obstructive tumor)
Previous spontaneous pneumothorax; spontaneous rupture of emphysematous bulla, subpleural bleb (COPD)

May exhibit:
Respirations: Rate increased/tachypnea
Increased work of breathing, use of accessory muscles in chest, neck; intercostal retractions, forced abdominal expiration
Breath sounds decreased or absent (involved side)
Fremitus decreased (involved site)
Chest percussion: Hyperresonance over air-filled area (pneumothorax); dullness over fluid-filled area (hemothorax)
Chest observation and palpation: Unequal (paradoxical) chest movement (if trauma, flail), reduced thoracic excursion (affected side)
Skin: Pallor, cyanosis, diaphoresis, subcutaneous crepitation (air in tissues on palpation)
Mentation: Anxiety, restlessness, confusion, stupor
Use of positive pressure mechanical ventilation/positive end-expiratory pressure (PEEP) therapy

SAFETY

May report:
Recent chest trauma (e.g., fractured ribs, penetrating wound)
Radiation/chemotherapy for malignancy
Presence of central IV line

TEACHING/LEARNING

May report: History of familial risk factors: Tuberculosis, cancer
Recent intrathoracic surgery/lung biopsy
Evidence of failure to improve

Discharge plan considerations: Temporary assistance with self-care, homemaker/maintenance tasks

Refer to section at end of plan for postdischarge considerations.

DIAGNOSTIC STUDIES

Chest x-ray: Initial study of choice in client with blunt trauma to chest. May show chest wall fractures, injuries to the heart or great vessels, and reveal air and/or fluid accumulation in the pleural space; may show shift of mediastinal structures (heart).

Thoracic CT: CT is more sensitive than x-rays in detecting thoracic injuries, lung contusion, hemothorax, and pneumothorax. Early CT may influence therapeutic management.

Thoracic ultrasound: Can be used in emergency department to quickly and reliably recognize hemothoraces associated with chest trauma.

ABGs: Variable depending on degree of compromised lung function, altered breathing mechanics, and ability to compensate. Pa_{CO_2} occasionally elevated. Pa_{O_2} may be normal or decreased; oxygen saturation usually decreased.

Thoracentesis: Presence of blood/serosanguineous fluid indicates hemothorax.

Hb: May be decreased, indicating blood loss.

NURSING PRIORITIES

1. Promote/maintain lung reexpansion for adequate oxygenation/ventilation.
2. Minimize/prevent complications.
3. Reduce discomfort/pain.
4. Provide information about disease process, treatment regimen, and prognosis.

DISCHARGE GOALS

1. Adequate ventilation/oxygenation maintained.
2. Complications prevented/resolved.
3. Pain absent/controlled.
4. Disease process/prognosis and therapy needs understood.
5. Plan in place to meet needs after discharge.

NURSING DIAGNOSIS: ineffective Breathing Pattern

May be related to

Decreased lung expansion (air/fluid accumulation)
Musculoskeletal impairment
Pain/anxiety
Inflammatory process

Possibly evidenced by

Dyspnea, tachypnea
Changes in depth/equality of respirations; altered chest excursion
Use of accessory muscles, nasal flaring
Cyanosis, abnormal ABGs

DESIRED OUTCOMES/EVALUATION CRITERIA—CLIENT WILL:

RESPIRATORY STATUS: Ventilation (NOC)

Establish a normal/effective respiratory pattern with ABGs within client's normal range.
Be free of cyanosis and other signs/symptoms of hypoxia.

ACTIONS/INTERVENTIONS	RATIONALE
Respiratory Monitoring (NIC)	
Independent	
Identify etiology/precipitating factors; e.g., spontaneous collapse, trauma, malignancy, infection, complication of mechanical ventilation.	Understanding the cause of lung collapse is necessary for proper chest tube placement and choice of other therapeutic measures.
Evaluate respiratory function, noting rapid/shallow respirations, dyspnea, reports of "air hunger," development of cyanosis, changes in vital signs.	Respiratory distress and changes in vital signs occur as a result of physiologic stress and pain, or may indicate development of shock due to hypoxia/hemorrhage.
Monitor for synchronous respiratory pattern when using mechanical ventilator. Note changes in airway pressures.	Difficulty breathing "with" ventilator and/or increasing airway pressures suggests worsening of condition/development of complications (e.g., spontaneous rupture of a bleb creating a new pneumothorax).
Auscultate breath sounds.	Breath sounds may be diminished or absent in a lobe, lung segment, or entire lung field (unilateral). Atelectatic area will have no breath sounds, and partially collapsed areas have decreased sounds. Regularly scheduled evaluation also helps determine areas of good air exchange and provides a baseline to evaluate resolution of pneumothorax.
Note chest excursion and position of trachea.	Chest excursion is unequal until lung re-expands. Trachea deviates away from affected side with tension pneumothorax.
Assess fremitus.	Voice and tactile fremitus (vibration) is reduced in fluid-filled/consolidated tissue.
Ventilation Assistance (NIC)	
Assist client with splinting painful area when coughing, deep breathing.	Supporting chest and abdominal muscles makes coughing more effective/less traumatic.
Maintain position of comfort, usually with head of bed elevated. Turn to affected side. Encourage client to sit up as much as possible.	Promotes maximal inspiration; enhances lung expansion and ventilation in unaffected side.
Maintain a calm attitude, assisting client to "take control" by using slower/deeper respirations.	Assists client to deal with the physiologic effects of hypoxia, which may be manifested as anxiety and/or fear.
TUBE CARE: Chest (NIC)	
Once chest tube is inserted:	
Check suction control chamber for correct amount of suction (determined by water level, wall/table regulator) at correct setting.	Maintains prescribed intrapleural negativity, which promotes optimum lung expansion and/or fluid drainage. *Note:* Dry-seal setups are also used with an automatic control valve (AVC), which provides a one-way valve seal similar to that achieved with the water-seal system.
Check fluid level in water-seal chamber; maintain at prescribed level.	Water in a sealed chamber serves as a barrier that prevents atmospheric air from entering the pleural space should the suction source be disconnected and aids in evaluating whether the chest drainage system is functioning appropriately. *Note:* Underfilling the water-seal chamber leaves it exposed to air, putting client at risk for pneumothorax or tension pneumothorax. Overfilling (a more common mistake) prevents air from easily exiting the pleural space, thus preventing resolution of pneumothorax and possibly creating a tension pneumothorax.
Observe water-seal chamber bubbling.	Bubbling during expiration reflects venting of pneumothorax (desired action). Bubbling usually decreases as the lung expands or may occur only during expiration or coughing as the pleural space diminishes. Absence of bubbling may indicate complete lung reexpansion (normal) or represent complications; e.g., obstruction in the tube.

ACTIONS/INTERVENTIONS	RATIONALE
Evaluate for abnormal/continuous water-seal chamber bubbling.	With suction applied, this indicates a persistent air leak that may be from a large pneumothorax at the chest insertion site (client centered) or chest drainage unit (system centered).
Determine location of air leak (client or system centered) by clamping thoracic catheter just distal to exit from chest.	If bubbling stops when catheter is clamped at insertion site, leak is client centered (at insertion site or within the client).
Place petrolatum gauze and/or other appropriate material around the insertion as indicated.	Usually corrects insertion site air leak.
Clamp tubing in stepwise fashion downward toward drainage unit if air leak continues.	Isolates location of a system-centered air leak. *Note:* Clamping for a suspected leak may be the only time that chest tube should be clamped.
Seal drainage tubing connection sites securely with lengthwise tape or bands according to established policy.	Prevents/corrects air leaks at connector sites.
Monitor water-seal chamber "tidaling." Note whether change is transient or permanent.	The water-seal chamber serves as an intrapleural manometer (gauges intrapleural pressure); therefore, fluctuation (tidaling) reflects pressure differences between inspiration and expiration. Tidaling of 2–6 cm during inspiration is normal and may increase briefly during coughing episodes. Continuation of excessive tidal fluctuations may indicate existence of airway obstruction or presence of a large pneumothorax.
Position drainage system tubing for optimal function; e.g., shorten tubing/coil extra tubing on bed, making sure tubing is not kinked or hanging below entrance to drainage container. Drain accumulated fluid as necessary.	Improper position, kinking, or accumulation of clots/fluid in the tubing changes the desired negative pressure and impedes air/fluid evacuation. *Note:* If a dependent loop in the drainage tube cannot be avoided, lifting and draining it every 15 min will maintain adequate drainage in the presence of a hemothorax.
Note character/amount of chest tube drainage, whether tube is warm and full of blood, and whether bloody fluid level in water-seal bottle is rising.	Useful in evaluating resolution of pneumothorax/development of hemorrhage requiring prompt intervention. *Note:* Some drainage systems are equipped with an autotransfusion device, which allows for salvage of shed blood.
Evaluate need for gentle "milking" of chest tube per protocol.	May be indicated to maintain drainage in the presence of fresh bleeding/large blood clots or purulent exudates (empyema). Caution is necessary to prevent undue discomfort or injury; e.g., invagination of tissue into catheter eyelets, rupture of small blood vessels.
If thoracic catheter is disconnected/dislodged:	
Observe for signs of respiratory distress. If possible, reconnect thoracic catheter to tubing/suction, using clean technique. If the catheter is dislodged from the chest, cover insertion site immediately with petrolatum dressing and apply firm pressure. Notify physician at once.	Pneumothorax may recur, requiring prompt intervention to prevent fatal pulmonary and circulatory impairment.
After thoracic catheter is removed:	
Cover insertion site with sterile occlusive dressing. Observe for signs/symptoms that may indicate recurrence of pneumothorax; e.g., shortness of breath, reports of pain. Inspect insertion site, note character of drainage.	Early detection of a developing complication is essential; e.g., recurrence of pneumothorax, presence of infection.

Collaborative

ACTIONS/INTERVENTIONS	RATIONALE
Assist with/prepare for reinflation procedures, (e.g., simple aspiration, Heimlich valve, chest tube placement with chest tube drainage unit [CDU]).	Treatment goals are air evacuation, lung reinflation, and prevention of recurrence. Although simple aspiration or Heimlich one-way valve procedures may be useful for small uncomplicated pneumothorax with little or no drainage, chest tube placement is the treatment of choice for traumatic hemopneumothoraces. Chest drainage units (CDUs) include a collection chamber, a water-seal chamber, and a suction-control regulator. Dry suction system can also be used. *Note*: Tension pneumothorax requires immediate needle depression, followed by chest tube placement.

ACTIONS/INTERVENTIONS	RATIONALE
Obtain postplacement x-rays and review serial chest x-rays.	Placement of tube(s) is determined by the cause of the problem (e.g., anterior chest near apex of lung, or one tube at the apex and one at posterior fifth to sixth intercostal space). X-rays confirm proper placement and monitor progress of reexpansion of lung.
Ventilation Assistance (NIC)	
Monitor/graph serial ABGs and pulse oximetry. Review vital capacity/tidal volume measurements.	Assesses status of gas exchange and ventilation, need for continuation or alterations in therapy.
Administer supplemental oxygen via cannula/mask/mechanical ventilation as indicated.	Aids in reducing work of breathing; promotes relief of respiratory distress and cyanosis associated with hypoxemia.
Administer analgesics/sedatives as indicated.	Given to manage pleuritic pain and reduce anxiety/tachycardia associated with impaired respiratory function, especially when client is on a ventilator.

NURSING DIAGNOSIS: risk for Trauma/Suffocation

Risk factors may include

Concurrent disease/injury process
Dependence on external device (chest drainage system)
Lack of safety education/precautions

Possibly evidenced by

[Not applicable; presence of signs and symptoms establishes an *actual* diagnosis.]

DESIRED OUTCOMES/EVALUATION CRITERIA—CLIENT WILL:

Risk Control (NOC)

Recognize need for/seek assistance to prevent complications.

CAREGIVER WILL:

Correct/avoid environmental and physical hazards.

ACTIONS/INTERVENTIONS	RATIONALE
TEACHING: Procedure/Treatment (NIC)	
Independent	
Review with client purpose/function of chest drainage unit, taking note of safety features.	Information on how system works provides reassurance, reducing client anxiety.
Instruct client to refrain from lying/pulling on tubing.	Reduces risk of obstructing drainage/inadvertently disconnecting tubing.
Identify changes/situations that should be reported to caregivers; e.g., change in sound of bubbling, sudden "air hunger" and chest pain, disconnection of equipment.	Timely intervention may prevent serious complications.
TUBE CARE: Chest (NIC)	
Anchor thoracic catheter to chest wall and provide extra length of tubing before turning or moving client.	Prevents thoracic catheter dislodgment or tubing disconnection and reduces pain/discomfort associated with pulling or jarring of tubing.

ACTIONS/INTERVENTIONS	RATIONALE
Secure tubing connection sites.	Prevents tubing disconnection.
Pad banding sites with gauze/tape.	Protects skin from irritation/pressure.
Secure drainage unit to client's bed or on stand/cart placed in low-traffic area.	Maintains upright position and reduces risk of accidental tipping/breaking of unit.
Provide safe transportation if client is sent off unit for diagnostic purposes. Before transporting: check water-seal chamber for correct fluid level, presence/absence of bubbling, presence/degree/timing of tidaling. Ascertain whether or not chest tube can be clamped or disconnected from suction source.	Promotes continuation of optimal evacuation of fluid/air during transport. If client is draining large amounts of chest fluid or air, tube should not be clamped or suction interrupted because of risk of reaccumulation of fluid/air, compromising respiratory status.
Monitor thoracic insertion site, noting condition of skin, presence/characteristics of drainage from around the catheter. Change/reapply sterile occlusive dressing as needed.	Provides for early recognition and treatment of developing skin/tissue erosion or infection.
Observe for signs of respiratory distress if thoracic catheter is disconnected/dislodged. (Refer to ND: ineffective Breathing Pattern.)	Pneumothorax may recur/worsen, compromising respiratory function and requiring emergency intervention.

NURSING DIAGNOSIS: deficient Knowledge [Learning Need] regarding condition, treatment regimen, self-care, and discharge needs

May be related to

Lack of exposure to information

Possibly evidenced by

Expressions of concern, request for information
Recurrence of problem

DESIRED OUTCOMES/EVALUATION CRITERIA—CLIENT WILL:

KNOWLEDGE: Disease Process (NOC)

Verbalize understanding of cause of problem (when known).
Identify signs/symptoms requiring medical follow-up.

KNOWLEDGE: Treatment Regimen (NOC)

Follow therapeutic regimen and demonstrate lifestyle changes if necessary to prevent recurrence.

ACTIONS/INTERVENTIONS	RATIONALE
TEACHING: Disease Process (NIC)	
Independent	
Review pathology of individual problem.	Information reduces fear of unknown. Provides knowledge base for understanding underlying dynamics of condition and significance of therapeutic interventions.
Identify likelihood for recurrence/long-term complications.	Certain underlying lung diseases such as severe COPD and malignancies may increase incidence of recurrence. In otherwise healthy clients who suffered a spontaneous pneumothorax, incidence of recurrence is 10%–50%. Those who have a second spontaneous episode are at high risk for a third incident (60%).

ACTIONS/INTERVENTIONS	RATIONALE
Review signs/symptoms requiring immediate medical evaluation; e.g., sudden chest pain, dyspnea/air hunger, progressive respiratory distress.	Recurrence of pneumothorax/hemothorax requires medical intervention to prevent/reduce potential complications.
Review significance of good health practices; e.g., adequate nutrition, rest, exercise.	Maintenance of general well-being promotes healing and may prevent/limit recurrences
Emphasize need for smoking cessation when indicated.	To prevent recurrence of pneumothorax or respiratory complications; e.g., fibrotic changes.

POTENTIAL CONSIDERATIONS following acute hospitalization (dependent on client's age, physical condition/presence of complications, personal resources, and life responsibilities)

risk for Infection—invasive procedure, traumatized tissue/broken skin, decreased ciliary action.

ineffective Breathing Pattern—recurrence of condition, inflammatory process.

RADICAL NECK SURGERY: LARYNGECTOMY (POSTOPERATIVE CARE)

Head and neck cancer refers to a malignancy that lies above the clavicle but excludes the brain, spinal cord, axial skeleton, and vertebrae. Although head and neck cancer accounts for 5% of all malignant disease, disability is great because of the potential loss of voice, disfigurement, and social consequences. The majority of the laryngeal neoplasms (95%) are squamous cell carcinomas that arise from the oral cavity. When cancer is limited to the vocal cords (intrinsic), spread may be slow. When the cancer involves the epiglottis (extrinsic), metastasis is more common.

Current treatment choices include surgery, radiation, and chemotherapy. Radiation alone is the most common treatment for early stages of certain types of head and neck cancers, such as that affecting the nasopharynx, larynx, oropharynx. Combinations of radiation and chemotherapies are also increasing in use in an effort to preserve structures. However, the mainstay of treatment for advanced-stage laryngeal cancer remains surgery, often in combination with radiation.

This plan of care focuses on nursing care of the client undergoing radical surgery of the neck, including laryngectomy.

Total laryngectomy (TL): Advanced cancers that involve a large portion of the larynx require removal of the entire larynx, the hyoid bone, the cricoid cartilage, two or three tracheal rings, and the strap muscles connected to the larynx. A permanent opening is created in the neck into the trachea, and a laryngectomy tube is inserted to keep the stoma open. The lower portion of the posterior pharynx is removed when the tumor extends beyond the epiglottis, with the remaining portion being sutured to the esophagus after a nasogastric tube is inserted. The client must breathe through a permanent tracheostomy, with normal speech and swallowing no longer being possible.

Near total laryngectomy (NTL): Also known by various terms depending on the procedure (e.g., partial or hemilaryngectomy [one vocal cord is retained], subtotal laryngectomy and conservation laryngeal surgery), NTL is an accepted alternative to TL for many persons with glottic, supraglottic, base of tongue, and hypopharyngeal cancers. In these procedures, the swallowing function and some voice may be retained.

CARE SETTINGS

Inpatient surgical and possibly subacute units.

RELATED CONCERNS

Cancer, page 857
Psychosocial aspects of care, page 770
Surgical intervention, page 788
Total nutritional support: parenteral/enteral feeding, page 478

Client Assessment Database (Preoperative and Postoperative)

Preoperative data presented here depend on the specific type/location of cancer process and underlying complications.

ACTIVITY/REST

Mary report: Weakness, fatigue, lethargy (postoperative)

EGO INTEGRITY

May report: Feelings of fear about loss of voice, dying, occurrence/recurrence of cancer
Concern about how surgery will affect family relationships, ability to work, and finances

May exhibit: Anxiety, depression, anger, and withdrawal
Denial

FOOD/FLUID

May report: Difficulty swallowing (dysphagia), chokes easily, taste changes (postoperative)

May exhibit: Difficulty handling oral secretions, or dry mouth (postoperative)
Swelling, ulcerations, masses may be noted depending on location of cancer
Oral inflammation/drainage, poor dental hygiene
Leukoplakia, erythroplasia of oral cavity
Halitosis
Swelling of tongue
Altered gag reflex and facial paralysis

HYGIENE

May exhibit: Neglect of dental hygiene
Need for assistance in basic care

NEUROSENSORY

May report: Diplopia (double vision)
Deafness
Tingling, paresthesia of facial muscles

May exhibit: Hemiparalysis of face (parotid and submandibular involvement), persistent hoarseness or loss of voice (dominant and earliest symptom of intrinsic laryngeal cancer)
Difficulty swallowing
Conduction deafness
Disruption of mucous membranes

PAIN/DISCOMFORT

May report: (Preoperatively) Chronic sore throat, "lump in throat"
Referred pain to ear, facial pain (late stage, probably metastatic)
Pain/burning sensation with swallowing (especially with hot liquids or citrus juices), local pain in oropharynx
Sore throat or mouth (pain is not usually reported as severe following head and neck surgery, as compared with pain noted before surgery)

May exhibit: Guarding behaviors
Restlessness
Facial mask of pain
Alteration in muscle tone

RESPIRATION

May report: History of smoking (including cigars)/chewing tobacco
Occupation working with hardwood sawdust, toxic chemicals/fumes, heavy metals
History of voice overuse; e.g., professional singer or auctioneer
History of chronic lung disease
Cough with/without sputum
Bloody nasal drainage

May exhibit: Blood-tinged sputum, hemoptysis
Dyspnea (late)

SAFETY

May report: Excessive sun exposure over a period of years or radiation therapy
Visual/hearing changes

May exhibit: Masses/enlarged nodes

SOCIAL INTERACTION

May report: Lack of family/support system (may be result of age group or behaviors; e.g., alcoholism)
Concerns about ability to communicate, engage in social interactions

May exhibit: Persistent hoarseness, change in voice pitch
Muffled/garbled speech, reluctance to speak
Hesitancy/reluctance of significant others to provide care/be involved in rehabilitation

TEACHING/LEARNING

May report: Nonhealing of oral lesions
Concurrent use of alcohol/history of alcohol abuse

Discharge plan considerations: Assistance with wound care, treatments, supplies, transportation, shopping, food preparation, self-care, homemaker/maintenance tasks

Refer to section at end of plan for postdischarge considerations.

DIAGNOSTIC STUDIES

Direct/indirect laryngoscopy; laryngeal tomography, biopsy, and needle biopsy: Are the most reliable diagnostic indicators for direct visualization or to detect local or regional spread/staging.
Laryngography: May be performed with contrast to study blood vessels and lymph nodes.
Pulmonary function studies: COPD is common in this group of clients. Abnormal findings may indicate need for additional interventions to improve pulmonary reserve prior to surgery
Chest x-ray: Done to establish baseline lung status and/or identify metastases.
CBC: May reveal anemia, which is a common problem. Folate deficiency is very common in clients with history of alcoholism and malnutrition.
Immunological surveys: May be done for clients receiving chemotherapy/immunotherapy.
Biochemical profile: Changes may occur in organ function as a result of cancer, metastasis, and therapies.
ABGs/pulse oximetry: May be done to establish baseline/monitor status of lungs (ventilation).

NURSING PRIORITIES

1. Maintain patent airway, adequate ventilation.
2. Assist client in developing alternative communication methods.
3. Restore/maintain skin integrity.
4. Reestablish/maintain adequate nutrition.
5. Provide emotional support for acceptance of altered body image.
6. Provide information about disease process/prognosis and treatment.

DISCHARGE GOALS

1. Ventilation/oxygenation adequate for individual needs.
2. Communicating effectively.
3. Complications prevented/minimized.
4. Beginning to cope with change in body image.
5. Disease process/prognosis and therapeutic regimen understood.
6. Plan in place to meet needs after discharge.

NURSING DIAGNOSIS: ineffective Airway Clearance/risk for Aspiration

May be related to

Partial/total removal of the glottis, altering ability to breathe, cough, and swallow
Temporary or permanent change to neck breathing (dependent on patent stoma)
Edema formation (surgical manipulation and lymphatic accumulation)
Copious and thick secretions

Possibly evidenced by (Airway Clearance)

Dyspnea/difficulty breathing
Changes in rate/depth of respiration; use of accessory respiratory muscles
Abnormal breath sounds
Cyanosis

Possibly evidenced by (Aspiration)

[Not applicable; presence of signs and symptoms establishes an *actual* diagnosis.]

DESIRED OUTCOMES/EVALUATION CRITERIA—CLIENT WILL:

RESPIRATORY STATUS: Airway Patency (NOC)

Maintain patent airway with breath sounds clear/clearing.
Expectorate/clear secretions and be free of aspiration.

Aspiration Prevention (NOC)

Demonstrate behaviors to improve/maintain airway clearance within level of ability/situation.

ACTIONS/INTERVENTIONS	RATIONALE
Airway Management (NIC)	
Independent	
Monitor respiratory rate/depth; note ease of breathing. Auscultate breath sounds. Investigate restlessness, dyspnea, development of cyanosis.	Changes in respirations, use of accessory muscles, and/or presence of crackles/wheezes suggest retention of secretions. Airway obstruction (even partial) can lead to ineffective breathing patterns and impaired gas exchange, resulting in complications; e.g., pneumonia, respiratory arrest.
Elevate head of bed 30–45 degrees.	Facilitates drainage of secretions, work of breathing, and lung expansion. *Note:* Increase elevation when oral intake is provided.
Encourage swallowing, if client is able.	Prevents pooling of oral secretions, reducing risk of aspiration. *Note:* Swallowing is impaired when the epiglottis is removed and/or significant postoperative edema and pain are present.
Encourage effective coughing and deep breathing.	Mobilizes secretions to clear airway and helps prevent respiratory complications.
Suction laryngectomy/tracheostomy tube, oral and nasal cavities. Note amount, color, and consistency of secretions.	Prevents secretions from obstructing airway, especially when swallowing ability is impaired and client cannot blow nose. Changes in character of secretions may indicate developing problems (e.g., dehydration, infection) and need for further evaluation/treatment.
Demonstrate and encourage client to begin self-suction procedures as soon as possible. Educate client in "clean" techniques.	Assists client to exercise some control in postoperative care and prevention of complications. Reduces anxiety associated with difficulty in breathing or inability to handle secretions when alone.
Maintain proper position of laryngectomy/tracheostomy tube. Check/adjust ties as indicated.	As edema develops/subsides, tube can be displaced, compromising airway. Ties should be snug but not constrictive to surrounding tissue or major blood vessels.
Observe tissues surrounding tube for bleeding. Change client's position to check for pooling of blood behind neck or on posterior dressings.	Small amount of oozing may be present; however, continued bleeding or sudden eruption of uncontrolled hemorrhage presents a sudden and real possibility of airway obstruction/suffocation.
Change tube/inner cannula as indicated. Instruct client in cleaning procedures.	Prevents accumulation of secretions and thick mucous plugs from obstructing airway. *Note:* This is a common cause of respiratory distress/arrest in later postoperative period.
Collaborative	
Provide supplemental humidification; e.g., compressed air/oxygen mist collar, increased fluid intake.	Normal physiologic (nose/nasal passages) means of filtering/humidifying air are bypassed. Supplemental humidity decreases mucous crusting and facilitates coughing/suctioning of secretions through stoma.
Resume oral intake with caution. (Refer to ND: imbalanced Nutrition: less than body requirements.)	Changes in muscle mass/strength and nerve innervation increase likelihood of aspiration.
Monitor serial ABGs/pulse oximetry; chest x-ray.	Pooling of secretions/presence of atelectasis may lead to pneumonia, requiring more aggressive therapeutic measures.

NURSING DIAGNOSIS: impaired verbal Communication

May be related to

Anatomical deficit (removal of vocal cords)
Physical barrier (tracheostomy tube)
Required voice rest

Possibly evidenced by

Inability to speak
Change in vocal characteristics

DESIRED OUTCOMES/EVALUATION CRITERIA—CLIENT WILL:

Communication (NOC)

Communicate needs in an effective manner.
Identify/plan for appropriate alternative speech methods after healing.

ACTIONS/INTERVENTIONS	RATIONALE
COMMUNICATION ENHANCEMENT: Speech Deficit (NIC)	
Independent	
Review preoperative instructions/discussion of why speech and breathing are altered, using anatomic drawings or models to assist in explanations.	Reinforces teaching at a time when fear of surviving surgery is past. *Note*: Following NTL procedure and the passage of time, the client may experience voice and ease of swallowing, although this depends entirely on multiple factors, including type and invasiveness of cancer, type and success of reconstructive surgery, and response to radiation and/or chemotherapies.
Determine whether client has other communication impairments; e.g., hearing, vision, literacy.	Presence of other problems influences plan for alternative communication.
Provide immediate and continual means to summon nurse; e.g., call light/bell. Let client know the summons will be answered immediately. Stop by to check on client periodically without being summoned. Post notice at central answering system/nursing station that client is unable to speak.	Client needs assurance that nurse is vigilant and will respond to summons. Trust and self-esteem are fostered when the nurse cares enough to come at times other than when called by client.
Prearrange signals for obtaining immediate help.	May decrease client's anxiety about inability to speak.
Provide alternative means of communication appropriate to client need; e.g., pad and pencil, magic slate, alphabet/picture board, sign language. Consider placement of IV.	Permits client to "express" needs/concerns. *Note:* IV positioned in hand/wrist may limit ability to write or sign.
Allow sufficient time for communication.	Loss of speech and stress of alternative communication can cause frustration and block expression, especially when caregivers seem "too busy" or preoccupied.
Provide nonverbal communication; e.g., touching and physical presence. Anticipate needs.	Communicates concern and meets need for contact with others. Touch is believed to generate complex biochemical events, with possible release of endorphins contributing to reduction of anxiety.
Encourage ongoing communication with "outside world"; e.g., newspapers, television, radio, calendar, clock.	Maintains contact with "normal lifestyle" and continued communication through other avenues.
Refer to loss of speech as temporary after a partial laryngectomy and/or depending on availability of voice prosthetics/vocal cord transplant.	Provides encouragement and hope for future with the thought that alternative means of communication and speech are available and possible. *Note*: Some procedures allow for return of voice function, either by means of an artificial larynx (neck or intraoral); a tracheoesophageal puncture (TEP) and prosthesis which allows lung-powered speech; or esophageal speech by air forced into the top of the esophagus does not require a prosthesis.
Caution client not to use voice until physician gives permission.	Promotes healing of vocal cord and limits potential for permanent cord dysfunction.

ACTIONS/INTERVENTIONS	RATIONALE
Arrange for meeting with other persons who have experienced this procedure, as appropriate.	Provides role model, enhancing motivation for problem solving and learning new ways to communicate.

Collaborative

Consult with appropriate health team members/therapists/rehabilitation agency (e.g., speech pathologist, social services, laryngectomee clubs) for hospital-based rehabilitation, and community resources such as Lost Chord/New Voice Club, International Association of Laryngectomees, American Cancer Society.	Ability to use alternative voice and speech methods (e.g., electrolarynx, tracheoesophageal puncture [TEP], voice prosthesis, esophageal speech) varies greatly, depending on extent of surgical procedures, client's age, emotional state, and motivation to return to an active life. Rehabilitation time may be lengthy and require a number of agencies/resources to facilitate/support learning process. *Note:* Some clients may be candidates for vocal cord transplant at a future date.

NURSING DIAGNOSIS: impaired Skin/Tissue Integrity

May be related to

Surgical removal of tissues/grafting
Radiation or chemotherapeutic agents
Altered circulation/reduced blood supply
Compromised nutritional status
Edema formation
Pooling/continuous drainage of secretions (oral, lymph, or chyle)

Possibly evidenced by

Disruption of skin/tissue surface
Destruction of skin/tissue layers

DESIRED OUTCOMES/EVALUATION CRITERIA—CLIENT WILL:

WOUND HEALING: Primary Intention (NOC)

Display timely wound healing without complications.
Demonstrate techniques to promote healing/prevent complications.

ACTIONS/INTERVENTIONS	RATIONALE
Skin Surveillance (NIC)	
Independent	
Assess skin color/temperature and capillary refill in operative and skin graft areas.	Skin should be pink or similar to color of surrounding skin. Skin graft flaps should be pink and warm and should blanch (when gentle finger pressure is applied), with return to color within seconds. Cyanosis and slow refill may indicate venous congestion, which can lead to tissue ischemia/necrosis.
Keep head of bed elevated 30–45 degrees. Monitor facial edema (usually peaks by third to fifth postoperative day).	Minimizes postoperative tissue congestion and edema related to excision of lymph channels.
Protect skin flaps and suture lines from tension or pressure. Provide pillows/rolls and instruct client to support head/neck during activity.	Pressure from tubings and tracheostomy tapes or tension on suture lines can alter circulation/cause tissue injury.

ACTIONS/INTERVENTIONS	RATIONALE
Monitor bloody drainage from surgical sites, suture lines, drains. Measure drainage from collection device (e.g., Hemovac) if used.	Bloody drainage usually declines steadily after first 24 hr. Steady oozing or frank bleeding indicates problem requiring medical attention.
Note/report any milky-appearing drainage.	Milky drainage may indicate thoracic lymph duct leakage (can result in depletion of body fluids and electrolytes). Such a leak may heal spontaneously or require surgical closure.

Wound Care (NIC)

Change dressings as indicated.	Damp dressings increase risk of tissue damage/infection. *Note:* Pressure dressings are not used over skin flaps because blood supply is easily compromised.
Cleanse incisions with sterile saline and peroxide (mixed 1:1) after dressings have been removed.	Prevents crust formation, which can trap purulent drainage, destroy skin edges, and increase size of wound. Peroxide is not used full strength because it may cauterize wound edges and impair healing.
Monitor donor site if graft performed; check dressings as indicated.	Donor site may be adjacent to operative site or a distant site (e.g., thigh). Pressure dressings are usually removed within 24–48 hr, and wound is left open to air to promote healing.
Cleanse thoroughly around stoma and neck tubes (if in place), avoiding soap or alcohol. Show client how to do self-stoma/tube care with clean water and peroxide, using soft, lint-free cloth, not tissue or cotton.	Keeping area clean promotes healing and comfort. Soap and other drying agents can lead to stomal irritation and possible inflammation. Materials other than cloth may leave fibers in stoma that can irritate or be inhaled into lungs.
Monitor all sites for signs of wound infection; e.g., unusual redness; increasing edema, pain, exudates; and temperature elevation.	Impedes healing, which may already be slow because of changes induced by cancer, cancer therapies, and/or malnutrition.

Collaborative

Cover donor sites with petroleum gauze or moisture-impermeable dressing.	Nonadherent dressing covers exposed sensory nerve endings and protects site from contamination.
Administer oral, IV, and topical antibiotics as indicated.	Prevents/controls infection.

NURSING DIAGNOSIS: impaired Oral Mucous Membrane

May be related to

Dehydration/absence of oral intake, decreased saliva production secondary to radiation (common) or surgical procedure (rare)
Poor/inadequate oral hygiene
Pathologic condition (oral cancer), mechanical trauma (oral surgery)
Difficulty swallowing and pooling of secretions/drooling
Nutritional deficits

Possibly evidenced by

Xerostomia (dry mouth), oral discomfort
Thick/mucoid saliva, decreased saliva production
Dry, crusted, coated tongue; inflamed lips
Absent teeth/gums, poor dental health, halitosis

DESIRED OUTCOMES/EVALUATION CRITERIA—CLIENT WILL:

TISSUE INTEGRITY: Skin and Mucous Membranes (NOC)

Report/demonstrate a decrease in symptoms.
Identify specific interventions to promote healthy oral mucosa.
Demonstrate techniques to restore/maintain mucosal integrity.

ACTIONS/INTERVENTIONS	RATIONALE
Oral Health Restoration (NIC)	
Independent	
Inspect oral cavity and note changes in:	
Saliva;	Damage to salivary glands may decrease production of saliva, resulting in dry mouth. Pooling and drooling of saliva may occur because of compromised swallowing capability or pain in throat and mouth.
Tongue;	Surgery may have included partial resection of tongue, soft palate, and pharynx. This client has decreased sensation and movement of tongue, with difficulty swallowing and increased risk of aspiration of secretions, as well as potential for hemorrhage.
Lips;	Surgical removal of part of lip may result in uncontrollable drooling.
Teeth and gums;	Teeth may not be intact (surgical) or may be in poor condition because of malnutrition, chemical therapies, and neglect. Gums may also be surgically altered or inflamed because of poor hygiene, long history of smoking/chewing tobacco, or chemical therapies.
Mucous membranes.	May be excessively dry, ulcerated, erythematous, edematous.
Suction oral cavity gently/frequently. Have client perform self-suctioning when possible or use gauze wick to drain secretions.	Saliva contains digestive enzymes that may be erosive to exposed tissues. Because drooling may be constant, client can promote own comfort and enhance oral hygiene by performing self-suctioning.
Show client how to brush inside of mouth, palate, tongue, and teeth.	Frequent oral care reduces bacteria and risk of infection; promotes tissue healing and comfort.
Apply lubrication to lips; provide oral irrigations as indicated.	Counteracts drying effects of therapeutic measures; negates erosive nature of secretions.
Avoid alcohol-based mouthwashes. Use normal saline or mixture of salt water and baking soda for rinsing. Suggest use of artificial saliva preparations (e.g., pilocarpine hydrochloride [Salagen]) if mucous membranes are dry.	Alcohol can be drying/irritating. Salt and soda rinses return mouth to neutral (rather than acidic) environment. Although drooling is often present and abundant immediately postoperatively, surgical/radiation damage to the parotid glands can drastically reduce saliva production on a permanent basis. Cholinergic effect of medication can increase saliva production.

NURSING DIAGNOSIS: acute Pain

May be related to

Surgical incisions
Tissue swelling
Presence of nasogastric/orogastric feeding tube

Possibly evidenced by

Discomfort in surgical areas/pain with swallowing
Facial mask of pain
Distraction behaviors, restlessness; guarding behavior

DESIRED OUTCOMES/EVALUATION CRITERIA—CLIENT WILL:

Pain Level (NOC)

Report/indicate pain is relieved/controlled.
Demonstrate relief of pain/discomfort by reduced tension and relaxed manner, sleeping/resting appropriately.

ACTIONS/INTERVENTIONS	RATIONALE
Pain Management (NIC)	
Independent	
Support head and neck with pillows. Show client how to support neck during activity.	Muscle weakness results from muscle and nerve resection in the structures of the neck and/or shoulders. Lack of support aggravates discomfort and may result in injury to suture areas.
Provide comfort measures (e.g., back rub, position change) and diversional activities such as television, visiting, reading.	Promotes relaxation and helps client refocus attention on something besides self/discomfort. May reduce analgesic dosage needs/frequency.
Encourage client to expectorate saliva or to suction mouth gently if unable to swallow.	Swallowing causes muscle activity that may be painful because of edema/strain on suture lines.
Investigate changes in characteristics of pain. Check mouth, throat suture lines for fresh trauma.	May reflect developing complications requiring further evaluation/intervention. Tissues are inflamed and congested and may be easily traumatized by suction catheter or feeding tube.
Note nonverbal indicators and autonomic responses to pain. Evaluate effects of analgesics.	Aids in determining presence of pain, need for/effectiveness of medication.
Medicate before activity/treatments as indicated.	May enhance cooperation and participation in therapeutic regimen.
Schedule care activities to balance with adequate periods of sleep/rest.	Prevents fatigue/exhaustion and may enhance coping with stress/discomfort.
Recommend use of stress management behaviors; e.g., relaxation techniques, guided imagery.	Promotes sense of well-being, may reduce analgesic needs and enhance healing.
Collaborative	
Provide oral irrigations, anesthetic sprays, and gargles. Instruct client in self-irrigations.	Improves comfort, promotes healing, and reduces halitosis. *Note:* Commercial mouthwashes containing alcohol or phenol are to be avoided because of their drying effect.
Administer analgesics (e.g., narcotics) on a scheduled basis and prn. Avoid medications containing aspirin.	Degree of pain is related to extent and psychologic impact of surgery, as well as general body condition. Giving medications on schedule rather than just prn minimizes chance that pain escalates "out of control." Products containing aspirin are contraindicated because they potentiate bleeding. *Note*: Studies appear to support the idea that many clients experience more pain before than after head and neck surgery.

NURSING DIAGNOSIS: imbalanced Nutrition: less than body requirements

May be related to

Temporary or permanent alteration in mode of food intake
Altered feedback mechanisms of desire to eat, taste, and smell because of surgical/structural changes, radiation, or chemotherapy

Possibly evidenced by

Inadequate food intake, perceived inability to ingest food
Aversion to eating, lack of interest in food, reported altered taste sensation
Weight loss
Weakness of muscles required for swallowing or mastication

DESIRED OUTCOMES/EVALUATION CRITERIA—CLIENT WILL:

Nutritional Status (NOC)

Indicate understanding of importance of nutrition to healing process and general well-being.
Make dietary choices to meet nutrient needs within individual situation.
Demonstrate progressive weight gain toward goal, with normalization of laboratory values and timely healing of tissues/incisions.

ACTIONS/INTERVENTIONS	RATIONALE
Nutrition Therapy (NIC)	
Independent	
Auscultate bowel sounds.	Feedings are usually begun after bowel sounds are restored postoperatively. *Note:* In more aggressive therapy, tube feeding may be started earlier if gastric residuals are closely monitored.
Maintain feeding tube; e.g., check for tube placement, flush with warm water as indicated.	Tube is inserted during surgery and usually sutured in place. Initially the tube may be attached to suction to reduce nausea and/or vomiting. Flushing aids in maintaining patency of tube.
Monitor intake and weigh as indicated. Show client how to monitor and record weight on a scheduled basis.	Provides information regarding nutritional needs and effectiveness of therapy.
Instruct client/SO in self-feeding techniques; e.g., bulb syringe, bag and funnel method, and blenderizing soft foods if client is to go home with a feeding tube. Make sure client and SO are able to perform this procedure before discharge and that appropriate food and equipment are available at home.	Helps promote nutritional success and preserves dignity in the adult who is now forced to depend on others for very basic needs in the social setting of meals.
Begin with small feedings and advance as tolerated. Note signs of gastric fullness, regurgitation, diarrhea.	Content of feeding may result in GI intolerance, requiring change in rate or type of formula.
Provide supplemental water by feeding tube or orally if client can swallow.	Keeps client hydrated to offset insensible losses and drainage from surgical areas. Meets free water needs associated with enteral feeding.
Encourage client when relearning swallowing; e.g., maintain quiet environment, have suction equipment on standby, and demonstrate appropriate breathing techniques.	Helps client deal with the frustration and safety concerns involved with swallowing. Provides reassurance that measures are available to prevent/limit aspiration.
Resume oral feedings when feasible. Stay with client during meals the first few days.	Oral feedings can usually resume after suture lines are healed (8–10 days) unless further reconstruction is required or client is going home with feeding tube. Client may experience pain or difficulty with chewing and swallowing initially and may require suctioning during meals in addition to support and encouragement.
Develop and encourage a pleasant environment for meals.	Promotes socialization and maximizes client comfort when eating difficulties cause embarrassment.
Help client/SO develop nutritionally balanced home meal plans.	Promotes understanding of individual needs and significance of nutrition in healing and recovery process.
Collaborative	
Consult with dietitian/nutritional support team as indicated. Incorporate and reinforce dietitian's teaching.	Useful in identifying individual nutritional needs to promote healing and tissue regeneration. Discharge teaching and follow-up by the dietitian may be needed to evaluate client needs for diet/equipment modifications and meal planning in the home setting.

ACTIONS/INTERVENTIONS	RATIONALE
Provide nutritionally balanced diet (e.g., semisolid/soft foods) or tube feedings (e.g., blended soft food or commercial preparations) as indicated.	Variations can be made to add or limit certain factors, such as fat and sugar, or to provide a food that client prefers.
Monitor laboratory studies; e.g., blood urea nitrogen (BUN), glucose, liver function, prealbumin/protein, electrolytes.	Indicators of utilization of nutrients and organ function.

NURSING DIAGNOSIS: disturbed Body Image/ineffective Role Performance

May be related to

Loss of voice
Changes in anatomical contour of face and neck (disfigurement and/or severe functional impairment)
Presence of chronic illness

Possibly evidenced by

Report of fear of rejection by/reaction of others; change in social involvement; discomfort in social situations
Negative feelings about body change
Refusal to verify actual change or preoccupation with change/loss, not looking at self in mirror
Change in self/others' perception of role
Anxiety, depression, lack of eye contact
Failure of family members to adapt to change or deal with experience constructively

DESIRED OUTCOMES/EVALUATION CRITERIA—CLIENT WILL:

Body Image (NOC)

Identify feelings and methods for coping with negative perception of self.
Demonstrate initial adaptation to body changes as evidenced by participating in self-care activities and positive interactions with others.

Role Performance (NOC)

Communicate with SO about changes in role that have occurred.
Begin to develop plans for altered lifestyle.
Participate in team efforts toward rehabilitation.

ACTIONS/INTERVENTIONS	RATIONALE
Body Image/Role Enhancement (NIC)	
Independent	
Discuss meaning of loss/change with client, identifying perceptions of current situation/future expectations.	Aids in identifying/defining the problem(s) to focus attention and interventions constructively.
Note nonverbal body language, negative attitudes/self-talk. Assess for self-destructive/suicidal behavior.	May indicate depression/despair, need for further assessment/more intense intervention.
Note emotional reactions; e.g., grieving, depression, anger. Allow client to progress at own rate.	Client may experience immediate depression after surgery or react with shock and denial. Acceptance of changes cannot be forced, and the grieving process needs time for resolution.

ACTIONS/INTERVENTIONS	RATIONALE
Maintain calm, reassuring manner. Acknowledge and accept expression of feelings of grief, hostility.	May help allay client's fears of dying, suffocation, inability to communicate, or mutilation. Client and SO need to feel supported and know that all feelings are appropriate for the type of experience they are going through.
Allow, but do not participate in, client's use of denial; e.g., when client is reluctant to participate in self-care such as suctioning stoma. Provide care in a nonjudgmental manner.	Denial may be the most helpful defense for client in the beginning, permitting the individual to begin to deal slowly with difficult adjustment.
Set limits on maladaptive behaviors, assisting client to identify positive behaviors that will aid recovery.	Acting out can result in lowered self-esteem and impede adjustment to new self-image.
Encourage SO to treat client normally and not as an invalid.	Distortions of body image may be unconsciously reinforced.
Alert staff that facial expressions and other nonverbal behaviors need to convey acceptance and not revulsion.	Client is very sensitive to nonverbal communication and may make negative assumptions about others' body language.
Encourage identification of anticipated personal/work conflicts that may arise.	Expressions of concern bring problems into the open where they can be examined/dealt with.
Recognize behavior indicative of overconcern with future lifestyle/relationship functioning.	Ruminating about anticipated losses/reactions of others is nonproductive and is a block to problem solving.
Encourage client to deal with situation in small steps.	May feel overwhelmed/have difficulty coping with larger picture but can manage one piece at a time.
Provide positive reinforcement for efforts/progress made.	Encourages client to feel a sense of movement toward recovery.
Encourage client/SO to communicate feelings to each other.	All those involved may have difficulty in this area (because of the loss of voice function and/or disfigurement) but need to understand that they may gain courage and help from one another.

Collaborative

Refer client/SO to supportive resources; e.g., psychotherapy, social worker, family counseling, pastoral care.	A multifaceted approach is required to assist client toward rehabilitation and wellness. Families need assistance in understanding the processes that client is going through and to help them with their own emotions. The goal is to enable them to guard against the tendency to withdraw from/isolate client from social contact.

NURSING DIAGNOSIS: deficient Knowledge [Learning Need] regarding prognosis, treatment, self-care, and discharge needs

May be related to

Lack of information/recall
Misinterpretation of information
Poor assimilation of material presented; lack of interest in learning

Possibly evidenced by

Indications of concern/request for information
Inaccurate follow-through of instructions
Inappropriate or exaggerated behavior; e.g., hostile, agitated, apathetic

DESIRED OUTCOMES/EVALUATION CRITERIA—CLIENT WILL:

KNOWLEDGE: Disease Process (NOC)

Indicate basic understanding of disease process, surgical intervention, prognosis.
Identify symptoms requiring medical evaluation/intervention.

KNOWLEDGE: Treatment Regimen (NOC)

Verbalize understanding of treatment regimen and rationale for actions.
Demonstrate ability to provide safe care.
Use resources (e.g., rehabilitation team members) appropriately.
Develop plan for/schedule follow-up appointments.

ACTIONS/INTERVENTIONS	RATIONALE
Learning Facilitation (NIC)	
Independent	
Ascertain amount of preoperative preparation and retention of information. Assess level of anxiety related to diagnosis and surgery.	Information can provide clues to client's postoperative reactions. Anxiety may have interfered with understanding of information given before surgery.
Provide/repeat explanations at client's level of acceptance.	Overwhelming stressors are present and may be coupled with limited knowledge.
Provide written directions for client/SO to read and have available for future reference.	Reinforces proper information and may be used as a home reference.
Discuss inaccuracies in perception of disease process and therapies with client and SO.	Misconceptions are inevitable, but failure to explore and correct them can result in client's failing to progress toward health.
Educate client and SO about basic care/safety regarding stoma; e.g.:	
Shower with stoma collar; shampoo by leaning forward; no swimming or water sports;	Although the extra humidity provided by a shower can be beneficial by loosening secretions and enhancing expectoration, excessive water entering airway/stoma is detrimental.
Cover stoma with foam or fiber filter (e.g., cotton or silk);	Prevents dust and particles from being inhaled.
Cover stoma when coughing or sneezing;	Normal airways are bypassed, and mucus will exit from stoma.
Clean and maintain valve/prosthesis as indicated.	Stoma may be fitted with a valve or other type of prosthesis for maintaining the stoma opening, and in preparation of future speech.
Reinforce necessity of not smoking.	Necessary to preserve lung function. *Note:* Client may need extra support and encouragement to understand that respiratory function and quality of life can be improved by cessation of smoking.
Discuss inability to smell and taste as before surgery.	Safety issues surround the inability to smell (e.g., smoke from fire or odor from infection in stoma). Also the loss of taste affects the desire to resume eating when client is otherwise able to do so.
Discuss importance of reporting to caregiver/physician immediately such symptoms as stoma narrowing, presence of "lump" in throat, dysphagia, or bleeding.	May be signs of tracheal stenosis, recurrent cancer, or carotid erosion.
Develop a means of emergency communication at home.	Permits client to summon assistance when needed.
Recommend wearing medical-alert identification tag/bracelet identifying client as a neck breather. Encourage family members to become certified in cardiopulmonary resuscitation (CPR) if they are interested/able to do so.	Provides for appropriate care if client becomes unconscious or suffers a cardiopulmonary arrest.
Give careful attention to the provision of needed rehabilitative measures; e.g., temporary/permanent prosthesis, dental care, speech therapy, surgical reconstruction; vocational, sexual/marital counseling, financial assistance.	These services can contribute to client's well-being and have a positive effect on client's quality of life.
Identify homecare needs and available resources (e.g., supplies, support, assistance).	Provides support for transition from hospital setting.

POTENTIAL CONSIDERATIONS following acute hospitalization (dependent on client's age, physical condition/presence of complications, personal resources, and life responsibilities)

risk for Aspiration—presence of tracheostomy, tube feedings, impaired swallowing, decreased muscle mass/strength (status after neck surgery).

impaired verbal Communication—anatomic presence of tracheostomy.

risk for Infection—broken skin/traumatized tissue, stasis of secretions, suppressed inflammatory response, chronic disease, malnutrition.

imbalanced Nutrition: less than body requirements—temporary alteration in mode of food intake, altered feedback mechanisms relative to senses of taste and smell.

Self-Care Deficit—decreased strength/endurance, presence of pain, depression.

VENTILATORY ASSISTANCE (MECHANICAL)

A mechanical ventilator provides ventilation support for clients whose pulmonary system cannot sustain ventilation on its own. This includes clients with (1) respiratory failure from various causes (e.g., severe pneumonia, pulmonary edema, acute respiratory distress syndrome [ARDS], COPD with respiratory muscle atrophy and malnutrition [inability to wean]); (2) neuromuscular deficits, such as quadriplegia with phrenic nerve injury or high C-spine injuries, Guillain-Barré syndrome, and amyotrophic lateral sclerosis (ALS); and (3) restrictive conditions of chest or lungs, such as kyphoscoliosis and interstitial fibrosis.

Mechanical ventilation can be invasive (client has artificial airway connected to a positive-pressure mechanical ventilator); or noninvasive (positive airway pressure ventilation is delivered using a bilevel positive airway pressure (BIPAP) machine, or continuous positive airway pressure (CPAP) machine via nasal mask, nasal pillow, full-face mask, or mouthpiece.

An order for mechanical ventilation specifies the main settings, such as (1) mode (e.g., positive-pressure ventilator modes include continuous mandatory ventilation [CMV], BIPAP, and CPAP); (2) ventilator rate (usually 8–16); (3) tidal volume (typically 8–12 mm/kg body weight); (4) oxygen (FIO_2 ranging from 21% to100%); (5) level of pressure support (PS) to deliver bigger breath with less work; and (6) level of positive end-expiratory pressure (PEEP) to apply positive pressure to airways and alveoli during exhalation to keep them open.

Types of Ventilators

Pressure-cycled ventilators are desirable for clients with relatively normal lung compliance who cannot initiate or sustain respiration because of muscular/phrenic nerve involvement (e.g., quadri/tetraplegia).
Volume-cycled ventilators are the primary choice for long-term ventilation of clients whose permanent changes in lung compliance and resistance require increased pressure to provide adequate ventilation (e.g., COPD).
Dual-control ventilators incorporate automated modes through microprocessors that use feedback mechanisms to individualize appropriate ventilator settings and alarms (e.g., mandatory minute ventilation [MMV] and pressure-regulated volume control [PRVC]).

CARE SETTING

The focus of this plan of care is the client with invasive mechanical ventilation who remains on a ventilator whether in an acute or post–acute care setting. The expectation is that the majority of clients will be weaned before discharge. However, some clients are either unsuccessful at weaning or are not candidates for weaning. For these clients, portions of this plan of care would need to be modified for the discharge care setting whether it be an extended care facility or home.

RELATED CONCERNS

Cardiac surgery: postoperative care, page 96
Chronic obstructive pulmonary disease (COPD) and asthma, page 117
Craniocerebral trauma (acute rehabilitative phase), page 218
Pneumothorax/hemothorax, page 150
Spinal cord injury (acute rehabilitative phase), page 271
Total nutritional support: parenteral/enteral feeding, page 478
Psychosocial aspects of care, page 770

Client Assessment Database

Gathered data depend on the underlying pathophysiology and/or reason for ventilatory support. Refer to the appropriate plan of care.

Discharge plan considerations: If ventilator-dependent, may require changes in physical layout of home, acquisition of equipment/supplies, provision of a back-up power source, instruction of SO/caregivers, provision for continuation of plan of care, assistance with transportation, and coordination of resources/support systems.

Refer to section at end of plan for postdischarge considerations.

DIAGNOSTIC STUDIES

Pulmonary function studies: Determine the ability of the lungs to exchange oxygen and carbon dioxide, and include but are not limited to the following:

Vital capacity (VC): Is reduced in restrictive chest or lung conditions, normal or increased in COPD, normal to decreased in neuromuscular diseases (e.g., Guillain-Barré syndrome), and decreased in conditions limiting thoracic movement (e.g., kyphoscoliosis).

Forced vital capacity (FVC): Measured by spirometry, is reduced in restrictive conditions and in asthma, and is normal to reduced in COPD.

Tidal volume (V_T): May be decreased in both restrictive and obstructive processes.

Negative inspiratory force (NIF): Can be substituted for vital capacity to help determine whether client can initiate a breath.

Minute ventilation (V_E): Measures volume of air inhaled and exhaled in 1 min of normal breathing. This reflects muscle endurance and is a major determinant of work of breathing.

Inspiratory pressure (Pi_{max}): Measures respiratory muscle strength (less than 20 cm H_2O is considered insufficient for weaning).

Forced expiratory volume (FEV): Usually decreased in COPD.

Flow-volume (F-V) loops: Abnormal loops are indicative of large and small airway obstructive disease and restrictive diseases when far advanced.

ABGs: Assesses status of oxygenation, ventilation, and acid-base balance. ABG results help determine the settings for the ventilator (e.g., partial pressure of arterial oxygen [Pao_2], arterial oxygen saturation [Sao_2], and partial pressure of arterial carbon dioxide $Paco_2$]).

Chest x-ray: Monitors resolution/progression of underlying condition (e.g., acute respiratory distress syndrome [ARDS]) or complications (e.g., atelectasis, pneumonia).

Nutritional assessment: Done to identify nutritional and electrolyte imbalances that might interfere with successful weaning.

NURSING PRIORITIES

1. Promote adequate ventilation and oxygenation.
2. Prevent complications.
3. Provide emotional support for client/SO.
4. Provide information about disease process/prognosis and treatment needs.

DISCHARGE GOALS

1. Respiratory function maximized/adequate to meet individual needs.
2. Complications prevented/minimized.
3. Effective means of communication established.
4. Disease process/prognosis and therapeutic regimen understood (including home ventilatory support if indicated).
5. Plan in place to meet needs after discharge.

NURSING DIAGNOSIS: ineffective Breathing Pattern/ impaired Spontaneous Ventilation

May be related to

Respiratory center depression
Respiratory muscle weakness/paralysis
Noncompliant lung tissue (decreased lung expansion)
Alteration of client's usual O_2/CO_2 ratio

Possibly evidenced by

Changes in rate and depth of respirations
Dyspnea/increased work of breathing, use of accessory muscles
Reduced VC/total lung volume
Tachypnea/bradypnea or cessation of respirations when off the ventilator
Cyanosis
Decreased Po_2 and Sao_2, increased Pco_2
Increased restlessness, apprehension, and metabolic rate

DESIRED OUTCOMES/EVALUATION CRITERIA—CLIENT WILL:

RESPIRATORY STATUS: Ventilation (NOC)

Reestablish/maintain effective respiratory pattern via ventilator with absence of retractions/use of accessory muscles, cyanosis, or other signs of hypoxia; ABGs/oxygen saturation within acceptable range.
Participate in efforts to wean (as appropriate) within individual ability.

CAREGIVER WILL:

Demonstrate behaviors necessary to maintain client's respiratory function.

ACTIONS/INTERVENTIONS	RATIONALE
Mechanical Ventilation (NIC)	
Independent	
Investigate etiology of respiratory failure.	Understanding the underlying cause of client's particular ventilatory problem is essential to the care of client; e.g., decisions about future capabilities/ventilation needs and most appropriate type of ventilatory support.
Observe overall breathing pattern. Note respiratory rate, distinguishing between spontaneous respirations and ventilator breaths.	Clients on ventilators can experience hyperventilation/hypoventilation, or dyspnea/"air hunger," and attempt to correct deficiency by overbreathing.
Auscultate chest periodically, noting presence/absence and equality of breath sounds, adventitious breath sounds, and symmetry of chest movement.	Provides information regarding airflow through the tracheobronchial tree and the presence/absence of fluid, mucous obstruction. *Note:* Frequent crackles or rhonchi that do not clear with coughing/suctioning may indicate developing complications (atelectasis, pneumonia, acute bronchospasm, pulmonary edema). Changes in chest symmetry may indicate improper placement of the ET tube, development of barotrauma.
Count client's respirations for 1 full minute and compare with desired/ventilator set rate.	Respirations vary depending on problem requiring ventilatory assistance; e.g., client may be totally ventilator dependent or be able to take breath(s) on own between ventilator-delivered breaths. Rapid client respirations can produce respiratory alkalosis and/or prevent desired volume from being delivered by ventilator. Slow client respirations/hypoventilation increases $Paco_2$ levels and may cause acidosis.
Verify that client's respirations are in phase with the ventilator.	Adjustments may be required in tidal volume, respiratory rate, and/or dead space of the ventilator, or client may need sedation to synchronize respirations and reduce work of breathing/energy expenditure.

ACTIONS/INTERVENTIONS	RATIONALE
Elevate head of bed or place in orthopedic chair if possible.	Elevation of client's head or getting out of bed while still on the ventilator is both physically and psychologically beneficial.
Place in prone position when tolerated.	Prone position relaxes abdominal muscles, improving diaphragmatic excursion, increasing PaO_2.
Inflate tracheal/ET tube cuff properly using minimal leak/occlusive technique. Check cuff inflation every 4–8 hr and whenever cuff is deflated/reinflated.	The cuff must be properly inflated to ensure adequate ventilation/delivery of desired tidal volume. *Note:* In long-term clients, the cuff may be deflated most of the time or a noncuffed tracheostomy tube used.
Check tubing for obstruction; e.g., kinking or accumulation of water. Drain tubing as indicated, avoiding draining toward client or back into the reservoir.	Kinks in tubing prevent adequate volume delivery and increase airway pressure. Condensation in tubing prevents proper gas distribution and predisposes to bacterial growth.
Check ventilator alarms for proper functioning. Do not turn off alarms, even for suctioning. Remove from ventilator and ventilate manually if source of ventilator alarm cannot be quickly identified and rectified. Ascertain that alarms can be heard in the nurses' station.	Ventilators have a series of visual and audible alarms; e.g., oxygen, low/high pressure, inspiratory: expiratory (I:E) ratio. Turning off/failure to reset alarms places client at risk for unobserved ventilator failure or respiratory distress/arrest.
Keep resuscitation bag at bedside and ventilate manually whenever indicated.	Provides/restores adequate ventilation when client or equipment problems require client to be temporarily removed from the ventilator.
Assist client in "taking control" of breathing if weaning is attempted/ventilatory support is interrupted during procedure/activity.	Coaching client to take slower, deeper breaths, practice abdominal/pursed-lip breathing, assume position of comfort, and use relaxation techniques can be helpful in maximizing respiratory function.

Collaborative

ACTIONS/INTERVENTIONS	RATIONALE
Assess ventilator settings routinely and readjust as indicated:	Controls/settings are adjusted according to client's primary disease and results of diagnostic testing to maintain parameters within appropriate limits.
Note operating mode of ventilation; that is, continuous mandatory ventilation (CMV), assist control (AC), intermittent mandatory (IM), pressure support (PS), or inverse ratio (IR);	Client's respiratory requirements, presence or absence of an underlying disease process, and the extent to which client can participate in ventilatory effort determine parameters of each setting. PS, a relatively new ventilation mode, has advantages for clients who are on long-term ventilation because it allows client to strengthen pulmonary musculature without compromising oxygenation and ventilation during the weaning process. Research suggests that intermittent trials of unassisted breathing work faster (for weaning) than methods involving partial ventilatory support.
Observe oxygen concentration percentage (Fio_2); verify that oxygen line is in proper outlet/tank; monitor in-line oxygen analyzer or perform periodic oxygen analysis;	FIO_2 is adjusted (21%–100%) to maintain an acceptable oxygen percentage and saturation (e.g., 90%) for client's condition. Because machine dials are not always accurate, an oxygen analyzer may be used to ascertain whether client is receiving the desired concentration of oxygen. *Note:* Fio_2 of 40% or below reduces risk of absorption atelectasis and surfactant inactivation.
Observe end-tidal CO_2 ($ETco_2$) values;	Measures the amount of exhaled CO_2 with each breath and is displayed graphically to spot CO_2 exchange problems early before they show up on ABGs. Values are affected by matching of ventilation in lung with perfusion of pulmonary capillaries.
Assess set respiratory frequency (f);	Respiratory rate of 10–15/min may be appropriate except for client with COPD and CO_2 retention. In these clients, rate and volume should be adjusted to achieve client's baseline $Paco_2$, not necessarily a "normal" $Paco_2$.

ACTIONS/INTERVENTIONS	RATIONALE
Assess tidal volume (V_T 10–15 mL/kg). Verify proper function of spirometer, bellows, or computer readout of delivered volume. Note alterations from desired volume delivery;	Monitors amount of air inspired and expired. Changes may indicate alteration in lung compliance or leakage through machine/around tube cuff (if used). *Note:* Smaller tidal volume may be required in clients with decreased lung compliance (e.g., ARDS).
Note airway pressure;	Airway pressure should remain relatively constant. Increased pressure alarm reading reflects (1) increased airway resistance as may occur with bronchospasm; (2) retained secretions; and/or (3) decreased lung compliance as may occur with obstruction of the ET tube, development of atelectasis, ARDS, pulmonary edema, worsening COPD, or pneumothorax. Low airway pressure alarms may be triggered by pathophysiologic conditions causing hypoventilation; e.g., disconnection from ventilator, low ET cuff pressure, ET tube displaced above the vocal cords, client "overbreathing" or out of phase with the ventilator.
Monitor I:E ratio;	Expiratory phase is usually twice the length of the inspiratory rate, but may be longer to compensate for air-trapping to improve gas exchange in the COPD client.
Check sigh rate intervals (usually 1 1/2 to two times V_T);	Sighing promotes maximal ventilation of alveoli to prevent/reduce atelectasis and enhances movement of secretions.
Note inspired humidity and temperature. Use heat moisture exchanger (HME) as indicated;	Usual warming and humidifying function of nasopharynx is bypassed with intubation. Dehydration can dry up normal pulmonary fluids, cause secretions to thicken, and increase risk of infection. Temperature should be maintained at about body temperature to reduce risk of damage to cilia and hyperthermia reactions. The introduction of a heated wire circuit to the traditional system significantly reduces the problem of "rainout" (condensation in the tubing).
Monitor serial ABGs and pulse oximetry.	Adjustments to ventilator settings may be required depending on client's response and trends in gas exchange parameters.

NURSING DIAGNOSIS: ineffective Airway Clearance

May be related to

Foreign body (artificial airway) in the trachea
Inability to cough/ineffective cough

Possibly evidenced by

Changes in rate or depth of respiration
Cyanosis
Abnormal breath sounds
Anxiety/restlessness

DESIRED OUTCOMES/EVALUATION CRITERIA—CLIENT WILL:

RESPIRATORY STATUS: Airway Patency (NOC)

Maintain patent airway with breath sounds clear.
Be free of aspiration.

CAREGIVER WILL:

Identify potential complications and initiate appropriate actions.

ACTIONS/INTERVENTIONS	RATIONALE
Artificial Airway Management (NIC)	
Independent	
Assess airway patency.	Obstruction may be caused by accumulation of secretions, mucous plugs, hemorrhage, bronchospasm, and/or problems with the position of tracheostomy/ET tube.
Evaluate chest movement and auscultate for bilateral breath sounds.	Symmetrical chest movement with breath sounds throughout lung fields indicates proper tube placement/unobstructed airflow. Lower airway obstruction (e.g., pneumonia/atelectasis) produces changes in breath sounds such as rhonchi, wheezing.
Monitor ET tube placement. Note lip line marking and compare with desired placement. Secure tube carefully with tape or tube holder. Obtain assistance when retaping or repositioning tube.	The ET tube may slip into the right main-stem bronchus, thereby obstructing airflow to the left lung and putting client at risk for a tension pneumothorax.
Note excessive coughing, increased dyspnea (using a 0–10 scale), high-pressure alarm sounding on ventilator, visible secretions in endotracheal/tracheostomy tube, increased rhonchi.	The intubated client often has an ineffective cough reflex, or client may have neuromuscular or neurosensory impairment, altering ability to cough. These clients are dependent on alternative means such as suctioning to remove secretions. *Note:* Research supports use of a dyspnea rating scale (like those used to measure pain) to more accurately quantify and measure changes in dyspnea as experienced by client.
Suction as needed when client is coughing or experiencing respiratory distress, limiting duration of suction to 15 sec or less. Choose appropriate suction catheter. Hyperventilate before and after each catheter pass, using 100% oxygen if appropriate (using vent rather than Ambu bag, which has an increased risk of barotrauma). Suction continuously or intermittently during withdrawal.	Suctioning should not be routine, and duration should be limited to reduce hazard of hypoxia. Suction catheter diameter should be less than 50% of the internal diameter of the endotracheal/tracheostomy tube for prevention of hypoxia. Hyperoxygenation with ventilator sigh on 100% oxygen may be desired to reduce atelectasis and to reduce accidental hypoxia. *Note:* Instilling normal saline (NS) is no longer recommended because research reveals that the fluid pools at the distal end of the endotracheal/tracheal tube, impairing oxygenation and increasing bronchospasm and the risk of infection.
Use inline catheter suction when available.	Reduces risk of infection for healthcare workers and helps maintain oxygen saturation and PEEP when used.
Instruct client in coughing techniques during suctioning; e.g., splinting, timing of breathing, and "quad cough" as indicated.	Enhances effectiveness of cough effort and secretion clearing.
Reposition/turn periodically.	Promotes drainage of secretions and ventilation to all lung segments, reducing risk of atelectasis.
Encourage/provide fluids within individual capability.	Helps liquefy secretions, enhancing expectoration.
Collaborative	
Provide chest physiotherapy as indicated; e.g., postural drainage, percussion.	Promotes ventilation of all lung segments and aids drainage of secretions.
Administer IV and aerosol bronchodilators as indicated; e.g., aminophylline, metaproterenol sulfate (Alupent), isoetharine hydrochloride (Bronkosol).	Promotes ventilation and removal of secretions by relaxation of smooth muscle/bronchospasm.
Assist with fiberoptic bronchoscopy, if indicated.	May be performed to remove secretions/mucous plugs.

NURSING DIAGNOSIS: impaired verbal Communication

May be related to

Physical barrier; e.g., endotracheal/tracheostomy tube
Neuromuscular weakness/paralysis

Possibly evidenced by

Inability to speak

DESIRED OUTCOMES/EVALUATION CRITERIA—CLIENT WILL:

COMMUNICATION: Expressive Ability (NOC)

Establish method of communication in which needs can be understood.

ACTIONS/INTERVENTIONS	RATIONALE
COMMUNICATION ENHANCEMENT: Speech Deficit (NIC)	
Independent	
Assess client's ability to communicate by alternative means.	Reasons for long-term ventilatory support are various; client may be alert and be adept at writing (e.g., chronic COPD with inability to be weaned) or may be lethargic, comatose, or paralyzed. Method of communicating with client is therefore highly individualized. *Note:* The inability to talk while intubated is a primary cause of feelings of fear.
Establish means of communication; e.g., maintain eye contact; ask yes/no questions; provide magic slate, paper/pencil, picture/alphabet board; use sign language as appropriate; validate meaning of attempted communications.	Eye contact assures client of interest in communicating; if client is able to move head, blink eyes, or is comfortable with simple gestures, a great deal can be done with yes/no questions. Pointing to letter boards or writing is often tiring to clients, who can then become frustrated with the effort needed to attempt conversations. Use of picture boards that express a concept or routine needs may simplify communication. Family members/other caregivers may be able to assist/interpret needs.
Consider form of communication when placing IV.	IV positioned in hand/wrist may limit ability to write or sign.
Place call light/bell within reach, making certain client is alert and physically capable of using it. Answer call light/bell immediately. Anticipate needs. Tell client that nurse is immediately available should assistance be required.	Ventilator-dependent client may be better able to relax, feel safe (not abandoned), and breathe with the ventilator knowing that nurse is vigilant and needs will be met.
Place note at central call station informing staff that client is unable to speak.	Alerts all staff members to respond to client at the bedside instead of over the intercom.
Encourage family/SO to talk with client, providing information about family and daily happenings.	SO may feel self-conscious in one-sided conversation, but knowledge that he or she is assisting client to regain/maintain contact with reality and enabling client to feel part of family unit can reduce feelings of awkwardness.
Collaborative	
Evaluate need for/appropriateness of talking tracheostomy tube.	Clients with adequate cognitive/muscular skills may have the ability to manipulate talking tracheostomy tube.

NURSING DIAGNOSIS: Fear/Anxiety [specify level]

May be related to

Situational crises; threat to self-concept
Threat of death/dependency on mechanical support
Change in health/socioeconomic status/role functioning
Interpersonal transmission/contagion

Possibly evidenced by

Increased muscle/facial tension
Insomnia; restlessness
Hypervigilance
Feelings of inadequacy
Fearfulness, uncertainty, apprehension
Focus on self/negative self-talk
Expressed concern regarding changes in life events

DESIRED OUTCOMES/EVALUATION CRITERIA—CLIENT WILL:

Fear Self-Control/Anxiety Self-Control (NOC)

Verbalize/communicate awareness of feelings and healthy ways to deal with them.
Demonstrate problem-solving skills/behaviors to cope with current situation.
Report that anxiety/fear is reduced to manageable level.
Appear relaxed and sleeping/resting appropriately.

ACTIONS/INTERVENTIONS	RATIONALE
Anxiety Reduction (NIC)	
Independent	
Identify client's perception of threat represented by situation. Determine current respiratory status/adequacy of ventilation.	Defines scope of individual problem separate from physiologic causes, and influences choice of interventions.
Observe/monitor physical responses; e.g., restlessness, changes in vital signs, repetitive movements. Note congruency of verbal/nonverbal communication.	Useful in evaluating extent/degree of concerns, especially when compared with "verbal" comments.
Encourage client/SO to acknowledge and express fears.	Provides opportunity for dealing with concerns, clarifies reality of fears, and reduces anxiety to a more manageable level.
Acknowledge the anxiety and fear of the situation. Avoid meaningless reassurance that everything will be all right.	Validates the reality of the situation without minimizing the emotional impact. Provides opportunity for client/SO to accept and begin to deal with what has happened, reducing anxiety.
Identify/review with client/SO the safety precautions being taken; e.g., backup power and oxygen supplies, emergency equipment at hand for suctioning. Discuss/review the meanings of alarm system.	Provides reassurance to help allay unnecessary anxiety, reduce concerns of the unknown, and preplan for response in emergency situation.
Note reactions of SO. Provide opportunity for discussion of personal feelings/concerns and future expectations.	Family members have individual responses to what is happening, and their anxiety may be communicated to client, intensifying these emotions.
Identify previous coping strengths of client/SO and current areas of control/ability.	Focuses attention on own capabilities, increasing sense of control.

ACTIONS/INTERVENTIONS	RATIONALE
Demonstrate/encourage use of relaxation techniques; e.g., focused breathing, guided imagery, progressive relaxation. Provide music therapy, biofeedback as appropriate.	Provides active management of situation to reduce feelings of helplessness.
Provide/encourage sedentary diversional activities within individual capabilities; e.g., handicrafts, writing, television.	Although handicapped by dependence on ventilator, activities that are normal/desired by the individual should be encouraged to enhance quality of life.

Collaborative

Refer to support individuals, groups, and therapy as needed.	May be necessary to provide additional assistance if client/SO are not managing anxiety or when client is "identified with the machine."

NURSING DIAGNOSIS: impaired Oral Mucous Membrane

Risk factors may include

Inability to swallow oral fluids
Presence of tube in mouth
Lack of or decreased salivation
Ineffective oral hygiene

Possibly evidenced by

[Not applicable; presence of signs and symptoms establishes an *actual* diagnosis.]

DESIRED OUTCOMES/EVALUATION CRITERIA—CLIENT WILL:

TISSUE INTEGRITY: Skin and Mucous Membrane (NOC)

Report/demonstrate a decrease in symptoms.

CAREGIVER WILL:

Identify specific interventions to promote healthy oral mucosa as appropriate.

ACTIONS/INTERVENTIONS — RATIONALE

Oral Health Maintenance (NIC)

Independent

ACTIONS/INTERVENTIONS	RATIONALE
Routinely inspect oral cavity, teeth, gums for sores, lesions, bleeding.	Early identification of problems provides opportunity for appropriate intervention/preventive measures.
Administer mouth care routinely and as needed, especially in client with an oral intubation tube; e.g., cleanse mouth with water, saline, or preferred alcohol-free mouthwash. Brush teeth with soft toothbrush, WaterPik, or moistened swab.	Prevents drying/ulceration of mucous membrane and reduces medium for bacterial growth. Promotes comfort.
Change position of ET tube/airway on a regular and prn schedule as appropriate.	Reduces risk of lip and oral mucous membrane ulceration.
Apply lip balm; administer oral lubricant solution.	Maintains moisture, prevents drying.

NURSING DIAGNOSIS: imbalanced Nutrition: less than body requirements

May be related to

Altered ability to ingest and properly digest food
Increased metabolic demands

Possibly evidenced by

Weight loss; poor muscle tone
Aversion to eating; reported altered taste sensation
Sore, inflamed buccal cavity
Absence of/hyperactive bowel sounds

DESIRED OUTCOMES/EVALUATION CRITERIA—CLIENT WILL:

Nutritional Status (NOC)

Indicate understanding of individual dietary needs.
Demonstrate progressive weight gain toward goal with normalization of laboratory values.

ACTIONS/INTERVENTIONS	RATIONALE
Nutrition Therapy (NIC)	
Independent	
Evaluate ability to eat.	Clients with a tracheostomy tube may be able to eat, but clients with ET tubes must be tube fed or parenterally nourished.
Observe/monitor for generalized muscle wasting, loss of subcutaneous fat.	These symptoms are indicative of depletion of muscle energy and can reduce respiratory muscle function.
Weigh as indicated.	Significant and recent weight loss (7%–10% body weight) and poor nutritional intake provide clues regarding catabolism, muscle glycogen stores, and ventilatory drive sensitivity.
Document oral intake if/when resumed. Offer foods that client enjoys.	Appetite is usually poor and intake of essential nutrients may be reduced. Offering favorite foods can enhance oral intake.
Provide small frequent feedings of soft/easily digested foods if able to swallow.	Prevents excessive fatigue, enhances intake, and reduces risk of gastric distress.
Encourage/administer fluid intake of at least 2500 mL/day within cardiac tolerance.	Prevents dehydration that can be exacerbated by increased insensible losses (e.g., ventilator/intubation) and reduces risk of constipation.
Assess GI function: presence/quality of bowel sounds; note changes in abdominal girth, nausea/vomiting. Observe/document changes in bowel movements; e.g., diarrhea/constipation. Test all stools for occult blood.	A functioning GI system is essential for the proper utilization of enteral feedings. Mechanically ventilated clients are at risk of developing abdominal distention (trapped air or ileus) and gastric bleeding (stress ulcers).
Collaborative	
Adjust diet to meet respiratory needs as indicated.	High intake of carbohydrates, protein, and calories may be desired/needed during ventilation to improve respiratory muscle function. Carbohydrates may be reduced and fat somewhat increased just before weaning attempts to prevent excessive CO_2 production and reduced respiratory drive.

ACTIONS/INTERVENTIONS	RATIONALE
Administer tube feeding/hyperalimentation as needed. (Refer to CP: Total Nutritional Support: Parenteral/Enteral Feeding.)	Provides adequate nutrients to meet individual needs when oral intake is insufficient/not appropriate.
Monitor laboratory studies as indicated; e.g., prealbumin, serum transferrin, BUN/creatinine (Cr), glucose.	Provides information about adequacy of nutritional support/need for change.

NURSING DIAGNOSIS: risk for Infection

Risk factors may include

Inadequate primary defenses (traumatized lung tissue, decreased ciliary action, stasis of body fluids)
Inadequate secondary defenses (immunosuppression)
Chronic disease, malnutrition
Invasive procedure (intubation)

Possibly evidenced by

[Not applicable; presence of signs and symptoms establishes an *actual* diagnosis.]

DESIRED OUTCOMES/EVALUATION CRITERIA—CLIENT/CAREGIVER WILL:

KNOWLEDGE: Infection Control (NOC)

Indicate understanding of individual risk factors.
Identify interventions to prevent/reduce risk of infection.
Demonstrate techniques to promote safe environment.

ACTIONS/INTERVENTIONS	RATIONALE
Infection Protection (NIC)	
Independent	
Note risk factors for occurrence of infection.	Intubation, prolonged mechanical ventilation, trauma, general debilitation, malnutrition, age, and invasive procedures are factors that potentiate client's risk of acquiring infection and prolonging recovery. Awareness of individual risk factors provides opportunity to limit effects and helps prevent ventilator-associated pneumonia (VAP), which is the primary cause of hospital-acquired pneumonia.
Observe color/odor/characteristics of sputum. Note drainage around tracheostomy tube.	Yellow/green, purulent odorous sputum is indicative of infection; thick, tenacious sputum suggests dehydration.
Reduce nosocomial risk factors via proper hand washing or alcohol-based hand rubs by all caregivers; maintaining sterile suction techniques in open system; use of closed-system ET tube allowing for continuous removal of secretions; reducing the number of times the ventilator tubes are open, and providing clean nebulizer/tubing changes.	These factors may be the simplest but are the most important keys to prevention of hospital-acquired infection. *Note:* Centers for Disease Control and Prevention (CDC) guidelines recommend changing tubing no more often than every 48 hr. Research indicates that less frequent tubing changes (every 5–7 days) may be acceptable.
Encourage deep breathing, coughing, and frequent position changes.	Maximizes lung expansion and mobilization of secretions to prevent/reduce atelectasis and accumulation of sticky, thick secretions.

ACTIONS/INTERVENTIONS	RATIONALE
Auscultate breath sounds.	Presence of rhonchi/wheezes suggests retained secretions requiring expectoration/suctioning.
Provide/instruct client/SO in proper oral care and secretion disposal; e.g., tissues, soiled tracheostomy dressings.	Reduces risk of pneumonia associated with aspiration of oral bacteria, as well as transmission of fluidborne organisms. *Note*: Chlorhexidine mouth rinse has been found to reduce plaque and gingival inflammation as a means of preventing VAP.
Monitor/screen visitors. Avoid contact with persons with respiratory infections.	Individual is already compromised and is at increased risk with exposure to infections.
Provide respiratory isolation when indicated.	Depending on specific diagnosis, client may require protection from others or must prevent transmission of infection to others (e.g., tuberculosis).
Maintain adequate hydration and nutrition. Encourage fluids to 2500 mL/day within cardiac tolerance.	Helps improve general resistance to disease and reduces risk of infection from static secretions.
Measure pH of gastric secretions, and monitor use of antacid medications as indicated.	Maintaining acid level of stomach around 7.2 pH may help reduce risk of nosocomial infection and stress ulcers and contamination of respiratory tract by means of reflux and aspiration.
Encourage self-care/activities to limit of tolerance. Assist with graded exercise program.	Improves general well-being and muscle strength and may stimulate immune system recovery.

Collaborative

Obtain sputum cultures as indicated.	May be needed to identify pathogens and appropriate antimicrobials. *Note*: Bacteria are the most frequently isolated pathogens for VAP.
Administer antimicrobials as indicated.	If infection does occur, one or more agents may be used depending on identified pathogen(s).

NURSING DIAGNOSIS: risk for dysfunctional Ventilatory Weaning Response

Risk factors may include

Sleep disturbance
Limited/insufficient energy stores
Pain or discomfort
Adverse environment (e.g., inadequate monitoring/support)
Client-perceived inability to wean; decreased motivation
History of extended weaning

Possibly evidenced by

[Not applicable; presence of signs and symptoms establishes an *actual* diagnosis.]

DESIRED OUTCOMES/EVALUATION CRITERIA—CLIENT WILL:

RESPIRATORY STATUS: Ventilation (NOC)

Actively participate in the weaning process.
Reestablish independent respiration with ABGs within acceptable range and free of signs of respiratory failure.
Demonstrate increased tolerance for activity/participate in self-care within level of ability.

ACTIONS/INTERVENTIONS	RATIONALE
Mechanical Ventilatory Weaning (NIC)	
Independent	
Assess physical factors involved in weaning; e.g.:	
Stable heart rate/rhythm, BP, and clear breath sounds;	The heart has to work harder to meet increased energy needs associated with weaning. Physician may defer weaning if tachycardia, pulmonary crackles, and/or hypertension are present.
Fever;	Increase of 1°F (0.6°C) in body temperature raises metabolic rate and oxygen demands by 7%.
Nutritional status and muscle strength.	Weaning is hard work. Client not only must be able to withstand the stress of weaning but also must have the stamina to breathe spontaneously for extended periods.
Determine psychologic readiness.	Weaning provokes anxiety for client regarding concerns about ability to breathe on own and long-term need of ventilator.
Explain weaning techniques; e.g., spontaneous breathing trial (SBT), T-piece, spontaneous intermittent maximal ventilation (SIMV), continuous positive airway pressure (CPAP), or nasal intermittent positive-pressure ventilation (NIPPV). Discuss individual plan and expectations.	Assists client to prepare for weaning process, helps limit fear of unknown, promotes cooperation, and enhances likelihood of a successful outcome. *Note:* Current guidelines recommend an SBT at least once each day for hemodynamically stable client. Pressure support ventilation unloads respiratory muscles, allowing client to "set" rate and volume and decelerating flow pattern because breath can be shaped to simulate a more normal respiratory pattern with higher gas flow on inspiration, then tapering off. This increases client comfort and is especially beneficial for clients at high risk for DVWR.
Provide undisturbed rest/sleep periods. Avoid stressful procedures/situations or nonessential activities.	Maximizes energy for weaning process; limits fatigue and oxygen consumption. *Note:* It takes approximately 12–14 hr of respiratory rest to rejuvenate tired respiratory muscles. For clients on assist/control, raising the rate to 20 breaths/min can also provide respiratory rest.
Evaluate/document client's progress. Note restlessness; changes in BP, heart rate, respiratory rate; use of accessory muscles; discoordinated breathing with ventilator; increased concentration on breathing (mild dysfunction); client's concerns about possible machine malfunction; inability to cooperate/respond to coaching; color changes.	Indicators that client may require slower weaning/opportunity to stabilize or may need to stop program. *Note:* Moving from pressure/volume (e.g., assist/control) ventilator to T-piece may precipitate a "flash" form of heart failure requiring prompt intervention.
Recognize/provide encouragement for client's efforts.	Positive feedback provides reassurance and support for continuation of weaning process.
Monitor cardiopulmonary response to activity.	Excessive oxygen consumption/demand increases the possibility of failure.
Collaborative	
Consult with dietitian, nutritional support team for adjustments in composition of diet.	Reduction of carbohydrates/fats may be required to prevent excessive production of CO_2, which could alter respiratory drive.
Monitor CBC, serum albumin and prealbumin, transferrin, total iron-binding capacity, and electrolytes (especially potassium, calcium, and phosphorus).	Verifies that nutrition is adequate to meet energy requirements for weaning.
Review chest x-ray and ABGs.	Chest x-rays should show clear lungs or marked improvement in pulmonary congestion or infiltrates. ABGs should document satisfactory oxygenation on an FIO_2 of 40% or less.

NURSING DIAGNOSIS: deficient Knowledge [Learning Need] regarding condition, prognosis and therapy, self-care and discharge needs

May be related to

Lack of exposure/recall
Misinterpretation of information; unfamiliarity with information resources
Stress of situational crisis

Possibly evidenced by

Questions about care, request for information
Reluctance to learn new skills
Inaccurate follow-through of instructions
Development of preventable complications

DESIRED OUTCOMES/EVALUATION CRITERIA—CLIENT/SO/CAREGIVER WILL:

Health-Seeking Behavior (NOC)

Participate in learning process.
Exhibit increased interest, shown by verbal/nonverbal cues.
Assume responsibility for own learning and begin to look for information and to ask questions.

KNOWLEDGE: Treatment Regimen (NOC)

Indicate understanding of mechanical ventilation therapy.
Demonstrate behaviors/new skills to meet individual needs/prevent complications.

ACTIONS/INTERVENTIONS	RATIONALE
Learning Facilitation (NIC)	
Independent	
Determine ability and willingness to learn.	Physical condition may preclude client involvement in care before and after discharge. SO/caregiver may feel inadequate and afraid of machinery and have reservations about ability to learn or deal with overall situation.
Schedule teaching sessions for quiet, nonstressful times when all participants are well rested.	Enhances learners' ability to focus on and absorb content provided.
Arrange information in logical sequence, progressing from simple to more complex material at learners' pace.	Allows learner to build on information learned in previous sessions; is less threatening/overwhelming.
KNOWLEDGE: Disease Process (NIC)	
Provide material in multiple formats (e.g., books/pamphlets, audiovisuals, hands-on demonstrations) and take-home instruction sheets as appropriate.	Uses multiple senses to stimulate learning/retention of information. Provides resources for review following discharge.
Discuss specific condition requiring ventilatory support, what measures are being tried for weaning, short- and long-term goals of treatment.	Provides knowledge base to aid client/SO in making informed decisions. Weaning efforts may continue for several weeks (extended period of time). Dependence is evidenced by repeatedly increased Pco_2 and/or decline in Pao_2 during weaning attempts, presence of dyspnea, anxiety, tachycardia, perspiration, cyanosis.

ACTIONS/INTERVENTIONS	RATIONALE
Encourage client/SO to evaluate impact of ventilatory dependence on their lifestyle and what changes they are willing or unwilling to make. Problem solve solutions to issues raised.	Quality of life must be resolved by the ventilator-dependent client and caregivers who need to understand that home ventilatory support is a 24-hr job that affects everyone.
Promote participation in self-care/diversional activities and socialization as appropriate.	Refocuses attention toward more normal life activities, increases endurance, and helps prevent depersonalization.
Review issues of general well-being: role of nutrition, assistance with feeding/meal preparation, graded exercise/specific restrictions, rest periods alternated with activity.	Enhances recuperation and ensures that individual needs will be met.
Recommend that SO/caregivers learn CPR.	Provides sense of security about ability to handle emergency situations that might arise until help can be obtained.
Schedule team conference. Establish in-hospital training for caregivers if client is to be discharged home on ventilator.	Team approach is needed to coordinate client's care and teaching program to meet individual needs.
Instruct caregiver and client in hand washing techniques, use of sterile technique for suctioning, tracheostomy/stoma care, and chest physiotherapy.	Reduces risk of infection and promotes optimal respiratory function.
Provide demonstration and "hands-on" sessions, as well as written material, about specific type of ventilator to be used, function, and care of equipment.	Enhances familiarity, reducing anxiety and promoting confidence in implementation of new tasks/skills.
Discuss what/when to report to the healthcare provider; e.g., signs of respiratory distress, infection.	Helps reduce general anxiety while promoting timely/appropriate evaluation and intervention to prevent complications.
Ascertain that all needed equipment is in place and that safety concerns have been addressed; e.g., alternative power source (generator, batteries), back-up equipment, client call/alarm system.	Predischarge preparations can ease the transfer process. Planning for potential problems increases sense of security for client/SO.
Contact community/hospital-based services.	Suppliers of home equipment, physical therapy, care providers, emergency power provider, social services; financial assistance, aid in procuring equipment/personnel, and facilitating transition to home.
Refer to vocational/occupational therapist.	Some ventilator-dependent clients are able to resume vocations either while on the ventilator or during the day (while ventilator dependent at night).

POTENTIAL CONSIDERATIONS following acute hospitalization (dependent on client's age, physical condition/presence of complications, personal resources, and life responsibilities)

If client is discharged on ventilator, the client's needs/concerns remain the same as noted in this plan of care, in addition to:

Self-Care Deficit—decreased strength/endurance, inability to perform ADLs, depression, restrictions imposed by therapeutic intervention.

interrupted Family Processes—situational crisis.

risk for Relocation Stress Syndrome—feelings of powerlessness, concern about adequacy of support, unpredictability of experiences.

risk for Caregiver Role Strain—severity of illness of care receiver, discharge of family member with significant home care needs, presence of situational stressors (economic vulnerability, changes in roles/responsibilities), duration of caregiving required, inexperience in caregiving.

PULMONARY TUBERCULOSIS (TB)

Although many still believe it to be a problem of the past, pulmonary tuberculosis (TB) is on the rise. Most frequently seen as a pulmonary disease, TB is a bacterial infection classified as (1) *latent* (body's immune system has encapsulated the bacteria into tiny capsules called tubercles) and cannot be spread to others; or (2) *active* (infection is spreading in the body and can be transmitted to others). TB can also be extrapulmonary, affecting organs and tissues other than the lungs.

In the United States, the incidence of TB is higher among persons with HIV infection, the homeless, drug-addicted, and impoverished populations, as well as among immigrants from or visitors to countries in which TB is endemic. In addition, persons at highest risk include those who may have been exposed to the tubercle bacillus in the past and those who are debilitated or have lowered immunity because of chronic conditions such as AIDS, cancer, advanced age, and malnutrition. When the immune system weakens, dormant TB organisms can reactivate and multiply. When this latent infection develops into active disease, it is known as reactivation TB, which is often drug resistant.

Multidrug-resistant tuberculosis (MDR-TB) is on the rise, especially in large cities, in those previously treated with antitubercular drugs, or in those who failed to follow or complete a drug regimen. It can progress from diagnosis to death in as little as 4–6 weeks. MDR tuberculosis can be primary or secondary. *Primary MDR-TB* is caused by person-to-person transmission of a drug-resistant organism; *secondary MDR-TB* is usually the result of nonadherence to therapy or inappropriate treatment.

CARE SETTING

Most clients are treated in community clinics, but may be hospitalized for diagnostic evaluation/initiation of therapy, adverse drug reactions, or severe illness/debilitation. This plan of care is intended to reflect care of the person with active (rather than latent) TB, although if latent TB is diagnosed, treatment will be initiated.

RELATED CONCERNS

Extended care, page 810
Pneumonia, page 128
Psychosocial aspects of care, page 770

Client Assessment Database

Data depend on stage of disease and degree of involvement.

ACTIVITY/REST

May report:
Generalized weakness and fatigue
Shortness of breath with exertion
Difficulty sleeping, with evening or night fever, chills, and/or sweats
Nightmares

May exhibit:
Tachycardia, tachypnea/dyspnea on exertion
Muscle wasting, pain, and stiffness (advanced stages)

EGO INTEGRITY

May report:
Recent/long-standing stress factors
Financial concerns, poverty
Feelings of helplessness/hopelessness
Cultural/ethnic populations: Native American, recent immigrants from Central America, Southeast Asia, Indian subcontinent

May exhibit:
Denial (especially during early stages)
Anxiety, apprehension, irritability

FOOD/FLUID

May report:
Loss of appetite
Indigestion
Weight loss
Night sweats

May exhibit:
Poor skin turgor, dry/flaky skin
Muscle wasting/loss of subcutaneous fat

PAIN/DISCOMFORT

May report:
Chest pain aggravated by recurrent cough

May exhibit:
Guarding of affected area
Distraction behaviors, restlessness

RESPIRATION

May report:
Persistent cough, productive or nonproductive
Shortness of breath
History of TB/exposure to infected individual

May exhibit: Increased respiratory rate (extensive disease or fibrosis of the lung parenchyma and pleura)
Asymmetry in respiratory excursion (pleural effusion)
Dullness to percussion and decreased fremitus (pleural fluid or pleural thickening)
Breath sounds diminished/absent bilaterally or unilaterally (pleural effusion/pneumothorax); tubular breath sounds and/or whispered pectoriloquies over large lesions; crackles may be noted over apex of lungs during quick inspiration after a short cough (posttussive crackles)
Sputum characteristics green/purulent, yellowish mucoid, or blood tinged
Tracheal deviation (bronchogenic spread)
Inattention, marked irritability, change in mentation (advanced stages)

SAFETY

May report: Presence of immunosuppressed conditions, e.g., AIDS, cancer
Positive HIV test/HIV infection
Visit to/immigration from or close contact with persons in countries with high prevalence of TB (e.g., Philippines, Vietnam, Cambodia, Laos, Puerto Rico, Haiti, Russia, Mexico); use of certain arthritis drugs (e.g., infliximab [Remicade], etanercept [Enbrel], adalimumab [Humira])

May exhibit: Low-grade fever or acute febrile illness
Enlarged lymph nodes in neck

SOCIAL INTERACTION

May report: Feelings of isolation/rejection because of communicable disease
Change in usual patterns of responsibility/change in physical capacity to resume role

TEACHING/LEARNING

May report: Familial history of TB
General debilitation/poor health status
Use/abuse of substances such as IV drugs, alcohol, cocaine, and crack
Failure to improve/reactivation of TB
Nonparticipation in therapy

Discharge plan considerations: May require assistance with/alteration in drug therapy and temporary assistance in self-care and homemaker/maintenance tasks

Refer to section at end of plan for postdischarge considerations.

DIAGNOSTIC STUDIES

Sputum culture: Positive for *Mycobacterium tuberculosis* in the active stage of the disease. Sensitivities will also be tested for isoniazid (INH), rifampin (RIF), and ethambutol (EMB). Sputum cultures will be repeated three months into therapy to evaluate for possible nonadherence to treatment or to identify drug-resistant bacilli.

Ziehl-Neelsen (acid-fast stain applied to a smear of body fluid): Positive for acid-fast bacilli (AFB).

Skin tests—purified protein derivative (PPD) administered by single-needle intradermal injection (Mantoux test), (multiple-puncture tests [e.g,. tine, Aplitest] using PPD or old tuberculin [OT] are not recommended for general screening): A positive reaction—area of induration 10 mm or greater, occurring 48–72 hr after interdermal injection of the antigen—indicates past infection and the presence of antibodies but is not necessarily indicative of active disease. Factors associated with a suppressed response to tuberculin skin tests include underlying viral or bacterial infections, malnutrition, lymphadenopathy, current use of corticosteroids/other immunosuppressants; live vaccine viruses (e.g., measles, mumps, rubella) within last 4–6 weeks. A significant reaction in a client who is clinically ill means that active TB cannot be dismissed as a diagnostic possibility. A significant reaction in healthy persons usually signifies dormant TB or an infection caused by a different mycobacterium.

Enzyme-linked immunosorbent assay (ELISA)/Western blot: May reveal presence of HIV (strong risk factor in development of TB).

Chest x-ray: May show small, patchy infiltrations of early lesions in the upper-lung field, calcium deposits of healed primary lesions, or fluid of an effusion. Changes indicating more advanced TB may include cavitation and scar tissue/fibrotic areas.

CT or MRI scan: Determines degree of lung damage and may confirm a difficult diagnosis.

Bronchoscopy: Shows inflammation and altered lung tissue. May also be performed to obtain sputum if client is unable to produce an adequate specimen.

Histologic or tissue cultures (including gastric washings; urine and cerebrospinal fluid [CSF]; skin biopsy): Positive for *M. tuberculosis* and may indicate extrapulmonary involvement.

Needle biopsy of lung tissue: Positive for granulomas of TB; presence of giant cells indicating necrosis.

Electrolytes: May be abnormal depending on the location and severity of infection; e.g., hyponatremia caused by abnormal water retention may be found in extensive chronic pulmonary TB.

ABGs: May be abnormal depending on location, severity, and residual damage to the lungs.

Pulmonary function studies: Decreased vital capacity, increased dead space, increased ratio of residual air to total lung capacity, and decreased oxygen saturation are secondary to parenchymal infiltration/fibrosis, loss of lung tissue, and pleural disease (extensive chronic pulmonary TB).

NURSING PRIORITIES

1. Achieve/maintain adequate ventilation/oxygenation.
2. Prevent spread of infection.
3. Support behaviors/tasks to maintain health.
4. Promote effective coping strategies.
5. Provide information about disease process/prognosis and treatment needs.

DISCHARGE GOALS

1. Respiratory function adequate to meet individual need.
2. Complications prevented.
3. Lifestyle/behavior changes adopted to prevent spread of infection.
4. Disease process/prognosis and therapeutic regimen understood.
5. Plan in place to meet needs after discharge.

NURSING DIAGNOSIS: risk for Infection [spread/reactivation]

Risk factors may include

Inadequate primary defenses, decreased ciliary action/stasis of secretions
Tissue destruction/extension of infection
Lowered resistance/suppressed inflammatory process
Malnutrition
Environmental exposure
Insufficient knowledge to avoid exposure to pathogens

Possibly evidenced by

[Not applicable; presence of signs and symptoms establishes an *actual* diagnosis.]

DESIRED OUTCOMES/EVALUATION CRITERIA—CLIENT WILL:

Risk Control (NOC)

Identify interventions to prevent/reduce risk of spread of infection.
Demonstrate techniques/initiate lifestyle changes to promote safe environment.

ACTIONS/INTERVENTIONS	RATIONALE
Infection Control (NIC)	
Independent	
Review pathology of disease (active/inactive phases; dissemination of infection through bronchi to adjacent tissues or via bloodstream/lymphatic system) and potential spread of infection via airborne droplet during coughing, sneezing, spitting, talking, laughing, singing.	Helps client realize/accept necessity of adhering to medication regimen to prevent reactivation/complication. Understanding of how the disease is passed and awareness of transmission possibilities help client/SO take steps to prevent infection of others.
Identify others at risk; e.g., household members, close associates/friends.	Those exposed may require a course of drug therapy to prevent spread/development of infection.

ACTIONS/INTERVENTIONS	RATIONALE
Instruct client to cough/sneeze and expectorate into tissue and to refrain from spitting. Review proper disposal of tissue and good hand-washing techniques. Request return demonstration.	Behaviors necessary to prevent spread of infection.
Review necessity of infection control measures; e.g., temporary respiratory isolation.	May help client understand need for protecting others while acknowledging client's sense of isolation and social stigma associated with communicable diseases. *Note:* AFB can pass through standard masks; therefore, particulate respirators are required.
Monitor temperature as indicated.	Febrile reactions are indicators of continuing presence of infection.
Identify individual risk factors for reactivation of tuberculosis; e.g., lowered resistance associated with alcoholism, malnutrition/intestinal bypass surgery, use of immunosuppression drugs/corticosteroids, presence of diabetes mellitus, cancer, postpartum.	Knowledge about these factors helps client alter lifestyle and avoid/reduce incidence of exacerbation.
Stress importance of uninterrupted drug therapy. Evaluate client's potential for cooperation.	Contagious period may last only 2–3 days after initiation of drug regimen, but in the presence of cavitation or moderately advanced disease, risk of spread of infection may continue up to 3 months. Compliance with multidrug regimens for prolonged periods is difficult, so directly observed therapy (DOT) should be considered.
Review importance of follow-up and periodic reculturing of sputum for the duration of therapy.	Aids in monitoring the effects of medications and client's response to therapy.
Encourage selection/ingestion of well-balanced meals. Provide frequent small "snacks" in place of large meals as appropriate.	Presence of anorexia and/or preexisting malnutrition lowers resistance to infectious process and impairs healing. Small snacks may enhance overall intake.

Collaborative

Administer anti-infective agents as indicated; e.g.:	The goals for treatment of TB are to cure the individual and to minimize transmission to other persons. It is essential that treatment be tailored, and supervision be based on each client's clinical and social circumstances. DOT may be the most effective way to maximize the completion of therapy.
Primary drugs: isoniazid (INF, Nidrazid), rifampin (RIF, Rifadin, Rimactane), pyrazinamide (PZA, Tebrazid), ethambutol (Myambutol), streptomycin, rifapentine (RPT, Priftin);	Initial therapy of uncomplicated pulmonary disease usually includes four primary drugs, (INH, RIF, PZA, [EMB]) or combination of drugs (e.g., INH and RIF [Rifamate]). INH is usually drug of choice for infected client and those exposed, who are at risk for developing TB. Extended therapy (up to 24 months) is indicated for reactivation cases, extrapulmonary reactivated TB, or in the presence of other medical problems, such as diabetes mellitus or silicosis. Prophylaxis with INH for 12 months should be considered in HIV-positive clients with positive PPD test.
Second-line drugs; e.g.: ethionamide (Trecator-SC), para-aminosalicylate (PAS), cycloserine (Seromycin), capreomycin (Capastat);	These second-line drugs may be required when infection is resistant to or intolerant of primary drugs or may be used concurrently with primary antitubercular drugs. *Note:* MDR-TB requires minimum of 18–24 months' therapy with at least three drugs in the regimen known to be effective against the specific infective organism and that client has not previously taken. Treatment is often extended to 24 months in clients with severe symptoms/HIV infection.
Investigational agent R207910.	Current research suggests a new antibiotic that cuts off the energy supply of the mycobacterium may be effective against even drug-resistant forms of TB with only 2–3 months of treatment.

ACTIONS/INTERVENTIONS	RATIONALE
Monitor laboratory studies; e.g., sputum smear results.	Client who has three consecutive negative sputum smears (takes 3–5 months), is adhering to drug regimen, and is asymptomatic will be classified as a nontransmitter.
Liver function studies; e.g., AST/ALT	The most common serious adverse effect of drug therapy (particularly RIF, but possibly others as well) is drug-induced hepatitis.
Notify local health department.	Required by law, and should be reported within 1 week of diagnosis. Helpful in identifying contacts to reduce spread of infection. Treatment course is long and usually handled in the community with public health nurse monitoring.

NURSING DIAGNOSIS: ineffective Airway Clearance

May be related to

Thick, viscous, or bloody secretions
Fatigue, poor cough effort
Tracheal/pharyngeal edema

Possibly evidenced by

Abnormal respiratory rate, rhythm, depth
Abnormal breath sounds (rhonchi, wheezes), stridor
Dyspnea

DESIRED OUTCOMES/EVALUATION CRITERIA—CLIENT WILL:

RESPIRATORY STATUS: Airway Patency (NOC)

Maintain patent airway.
Expectorate secretions without assistance.
Demonstrate behaviors to improve/maintain airway clearance.
Participate in treatment regimen, within the level of ability/situation.
Identify potential complications and initiate appropriate actions.

Airway Management (NIC)

Independent

ACTIONS/INTERVENTIONS	RATIONALE
Assess respiratory function; e.g., breath sounds, rate, rhythm, and depth, and use of accessory muscles.	Diminished breath sounds may reflect atelectasis. Rhonchi, wheezes indicate accumulation of secretions/inability to clear airways that may lead to use of accessory muscles and increased work of breathing.
Note ability to expectorate mucus/cough effectively; document character, amount of sputum, presence of hemoptysis.	Expectoration may be difficult when secretions are very thick as a result of infection and/or inadequate hydration. Blood-tinged or frankly bloody sputum results from tissue breakdown (cavitation) in the lungs or from bronchial ulceration and may require further evaluation/intervention.
Place client in semi- or high-Fowler's position. Assist client with coughing and deep-breathing exercises.	Positioning helps maximize lung expansion and decreases respiratory effort. Maximal ventilation may open atelectatic areas and promote movement of secretions into larger airways for expectoration.

ACTIONS/INTERVENTIONS	RATIONALE
Clear secretions from mouth and trachea; suction as necessary.	Prevents obstruction/aspiration. Suctioning may be necessary if client is unable to expectorate secretions.
Maintain fluid intake of at least 2500 mL/day unless contraindicated.	High fluid intake helps thin secretions, making them easier to expectorate.

Collaborative

Humidify inspired air/oxygen.	Prevents drying of mucous membranes; helps thin secretions.
Administer medications as indicated:	
Mucolytic agents; e.g., acetylcysteine (Mucomyst);	Reduces the thickness and stickiness of pulmonary secretions to facilitate clearance.
Bronchodilators; e.g., oxtriphylline (Choledyl), theophylline (Theo-Dur);	Increases lumen size of the tracheobronchial tree, thus decreasing resistance to airflow and improving oxygen delivery.
Corticosteroids (prednisone).	May be useful in the presence of extensive involvement with profound hypoxemia and when inflammatory response is life-threatening.
Be prepared for/assist with emergency intubation.	Intubation may be necessary in rare cases of bronchogenic TB accompanied by laryngeal edema or acute pulmonary bleeding.

NURSING DIAGNOSIS: risk for impaired Gas Exchange

Risk factors may include

Decrease in effective lung surface, atelectasis
Destruction of alveolar-capillary membrane
Thick, viscous secretions
Bronchial edema

Possibly evidenced by

[Not applicable; presence of signs and symptoms establishes an *actual* diagnosis.]

DESIRED OUTCOMES/EVALUATION CRITERIA—CLIENT WILL:

RESPIRATORY STATUS: Gas Exchange (NOC)

Report absence of/decreased dyspnea.
Demonstrate improved ventilation and adequate oxygenation of tissues by ABGs within acceptable ranges.
Be free of symptoms of respiratory distress.

Respiratory Monitoring (NIC)

Independent

ACTIONS/INTERVENTIONS	RATIONALE
Assess for dyspnea (using 0–10 scale), tachypnea, abnormal/diminished breath sounds, increased respiratory effort, limited chest wall expansion, and fatigue.	Pulmonary TB can cause a wide range of effects in the lungs, ranging from a small patch of bronchopneumonia to diffuse intense inflammation, caseous necrosis, pleural effusion, and extensive fibrosis. Respiratory effects can range from mild dyspnea to profound respiratory distress. *Note:* Use of a scale to evaluate dyspnea helps clarify degree of difficulty and changes in condition.

ACTIONS/INTERVENTIONS	RATIONALE
Evaluate change in level of mentation. Note cyanosis and/or change in skin color, including mucous membranes and nail beds.	Accumulation of secretions/airway compromise can impair oxygenation of vital organs and tissues. (Refer to ND: ineffective Airway Clearance.)
Demonstrate/encourage pursed-lip breathing during exhalation, especially for clients with fibrosis or parenchymal destruction.	Creates resistance against outflowing air to prevent collapse/narrowing of the airways, thereby helping distribute air throughout the lungs and relieve/reduce shortness of breath.
Promote bed rest/limit activity and assist with self-care activities as necessary.	Reducing oxygen consumption/demand during periods of respiratory compromise may reduce severity of symptoms.

Collaborative

Monitor serial ABGs/pulse oximetry.	Decreased oxygen content (Pao_2) and/or saturation or increased $Paco_2$ indicate need for intervention/change in therapeutic regimen.
Provide supplemental oxygen as appropriate.	Aids in correcting the hypoxemia that may occur secondary to decreased ventilation/diminished alveolar lung surface.

NURSING DIAGNOSIS: imbalanced Nutrition: less than body requirements

May be related to

Fatigue
Frequent cough/sputum production; dyspnea
Anorexia
Insufficient financial resources

Possibly evidenced by

Weight 10%–20% below ideal for frame and height
Reported lack of interest in food, altered taste sensation
Poor muscle tone

DESIRED OUTCOMES/EVALUATION CRITERIA—CLIENT WILL:

Nutritional Status (NOC)

Demonstrate progressive weight gain toward goal with normalization of laboratory values and be free of signs of malnutrition.
Initiate behaviors/lifestyle changes to regain and/or to maintain appropriate weight.

ACTIONS/INTERVENTIONS — RATIONALE

Nutrition Management (NIC)

Independent

ACTIONS/INTERVENTIONS	RATIONALE
Document client's nutritional status on admission, noting skin turgor, current weight and degree of weight loss, integrity of oral mucosa, ability/inability to swallow, presence of bowel tones, history of nausea/vomiting or diarrhea.	Useful in defining degree/extent of problem and appropriate choice of interventions.
Ascertain client's usual dietary pattern, likes/dislikes.	Helpful in identifying specific needs/strengths. Consideration of individual preferences may improve dietary intake.

ACTIONS/INTERVENTIONS	RATIONALE
Monitor I&O and weight periodically.	Useful in measuring effectiveness of nutritional and fluid support.
Investigate anorexia and nausea/vomiting, and note possible correlation to medications. Monitor frequency, volume, consistency of stools.	May affect dietary choices and identify areas for problem solving to enhance intake/utilization of nutrients.
Encourage and provide for frequent rest periods.	Helps conserve energy, especially when metabolic requirements are increased by fever.
Provide oral care before and after respiratory treatments.	Reduces bad taste left from sputum or medications used for respiratory treatments that can stimulate the vomiting center.
Encourage small, frequent meals with foods high in protein and carbohydrates.	Maximizes nutrient intake without undue fatigue/energy expenditure from eating large meals, and reduces gastric irritation.
Encourage SO to bring foods from home and to share meals with client unless contraindicated.	Creates a more normal social environment during mealtime, and helps meet personal, cultural preferences.

Collaborative

ACTIONS/INTERVENTIONS	RATIONALE
Refer to dietitian for adjustments in dietary composition.	Provides assistance in planning a diet with nutrients adequate to meet client's metabolic requirements, dietary preferences, and financial resources post/discharge.
Consult with respiratory therapy to schedule treatments 1–2 hr before/after meals.	May help reduce the incidence of nausea and vomiting associated with medications or the effects of respiratory treatments on a full stomach.
Monitor laboratory studies; e.g., BUN, serum protein, and prealbumin/albumin.	Low values reflect malnutrition and indicate need for intervention/change in therapeutic regimen.
Administer antipyretics as appropriate.	Fever increases metabolic needs and therefore calorie consumption.

NURSING DIAGNOSIS: deficient Knowledge [Learning Need] regarding condition, treatment, prevention, self-care, and discharge needs

May be related to

Lack of exposure to/misinterpretation of information
Cognitive limitations
Inaccurate/incomplete information presented

Possibly evidenced by

Request for information
Expressed misconceptions about health status
Lack of or inaccurate follow-through of instructions/behaviors
Expressing or exhibiting feelings of being overwhelmed

DESIRED OUTCOMES/EVALUATION CRITERIA—CLIENT WILL:

KNOWLEDGE: Illness Care (NOC)

Verbalize understanding of disease process/prognosis and prevention.
Initiate behaviors/lifestyle changes to improve general well-being and reduce risk of reactivation of TB.
Identify symptoms requiring evaluation/intervention.
Describe a plan for receiving adequate follow-up care.
Verbalize understanding of therapeutic regimen and rationale for actions.

ACTIONS/INTERVENTIONS	RATIONALE
Learning Facilitation (NIC)	
Independent	
Assess client's ability to learn (e.g., level of fear, concern, fatigue, participation level); best environment in which client can learn; how much content; best media and language; who should be included.	Learning depends on emotional and physical readiness and is achieved at an individual pace.
Provide instruction and specific written information for client to refer to; e.g., schedule for medications and follow-up sputum testing for documenting response to therapy.	Written information relieves client of the burden of having to remember large amounts of information. Repetition strengthens learning.
Encourage client/SO to verbalize fears/concerns. Answer questions factually. Note prolonged use of denial.	Provides opportunity to correct misconceptions/alleviate anxiety. Inadequate finances/prolonged denial may affect coping with/managing the tasks necessary to regain/maintain health.
TEACHING: Disease Process (NIC)	
Identify symptoms that should be reported to healthcare provider; e.g., hemoptysis, chest pain, fever, difficulty breathing, hearing loss, vertigo.	May indicate progression or reactivation of disease or side effects of medications, requiring further evaluation.
Emphasize the importance of maintaining high-protein and carbohydrate diet and adequate fluid intake. (Refer to ND: imbalanced Nutrition: less than body requirements.)	Meeting metabolic needs helps minimize fatigue and promote recovery. Fluids aid in liquefying/expectorating secretions.
Explain medication dosage, frequency of administration, expected action, and the reason for long treatment period. Review potential interactions with other drugs/substances and reportable side effects.	Enhances cooperation with therapeutic regimen and may prevent client from discontinuing medication before cure is truly effected. DOT is the treatment of choice when client is unable or unwilling to take medications as prescribed. *Note*: Clients with HIV infection and TB are particularly susceptible to drug interactions because they are typically taking numerous medications, some of which react with antituburculosis medications.
Review potential side effects of treatment (e.g., dryness of mouth, nausea/GI upset; constipation, visual disturbances, headache, orthostatic hypertension) and problem-solve solutions.	It is important that antituburculosis drugs not be discontinued because of "nuisance" side effects. Problem-solving (e.g., taking medication with food, changing the hour of dosing) may prevent/reduce discomfort associated with therapy and enhance cooperation with regimen. Severe reactions must be reported to physician.
Stress need to abstain from alcohol while on INH.	Combination of INH and alcohol has been linked with increased incidence of hepatitis.
Refer for eye examination after starting and then monthly while taking EMB.	Major side effect is reduced visual acuity; initial sign may be decreased ability to perceive green.
Encourage abstaining from smoking.	Although smoking does not stimulate recurrence of TB, it does increase the likelihood of respiratory dysfunction/bronchitis.
Review how TB is transmitted (e.g., primarily by inhalation of airborne organisms, but may also spread through stools or urine if infection is present in these systems) and hazards of reactivation.	Knowledge may reduce risk of transmission/reactivation. Complications associated with reactivation include cavitation, abscess formation, destructive emphysema, spontaneous pneumothorax, diffuse interstitial fibrosis, serous effusion, empyema, bronchiectasis, hemoptysis, GI ulceration, bronchopleural fistula, tuberculosis laryngitis, and miliary spread.
Discuss/reinforce concerns (e.g., treatment failure, drug resistant TB and relapse).	Treatment failure most often occurs because client is not adhering to treatment regimen, but can also be due to drug resistance, malabsorption of drugs, laboratory error, and extreme biologic variation in response. Most relapses (recurrence of positive cultures or radiographic deterioration) occur 6–12 months after completion of therapy. Continuous monitoring by healthcare providers can identify these concerns early and alter the plan accordingly.

ACTIONS/INTERVENTIONS	RATIONALE
Refer to public health agency as appropriate.	DOT by community nurses is often the most effective way to ensure client adherence to therapy. Monitoring can include pill counts and urine dipstick testing for presence of antitubercular drug. Clients with MDR-TB may be monitored with monthly sputum specimens for AFB smear and culture. *Note:* In some states, there are legal means for involuntary confinement for care if efforts to ensure client adherence are ineffective.

POTENTIAL CONSIDERATIONS following acute hospitalization (dependent on client's age, physical condition/presence of complications, personal resources, and life responsibilities)

ineffective Therapeutic Regimen Management—complexity of therapeutic regimen, economic difficulties, family patterns of health care, perceived seriousness/benefits.

risk for Infection (secondary)—decrease in ciliary action, stasis of body fluids, suppressed inflammatory response, tissue destruction, chronic disease, malnutrition, increased environmental exposure.

Fatigue—increased energy requirements to perform ADLs, discomfort.

ineffective Family Therapeutic Regimen Management—complexity of therapeutic regimen, decisional conflicts, economic difficulties, family conflict.

RESPIRATORY ACID-BASE IMBALANCES

The body has the remarkable ability to maintain plasma pH within a narrow range of 7.35–7.45. It does so by means of chemical buffering mechanisms involving the lungs and kidneys. Although simple acid-base imbalances (e.g., respiratory acidosis) do occur, mixed acid-base imbalances are more common (e.g., the respiratory acidosis/metabolic acidosis that occur with cardiac arrest).

RESPIRATORY ACIDOSIS (PRIMARY CARBONIC ACID EXCESS)

Respiratory acidosis (elevated $Pa{CO_2}$ level) is due to alveolar hypoventilation with resultant excess carbonic acid (H_2CO_3). Acidosis can be due to/associated with primary defects in lung function or changes in normal respiratory pattern. The disorder may be acute or chronic.

Compensatory mechanisms include (1) an increased respiratory rate; (2) hemoglobin (Hgb) buffering, forming bicarbonate ions and deoxygenated Hgb; and (3) increased renal ammonia acid excretions with reabsorption of bicarbonate.

Acute respiratory acidosis: $Pa{CO_2}$ >47 mm Hg with accompanying acidemia (pH 7.25). Occurs when an abrupt failure of ventilation occurs, which may be caused by (1) depression of the central respiratory center by brain disorders (e.g., brainstem disease/trauma, tumors, encephalitis, cerebral vascular accident [CVA] or drugs (e.g., overdose of sedatives/barbiturate poisoning); (2) inability to ventilate adequately such as may occur with neuromuscular diseases (e.g., myasthenia gravis, amyotrophic lateral sclerosis [ALS], Guillain-Barré syndrome, muscular dystrophy), hemothorax/pneumothorax, atelectasis, adult respiratory distress syndrome (ARDS), anesthesia/surgery; or (3) airway obstruction (e.g., asthma or COPD exacerbation, aspiration of foreign body, acute pulmonary edema, acute laryngospasm, smoke inhalation, excessive CO_2 intake (e.g., use of rebreathing mask, CO_2 therapy).

Chronic respiratory acidosis: $Pa{CO_2}$ >47 mm Hg, normal or near normal pH, and elevated serum bicarbonate (HCO_3 >30 mm Hg) reflecting renal compensation. Chronic respiratory acidosis may be secondary to many disorders (e.g., hypoventilation in COPD that involves multiple mechanisms—decreased responsiveness to hypoxia and hypercapnia, increased ventilation-perfusion mismatch leading to increased dead space ventilation and decreased diaphragm function secondary to fatigue and hyperinflation). This condition is associated with emphysema, asthma, bronchiectasis, and severe restrictive ventilatory defects (e.g., interstitial fibrosis and thoracic deformities, neuromuscular disorders [such as Guillain-Barré syndrome, ALS], obesity [Pickwickian syndrome], botulism, spinal cord injuries).

CARE SETTING

This condition does not occur in isolation, but rather is a complication of a broader health problem/disease or condition for which the severely compromised client requires admission to a medical-surgical or subacute unit.

RELATED CONCERNS

Plans of care specific to predisposing factors/disease or medical condition; e.g.:

Cerebrovascular accident (CVA)/stroke, page 236
Chronic obstructive pulmonary disease (COPD) and asthma, page 117
Craniocerebral trauma (acute rehabilitative phase), page 218
Eating disorders: obesity, page 393
Alcohol: acute withdrawal, page 831
Spinal cord injury (acute rehabilitative phase), page 271
Surgical intervention, page 788
Ventilatory assistance (mechanical), page 170

OTHER CONCERNS

Fluid and electrolyte imbalances page 919
Metabolic acidosis page 492
Metabolic alkalosis page 495

Client Assessment Database

Dependent on underlying cause. Findings vary widely.

ACTIVITY/REST

May report: Fatigue, mild to profound; sleep disturbances

May exhibit: Generalized weakness, ataxia/staggering, loss of coordination (chronic), to stupor

CIRCULATION

May exhibit: Low BP/hypotension with bounding pulses, pinkish color, warm skin; dilation of conjunctival and superficial facial blood vessels (reflects vasodilation of severe acidosis)

Tachycardia, irregular pulse (other/various dysrhythmias)

Diaphoresis, pallor, and cyanosis (late stage)

FOOD/FLUID

May report: Nausea/vomiting

NEUROSENSORY

May report: Feeling of fullness in head (acute—associated with vasodilation)

Headache, dizziness, visual disturbances

May exhibit: Anxiety, confusion, apprehension, agitation, restlessness, delirium, depressed mental status, somnolence (CO_2 narcosis), coma (acute)

Tremors, decreased reflexes; or asterixis, myoclonus, and seizures (severe)

RESPIRATION

May report: Shortness of breath, dyspnea with exertion

May exhibit: Respiratory rate dependent on underlying cause; that is, decrease in respiratory center depression/muscle paralysis; otherwise rate is rapid/shallow, often with prolonged expiration

Increased respiratory effort with nasal flaring/yawning, use of neck and upper body muscles

Decreased respiratory rate/hypoventilation (associated with decreased function of respiratory center as in head trauma, oversedation, general anesthesia, metabolic alkalosis)

Decreased breath sounds.

Hyperresonance on percussion

Adventitious breath sounds (wheezes); stridor, crowing

TEACHING/LEARNING

Refer to specific plans of care reflecting individual predisposing/contributing factors.

Discharge plan considerations: May require assistance with changes in therapies for underlying disease process/condition

Refer to section at end of plan for postdischarge considerations.

DIAGNOSTIC STUDIES

ABGs: *Pa_{O_2}:* Normal or may be low. Oxygen saturation (SaO_2) decreased.
Pa_{CO_2}: Increased, greater than 45 mm Hg (primary acidosis).
Bicarbonate (HCO_3): Normal or increased, greater than 26 mEq/L (compensated/chronic stage).
Arterial pH: Decreased, less than 7.35.

Electrolytes: *Serum potassium:* Typically increased.
Serum chloride: Decreased.
Serum calcium: Increased.

Lactic acid: May be elevated.

Urinalysis: Urine pH decreased.

Other screening tests: As indicated by underlying illness/condition to determine underlying cause (including chest x-ray, chest CT, brain MRI, pulmonary function studies, drug and toxicology screens, tests to measure diaphragmatic function).

NURSING PRIORITIES

1. Achieve homeostasis.
2. Prevent/minimize complications.
3. Provide information about condition/prognosis and treatment needs as appropriate.

DISCHARGE GOALS

1. Physiological balance restored.
2. Free of complications.
3. Condition, prognosis, and treatment needs understood.
4. Plan in place to meet needs after discharge.

NURSING DIAGNOSIS: impaired Gas Exchange

May be related to

Ventilation perfusion imbalance (e.g., altered oxygen-carrying capacity of blood, altered oxygen supply, alveolar-capillary membrane changes, or altered blood flow)

Possibly evidenced by

Dyspnea with exertion, tachypnea
Changes in mentation, irritability
Tachycardia
Hypoxia, hypercapnia

DESIRED OUTCOMES/EVALUATION CRITERIA—CLIENT WILL:

Electrolyte and Acid-Base Balance (NOC)

Demonstrate improved ventilation and adequate oxygenation of tissues as evidenced by ABGs within client's acceptable limits and absence of symptoms of respiratory distress.

KNOWLEDGE: Disease Process (NOC)

Verbalize understanding of causative factors and appropriate interventions.
Participate in treatment regimen within level of ability/situation.

ACTIONS/INTERVENTIONS	RATIONALE
ACID-BASE MANAGEMENT: Respiratory Acidosis (NIC)	
Independent	
Monitor respiratory rate, depth, and effort.	Alveolar hypoventilation and associated hypoxemia lead to respiratory failure.
Auscultate breath sounds.	Identifies area(s) of decreased ventilation (e.g., atelectasis) or airway obstruction and changes as client deteriorates or improves, reflecting effectiveness of treatment, dictating therapy needs.
Note declining level of awareness/consciousness.	Signals severe acidotic state, which requires immediate attention. *Note:* In recovery, sensorium clears slowly because hydrogen ions are slow to cross the blood-brain barrier and clear from cerebrospinal fluid and brain cells.
Monitor heart rate/rhythm.	Tachycardia develops early because the sympathetic nervous system is stimulated, resulting in the release of catecholamines, epinephrine, and norepinephrine in an attempt to increase oxygen delivery to the tissues. Dysrhythmias that may occur are due to hypoxia (myocardial ischemia) and electrolyte imbalances.
Note skin color, temperature, moisture.	Diaphoresis, pallor, cool/clammy skin are late changes associated with severe or advancing hypoxemia.
Encourage/assist with deep-breathing exercises, turning, and coughing. Suction as necessary. Provide airway adjunct as indicated. Place in semi-Fowler's position.	These measures improve lung ventilation and reduce/prevent airway obstruction associated with accumulation of mucus.
Restrict use of hypnotic sedatives or tranquilizers.	In the presence of hypoventilation, respiratory depression and CO_2 narcosis may develop.
Discuss cause of chronic condition (when known) and appropriate interventions/self-care activities.	Promotes participation in therapeutic regimen, and may reduce recurrence of disorder.
Collaborative	
Assist with identification/treatment of underlying cause.	Treatment of disorder is directed at improving alveolar ventilation. Multiple team management may be required (e.g., physicians, pulmonologist and respiratory therapists, or neurologists) to address the underlying condition (e.g., oversedation, brain trauma, COPD, pulmonary edema, aspiration) and promote correction of the acid-base disorder.
Monitor/graph serial ABGs, pulse oximetry readings; Hgb, serum electrolyte levels.	Evaluates therapy needs/effectiveness. *Note:* Pulse oximetry monitoring is used to monitor and show early changes in oxygenation, which can occur before other signs or symptoms are observed.
Administer oxygen as indicated, using appropriate delivery means (e.g., endotracheal intubation with mechanical ventilation or nasal continuous positive pressure ventilation; or nasal bilevel ventilation).	Prevents/corrects hypoxemia and pulmonary hypertension, and its use prevents the consequences of longstanding hypoxemia. *Note:* Although oxygen must be used with caution in presence of emphysema (can worsen hypercapnia), oxygen therapy has been shown to have decreased morality in clients with COPD.
Increase respiratory rate or tidal volume of ventilator if used.	Increases lung expansion and opens airways to improve ventilation and gas diffusion, preventing respiratory failure.
Assist with ventilatory aids; e.g., IPPB in conjunction with bronchodilators. Monitor peak flow pressure.	Assists in correction of acidity and thinning/mobilization of respiratory secretions.
Maintain hydration (IV/PO)/provide humidification.	Aids in clearing secretions, which improves ventilation, allowing excess CO_2 to be eliminated.

ACTIONS/INTERVENTIONS	RATIONALE
Administer medications as indicated,;e.g.:	
Opioid antagonist, such as naloxone hydrochloride (Narcan), flumazenil (Romazicon);	Can be useful in reversing the effects of certain opiates and sedative drugs on the respiratory center, stimulating ventilation in presence of drug overdose/sedation, or acidosis resulting from cardiac arrest.
Bonchodilators such as β-agonists (e.g., albuterol [Proventil, Ventolin], salmeterol [Serevent]); anticholinergic agents (e.g., ipratropium bromide [Atrovent]) methylxanthines (e.g., theophylline);	Helpful in treating client with acidosis secondary to obstructive lung disease and severe bronchospasm. Theophylline may improve diaphragm muscle contractility and may stimulate the respiratory center.
Electrolytes, e.g., KCl, as indicated;	Respiratory acidosis does not have a great effect on electrolyte levels, although some effects occur on calcium and potassium levels. Acidemia causes an extracellular shift of potassium. Correction of the acidosis may cause a relative serum hypokalemia as potassium shifts back into cells. Potassium imbalance can impair neuromuscular/respiratory function, causing generalized muscle weakness and cardiac dysrhythmias. *Note*: Infusion of sodium bicarbonate is rarely indicated, although it may be considered in cardiopulmonary arrest when pH is <7.0.
Provide/refer for pulmonary rehabilitation as indicated.	Provides restorative and preventative care to reverse respiratory acidosis secondary to underlying conditions (e.g., bronchial hygiene, breathing retraining, exercise conditioning). Therapy modalities and length of intervention may vary depending on whether the respiratory acidosis is acute or chronic.
Provide low-carbohydrate, high-fat diet (e.g., Pulmocare feedings) if indicated.	Helps reduce CO_2 production and improves respiratory muscle function and metabolic homeostasis.

POTENTIAL CONSIDERATIONS following acute hospitalization (dependent on client's age, physical condition/presence of complications, personal resources, and life responsibilities)

Refer to Potential Considerations relative to underlying cause of acid-base disorder.

RESPIRATORY ALKALOSIS (PRIMARY CARBONIC ACID DEFICIT)

Respiratory alkalosis is the most common acid-base abnormality in critically ill persons and is associated with numerous illnesses. It is the most frequently occurring acid-base imbalance in hospitalized clients, with the elderly being at increased risk because of the high incidence of pulmonary disorders and alterations in neurologic status.

Respiratory alkalosis is a clinical disturbance due to alveolar hyperventilation, which leads to hypocapnea ($Paco_2$ <35 mm Hg), increases the ratio of bicarbonate concentration to $Paco_2$, and raises pH. Compensatory mechanisms include decreased respiratory rate (if the body is able to respond to the drop in $Paco_2$), increased renal excretion of bicarbonate, and retention of hydrogen.

Causes of respiratory alkalosis include (1) central nervous system (e.g., CVA, meningitis, encephalits, brain trauma/tumor, pain, hyperventilation, anxiety, psychosis, fever); (2) hypoxemia (e.g., severe anemia, right-to-left shunts, high altitude); (3) drugs (e.g., salicylates, nicotine, methalyxanthines, catecholamines); (4) endocrine (e.g., pregnancy, increased progesterone levels, hyperthyroidism); (5) stimulation of chest receptors (e.g., pulmonary embolus, pulmomary edema, aspiration, hemo-pneumothorax); and (6) miscellaneous (e.g., sepsis, liver failure, heat exhaustion, mechanical ventilation). The two primary mechanisms that trigger hyperventilation are (1) hypoxemia and (2) direct stimulation of the central respiratory center of the brain (such as occurs with high fever, head trauma/CNS lesions, early salicylate intoxication).

Respiratory alkalosis can be acute ($Paco_2$ is below lower limit of normal, serum pH is alkalemic due to loss of potassium, and phosphate secondary to cellular uptake) or chronic ($Paco_2$ is below the lower limit of normal, but pH is normal or near normal because of renal compensation).

CARE SETTING

This condition does not occur in isolation, but rather is a complication of a broader problem. Treatment is primarily directed at correcting the underlying disorder causing respiratory alkalosis, and is usually found in clients requiring care in a medical/surgical or subacute unit.

RELATED CONCERNS

Plans of care specific to predisposing factors, e.g.:

Anemias (iron deficiency, pernicious, aplastic, hemolytic), page 499
Cirrhosis of the liver, page 453
Craniocerebral trauma, page 218
Hyperthyroidism, page 426
Fluid and electrolyte imbalance, page 919
Heart failure: chronic, page 47
Pneumonia, page 128
Sepsis/septicemia, page 701
Ventilatory assistance (mechanical), page 170

OTHER CONCERNS

Metabolic acidosis, page 492
Metabolic alkalosis, page 495

Client Assessment Database

Dependent on underlying cause.

CIRCULATION

May report: History/presence of anemia
Palpitations

May exhibit: Hypotension
Tachycardia, irregular pulse/dysrhythmias

EGO INTEGRITY

May exhibit: Extreme anxiety (most common cause of hyperventilation)

FOOD/FLUID

May report: Dry mouth
Nausea/vomiting

May exhibit: Abdominal distention (elevating diaphragm as with ascites, pregnancy)
Vomiting

NEUROSENSORY

May report: Headache, tinnitus
Numbness/tingling of face, hands, and toes; circumoral numbness and generalized paresthesia
Lightheadedness, syncope, vertigo, blurred vision

May exhibit: Confusion, restlessness, obtunded responses, coma
Hyperactive reflexes, positive Chvostek's and Trousseau signs; tetany, seizures
Heightened sensitivity to environmental noise and activity
Muscle weakness, unsteady gait

PAIN/DISCOMFORT

May report: Muscle spasms/cramps, epigastric pain, precordial pain (tightness)

RESPIRATION

May report: Dyspnea
History of asthma, pulmonary fibrosis
Recent move/visit to location at high altitude

May exhibit: Tachypnea; rapid, shallow breathing; hyperventilation (often 40 or more respirations/min)
Intermittent periods of apnea

SAFETY

May exhibit Fever

TEACHING/LEARNING

May report: Use of salicylates/salicylate overdose, catecholamines, theophylline

Discharge plan considerations: May require change in treatment/therapy of underlying disease process/condition

Refer to section at end of plan for postdischarge considerations.

DIAGNOSTIC STUDIES

Arterial pH: > 7.44 (may be near normal in chronic stage).
Bicarbonate (HCO_3): Normal or decreased; <25 mEq/L (compensatory mechanism).
$Paco_2$: Decreased, <36 mm Hg (primary).
Electrolytes: Minor shifts usually occur, e.g. serum sodium, potassium, and phosphate decreased due to intracellular shifts; serum chloride increased; serum calcium decreased.
Screening tests as indicated to determine underlying cause; e.g.:

- *CBC:* May reveal severe anemia (decreasing oxygen-carrying capacity) or elevated WBCs (early sepsis)
- *Blood cultures:* May identify sepsis (usually gram negative).
- *Blood alcohol:* Marked elevation (acute alcoholic intoxication).
- *Toxicology screen:* May reveal early salicylate poisoning.
- *Chest x-ray/lung scan:* May reveal pulmonary disease as cause of hypocapnea or may reveal pneumonia, pulmonary emboli, aspiration pneumonitis, pnemothorax, interstitial disease.
- *CT scan and ventilation/perfusion studes:* May be done to diagnose pulmonary disorders.
- *MRI and/or CT scan:* May be done if a central cause for hyperventilation and respiratory alkalosis is suspected.

NURSING PRIORITIES

1. Achieve homeostatis.
2. Prevent/minimize complications.
3. Provide information about condition/prognosis and treatment needs as appropriate.

DISCHARGE GOALS

1. Physiological balance restored.
2. Free of complications.
3. Condition, prognosis, and treatment needs understood.
4. Plan in place to meet needs after discharge.

NURSING DIAGNOSIS: impaired Gas Exchange

May be related to

Ventilation perfusion imbalance (e.g., altered oxygen supply, altered blood flow, altered oxygen-carrying capacity of blood, alveolar-capillary membrane changes)

Possibly evidenced by

Dyspnea, tachypnea
Changes in mentation
Hypocapnia, tachycardia
Hypoxia

DESIRED OUTCOMES/EVALUATION CRITERIA—CLIENT WILL:

Electrolyte and Acid-Base Balance (NOC)

Demonstrate improved ventilation and adequate oxygenation of tissue as evidenced by ABGs within client's acceptable limits and absence of symptoms of respiratory distress.
Verbalize understanding of causative factors and appropriate interventions.
Participate in treatment regimen within level of ability/situation.

ACTIONS/INTERVENTIONS	RATIONALE
ACID-BASE MANAGEMENT: Respiratory Alkalosis (NIC)	
Independent	
Monitor respiratory rate, depth, and effort; ascertain cause of hyperventilation if possible; e.g., anxiety, pain, improper ventilator settings.	Identifies alterations from usual breathing pattern and influences choice of intervention.
Assess level of awareness/cognition and note neuromuscular status; e.g., strength, tone, reflexes, sensation, and presence of tremors.	Decreased mentation (mild to severe) and tetany or seizures may occur when alkalosis is severe owing to shifts in calcium.
Instruct/encourage client to breathe slowly and deeply. Speak in a low, calm tone of voice; provide safe environment.	May help reassure and calm the agitated client, thereby aiding the reduction of respiratory rate. Assists client to regain control. *Note:* Clients with hyperventilation syndrome as a cause of their respiratory alkalosis may particularly benefit from reassurance and client education in breathing techniques.
Demonstrate appropriate breathing patterns, if appropriate, and assist with respiratory aids; e.g., rebreathing mask/bag.	Decreasing the rate of respirations can halt the "blowing off" of CO_2, elevating Pco_2 level and normalizing pH.
Provide comfort measures; encourage use of meditation and visualization. Use tepid sponge bath/cool cloths.	Promotes relaxation and reduces stress. Control and reduction of fever reduces potential for seizures and helps reduce respiration rate.
Provide safety/seizure precautions; e.g., bed in low position, padded side rails, frequent observation.	Changes in mentation/CNS and neuromuscular hyperirritability may result in client harm, especially if tetany/convulsions occur.
Discuss cause of condition (if known) and appropriate interventions/self-care activities.	Promotes participation in therapeutic regimen and may reduce recurrence of disorder.
Collaborative	
Assist with identification/treatment of underlying cause.	Respiratory alkalosis is a complication, not an isolated occurrence and rarely requires emergent treatment (unless pH is >7.5); thus correction of alkalosis is undertaken by addressing the primary condition (e.g., hyperventilation of panic attack, organ failure, severe anemia, drug effect). Because respiratory alkalosis usually occurs in response to some stimulus, treatment is unsuccessful unless the stimulus is controlled.
Monitor/graph serial ABGs, and pulse oximetry.	Identifies therapy needs/effectiveness. *Note*: Rapid correction of $Paco_2$ in individual with chronic respiratory alkalosis (has a lower serum bicarbonate) may cause metabolic acidosis to develop.
Monitor serum potassium. Replace as indicated.	Hypokalemia may occur as potassium is lost (via urine) or shifted into the cell in exchange for hydrogen in an attempt to correct alkalosis.
Provide sedation/pain medication as indicated.	Control of pain and/or sedation may be needed to reduce cause of hyperventilation if client is not responding to conservative measures.
Administer CO_2 (by rebreathing bag or mask) as indicated. Reduce respiratory rate and tidal volume, or add additional dead space (tubing) to mechanical ventilator.	Increasing CO_2 retention may correct carbonic acid deficit, leading to improvement and resolution of alkalotic state.

POTENTIAL CONSIDERATIONS following acute hospitalization (dependent on client's age, physical condition/presence of complications, personal resources, and life responsibilities)

Refer to Potential Considerations relative to underlying cause of acid-base disorder.

6

CHAPTER

Neurologic/Sensory Disorders

GLAUCOMA

The term *glaucoma* encompasses a group of eye diseases in which blindness occurs gradually without warning and often without symptoms. Vision loss is caused by damage to the optic nerve. It was once thought that high intraocular pressure (IOP) was the main cause of this optic nerve damage. Although IOP is statistically linked (and clearly a risk factor), it is now know that other factors must also be involved because people with normal IOP can develop glaucoma. Elevated IOP is the result of inadequate drainage of aqueous humor from the anterior chamber of the eye. The increased pressure causes atrophy of the optic nerve and, if untreated, blindness.

There are two primary categories of glaucoma: (1) *open-angle* and (2) *closed-angle* (or *narrow-angle*). Chronic open-angle glaucoma is the most common type, accounting for 90% of all glaucoma cases. It develops slowly, may be associated with diabetes and myopia, and usually develops in both eyes simultaneously, or in one eye following the other in a short time period. Chronic glaucoma has no early warning signs, and the loss of peripheral vision occurs so gradually that substantial optic nerve damage can occur before glaucoma is detected. It usually responds well to medication if detected early and treated.

Primary narrow-angle (or angle-closure) glaucoma is the less common form, and may be associated with eye trauma, various inflammatory processes, and pupillary dilation after the instillation of mydriatic drops. Acute angle-closure glaucoma is manifested by sudden excruciating pain in or around the eye, blurred vision, and ocular redness. This condition constitutes a medical emergency because blindness may suddenly ensue. Treatment is usually surgical, is usually successful, and is long lasting.

Secondary glaucoma can occur as a result of an eye injury. This might be direct trauma to the eye, such as might occur with a blow to the head or a direct blow to eye (e.g., hit by baseball, blunt trauma, boxing injury); inflammation, tumor, or in advanced cases of cataract or diabetes. It may be mild or severe, and treatment will depend on whether it is open-angle or angle-closure glaucoma. Pigmentary glaucoma is a form of secondary glaucoma in which pigment granules in the back of the iris break into the aqueous humor and clog the drainage canals. Treatment usually includes drug therapy or surgery.

Normal-tension glaucoma (NTG), also known as low-tension or normal-pressure glaucoma, occurs when the optic nerve is damaged even though IOP is not elevated. The cause is unknown, although it has been linked to systemic heart disease, and has been found to have a higher incidence in people of Japanese ancestry. Treatment is aimed at keeping eye pressures as low as possible with drugs or laser or filtering surgery.

Glaucoma and cataracts can be a natural part of the aging process. Many people over age 60 years have both conditions. Otherwise, the two are not associated. Loss of vision from glaucoma (unlike that of cataracts) is not reversible.

CARE SETTING

Community, unless sudden increase in IOP requires emergency intervention and close monitoring.

RELATED CONCERNS

Psychosocial aspects of care, page 770

Client Assessment Database

ACTIVITY/REST

May report: Change in usual activities/hobbies due to altered vision

FOOD/FLUID

May report: Nausea/vomiting (acute glaucoma)

NEUROSENSORY

May report: Gradual loss of peripheral vision, Frequent change of glasses, difficulty adjusting to darkened room, halos around lights, mild headache (chronic glaucoma)
Cloudy/blurred vision, appearance of halos/rainbows around lights, sudden loss of peripheral vision, photophobia (acute glaucoma)
Glasses/treatment change does not improve vision

May exhibit: Dilated, fixed, cloudy pupils (acute glaucoma)
Fixed pupil and red/hard eye with cloudy cornea (glaucoma emergency)
Increased tearing
Intumescent cataracts, intraocular hemorrhage (glaucoma secondary to trauma)

PAIN/DISCOMFORT

May report: Mild discomfort or aching/tired eyes (chronic glaucoma)
Sudden/persistent severe pain or pressure in and around eye(s), headache (acute glaucoma)

SAFETY

May report: History of hemorrhage, trauma, ocular disease, tumor (secondary to trauma)
Difficulty seeing, managing activities

May exhibit: Inflammatory disease of eye (glaucoma secondary to trauma)

TEACHING/LEARNING

May report: Family history of glaucoma, diabetes, systemic vascular disorders
History of stress, allergies, vasomotor disturbances (e.g., increased venous pressure), endocrine imbalance, diabetes
History of ocular surgery/cataract removal, steroid use

Discharge plan considerations: May require assistance with transportation, meal preparation, self-care, homemaker/maintenance tasks

Refer to section at end of plan for postdischarge considerations.

DIAGNOSTIC STUDIES

Ophthalmoscopy examination: Assesses internal ocular structures, noting optic nerve shape and color, optic disc atrophy, papilledema, retinal hemorrhage, and microaneurysms. Slit-lamp examination provides three-dimensional view of eye structures, identifies corneal abnormalities/change in shape, increased IOP, and general vision deficits associated with glaucoma.

Visual acuity tests (e.g., Snellen, Jayer): Vision may be impaired by defects in cornea, lens, aqueous or vitreous humor, refraction, or disease of the nervous or vascular system supplying the retina or optic pathway.

Visual fields (e.g., confrontation, tangent screen, automated or manual perimetry): Assesses vision when client looks forward while a light passes through peripheral vision fields. Reduction of peripheral vision may be caused by glaucoma or other conditions such as cerebrovascular accident (CVA), pituitary/brain tumor mass, or carotid or cerebral artery pathology.

Tonometry measurement: Assesses intraocular pressure (normal: 10–21 mm Hg). In acute angle-closure glaucoma, IOP may be 50 mm Hg or higher.

Gonioscopy measurement: Helps differentiate open-angle from angle-closure glaucoma.

Provocative tests: May be useful in establishing presence/type of glaucoma when IOP is normal or only mildly elevated.

Imaging studies

Ultrasound biomicroscopy (UBM): Ultrasound probe passed over surface of eye, recording images of the front portion of the eye (e.g., cornea, anterior chamber, posterior chamber, ciliary body, sclera, anterior lens capsule).

Heidelberg retina tomograph (HRT): Laser-scanning microscope for acquiring and analyzing the posterior segment of the retina.

Scanning laser polarimetry (SLP): Measures retinal nerve fiber layer (RNFL) directly.

Glucose tolerance test/fasting blood sugar (FBS): Determines presence/control of diabetes, which is implicated at times in secondary glaucoma.

NURSING PRIORITIES

1. Prevent further visual deterioration.
2. Promote adaptation to changes in/reduced visual acuity.

3. Prevent complications.
4. Provide information about disease process/prognosis and treatment needs.

DISCHARGE GOALS

1. Vision maintained at highest possible level.
2. Client coping with situation in a positive manner.
3. Complications prevented/minimized.
4. Disease process/prognosis and therapeutic regimen understood.
5. Plan in place to meet needs after discharge.

NURSING DIAGNOSIS: disturbed visual Sensory Perception

May be related to

Altered sensory reception: altered status of sense organs

Possibly evidenced by

Reported change in sensory acuity (e.g., photosensitivity, visual distortions)
Progressive loss of visual field; measured change in sensory acuity

DESIRED OUTCOMES/EVALUATION CRITERIA—CLIENT WILL:

SENSORY FUNCTION: Vision (NOC)

Participate in therapeutic regimen.
Maintain current visual field/acuity without further loss.

ACTIONS/INTERVENTIONS	RATIONALE
COMMUNICATION ENHANCEMENT: Visual Deficit (NIC)	
Independent	
Ascertain type/degree of visual loss.	Affects choice of interventions and client's future expectations.
Encourage expression of feelings about loss/possibility of loss of vision.	Although early intervention can prevent blindness, client faces the possibility or may have already experienced partial or complete loss of vision. Although vision loss cannot be restored (even with treatment), further loss can be prevented.
Recommend measures to assist client to manage visual limitations; e.g., reducing clutter, arranging furniture out of travel path, turning head to view subjects or objects, correcting for dim light and problems of night vision.	Reduces safety hazards related to changes in visual fields/loss of vision and papillary accommodation to environmental light.
MEDICATION ADMINISTRATION: Eye (NIC)	
Demonstrate/have client/significant other (SO) administer eye drops using correct procedures; e.g., placement of drop, counting drops, adhering to schedule, not missing doses.	Although burdensome, lifelong eyedrop treatment is needed to control IOP and prevent further loss of vision.
Collaborative	
Assist with administration of medications as indicated:	

ACTIONS/INTERVENTIONS	RATIONALE
Chronic, open-angle type:	
Miotics: e.g., pilocarpine (Isopto Carpine, Ocusert [disc], Pilopine HS gel);	These direct-acting topical myotic drugs cause pupillary constriction, facilitating the outflow of aqueous humor and lowering IOP. *Note:* Ocusert is a disc (similar to a contact) that is placed in the lower eyelid, where it can remain for up to 1 wk before being replaced.
Timolol (Timoptic, Betamol), betaxolol (Betoptic), levobetaxolol (Betaxin), carteolol (Ocupress), metipranolol (OptiPranolol), levobunolol (Betagan);	β-Blockers decrease formation of aqueous humor without changing pupil size, vision, or accommodation. *Note:* These drugs may be contraindicated or require close monitoring for systemic effects in the presence of bradycardia or asthma.
Brinzolamide (Azopt), methazolamide (Neptazane), dorzolamide (Trusopt);	Carbonic anhydrase inhibitors decrease the amount and rate of production of aqueous humor. *Note:* Systemic adverse effects are common, including mood disturbances, gastrointestinal (GI) upset, and fatigue.
Bimataprost (Lumigan), Latanaprost (Xalatan), travapost (Travatan), unoprostone (Rescular).	Prostoglandin agonists are now being trialed for management of IOP by working near the drainage area of the eye to increase outflow of aqueous humor.
Narrow-angle (angle-closure) type:	
Myotics (see preceding);	Contract the sphincter muscles of the iris, deepen anterior chamber, and dilate vessels of outflow tract during acute attack or before surgery.
Sympathomimetics: e.g., dipivefrin (Propine), bromonidine (Alphagan), epinephrine (Epifrin), apraclonidine (Lopidine), latanoprost (Xalatan);	Adrenergic drops decrease formation of aqueous humor and may be beneficial when client is unresponsive to other medications. Although free of side effects such as miosis, blurred vision, and night blindness, they have potential for additive adverse cardiovascular effects in combination with other cardiovascular agents. *Note:* Light-colored eyes are more responsive to these drugs than dark-colored eyes, necessitating added considerations when determining appropriate dosage.
Hyperosmotic agents: e.g., mannitol (Osmitrol), glycerin (Ophthalgan, Osmoglyn oral); isosorbide (Ismotic).	Used to decrease circulating fluid volume, which will decrease production of aqueous humor if other treatments have not been successful.
Provide sedation, analgesics as necessary.	Acute glaucoma attack is associated with sudden pain, which can precipitate anxiety/agitation, further elevating IOP. Medical management may be required before IOP decreases and pain subsides.
Prepare for surgical intervention as indicated; e.g.:	
Laser therapy (e.g., argon laser trabeculoplasty [ALT]), laser cyclophotocoagulation [CPC], or trabeculectomy/trephination with Malento valve implant or aqueous-venous shunt;	Surgical treatment may be performed before or after attempts to reduce IOP with medications, and include incisional or laser procedures. Filtering operations (laser surgery) are highly successful procedures for reducing IOP by creating an opening between the anterior chamber and the subjunctival spaces so that aqueous humor can bypass the trabecular mesh block. CPC separates ciliary body from the sclera by freezing to facilitate outflow of aqueous humor. *Note:* Apraclonidine (Lopidine) eye drops may be used in conjunction with laser therapy to lessen/prevent postprocedure elevations of IOP. A Malento valve implant or an aqueous venous shunt may be used to correct or prevent scarring over/closure of drainage sac created by trabeculectomy.
Iridotomy;	Surgical removal of a portion of the iris facilitates drainage of aqueous humor through a newly created opening in the iris connecting to normal outflow channels. *Note:* Bilateral iridectomy is performed because glaucoma usually develops in the other eye.
Diathermy/cryosurgery.	Destroys the ciliary body, and thereby reduces formation of aqueous humor.

NURSING DIAGNOSIS: Anxiety [specify level]

May be related to

Physiologic factors, change in health status, presence of pain, possibility/reality of loss of vision
Unmet needs
Negative self-talk

Possibly evidenced by

Apprehension, uncertainty
Expressed concern regarding changes in life events

DESIRED OUTCOMES/EVALUATION CRITERIA—CLIENT WILL:

Anxiety Self-Control (NOC)

Appear relaxed and report anxiety is reduced to a manageable level.
Demonstrate problem-solving skills.
Use resources effectively.

ACTIONS/INTERVENTIONS	RATIONALE
Anxiety Reduction (NIC)	
Independent	
Assess anxiety level, degree of pain experienced/suddenness of onset of symptoms, and current knowledge of condition.	These factors affect client's perception of threat to self, potentiate the cycle of anxiety, and may interfere with medical attempts to control IOP.
Provide accurate, honest information. Discuss probability that careful monitoring and treatment can prevent additional visual loss.	Reduces anxiety related to unknown/future expectations, and provides factual basis for making informed choices about treatment.
Encourage client to acknowledge concerns and express feelings.	Provides opportunity for client to deal with reality of situation, clarify misconceptions, and problem solve concerns.
Identify helpful resources/people.	Provides reassurance that client is not alone in dealing with problems.

NURSING DIAGNOSIS: deficient Knowledge [Learning Need] regarding condition, prognosis, treatment, self-care needs

May be related to

Lack of exposure/unfamiliarity with resources
Lack of recall, information misinterpretation

Possibly evidenced by

Questions; statement of misconception
Inaccurate follow-through of instruction
Development of preventable complications

DESIRED OUTCOMES/EVALUATION CRITERIA—CLIENT WILL:

KNOWLEDGE: Illness Care (NOC)

Verbalize understanding of condition, prognosis, and treatment.
Identify relationship of signs/symptoms to the disease process.
Verbalize understanding of treatment needs.
Correctly perform necessary procedures and explain reasons for the actions.

ACTIONS/INTERVENTIONS	RATIONALE
TEACHING: Disease Process (NIC)	
Independent	
Review pathology/prognosis of condition and lifelong need for treatment.	Provides opportunity to clarify/dispel misconceptions and present condition as something that is manageable.
Discuss necessity of wearing identification/Medical Alert bracelet.	Vital to provide information for caregivers in case of emergency to reduce risk of receiving contraindicated drugs (e.g., atropine).
Demonstrate proper technique for administration of eye drops, gels, or discs. Have client perform return demonstration.	Enhances effectiveness of treatment. Provides opportunity for client to show competence and ask questions.
Review importance of maintaining eye drop schedule.	This disease can be controlled, not cured, and maintaining a consistent medication regimen is vital to control.
Discuss medications that should be avoided; e.g., mydriatic drops (atropine/propantheline bromide), overuse of topical steroids, and additive effects of β-blocking when systemic β-blocking agents are used.	Some drugs cause pupil dilation, increasing IOP and potentiating additional loss of vision. *Note:* All β-blocking glaucoma medications are contraindicated in client with greater than first-degree heart block, cardiogenic shock, or overt heart failure.
Identify potential side effects/adverse reactions of treatment; e.g., decreased appetite, nausea/vomiting, diarrhea, fatigue, "drugged" feeling, decreased libido, impotence, cardiac irregularities, syncope, heart failure (HF).	Drug side/adverse effects range from uncomfortable to severe or health threatening. Approximately 50% of clients develop sensitivity/allergy to parasympathomimetics (e.g., pilocarpine) or anticholinesterase drugs. These problems require medical evaluation and possible change in therapeutic regimen.
Encourage client to make necessary changes in lifestyle.	A tranquil lifestyle decreases the emotional response to stress, preventing ocular changes that push the iris forward, which may precipitate an acute attack.
Reinforce avoidance of activities such as heavy lifting/pushing, snow shoveling, wearing tight/constricting clothing.	May increase IOP, precipitating acute attack. *Note:* When client is not experiencing pain, cooperation with drug regimen and acceptance of lifestyle changes are often difficult to sustain.
Discuss dietary considerations; e.g., adequate fluid, bulk/fiber intake.	Measures to maintain consistency of stool to avoid constipation/straining during defecation.
Stress importance of routine checkups.	Important to monitor progression/maintenance of disease to allow for early intervention and prevent further loss of vision.
Advise client to immediately report severe eye pain, inflammation, increased photophobia, increased lacrimation, changes in visual field/veil-like curtain, blurred vision, flashes of light/particles floating in visual field.	Prompt action may be necessary to prevent further vision loss/other complications; e.g., detached retina.

ACTIONS/INTERVENTIONS	RATIONALE
Recommend family members be examined regularly for signs of glaucoma.	Hereditary tendency for shallow anterior chambers places family members at increased risk for developing the condition. *Note:* African-Americans in every age category should have periodic examinations because of increased incidence and more aggressive course of glaucoma in these individuals.
Identify strategies/resources for socialization; e.g., support groups, Visually Impaired Society, local library, and transportation services.	Decreased visual acuity may limit client's ability to drive/cause client to withdraw from usual activities.

POTENTIAL CONSIDERATIONS long-term/chronic concerns (dependent on client's age, physical condition/presence of complications, personal resources, and life responsibilities)

risk for Trauma—poor vision.

impaired Social Interaction—limited physical mobility (poor vision), inadequate support system.

ineffective Therapeutic Regimen Management—complexity of therapeutic regimen, economic difficulties, inadequate number and type of cues to action, perceived seriousness (of condition) or benefit (versus side effects).

SEIZURE DISORDERS

Seizures are sudden, abnormal, and excessive electrical discharges from the brain that can change motor or autonomic function, consciousness, or sensation. Seizures can be associated with a variety of cerebral or systemic disorders, or can occur in response to a stimulus outside the central nervous system (e.g., alcohol withdrawal, fever, hypoxia, drug intoxication, and poisoning). Seizures can develop at any time during a person's life, and can occur at any time. Seizures may occur as a one-time incident, or become a disorder, with recurrent episodes occurring throughout life.

There are many types of seizures, with the type depending primarily on what part of the brain is involved. One term used for seizures is epilepsy; however, a stricter definition of epilepsy requires that the seizures, although recurrent, have no known underlying cause. All types of seizures can present as status epilepticus (SE), which is defined as seizure activity lasting more than 30 minutes. Most frequently seen in the hospital setting is the generalized tonic-clonic SE.

The known causes for seizures can be divided into six categories:

Cerebral pathology: Resulting from traumatic head injury, stroke, infections, hypoxia, expanding brain lesions, and increased intracranial pressure.

Toxic agents: Poisons, alcohol, overdoses of prescription/nonprescription drugs and drugs of abuse (with drugs being the leading cause)

Chemical imbalances: Hypoglycemia, hypokalemia, hyponatremia, hypomagnesemia, and acidosis

Fever: Acute infections, heatstroke

Eclampsia: Prenatal hypertension/toxemia of pregnancy

Idiopathic: Unknown origin (also known as epilepsy)

Seizures can be divided into two major classifications (generalized and partial). *Generalized seizures* include tonic-clonic, myoclonic, clonic, tonic, atonic, and absence seizures. In myoclonic and absence seizures (also known as petit mal seizures), there are no convulsions. In generalized tonic-clonic seziures, all areas of the cortex are involved, convulsions occur, and they are sometimes called grand mal seizures. Consciousness is lost, and breathing may seem to stop.

Partial (focal) seizures are the most common type of seizures in adults, and are categorized as either (1) *simple* (partial motor, partial sensory) or (2) *complex*. In partial seizures, a specific part of the brain is involved, so a specific part of the body is affected, (e.g., a simple partial motor seizure may manifest as a rhythmic jerking of one hand; or a person experiencing a partial complex seizure might appear dazed and confused with no motor activity being apparent). Consciousness is not impaired in simple seizures, but the client cannot control what is occurring. In complex seizures, the client loses consciousness.

Seizure phases are known as *prodromal,* in which the client can experience *auras* (pre-seizure event or symptom such as an odd odor, taste, or sensation); *ictal* (the seizure); and *postictal* (period following the seizure in which the client may be confused, tired, and unaware of previous event).

CARE SETTING

Community; however, client with convulsive seizures may require brief inpatient care on a medical or subacute unit for stabilization; or for treatment of status epilepticus (a life-threatening emergency).

RELATED CONCERNS

Cerebrovascular accident (CVA)/stroke, page 236
Craniocerebral trauma (acute rehabilitative phase), page 218
Psychosocial aspects of care, page 770
Substance dependence/abuse rehabilitation, page 848

Client Assessment Database

ACTIVITY/REST

May report: Fatigue, general weakness
Limitation of activities/occupation imposed by self/SO/healthcare provider or others

May exhibit: Altered muscle tone/strength
Involuntary movement/contractions of muscles or muscle groups (generalized tonic-clonic seizures)

CIRCULATION

May exhibit: Ictal: Hypertension, increased pulse, cyanosis
Postictal: Vital signs normal or depressed with decreased pulse and respiration

EGO INTEGRITY

May report: Internal/external stressors related to condition and/or treatment
Irritability, sense of helplessness/hopelessness
Changes in relationships

May exhibit: Wide range of emotional responses (especially when temporal lobe is involved)

ELIMINATION

May report: Episodic incontinence

May exhibit: Ictal: Increased bladder pressure and sphincter tone
Postictal: Muscles relaxed, resulting in incontinence (urinary/fecal)

FOOD/FLUID

May report: Food sensitivity nausea/vomiting correlating with seizure activity

May exhibit: Dental/soft-tissue damage (injury during seizure)
Gingival hyperplasia (side effect of long-term phenytoin [Dilantin] use)

NEUROSENSORY

May report: History of headaches, recurring seizure activity, fainting, dizziness
History of head trauma, anoxia, cerebral infections
Prodromal phase: Vague changes in emotional reactivity or affective response preceding aura in some cases and lasting minutes to hours
Presence of aura (stimulation of visual, auditory, hallucinogenic areas)
Postictal: Weakness, muscle pain, areas of paresthesia/paralysis

May exhibit: Seizure characteristics: (ictal, postictal)

Convulsive generalized seizures:

Tonic-clonic (grand mal): Rigidity and jerking, posturing, vocalization, loss of consciousness, dilated pupils, stertorous respiration, excessive salivation (froth), fecal/urinary incontinence, and biting of the tongue may occur and last 2–5 min. Postictal phase: Client is exhausted, may sleep several hours, then may be weak, confused, and amnesic concerning the episode, with nausea and stiff, sore muscles

Tonic phase: Abrupt increase in muscle tone of torso/face, flexion of arms, extension of legs; lasts seconds

Clonic phase: Muscle contraction with relaxation occurring between tonic muscle contractions. Client lies still with flaccid muscles, may have stridorous breathing and excessive salivation. This phase lengthens as tonic muscle activity subsides

Status epilepticus: Defined as 30 or more minutes of continuous generalized seizure activity, or two or more sequential seizures without full recovery of consciousness in between, possibly related to abrupt withdrawal of anticonvulsants and other metabolic phenomena. If absence seizures are the pattern, problem may go undetected for a period of time because client does not lose consciousness

Partial seizures:

Complex (psychomotor/temporal lobe): Client generally remains conscious, with reactions such as dream state, staring, wandering, irritability, hallucinations, hostility, or fear. May display involuntary motor symptoms (lip smacking) and behaviors that appear purposeful but are inappropriate (automatism) and include impaired judgment and, on occasion, antisocial acts; lasts 1–3 min. Postictal phase: Absence of memory for these events, mild to moderate confusion

Simple (focal-motor/Jacksonian): Often preceded by aura (may report deja vu or fearful feeling); no loss of consciousness (unilateral) or loss of consciousness (bilateral); convulsive movements and temporary disturbance in part controlled by the brain region involved (e.g., frontal lobe [motor dysfunction], parietal [numbness, tingling], occipital [bright, flashing lights], posterotemporal [difficulty speaking]). Convulsions may march along limb or side of body in orderly progression. If restrained during seizure, client may exhibit combative and uncooperative behavior; lasts seconds to minutes

PAIN/DISCOMFORT

May report: Headache, muscle/back soreness postictally
Paroxysmal abdominal pain during ictal phase (may occur during some partial/focal seizures without loss of consciousness)

May exhibit: Guarding behavior
Alteration in muscle tone
Distraction behavior/restlessness

RESPIRATION

May exhibit: Ictal: Clenched teeth, cyanosis, decreased or rapid respirations; increased mucous secretions
Postictal: Apnea

SAFETY

May report: History of accidental falls/injuries, fractures
Presence of allergies

May exhibit: Soft-tissue injury/ecchymosis
Decreased general strength/muscle tone

SOCIAL INTERACTION

May report: Problems with interpersonal relationships within family/socially
Limitation/avoidance of social contacts

TEACHING/LEARNING

May report: Familial history of epilepsy
Drug (including alcohol) use/misuse
Use of herbal supplements (e.g., aloe, betony, blue cohash, kava)
Increased frequency of episodes/difficulty with learning resulting in failure to improve

Discharge plan considerations: May require changes in medications, assistance with some homemaker/maintenance tasks relative to issues of safety, and transportation

Refer to section at end of plan for postdischarge considerations.

DIAGNOSTIC STUDIES

May vary depending upon whether or not the client has a known seizure disorder.

Electrolytes: Imbalances (e.g., low sodium, calcium, magnesium) may affect/predispose to seizure activity.

Glucose: Hypoglycemia may precipitate seizure activity.

Blood urea nitrogen (BUN): May potentiate seizure activity or may indicate nephrotoxicity related to medication regimen.

Liver function tests (LFTs): May be elevated due to alcohol, drugs, and poisoning, metabolic abnormalities (potentiates seizures); or reflect drug reaction/interaction.

Complete blood count (CBC): Aplastic anemia may result from drug therapy. Elevated WBCs may indicate presence of infection (can be a precipitator of SE)

Serum drug levels: To verify antiepileptic drug (AEDs) levels.

Toxicology screen: Determines potentiating factors, such as alcohol or other drug use.

Skull x-rays: Identifies presence of space-occupying lesions, fractures.

Electroencephalogram (EEG) may be done serially: Most definitive test, locating area of cerebral dysfunction and measuring brain activity. Brain waves take on characteristic spikes in each type of seizure activity; however, up to 40% of seizure clients have normal EEGs because the paroxysmal abnormalities occur intermittently.

Video–EEG monitoring, 24 hours (video picture obtained at same time as EEG): May identify exact focus of seizure activity (advantage of repeated viewing of event with EEG recording).
Computed tomography (CT) scan: Identifies localized cerebral lesions, infarcts, hematomas, cerebral edema, trauma, abscesses, tumor; can be done with or without contrast medium.
Magnetic resonance imaging (MRI): Localizes focal lesions.
Positron emission tomography (PET): Demonstrates metabolic alterations; e.g., decreased metabolism of glucose at site of lesion.
Single photon emission computed tomography (SPECT): May show local areas of brain dysfunction when CT and MRI are normal.
Magnetoencephalogram: Maps the electrical impulses/potential of brain for abnormal discharge patterns.
Lumbar puncture: Detects abnormal cerebrospinal fluid (CSF) pressure, signs of infections or bleeding (i.e., subarachnoid, subdural hemorrhage) as a cause of seizure activity (rarely required).
Wada's test: Determines hemispheric dominance (done as a presurgical evaluation before temporal lobectomy).

NURSING PRIORITIES

1. Prevent/control seizure activity.
2. Protect client from injury.
3. Maintain airway/respiratory function.
4. Promote positive self-esteem.
5. Provide information about disease process, prognosis, and treatment needs.

DISCHARGE GOALS

1. Seizure activity controlled.
2. Complications/injury prevented.
3. Capable/competent self-image displayed.
4. Disease process/prognosis, therapeutic regimen, and limitations understood.
5. Plan in place to meet needs after discharge.

NURSING DIAGNOSIS: risk for Trauma/Suffocation

Risk factors may include

Weakness, balancing difficulties
Cognitive limitations/altered consciousness
Loss of large or small muscle coordination
Emotional difficulties

Possibly evidenced by

[Not applicable; presence of signs and symptoms establishes an *actual* diagnosis.]

DESIRED OUTCOMES/EVALUATION CRITERIA—CLIENT WILL:

Risk Detection (NOC)

Verbalize understanding of factors that contribute to possibility of trauma and/or suffocation and take steps to correct situation.

Risk Control (NOC)

Demonstrate behaviors, lifestyle changes to reduce risk factors and protect self from future seizure events and injury.
Modify environment as indicated to enhance safety.
Maintain treatment regimen to control/eliminate seizure activity.

SO/CAREGIVERS WILL:

KNOWLEDGE: Personal Safety (NOC)

Identify actions/measures to take when seizure activity occurs.

ACTIONS/INTERVENTIONS	RATIONALE
Seizure Precautions (NIC)	
Independent	
Explore with client the various stimuli that may precipitate seizure activity.	Alcohol, various drugs, and other stimuli (e.g., loss of sleep, flashing lights, prolonged television viewing) may increase the potential for seizure activity. Client may or may not have control over many precipitating factors, but may benefit from becoming aware of risks.
Discuss seizure warning signs (if appropriate) and usual seizure pattern. Teach SO to recognize warning signs and how to care for client during and after seizure.	Can enable client/SO to protect individual from injury, and to recognize changes that require notification of physician/further intervention. Knowing what to do when seizure occurs can prevent injury/complications and decreases SO's feelings of helplessness.
Seizure Management (NIC)	
In hospitalized client:	
Keep padded side rails up with bed in lowest position, or place bed up against wall, and place in padded floor bed if rails not available/appropriate.	Minimizes injury should seizures (frequent/generalized) occur while client is in bed.
Maintain strict bed rest if prodromal signs/aura experienced. Explain necessity for these actions.	Client may feel restless/need to ambulate or even defecate during aural phase, thereby inadvertently removing self from safe environment and easy observation. Understanding importance of providing for own safety needs may enhance client cooperation.
Stay with client during/after seizure.	Promotes client safety and reduces sense of isolation during event.
Turn head to side/suction airway as indicated. Insert plastic bite block per facility protocol only if jaw relaxed.	Helps maintain airway and reduces risk of oral trauma but should not be "forced" or inserted when teeth are clenched because dental and soft-tissue damage may result. *Note*: Current practice is mixed regarding the use of airways during seizure activity. (Refer to ND: risk for ineffective Airway Clearance/Breathing Pattern.)
Cradle head, place on soft area, or assist to floor if out of bed. Do not attempt to restrain.	Gentle guiding of extremities reduces risk of physical injury when client lacks voluntary muscle control. *Note:* If attempt is made to restrain client during seizure, erratic movements may increase, and client may injure self or others.
Perform neurologic/vital sign check after seizure; e.g., level of consciousness, orientation, ability to comply with simple commands, ability to speak, memory of incident, weakness/motor deficits, blood pressure (BP), pulse/respiratory rate.	Documents postictal state and time/completeness of recovery to normal state. May identify additional safety concerns to be addressed.
Reorient client following seizure activity.	Client may be confused, disoriented, and possibly amnesic after the seizure and need help to regain control and alleviate anxiety.
Allow postictal "automatic" behavior without interfering while providing environmental protection.	May display behavior (of motor or psychic origin) that seems inappropriate/irrelevant for time and place. Attempts to control or prevent activity may result in client becoming aggressive/combative.
Investigate reports of pain.	May be result of repetitive muscle contractions or symptom of injury incurred, requiring further evaluation/intervention.

ACTIONS/INTERVENTIONS	RATIONALE
Observe for status epilepticus (SE); that is, one tonic-clonic seizure after another in rapid succession.	This is a life-threatening emergency that if left untreated could cause metabolic acidosis, hyperthermia, hypoglycemia, arrhythmias, hypoxia, increased intracranial pressure, airway obstruction, and respiratory arrest. Immediate intervention is required to control seizure activity and prevent permanent injury/death. *Note:* Although absence seizures may become static, they are not usually life threatening.
Document: preseizure activity, presence of aura or unusual behavior, type of seizure activity (e.g., location/duration of motor activity, loss of consciousness, incontinence, eye activity, respiratory impairment/cyanosis), and frequency/recurrence. Note whether client fell, expressed vocalizations, drooled, or had automatisms (e.g., lip smacking, chewing, picking at clothes).	Helps localize the cerebral area of involvement, and may be useful in chronic conditions in helping client/SO prepare for/manage seizure activity.

Collaborative

ACTIONS/INTERVENTIONS	RATIONALE
Administer medications as indicated:	Choice of drug therapy and route of administration depends on seizure type and current severity of seizure activity. Some clients require multiple medications or frequent medication adjustments to control seizure activity. This increases the risk of adverse reactions and problems with adherence.
Antiepileptic drugs (AEDs); e.g., phenytoin (Dilantin), fosphenytoin (Cerebyx), primidone (Mysoline), carbamazepine (Carbatrol, Tegretol), clonazepam (Klonopin), valproic acid (Depakene), divalproex (Depakote), acetazolamide (Diamox), ethotoin (Peganone), methsuximide (Celotin);	AEDs treat and/or prevent seizures by raising the seizure threshold, stabilizing nerve cell membranes, reducing the excitability of the neurons, or through direct action on the limbic system, thalamus, and hypothalamus. Goal is optimal suppression of seizure activity with lowest possible dose of drug and with fewest side effects. Long-term drug treatment is required for clients who have recurrent seizures, seizures with an unknown cause, or a cause that can't be reversed.
Oxycarbazepine (Trileptal), Topiramate (Topamax), ethosuximide (Zarontin), clorazepate (Apo-Clorazepate), lamotrigine (Lamictal), gabapentin (Neurontin);	Adjunctive therapy for prevention and treatment of partial seizures, or an alternative for clients when seizures are not adequately controlled by other drugs.
Phenobarbital (Luminal);	May be given in emergent situation to potentiate/enhance effects of other AEDs, and allow for lower dosage to reduce side effects.
Lorazepam (Ativan);	Used to abort status seizure activity because it is shorter acting than diazepam (Valium) and less likely to prolong postseizure sedation.
Diazepam (Valium, Diastat rectal gel);	May be used alone (or in combination with phenobarbital) to suppress status seizure activity. Diastat, a gel, may be administered rectally, even in the home setting, to reduce frequency of seizures and need for additional medical care.
Glucose, thiamine.	May be given to restore metabolic balance if seizure is induced by hypoglycemia or alcohol.
Monitor/document AED drug levels, corresponding side effects, and frequency of seizure activity.	Blood levels of the various AEDs should be evaluated on a regular basis; e.g. weekly for a period of time, then monthly, annually. Blood levels should also be done when breakthrough seizures occur, or any change occurs in the client's status. Standard therapeutic level may not be optimal for individual client if untoward side effects develop or seizures are not controlled.

ACTIONS/INTERVENTIONS	RATIONALE
Monitor CBC, electrolytes, glucose levels.	Identifies factors that aggravate/decrease seizure threshold.
Prepare for surgery/electrode implantation as indicated.	Vagal nerve stimulator, magnetic beam therapy, or other surgical intervention (e.g., temporal lobectomy) may be done for intractable seizures or well-localized epileptogenic lesions when client is disabled and at high risk for serious injury. Success has been reported with gamma ray radiosurgery for the treatment of multiple seizure activity that has otherwise been difficult to control.

NURSING DIAGNOSIS: risk for ineffective Airway Clearance/Breathing Pattern

Risk factors may include

Neuromuscular impairment
Tracheobronchial obstruction
Perceptual/cognitive impairment

Possibly evidenced by

[Not applicable; presence of signs and symptoms establishes an *actual* diagnosis.]

DESIRED OUTCOMES/EVALUATION CRITERIA—CLIENT WILL:

RESPIRATORY STATUS: Ventilation (NOC)

Maintain effective respiratory pattern with airway patent/aspiration prevented.

ACTIONS/INTERVENTIONS	RATIONALE
Airway Management (NIC)	
Independent	
Encourage client to empty mouth of dentures/foreign objects if aura occurs and to avoid chewing gum/sucking lozenges if seizures occur without warning.	Reduces risk of aspiration/foreign bodies lodging in pharynx.
Place in lying position, flat surface; turn head to side during seizure activity.	Promotes drainage of secretions; prevents tongue from obstructing airway.
Loosen clothing from neck/chest and abdominal areas.	Facilitates breathing/chest expansion.
Insert plastic airway as indicated per facility protocol and only if jaw is relaxed.	If inserted before jaw is tightened, these devices may prevent biting of tongue and facilitate suctioning/respiratory support if required. Airway adjunct may be indicated after cessation of seizure activity if client is unconscious and unable to maintain safe position of tongue. *Note*: Current practice is mixed regarding the use of airways during seizure activity.
Suction as needed.	Reduces risk of aspiration/asphyxiation. *Note:* Risk of aspiration is low unless individual has eaten within the last 40 min.

ACTIONS/INTERVENTIONS	RATIONALE
Collaborative	
Administer supplemental oxygen/bag ventilation as needed postictally.	May reduce cerebral hypoxia resulting from decreased circulation/oxygenation secondary to vascular spasm during seizure. *Note:* Artificial ventilation during general seizure activity is of limited or no benefit because it is not possible to move air in/out of lungs during sustained contraction of respiratory musculature. As seizure abates, respiratory function will return unless a secondary problem exists (e.g., foreign body/aspiration).
Prepare for/assist with intubation, if indicated.	Presence of prolonged apnea postictally may require ventilatory support.

NURSING DIAGNOSIS: Self-Esteem [specify situational or chronic low]

May be related to

Stigma associated with condition
Perception of helplessness

Possibly evidenced by

Verbalization about changed lifestyle
Fear of rejection; negative feelings about body (self image)
Potential change in perception of role
Change in usual patterns of responsibility
Denial of problem resulting in lack of follow-through/nonparticipation in therapy

DESIRED OUTCOMES/EVALUATION CRITERIA—CLIENT WILL:

Self-Esteem (NOC)

Identify feelings and methods for coping with negative perception of self.
Verbalize increased sense of self-esteem in relation to diagnosis.
Verbalize realistic perception and acceptance of self in changed role/lifestyle.

ACTIONS/INTERVENTIONS	RATIONALE
Self-Esteem Enhancement (NIC)	
Independent	
Discuss feelings about diagnosis, perception of threat to self. Encourage expression of feelings.	Reactions vary among individuals, and previous knowledge/experience with this condition affects acceptance of therapeutic regimen. Verbalization of fears, anger, and concerns about future implications can help client begin to accept/deal with situation.
Identify possible/anticipated public reaction to condition. Encourage client to refrain from concealing problem.	Provides opportunity to problem-solve response, and provides measure of control over situation. Concealment is destructive to self-esteem (potentiates denial), blocking progress in dealing with problem, and may actually increase risk of injury/negative response when seizure does occur.

ACTIONS/INTERVENTIONS	RATIONALE
Explore with client current/past successes and strengths.	Focusing on positive aspects can help alleviate feelings of guilt/self-consciousness and help client begin to accept manageability of condition.
Avoid overprotecting client; encourage activities, providing supervision/monitoring when indicated.	Participation in as many experiences as possible can lessen depression about limitations. Observation/supervision may need to be provided for such activities as gymnastics, climbing, and water sports.
Determine attitudes/capabilities of SO. Help individual realize that client's feelings are normal; however, guilt and blame are not helpful.	Negative expectations from SO may affect client's sense of competency/self-esteem and interfere with support received from SO, limiting potential for optimal management/personal growth.
Stress importance of staff/SO remaining calm during seizure activity.	Anxiety of caregivers is contagious and can be conveyed to the client, increasing/multiplying individual's own negative perceptions of situation/self.
Refer client/SO to support groups; e.g., Epilepsy Foundation of America, National Association of Epilepsy Centers, and Delta Society's National Service Dog Center.	Provides opportunity to gain information, support, and ideas for dealing with problems from others who share similar experiences. *Note:* Some service dogs have ability to sense/predict seizure activity, allowing client to institute safety measures, increasing independence and personal sense of control.
Discuss referral for psychotherapy with client/SO.	Seizures have a profound effect on personal self-esteem, and client/SO may feel guilt over perceived limitations and public stigma. Counseling can help overcome feelings of inferiority/self-consciousness.

NURSING DIAGNOSIS: deficient Knowledge [Learning Need] regarding condition, prognosis, treatment regimen, self-care, and discharge needs

May be related to

Lack of exposure, unfamiliarity with resources
Information misinterpretation
Lack of recall; cognitive limitation

Possibly evidenced by

Questions, statement of concerns
Increased frequency/lack of control of seizure activity
Lack of follow-through of drug regimen

DESIRED OUTCOMES/EVALUATION CRITERIA—CLIENT WILL:

KNOWLEDGE: Illness Care (NOC)

Verbalize understanding of disorder and various stimuli that may increase/potentiate seizure activity.
Adhere to prescribed drug regimen.

KNOWLEDGE: Personal Safety (NOC)

Initiate necessary lifestyle/behavior changes as indicated.

ACTIONS/INTERVENTIONS	RATIONALE
TEACHING: Disease Process (NIC)	
Independent	
Review pathology/prognosis of condition and lifelong need for treatments as indicated. Discuss client's particular trigger factors (e.g., flashing lights, hyperventilation, loud noises, video games, TV viewing) if known.	Provides opportunity to clarify/dispel misconceptions and present condition as something that is manageable within a normal lifestyle.
Review possible effects of female hormonal changes.	Alterations in hormonal levels that occur during menstruation and pregnancy may increase risk of seizure breakthrough.
Discuss significance of maintaining good general health; e.g., adequate diet, rest, moderate exercise, and avoidance of exhaustion, alcohol, caffeine, and stimulant drugs.	Regularity and moderation in activities may aid in reducing/controlling precipitating factors, enhancing sense of general well-being, and strengthening coping ability and self-esteem. *Note:* Too little sleep or too much alcohol can precipitate seizure activity in some people.
Review importance of good oral hygiene and regular dental care.	Reduces risk of oral infections and gingival hyperplasia.
Encourage client who smokes to refrain from smoking except while supervised.	May cause burns if cigarette is accidentally dropped during aura/seizure activity.
Evaluate need for/provide protective headgear.	Use of helmet may provide added protection for individuals who suffer recurrent/severe seizures.
Identify necessity/promote acceptance of actual limitations; discuss safety measures regarding driving, using mechanical equipment, climbing ladders, swimming, and hobbies.	Reduces risk of injury to self or others, especially if seizures occur without warning.
Discuss local laws/restrictions pertaining to persons with epilepsy/seizure disorder. Encourage awareness but not necessarily acceptance of these policies.	Although legal/civil rights of persons with epilepsy have improved during the past decade, restrictions still exist in some states pertaining to obtaining a driver's license, sterilization, workers' compensation, and required reportability to state agencies.
TEACHING: Prescribed Medication (NIC)	
Review medication regimen, necessity of taking drugs as ordered, and not discontinuing therapy without physician supervision. Include directions for missed dose.	Lack of cooperation with medication regimen is a leading cause of seizure breakthrough. Client needs to know risks of status epilepticus resulting from abrupt withdrawal of anticonvulsants. Depending on the drug dose and frequency, client may be instructed to take missed dose if remembered within a predetermined time frame.
Recommend taking drugs with meals if appropriate.	May reduce incidence of gastric irritation, nausea/vomiting.
Discuss nuisance and adverse side effects of particular drugs; e.g., drowsiness, fatigue, lethargy, hyperactivity, sleep disturbances, gingival hypertrophy, visual disturbances, nausea/vomiting, rashes, syncope/ataxia, birth defects, aplastic anemia.	May indicate need for change in dosage/choice of drug therapy. Promotes involvement/participation in decision-making process and awareness of potential long-term effects of drug therapy, and provides opportunity to minimize/prevent complications.
Provide information about potential drug interactions and necessity of notifying other healthcare providers of drug regimen.	Knowledge of anticonvulsant use reduces risk of prescribing drugs that may interact, thus altering seizure threshold or therapeutic effect. For example, phenytoin (Dilantin) potentiates anticoagulant effect of warfarin (Coumadin), whereas isoniazid (INH) and chloramphenicol (Chloromycetin) increase the effect of Dilantin, and some antibiotics (e.g., erythromycin) can cause elevation of serum level of carbamazepine (Tegretol), possibly to toxic levels.

ACTIONS/INTERVENTIONS	RATIONALE
Review proper use of diazepam rectal gel (Diastat) with client and SO/caregiver as appropriate.	Useful in controlling serial or cluster seizures. Can be administered in any setting and is effective usually within 15 min. May reduce dependence on emergency department visits.
Discuss use of over-the-counter (OTC) medications and supplements/herbals.	Anticonvulsant drugs can interact with many other medications and substances. Some medications can decrease the effectiveness of anticonvulsant drugs, or the client may choose a folk-remedy or herbal supplement without being aware of its effect.
Encourage client to wear identification tag/bracelet stating the presence of a seizure disorder.	Expedites treatment and diagnosis in emergency situations.
Stress need for routine follow-up care/laboratory testing as indicated; e.g., CBC should be monitored biannually and in presence of sore throat/fever, signs of other infection.	Therapeutic needs may change and/or serious drug side effects (e.g., agranulocytosis or toxicity) may develop.

POTENTIAL CONSIDERATIONS following acute hospitalization (dependent on client's age, physical condition/presence of complications, personal resources, and life responsibilities)

risk for Injury—weakness, balancing difficulties, cognitive limitations/altered consciousness, loss of large or small muscle coordination.

Self-Esteem (specify)—stigma associated with condition, perception of being out of control, personal vulnerability, negative evaluation of self/capabilities.

ineffective Therapeutic Regimen Management—social support deficits, perceived benefit (versus side effects of medication), perceived susceptibility (possible long periods of remission).

CRANIOCEREBRAL TRAUMA (ACUTE REHABILITATIVE PHASE)

Craniocerebral trauma, also called traumatic head or brain injury (open or closed), includes skull fractures, brain concussion, cerebral contusion/laceration, and hemorrhage (subarachnoid, subdural, epidural, intracerebral, brainstem). Primary injury occurs from a direct or indirect blow to the head, causing acceleration/deceleration of the brain. Secondary brain injury results from diffuse intracerebral axonal injury, intracranial hypertension, hypoxemia, hypercapnia, or systemic hypotension. Cerebral concussion is the most minor and the most common form of head injury

Common causes of traumatic brain injury include motor vehicle crashes (e.g., collisions between vehicles, pedestrians struck by motor vehicles, bicycle and motorcycle accidents), falls, assaults, sports-related injuries, and penetrating trauma.

Consequences of brain injury range from no apparent neurologic disturbance to a persistent vegetative state or death. Therefore, every head injury must be considered potentially dangerous. Individuals who experience mild to severe brain injury often require specialized rehabilitation to regain skills and abilities, and to address new problems associated with their injuries.

The incidence of traumatic brain injury (TBI) in the United States is estimated at approximately 600,000 new cases per year, with an annual direct cost at more than $25 billion, excluding inpatient care. The cost to society is enormous, considering that most severe head injures occur in adolescents and young adults, and that almost 100% of persons with severe TBI and 66% of persons with moderate TBI will be permanently disabled and will not be able to return to their preinjury level of function.

CARE SETTING

This plan of care focuses on acute care and acute inpatient rehabilitation. Brain injury care for those experiencing moderate to severe trauma progresses along a continuum of care, beginning with acute hospital care and inpatient rehabilitation to subacute and outpatient rehabilitation, as well as home- and community-based services.

RELATED CONCERNS

Cerebrovascular accident (CVA)/stroke, page 236
Psychosocial aspects of care, page 770
Seizure disorders/epilepsy, page 208
Surgical intervention, page 788
Thrombophlebitis: deep vein thrombosis, page 108

Total nutritional support: parenteral/enteral feeding, page 478
Upper gastrointestinal/esophageal bleeding, page 309

Client Assessment Database

Data depend on type, location, and severity of injury and may be complicated by additional injury to other vital organs.

ACTIVITY/REST

May report: Weakness, fatigue, clumsiness, loss of balance

May exhibit: Altered consciousness, lethargy
Hemiparesis, quadriparesis
Unsteady gait (ataxia); balance problems
Orthopedic injuries (trauma)
Loss of muscle tone, muscle spasticity

CIRCULATION

May exhibit: Normal or altered BP (hypotension or hypertension)
Changes in heart rate (bradycardia, tachycardia alternating with bradycardia, other dysrhythmias)

EGO INTEGRITY

May report: Behavior or personality changes (subtle to dramatic)

May exhibit: Anxiety, irritability, delirium, agitation, confusion, depression, impulsivity

ELIMINATION

May exhibit: Bowel/bladder incontinence or dysfunction

FOOD/FLUID

May report: Nausea/vomiting, changes in appetite

May exhibit: Vomiting (may be projectile)
Swallowing problems (coughing, drooling, dysphagia)

NEUROSENSORY

May report: Loss of consciousness, variable levels of awareness, amnesia surrounding trauma events
Vertigo, syncope, tinnitus, hearing loss
Tingling, numbness in extremity
Visual changes; e.g., decreased acuity, diplopia, photophobia, loss of part of visual field
Loss of/changes in senses of taste or smell

May exhibit: Alteration in consciousness from lethargy to coma
Mental status changes (orientation, alertness/responsiveness, attention, concentration, problem-solving, emotional affect/behavior, memory)
Pupillary changes (response to light, symmetry), deviation of eyes, inability to follow
Loss of senses; e.g., taste, smell, hearing
Facial asymmetry
Unequal, weak handgrip
Absent/weak deep tendon reflexes
Apraxia, hemiparesis, quadriparesis
Posturing (decorticate, decerebrate); seizure activity
Heightened sensitivity to touch and movement
Altered sensation to parts of body
Difficulty in understanding self/limbs in relation to environment (proprioception)

PAIN/DISCOMFORT

May report: Headache of variable intensity and location (usually persistent/long-lasting)

May exhibit: Facial grimacing, withdrawal response to painful stimuli, restlessness, moaning

RESPIRATION

May exhibit: Changes in breathing patterns (e.g., periods of apnea alternating with hyperventilation)
Noisy respirations, stridor, choking
Rhonchi, wheezes (possible aspiration)

SAFETY

May report:	Recent trauma/accidental injuries
May exhibit:	Fractures/dislocations Impaired vision, visual field disturbances, abnormal eye movements Skin: Head/facial lacerations, abrasions, discoloration; e.g., raccoon eyes. Battle's sign around ears (trauma signs) Drainage from ears/nose (CSF) Impaired cognition Range of motion (ROM) impairment, loss of muscle tone, general strength, paralysis Fever, instability in internal regulation of body temperature

SOCIAL INTERACTION

May exhibit:	Expressive or receptive aphasia, unintelligible speech, repetitive speech, dysarthria, anomia Difficulty dealing with noisy environment, interacting with more than one or two individuals at a time Changes in role/family structure related to condition

TEACHING/LEARNING

May report:	Use of alcohol/other drugs
Discharge plan considerations:	May require assistance with self-care, ambulation, transportation, food preparation, shopping, treatments, medications, homemaker/maintenance tasks, change in physical layout of home or placement in living facility other than home

Refer to section at end of plan for postdischarge considerations.

DIAGNOSTIC STUDIES

CT scan (with/without contrast): Screening image of choice in acute brain injury. Identifies space-occupying lesions, hematomas, contusions, hemorrhage, skull fractures, brain tissue swelling and shift.

MRI: Uses similar to those of CT scan but more sensitive than CT for detecting cerebral trauma, determining neurologic deficits not explained by CT, evaluating prolonged interval of disturbed consciousness, defining evidence of previous trauma superimposed on acute trauma. *Note*: MRI has limited role in evaluation of acute head injury because of longer procedure time and difficulty obtaining MRI in an acutely injured person.

Cerebral angiography: Demonstrates cerebral circulatory anomalies; e.g., brain tissue shifts secondary to edema, hemorrhage, trauma. *Note*: Rarely used in acute head injury, but can be done when subarachnoid or parenchymal hemorrhage is known or suspected.

Serial EEG: May reveal presence or development of pathologic waves. EEG is not generally indicated in the immediate period of emergency response, evaluation, and treatment. If the client fails to improve, EEG may help in diagnostic evaluation for seizures, focal or diffuse encephalopathy.

Skull x-rays: Although largely replaced by CT scan, can be used to detect changes in bony structure (fractures), shifts of midline structures (bleeding/edema); assess degree of, e.g., foreign body penetration, bone fragments

Brainstem auditory evoked responses (BAER): Determines levels of cortical and brainstem function.

PET/SPECT tomography: Detects changes in metabolic activity in the brain and may be used for differentiation of head injuries. (These procedures are not in widespread clinical use, but are more often used for research.)

Lumbar puncture and CSF analysis: May be performed in client with suspected or known increased intracranial pressure when CT or MRI is not diagnostic. Generally contraindicated in acute trauma.

ABGs: Determines presence of ventilation or oxygenation problems that may exacerbate/increase intracranial pressure.

Serum chemistry/electrolytes: May reveal imbalances that contribute to increased intracranial pressure (ICP)/changes in mentation.

Toxicology screen: Detects drugs that may be responsible for/potentiate loss of consciousness.

Serum anticonvulsant levels: May be done to ensure that therapeutic level is adequate to prevent seizure activity.

NURSING PRIORITIES

1. Maximize cerebral perfusion/function.
2. Prevent/minimize complications.
3. Promote optimal functioning/return to pre-injury level.
4. Support coping process and family recovery.
5. Provide information about condition/prognosis, potential complications, treatment plan, and resources.

DISCHARGE GOALS

1. Cerebral function improved; neurologic deficits resolving/stabilized.
2. Complications prevented or minimized.

3. Activities of daily living (ADLs) met by self or with assistance of other(s).
4. Family acknowledging reality of situation and involved in recovery program.
5. Condition/prognosis, complications, and treatment regimen understood and available resources identified.
6. Plan in place to meet needs after discharge.

NURSING DIAGNOSIS: ineffective cerebral Tissue Perfusion

May be related to

Interruption of blood flow by space-occupying lesions (hemorrhage, hematoma), cerebral edema (localized or generalized response to injury, metabolic alterations, drug/alcohol overdose), decreased systemic BP/hypoxia (hypovolemia, cardiac dysrhythmias)

Possibly evidenced by

Altered level of consciousness, memory loss
Changes in motor/sensory responses, restlessness
Changes in vital signs

DESIRED OUTCOMES/EVALUATION CRITERIA—CLIENT WILL:

Neurologic Status (NOC)

Maintain usual/improved level of consciousness, cognition, and motor/sensory function.
Demonstrate stable vital signs and absence of signs of increased ICP.

ACTIONS/INTERVENTIONS	RATIONALE
Neurologic Monitoring (NIC)	
Independent	
Determine factors related to individual situation, cause for coma/decreased cerebral perfusion, and potential for increased ICP.	Influences choice of interventions. Deterioration in neurologic signs/symptoms or failure to improve after initial insult may reflect decreased intracranial adaptive capacity, requiring the client be transferred to critical care for monitoring of ICP and/or surgical intervention.
Monitor/document neurologic status frequently and compare with baseline; e.g., Glasgow Coma Scale during first 48 hr:	Measures best responses in eye opening, motor and verbal responses (1–5 in each category). Assesses trends and potential for increased ICP and is useful in determining location, extent, and progression/resolution of CNS damage. *Note:* The Rancho Los Amigos Scale (or Rancho Levels) may also be used. These levels do not require cooperation from the client, are based on client's response to environmental stimuli and a range of behavioral responses, (e g., no response, confused-agitated, purposeful-appropriate)
Evaluate eye opening; e.g., spontaneous (awake), opens only to painful stimuli, keeps eyes closed (coma);	Determines arousal ability/level of consciousness.
Assess verbal response; note whether client is alert; oriented to person, place, and time; or is confused; uses inappropriate words/phrases that make little sense;	Measures appropriateness of speech and content of consciousness. If minimal damage has occurred in the cerebral cortex, client may be aroused by verbal stimuli but may appear drowsy or uncooperative. More extensive damage to the cerebral cortex may be displayed by slow response to commands, lapsing into sleep when not stimulated, disorientation, and stupor. Damage to midbrain, pons, and medulla is manifested by lack of appropriate responses to stimuli.

ACTIONS/INTERVENTIONS	RATIONALE
Assess motor response to simple commands, noting purposeful (obeys command, attempts to push stimulus away) and nonpurposeful (posturing) movement. Note limb movement and document right and left sides separately.	Measures overall awareness and ability to respond to external stimuli, and best indicates state of consciousness in the client whose eyes are closed because of trauma or who is aphasic. Consciousness and involuntary movement are integrated if client can both grasp and release the tester's hand or hold up two fingers on command. Purposeful movement can include grimacing or withdrawing from painful stimuli or movements that the client desires; e.g., sitting up. Other movements (posturing and abnormal flexion of extremities) usually indicate diffuse cortical damage. Absence of spontaneous movement on one side of the body indicates damage to the motor tracts in the opposite cerebral hemisphere.
Monitor vital signs; e.g.:	
BP, noting onset of/continuing systolic hypertension and widening pulse pressure; observe for hypotension in multiple trauma client;	Normally, autoregulation maintains constant cerebral blood flow despite fluctuations in systemic BP. Loss of autoregulation may follow local or diffuse cerebrovascular damage. Elevating systolic BP accompanied by decreasing diastolic BP (widening pulse pressure) is an ominous sign of increased ICP when accompanied by decreased level of consciousness. Hypovolemia/hypotension (associated with multiple trauma) may also result in cerebral ischemia/damage.
Heart rate/rhythm, noting bradycardia, alternating bradycardia/tachycardia, other dysrhythmias;	Changes in rate (most often bradycardia) and dysrhythmias may develop, reflecting brainstem pressure/injury in the absence of underlying cardiac disease.
Respirations, noting patterns and rhythm; e.g., periods of apnea after hyperventilation, Cheyne-Stokes respiration.	Irregularities can suggest location of cerebral insult/increasing ICP and need for further intervention, including possible respiratory support. (Refer to ND: risk for ineffective Breathing Pattern following.)
Evaluate pupils, noting size, shape, equality, light reactivity.	Pupil reactions are regulated by the oculomotor (III) cranial nerve and are useful in determining whether the brainstem is intact. Pupil size/equality is determined by balance between parasympathetic and sympathetic innervation. Response to light reflects combined function of optic (II) and oculomotor (III) cranial nerves.
Assess position/movement of eyes, noting whether in midposition or deviated to side or downward. Note loss of doll's eyes (oculocephalic reflex).	Position and movement of eyes help localize area of brain involvement. An early sign of increased ICP is impaired abduction of eyes, indicating pressure/injury to the fifth cranial nerve. Loss of doll's eyes indicates deterioration in brainstem function and poor prognosis.
Note presence/absence of reflexes (e.g., blink, cough, gag, Babinski).	Altered reflexes reflect injury at level of midbrain or brainstem and have direct implications for client safety. Loss of blink reflex suggests damage to the pons and medulla. Absence of cough and gag reflexes reflects damage to medulla. Presence of Babinski reflex indicates injury along pyramidal pathways in the brain.
Cerebral Perfusion Promotion (NIC)	
Monitor temperature and regulate environmental temperature as indicated. Limit use of blankets; administer tepid sponge bath in presence of fever. Wrap extremities in blankets when hypothermia blanket is used.	Fever may reflect damage to hypothalamus. Increased metabolic needs and oxygen consumption occur (especially with fever and shivering), which can further increase ICP.
Monitor I&O. Weigh as indicated. Note skin turgor, status of mucous membranes.	Useful indicators of total body water, which is an integral part of tissue perfusion. Cerebral trauma/ischemia can result in diabetes insipidus (DI) or syndrome of inappropriate antidiuretic hormone (SIADH). Alterations may lead to hypovolemia or vascular engorgement, either of which can negatively affect cerebral pressure.

ACTIONS/INTERVENTIONS	RATIONALE
Maintain head/neck in midline or neutral position, support with small towel rolls and pillows. Avoid placing head on large pillows. Periodically check position/fit of cervical collar or tracheostomy ties when used.	Turning head to one side compresses the jugular veins and inhibits cerebral venous drainage, thereby increasing ICP. Tight- fitting collar/ties can also limit jugular venous drainage.
Provide rest periods between care activities and limit duration of procedures.	Continual activity can increase ICP by producing a cumulative stimulant effect.
Decrease extraneous stimuli and provide comfort measures; e.g., back massage, quiet environment, soft voice, gentle touch.	Provides calming effect, reduces adverse physiologic response, and promotes rest to maintain/lower ICP.
Help client avoid/limit coughing, vomiting, straining at stool/bearing down, when possible. Reposition client slowly; prevent client from bending knees and pushing heels against mattress to move up in bed.	These activities increase intrathoracic and intra-abdominal pressures, which can increase ICP.
Avoid/limit use of restraints.	Mechanical restraints may enhance fight response, increasing ICP. *Note:* Cautious use may be indicated to prevent injury to client when other measures including medications are ineffective.
Limit number and duration of suctioning passes (e.g., two passes less than 10 sec each). Hyperventilate only when indicated.	Prevents hypoxia and associated vasoconstriction that can impair cerebral perfusion. *Note*: The use of prophylactic hyperventilation prior to suctioning or as a stand-alone treatment should be avoided during the first 24 hr, as it can compromise cerebral perfusion. It may be used for brief periods when there is neurologic deterioration, ICP is refractory to sedation.
Encourage SO to talk to client.	Familiar voices of family/SO appear to have a relaxing effect on many comatose clients, which can reduce ICP.
Investigate increasing restlessness, moaning, guarding behaviors.	These nonverbal cues may indicate increasing ICP or reflect presence of pain when client is unable to verbalize complaints. Unrelieved pain can in turn aggravate/potentiate increased ICP.
Palpate for bladder distention; maintain patency of urinary drainage if used. Monitor for constipation.	May trigger autonomic responses, potentiating elevation of ICP.
Observe for seizure activity and protect client from injury.	Seizures can occur as a result of cerebral irritation, hypoxia, or increased ICP; additionally, seizures can further elevate ICP, compounding cerebral damage.
Assess for nuchal rigidity, twitching, increased restlessness, irritability, onset of seizure activity.	Indicative of meningeal irritation, which may occur because of interruption of dura, and/or development of infection during acute or recovery period of brain injury.

Collaborative

Elevate head of bed gradually to 20–30 degrees as tolerated/indicated. Avoid hip flexion greater than 90 degrees.	Promotes venous drainage from head, thereby reducing cerebral congestion and edema/risk of increased ICP. *Note:* Presence of hypotension can compromise cerebral perfusion pressure, negating beneficial effect of elevating head of bed.
Administer isotonic IV fluids (e.g., 0.9% sodium chloride) with control device.	Fluids should not be routinely restricted, but should be administered to maintain normal intravascular volume, systemic blood pressure, and cardiac output in order to maintain brain perfusion and decrease risk of cerebral edema and ICP.
Administer supplemental oxygen via appropriate route (e.g., mechanical ventilator, mask) to maintain O_2 saturation >94% as indicated.	Reduces hypoxemia, which is known to increase cerebral vasodilation and blood volume, elevating ICP.
Monitor ABGs/pulse oximetry.	Determines respiratory sufficiency (presence of hypoxia/acidosis) and indicates therapy needs.

ACTIONS/INTERVENTIONS	RATIONALE
Administer medications as indicated:	
Diuretics; e.g., mannitol (Osmitrol), furosemide (Lasix);	Diuretics may be used in acute phase to draw water from brain cells, reducing cerebral edema and ICP. *Note:* Loop diuretics (e.g., Lasix) also reduce production of CSF, which can contribute to increased ICP when cerebral edema impairs CSF circulation.
Barbiturates; e.g. pentobarbital;	Barbiturates are the most common class of drugs used to suppress cerebral metabolism and reduce ICP. Barbiturates are typically continued for 48 hours, and then the client is weaned.
Steroids; e.g., dexamethasone (Decadron), methylprednisolone (Medrol);	May be effective for treating vasogenic edema—decreasing inflammation, reducing tissue edema. *Note:* Use and efficacy of steroids continues to be debated in this condition.
Anticonvulsant; e.g., phenytoin (Dilantin);	Dilantin is the drug of choice for treatment and prevention of seizure activity in immediate posttraumatic period to reduce risk of secondary injury from associated increased ICP. Prophylactic anticonvulsive therapy may be continued for an indeterminate period of time.
Chlorpromazine (Thorazine);	Useful in treating posturing and shivering, which can increase ICP. *Note:* This drug can lower the seizure threshold or precipitate Dilantin toxicity.
Mild analgesics and sedatives; e.g., lorazepam (Ativan);	May be indicated to relieve pain and agitation and their negative effects on ICP. Client on ventilator will be sedated, and possibly require deep sedation.
Antipyretics; e.g., acetaminophen (Tylenol).	Reduces/controls fever and its deleterious effect on cerebral metabolism/oxygen needs and insensible fluid losses.
Initiate cooling measures, as indicated	May be needed to regain/maintain normal core body temperature (hyperthermia exacerbates a hypermetabolic state).
Prepare for surgical intervention if indicated.	Client may require craniotomy to remove bone fragments, elevate depressed fractures, evacuate hematoma, control hemorrhage, and debride necrotic tissue. Intracranial pressure monitoring devices (e.g., intraparenchymal, intraventricular, or epidural) can be surgically placed, and are usually done in conjunction with other cranial surgery procedures, but may be placed in any client with Glasow Coma Scale (GCS) score less than 9, with an abnormal CT scan.

NURSING DIAGNOSIS: risk for ineffective Breathing Pattern

Risk factors may include

Neuromuscular impairment (injury to respiratory center of brain)
Perception or cognitive impairment
Tracheobronchial obstruction

Possibly evidenced by

[Not applicable; presence of signs and symptoms establishes an *actual* diagnosis.]

DESIRED OUTCOMES/EVALUATION CRITERIA—CLIENT WILL:

RESPIRATORY STATUS: Ventilation (NOC)

Maintain a normal/effective respiratory pattern, free of cyanosis, with ABGs/pulse oximetry within client's acceptable range.

ACTIONS/INTERVENTIONS	RATIONALE
Airway Management (NIC)	
Independent	
Monitor rate, rhythm, depth of respiration. Note breathing irregularities; e.g., apneustic, ataxic, or cluster breathing.	Changes may indicate onset of pulmonary complications (common following brain injury) or indicate location/extent of brain involvement. Slow respiration and periods of apnea (apneustic, ataxic, or cluster breathing patterns) are signs of brainstem injury and warn of impending respiratory arrest.
Note competence of gag/swallow reflexes and client's ability to protect own airway. Insert airway adjunct as indicated.	Ability to mobilize or clear secretions is important to airway maintenance. Loss of swallow or cough reflex may indicate need for artificial airway/intubation. *Note:* Soft nasopharyngeal airways may be preferred to prevent stimulation of the gag reflex caused by hard oropharyngeal airway, which can lead to excessive coughing and increased ICP.
Elevate head of bed as permitted, position on sides as indicated.	Facilitates lung expansion/ventilation and reduces risk of airway obstruction by tongue.
Encourage deep breathing if client is conscious.	Prevents/reduces atelectasis.
Suction with extreme caution; no longer than 10–15 sec. Note character, color, odor of secretions.	Suctioning is usually required if client is comatose or immobile and unable to clear own airway. Deep tracheal suctioning should be done with caution because it can cause or aggravate hypoxia, which produces vasoconstriction, adversely affecting cerebral perfusion. *Note:* Administration of intratracheal or IV lidocaine 1–2 min before suctioning can suppress cough reflex and minimize Valsalva maneuver, limiting impact on ICP.
Auscultate breath sounds, noting areas of hypoventilation and presence of adventitious sounds (crackles, rhonchi, wheezes).	Identifies pulmonary problems such as atelectasis, congestion, and airway obstruction, which may jeopardize cerebral oxygenation and/or indicate onset of pulmonary infection (common complication of head injury).
Monitor use of respiratory depressant drugs; e.g., sedatives.	Can increase respiratory embarrassment/complications.
Collaborative	
Monitor/graph serial ABGs, pulse oximetry.	Determines respiratory sufficiency, acid-base balance, and therapy needs.
Review chest x-rays.	Reveals ventilatory state and signs of developing complications (e.g., atelectasis, pneumonia).
Administer supplemental oxygen.	Maximizes arterial oxygenation and aids in prevention of cerebral hypoxia. If respiratory center is depressed, mechanical ventilation may be required.
Assist with chest physiotherapy when indicated.	Although contraindicated in client with acutely elevated ICP, these measures are often necessary in acute rehabilitation phase to mobilize and clear lung fields and reduce atelectasis/pulmonary complications.

NURSING DIAGNOSIS: disturbed Sensory Perception [specify]

May be related to

Altered sensory reception, transmission and/or integration (neurologic trauma or deficit)

Possibly evidenced by

Disorientation to time, place, person
Change in usual response to stimuli

Motor incoordination, alterations in posture, inability to tell position of body parts (proprioception)
Altered communication patterns
Visual and auditory distortions
Poor concentration, altered thought processes/bizarre thinking
Exaggerated emotional responses, change in behavior pattern

DESIRED OUTCOMES/EVALUATION CRITERIA—CLIENT WILL:

Cognition (NOC)

Regain/maintain usual level of consciousness and perceptual functioning.
Acknowledge changes in ability and presence of residual involvement.
Demonstrate behaviors/lifestyle changes to compensate for/overcome deficit.

ACTIONS/INTERVENTIONS	RATIONALE
Reality Orientation (NIC)	
Independent	
Evaluate/continually monitor changes in orientation, ability to speak, mood/affect, sensorium, thought process.	Upper cerebral functions are often the first to be affected by altered circulation/oxygenation. Damage may occur at time of initial injury or develop later because of swelling or bleeding. Motor, perceptual, cognitive, and personality changes may develop and persist, with gradual normalization of responses, or changes may remain permanently to some degree.
Assess sensory awareness; e.g., response to touch, hot/cold, dull/sharp, and awareness of motion and location of body parts. Note problems with vision, other senses.	Information is essential to client safety. All sensory systems may be affected, with changes involving increased or decreased sensitivity or loss of sensation and/or the ability to perceive and respond appropriately to stimuli.
Observe behavioral responses; e.g., hostility, crying, inappropriate affect, agitation, hallucinations. (Refer to ND: disturbed Thought Processes, following.)	Individual responses may be variable, but commonalities, such as emotional lability, increased irritability/frustration, apathy, and impulsiveness, exist during recovery from brain injury. Documentation of behavior provides information needed for development of structured rehabilitation.
Document specific changes in abilities; e.g., focusing/tracking with both eyes, following simple verbal instructions, answering "yes" or "no" to questions, feeding self with dominant hand.	Helps localize areas of cerebral dysfunction, and identifies signs of progress toward improved neurologic function.
Eliminate extraneous noise/stimuli as necessary.	Reduces anxiety, exaggerated emotional responses/confusion associated with sensory overload.
Speak in calm, quiet voice. Use short, simple sentences. Maintain eye contact.	Client may have limited attention span/understanding during acute and recovery stages, and these measures can help client attend to communication.
Ascertain/validate client's perceptions, provide feedback. Reorient client frequently to environment, staff, and procedures, especially if vision is impaired.	Assists client to differentiate reality in the presence of altered perceptions. Cognitive dysfunction and/or visual deficits potentiate disorientation and anxiety.
Provide meaningful stimulation: verbal (talk to client), olfactory (e.g., oil of clove, coffee), tactile (touch, hand holding), and auditory (tapes, television, radio, visitors). Avoid physical or emotional isolation of client.	Carefully selected sensory input may be useful for coma stimulation as well as for documenting progress during cognitive retraining.
Provide structured therapies, activities, and environment. Provide written schedule for client to refer to on a regular basis.	Promotes consistency and reassurance, reducing anxiety associated with the unknown. Promotes sense of control/cognitive retraining.

ACTIONS/INTERVENTIONS	RATIONALE
Schedule adequate rest/uninterrupted sleep periods.	Reduces fatigue, prevents exhaustion, and improves sleep. *Note:* Absence of rapid eye movement (REM) sleep is known to aggravate sensory perception deficits.
Use day/night lighting.	Provides for normal sense of passage of time and sleep/wake pattern.
Allow adequate time for communication and performance of activities.	Reduces frustration associated with altered abilities/delayed response pattern.
Provide client safety; e.g., padded side rails, assistance with ambulation, protection from hot/sharp objects. Document perceptual deficit and compensatory activities on chart and at bedside.	Agitation, impaired judgment, poor balance, and sensory deficits increase risk of client injury.
Identify alternative ways of dealing with perceptual deficits; e.g., arrange bed, personal articles, food to take advantage of functional vision; describe where affected body parts are located.	Enables client to progress toward independence, enhancing sense of control, while compensating for neurologic deficits.

Collaborative

Refer to physical, occupational, speech, and cognitive therapists.	Interdisciplinary approach can create an integrated treatment plan based on the individual's unique combination of abilities/disabilities with focus on evaluation and functional improvement in physical, cognitive, and perceptual skills.

NURSING DIAGNOSIS: disturbed Thought Processes

May be related to

Physiologic changes, psychologic conflicts

Possibly evidenced by

Memory deficit/changes in remote, recent, immediate memory
Distractibility, altered attention span/concentration
Disorientation to time, place, person, circumstances, and events
Impaired ability to make decisions, problem solve, reason, abstract, or conceptualize
Personality changes; inappropriate social behavior

DESIRED OUTCOMES/EVALUATION CRITERIA—CLIENT WILL:

Distorted Thought Self-Control (NOC)

Maintain/regain usual mentation and reality orientation.
Recognize changes in thinking/behavior.
Participate in therapeutic regimen/cognitive retraining.

ACTIONS/INTERVENTIONS — RATIONALE

Cognitive Stimulation (NIC)

Independent

ACTIONS/INTERVENTIONS	RATIONALE
Assess attention span, distractibility. Note level of anxiety.	Attention span/ability to attend/concentrate may be severely shortened, which both causes and potentiates anxiety, affecting thought processes.

ACTIONS/INTERVENTIONS	RATIONALE
Confer with SO to compare past behaviors/preinjury personality with current responses.	Recovery from head injury includes a phase of agitation, angry responses, and disordered thought sequences/conversation. Hallucinations or altered interpretation of stimuli may have been present before the head injury or be part of developing sequelae of brain injury. *Note:* SOs often have difficulty accepting and dealing with client's aberrant behavior and may require assistance in coping with situation.
Maintain consistency in staff assigned to client to the extent possible.	Provides client with feelings of stability, familiarity, and control of situation.
Present reality concisely and briefly; avoid challenging illogical thinking.	Client may be totally unaware of injury (amnesic) or of extent of injury and therefore deny reality of injury. Structured reality orientation can reduce defensive reactions.
Provide information about injury process in relationship to symptoms. Explain procedures and reinforce explanations given by others.	Loss of internal structure (changes in memory, reasoning, and ability to conceptualize) and fear of the unknown affect processing and retention of information and can compound anxiety, confusion, and disorientation.
Review necessity of recurrent neurologic evaluations.	Understanding that assessments are done frequently to prevent/limit complications, and do not necessarily reflect seriousness of client's condition, may help reduce anxiety.
Reduce provocative stimuli, negative criticism, arguments, and confrontations.	Reduces risk of triggering fight/flight response. Aggression, anger, and self-control are common problems in brain-injured clients, who may become violent or physically/verbally abusive.
Listen with regard to client's verbalizations in spite of speech pattern/content.	Conveys interest and worth to individual, enhancing self-esteem and encouraging continued efforts.
Promote socialization within individual limitations.	Reinforcement of positive behaviors (e.g., appropriate interaction with others) may be helpful in relearning internal structure.
Encourage SO to provide current news/family happenings.	Promotes maintenance of contact with usual events, enhancing reality orientation and normalization of thinking.
Instruct in relaxation techniques. Provide diversional activities.	Can help refocus attention and reduce anxiety to manageable levels.
Maintain realistic expectations of client's ability to control own behavior, comprehend, remember information.	It is important to maintain an expectation of the ability to improve and progress to a higher level of functioning, to maintain hope, and promote continued work of rehabilitation.
Avoid leaving client alone when agitated, frightened.	Anxiety can lead to loss of control and escalate to panic. Support may provide calming effect, reducing anxiety and risk of injury.
Implement measures to control emotional outbursts/aggressive behavior if needed; e.g., tell client to "stop," speak in a calm voice, remove client from the situation, provide distraction, restrain for brief periods of time.	Client may need help/external control to protect self or others from harm until internal control is regained. Restraints (physical holding, mechanical, pharmacologic) should be used judiciously to avoid escalating violent, irrational behavior.
Inform client/SO that intellectual function, behavior, and emotional functioning will gradually improve but that some effects may persist for months or even be permanent.	Most brain-injured clients have persistent problems with concentration, memory, and problem solving. If brain injury was moderate to severe, recovery may be complete or residual effects may remain.
Collaborative	
Refer for neuropsychologic evaluation as indicated.	Useful for determining therapeutic interventions for cognitive and neurobehavioral disturbances.

ACTIONS/INTERVENTIONS	RATIONALE
Coordinate participation in cognitive retraining or rehabilitation program as indicated.	Assists client with learning methods to compensate for disruption of cognitive skills. Addresses problems in concentration, memory, judgment, sequencing, and problem-solving. *Note:* New developments in technology and computer software allow for the creation of interactive sensory-motor virtual reality environments. This provides an opportunity for safe interaction between client and naturalistic environments for the purpose of practicing/establishing effective behavioral responses.
Refer to support groups; e.g., Brain Injury Association, social services, visiting nurse, and counseling/therapy as needed.	Additional long-term assistance may be helpful in supporting/sustaining recovery.

NURSING DIAGNOSIS: impaired physical Mobility

May be related to

Perceptual or cognitive impairment
Decreased strength/endurance
Restrictive therapies/safety precautions; e.g., bedrest, immobilization

Possibly evidenced by

Inability to purposefully move within the physical environment, including bed mobility, transfer, ambulation
Impaired coordination, limited range of motion, decreased muscle strength/control

DESIRED OUTCOMES/EVALUATION CRITERIA—CLIENT WILL:

IMMOBILITY CONSEQUENCES: Physiological (NOC)

Maintain/increase strength and function of affected and/or compensatory body part(s).
Regain/maintain optimal position of function, as evidenced by absence of contractures, footdrop.

Mobility (NOC)

Demonstrate techniques/behaviors that enable resumption of activities.
Maintain skin integrity, bladder and bowel function.

ACTIONS/INTERVENTIONS — RATIONALE

EXERCISE THERAPY: Muscle Control (NIC)

Independent

ACTIONS/INTERVENTIONS	RATIONALE
Review functional ability and reasons for impairment.	Identifies probable functional impairments and influences choice of interventions.
Assess degree of immobility, using a scale to rate dependence (0–4).	The client may be completely independent (0), may require minimal assistance/equipment (1), moderate assistance/supervision/teaching (2), extensive assistance/equipment and devices (3), or be completely dependent on caregivers (4). Persons in all categories are at risk for injury, but those in categories 2–4 are at greatest risk.
Provide/assist with ROM exercises.	Maintains mobility and function of joints/functional alignment of extremities and reduces venous stasis.

ACTIONS/INTERVENTIONS	RATIONALE
Instruct/assist client with exercise program and use of mobility aids. Increase activity and participation in self-care as tolerated.	Lengthy convalescence often follows brain injury, and physical reconditioning is an essential part of the program.

BedRest Care (NIC)

Position client to avoid skin/tissue pressure damage. Turn at regular intervals, and make small position changes between turns.	Regular turning more normally distributes body weight and promotes circulation to all areas. If paralysis or limited cognition is present, client should be repositioned frequently.
Provide meticulous skin care, massaging with emollients. Remove wet linen/clothing, keep bedding free of wrinkles.	Promotes circulation and skin elasticity and reduces risk of skin excoriation.
Maintain functional body alignment; e.g., hips, feet, hands. Monitor for proper placement of devices and/or signs of pressure from devices.	Use of high-top tennis shoes, "space boots," and T-bar sheepskin devices can help prevent footdrop. Hand splints are variable and designed to prevent hand deformities and promote optimal function. Use of pillows, bedrolls, and sandbags can help prevent abnormal hip rotation.
Support head and trunk, arms and shoulders, feet and legs when client is in wheelchair/recliner. Pad chair seat with foam or water-filled cushion, and assist client to shift weight at frequent intervals.	Maintains comfortable, safe, and functional posture, and prevents/reduces risk of skin breakdown.
Provide eye care, artificial tears; patch eyes as indicated.	Protects delicate eye tissues from drying. Client may require patches during sleep to protect eyes from trauma if unable to keep eyes closed.
Monitor urinary output. Note color and odor of urine. Assist with bladder retraining when appropriate.	Indwelling catheter used during the acute phase of injury may be needed for an extended period of time before bladder retraining is possible. Once the catheter is removed, several methods of continence control may be tried, e.g., intermittent catheterization (for residual and complete emptying), external catheter, planned intervals on commode, incontinence pads.
Provide fluids, including 8 oz cranberry juice, within individual tolerance (i.e., regarding neurologic and cardiac concerns) as indicated.	Once past the acute phase of head injury and if client has no other contraindicating factors, forcing fluids decreases risk of urinary tract infections/stone formation and provides other positive effects such as normal stool consistency and optimal skin turgor.
Monitor bowel elimination and provide for/assist with a regular bowel routine. Check for impacted stool; use digital stimulation as indicated. Sit client upright on commode or stool at regular intervals. Add fiber/bulk/fruit juice to diet as appropriate.	A regular bowel routine requires simple but diligent measures to prevent complications. Stimulation of the internal rectal sphincter stimulates the bowel to empty automatically if stool is soft enough to do so. Upright position aids evacuation.
Inspect for localized tenderness, redness, skin warmth, muscle tension, and/or ropy veins in calves of legs. Observe for sudden dyspnea, tachypnea, fever, respiratory distress, chest pain.	Client is at risk for development of deep vein thrombosis (DVT) and pulmonary embolus (PE), requiring prompt medical evaluation/intervention to prevent serious complications.

Collaborative

Provide air/water mattress, kinetic therapy as appropriate.	Equalizes tissue pressure, enhances circulation, and helps reduce venous stasis to decrease risk of tissue injury.
Apply/monitor use of sequential compression device to legs.	SCD may be used to reduce risk of deep vein thrombosis associated with bedrest/limited mobility.

EXERCISE THERAPY: Muscle Control (NIC)

Refer to physical/occupational therapists as indicated.	Useful in determining individual needs, therapeutic activities, and assistive devices.

NURSING DIAGNOSIS: risk for Infection

Risk factors may include

Traumatized tissues, broken skin, invasive procedures
Decreased ciliary action, stasis of body fluids
Nutritional deficits
Suppressed inflammatory response (steroid use)
Altered integrity of closed system (CSF leak)

Possibly evidenced by

[Not applicable; presence of signs and symptoms establishes an *actual* diagnosis.]

DESIRED OUTCOMES/EVALUATION CRITERIA—CLIENT WILL:

Immune Status (NOC)

Maintain normothermia, free of signs of infection.
Achieve timely wound healing when present.

ACTIONS/INTERVENTIONS	RATIONALE
Infection Protection (NIC)	
Independent	
Provide meticulous/aseptic care, maintain good handwashing techniques.	First-line defense against nosocomial infections.
Observe areas of impaired skin integrity (e.g., wounds, suture lines, invasive line insertion sites), noting drainage characteristics and presence of inflammation.	Early identification of developing infection permits prompt intervention and prevention of further complications.
Monitor temperature routinely. Note presence of chills, diaphoresis, changes in mentation.	May indicate developing sepsis requiring further evaluation/intervention.
Encourage deep breathing, aggressive pulmonary toilet. Observe sputum characteristics.	Enhances mobilization and clearing of pulmonary secretions to reduce risk of pneumonia, atelectasis. *Note:* Postural drainage should be used with caution if risk of increased ICP exists.
Provide perineal care. Maintain integrity of closed urinary drainage system if used. Encourage adequate fluid intake.	Reduces potential for bacterial growth/ascending infection.
Observe color/clarity of urine. Note presence of foul odor.	Indicators of developing urinary tract infection (UTI) requiring prompt intervention.
Screen/restrict access of visitors or caregivers with upper respiratory infections (URIs).	Reduces exposure of "compromised host."
Infection Control (NIC)	
Collaborative	
Obtain specimens as indicated.	Culture/sensitivity, Gram's stain may be done to verify presence of infection and identify causative organism and appropriate treatment choices.

NURSING DIAGNOSIS: risk for imbalanced Nutrition: less than body requirements

Risk factors may include

Altered ability to ingest nutrients (decreased level of consciousness)
Weakness of muscles required for chewing, swallowing
Hypermetabolic state

Possibly evidenced by

[Not applicable; presence of signs and symptoms establishes an *actual* diagnosis.]

DESIRED OUTCOMES/EVALUATION CRITERIA—CLIENT WILL:

Nutritional Status (NOC)

Demonstrate maintenance of desired weight/progressive weight gain toward goal.
Experience no signs of malnutrition, with laboratory values within normal range.

ACTIONS/INTERVENTIONS	RATIONALE
Nutrition Therapy (NIC)	
Independent	
Assess ability to chew, swallow, cough, handle secretions.	These factors determine choice of feeding options because client must be protected from aspiration.
Auscultate bowel sounds, noting decreased/absent or hyperactive sounds.	GI functioning is usually preserved in brain-injured clients, so bowel sounds help in determining response to feeding or development of complications; e.g., ileus.
Weigh as indicated.	Evaluates effectiveness or need for changes in nutritional therapy.
Provide for feeding safety; e.g., elevate head of bed while eating or during tube feeding.	Reduces risk of regurgitation and/or aspiration.
Divide feedings into small amounts and give frequently.	Enhances digestion and client's tolerance of nutrients and can improve client cooperation in eating.
Promote pleasant, relaxing environment, including socialization during meals. Encourage SO to bring in food that client enjoys.	Although the recovering client may require assistance with feeding and/or use of assistive devices, mealtime socialization with SO or friends can improve intake and normalize the life function of eating.
Check stools, gastric aspirant, vomitus for blood.	Acute/subacute bleeding may occur (Cushing's ulcer), requiring intervention and alternative method of providing nutrition.
Collaborative	
Consult with dietitian/nutritional support team.	Effective resource for identifying caloric/nutrient needs, depending on age, body size, desired weight, concurrent conditions (trauma, cardiac/metabolic problems).
Monitor laboratory studies; e.g., prealbumin/albumin, transferrin, amino acid profile, iron, BUN, nitrogen balance studies, glucose, AST/ALT, electrolytes.	Identifies nutritional deficiencies, organ function, and response to nutritional therapy.
Administer feedings by appropriate means; e.g., IV/tube feeding, oral feedings with soft foods and thick liquids (Refer to CP: Total Nutritional Support: Parenteral/Enteral Feeding.)	Choice of route depends on client needs/capabilities. Tube feedings (nasogastric, jejunostomy) may be required initially, or parenteral route may be indicated in presence of gastric/intestinal pathology. If client is able to swallow, soft foods or semiliquid foods may be more easily managed without aspiration.

ACTIONS/INTERVENTIONS	RATIONALE
Involve speech/occupational/physical therapists when mechanical problem exists; e.g., impaired swallow reflexes, wired jaws, contractures of hands, paralysis.	Individual strategies/devices may be needed to improve ability to eat.

NURSING DIAGNOSIS: interrupted Family Processes

May be related to

Situational transition and crisis
Uncertainty about outcomes/expectations

Possibly evidenced by

Difficulty adapting to change or dealing with traumatic experience constructively
Family not meeting needs of its members
Difficulty accepting or receiving help appropriately
Inability to express or to accept feelings of members

DESIRED OUTCOMES/EVALUATION CRITERIA—FAMILY WILL:

Family Coping (NOC)

Begin to express feelings freely and appropriately.
Identify internal and external resources to deal with the situation.
Direct energies in a purposeful manner to plan for resolution of crisis.
Encourage and allow injured member to progress toward independence.

ACTIONS/INTERVENTIONS	RATIONALE
Family Integrity Promotion (NIC)	
Independent	
Note components of family unit, availability/involvement of support systems.	Defines family resources and identifies areas of need.
Encourage expression of concerns about seriousness of condition, possibility of death, or incapacitation.	Verbalization of fears gets concerns out in the open and can decrease anxiety and enhance coping with reality.
Listen for expressions of helplessness/hopelessness.	Joy of survival of victim is replaced by grief/anger at "loss" and necessity of dealing with "new person that family does not know and may not even like." Prolongation of these feelings may result in depression.
Encourage expression of/acknowledge feelings. Do not deny or reassure client/SO that everything will be all right.	Because it is not possible to predict the outcome, it is more helpful to assist the person to deal with feelings about what is happening instead of giving false reassurance.
Support family grieving for "loss" of member. Acknowledge normality of wide range of feelings and ongoing nature of process.	Although grief may never be fully resolved and family may vacillate among various stages, understanding that this is typical may help members accept/cope with the situation.
Stress importance of continuous open dialogue between family members.	Provides opportunity to get feelings out in the open. Recognition and awareness promotes resolution of guilt, anger.
Help family recognize needs of all members.	Attention may be so focused on injured member that other members feel isolated/abandoned, which can compromise family growth and unity.

ACTIONS/INTERVENTIONS	RATIONALE
Family Mobilization (NIC)	
Evaluate/discuss family goals and expectations.	Family may believe that if client is going to live, rehabilitation will bring about a cure. Despite accurate information, expectations may be unrealistic. Also, client's early recovery may be rapid, then plateau, resulting in disappointment/frustration.
Reinforce previous explanations about extent of injury, treatment plan, and prognosis. Provide accurate information at current level of understanding/ability to accept.	Client/SO are unable to absorb/recall all information, and blocking can occur because of emotional trauma. As time goes by, reinforcement of information can help reduce misconceptions, fear about the unknown/future expectations.
Identify individual roles and anticipated/perceived changes.	Responsibilities/roles may have to be partially or completely assumed by others, which can further complicate family coping.
Assess energy direction; e.g., whether efforts at resolution/problem solving are purposeful or scattered.	May need assistance to focus energies in an effective way/enhance coping.
Identify and encourage use of previously successful coping behaviors.	Focuses on strengths and reaffirms individual's ability to deal with current crisis.
Demonstrate and encourage use of stress management skills; e.g., relaxation techniques, breathing exercises, visualization.	Helps redirect attention toward revitalizing self to enhance coping ability.

Collaborative

Include family in rehabilitation team meetings and care planning/placement decisions.	Facilitates communication, enables family to be an integral part of the rehabilitation, and provides sense of control.
Identify community resources; e.g., visiting nurse, homemaker service, day care/respite facility, legal/financial counselor.	Provides assistance with problems that may arise because of altered role function. Also, as family structure changes over time and client's needs increase with age, additional resources/support are often required.
Refer to family therapy, support groups.	Cognitive/personality changes are usually very difficult for family to deal with. Decreased impulse control, emotional lability, inappropriate sexual or aggressive/violent behavior can disrupt family and result in abandonment/divorce. Trained therapists and peer role models may assist family to deal with feelings/reality of situation and provide support for decisions that are made.

NURSING DIAGNOSIS: deficient Knowledge [Learning Need] regarding condition, prognosis, potential complications, treatment, self-care, and discharge needs

May be related to

Lack of exposure, unfamiliarity with information/resources
Lack of recall/cognitive limitation

Possibly evidenced by

Request for information, statement of misconception
Inaccurate follow-through of instructions

DESIRED OUTCOMES/EVALUATION CRITERIA—CLIENT/SO WILL:

KNOWLEDGE: Disease Process (NOC)

Participate in learning process.
Verbalize understanding of condition, prognosis, potential complications.

KNOWLEDGE: Treatment Regimen (NOC)

Verbalize understanding of therapeutic regimen and rationale for actions.
Initiate necessary lifestyle changes and/or involvement in rehabilitation program.
Correctly perform necessary procedures.

ACTIONS/INTERVENTIONS	RATIONALE
TEACHING: Disease Process (NIC)	
Independent	
Evaluate capabilities and readiness to learn of both client and SO.	Permits presentation of material based on individual needs. *Note:* Client may not be emotionally/mentally capable of assimilating information.
Review information regarding injury process and aftereffects.	Aids in establishing realistic expectations and promotes understanding of current situation and needs.
Review/reinforce current therapeutic regimen. Identify ways of continuing program after discharge.	Recommended activities, limitations, medication/therapy needs have been established on the basis of a coordinated interdisciplinary approach, and follow-through is essential to progression of recovery/prevention of complications.
Discuss plans for meeting self-care needs.	Varying levels of assistance may be required/need to be planned based on individual situation.
Provide written instructions and schedules for activity, medication, important facts.	Provides visual reinforcement and reference source after discharge.
Identify signs/symptoms of individual risks; e.g., delayed CSF leak, posttraumatic seizures, headache/chronic pain.	Recognizing developing problems provides opportunity for prompt evaluation and intervention to prevent serious complications.
Discuss with client/SO development of symptoms, such as reexperiencing traumatic event (flashbacks, intrusive thoughts, repetitive dreams/nightmares); psychic/emotional numbness; changes in lifestyle, including adoption of self-destructive behaviors.	May indicate occurrence/exacerbation of posttrauma response, which can occur months to years after injury, requiring further evaluation and supportive interventions.
Identify community resources; e.g., head injury support groups, social services, rehabilitation facilities, outpatient programs, home care/visiting nurse.	May be needed to provide assistance with physical care, home management, adjustment to lifestyle changes, and emotional and financial concerns. *Note:* Studies suggest an increased risk of developing Alzheimer's disease and the possibility of acceleration of the aging process in brain injury survivors. SO/families will require continued support to meet these challenges.
Refer/reinforce importance of follow-up care by rehabilitation team; e.g., physical/occupational/speech/vocational therapists, cognitive retrainers.	With diligent work (often for several years with these providers), the client may eventually overcome residual neurologic deficits and/or be able to resume desired/productive lifestyle.

POTENTIAL CONSIDERATIONS following acute hospitalization (dependent on client's age, physical condition/presence of complications, personal resources, and life responsibilities)

impaired Memory—neurologic disturbances, anemia, fluid/electrolyte imbalances.

ineffective Health Maintenance/impaired Home Maintenance—significant alteration in communication skills, lack of ability to make deliberate/thoughtful judgments, perceptual/cognitive impairments, insufficient finances, unfamiliarity with neighborhood resources, inadequate support systems.

acute/chronic Pain—tissue injury/neuronal damage, stress/anxiety.

chronic Confusion—head injury.

CEREBROVASCULAR ACCIDENT (CVA)/STROKE

Cerebrovascular disease refers to any functional or structural abnormality of the brain caused by a pathologic condition of the cerebral vessels or of the entire cerebrovascular system. This pathology either (1) causes hemorrhage as a result of a vessel wall rupture and bleeding into the brain or (2) impairs the cerebral circulation by a partial or complete occlusion of the vessel lumen with transient or permanent effects. Each year, over 700,000 Americans are affected by a new or recurrent stroke. In addition, CVA is the third leading cause of death after heart disease and cancer and is the leading cause of disability cost to the nation (direct and indirect cost is approximately $53.6 billion/year [Harvey, 2004]).

Ischemia (as a result of thrombosis or embolism) and hemorrhage are the primary causes for CVA, with thrombosis being the main cause of both CVAs and transient ischemic attacks (TIAs). The most common vessels involved are the carotid arteries and those of the vertebrobasilar system at the base of the brain. A thrombotic CVA causes a slow evolution of symptoms, usually over several hours, and is "completed" when the condition stabilizes. An embolic CVA occurs when a clot is carried into cerebral circulation and causes a localized cerebral infarct. Hemorrhagic CVA is caused by other conditions such as a ruptured aneurysm, hypertension, arteriovenous (AV) malformations, or a bleeding disorder. Symptoms depend on distribution of the cerebral vessel(s) involved. Ischemia may (1) be transient and resolve within 24 hours, (2) be reversible with resolution of symptoms over a period of 1 week (reversible ischemic neurologic deficit [RIND]), or (3) progress to cerebral infarction with variable effects and degrees of recovery.

CARE SETTING

Although the client may initially be cared for in the intensive care unit (ICU) for severe/evolving deficits, this plan of care focuses on the step-down or medical unit and subacute/rehabilitation units to the community level.

RELATED CONCERNS

Hypertension: severe, page 35
Craniocerebral trauma (acute rehabilitative phase), page 218
Psychosocial aspects of care, page 770
Seizure disorders, page 208
Total nutritional support: parenteral/enteral feeding, page 478

Client Assessment Database

Collected data are determined by location, severity, and duration of pathology.

ACTIVITY/REST

May report: Difficulties with activity due to weakness, loss of sensation, or paralysis (hemiplegia); tires easily; difficulty resting (pain or muscle twitching)

May exhibit: Altered muscle tone (flaccid or spastic), paralysis (hemiplegia), generalized weakness
Visual disturbances
Altered level of consciousness

CIRCULATORY

May report: History of postural hypotension, cardiac disease (e.g., myocardial infarction [MI], rheumatic/valvular heart disease, HF, bacterial endocarditis), polycythemia

May exhibit: Arterial hypertension (common unless CVA is due to embolism or vascular malformation)
Pulse rate may vary (preexisting heart conditions, medications, effect of stroke on vasomotor center)
Dysrhythmias, electrocardiographic (ECG) changes
Bruit in carotid, femoral, or iliac arteries or abdominal aorta

EGO INTEGRITY

May report: Feelings of helplessness, hopelessness

May exhibit: Emotional lability and inappropriate response to anger, sadness, happiness
Difficulty expressing self

ELIMINATION

May exhibit: Change in voiding patterns; e.g., incontinence, anuria
Distended abdomen (overdistended bladder), absent bowel sounds (paralytic ileus)

FOOD/FLUID

May report: Lack of appetite
Nausea/vomiting during acute event (increased ICP)

Loss of sensation in tongue, cheek, and throat; dysphagia
History of diabetes, elevated serum lipids

May exhibit: Mastication/swallowing problems (palatal and pharyngeal reflex involvement)
Obesity (risk factor)

NEUROSENSORY

May report: Dizziness/syncope (before CVA/transient during TIA)
Severe headache (intracerebral or subarachnoid hemorrhage)
Tingling/numbness/weakness (commonly reported during TIAs, found in varying degrees in other types of stroke); involved side seems "dead"
Visual deficits; e.g., blurred vision, partial loss of vision (monocular blindness), double vision (diplopia), or other disturbances in visual fields
Touch: Sensory loss on contralateral side (opposite side) in extremities and sometimes in ipsilateral side (same side) of face
Disturbance in senses of taste, smell
History of TIA, RIND (predisposing factor for subsequent infarction)

May exhibit: Mental status/LOC: Coma usually presents in the initial stages of hemorrhagic disturbances; consciousness is usually preserved when the etiology is thrombotic in nature; altered behavior (e.g., lethargy, apathy, combativeness); altered cognitive function (e.g., memory, problem solving, sequencing)
Extremities: Weakness/paralysis (contralateral with all kinds of stroke), unequal hand grasp; diminished deep tendon reflexes (contralateral)
Facial paralysis or paresis (ipsilateral)
Aphasia: Defect or loss of language function may be expressive (difficulty producing speech), receptive (difficulty comprehending speech), or global (combination of the two)
Loss of ability to recognize or appreciate import of visual, auditory, tactile stimuli (agnosia); e.g., altered body image awareness, neglect or denial of contralateral side of body, disturbances in perception
Loss of ability to execute purposeful motor acts despite physical ability and willingness to do so (apraxis)
Pupil size/reaction: Inequality; dilated and fixed pupil on the ipsilateral side (hemorrhage/herniation)
Nuchal rigidity (common in hemorrhagic etiology), seizures (common in hemorrhagic etiology)

PAIN/DISCOMFORT

May report: Headache of varying intensity (carotid artery involvement)
May exhibit: Guarding/distraction behaviors, restlessness, muscle/facial tension

RESPIRATION

May report: Smoking (risk factor)
May exhibit: Inability to swallow/cough/protect airway
Labored and/or irregular respirations
Noisy respirations/rhonchi (aspiration of secretions)

SAFETY

May exhibit: Motor/sensory: Problems with vision
Changes in perception of body spatial orientation (right CVA) neglect
Difficulty seeing objects on left side (right CVA)
Being unaware of affected side
Inability to recognize familiar objects, colors, words, faces
Diminished response to heat and cold/altered body temperature regulation
Swallowing difficulty, inability to meet own nutritional needs
Impaired judgment, little concern for safety, impatience, lack of insight (right CVA)

SOCIAL INTERACTION

May exhibit: Speech problems, inability to communicate, inappropriate behavior

TEACHING/LEARNING

May report: Family history of hypertension, strokes; African heritage (risk factor)
Use of oral contraceptives, alcohol abuse (risk factors)

Discharge plan considerations:

May require medication regimen/therapeutic treatments

Assistance with transportation, shopping, food preparation, self-care, and homemaker/maintenance tasks

Changes in physical layout of home; transition placement before return to home setting

Refer to section at end of plan for postdischarge considerations.

DIAGNOSTIC STUDIES

CT scan (with/without enhancement): Demonstrates structural abnormalities, edema, hematomas, ischemia, and infarctions. *Note:* May not immediately reveal all changes; e.g., ischemic infarcts are not evident on CT for 8–12 hr. However, intracerebral hemorrhage is immediately apparent; therefore, emergency CT is always done before administering tissue plasminogen activator (t-PA). In addition, clients with TIA commonly have a normal CT scan.

MRI: Can show evidence of stroke within minutes of occurrence, and is especially beneficial for assessing smaller strokes deep within the brain.

PET scan: Provides data on cerebral metabolism and blood flow changes, especially in ischemic stroke.

Cerebral angiography: Helps determine specific cause of stroke; e.g., hemorrhage or obstructed artery, pinpoints site of occlusion or rupture. Digital subtraction angiography evaluates patency of cerebral vessels, identifies their position in head and neck, and detects/evaluates lesions and vascular abnormalities.

Lumbar puncture (LP): Pressure is usually normal and CSF is clear in cerebral thrombosis, embolism, and TIA. Pressure elevation and grossly bloody fluid suggest subarachnoid and intracerebral hemorrhage. CSF total protein level may be elevated in cases of thrombosis because of inflammatory process. LP should be performed if septic embolism from bacterial endocarditis is suspected.

Transcranial Doppler ultrasonography: Evaluates the velocity of blood flow through major intracranial vessels, and identifies AV disease; e.g., problems with carotid system (blood flow/presence of atherosclerotic plaques).

EEG: Identifies problems based on reduced electrical activity in specific areas of infarction; and can differentiate seizure activity from CVA damage.

X-rays (skull): May show shift of pineal gland to the opposite side from an expanding mass; calcifications of the internal carotid may be visible in cerebral thrombosis; partial calcification of walls of an aneurysm may be noted in subarachnoid hemorrhage.

Laboratory studies to rule out systemic causes: CBC, platelet and clotting studies, VDRL/RPR, erythrocyte sedimentation rate (ESR); metabolic panel (e.g. renalytes, glucose).

ECG, chest x-ray, and echocardiography: To rule out cardiac origin as source of embolus (20% of strokes are the result of blood or vegetative emboli associated with valvular disease, dysrhythmias, or endocarditis).

NURSING PRIORITIES

1. Promote adequate cerebral perfusion and oxygenation.
2. Prevent/minimize complications and permanent disabilities.
3. Assist client to gain independence in ADLs.
4. Support coping process and integration of changes into self-concept.
5. Provide information about disease process/prognosis and treatment/rehabilitation needs.

DISCHARGE GOALS

1. Cerebral function improved, neurologic deficits resolving/stabilized.
2. Complications prevented or minimized.
3. ADL needs met by self or with assistance of other(s).
4. Coping with situation in positive manner, planning for the future.
5. Disease process/prognosis and therapeutic regimen understood.
6. Plan in place to meet needs after discharge.

NURSING DIAGNOSIS: ineffective cerebral Tissue Perfusion

May be related to

Interruption of blood flow: occlusive disorder, hemorrhage; cerebral vasospasm, cerebral edema

Possibly evidenced by

Altered level of consciousness; memory loss

Changes in motor/sensory responses; restlessness

Sensory, language, intellectual, and emotional deficits
Changes in vital signs

DESIRED OUTCOMES/EVALUATION CRITERIA—CLIENT WILL:

Neurologic Status (NOC)

Maintain usual/improved level of consciousness, cognition, and motor/sensory function.
Demonstrate stable vital signs and absence of signs of increased ICP.
Display no further deterioration/recurrence of deficits

ACTIONS/INTERVENTIONS	RATIONALE
Cerebral Perfusion Promotion (NIC)	
Independent	
Determine factors related to individual situation/cause for coma/decreased cerebral perfusion and potential for increased ICP.	Influences choice of interventions. Deterioration in neurologic signs/symptoms or failure to improve after initial insult may reflect decreased intracranial adaptive capacity requiring client to be transferred to critical care area for monitoring of ICP, other therapies. If the stroke is evolving, client can deteriorate quickly and require repeated assessment and progressive treatment. If the stroke is "completed," the neurologic deficit is nonprogressive, and treatment is geared toward rehabilitation and preventing recurrence.
Monitor/document neurologic status frequently and compare with baseline. (Refer to CP: Craniocerebral Trauma [Acute Rehabilitative Phase], ND: ineffective cerebral Tissue Perfusion for complete neurologic evaluation.)	Assesses trends in level of consciousness (LOC) and potential for increased ICP and is useful in determining location, extent, and progression/resolution of CNS damage. May also reveal presence of TIA, which may warn of impending thrombotic CVA.
Monitor vital signs; that is, note:	
Hypertension/hypotension, compare BP readings in both arms;	Fluctuations in pressure may occur because of cerebral pressure/injury in vasomotor area of the brain. Hypertension or postural hypotension may have been a precipitating factor. Hypotension may occur because of shock (circulatory collapse). Increased ICP may occur because of tissue edema or clot formation. Subclavian artery blockage may be revealed by difference in pressure readings between arms.
Heart rate and rhythm; auscultate for murmurs;	Changes in rate, especially bradycardia, can occur because of the brain damage. Dysrhythmias and murmurs may reflect cardiac disease, which may have precipitated CVA (e.g., stroke after MI or from valve dysfunction).
Respirations, noting patterns and rhythm; e.g., periods of apnea after hyperventilation, Cheyne-Stokes respiration.	Irregularities can suggest location of cerebral insult/increasing ICP and need for further intervention, including possible respiratory support. (Refer to CP: Craniocerebral Trauma [Acute Rehabilitative Phase], ND: risk for ineffective Breathing Pattern.)
Evaluate pupils, noting size, shape, equality, light reactivity.	Pupil reactions are regulated by the oculomotor (III) cranial nerve and are useful in determining whether the brainstem is intact. Pupil size/equality is determined by balance between parasympathetic and sympathetic enervation. Response to light reflects combined function of the optic (II) and oculomotor (III) cranial nerves.

ACTIONS/INTERVENTIONS	RATIONALE
Document changes in vision; e.g., reports of blurred vision, alterations in visual field/depth perception.	Specific visual alterations reflect area of brain involved, indicate safety concerns, and influence choice of interventions.
Assess higher functions, including speech, if client is alert. (Refer to ND: impaired verbal [and/or written] Communication.)	Changes in cognition and speech content are an indicator of location/degree of cerebral involvement and may indicate deterioration/increased ICP.
Position with head slightly elevated and in neutral position.	Reduces arterial pressure by promoting venous drainage and may improve cerebral circulation/perfusion.
Maintain bedrest, provide quiet environment, restrict visitors/activities as indicated. Provide rest periods between care activities, limit duration of procedures.	Continual stimulation/activity can increase ICP. Absolute rest and quiet may be needed to prevent rebleeding in the case of hemorrhage.
Prevent straining at stool or holding breath.	Valsalva maneuver increases ICP and potentiates risk of rebleeding.
Assess for nuchal rigidity, twitching, increased restlessness, irritability, onset of seizure activity.	Indicative of meningeal irritation, especially in hemorrhagic disorders. Seizures may reflect increased ICP/cerebral injury, requiring further evaluation and intervention.

Collaborative

ACTIONS/INTERVENTIONS	RATIONALE
Administer supplemental oxygen as indicated.	Reduces hypoxemia, which can cause cerebral vasodilation and increase pressure/edema formation.
Administer medications as indicated:	
Intravenous thrombolytics; e.g., tissue plasminogen activator (tPA), alteplase (Activase), recombinant prourokinase (Prourokinase);	As the only proven therapy for acute stroke, t-PA is useful in minimizing the size of the infarcted area by opening blocked vessels that are occluded with clot. Treatment must be started within 3 hr of initial symptoms to improve outcomes. *Note:* These agents are contraindicated in several instances (e.g., intracranial hemorrhage as diagnosed by CT scan., recent intracranial surgery, serious head trauma, uncontrolled hypertension).
Anticoagulants; e.g., warfarin sodium (Coumadin), low-molecular-weight heparin (e.g., enoxaparin [Lovenox], dalteparin [Fragmin]), direct thrombin inhibitor (e.g. ximelagatran [Exanta]);	May be used to improve cerebral blood flow and prevent further clotting when embolus/thrombosis is the problem.
Antiplatelet agents; e.g., aspirin (ASA), ticlopidine (Ticlid), clopidogrel (Plavix);	May be used to prevent further clotting/reduce risk of recurrence of stroke.
Antihypertensives;	Preexisting/chronic hypertension requires cautious treatment because aggressive management increases the risk of extension of tissue damage. Transient hypertension often occurs during acute stroke and resolves often without therapeutic intervention.
Peripheral vasodilators; e.g., cyclandelate (Cyclospasmol), papaverine (Pavabid), isoxsuprine (Vasodilan);	Used to improve collateral circulation or decrease vasospasm.
Neuroprotective agents; e.g., calcium channel blockers, excitatory amino acid inhibitors, gangliosides;	These agents are being researched as a means to protect the brain by interrupting the destructive cascade of biochemical events (e.g., influx of calcium into cells, release of excitatory neurotransmitters, buildup of lactic acid) to limit ischemic injury.
Phenytoin (Dilantin), phenobarbital.	May be used to control seizures and/or for sedative action. *Note:* Phenobarbital enhances action of antiepileptics.
Prepare for surgery as appropriate; e.g., carotid endarterectomy, microvascular bypass, cerebral angioplasty.	May be necessary to resolve situation, reduce neurologic symptoms/risk of recurrent stroke.
Monitor laboratory studies as indicated; e.g., prothrombin time (PT)/activated partial thromboplastin time (aPTT), Dilantin level.	Provides information about drug effectiveness/therapeutic level.

NURSING DIAGNOSIS: impaired physical Mobility

May be related to

Neuromuscular involvement: weakness, paresthesia; flaccid/hypotonic paralysis (initially); spastic paralysis
Perceptual/cognitive impairment

Possibly evidenced by

Inability to purposefully move within the physical environment, impaired coordination, limited ROM, decreased muscle strength/control

DESIRED OUTCOMES/EVALUATION CRITERIA—CLIENT WILL:

IMMOBILITY CONSEQUENCES: Physiologic (NOC)

Maintain/increase strength and function of affected or compensatory body part.
Maintain optimal position of function as evidenced by absence of contractures, footdrop.
Demonstrate techniques/behaviors that enable resumption of activities.
Maintain skin integrity.

ACTIONS/INTERVENTIONS	RATIONALE
Positioning (NIC)	
Independent	
Assess functional ability/extent of impairment initially and on a regular basis. Classify according to 0–4 scale. (Refer to CP: Craniocerebral Trauma [Acute Rehabilitative Phase], ND: impaired physical Mobility.)	Identifies strengths/deficiencies and may provide information regarding recovery. Assists in choice of interventions because different techniques are used for flaccid and spastic types of paralysis.
Change positions at least every 2 hr (supine, side lying) and possibly more often if placed on affected side.	Reduces risk of tissue ischemia/injury. Affected side has poorer circulation and reduced sensation and is more predisposed to skin breakdown/decubitus ulcer.
Position in prone position once or twice a day if client can tolerate.	Helps maintain functional hip extension; however, may increase anxiety, especially about ability to breathe.
Prop extremities in functional position; use footboard during the period of flaccid paralysis. Maintain neutral position of head.	Prevents contractures/footdrop and facilitates use when/if function returns. Flaccid paralysis may interfere with ability to support head, whereas spastic paralysis may lead to deviation of head to one side.
Use arm sling when client is in upright position as indicated.	During flaccid paralysis, use of sling may reduce risk of shoulder subluxation and shoulder-hand syndrome.
Evaluate use of/need for positional aids and/or splints during spastic paralysis:	Flexion contractures occur because flexor muscles are stronger than extensors.
Place pillow under axilla to abduct arm;	Prevents adduction of shoulder and flexion of elbow.
Elevate arm and hand;	Promotes venous return and helps prevent edema formation.
Place hard hand-rolls in the palm with fingers and thumb opposed;	Hard cones decrease the stimulation of finger flexion, maintaining finger and thumb in a functional position.
Place knee and hip in extended position;	Maintains functional position.
Maintain leg in neutral position with a trochanter roll;	Prevents external hip rotation.
Discontinue use of footboard, when appropriate.	Continued use (after change from flaccid to spastic paralysis) can cause excessive pressure on the ball of the foot, enhance spasticity, and actually increase plantar flexion.

ACTIONS/INTERVENTIONS	RATIONALE
Observe affected side for color, edema, or other signs of compromised circulation.	Edematous tissue is more easily traumatized and heals more slowly.
Inspect skin regularly, particularly over bony prominences. Gently massage any reddened areas and provide aids such as sheepskin pads as necessary.	Pressure points over bony prominences are most at risk for decreased perfusion/ischemia. Circulatory stimulation and padding help prevent skin breakdown and decubitus ulcer development.

EXERCISE THERAPY: Muscle Control (NIC)

Begin active/passive ROM to all extremities (including splinted) on admission. Encourage exercises such as quadriceps/gluteal exercise, squeezing rubber ball, extension of fingers and legs/feet.	Minimizes muscle atrophy, promotes circulation, and helps prevent contractures. Reduces risk of hypercalciuria and osteoporosis if underlying problem is hemorrhage. *Note:* Excessive/imprudent stimulation can predispose to rebleeding.
Assist to develop sitting balance (e.g., raise head of bed; assist to sit on edge of bed, having client use the strong arm to support body weight and strong leg to move affected leg; increase sitting time) and standing balance (e.g., put flat walking shoes on client, support client's lower back with hands while positioning own knees outside client's knees, assist in using parallel bars/walker).	Aids in retraining neuronal pathways, enhancing proprioception and motor response.
Get client up in chair as soon as vital signs are stable except following cerebral hemorrhage.	Helps stabilize BP (restores vasomotor tone), promotes maintenance of extremities in a functional position and emptying of bladder/kidneys, reducing risk of urinary stones and infections from stasis. *Note:* If stroke is not completed, activity increases risk of additional bleed/infarction.
Pad chair seat with foam or water-filled cushion, and assist client to shift weight at frequent intervals.	Prevents/reduces pressure on the coccyx/skin breakdown.
Set goals with client/SO for increasing participation in activities/exercise and position changes.	Promotes sense of expectation of progress/improvement, and provides some sense of control/independence.
Encourage client to assist with movement and exercises using unaffected extremity to support/move weaker side.	May respond as if affected side is no longer part of body and needs encouragement and active training to "reincorporate" it as a part of own body.

Positioning (NIC)

Collaborative

Provide egg-crate mattress, water bed, flotation device, or specialized bed (e.g., kinetic) as indicated.	Promotes even weight distribution, decreasing pressure on bony points and helping to prevent skin breakdown/decubitus ulcer formation. Specialized beds help with positioning, enhance circulation, and reduce venous stasis to decrease risk of tissue injury and complications such as orthostatic pneumonia.

EXERCISE THERAPY: Muscle Control (NIC)

Consult with physical therapist regarding active, resistive exercises and client ambulation.	Individualized program can be developed to meet particular needs/deal with deficits in balance, coordination, strength.
Assist with electrical stimulation, e.g., transcutaneous electrical nerve stimulator (TENS) unit, as indicated.	May assist with muscle strengthening and increase voluntary muscle control, as well as pain control.
Administer muscle relaxants, antispasmodics as indicated; e.g., baclofen (Lioresal), dantrolene (Dantrium).	May be required to relieve spasticity in affected extremities.

NURSING DIAGNOSIS: impaired verbal [and/or written] Communication

May be related to

Impaired cerebral circulation; neuromuscular impairment, loss of facial/oral muscle tone/control; generalized weakness/fatigue

Possibly evidenced by

Impaired articulation; soft speech or does not/cannot speak (dysarthria)
Inability to modulate speech, find and name words, identify objects; inability to comprehend written/spoken language, global aphasia
Inability to produce written communication, expressive aphasia

DESIRED OUTCOMES/EVALUATION CRITERIA—CLIENT WILL:

Communication (NOC)

Indicate an understanding of the communication problems.
Establish method of communication in which needs can be expressed.
Use resources appropriately.

ACTIONS/INTERVENTIONS	RATIONALE
COMMUNICATION ENHANCEMENT: Speech Deficit (NIC)	
Independent	
Assess type/degree of dysfunction: e.g., receptive aphasia, client does not seem to understand words or has trouble speaking or making self understood, expressive aphasia:	Helps determine area and degree of brain involvement and difficulty client has with any or all steps of the communication process. Client may have trouble understanding spoken words (receptive aphasia/damage to Wernicke's speech area), speaking words correctly (expressive aphasia/damage to Broca's speech areas), or may experience damage to both areas.
Differentiate aphasia from dysarthria;	Choice of interventions depends on type of impairment. Aphasia is a defect in using and interpreting symbols of language and may involve sensory and/or motor components; e.g., inability to comprehend written/spoken words or to write, make signs, speak. A dysarthric person can understand, read, and write language but has difficulty forming/pronouncing words because of weakness and paralysis of oral musculature, resulting in softly spoken speech.
Listen for errors in conversation and provide feedback;	Client may lose ability to monitor verbal output and be unaware that communication is not sensible. Feedback helps client realize why caregivers are not understanding/responding appropriately and provides opportunity to clarify content/meaning.
Ask client to follow simple commands (e.g., "Shut your eyes"; "Point to the door"); repeat simple words/ sentences;	Tests for receptive aphasia.
Point to objects and ask client to name them;	Tests for expressive aphasia; e.g., client may recognize item but not be able to name it.
Have client produce simple sounds; e.g., "sh," "cat";	Identifies dysarthria because motor components of speech (tongue, lip movement, breath control) can affect articulation and may/may not be accompanied by expressive aphasia.

ACTIONS/INTERVENTIONS	RATIONALE
Ask client to write name and/or a short sentence. If unable to write, have client read a short sentence.	Tests for writing disability (agraphia) and deficits in reading comprehension (alexia), which are also part of receptive and expressive aphasia.
Post notice at nurses' station and client's room about speech impairment. Provide special call bell if necessary.	Allays anxiety related to inability to communicate and fear that needs will not be met promptly. Call bell that is activated by minimal pressure is useful when client is unable to use regular call system.
Provide alternative methods of communication; e.g., writing or felt board, pictures. Provide visual clues (gestures, pictures, "needs" list, demonstration).	Provides for communication of needs/desires based on individual situation/underlying deficit.
Anticipate and provide for client's needs.	Helpful in decreasing frustration when dependent on others and unable to communicate desires.
Talk directly to client, speaking slowly and distinctly. Use yes/no questions to begin with, progressing in complexity as client responds.	Reduces confusion/anxiety at having to process and respond to large amount of information at one time. As retraining progresses, advancing complexity of communication stimulates memory and further enhances word/idea association.
Speak with normal volume and avoid talking too fast. Give client ample time to respond. Talk without pressing for a response.	Client is not necessarily hearing impaired, and raising voice may irritate or anger client. Forcing responses can result in frustration and may cause client to resort to "automatic" speech; e.g., garbled speech, obscenities.
Encourage SO/visitors to persist in efforts to communicate with client; e.g., reading mail, discussing family happenings even if client is unable to respond appropriately.	It is important for family members to continue talking to client to reduce client's isolation, promote establishment of effective communication, and maintain sense of connectedness with family.
Discuss familiar topics; e.g., job, family, hobbies.	Promotes meaningful conversation and provides opportunity to practice skills.
Respect client's preinjury capabilities; avoid "speaking down" to client or making patronizing remarks.	Enables client to feel esteemed because intellectual abilities often remain intact.

Collaborative

Consult with/refer to speech therapist.	Assesses individual verbal capabilities and sensory, motor, and cognitive functioning to identify deficits/therapy needs.

NURSING DIAGNOSIS: disturbed Sensory Perception [specify]

May be related to

Altered sensory reception, transmission, integration (neurologic trauma or deficit)
Psychologic stress (narrowed perceptual fields caused by anxiety)

Possibly evidenced by

Disorientation to time, place, person
Change in behavior pattern/usual response to stimuli; exaggerated emotional responses
Poor concentration, altered thought processes/bizarre thinking
Reported/measured change in sensory acuity: hypoparesthesia; altered sense of taste/smell
Inability to tell position of body parts (proprioception)
Inability to recognize/attach meaning to objects (visual agnosia)
Altered communication patterns
Motor incoordination

DESIRED OUTCOMES/EVALUATION CRITERIA—CLIENT WILL:

Cognition (NOC)

Regain/maintain usual level of consciousness and perceptual functioning.
Acknowledge changes in ability and presence of residual involvement.
Demonstrate behaviors to compensate for/overcome deficits.

ACTIONS/INTERVENTIONS	RATIONALE
Environmental Management (NIC)	
Independent	
Review pathology of individual condition.	Awareness of type/area of involvement aids in assessing for/anticipating specific deficits and planning care.
Observe behavioral responses, e.g., hostility, crying, inappropriate affect, agitation, hallucination (use Los Ranchos Scale as appropriate). (Refer to CP: Craniocerebral Trauma [Acute Rehabilitative Phase], ND: disturbed Thought Processes.)	Individual responses are variable, but commonalities such as emotional lability, lowered frustration threshold, apathy, and impulsiveness may complicate care. Eight-level Los Ranchos Scale aids in documenting progress during initial weeks following insult.
Eliminate extraneous noise/stimuli as necessary.	Reduces anxiety and exaggerated emotional responses/confusion associated with sensory overload.
Speak in calm, quiet voice, using short sentences. Maintain eye contact.	Client may have limited attention span or problems with comprehension. These measures can help client attend to communication.
Ascertain/validate client's perceptions. Reorient client frequently to environment, staff, and procedures.	Assists client to identify inconsistencies in reception and integration of stimuli and may reduce perceptual distortion of reality.
Evaluate for visual deficits. Note loss of visual field, changes in depth perception (horizontal/vertical planes), presence of diplopia (double vision).	Presence of visual disorders can negatively affect client's ability to perceive environment and relearn motor skills and increases risk of accident/injury.
Approach client from visually intact side. Leave light on; position objects to take advantage of intact visual fields. Patch affected eye or encourage wearing of prism glasses if indicated.	Provides for recognition of the presence of persons/objects; may help with depth perception problems; prevents client from being startled. Patching may decrease the sensory confusion of double vision, and prism glasses may enhance vision across midline, decreasing neglect of affected side.
Peripheral Sensation Management (NIC)	
Assess sensory awareness (e.g., differentiation of hot/cold, dull/sharp), position of body parts/muscle, joint sense.	Diminished sensory awareness and impairment of kinesthetic sense negatively affects balance/positioning (proprioception) and appropriateness of movement, which interferes with ambulation, increasing risk of trauma.
Stimulate sense of touch; e.g., give client objects to touch, grasp. Have client practice touching walls/other boundaries.	Aids in retraining sensory pathways to integrate reception and interpretation of stimuli. Helps client orient self spatially and strengthens use of affected side.
Protect from temperature extremes; assess environment for hazards. Recommend testing warm water with unaffected hand.	Promotes client safety, reducing risk of injury.
Note inattention to body parts, segments of environment; lack of recognition of familiar objects/persons.	Presence of agnosia (loss of comprehension of auditory, visual, or other sensations, although sensory sphere is intact) may lead to/result in unilateral neglect, inability to recognize environmental cues/meaning of commonplace objects, considerable self-care deficits, and disorientation or bizarre behavior.

ACTIONS/INTERVENTIONS	RATIONALE
Encourage client to watch feet when appropriate and consciously position body parts. Make client aware of all neglected body parts; e.g., sensory stimulation to affected side, exercises that bring affected side across midline, reminding person to dress/care for affected ("blind") side.	Use of visual and tactile stimuli assists in reintegration of affected side and allows client to experience forgotten sensations of normal movement patterns.

NURSING DIAGNOSIS: Self-Care Deficit [specify]

May be related to

Neuromuscular impairment, decreased strength and endurance, loss of muscle control/coordination
Perceptual/cognitive impairment
Pain/discomfort
Depression

Possibly evidenced by

Impaired ability to perform ADLs: e.g., inability to bring food from receptacle to mouth; inability to wash body part(s), regulate temperature of water; impaired ability to put on/take off clothing; difficulty completing toileting tasks

DESIRED OUTCOMES/EVALUATION CRITERIA—CLIENT WILL:

SELF-CARE: Activities of Daily Living (ADL) (NOC)

Demonstrate techniques/lifestyle changes to meet self-care needs.
Perform self-care activities within level of own ability.
Identify personal/community resources that can provide assistance as needed.

ACTIONS/INTERVENTIONS — RATIONALE

Self-Care Assistance (NIC)

Independent

ACTIONS/INTERVENTIONS	RATIONALE
Assess abilities and level of deficit (0–4 scale) for performing ADLs.	Aids in anticipating/planning for meeting individual needs.
Avoid doing things for client that client can do for self, providing assistance as necessary.	These clients may become fearful and dependent, and although assistance is helpful in preventing frustration, it is important for client to do as much as possible for self to maintain self-esteem and promote recovery.
Be aware of impulsive behavior/actions suggestive of impaired judgment.	May indicate need for additional interventions and supervision to promote client safety.
Maintain a supportive, firm attitude. Allow client sufficient time to accomplish tasks.	Clients need empathy and to know caregivers will be consistent in their assistance.
Provide positive feedback for efforts and accomplishments.	Enhances sense of self-worth, promotes independence, and encourages client to continue endeavors.
Create plan for visual deficits that are present; e.g.:	
Place food and utensils on the tray related to client's unaffected side;	Client will be able to see to eat the food.
Situate the bed so that client's unaffected side is facing the room with the affected side to the wall;	Will be able to see when getting in/out of bed and observe anyone who comes into the room.

ACTIONS/INTERVENTIONS	RATIONALE
Position furniture against wall/out of travel path.	Provides for safety when client is able to move around the room, reducing risk of tripping/falling over furniture.
Provide self-help devices; e.g., button/zipper hook, knife-fork combinations, long-handled brushes, extensions for picking things up from floor, toilet riser, leg bag for catheter, shower chair. Assist and encourage good grooming and makeup habits.	Enables client to manage for self, enhancing independence and self-esteem; reduces reliance on others for meeting own needs; and enables client to be more socially active.
Encourage SO to allow client to do as much as possible for self.	Reestablishes sense of independence and fosters self-worth and enhances rehabilitation process. *Note:* This may be very difficult and frustrating for the SO/caregiver, depending on degree of disability and time required for client to complete activity.
Assess client's ability to communicate the need to void and/or ability to use urinal, bedpan. Take client to the bathroom at frequent/scheduled intervals for voiding if appropriate.	Client may have neurogenic bladder, be inattentive, or be unable to communicate needs in acute recovery phase, but usually is able to regain independent control of this function as recovery progresses.
Identify previous bowel habits and reestablish normal regimen. Increase bulk in diet; encourage fluid intake, increased activity.	Assists in development of retraining program (independence) and aids in preventing constipation and impaction (long-term effects).

Collaborative

Administer suppositories and stool softeners.	May be necessary at first to aid in establishing regular bowel function.
Consult with rehabilitation team/physical/occupational therapists.	Provides assistance in developing a comprehensive therapy program and identifying special equipment needs that can increase client's participation in self-care.

NURSING DIAGNOSIS: ineffective Coping

May be related to

Situational crises, vulnerability, cognitive perceptual changes

Possibly evidenced by

Inappropriate use of defense mechanisms
Inability to cope/difficulty asking for help
Change in usual communication patterns
Inability to meet basic needs/role expectations
Difficulty problem solving

DESIRED OUTCOMES/EVALUATION CRITERIA—CLIENT WILL:

Coping (NOC)

Verbalize acceptance of self in situation.
Talk/communicate with SO about situation and changes that have occurred.
Verbalize awareness of own coping abilities.
Meet psychologic needs as evidenced by appropriate expression of feelings, identification of options, and use of resources.

ACTIONS/INTERVENTIONS	RATIONALE
Coping Enhancement (NIC)	
Independent	
Assess extent of altered perception and related degree of disability. Determine Functional Independence Measure score.	Determination of individual factors aids in developing plan of care/choice of interventions and discharge expectations.
Identify meaning of the loss/dysfunction/change to client. Note ability to understand events, provide realistic appraisal of situation.	Independence/ability is highly valued in American society but is not as significant in some other cultures. Some clients accept and manage altered function effectively with little adjustment, whereas others have considerable difficulty recognizing and adjusting to deficits. In order to provide meaningful support and appropriate problem solving, healthcare providers need to understand the meaning of the stroke/limitations to the client.
Determine outside stressors; e.g., family, work, social, future nursing/healthcare needs.	Helps identify specific needs, provides opportunity to offer information/support and begin problem solving. Consideration of social factors, in addition to functional status, is important in determining appropriate discharge destination.
Encourage client to express feelings, including hostility or anger, denial, depression, sense of disconnectedness.	Demonstrates acceptance of/assists client in recognizing and beginning to deal with these feelings.
Note whether client refers to affected side as "it" or denies affected side and says it is "dead."	Suggests rejection of body part/negative feelings about body image and abilities, indicating need for intervention and emotional support.
Acknowledge statement of feelings about betrayal of body; remain matter-of-fact about reality that client can still use unaffected side and learn to control affected side. Use words (e.g., weak, affected, right-left) that incorporate that side as part of the whole body.	Helps client see that the nurse accepts both sides as part of the whole individual. Allows client to feel hopeful and begin to accept current situation.
Identify previous methods of dealing with life problems. Determine presence/quality of support systems.	Provides opportunity to use behaviors previously effective, build on past successes, and mobilize resources.
Emphasize and provide positive I-messages for small gains either in recovery of function or independence.	Consolidates gains, helps reduce feelings of anger and helplessness, and conveys sense of progress.
Support behaviors/efforts such as increased interest/participation in rehabilitation activities.	Suggests possible adaptation to changes and understanding about own role in future lifestyle.
Monitor for sleep disturbance, increased difficulty concentrating, statements of inability to cope, lethargy, withdrawal.	May indicate onset of depression (common aftereffect of stroke), which may require further evaluation and intervention.
Collaborative	
Refer for neuropsychologic evaluation and/or counseling if indicated.	May facilitate adaptation to role changes that are necessary for a sense of feeling/being a productive person. *Note:* Depression is common in stroke survivors and may be a direct result of the brain damage and/or an emotional reaction to sudden-onset disability.

NURSING DIAGNOSIS: risk for impaired Swallowing

Risk factors may include

Neuromuscular/perceptual impairment

Possibly evidenced by

[Not applicable; presence of signs and symptoms establishes an *actual* diagnosis.]

DESIRED OUTCOMES/EVALUATION CRITERIA—CLIENT WILL:

Swallowing Status (NOC)

Demonstrate feeding methods appropriate to individual situation with aspiration prevented.
Maintain desired body weight.

ACTIONS/INTERVENTIONS	RATIONALE
Swallowing Therapy (NIC)	
Independent	
Review individual pathology/ability to swallow, noting extent of paralysis; clarity of speech; facial, tongue involvement; ability to protect airway/episodes of coughing or choking; presence of adventitious breath sounds; amount/character of oral secretions. Weigh periodically as indicated.	Nutritional interventions/choice of feeding route is determined by these factors.
Have suction equipment available at bedside, especially during early feeding efforts.	Timely intervention may limit amount/untoward effect of aspiration.
Promote effective swallowing; e.g.:	
Schedule activities/medications to provide a minimum of 30 min rest before eating;	Promotes optimal muscle function, helps to limit fatigue.
Provide pleasant environment free of distractions (e.g., TV);	Promotes relaxation and allows client to focus on task of eating/swallowing.
Assist client with head control/support, and position based on specific dysfunction;	Counteracts hyperextension, aiding in prevention of aspiration and enhancing ability to swallow. Optimal positioning can facilitate intake/reduce risk of aspiration; e.g., head back for decreased posterior propulsion of tongue, head turned to weak side for unilateral pharyngeal paralysis, lying down on either side for reduced pharyngeal contraction.
Place client in upright position during/after feeding as appropriate;	Uses gravity to facilitate swallowing and reduces risk of aspiration.
Provide oral care based on individual need prior to meal;	Clients with dry mouth require a moisturizing agent (e.g., artificial saliva or alcohol-free mouthwash) before and after eating; clients with excess saliva will benefit from use of a drying agent (e.g., lemon or glycerin swabs) before meal and a moisturizing agent afterward.
Season food with herbs, spices, lemon juice according to client's preference, within dietary restrictions;	Increases salivation, improving bolus formation and swallowing effort.
Serve foods at customary temperature and water always chilled;	Lukewarm temperatures are less likely to stimulate salivation so foods/fluids should be served cold or warm as appropriate. *Note:* Water is the most difficult to swallow.
Stimulate lips to close or manually open mouth by light pressure on lips/under chin if needed;	Aids in sensory retraining and promotes muscular control.
Place food of appropriate consistency in unaffected side of mouth;	Provides sensory stimulation (including taste), which may increase salivation and trigger swallowing efforts, enhancing intake. Food consistency is determined by individual deficit. *For example:* Clients with decreased range of tongue motion require thick liquids initially, progressing to thin liquids, whereas clients with delayed pharyngeal swallow will handle thick liquids and thicker foods better. *Note:* Pureed food is not recommended because client may not be able to recognize what is being eaten; and most milk products, peanut butter, syrup, and bananas are avoided because they produce mucus/are sticky.

ACTIONS/INTERVENTIONS	RATIONALE
Touch parts of the cheek with tongue blade/apply ice to weak tongue;	Can improve tongue movement and control (necessary for swallowing), and inhibits tongue protrusion.
Feed slowly, allowing 30–45 min for meals;	Feeling rushed can increase stress/level of frustration, may increase risk of aspiration, and may result in client's terminating meal early.
Offer solid foods and liquids at different times;	Prevents client from swallowing food before it is thoroughly chewed. In general, liquids should be offered only after client has finished eating solids.
Limit/avoid use of drinking straw for liquids;	Although use may strengthen facial and swallowing muscles, if client lacks tight lip closure to accommodate straw or if liquid is deposited too far back in mouth, risk of aspiration may be increased.
Encourage SO to bring favorite foods.	Provides familiar tastes and preferences. Stimulates feeding efforts and may enhance swallowing/intake.
Maintain upright position for 45–60 min after eating.	Helps client manage oral secretions and reduces risk of regurgitation.
Maintain accurate I&O; record calorie count.	If swallowing efforts are not sufficient to meet fluid/nutrition needs, alternative methods of feeding must be pursued.
Encourage participation in exercise/activity program.	May increase release of endorphins in the brain, promoting a sense of general well-being and increasing appetite.

Collaborative

Review results of radiographic studies; e.g., video fluoroscopy.	Aids in determining phase of swallowing difficulties (i.e., oral preparatory, oral, pharyngeal, or esophageal phase).
Administer IV fluids and/or tube feedings.	May be necessary for fluid replacement and nutrition if client is unable to take anything orally.
Coordinate multidisciplinary approach to develop treatment plan that meets individual needs.	Inclusion of dietitian, speech, and occupational therapists can increase effectiveness of long-term plan and significantly reduce risk of silent aspiration.

NURSING DIAGNOSIS: deficient Knowledge [Learning Need] regarding condition, prognosis, treatment, self-care, and discharge needs

May be related to

Lack of exposure, unfamiliarity with information resources
Cognitive limitation, information misinterpretation, lack of recall

Possibly evidenced by

Request for information
Statement of misconception
Inaccurate follow-through of instructions
Development of preventable complications

DESIRED OUTCOMES/EVALUATION CRITERIA—CLIENT/SO WILL:

KNOWLEDGE: Disease Process (NOC)

Participate in learning process.
Verbalize understanding of condition/prognosis and potential complications.

KNOWLEDGE: Treatment Regimen (NOC)

Verbalize understanding of therapeutic regimen and rationale for actions.
Initiate necessary lifestyle changes.

ACTIONS/INTERVENTIONS	RATIONALE
TEACHING: Disease Process (NIC)	
Independent	
Evaluate type/degree of sensory-perceptual involvement.	Deficits affect the choice of teaching methods and content/complexity of instruction.
Include SO/family in discussions and teaching.	These individuals will be providing support/care and have great impact on client's quality of life.
Discuss specific pathology and individual potentials.	Aids in establishing realistic expectations and promotes understanding of current situation and needs.
Identify signs/symptoms requiring further follow-up; e.g., changes/decline in visual, motor, sensory functions; alteration in mentation or behavioral responses; severe headache.	Prompt evaluation and intervention reduces risk of complications/further loss of function.
Review current restrictions/limitations and discuss planned/potential resumption of activities (including sexual relations).	Promotes understanding, provides hope for future, and creates expectation of resumption of more "normal" life.
Review/reinforce current therapeutic regimen, including use of medications to control hypertension, hypercholesterolemia, diabetes as indicated; aspirin or similar-acting drug; e.g., ticlopidine (Ticlid), warfarin sodium (Coumadin). Identify ways of continuing program after discharge.	Recommended activities, limitations, and medication/therapy needs are established on the basis of a coordinated interdisciplinary approach. Follow-through is essential to progression of recovery/prevention of complications. *Note:* Long-term anticoagulation may be beneficial for clients older than 45 years of age who are prone to clot formation; however, use of these drugs is not effective for CVA resulting from vascular aneurysm/vessel rupture.
Provide written instructions and schedules for activity, medication, important facts.	Provides visual reinforcement and reference source after discharge.
Encourage client to refer to lists/written communications or notes; that is, memory book.	Provides aids to support memory and promotes improvement in cognitive skills.
Discuss plans for meeting self-care needs.	Varying levels of assistance may be required/need to be planned for based on individual situation.
Refer to discharge planner/home care supervisor, visiting nurse.	Home environment may require evaluation and modifications to meet individual needs.
Identify community resources; e.g., National Stroke Association, American Heart Association's Stroke Connection, stroke support clubs, senior services, Meals on Wheels, adult day care/respite program, and visiting nurse.	Enhances coping abilities and promotes home management and adjustment to impairments for both stroke survivors and caregivers. *Note:* Recent innovations include such programs as Menu-Direct, which provides fully prepared meal programs with nutrition-rich foods. Some entrees have soufflé-like consistency to help trigger swallowing response.
Suggest client reduce/limit environmental stimuli, especially during cognitive activities.	Multiple/concomitant stimuli may aggravate confusion and impair mental abilities.
Recommend client seek assistance in problem-solving process and validate decisions as indicated.	Some clients (especially those with right CVA) may display impaired judgment and impulsive behavior, compromising ability to make sound decisions.
Identify individual risk factors (e.g., hypertension, cardiac dysrhythmias, obesity, smoking, heavy alcohol use, atherosclerosis, poor control of diabetes, use of oral contraceptives) and discuss necessary lifestyle changes.	Promotes general well-being and may reduce risk of recurrence. *Note:* Obesity in women has been found to have a high correlation with ischemic stroke.
Review importance of balanced diet, low in cholesterol and sodium if indicated. Discuss role of vitamins and other supplements.	Improves general health and well-being and provides energy for life activities.
Refer to/reinforce importance of follow-up care by rehabilitation team; e.g., physical/occupational/speech/vocational therapists.	Diligent work may eventually overcome/minimize residual deficits.

POTENTIAL CONSIDERATIONS following acute hospitalization (dependent on client's age, physical condition/presence of complications, personal resources, and life responsibilities)

risk for Injury—general weakness, visual deficits, balancing difficulties, reduced large/small muscle or hand-eye coordination, cognitive impairment.

imbalanced Nutrition: less than body requirements—inability to prepare/ingest food, cognitive limitations, limited financial resources.

Self-Care Deficit—decreased strength/endurance, perceptual/cognitive impairment, neuromuscular impairment, muscular pain, depression.

impaired Home Maintenance—individual physical limitations, inadequate support systems, insufficient finances, unfamiliarity with neighborhood resources.

situational low Self-Esteem—cognitive/perceptual impairment, perceived loss of control in some aspect of life, loss of independent functioning.

risk for Caregiver Role Strain—severity of illness/deficits of care receiver, duration of caregiving required, complexity/amount of caregiving task, caregiver isolation/lack of respite.

HERNIATED NUCLEUS PULPOSUS (RUPTURED INTERVERTEBRAL DISC)

A *herniated disc (herniated nucleus pulposus)* (HNP) is a major cause of severe, chronic, and recurrent back pain. Herniation (either complete or partial) most often occurs in discs of the lumbar vertebral areas of L-4 to L-5, L-5 to S-1, and cervical vertebral areas of C-5 to C-6, C-6 to C-7. Disc herniation occurs more frequently in middle-aged (30s and 40s) and older men, especially those involved in strenuous physical activity. Other causes include trauma, occupations requiring lifting of heavy objects and/or repetitive lifting, congenital conditions affecting the size of the spinal canal, and degenerative changes associated with the aging process.

CARE SETTING

Most disc problems are treated conservatively at the community level, although diagnostics and therapy services may be provided through outpatient facilities. Brief hospitalization is restricted to episodes of severe debilitating pain/neurologic deficit.

RELATED CONCERNS

Disc surgery, page 260
Psychosocial aspects of care, page 770

Client Assessment Database

Data depend on site, severity, whether acute/chronic, effects on surrounding structures and degree of nerve root compression.

ACTIVITY/REST:

May report: History of occupation requiring heavy lifting, sitting, driving for long periods
Need to sleep on bedboard/firm mattress, difficulty falling asleep/staying asleep
Decreased ROM of affected extremity/extremities
Inability to perform usual/desired activities

May exhibit: Atrophy of muscles on the affected side
Gait disturbances

ELIMINATION

May report: Constipation, difficulty in defecation
Urinary incontinence/retention

EGO INTEGRITY

May report: Fear of paralysis
Financial, employment concerns

May exhibit: Anxiety, depression, withdrawal from family/SO

NEUROSENSORY

May report: Tingling, numbness, weakness of affected extremity/extremities

May exhibit: Decreased deep tendon reflexes; muscle weakness, hypotonia
Tenderness/spasm of paravertebral muscles
Decreased pain perception (sensory)

PAIN/DISCOMFORT

May report: Pain knifelike, aggravated by coughing, sneezing, bending, lifting, defecation, straight leg raising
Unremitting pain or intermittent episodes of more severe pain
Radiation into legs/feet, buttocks area (lumbar), shoulder, shoulder blade area, arms, head/face, neck (cervical)
May have heard "snapping" sound at time of initial pain/trauma or felt "back giving way"
Limited mobility/forward bending

May exhibit: Stance: Leans away from affected area
Altered gait, walking with a limp, elevated hip on affected side
Pain on palpation

SAFETY

May report: History of previous back problems

TEACHING/LEARNING

May report: Lifestyle sedentary or overactive
Use of herbal supplements for backache (e.g., ashwaganda, burdock, cayenne, ginger, kava-kava, yarrow)

Discharge plan considerations: May require assistance with transportation, self-care, and homemaker/maintenance tasks

Refer to section at end of plan for postdischarge. considerations.

DIAGNOSTIC STUDIES

MRI: Diagnostic test of choice in chronic, unremitting back pain. Can reveal changes in bone, discs, and soft tissues, and can validate disc herniation/surgical decisions.

Spinal radiographs: May show degenerative changes in spine/intravertebral space, or be used to rule out other suspected pathology; e.g., tumors, osteomyelitis.

CT scan with/without enhancement: May reveal spinal canal narrowing, disc protrusion.

Provocative tests (discography, nerve root blocks): Determines site of origin of pain by replicating and then relieving symptoms, particularly in lumbar disc pain. The validity, specificity, and sensitivity of facet joint diagnostic blocking are considered strong in the diagnosis of facet joint pain. Sacroiliac joint blocks can also be used to rule out sacroiliac joint involvement, but are less reliable.

Electrophysiologic studies—electromyoneurography (EMG) and nerve conduction studies (NCS): Can localize lesion to level of particular spinal nerve root involved; nerve conduction and velocity study usually done in conjunction with study of muscle response to assist in diagnosis of peripheral nerve impairment and effect on skeletal muscle.

Myelogram: Rarely performed, but when done, may be normal or show "narrowing" of disc space, specific location and size of herniation.

Epidural venogram: May be done for cases where myelogram accuracy is limited.

NURSING PRIORITIES

1. Reduce back stress, muscle spasm, and pain.
2. Promote optimal functioning.
3. Support client/SO in rehabilitation process.
4. Provide information concerning condition/prognosis and treatment needs.

DISCHARGE GOALS

1. Pain relieved/manageable.
2. Proper lifting, posture, exercises demonstrated.
3. Motor function/sensation restored to optimal level.
4. Disease/injury process, prognosis, and therapeutic regimen understood.
5. Plan in place to meet needs after discharge.

NURSING DIAGNOSIS: acute/chronic Pain

May be related to

Physical injury agents: nerve compression, muscle spasm

Possibly evidenced by

Reports of back pain, stiff neck, decreased tolerance for activity
Walking with a limp, inability to walk, preoccupation with pain, self/narrowed focus
Guarding behavior, leans toward affected side when standing
Altered muscle tone
Facial mask of pain, distraction
Autonomic responses (when pain is acute)
Changes in sleep patterns; physical/social withdrawal

DESIRED OUTCOMES/EVALUATION CRITERIA—CLIENT WILL:

Pain Control (NOC)

Report pain is relieved/controlled.
Verbalize methods that provide relief.
Demonstrate use of therapeutic interventions (e.g., relaxation skills, behavior modification) to relieve pain.

ACTIONS/INTERVENTIONS	RATIONALE
Pain Management (NIC)	
Independent	
Assess client's perceptions of pain, and attitude toward pain and use of specific pain medications	Perception of pain is influenced by age and developmental stage, underlying problem causing the pain, and cognitive, behavioral, and sociocutural factors. Client may have beliefs about medications, have high or low tolerance for pain and pain medications.
Perform comprehensive assessment of pain, noting location, duration, precipitating/aggravating factors, and severity. Ask client to rate on scale of 0–10 (or other scale as appropriate). Accept client's description of pain.	Helps determine choice of interventions and provides basis for comparison and evaluation of therapy.
Note presence of behaviors associated with pain; e.g., changes in vital signs (with acute pain), crying, grimacing, sleep disturbances, withdrawal, narrowed focus. Evaluate current and past medication use.	Nonverbal evidence of pain. Observations may or may not be congruent with verbal reports, indicating need for further evaluation; e.g., stoic client reporting a 3/10 pain scale, may also be restless, agitated, and sleepless.
Maintain bedrest briefly during acute phase. Place client in semi-Fowler's position with spine, hips, and knees flexed; supine with/without head elevated 10–30 degrees; or lateral position.	Bedrest (usually prescribed for a very short time; e.g., 48 hr) in position of comfort decreases muscle spasm, reduces stress on structures, and facilitates reduction of disc protrusion.
Instruct in logrolling technique for position change if condition requires.	Reduces flexion, twisting, and strain on back, especially when nerve impingement impairs client's ability to move legs.
Assist with application of brace/corset. Instruct client in how to self-place brace with assistance, then independently.	Often used briefly during acute phase of ruptured disc or after surgery to provide support and limit flexion/twisting. *Note:* Prolonged use can increase muscle weakness and cause further disc degeneration, nerve impairment.
Limit activity during acute phase as indicated. Intersperse rest periods, shortening rest interval and length as client improves.	Decreases forces of gravity and motion, which can relieve muscle spasms and reduce edema and stress on structures around affected disc.

ACTIONS/INTERVENTIONS	RATIONALE
Place needed items, call bell/phone within easy reach.	Reduces risk of straining to reach.
Provide comfort measures; e.g., backrub, positional and stretching exercises, therapeutic touch (TT), quiet environment.	Nonpharmacologic pain management is an essential nursing function in assisting the client to achieve pain-free periods.
Instruct in/assist with relaxation/visualization techniques, progressive muscle relaxation, breathing exercises.	Refocuses attention away from pain, aids in reducing muscle spasm/tension; and promotes tissue oxygenation/healing.
Instruct in modification of activities; encourage correct body mechanics/body posture.	Alleviates stress on muscles and prevents further aggravation of injury.
Evaluate emotional/physical components of individual situation.	Individuals with certain psychologic syndromes (e.g., major depression, somatization disorder, hypochondriasis) are at increased risk of developing chronic pain syndrome. Any painful condition, such as back pain, can cause or exacerbate emotional responses (e.g., depression, withdrawal, agitation, anger).
Provide opportunities to talk/listen to concerns.	Verbalization of worries can help decrease stress factors present in illness/hospitalization. Provides opportunity to give information/correct misinformation.

Collaborative

ACTIONS/INTERVENTIONS	RATIONALE
Provide orthopedic bed or firm mattress.	Increases support and reduces spinal flexion, decreasing spasms.
Administer medications as indicated:	Pain management may be complex and should be geared to providing consistent and sufficient medication for pain relief while managing side effects.
Nonsteroidal anti-inflammatory drugs (NSAIDs); e.g., indomethacin (Indocin), ibuprofen (Motrin, Advil), naproxen (Aleve, Anaprox) etodolac (Lodine), diflunisal (Dolobid), ketoprofen (Orudis);	Suppress pain and inflammation, decrease edema and pressure on nerve root(s). *Note:* Epidural or facet joint injection of anti-inflammatory drugs has been found to be helpful in providing short-term pain relief in some clients if other interventions fail to alleviate pain.
Muscle relaxants; e.g., cyclobenzaprine (Flexeril), baclofen (Lioresal), diazepam (Valium), carisoprodol (Soma), methocarbamol (Robaxin), metaxalone (Skelaxin);	Relaxes striated muscles, decreasing pain. *Note:* Because these drugs act centrally on the brain, drowsiness, dizziness, and lightheadedness may occur, especially during initial therapy, raising safety concerns.
Analgesics; e.g., acetaminophen (Tylenol) with codeine (Tylenol #3), hydrocodone (Vicodin, Lortab), oxycodone compound (Oxycontin, Roxicet), propoxyphene (Darvon N, Darvocet), butorphanol (Stadol), fentanyl (Duragesic), meperidine (Demerol) morphine; hydromorphone (Dilaudid).	May be required for relief of moderate to severe pain, usually during periods of exacerbation of symptoms. Used with caution for relief of chronic pain because concerns of dependency must be balanced with client's functional abilities/quality of life needs.
Apply physical supports; e.g., lumbar brace, cervical collar.	Support of structures decreases muscle stress/spasms and reduces pain.
Maintain traction if indicated.	May occasionally be used to remove weight bearing from affected disc area, increasing intravertebral separation and allowing disc bulge to move away from nerve root.
Consult with physical therapist.	Individualized conservative care program (including hot and cold packs, ultrasound, massage, transcutaneous electrical nerve stimulation [TENS], therapeutic exercises, and pool therapy) can be implemented to relieve muscle spasm and strengthen back, extensor, abdominal, and quadriceps muscles to increase support to lumbar area.
Apply/monitor use and effects of cold or moist hot packs.	Increases circulation to affected muscles, promotes relief of spasms, and enhances client's relaxation. However, prolonged use may result in thermal injury to skin.

ACTIONS/INTERVENTIONS	RATIONALE
Instruct in postmyelogram/postepidural block care when appropriate; e.g., force fluids and lie flat or at 30-degree elevation as indicated for specified period of time.	Decreases risk of postprocedure headache/spinal fluid leak.
Assist with/instruct in use of electrical stimulation; e.g., TENS unit.	Decreases stimuli by blocking pain transmission.
Refer to rehabilitation/pain management clinic.	Coordinated team efforts may include physical, occupational, and psychologic therapy to deal with all aspects of chronic pain and allow client to increase activity and productivity.
Refer for alternative therapies as appropriate.	Client may require surgery, or may be candidate for other therapies; e.g., spinal manipulation, spinal cord stimulation, implantable intrathecal drug administration system, percutaneous lysis of adhesions.

NURSING DIAGNOSIS: impaired physical Mobility

May be related to

Pain and discomfort, muscle spasms
Restrictive therapies, e.g., bedrest, traction
Neuromuscular impairment

Possibly evidenced by

Reports of pain on movement
Reluctance to attempt/difficulty with purposeful movement
Impaired coordination, limited ROM, decreased muscle strength

DESIRED OUTCOMES/EVALUATION CRITERIA—CLIENT WILL:

IMMOBILITY CONSEQUENCES: Physiologic (NOC)

Verbalize understanding of situation/risk factors and individual treatment regimen.
Be free of complications.
Demonstrate techniques/behaviors that enable resumption of activities.

Mobility (NOC)

Maintain or increase strength and function of affected and/or compensatory body part.

ACTIONS/INTERVENTIONS	RATIONALE
Bed Rest Care (NIC)	
Independent	
Perform/assist with passive and active ROM exercises.	Strengthens abdominal muscles and flexors of spine; promotes good body mechanics.
Encourage lower leg/ankle exercises. Evaluate for edema, erythema of lower extremities, calf pain/tenderness.	Stimulates venous circulation/return, decreasing venous stasis and possible thrombus formation.
Provide good skin care; gently massage pressure points after each position change. Check skin under brace periodically.	Reduces risk of skin irritation/breakdown.

ACTIONS/INTERVENTIONS	RATIONALE
Encourage diet high in fiber and adequate fluid intake.	Reduces risk of constipation related to decreased level of activity.
Note emotional/behavioral responses to immobility. Provide diversional activities.	Forced immobility may heighten restlessness, irritability. Diversional activity aids in refocusing attention and enhances coping with limitations.

EXERCISE THERAPY: Ambulation (NIC)

ACTIONS/INTERVENTIONS	RATIONALE
Provide for safety measures as indicated by individual situation.	Depending on area of involvement/type of procedure, imprudent activity increases chance of spinal injury. (Refer to CP: Disc Surgery, ND: risk for spinal Trauma.)
Assist with activity/progressive ambulation and therapeutic exercises.	Activity depends on individual situation but should begin as early as possible and usually progresses slowly according to tolerance.
Demonstrate use of adjunctive devices; e.g., walker, cane.	Provides stability and support to compensate for altered muscle tone/strength and balance.

Collaborative

ACTIONS/INTERVENTIONS	RATIONALE
Administer medication for pain on a regular schedule, or approximately 30 min before anticipated painful procedures or activities as indicated.	Anticipation of pain can increase muscle tension. Medication can relax client, enhance comfort and cooperation during activity.
Apply antiembolism stockings as indicated.	Promotes venous return, reducing risk of DVT.

NURSING DIAGNOSIS: Anxiety (specify level)/ ineffective Coping

May be related to

Situational crisis
Threat to/change in health status, socioeconomic status, role functioning
Recurrent disorder with continuing pain
Inadequate relaxation, little or no exercise
Inadequate coping methods

Possibly evidenced by

Apprehension, uncertainty, helplessness
Expressed concerns regarding changes in life events
Verbalization of inability to cope
Muscular tension, general irritability, restlessness; insomnia/fatigue
Inability to meet role expectations

DESIRED OUTCOMES/EVALUATION CRITERIA—CLIENT WILL:

Anxiety Self-Control (NOC)

Appear relaxed and report anxiety is reduced to a manageable level.
Identify ineffective coping behaviors and consequences.
Assess the current situation accurately.
Demonstrate effective problem-solving skills.
Develop plan for necessary lifestyle changes.

ACTIONS/INTERVENTIONS	RATIONALE
Coping Enhancement (NIC)	
Independent	
Assess level of anxiety. Determine how client had dealt with problems in the past and how he or she is coping with current situation.	Aids in identifying strengths and skills that may help client deal with current situation and/or enable others to provide appropriate assistance.
Provide accurate information and honest answers.	Helpful in clarifying misconceptions, identifying actual risk. Enables client to make decisions based on knowledge.
Provide opportunity for expression of concerns; e.g., possible permanent nerve damage/paralysis, effect on sexual ability, changes in employment/finances, altered role responsibilities.	Most clients have concerns that need to be expressed and responded to with accurate information to promote coping with situation.
Assess presence of secondary gains that may impede recovery.	Client may unconsciously experience advantages such as attention, control of others, relief from responsibilities. These need to be dealt with positively to promote recovery.
Note behaviors of SO that promote "sick role" for client.	SO may unconsciously enable client to remain dependent by doing things that client should do for self.
Collaborative	
Refer to community support groups, social services, financial/vocational counselor, marital therapy/psychotherapy, as appropriate.	Provides support for adapting to changes and provides resources to deal with problems.

NURSING DIAGNOSIS: deficient Knowledge [Learning Need] regarding condition, prognosis, treatment, self-care, and discharge needs

May be related to

Misinformation/lack of knowledge
Information misinterpretation, lack of recall
Unfamiliarity with information resources

Possibly evidenced by

Verbalization of problems, statement of misconception
Inaccurate return demonstration
Development of preventable complications

DESIRED OUTCOMES/EVALUATION CRITERIA—CLIENT WILL:

KNOWLEDGE: Disease Process (NOC)

Verbalize understanding of condition, prognosis, and treatment.

KNOWLEDGE: Treatment Regimen (NOC)

Initiate necessary lifestyle changes.
Participate in therapeutic regimen.

ACTIONS/INTERVENTIONS	RATIONALE
TEACHING: Disease Process (NIC)	
Independent	
Review disease/injury process and prognosis. Stress activity restrictions/limitations; e.g., avoid riding in car for long periods, refrain from participation in aggressive sports.	Helpful in clarifying and developing understanding and acceptance of necessary lifestyle modifications. Full knowledge base provides opportunity for client to make informed choices. May enhance cooperation with treatment program and achievement of optimal recovery.
Give information about and instruct in proper body mechanics, back school, ergonomics, and home exercises. Include information about proper posture/body mechanics for standing, sitting, and lifting and use of supportive shoes.	Reduces risk of reinjuring back/neck area by using muscles of thighs/buttocks.
Investigate appropriateness of using pneumatic continuous passive motion (CPM) supports when sitting.	Many individuals with low back pain have difficulty sitting for any length of time. This has a direct negative impact on work and leisure activities. The superficial soft-tissue effects of massage and vibration are usually short lived. CPM slowly moves the spine through the ranges of lordosis on a continuous basis while the individual is seated, whether riding in/driving a car, sitting at a desk, or reclining at home.
Discuss medications and side effects; e.g., some medications cause drowsiness (analgesics, muscle relaxants), whereas others can irritate gastric mucosa/aggravate ulcer disease (NSAIDs).	Reduces risk of complications/injury.
Recommend use of bedboards/firm mattress, small flat pillow under neck, sleeping on side with knees flexed, avoiding prone position.	May decrease muscle strain through structural support and prevention of hyperextension of spine.
Discuss dietary needs/goals.	High-fiber diet can reduce constipation (may be present because of inactivity and use of opoid analgesics). Caloric restrictions promote weight control/reduction (when obesity is aggravating back pain), which can decrease pressure on disc.
Instruct client to avoid prolonged heat application, and to alternate heat and cold.	Heat over a long period of time can increase local tissue congestion, and impaired sensitivity to heat can result in thermal injury. Alternating heat and cold during acute pain episodes helps to bring fresh circulation to the area and carry away toxins (heat), whereas cold helps reduce nerve pain.
Review use of soft cervical collar.	Maintaining slight flexion of head (allowing maximal opening of intravertebral foramina) may be useful for relieving pressure in mild to moderate cervical disc disease. *Note*: Hyperextension should be avoided.
Encourage regular medical follow-up.	Evaluates resolution/progression of degenerative process, monitors development of side effects/complications of drug therapy; may indicate need for change in therapeutic regimen.
Provide information about what symptoms need to be reported to primary provider; e.g., sharp pain, loss of sensation/ability to walk, change in bowel/bladder control.	Progression of the process requires further evaluation; may necessitate additional treatment/surgery.
Answer questions about treatment alternatives; e.g.:	
Chemonucleolysis;	As an alternative to surgery, the enzyme chymopapain or similar proteolytic agent (e.g., collagenase) may be injected into the disc to dissolve the mucoprotein disc material. Although many clients experience relief, the procedure is not widely done because of side effects, including allergic reaction to the enzyme, transverse myelitis, and possible paraplegia.

ACTIONS/INTERVENTIONS	RATIONALE
Surgical interventions.	*Microdiscetomy* may be performed to excise fragments of the disc with a comparatively lower risk than more invasive surgery. *Laminectomy* with/without spinal fusion may be performed when conservative treatment is ineffective or when neurologic deficits persist. (See CP: Disc surgery, page 260.)

POTENTIAL CONSIDERATIONS following acute hospitalization (dependent on client's age, physical condition/presence of complications, personal resources, and life responsibilities)

impaired Adjustment—disability, requiring change in lifestyle, assault to self-esteem, altered locus of control.

chronic Pain—prolonged physical/psychosocial disability.

ineffective Therapeutic Regimen Management—complexity of therapeutic regimen, decisional conflicts, economic difficulties, perceived benefits, powerlessness.

risk for Disuse Syndrome—severe pain, periods of immobility.

DISC SURGERY

Laminectomy is the surgical excision of a vertebral posterior arch and is commonly performed for injury to the spinal column, to relieve pressure on the spinal cord, and to remove a source of pain in the presence of a herniated disc. Open surgery is performed as an inpatient procedure under general anesthesia. Skin, muscles, and ligaments are cut, bone is permanently removed, and a longer recovery period is expected.

The procedure may be done with or without removal of disc material, and with or without fusion of vertebrae. If several discs or nerves are involved, the vertebrae may be fused together with bone grafts or other synthetic materials. Damaged discs may be replaced with an artificial disc. (Additionally, a possible technique using a genetically designed version of a natural body chemical called OP-1 is currently being tested. This "gene putty" acts as a bone spackle that fuses diseased vertebrae, negating the need for bone graft harvesting.)

Minimally invasive procedures are taking precedence over laminectomy in many areas of the world. These include *microdiscetomy, endoscopic lumbar* and *cervical discectomy,* and *intradiscal electrothermal therapy (IDET),* also known as *thermal discoplasty.* These procedures cause no damage to muscles, no bone is removed, and no large incisions are made, so they can be performed in an outpatient setting. *Endoscopic surgery* can be performed as an outpatient procedure: Surgical tools are inserted into a small incision, and the herniated disc is removed or remodeled. *Microdisectomy* is an outpatient minimally invasive procedure in which disc material is removed through a small puncture in the skin, using a microscope for guidance. These procedures do not require general anesthesia, and a short recovery period is expected.

This plan of care relates to the open surgery procedures where the client experiences a hospital stay.

CARE SETTING

Inpatient or outpatient surgical or orthopedic unit.

RELATED CONCERNS

Psychosocial aspects of care, page 770
Surgical intervention, page 788

Client Assessment Database

Refer to CP: Herniated Nucleus Pulposus (Ruptured Intervertebral Disc).

TEACHING/LEARNING

Discharge plan considerations: May require assistance with ADLs, transportation, homemaker/maintenance tasks, vocational counseling, possible changes in layout of home

Refer to section at end of plan for postdischarge considerations.

DIAGNOSTIC STUDIES

Refer to CP: Herniated Nucleus Pulposus (Ruptured Intervertebral Disc).

NURSING PRIORITIES

1. Maintain tissue perfusion/neurologic function.
2. Promote comfort and healing.
3. Prevent/minimize complications.
4. Assist with return to normal mobility.
5. Provide information about condition/prognosis, treatment needs, and limitations.

DISCHARGE GOALS

1. Neurologic function maintained/improved.
2. Complications prevented.
3. Limited mobility achieved with potential for increasing mobility.
4. Condition/prognosis, therapeutic regimen, and behavior/lifestyle changes are understood.
5. Plan in place to meet needs after discharge.

NURSING DIAGNOSIS: ineffective Tissue Perfusion, [specify]

May be related to

Diminished/interrupted blood flow (e.g., edema of operative site, hematoma formation)
Hypovolemia

Possibly evidenced by

Paresthesia, numbness
Decreased ROM, muscle strength

DESIRED OUTCOMES/EVALUATION CRITERIA—CLIENT WILL:

Neurologic Status (NOC)

Report/demonstrate normal sensations and movement as appropriate.

ACTIONS/INTERVENTIONS	RATIONALE
Surveillance (NIC)	
Independent	
Check neurologic signs periodically and compare with baseline. Assess movement/sensation of lower extremities and feet (lumbar) and hands/arms (cervical).	Although some degree of sensory impairment is usually present, changes may reflect development or resolution of spinal cord edema, and/or inflammation of the tissues secondary to damage to motor nerve roots from surgical manipulation; or tissue hemorrhage compressing the spinal cord, requiring prompt medical evaluation and intervention.
Keep client flat on back for several hours.	Pressure to operative site reduces risk of hematoma.
Monitor vital signs. Note color, warmth, capillary refill.	Hypotension (especially postural) with corresponding changes in pulse rate may reflect hypovolemia from blood loss, restriction of oral intake, nausea/vomiting.

ACTIONS/INTERVENTIONS	RATIONALE
Monitor I&O and Hemovac drainage (if used).	Provides information about circulatory status and replacement needs. Excessive/prolonged blood loss requires further evaluation to determine appropriate intervention.
Visually check and/or gently palpate operative site for swelling. Inspect dressing for excess drainage and test for glucose if indicated.	Change in contour of operative site suggests hematoma/edema formation. Inspection may reveal frank bleeding or dura leak of CSF (will test glucose positive), requiring prompt intervention.
Assess extremities (particularly lower) for redness, swelling, pain.	Suggests complications associated with immobility and clotting/development of DVT.

Collaborative

Administer IV fluids/blood as indicated.	Fluid replacement depends on the degree of hypovolemia and duration of oozing/bleeding/CSF leaking.
Monitor blood counts; e.g., hemoglobin (Hb), hematocrit (Hct), and red blood cells (RBCs).	Aids in establishing replacement needs, and monitors effectiveness of therapy.
Apply/maintain schedule for wearing antiembolic hose/sequential compression devices.	Reduces risks associated with venous stasis in lower extremities.

NURSING DIAGNOSIS: risk for spinal Trauma

Risk factors may include

Temporary weakness of vertebral column
Balancing difficulties, changes in muscle coordination

Possibly evidenced by

[Not applicable; presence of signs and symptoms establishes an *actual* diagnosis.]

DESIRED OUTCOMES/EVALUATION CRITERIA—CLIENT WILL:

Risk Control (NOC)

Maintain proper alignment of spine.
Recognize need for/seek assistance with activity as appropriate.

ACTIONS/INTERVENTIONS	RATIONALE
POSITIONING: Neurologic (NIC)	
Independent	
Post sign at bedside regarding prescribed position.	Reduces risk of inadvertent strain/flexion of operative area.
Provide bedboard/firm mattress.	Aids in stabilizing back.
Maintain brace wearing schedule, as indicated.	May be used to decrease muscle spasm and support the surrounding structures during healing, and allow more normal sensory stimulation to occur.
Limit activities as prescribed when client has had a spinal fusion.	Following surgery, spinal movement is restricted to promote healing of fusion, requiring a longer recuperation time.
Logroll client from side-to-side. Have client fold arms across chest; tighten long back muscles, keeping shoulders and pelvis straight. Use pillows between knees during position change and when on side. Use turning sheet and sufficient personnel when turning, especially on the first postoperative day. Instruct client in these movements as self-care progresses.	Maintains body alignment while turning, preventing twisting motion, which may interfere with healing process.

ACTIONS/INTERVENTIONS	RATIONALE
Assist out of bed: logroll to side of bed, splint back, and raise to sitting position. Avoid prolonged sitting. Move to standing position in single smooth motion.	Avoids twisting and flexing of back while arising from bed/chair, protecting surgical area.
Avoid sudden stretching, twisting, flexing, or jarring of spine.	May cause vertebral collapse, shifting of bone graft, delayed hematoma formation, or subcutaneous wound dehiscence.
Monitor BP; note reports of dizziness or weakness. Recommend client change position slowly.	Presence of postural hypotension may result in fainting/falling and possible injury to surgical site.
Have client wear firm/flat walking shoes when ambulating.	Reduces risk of falls.

Collaborative

Apply lumbar brace/cervical collar as appropriate.	Brace/corset may be used in and/or out of bed during postoperative phase to support spine and surrounding structures until muscle strength improves. Brace is applied while client is supine in bed. Spinal fusion generally requires a lengthy recuperation period in a corset/collar.
Refer to physical therapy. Implement program as outlined.	Strengthening exercises may be initiated during the rehabilitative phase to decrease muscle spasm and strain on the vertebral disc area.

NURSING DIAGNOSIS: risk for ineffective Breathing Pattern/Airway Clearance

Risk factors may include

Tracheal/bronchial obstruction/edema
Decreased lung expansion, pain

Possibly evidenced by

[Not applicable; presence of signs and symptoms establishes an *actual* diagnosis.]

DESIRED OUTCOMES/EVALUATION CRITERIA—CLIENT WILL:

RESPIRATORY STATUS: Ventilation (NOC)

Maintain a normal/effective respiratory pattern free of cyanosis and other signs of hypoxia, with ABGs within acceptable range.

ACTIONS/INTERVENTIONS — RATIONALE

Respiratory Monitoring (NIC)

Independent

ACTIONS/INTERVENTIONS	RATIONALE
Inspect for edema of face/neck (cervical laminectomy), especially first 24–48 hr after surgery.	Tracheal edema/compression or nerve injury can compromise respiratory function.
Listen for hoarseness. Encourage voice rest.	May indicate laryngeal nerve injury or edema of surgical area, which can negatively affect cough (ability to clear airway).
Auscultate breath sounds, note presence of wheezes/rhonchi.	Suggests accumulation of secretions/need to engage in more aggressive therapeutic actions to clear airway.
Assist with coughing, turning, and deep breathing. Encourage client's use of incentive spirometry/other deep breathing devices.	Facilitates movement of secretions and clearing of lungs; reduces risk of respiratory complications (pneumonia, pulmonary embolus).

ACTIONS/INTERVENTIONS	RATIONALE
Collaborative	
Administer supplemental oxygen if indicated.	May be necessary for periods of respiratory distress or evidence of hypoxia.
Monitor/graph ABGs or pulse oximetry.	Monitors effectiveness of breathing pattern/therapy.

NURSING DIAGNOSIS: acute Pain

May be related to

Physical agent: surgical manipulation, edema, inflammation, harvesting of bone graft

Possibly evidenced by

Reports of pain
Autonomic responses: diaphoresis, changes in vital signs, pallor
Alteration in muscle tone
Guarding, distraction behaviors/restlessness

DESIRED OUTCOMES/EVALUATION CRITERIA—CLIENT WILL:

Pain Self-Control (NOC)

Report pain is relieved/controlled.
Verbalize methods that provide relief.
Demonstrate use of relaxation skills and diversional activities.

ACTIONS/INTERVENTIONS	RATIONALE
Pain Management (NIC)	
Independent	
Assess intensity, description, and location/radiation of pain, changes in sensation.	May be mild to severe with radiation to shoulders/occipital area (cervical) or hips/buttocks (lumbar). If bone graft has been taken from the iliac crest, pain may be more severe at the donor site. Numbness/tingling discomfort may reflect return of sensation after nerve root decompression, or result from developing edema causing nerve compression.
Instruct in regular use of rating scale (e.g., 0–10).	Standardized tool for rating pain helps in characterizing pain and in documenting pain and pain management.
Review expected manifestations/changes in intensity of pain.	Development/resolution of edema and inflammation in the immediate postoperative phase can affect pressure on various nerves and cause changes in degree of pain (especially 3 days after procedure, when muscle spasms/improved nerve root sensation intensify pain).
Encourage client to assume position of comfort, as indicated. Use logrolling for position change.	Positioning is dictated by physical preference, type of operation (e.g., head of bed may be slightly elevated after cervical laminectomy). Readjustment of position aids in relieving muscle fatigue and discomfort. Logrolling avoids tension in the operative areas, maintains straight spinal alignment, and reduces risk of displacing epidural client-controlled analgesia (PCA) when used.

ACTIONS/INTERVENTIONS	RATIONALE
Provide back rub/massage, avoiding operative site.	Relieves/reduces pain by alteration of sensory neurons, muscle relaxation.
Demonstrate/encourage use of relaxation skills; e.g., deep breathing, visualization.	Refocuses attention, reduces muscle tension, promotes sense of well-being, and controls/decreases discomfort.
Provide liquid and/or soft diet, room humidifier; encourage voice rest following anterior cervical laminectomy.	Reduces discomfort associated with sore throat and difficulty swallowing.
Investigate client reports of return of radicular pain.	Suggests complications (e.g., collapsing of disc space, shifting of bone graft) requiring further medical evaluation and intervention. *Note:* Sciatica and muscle spasms often recur after laminectomy but should resolve within several days or weeks.

Collaborative

Administer analgesics, as indicated:	
Narcotics; e.g., morphine (MS), codeine, meperidine (Demerol), butorphanol (Stadol), fentanyl (Duragesic), hydromorphone (Dilaudid), oxycodone (Tylox, Percocet), oxycodone compound (Oxycontin, Roxicet) hydrocodone (Vicodin, Lortab);	Narcotics are used during the first few postoperative days, and then nonnarcotic agents are incorporated as intensity of pain diminishes. *Note:* Narcotics may be administered via epidural catheter and patient-controlled analgesia (PCA).
Muscle relaxants; e.g., cyclobenzaprine (Flexeril), diazepam (Valium).	May be used to relieve muscle spasms resulting from intraoperative nerve irritation.
Instruct client in use of/maintain PCA.	Gives client control of medication administration (usually narcotics) to achieve a more constant level of comfort, which may enhance healing and sense of well-being.
Provide throat sprays/lozenges, viscous lidocaine (Xylocaine).	Sore throat may be a major complaint following cervical laminectomy.
Apply TENS unit as needed.	TENS may be used for incisional pain or when nerve involvement continues after discharge. Decreases level of pain by blocking nerve transmission of pain.

NURSING DIAGNOSIS: impaired physical Mobility

May be related to

Neuromusclar impairment
Limitations imposed by condition; pain

Possibly evidenced by

Impaired coordination, limited ROM
Reluctance to attempt movement
Decreased muscle strength/control

DESIRED OUTCOMES/EVALUATION CRITERIA—CLIENT WILL:

KNOWLEDGE: Personal Safety (NOC)

Demonstrate techniques/behaviors that enable resumption of activities.

Mobility (NOC)

Maintain or increase strength and function of affected body part.

ACTIONS/INTERVENTIONS	RATIONALE
Body Mechanics Promotion (NIC)	
Independent	
Schedule activity/procedures with rest periods. Encourage participation in ADLs within individual limitations.	Enhances healing and builds muscle strength and endurance. Client participation promotes independence and sense of control.
Provide/assist with passive and active range of motion and strengthening exercises, depending on surgical procedure.	Strengthens abdominal muscles and flexors of spine; promotes good body mechanics.
Assist with activity/progressive ambulation.	Until healing occurs, activity is limited and advanced slowly according to individual tolerance.
Review proper body mechanics/techniques for participation in activities.	Reduces risk of muscle strain/injury/pain and increases likelihood of client involvement in progressive activity.

Refer to CP: Herniated Nucleus Pulposus (Ruptured Intervertebral Disc), ND: impaired physical Mobility, for further considerations.

NURSING DIAGNOSIS: Constipation

May be related to

Pain and swelling in surgical area
Immobilization, decreased physical activity
Altered nerve stimulation, ileus
Emotional stress, lack of privacy
Changes/restriction of dietary intake

Possibly evidenced by

Decreased bowel sounds
Increased abdominal girth
Abdominal pain/rectal fullness, nausea
Change in frequency, consistency, and amount of stool

DESIRED OUTCOMES/EVALUATION CRITERIA—CLIENT WILL:

Bowel Elimination (NOC)

Reestablish normal patterns of bowel functioning.
Pass stool of soft/semiformed consistency without straining.

ACTIONS/INTERVENTIONS	RATIONALE
Constipation/Impaction Management (NIC)	
Independent	
Note abdominal distention and auscultate bowel sounds.	Distention and absence of bowel sounds indicate that bowel is not functioning, possibly because of sudden loss of parasympathetic enervation of the bowel.
Use fraction or child-size bedpan until allowed out of bed.	Promotes comfort, reduces muscle tension.

ACTIONS/INTERVENTIONS	RATIONALE
Provide privacy.	Promotes psychologic comfort.
Encourage early ambulation.	Stimulates peristalsis, facilitating passage of flatus.

Collaborative

Begin progressive diet as tolerated.	Solid foods are not started until bowel sounds have returned/flatus has been passed and danger of ileus formation has abated.
Provide rectal tube, suppositories, and enemas as needed.	May be necessary to relieve abdominal distention, promote resumption of normal bowel habits.
Administer laxatives, stool softeners as indicated.	Softens stools, promotes normal bowel habits/evacuation, decreases straining.

NURSING DIAGNOSIS: risk for Urinary Retention

Risk factors may include

Pain and swelling in operative area
Need for remaining flat in bed

Possibly evidenced by

[Not applicable; presence of signs and symptoms establishes an *actual* diagnosis.]

DESIRED OUTCOMES/EVALUATION CRITERIA—CLIENT WILL:

Urinary Continence (NOC)

Empty bladder in sufficient amounts.
Be free of bladder distention, with postvoid residuals within normal limits (WNL).

ACTIONS/INTERVENTIONS — RATIONALE

Urinary Retention Care (NIC)

Independent

ACTIONS/INTERVENTIONS	RATIONALE
Observe and record amount/time of voiding.	Determines whether bladder is being emptied and when interventions may be necessary.
Palpate for bladder distention.	May indicate urine retention.
Force fluids.	Maintains kidney function.
Stimulate bladder emptying by running water, pouring warm water over peritoneum, or having client put hand in warm water as needed.	Promotes urination by relaxing urinary sphincter.

Collaborative

Perform ultrasound bladder scan or catheterize for bladder residual after voiding when indicated. Insert/maintain indwelling catheter as needed.	Intermittent or continuous catheterization may be necessary for several days postoperatively until swelling is decreased.

NURSING DIAGNOSIS: deficient Knowledge [Learning Need] regarding condition, prognosis, treatment, self-care, and discharge needs

May be related to

Lack of exposure
Information misinterpretation, lack of recall
Unfamiliarity with information resources

Possibly evidenced by

Request for information, statement of misconception
Inaccurate follow-through of instruction

DESIRED OUTCOMES/EVALUATION CRITERIA—CLIENT WILL:

KNOWLEDGE: Disease Process (NOC)

Verbalize understanding of condition, prognosis, and potential complications.
List signs/symptoms requiring medical follow-up.

KNOWLEDGE: Treatment Regimen (NOC)

Verbalize understanding of therapeutic regimen.
Initiate necessary lifestyle changes.

ACTIONS/INTERVENTIONS	RATIONALE
TEACHING: Disease Process (NIC)	
Independent	
Review particular condition/prognosis.	Individual needs dictate tolerance levels/limitations of activity.
Discuss possibility of unrelieved/renewed pain.	Some pain may continue for several months as activity level increases and scar tissue stretches. Pain relief from surgical procedure could be temporary if other discs in the area have similar amount of degeneration.
Discuss use of heat; e.g., warm packs, heating pad, or showers.	Increased circulation to the back/surgical area transports nutrients for healing to the area and aids in resolution of pathogens/exudates out of the area. Decreases muscle spasms that may result from nerve root irritation during healing process.
Discuss judicious use of cold packs before/after stretching activity if indicated.	May decrease muscle spasm in some instances more effectively than heat.
Avoid tub baths for 3–4 wk, depending on physician recommendation.	Tub baths increase risk of falls and flexing/twisting of spine.
Review dietary/fluid needs.	Should be tailored to reduce risk of constipation, reduce obesity, avoid weight gain, while meeting nutrient needs to facilitate healing. Note: Some sources recommend intake of structural raw materials (e.g., glucosamine, chondroitin, and methylsulfonylmethane [MSM]) for uptake by bone to promote a healthy spine.
Review/reinforce incisional care.	Correct incisional care promotes healing, reduces risk of wound infection. *Note:* This information is especially critical for the client's SO/caregiver in this era of early discharge (sometimes 24 hr after surgery).

ACTIONS/INTERVENTIONS	RATIONALE
Identify signs/symptoms requiring notification of healthcare provider; e.g., fever, increased incisional pain, inflammation, wound drainage, decreased sensation/motor activity in extremities.	Prompt evaluation and intervention may prevent complications/permanent injury.
Discuss necessity of follow-up care.	Long-term medical supervision may be needed to manage problems/complications and to reincorporate individual into desired/altered lifestyle and activities.
Review need for/use of immobilization device, as indicated.	Correct application and wearing time is important to gaining the most benefit from the brace.
Assess current lifestyle/job, finances, activities at home and leisure.	Knowledge of current situation allows nurse to highlight areas for possible intervention, such as referral for occupational/vocational testing and counseling.
Listen/communicate with client regarding alternatives and lifestyle changes. Be sensitive to client's needs.	Low back pain is a frequent cause of chronic disability. Many clients may have to stop/modify work and have had long-term/chronic pain creating relationship and financial crises. Client may be viewed as being a malingerer, which creates further problems in social/work relationships.
Note overt/covert expressions of concern about sexuality.	Although client may not ask directly, there may be concerns about the effect of this surgery on both the ability to cope with usual role in the family/community and ability to perform sexually.
Provide written copy of all instructions.	Useful as a reference after discharge.
Identify community resources as indicated; e.g., social services, rehabilitation/vocational counseling services.	A team effort can be helpful in providing support during recuperative period.
Recommend counseling, sex therapy, psychotherapy as appropriate.	Depression is common in conditions for which a lengthy recuperative time (2–9 months) is expected. Therapy may alleviate anxiety, assist client to cope effectively, and enhance healing process. Presence of physical limitations, pain, and depression may negatively impact sexual desire/performance and add additional stress to relationship.

TEACHING: Prescribed Activity/Exercise (NIC)

ACTIONS/INTERVENTIONS	RATIONALE
Discuss return to activities, stressing importance of increasing as tolerated.	Although the recuperative period may be lengthy, following prescribed activity program promotes muscle and tissue circulation, healing, and strengthening.
Encourage development of regular exercise program; e.g., walking, stretching.	Promotes healing, strengthens abdominal and erector muscles to provide support to the spinal column, and enhances general physical and emotional well-being.
Discuss importance of good posture and avoidance of prolonged standing/sitting. Recommend sitting in straight-backed chair with feet on a footstool or flat on the floor.	Prevents further injuries/stress by maintaining proper alignment of spine.
Stress importance of avoiding activities that increase the flexion of the spine; e.g., climbing stairs, automobile driving/riding, bending at the waist with knees straight, lifting more than 5 lb, engaging in strenuous exercise/sports. Discuss limitations on sexual relations/positions.	Flexing/twisting of the spine aggravates the healing process and increases risk of injury to spinal cord.
Encourage lying-down rest periods, balanced with activity.	Reduces general and spinal fatigue and assists in the healing/recuperative process.
Explore limitations/abilities.	Placing limitations into perspective with abilities allows client to understand own situation and exercise choice.

POTENTIAL CONSIDERATIONS following acute hospitalization (dependent on client's age, physical condition/presence of complications, personal resources, and life responsibilities)

impaired Physical Mobility—decreased strength/endurance, pain, immobilizing device.

Self-Care Deficit—decreased strength/endurance, pain, immobilizing device.

risk for Trauma/Falls—weakness, balancing difficulties, decreased muscle coordination, reduced temperature/tactile sensation.

compromised family Coping—temporary family disorganization and role changes.

CP 6-1 Sample CP: Cervical Laminectomy with Fusion. ELOS: 3 Days Orthopedic or Surgical Unit

ND and Categories of Care	Day 1 Day of Surgery ____	Day 2 POD #1 ____	Day 3 POD #2 ____
Ineffective tissue perfusion, R/T altered blood flow (operative site edema, hematoma formation, hypovolemia)	Goals: Maintain proper alignment of cervical spine Display stable/improved sensation in affected limbs	Display normal sensory/motor response Identify appropriate safety measures	
Diagnostic studies		Hb/Hct, RBC Electrolytes	C-spine-PA/lat
Additional assessments	VS q1h × 4 then q4h	→ qid	→
	Neurovascular checks UE, q1h × 4 then q4h	→ qid	→ q8h
	Dressings/drainage q4h	→	→ q8h
	I&O q8h	→	→ bid
	Hemovac (if used) q8h	→	→ D/C
	Palpate operative site for swelling, inspect face/neck for edema qh × 4	→ q8h	→ D/C
Medications	IV fluids/blood as indicated	→ D/C or convert to NS lock	
Client education	Purpose/necessity of cervical collar	Cessation of smoking if indicated	Use of heat
	Protocol for position change		Signs/symptoms to be reported to healthcare provider
Additional nursing actions	Position per protocol/HOB elevated 30°	→	→
	Logroll q2h	→ Chair ×3	→ Ambulate as tolerated
	Cervical collar in place	→	
	BRP w/assistance (tennis shoes—not slippers)	→	→ Per self as tolerated
	Fluids as tolerated	→ Advanced diet as tolerated	→
Pain R/T surgical intervention	Report pain controlled	→	
		Participate in activities to increase comfort	→ Verbalize understanding of therapeutic interventions
Additional assessments	Pain characteristics/change	→	→
	Response to interventions	→	→
Medications Allergies:____	Analgesics—PCA or IM	→ D/C PCA	→ D/C IM
	Throat spray/lozenges	→ PO analgesics	→
		→	→ D/C
Client education	Orient to unit/room	Relaxation techniques	Use of TENS as indicated
	Reporting of pain/effects of interventions	Medication dose, frequency, purpose, side effects	Signs/symptoms to report to healthcare provider
	Proper use of PCA		

CP 6–1 Sample CP: Cervical Laminectomy with Fusion. ELOS: 3 Days Orthopedic or Surgical Unit

ND and Categories of Care	Day 1 Day of Surgery ___	Day 2 POD #1 ___	Day 3 POD #2 ___
	Recovery/rehabilitation expectations Limitations of movement (e.g., twisting, flexing, pulling) Voice rest (anterior approach)		
Additional nursing actions	Provide firm mattress Comfort measures	→ →	→ →
Impaired physical mobility R/T musculoskeletal impairment; pain and therapeutic restriction		Reestablish normal bowel/bladder elimination	Verbalize understanding of activity program/restrictions Report plan in place to meet needs postdischarge
Referrals	Social Services	Home Care	
Additional assessments	General muscle tone/strength Level of functional ability Breath sounds q4h Bowel sounds q4h Amount/time of voids	→ Ability to perform ADLs → independently → q8h → q8h → D/C Edema, pain lower extremities, Homans' sign q8h	 → → →
Medications		Stool softener	→ Fleets if no BM
Client education	Activity level/progression Bed exercises Skin care needs	General wellness—diet, exercise, adequate rest Home exercise program Proper body mechanics Use of assistive devices as required	Activity restrictions e.g., shower instead of tub bath, no lifting, resumption of work, hobbies, sexual activity Provide written copy of instructions
Additional nursing actions	Assist w/passive and active ROM exercises Encourage participation of ADLs w/in level of ability T, C, DB, q2h Incentive spirometry q4h Thigh-high TEDs Skin care per Risk Protocol	→ → → → q4h while awake → Remove q8h →	→ → Per self → Per self → D/C → D/C →

SPINAL CORD INJURY (ACUTE REHABILITATIVE PHASE)

The leading causes of *spinal cord injury* (SCI) include motor vehicle crashes, falls, acts of violence, and sporting injuries. The mechanism of injury influences the type of SCI and the degree of neurologic deficit. Spinal cord lesions are classified as complete (total loss of sensation and voluntary motor function) or incomplete (mixed loss of sensation and voluntary motor function).

Physical findings vary depending on the level of injury, degree of spinal shock, and phase and degree of recovery, but, in general, are classified as follows:

C-1 to C-3: Tetraplegia with total loss of muscular/respiratory function.

C-4 to C-5: Tetraplegia with impairment, poor pulmonary capacity, complete dependency for ADLs.

C-6 to C-7: Tetraplegia with some arm/hand movement allowing some independence in upper body ADLs.

C-7 to T-1: Tetraplegia with limited use of thumb/fingers, increasing independence.

T-2 to L-1: Paraplegia with intact arm function, varying function of intercostal and abdominal muscles, and loss of function below level of injury.

L-1 to L-2 or below: Mixed motor-sensory loss; bowel and bladder dysfunction.

CARE SETTING

Inpatient medical/surgical and subacute/rehabilitation units.

RELATED CONCERNS

Disc surgery, page 260
Fractures, page 442
Pneumonia, page 128
Psychosocial aspects of care, page 770
Thrombophlebitis: deep vein thrombosis, page 108
Total nutritional support: parenteral/enteral feeding, page 478
Upper gastrointestinal/esophageal bleeding, page 309
Ventilatory assistance (mechanical), page 170

Client Assessment Database

ACTIVITY/REST

May exhibit: Paralysis of muscles (flaccid during spinal shock) at/below level of lesion
Muscle/generalized weakness (cord contusion and compression)

CIRCULATION:

May report: Palpitations
Dizziness with position changes

May exhibit: Low BP, postural BP changes, bradycardia
Cool, pale extremities
Absence of perspiration in affected area

ELIMINATION

May exhibit: Incontinence of bladder and bowel
Urinary retention
Abdominal distention; loss of bowel sounds
Melena, coffee-ground emesis/hematemesis

EGO INTEGRITY

May report: Denial, disbelief, sadness, anger

May exhibit: Fear, anxiety, irritability, withdrawal

FOOD/FLUID

May exhibit: Abdominal distention, loss of bowel sounds (paralytic ileus)

HYGIENE

May exhibit: Variable level of dependence in ADLs

NEUROSENSORY

May report: Absence of sensation below area of injury or opposite side sensation
Numbness, tingling, burning, twitching of arms/legs

May exhibit: Flaccid paralysis (spasticity may develop as spinal shock resolves, depending on area of cord involvement)
Loss of sensation (varying degrees may return after spinal shock resolves)
Loss of muscle/vasomotor tone
Loss of/asymmetrical reflexes, including deep tendon reflexes
Changes in pupil reaction, ptosis of upper eyelid
Loss of sweating in affected area

PAIN/DISCOMFORT

May report: Pain/tenderness in muscles
Hyperesthesia immediately above level of injury

May exhibit: Vertebral tenderness, deformity

RESPIRATION

May report: Shortness of breath, "air hunger," inability to breathe

May exhibit: Shallow/labored respirations, periods of apnea
Diminished breath sounds, rhonchi
Pallor, cyanosis

SAFETY

May exhibit: Temperature fluctuations (taking on temperature of environment)

SEXUALITY

May report: Expressions of concern about return to normal functioning

May exhibit: Uncontrolled erection (priapism)
Menstrual irregularities

TEACHING/LEARNING

Discharge plan considerations: Will require varying degrees of assistance with transportation, shopping, food preparation, self-care, finances, medications/treatment, and homemaker/maintenance tasks
May require changes in physical layout of home and/or placement in a rehabilitative center

Refer to section at end of plan for postdischarge considerations.

DIAGNOSTIC STUDIES

Spinal radiograph: Locates level and type of bony injury (fracture, dislocation); determines alignment and reduction after traction or surgery.

CT scan: Done emergently to locate injury, and evaluates structural alterations. Useful for rapid screening and providing additional information if x-rays questionable for fracture/cord status. Scanning should include the entire spine.

MRI: Identifies spinal cord lesions, edema, and compression.

Myelogram: May be done to visualize spinal column if pathology is unclear or if occlusion of spinal subarachnoid space is suspected (not usually done after penetrating injuries).

Somatosensory evoked potential (SEP): Elicited by presenting a peripheral stimulus and measuring degree of latency in cortical response to evaluate spinal cord functioning/potential for recovery.

Chest x-ray: Demonstrates pulmonary status (e.g., changes in level of diaphragm, atelectasis).

Pulmonary function studies (vital capacity, tidal volume): Measures maximum volume of inspiration and expiration; especially important in clients with low cervical lesions or thoracic lesions with possible phrenic nerve and intercostal muscle involvement.

ABGs: Indicates effectiveness of gas exchange and ventilatory effort.

NURSING PRIORITIES

1. Maximize respiratory function.
2. Prevent further injury to spinal cord.
3. Promote mobility/independence.
4. Prevent or minimize complications.
5. Support psychological adjustment of client/SO.
6. Provide information about injury, prognosis and expectations, treatment needs, possible and preventable complications.

DISCHARGE GOALS

1. Ventilatory effort adequate for individual needs.
2. Spinal injury stabilized.
3. Complications prevented/controlled.
4. Self-care needs met by self/with assistance, depending on specific situation.
5. Beginning to cope with current situation and planning for future.
6. Condition/prognosis, therapeutic regimen, and possible complications understood.
7. Plan in place to meet needs after discharge.

NURSING DIAGNOSIS: risk for ineffective Breathing Pattern

Risk factors may include

Impairment of innervation of diaphragm (lesions at or above C-5)
Complete or mixed loss of intercostal muscle function
Reflex abdominal spasms; gastric distention

Possibly evidenced by

[Not applicable; presence of signs and symptoms establishes an *actual* diagnosis.]

DESIRED OUTCOMES/EVALUATION CRITERIA—CLIENT WILL:

RESPIRATORY STATUS: Ventilation (NOC)

Maintain adequate ventilation as evidenced by absence of respiratory distress and ABGs within acceptable limits, pulse oximetry maintained at 90% or greater.
Demonstrate appropriate behaviors to support respiratory effort.

ACTIONS/INTERVENTIONS	RATIONALE
Respiratory Monitoring (NIC)	
Independent	
Note client's level of injury when assessing respiratory function. Note presence or absence of spontaneous effort and quality of respirations; e.g., labored, using accessory muscles.	C-1 to C-3 injuries result in complete loss of respiratory function. Injuries at C-4 or C-5 can result in variable loss of respiratory function, depending on phrenic nerve involvement and diaphragmatic function, but generally cause decreased vital capacity and inspiratory effort. For injuries below C-6 or C-7, respiratory muscle function is preserved; however, weakness/impairment of intercostal muscles may impair effectiveness of cough and the ability to sigh, deep breathe.
Auscultate breath sounds. Note areas of absent or decreased breath sounds or development of adventitious sounds (e.g., rhonchi).	Hypoventilation is common and leads to accumulation of secretions, atelectasis, and pneumonia (frequent complications). *Note:* Respiratory compromise is one of the leading causes of mortality, especially during the acute stage as well as later in life.
Note strength/effectiveness of cough.	Level of injury determines function of intercostal muscles and ability to cough spontaneously/move secretions. High-level paraplegics and all tetraplegics lose the ability to cough, and are at greatest risk of developing atelectasis and respiratory failure.
Observe skin color for developing cyanosis, duskiness.	May reveal impending respiratory failure, need for immediate medical evaluation and intervention.
Assess for abdominal distention and muscle spasm.	Abdominal fullness may impede diaphragmatic excursion, reducing lung expansion and further compromising respiratory function.
Monitor/limit visitors as indicated.	General debilitation and respiratory compromise place client at increased risk for acquiring URIs.
Monitor diaphragmatic movement if phrenic pacemaker is implanted.	Stimulation of phrenic nerve may enhance respiratory effort, decreasing dependency on mechanical ventilator.
Elicit concerns/questions regarding mechanical ventilation devices.	Acknowledges reality of situation. (Refer to CP: Ventilatory Assistance [Mechanical].)
Provide honest answers.	Future respiratory function/support needs will not be totally known until spinal shock resolves and acute rehabilitative phase is completed. Even though respiratory support may be required, alternative devices/techniques may be used to enhance mobility and promote independence.
Maintain client airway: keep head in neutral position, elevate head of bed slightly if tolerated, and use airway adjuncts as indicated.	Clients with high cervical injury and impaired gag/cough reflex require assistance in preventing aspiration/maintaining patent airway.
Assist client in "taking control" of respirations as indicated. Instruct in and encourage deep breathing, focusing attention on steps of breathing.	Breathing may no longer be a totally involuntary activity but require conscious effort, depending on level of injury/involvement of respiratory muscles.
Assist with coughing as indicated for level of injury; e.g., have client take deep breath and hold for 2 sec before coughing, or inhale deeply, then cough at the end of a slow exhalation. Alternatively, assist by placing hands below diaphragm and pushing upward as client exhales (quad cough).	Adds volume to cough and facilitates expectoration of secretions or helps move them high enough to be suctioned out. *Note:* Quad cough procedure is generally reserved for clients with stable injuries once they are in the rehabilitation stage.

ACTIONS/INTERVENTIONS	RATIONALE
Suction as necessary. Monitor pulse oximetry and heart rate during suctioning. Document quality and quantity of secretions.	If cough is ineffective, suctioning may be needed to remove secretions, enhance gas exchange, and reduce risk of respiratory infections. *Note:* "Routine" suctioning increases risk of hypoxia and bradycardia (especially with higher level tetraplegia). Heart rate should ideally be between 60 and 100. Therefore, suctioning needs are based on presence of/inability to move secretions.
Reposition/turn periodically. Avoid/limit prone position when indicated.	Enhances ventilation of all lung segments, mobilizes secretions, reducing risk of complications such as atelectasis and pneumonia. *Note:* Prone position significantly decreases vital capacity, increasing risk of respiratory compromise/failure.
Encourage fluids (at least 2000 mL/day).	Aids in liquefying secretions, promoting mobilization/expectoration.

Collaborative

Measure/graph:	
Vital capacity (VC), tidal volume (V_T), inspiratory force;	Determines level of respiratory muscle function. Serial measurements may be done to predict impending respiratory failure (acute injury) or determine level of function after spinal shock phase and/or while weaning from ventilatory support.
Serial ABGs and/or pulse oximetry.	Documents status of ventilation and oxygenation identifies respiratory problems; e.g., hypoventilation (low PaO_2/elevated $PaCO_2$) and pulmonary complications.

Airway Management (NIC)

Administer oxygen by appropriate method; e.g., nasal prongs, mask, intubation/ventilator.	Method is determined by level of injury, degree of respiratory insufficiency, and amount of recovery of respiratory muscle function after spinal shock phase.
Assist with use of respiratory adjuncts (e.g., incentive spirometer, blow bottles) and aggressive chest physiotherapy (e.g., chest percussion).	Preventing retained secretions is essential to maximize gas diffusion and to reduce risk of pneumonia.
Refer to/consult with respiratory and physical therapists.	Helpful in identifying individually appropriate therapies/mechanisms to stimulate or strengthen respiratory muscles/effort. For example, glossopharyngeal breathing uses muscles of mouth, pharynx, and larynx to swallow air into lungs, thereby enhancing VC and chest expansion.

NURSING DIAGNOSIS: risk for [additional spinal] Trauma

Risk factors may include

Temporary weakness/instability of spinal column

Possibly evidenced by

[Not applicable; presence of signs and symptoms establishes an *actual* diagnosis.]

DESIRED OUTCOMES/EVALUATION CRITERIA—CLIENT WILL:

Bone Healing (NOC)

Maintain proper alignment of spine without further spinal cord damage.

ACTIONS/INTERVENTIONS	RATIONALE
Traction/Immobilization Care (NIC)	
Independent	
Maintain bedrest and immobilization device(s); e.g., sandbags, traction, halo, hard/soft cervical collars, brace.	Immobilization prevents vertebral column instability and aids healing. *Note:* Traction is used only for cervical spine stabilization.
Check external stabilization device; e.g., Gardner-Wells tongs or skeletal traction apparatus.	These devices are used for decompression of spinal fractures and stabilization of vertebral column during the early acute phase of injury to prevent further spinal cord damage.
Elevate head of traction frame or bed as indicated. Ensure that traction frames are secure, pulleys aligned, weights hanging free.	Creates safe, effective counterbalance to maintain both client's alignment and traction pull.
Check weights for ordered traction pull (usually 10–20 lb).	Weight pull depends on client's size and amount of reduction needed to maintain vertebral column alignment.
Reposition at intervals, using adjuncts for turning and support; e.g., turn sheets, foam wedges, blanket rolls, pillows. Use several staff members when turning/logrolling client. Follow special instructions for traction equipment, kinetic bed, and frames once halo is in place.	Maintains proper spinal column alignment, reducing risk of further trauma. *Note:* Grasping the brace/halo vest to turn or reposition client may cause additional injury.
Collaborative	
Assist with preparation/maintain skeletal traction via tongs, calipers, halo/vest, as indicated.	Reduces vertebral fracture/dislocation.
Prepare for internal stabilization surgery, e.g., spinal laminectomy or fusion, if indicated.	Surgery may be indicated for spinal stabilization/cord decompression or removal of bony fragments.
Administer medications as indicated; e.g., dexamethasone (Decadron), methylprednisolone (Depo-Medrol)	Although many experts recommend the use of high-dose cortisone within 8 hr of non-penetrating SCI as the Standard of Care, many national organizations are now changing their recommendations to include this therapy for the improvement of neurologic outcome, but are not requiring it, suggesting that its benefits be weighed against the client's potential for developing sepsis.

NURSING DIAGNOSIS: impaired physical Mobility

May be related to

Neuromuscular impairment
Immobilization by traction

Possibly evidenced by

Inability to purposefully move, paralysis
Muscle atrophy, contractures

DESIRED OUTCOMES/EVALUATION CRITERIA—CLIENT WILL:

IMMOBILITY CONSEQUENCES: Physiologic (NOC)

Maintain position of function as evidenced by absence of contractures, footdrop.

NEUROLOGIC STATUS: Spinal Sensory/Motor Function (NOC)

Increase strength of unaffected/compensatory body parts.
Demonstrate techniques/behaviors that enable resumption of activity.

ACTIONS/INTERVENTIONS	RATIONALE
Bed Rest Care (NIC)	
Independent	
Continually assess motor function (as spinal shock/edema resolves) by requesting client to perform certain actions; e.g., shrug shoulders, spread fingers, squeeze/release examiner's hands.	Evaluates status of individual situation (motor-sensory impairment may be mixed and/or not clear) for a specific level of injury, affecting type and choice of interventions.
Provide means to summon help; e.g., special sensitive call light.	Enables client to have a sense of control, and reduces fear of being left alone. *Note:* Tetradriplegic on ventilator requires continuous observation in early management.
Perform/assist with full ROM exercises on all extremities and joints, using slow, smooth movements. Hyperextend hips periodically.	Enhances circulation, restores/maintains muscle tone and joint mobility, and prevents disuse contractures and muscle atrophy.
Position arms at 90-degree angle at regular intervals.	Prevents frozen shoulder contractures.
Maintain ankles at 90 degrees with footboard, high-top tennis shoes, and so on. Place trochanter rolls along thighs when in bed.	Prevents footdrop and external rotation of hips.
Elevate lower extremities at intervals when in chair, or raise foot of bed when permitted in individual situation. Assess for edema of feet/ankles.	Loss of vascular tone and "muscle action" results in pooling of blood and venous stasis in the lower abdomen and lower extremities, with increased risk of hypotension and thrombus formation.
Plan activities to provide uninterrupted rest periods. Encourage involvement within individual tolerance/ability.	Prevents fatigue, allowing opportunity for maximal efforts/participation by client.
Measure/monitor BP before and after activity in acute phases or until stable. Change position slowly. Use cardiac bed or tilt table/CircOlectric bed as activity level is advanced.	Orthostatic hypotension may occur as a result of venous pooling (secondary to loss of sympathetic innervation, when injury is at T-6 and higher). Side-to-side movement or elevation of head can aggravate hypotension and cause syncope.
Reposition periodically even when sitting in chair. Teach client how to use weight-shifting techniques.	Reduces pressure areas, promotes peripheral circulation.
Prepare for weight-bearing activities; e.g., use of tilt table for upright position, strengthening/conditioning exercises for unaffected body parts.	Early weight bearing reduces osteoporotic changes in long bones and reduces incidence of urinary infections and kidney stones. *Note:* Fifty percent of clients develop heterotopic ossification that can lead to pain and decreased joint flexibility
Encourage use of relaxation techniques.	Reduces muscle tension/fatigue, may help limit pain of muscle spasms, spasticity.
Inspect skin daily. Observe for pressure areas, and provide meticulous skin care. Teach client to inspect skin surfaces and to use a mirror to look at hard-to-see-areas.	Altered circulation, loss of sensation, and paralysis potentiate pressure sore formation. This is a lifelong consideration. (Refer to ND: risk for impaired Skin Integrity.)
Assist with/encourage pulmonary hygiene; e.g., deep breathing, coughing, suctioning. (Refer to ND: risk for ineffective Breathing Pattern.)	Immobility and bedrest increase risk of pulmonary infection.
Assess for redness, swelling/muscle tension of calf tissues. Record calf and thigh measurements as indicated.	In a high percentage of clients with cervical cord injury, thrombi develop because of altered peripheral circulation, immobilization, and flaccid paralysis. Risk is greatest during the 2 weeks immediately following injury, but risk persists throughout lifespan.
Investigate sudden onset of dyspnea, cyanosis, and/or other signs of respiratory distress.	Development of pulmonary emboli may be "silent" because pain perception is altered and/or DVT is not readily recognized.
Collaborative	
Place client in kinetic therapy bed when appropriate.	Effectively immobilizes unstable spinal column and improves systemic circulation, which is thought to decrease complications associated with immobility.
Apply antiembolic hose/leotard or sequential compression devices (SCDs) to legs as appropriate.	Limits pooling of blood in lower extremities or abdomen, thus improving vasomotor tone and reducing incidence of thrombus formation and pulmonary emboli.

ACTIONS/INTERVENTIONS	RATIONALE
Consult with physical/occupational therapists/rehabilitation team.	Helpful in planning and implementing individualized exercise program and identifying/developing assistive devices to maintain function, enhance mobility and independence.
Administer medications as indicated:	
Vasopressors; e.g., dobutamine (Dobutrex);	May be indicated in acute phase to maintain systolic blood pressure greater than 100. Client requiring this level of support will likely be in an ICU.
Muscle relaxants/antispasticity agents as indicated; e.g., diazepam (Valium), baclofen (Lioresal), dantrolene (Dantrium);	May be useful (after spinal shock phase) in limiting or reducing pain associated with spasticity. *Note:* Baclofen may be delivered via implanted intrathecal pump on a long-term basis as appropriate.
Tizanidine (Zanaflex).	Centrally acting α_2-adrenergic agonist reduces spasticity. Short duration of action requires careful dosage monitoring to achieve maximum effect. May have additive effect with baclofen, but needs to be used with caution because both drugs have similar side effects.

NURSING DIAGNOSIS: disturbed Sensory Perception

May be related to

Destruction of sensory tracts with altered sensory reception, transmission, and integration
Reduced environmental stimuli
Psychologic stress (narrowed perceptual fields caused by anxiety)

Possibly evidenced by

Measured change in sensory acuity, including position of body parts/proprioception
Change in usual response to stimuli
Motor incoordination
Anxiety, disorientation, bizarre thinking; exaggerated emotional responses

DESIRED OUTCOMES/EVALUATION CRITERIA—CLIENT WILL:

NEUROLOGIC STATUS: Spinal Sensory/Motor Function (NOC)

Recognize sensory impairments.

KNOWLEDGE: Personal Safety (NOC)

Identify behaviors to compensate for deficits.
Verbalize awareness of sensory needs and potential for deprivation/overload.

ACTIONS/INTERVENTIONS	RATIONALE
Peripheral Sensation Management (NIC)	
Independent	
Assess/document sensory function or deficit (e.g., by means of touch, pinprick, hot/cold), progressing from area of deficit to neurologically intact area.	Changes may not occur during acute phase, but as spinal shock resolves, changes should be documented by dermatome charts or anatomic landmarks; e.g., "2 inches above nipple line."
Protect from bodily harm; e.g., falls, burns, positioning of arm or objects.	Client may not sense pain or be aware of body position.

ACTIONS/INTERVENTIONS	RATIONALE
Assist client to recognize and compensate for alterations in sensation.	May help reduce anxiety of the unknown and prevent injury.
Explain procedures before and during care, identifying the body part involved.	Enhances client perception of "whole" body.
Provide tactile stimulation, touching client in intact sensory areas; e.g., shoulders, face, head.	Touching conveys caring and fulfills normal physiologic and psychologic needs.
Position client to see surroundings and activities. Provide prism glasses when prone on turning frame. Talk to client frequently.	Provides sensory input, which may be severely limited, especially when client is in prone position.
Provide diversional activities; e.g., television, radio, music, liberal visitation. Use clocks, calendars, pictures, bulletin boards, and so on. Encourage SO/family to discuss general and personal news.	Aids in maintaining reality orientation and provides some sense of normality in daily passage of time.
Provide uninterrupted sleep and rest periods.	Reduces sensory overload, enhances orientation and coping abilities, and aids in reestablishing natural sleep patterns.
Note presence of exaggerated emotional responses, altered thought processes; e.g., disorientation, bizarre thinking.	Indicative of damage to sensory tracts and/or psychologic stress, requiring further assessment and intervention.

NURSING DIAGNOSIS: acute Pain

May be related to

Physical injury
Traction apparatus

Possibly evidenced by

Hyperesthesia immediately above level of injury
Burning pain below level of injury (paraplegia)
Muscle spasm/spasticity
Phantom pain, headaches

DESIRED OUTCOMES/EVALUATION CRITERIA—CLIENT WILL:

Pain Level (NOC)

Report relief or control of pain/discomfort.

Pain Control (NOC)

Identify ways to manage pain.
Demonstrate use of relaxation skills and diversional activities as individually indicated.

ACTIONS/INTERVENTIONS	RATIONALE
Pain Management (NIC)	
Independent	
Assess for presence of pain. Help client identify and quantify pain; e.g., location, type of pain, intensity on scale of 0–10.	Client usually reports pain above the level of injury (e.g., chest/back or headache possibly from stabilizer apparatus). After resolution of spinal shock phase, client may also report muscle spasms and radicular pain, described as a burning or stabbing pain (associated with injury to peripheral nerves and radiating in a dermatomal pattern). Onset of this pain is within days to weeks after SCI and may become chronic.

ACTIONS/INTERVENTIONS	RATIONALE
Evaluate increased irritability, muscle tension, restlessness, unexplained vital sign changes.	Nonverbal cues indicative of pain/discomfort requiring intervention.
Assist client in identifying precipitating factors.	Burning pain and muscle spasms can be precipitated/aggravated by multiple factors; e.g., anxiety, tension, external temperature extremes, sitting for long periods, bladder distention.
Provide comfort measures, e.g., position changes, massage, ROM exercises, warm/cold packs, as indicated.	Alternative measures for pain control are desirable for emotional benefit, in addition to reducing pain medication needs/undesirable effects on respiratory function.
Encourage use of relaxation techniques; e.g., guided imagery, visualization, deep-breathing exercises. Provide diversional activities, e.g., television, radio, telephone, unlimited visitors, as appropriate.	Refocuses attention, promotes sense of control, and may enhance coping abilities.
Collaborative	
Administer medications as indicated: muscle relaxants (e.g., dantrolene {Dantrium], baclofen [Lioresal]); analgesics; antianxiety agents (e.g., diazepam [Valium]).	May be desired to relieve muscle spasm/pain associated with spasticity or to alleviate anxiety and promote rest.

NURSING DIAGNOSIS: anticipatory Grieving

May be related to

Perceived/actual loss of physiopsychosocial well-being

Possibly evidenced by

Altered communication patterns
Expression of distress, choked feelings, e.g., denial, guilt, fear, sadness; altered affect
Alterations in sleep patterns

DESIRED OUTCOMES/EVALUATION CRITERIA—CLIENT WILL:

Grief Resolution (NOC)

Express feelings freely/effectively.
Begin to progress through recognized stages of grief, focusing on 1 day at a time.

ACTIONS/INTERVENTIONS	RATIONALE
Grief Work Facilitation (NIC)	
Independent	
Identify signs of grieving (e.g., shock, denial, anger, depression).	Client experiences a wide range of emotional reactions to the injury and its actual/potential impact on life. These stages are not static, and the rate at which client progresses through them is variable.
Shock Note lack of communication or emotional response, absence of questions.	Shock is the initial reaction associated with overwhelming injury. Primary concern is to maintain life, and client may be too ill to express feelings.

ACTIONS/INTERVENTIONS	RATIONALE
Provide simple, accurate information to client and SO regarding diagnosis and care. Be honest; do not give false reassurance while providing emotional support.	Client's awareness of surroundings and activity may be blocked initially, and attention span may be limited. Little is actually known about the final outcome of client's injuries during acute phase, and lack of knowledge may add to frustration and grief of family. Therefore, early focus of emotional support may be directed toward SO.
Encourage expressions of sadness, grief, guilt, and fear among client/SO/friends.	Knowledge that these are appropriate feelings that should be expressed may be very supportive to client/SO.
Incorporate SO into problem solving and planning for client's care.	Assists in establishing therapeutic relationships. Provides some sense of control of situation of many losses/forced changes, and promotes well-being of client.
Denial	
Assist client/SO to verbalize feelings about situation, avoiding judgment about what is expressed.	Important beginning step to deal with what has happened. Helpful in identifying client's coping mechanisms.
Note comments indicating that client expects to walk shortly and/or is making a bargain with God. Do not confront these comments in early phases of rehabilitation.	Client may not deny entire disability but may deny its permanency. Situation is compounded by actual uncertainty of outcome, and denial may be useful for coping at this time.
Focus on present needs (e.g., ROM exercises, skin care).	Attention on "here and now" reduces frustration and hopelessness of uncertain future and may make dealing with today's problems more manageable.
Anger	
Identify use of manipulative behavior and reactions to caregivers.	Client may express anger verbally or physically (e.g., spitting, biting). Client may say that nothing is done right by caregivers/SO or may pit one caregiver against another.
Encourage client to take control when possible; e.g., establishing care routines, dietary choices, diversional activities.	Helps reduce anger associated with powerlessness, and provides client with some sense of control and expectation of responsibility for own behavior.
Accept expressions of anger and hopelessness (e.g., "let me die"). Avoid arguing. Show concern for client.	Client is acknowledged as a worthwhile individual, and compassionate, nonjudgmental care is provided.
Set limits on acting out and unacceptable behavior when necessary (e.g., abusive language, sexually aggressive or suggestive behavior).	Although it is important to express negative feelings, client and staff need to be protected from violence and embarrassment. This phase is traumatic for all involved, and support of family is essential.
Depression	
Note loss of interest in living, sleep disturbance, suicidal thoughts, hopelessness. Listen to, but do not confront, these expressions. Let client know nurse is available for support.	Phase may last weeks, months, or even years. Acceptance of these feelings and consistent support during this phase are important to a satisfactory resolution. May need psychologic counseling.
Arrange visit by individual similarly affected as appropriate.	Talking with another person who has shared similar feelings/fears and survived may help client reach acceptance of reality of condition and deal with perceived/actual losses.

Collaborative

Consult with/refer to psychiatric nurse, social worker, psychiatrist, pastor.	Client/SO need assistance to work through feelings of alienation, guilt, and resentment concerning lifestyle and role changes. The family (required to make adaptive changes to a member who may be permanently "different") benefit from supportive, long-term assistance and/or counseling in coping with these changes and the future. Client and SO may suffer great spiritual distress, including feelings of guilt, deprivation of peace, and anger at God, which may interfere with progression through/resolution of grief process.

NURSING DIAGNOSIS: situational low Self-Esteem

May be related to

Traumatic injury, situational crisis, forced crisis

Possibly evidenced by

Verbalization of forced change in lifestyle
Fear of rejection/reaction by others
Focus on past strength, function, or appearance
Negative feelings about body
Feelings of helplessness, hopelessness, or powerlessness
Actual change in structure and/or function
Lack of eye contact
Change in physical capacity to resume role
Confusion about self, purpose, or direction of life

DESIRED OUTCOMES/EVALUATION CRITERIA—CLIENT WILL:

PSYCHOSOCIAL ADJUSTMENT: Life Change (NOC)

Verbalize acceptance of self in situation.
Recognize and incorporate changes into self-concept in accurate manner without negating self-esteem.
Develop realistic plans for adapting to new role/role changes.

ACTIONS/INTERVENTIONS	RATIONALE
Self-Esteem Enhancement (NIC)	
Independent	
Acknowledge difficulty in determining degree of functional incapacity and/or chance of functional improvement.	During acute phase of injury, long-term effects are unknown, which delays the client's ability to integrate situation into self-concept.
Listen to client's comments and responses to situation.	Provides clues to view of self, role changes, and needs and is useful for providing information at client's level of acceptance.
Assess dynamics of client and SOs (e.g., client's role in family, cultural factors).	Client's previous role in family unit is disrupted or altered by injury, adding to difficulty in integrating self-concept. In addition, issues of independence/dependence need to be addressed.
Encourage SO to treat client as normally as possible (e.g., discussing home situations, family news).	Involving client in family unit reduces feelings of social isolation, helplessness, and uselessness and provides opportunity for SO to contribute to client's welfare.
Provide accurate information. Discuss concerns about prognosis and treatment honestly at client's level of acceptance.	Focus of information should be on present and immediate needs initially and incorporated into long-term rehabilitation goals. Information should be repeated until client has assimilated or integrated information.
Discuss meaning of loss or change with client/SO. Assess interactions between client and SO.	Actual change in body image may be different from that perceived by client. Distortions may be unconsciously reinforced by SO.
Accept client, show concern for individual as a person. Identify and build on client's strengths, give positive reinforcement for progress noted.	Establishes therapeutic atmosphere for client to begin self-acceptance. Provides encouragement.

ACTIONS/INTERVENTIONS	RATIONALE
Include client/SO in care, allowing client to make decisions and participate in self-care activities as possible.	Recognizes that client is still responsible for own life and provides some sense of control over situation. Sets stage for future lifestyle, pattern, and interaction required in daily care. *Note:* Client may reject all help or may be completely dependent during this phase.
Be alert to sexually oriented jokes/flirting or aggressive behavior. Elicit concerns, fears, and feelings about current situation/future expectations.	Anxiety develops as a result of perceived loss/change in masculine/feminine self-image and role. Forced dependency is often devastating, especially in light of change in function/appearance.
Be aware of own feelings/reaction to client's sexual anxiety.	Behavior may be disruptive, creating conflict between client/staff, further reinforcing negative feelings and possibly eliminating client's desire to work through situation/participate in rehabilitation.
Arrange visit by similarly affected person if client desires and/or situation allows.	May be helpful to client by providing hope for the future/role model. Can be a vital postdischarge resource during the difficult period of adjustment after injury.

Collaborative

Refer to counseling/psychotherapy as indicated; e.g., psychiatric clinical nurse specialist, psychiatrist, social worker, sex therapist.	May need additional assistance to adjust to change in body image/life.

NURSING DIAGNOSIS: Bowel Incontinence/Constipation

May be related to

Disruption of innervation to bowel and rectum
Perceptual impairment
Altered dietary and fluid intake
Change in activity level
Medications

Possibly evidenced by

Loss of ability to evacuate bowel voluntarily
Constipation
Gastric dilation, ileus

DESIRED OUTCOMES/EVALUATION CRITERIA—CLIENT WILL:

Bowel Continence (NOC)

Verbalize behaviors/techniques for individual bowel program.
Reestablish satisfactory bowel elimination pattern.

ACTIONS/INTERVENTIONS	RATIONALE
Bowel Management (NIC)	
Independent	
Auscultate bowel sounds, noting location and characteristics.	Bowel sounds may be absent during spinal shock phase. High tinkling sounds may indicate presence of ileus.

ACTIONS/INTERVENTIONS	RATIONALE
Observe for abdominal distention if bowel sounds are decreased or absent.	Loss of peristalsis (related to impaired innervation) paralyzes the bowel, creating ileus and bowel distention. *Note:* Overdistention of the bowel is a precipitator of autonomic dysreflexia once spinal shock subsides. (Refer to ND: risk for Autonomic Dysreflexia.)
Note reports of nausea, onset of vomiting. Check vomitus or gastric secretions (if tube in place) and stools for occult blood.	GI bleeding may occur in response to injury (Curling's ulcer) or as a side effect of certain therapies (steroids or anticoagulants).
Record frequency, characteristics, and amount of stool.	Identifies degree of impairment/dysfunction and level of assistance required.
Recognize signs of/check for presence of impaction; e.g., no formed stool for several days, semiliquid stool, restlessness, increased feelings of fullness in/distention of abdomen, presence of nausea, vomiting, and possibly urinary retention.	Early intervention is necessary to effectively treat constipation/retained stool and reduce risk of complications.
Establish regular daily bowel program; e.g., digital stimulation, prune juice and/or warm beverage, and use of stool softeners/suppositories at set intervals. Determine a time/routine of bowel evacuation, so it is the same every day.	A lifelong program is necessary to routinely evacuate the bowel because the ability to control bowel evacuation is important to the client's physical independence and social acceptance. *Note:* Bowel movements in clients with upper motor neuron damage are generally regulated with suppositories or digital stimulation. Lower motor neurogenic bowel is more difficult to regulate and usually requires manual disimpaction. Incorporating elements of client's usual routine may enhance cooperation and success of program. *Note:* Many clients prefer morning program rather than evening schedule often practiced in acute/rehab setting.
Encourage well-balanced diet that includes bulk and roughage and increased fluid intake (at least 2000 mL/day), including fruit juices.	Improves consistency of stool for transit through the bowel. *Note:* Mixture of prune juice, applesauce, and bran often provides adequate fiber for effective bowel management, or an OTC fiber-containing product.
Assist with/encourage exercise and activity within individual ability and up in chair as tolerated.	Improves appetite and muscle tone, enhancing GI motility.
Observe for incontinence and help client relate incontinence to change in diet or routine.	Client can eventually achieve fairly normal routine bowel habits, which enhance independence, self-esteem, and socialization.
Restrict intake of grapefruit juice and caffeinated beverages (e.g., coffee, tea, cola, chocolate).	Diuretic effect can reduce fluid available in the bowel, increasing risk of dry/hard formed stool.
Provide meticulous skin care.	Loss of sphincter control and innervation in the area potentiates risk of skin irritation/breakdown.

Collaborative

ACTIONS/INTERVENTIONS	RATIONALE
Insert/maintain nasogastric tube and attach to suction if appropriate.	May be used initially to reduce gastric distention and prevent vomiting (reduces risk of aspiration).
Consult with dietitian/nutritional support team.	Aids in creating dietary plan to meet individual nutritional needs with consideration of state of digestion/bowel function.
Administer medications as indicated; e.g.:	
Stool softeners, laxatives, suppositories, enemas (e.g., Therevac-SB);	Stimulates peristalsis and routine bowel evacuation when necessary. Suppositories should be warmed to room temperature and lubricated before insertion. Therevac-SB is a 4-mL minienema of docusate and glycerin that may reduce time for bowel care by as much as 1 hr.
Antacids, and/or histamine H_2 antagonists; e.g., cimetidine (Tagamet), ranitidine (Zantac).	Reduces or neutralizes gastric acid to lessen gastric irritation and risk of bleeding.

NURSING DIAGNOSIS: impaired Urinary Elimination

May be related to

Disruption in bladder innervation
Bladder atony
Fecal impaction

Possibly evidenced by

Bladder distention; incontinence/overflow, retention
Urinary tract infections
Bladder, kidney stone formation
Renal dysfunction

DESIRED OUTCOMES/EVALUATION CRITERIA—CLIENT WILL:

Urinary Continence (NOC)

Verbalize understanding of condition.
Maintain balanced I&O with clear, odor-free urine, free of bladder distention/urinary leakage.
Verbalize/demonstrate behaviors and techniques to prevent retention/urinary infection.

ACTIONS/INTERVENTIONS	RATIONALE
Urinary Elimination Management (NIC)	
Independent	
Assess voiding pattern; e.g., frequency and amount. Compare urine output with fluid intake. Note specific gravity.	Identifies characteristics of bladder function (e.g., effectiveness of bladder emptying, renal function, and fluid balance). *Note:* Urinary complications are a major cause of mortality.
Palpate for bladder distention and observe for overflow.	Bladder dysfunction is variable but may include loss of bladder contraction/inability to relax urinary sphincter, resulting in urine retention and reflux incontinence. *Note:* Bladder distention can precipitate autonomic dysreflexia. (Refer to ND: risk for Autonomic Dysreflexia, following.)
Encourage intake (2–4 L/day), including acid ash juices (e.g., cranberry).	Helps maintain renal function, prevents infection and formation of urinary stones. *Note:* Fluid may be restricted for a period during initiation of intermittent catheterization.
Begin bladder retraining per protocol when appropriate; e.g., fluids between certain hours, digital stimulation of trigger area, contraction of abdominal muscles, Credé's maneuver.	Timing and type of bladder program depend on type of injury (upper or lower neuron involvement). *Note:* Credé's maneuver should be used with caution because it may precipitate autonomic dysreflexia.
Observe for cloudy or bloody urine, foul odor. Dipstick urine as indicated.	Signs of urinary tract or kidney infection that can potentiate sepsis. Multistrip dipsticks can provide a quick determination of pH, nitrite, and leukocyte esterase, suggesting presence of infection.
Cleanse perineal area and keep dry. Provide catheter care as appropriate.	Decreases risk of skin irritation/breakdown and development of ascending infection.

ACTIONS/INTERVENTIONS	RATIONALE
URINARY CATHETERIZATION: [Indwelling/] Intermittent (NIC)	
Collaborative	
Monitor BUN, creatinine, white blood cell (WBC) count, urinalysis.	Reflects renal function, identifies complications.
Administer medications as indicated (e.g., vitamin C) and/or urinary antiseptics (e.g., methenamine mandelate [Mandelamine]).	Maintains acidic environment and discourages bacterial growth.
Refer for further evaluation for bladder/bowel stimulation.	Clinical research is being conducted on the technology of electronic bladder control. The implantable device sends electrical signals to the spinal nerves that control the bladder and bowel.
Keep bladder deflated by means of indwelling catheter initially. Begin intermittent catheterization program when appropriate, after bladder scan to determine postvoid residual.	Indwelling catheter is used during acute phase for prevention of urinary retention and for monitoring output. Intermittent catheterization may be implemented to reduce complications usually associated with long-term use of indwelling catheters. A suprapubic catheter may also be inserted for long-term management.
Measure residual urine via postvoid catheterization or ultrasound.	Helpful in detecting presence of urinary retention/effectiveness of bladder training program. *Note:* Use of ultrasound is noninvasive, reducing risk of colonization of bladder.

NURSING DIAGNOSIS: risk for Autonomic Dysreflexia

Risk factors may include

Altered nerve function (spinal cord injury at T-8 and above)
Bladder/bowel/skin stimulation (tactile, pain, thermal)

Possibly evidenced by

[Not applicable; presence of signs and symptoms establishes an *actual* diagnosis.]

DESIRED OUTCOMES/EVALUATION CRITERIA—CLIENT WILL:

Symptom Control (NOC)

Recognize signs/symptoms of syndrome.
Identify preventive/corrective measures.

NEUROLOGIC STATUS: Autonomic (NOC)

Experience no episodes of dysreflexia.

ACTIONS/INTERVENTIONS	RATIONALE
Dysreflexia Management (NIC)	
Independent	
Identify/monitor precipitating risk factors; e.g., bladder/bowel distention or manipulation; bladder spasms, stones, infection; skin/tissue pressure areas, prolonged sitting position; temperature extremes/drafts.	Visceral distention is the most common cause of autonomic dysreflexia, which is considered an emergency. Treatment of acute episode must be carried out immediately (removing stimulus, treating unresolved symptoms), then interventions must be geared toward prevention.

ACTIONS/INTERVENTIONS	RATIONALE
Observe for signs/symptoms of syndrome; e.g., changes in VS, paroxysmal hypertension, tachycardia/ bradycardia; autonomic responses: sweating, flushing above level of lesion; pallor below injury, chills, goose flesh, piloerection, nasal stuffiness, severe pounding headache, especially in occiput and frontal regions. Note associated symptoms; e.g., chest pains, blurred vision, nausea, metallic taste, Horner's syndrome (contraction of pupil, partial stasis of eyelid, enophthalmos [recession of eyeball into the orbit], and sometimes loss of sweating over one side of the face).	Early detection and immediate intervention is essential to prevent serious consequences/complications. *Note:* Average systolic BP in tetraplegic client after spinal shock has resolved is 120; therefore, readings of 140+ are considered high.
Stay with client during episode.	This is a potentially fatal complication. Continuous monitoring/intervention may reduce client's level of anxiety.
Monitor BP frequently (every 3–5 min) during acute autonomic dysreflexia and take action to eliminate stimulus. Continue to monitor BP at intervals after symptoms subside.	Aggressive therapy/removal of stimulus may drop BP rapidly, resulting in a hypotensive crisis, especially in those clients who routinely have low BP. In addition, autonomic dysreflexia may recur, particularly if stimulus is not eliminated.
Elevate head of bed to 45-degree angle or place client in sitting position.	Lowers BP to prevent intracranial hemorrhage, seizures, or even death. *Note:* Placing tetraplegic in sitting position automatically lowers BP.
Correct/eliminate causative stimulus as able; e.g., bladder, bowel, skin pressure (including loosening tight leg bands/clothing, removing abdominal binder/elastic stockings); temperature extremes.	Removing noxious stimulus usually terminates episode and may prevent more serious autonomic dysreflexia; e.g., in the presence of sunburn, topical anesthetic should be applied. Removal of constrictive clothing/vascular support also promotes venous pooling to help lower BP. *Note:* Removal of bowel impaction must be delayed until cardiovascular condition is stabilized.
Inform client/SO of warning signals and how to avoid onset of syndrome; e.g., goose flesh, sweating, piloerection may indicate full bowel; sunburn may precipitate episode.	This lifelong problem can be largely controlled by avoiding pressure from overdistention of visceral organs or pressure on the skin.

Collaborative

ACTIONS/INTERVENTIONS	RATIONALE
Administer medications as indicated (IV, parenteral, oral, or transdermal) and monitor response:	
Diazoxide (Hyperstat), hydralazine (Apresoline);	Reduces BP if severe/sustained hypertension occurs.
Nifedipine (Procardia), 2% nitroglycerin ointment (Nitrostat);	Sublingual administration usually effective in absence of IV access for diazoxide (Hyperstat), but may require repeat dose in 30–60 min. May be used in conjunction with topical nitroglycerin.
Morphine sulfate;	Relaxes smooth muscle to aid in lowering blood pressure and muscle tension.
Adrenergic blockers; e.g., methysergide maleate (Sansert);	May be used prophylactically if problem persists/recurs frequently.
Antihypertensives; e.g., prazosin (Minipress), phenoxybenzamine (Dibenzyline), clonidine (Catapress).	Long-term use may relax bladder neck and enhance bladder emptying, alleviating the most common cause of chronic autonomic dysreflexia.
Obtain urinary culture as indicated.	Presence of infection may trigger autonomic dysreflexia episode.
Apply local anesthetic ointment to rectum. Remove impaction if indicated after symptoms subside.	Ointment blocks further autonomic stimulation and eases later removal of impaction without aggravating symptoms.
Prepare client for pelvic/pudendal nerve block or posterior rhizotomy if indicated.	Procedures may be considered if autonomic dysreflexia does not respond to other therapies.

NURSING DIAGNOSIS: risk for impaired Skin/Tissue Integrity

Risk factors may include

Altered/inadequate peripheral circulation, sensation
Presence of edema, tissue pressure
Altered metabolic state
Immobility, traction apparatus

Possibly evidenced by

[Not applicable; presence of signs and symptoms establishes an *actual* diagnosis.]

DESIRED OUTCOMES/EVALUATION CRITERIA—CLIENT WILL:

Risk Control (NOC)

Identify individual risk factors.
Verbalize understanding of treatment needs.
Participate to level of ability to prevent skin breakdown.

ACTIONS/INTERVENTIONS	RATIONALE
Skin Surveillance (NIC)	
Independent	
Inspect all skin areas, noting capillary blanching/refill, redness, swelling. Pay particular attention to back of head, skin under halo frame or vest, and folds where skin continuously touches.	Skin is especially prone to breakdown because of changes in peripheral circulation, inability to sense pressure, immobility, altered temperature regulation.
Observe halo and tong insertion sites. Note swelling, redness, drainage.	These sites are prone to inflammation and infection and provide route for pathologic microorganisms to enter cranial cavity. *Note:* New style of halo frame does not require screws or pins.
Encourage continuation of regular exercise program.	Stimulates circulation, enhancing cellular nutrition/oxygenation to improve tissue health.
Elevate lower extremities periodically if tolerated.	Enhances venous return, reduces edema formation.
Avoid/limit injection of medication below the level of injury.	Reduced circulation and sensation increase risk of delayed absorption, local reaction, and tissue necrosis.
SKIN CARE: Topical Treatments (NIC)	
Massage and lubricate skin with bland lotion/oil. Protect pressure points by use of heel/elbow pads, lamb's wool, foam padding, egg-crate mattress. Use skin-hardening agents; e.g., tincture of benzoin, karaya, Sween cream.	Enhances circulation and protects skin surfaces, reducing risk of ulceration. Tetraplegic and paraplegic clients require lifelong protection from decubitus ulcer formation, which can cause extensive tissue necrosis and sepsis.
Reposition frequently, whether in bed or in sitting position. Place in prone position periodically.	Improves skin circulation and reduces pressure time on bony prominences.
Wash and dry skin, especially in high-moisture areas such as perineum. Take care to avoid wetting lining of brace/halo vest.	Clean, dry skin is less prone to excoriation/breakdown.
Keep bedclothes dry and free of wrinkles, crumbs.	Reduces/prevents skin irritation.
Cleanse halo/tong insertion sites routinely and apply antibiotic ointment per protocol.	Helpful in preventing local infection and reducing risk of cranial infection.
Collaborative	
Provide kinetic therapy or alternating-pressure mattress as indicated.	Improves systemic and peripheral circulation and decreases pressure on skin, reducing risk of breakdown.

NURSING DIAGNOSIS: deficient Knowledge [Learning Need] regarding condition, prognosis, potential complications, treatment, self-care, and discharge needs

May be related to

Lack of exposure/recall
Information misinterpretation
Unfamiliarity with information resources

Possibly evidenced by

Questions, statement of misconception, request for information
Inadequate follow-through of instruction
Inappropriate or exaggerated behaviors; e.g., hostile, agitated, apathetic
Development of preventable complication(s)

DESIRED OUTCOMES/EVALUATION CRITERIA—CLIENT WILL:

KNOWLEDGE: Disease Process (NOC)

Verbalize understanding of condition, prognosis, and treatment.

KNOWLEDGE: Treatment Regimen (NOC)

Correctly perform necessary procedures and explain reasons for the actions.
Initiate necessary lifestyle changes and participate in treatment regimen.

ACTIONS/INTERVENTIONS	RATIONALE
TEACHING: Disease Process (NIC)	
Independent	
Discuss injury process, current prognosis, and future expectations.	Provides common knowledge base necessary for making informed choices and commitment to the therapeutic regimen. *Note:* Improvement in managing effects of SCI has increased life expectancy of clients to only about 5 yr below norm for specific age group. New treatment options (e.g., Procord, GM-1, minocycline) are in clinical trials to determine if they can improve neurologic outcomes.
Provide information and demonstrate:	
Positioning and weight shifting;	Promotes circulation, reduces tissue pressure and risk of complications.
Use of pillows/supports, splints.	Keeps spine aligned and prevents/limits contractures, thus improving function and independence.
Encourage continued participation in daily exercise and conditioning program and avoidance of fatigue/chills.	Reduces spasticity complications and risk of thrombogenesis (common complication). Increases mobility, muscle strength and tone for improving organ/body function; e.g., squeezing rubber ball and arm exercises enhance upper body strength to increase independence in transfers/wheelchair mobility, tightening/contracting rectum or vaginal muscles improves bladder control, pushing abdomen up, bearing down, contracting abdomen strengthens trunk and improves GI function (paraplegic).
Identify energy conservation techniques and stress importance of pacing activities/adequate rest.	Fatigue is common and limits client's ability to participate in/manage care, decreasing quality of life, and increasing feelings of helplessness/hopelessness.

ACTIONS/INTERVENTIONS	RATIONALE
Review drug regimen, noting desired effects and expected side effects, as well as medication interactions.	Medications used to treat spasticity can exacerbate fatigue, necessitating a change in drug choice/dosage. *Note:* Amantadine (Symmetrel) and fluoxetine (Prozac) may be added to decrease sense of fatigue by potentiating the action of dopamine or selectively inhibiting serotonin uptake in the CNS.
Have SO/caregivers participate in client care and demonstrate proper procedures; e.g., applications of splints, braces, suctioning, positioning, skin care, transfers, bowel/bladder program, checking temperature of bath water and food.	Allows home caregivers to become adept and more comfortable with the care tasks they are called on to provide, and reduces risk of injury/complications.
Instruct caregiver in techniques to facilitate cough as appropriate.	Quad coughing is performed to facilitate expectoration of secretions or to move them high enough to be suctioned out.
Recommend applying abdominal binder before arising (tetraplegic) and remind to change position slowly. Use safety belt and adequate number of people during bed-to-wheelchair transfers.	Reduces pooling of blood in abdomen/pelvis, minimizing postural hypotension. Protects client from falls and/or injury to caregivers.
Instruct in proper skin care, inspecting all skin areas daily, using adequate padding (foam, silicone gel, water pads) in bed and chair, and keeping skin dry. Stress importance of regularly monitoring condition and positioning of support surfaces (e.g., cushions, mattresses, and overlays).	Reduces skin irritation, decreasing incidence of decubitus ulcers (client must manage this throughout life). Timely recognition of product fatigue, improper orientation, or other misuse can reduce risk of pressure ulcer formation.
Discuss necessity of preventing or managing excessive diaphoresis by using tepid bath water, providing comfortable environment (e.g., fans), removing excess clothing.	Promotes cooling, reduces skin irritation/possible breakdown.
Review dietary needs, including adequate bulk and roughage. Problem-solve solutions to alterations in muscular strength/tone and GI function.	Provides adequate nutrition to meet energy needs and promote healing, prevent complications (e.g., constipation, abdominal distention/gas formation).
Review pain-management techniques. Discuss the potential for future pain-management therapies if pain becomes chronic. Recommend avoidance of OTC drugs without approval of healthcare provider.	Enhances client safety and may improve cooperation with specific regimen. *Note:* Pain often becomes chronic in clients with spinal cord injury and may be mechanical (e.g., overuse syndrome involving joints); radicular (from injury to peripheral nerves); or cervical (burning, aching just below level of injury). Dysesthetic pain (distal to site of injury) is extremely disabling (similar to phantom pain). Treatment for these painful conditions may include a team pain-management approach, medications (e.g., gabapentin [Neurontin], clonazepam [Klonopin], amitriptyline [Elavil]), or electrical stimulation.
Discuss ways to identify and manage autonomic dysreflexia.	Client may be able to recognize signs, but caregivers need to understand how to prevent precipitating factors and know what to do if autonomic dysreflexia occurs. (Refer to ND: risk for Autonomic Dysreflexia.)
Identify symptoms to report immediately to healthcare provider; e.g., infection of any kind, especially urinary, respiratory; skin breakdown; unresolved autonomic dysreflexia; suspected pregnancy.	Early identification allows for intervention to prevent/minimize complications.
Stress importance of continuing with rehabilitation team to achieve specific functional goals and continue long-term monitoring of therapy needs.	No matter what the level of injury, individual may ultimately be able to exercise some independence; e.g., manipulating electric wheelchair with mouth stick (C-3/C-4); being independent for dressing, transfers to bed, car, toilet (C-7); or achieving total wheelchair independence (C-8 to T-4). Over time, new discoveries continue to modify equipment/therapy needs and increase client's potential.
Evaluate home layout and make recommendations for necessary changes. Identify equipment/medical supply needs and resources.	Physical changes may be required to accommodate client and support equipment. Prior arrangements facilitate the transfer to the home setting.

ACTIONS/INTERVENTIONS	RATIONALE
Discuss sexual activity and reproductive concerns. Review alternative sexual activities/positions and spasticity management as indicated (e.g., opposing pressure on area of spasm, using pillows for support, regular stretching/ROM exercises, appropriate medications).	Concerns about individual sexuality/resumption of activity are frequently an unspoken concern that needs to be addressed. Spinal cord injury affects all areas of sexual functioning. In addition, choice of contraception is impacted by level of spinal cord injury and side effects/adverse complications of specific method. Finally, some female clients may develop autonomic dysreflexia during intercourse or labor/delivery.
Identify community resources/supports; e.g., health agencies, visiting nurse, financial counselor, service organizations, Spinal Cord Injury Foundation.	Enhances independence, assisting with home management and providing respite for caregivers.
Coordinate cooperation among community/rehabilitation resources.	Various agencies/therapists/individuals in community may be involved in the long-term care and safety of client, and coordination can ensure that needs are not overlooked and optimal level of rehabilitation is achieved. *Note:* Individuals with SCI are living longer, and more injuries are occurring at advanced ages, creating new challenges in care as SCI clients deal with the effects of aging.
Arrange for transmitter/emergency call system.	Provides for safety and access to emergency assistance and equipment.
Plan for alternate caregivers, identify respite services as needed.	May be needed to provide respite if regular caregivers are ill, unplanned emergencies arise.

POTENTIAL CONSIDERATIONS following acute hospitalization (dependent on client's age, physical condition/presence of complications, personal resources, and life responsibilities)

risk for Disuse Syndrome—paralysis/mechanical immobilization.

Autonomic Dysreflexia—bladder/bowel distention, skin irritation, lack of caregiver knowledge.

Self-Care Deficit—neuromuscular impairment, decreased strength/endurance, pain, depression.

risk for imbalanced Nutrition (specify)—dysfunctional eating pattern, excessive/inadequate intake in relation to metabolic need.

ineffective Role Performance/Sexual Dysfunction—situational crisis and transition, altered body function.

interrupted Family Processes—situational crisis and transition.

Caregiver Role Strain—discharge of family member with significant home care needs, situational stressors, such as significant loss, economic vulnerability; duration of caregiving required, lack of respite for caregiver, inexperience with caregiving, caregiver's competing role commitments.

MULTIPLE SCLEROSIS

Multiple sclerosis (MS) is the most common of the demyelinating disorders and the predominant central nervous system (CNS) disease among young adults. It is a chronic disorder in which irregular demyelination of the CNS (brain and spinal cord) results in emotional changes and varying degree of cognitive, motor, and sensory dysfunction at the central and peripheral levels. It is a perivascular inflammatory response, possibly related to chronic viral infection in genetically susceptible individuals, producing a limited disruption in the blood-brain barrier, allowing β-lymphocyte clones to colonize the CNS. Research suggests that, in addition to destruction of myelin sheaths (which facilitate the movement of nerve impulses), some underlying nerve fibers are also damaged or severed, which may account for the permanent neurologic impairment.

MS is difficult to categorize, but can generally be grouped into the following four types:

Relapsing-remitting: Periods of neurologic dysfunction in which neurologic deficits occur in different parts of the body, followed by partial or full recovery, leaving little residual deficit (accounts for approximately 85% of persons with MS).

Primary-progressive: Function declines steadily with periods of minimal recovery and increasing disability (about 10% of cases).

Secondary-progressive: Person with relapsing-remitting MS may convert after a period of time to a secondary progressive pattern characterized by continued progression with increasing disability (approximately 50%).
Progressive-relapsing: Progressive from onset with clear exacerbations (rare).

In most people, MS is characterized by periods of exacerbations and remissions, and is progressive in approximately 50% of clients. It is difficult to diagnose, and cannot be diagnosed after only one presentation of symptoms, but rather over time. Individual prognosis is variable and unpredictable, presenting complex physical, psychosocial, and rehabilitative issues.

CARE SETTING

Community or long-term care with intermittent hospitalization for disease-related exacerbations/complications.

RELATED CONCERNS

Extended care, page 810
Pneumonia, page 128
Psychosocial aspects of care, page 770
Sepsis/Septicemia, page 701

Client Assessment Database

Symptomatology depends on the stage and extent of disease and areas of neuronal involvement. For example, common signs associated with motor systems of the cerebellum include (and are not limited to) ataxia, diplopia, dizziness, dysphagia, fatigability, and tremors. Signs associated with motor systems of the corticospinal tract include (but are not limited to) Babinski's sign, bladder dysfunction, fatigue, heat sensitivity, paralysis, and trigeminal neuralgia. The following represents a range of symptoms that may be present at a given time or over time.

ACTIVITY/REST

May report:
Extreme fatigue/weakness, exaggerated intolerance to activity, needing to rest after even simple activities such as shaving/showering; increased weakness/intolerance to temperature extremes, especially heat (e.g., summer weather, hot tubs)
Limitation in usual activities, employment, hobbies
Numbness, tingling in the extremities
Sleep disturbances, may awaken early or frequently for multiple reasons (e.g., nocturia, nocturnal spasticity, pain, worry, depression)

May exhibit:
Absence of predictable pattern of symptoms
Generalized weakness, decreased muscle tone/mass (disuse), spasticity, tremors
Staggering, dragging of feet, ataxia
Intention tremors, decreased fine motor skills

CIRCULATION

May report: Dependent edema (steroid therapy or inactivity)

May exhibit:
Blue/mottled, puffy extremities (inactivity)
Capillary fragility (especially on face)

EGO INTEGRITY

May report:
Statements of reflecting loss of self-esteem/body image
Expressions of grief
Anxiety/fear of exacerbations/progression of symptoms, pain, disability, rejection, pity
Keeping illness confidential
Feelings of helplessness, hopelessness, powerlessness (loss of control)
Personal tragedies (divorce, abandonment by SO/friends)

May exhibit:
Denial, rejection
Mood changes, irritability, restlessness, lethargy, euphoria, depression, anger

ELIMINATION

May report:
Nocturia
Incomplete bladder emptying, retention with overflow
Urinary/bowel hesitancy or urgency, incontinence of varying severity
Irregular bowel habits, constipation
Recurrent UTIs

May exhibit:
Loss of sphincter control
Kidney stone formation, kidney damage

FOOD/FLUID

May report: Difficulty chewing, swallowing (weak throat muscles), sense of food sticking in throat, coughing after swallowing

Problems getting food to mouth (related to intentional tremors of upper extremities)

Hiccups, possibly lasting for extended periods

May exhibit: Difficulty feeding self

Weight loss

Decreased bowel sounds (slowed peristalsis)

Abdominal bloating

HYGIENE

May report: Difficulty with/dependence in some/all ADLs

Use of assistive devices/individual caregiver

May exhibit: Poor personal habits, disheveled appearance, signs of incontinence

NEUROSENSORY

May report: Weakness, nonsymmetrical paralysis of muscles (may affect one, two, or three limbs, usually worse in lower extremities or may be unilateral), numbness, tingling (prickling sensations in parts of the body)

Change in visual acuity (diplopia), scotomas (holes in vision), eye pain (optic neuritis)

Moving head back and forth while watching television, difficulty driving (distorted visual field), blurred vision (difficulty focusing)

Cognitive changes; i.e., attention, comprehension, use of speech, problem-solving, difficulty retrieving/recalling, sorting out information (cerebral involvement)

Difficulty making decisions

Communication difficulties, such as coining words

Seizures

May exhibit: Mental status: Mood swings, depression, euphoria, irritability, apathy, lack of judgment, impairment of short-term memory, disorientation/confusion

Scanning speech, slow hesitant speech, poor articulation

Partial/total loss of vision in one eye, vision disturbances

Positional/vibratory sense impaired or absent

Impaired touch/pain sensation

Facial/trigeminal nerve involvement, nystagmus, diplopia (brainstem involvement)

Loss of motor skills (major/fine), changes in muscle tone, spastic paresis/total immobility (advanced stages)

Ataxia, decreased coordination, tremors (may be originally misinterpreted as intoxication), intention tremor

Hyperreflexia, positive Babinski's sign, ankle clonus, absent superficial reflexes (especially abdominal)

PAIN/DISCOMFORT

May report: Painful spasms, burning pain along nerve path (some clients do not experience normal pain sensations)

Frequency varied may be sporadic/intermittent (possibly once a day) or may be constant

Duration lightning-like, repetitive, intermittent; persistent long-term painful spasms of extremity or back

Facial neuralgia

Dull back pain

May exhibit: Distraction behaviors (restlessness, moaning), guarding

Self-focusing

SAFETY

May report: Uneasiness around small children or moving objects, fear of falling (weakness, decreased vision, slowed reflexes, loss of position sense, decreased judgment)

History of falls/accidental injuries

Use of ambulation devices

Vision impairment

Suicidal ideation

May exhibit: Wall/furniture walking

SEXUALITY

May report:

Relationship stresses
Enhanced or decreased sexual desire
Problems with positioning
Genital anesthesia/hyperesthesia, decreased lubrication (female)
Impotence/nocturnal erections or ejaculatory difficulties (male)
Disturbances in sexual functioning (affected by nerve impairment, fatigue, bowel and bladder control, sense of vulnerability, and effects of medications)

SOCIAL INTERACTION

May report:

Lack of social activities/involvement
Withdrawal from interactions with others/isolation behaviors (e.g., stays at home/in room, watches TV all day)
Feelings of isolation (increased divorce rate/loss of friends)
Difficult time with employment because of excessive fatigue/cognitive dysfunction, physical limitations

May exhibit:

Speech impairment

TEACHING/LEARNING

May report:

Use of prescription/OTC medications, may forget to take regularly
Difficulty retaining information
Family history of disease (possibly due to common environmental/inherited factors)
Use of "holistic"/natural products/healthcare practices, "trying out cures," "doctor shopping"

Discharge plan considerations:

May require assistance in any or all areas, depending on individual situation
May eventually need total care/placement in assisted living/extended care facility

Refer to section at end of plan for postdischarge considerations.

DIAGNOSTIC STUDIES

There are no tests specific for MS and no single test is 100% conclusive. However, the following tests may be done to support a clinical diagnosis.

Brain MRI: Detects presence of certain macroscopic plaques characteristic of MS that are due to nerve sheath demyelination, but is not diagnostic without supporting clinical symptoms, and does not correlate well with impairment or disability. However, MRI remains the imaging procedure of choice for diagnosing and monitoring disease progression, as it can show brain abnormalities in up to 90%–95% of clients and spinal cord lesions in up to 75% of cases, especially in the elderly.

CT scan with enhancement: Demonstrates acute brain lesions, ventricular enlargement or thinning. Not helpful for client with stable disease as lesions do not enhance.

Magnetic Resonance Spectroscopy: Newer neuroimaging technique useful in following N-acetyl-aspartate (NAA) levels, found to be reduced in clients with MS.

Evoked Potential tests (EVPs): Visual evoked responses (VER), brainstem auditory evoked responses (BAER), and somatosensory evoked responses (SSER) are abnormal early in a high percentage of clients with clinically definite MS (CDMS) or suspected MS.

Lumbar puncture: CSF may show elevated levels of IgG (occurs with progressive MS, usually negative in relapsing MS) and IgM. Fluid is also tested for presence of antibodies, oligoclonal bands (OCBs) found in 90%–95% of clients with MS, and myelin-basic protein (MBP), which may be noted during active demyelination process.

EEG: May be mildly abnormal in some cases.

NURSING PRIORITIES

1. Maintain optimal functioning.
2. Assist with/provide for maintenance of ADLs.
3. Support acceptance of changes in body image/self-esteem and role performance.
4. Provide information about disease process/prognosis, therapeutic needs, and available resources.

DISCHARGE GOALS

1. Remain active within limits of individual situation.
2. ADLs are managed by client/caregivers.
3. Changes in self-concept are acknowledged and being dealt with.
4. Disease process/prognosis, therapeutic regimen are understood and resources identified.
5. Plan in place to meet needs after discharge.

NURSING DIAGNOSIS: Fatigue

May be related to

Decreased energy production, increased energy requirements to perform activities
Psychologic/emotional demands
Pain/discomfort
Medication side effects

Possibly evidenced by

Verbalization of overwhelming lack of energy
Inability to maintain usual routines; decreased performance
Impaired ability to concentrate; disinterest in surroundings
Increase in physical complaints

DESIRED OUTCOMES/EVALUATION CRITERIA—CLIENT WILL:

Energy Conservation (NOC)

Identify risk factors and individual actions affecting fatigue.
Identify alternatives to help maintain desired activity level.
Participate in recommended treatment program.
Report improved sense of energy.

ACTIONS/INTERVENTIONS	RATIONALE
Energy Management (NIC)	
Independent	
Note and accept presence of fatigue.	Fatigue is the most persistent and commonly reported symptom of MS. Studies indicate that the fatigue encountered by clients with MS occurs with expenditure of minimal energy, is more frequent and severe than "normal" fatigue, has a disproportionate impact on ADLs, has a slower recovery time, and may show no direct relationship between fatigue severity and client's clinical neurologic status.
Identify/review factors affecting ability to be active; e.g., temperature extremes, inadequate food intake, insomnia, use of medications, time of day.	Provides opportunity to problem solve to maintain/improve mobility.
Accept when client is unable to do activities.	Ability can vary from moment to moment. Nonjudgmental acceptance of client's evaluation of day-to-day variations in capabilities provides opportunity to promote independence while supporting fluctuations in level of required care.
Determine need for mobility aids; e.g., Canadian canes, braces, walker, wheelchair, scooter. Review safety considerations.	Can decrease fatigue, enhancing independence and comfort, as well as safety. However, individual may display poor judgment about ability to safely engage in activity/operate scooter.
Schedule ADLs and outside activities in the morning or over time/throughout the course of the day. Investigate use of air conditioning, cooling vest, light-colored clothing, and wide-brimmed hats if appropriate	Fatigue commonly worsens when exposed to high temperatures due to weather, environmental heat, exercise, or fever. Some clients report lessening of fatigue with stabilization of body temperature.
Plan care with consistent rest periods between activities. Encourage afternoon nap.	Reduces fatigue, aggravation of muscle weakness.
Stress need for stopping exercise/activity just short of fatigue.	Pushing self beyond individual physical limits can result in excessive/prolonged fatigue and discouragement. In time, client can become very adept at knowing limitations.

ACTIONS/INTERVENTIONS	RATIONALE
Investigate appropriateness of obtaining a service dog.	Service dogs not only can increase client's level of independence (e.g., balance/mobility assistance), but also can assist in energy conservation by carrying items in "saddle" bags, fetching/retrieving, and performing tasks (e.g., turning lights on/off).

Collaborative

ACTIONS/INTERVENTIONS	RATIONALE
Recommend participation in groups involved in fitness/exercise and/or the Multiple Sclerosis Society.	Can help client to stay motivated to remain active within the limits of the disability/condition. Group activities need to be selected carefully to meet client's need(s) and prevent discouragement or anxiety.
Administer medications as indicated; e.g.:	
Amantadine (Symmetrel), pemoline (Cylert);	Useful in treatment of fatigue. Use may be limited by side effects of increased spasticity, insomnia, paresthesias of hands/feet.
Methylphenidate (Ritalin), modafinil (Provigil);	CNS stimulants that may reduce fatigue but may also cause side effects of nervousness, restlessness, and insomnia.
Sertraline (Zoloft), fluoxetine (Prozac);	Antidepressants useful in lifting mood, and "energizing" client (especially when depression is a factor) and when client is free of anticholinergic side effects.
Tricyclic antidepressants; e.g., amitriptyline (Elavil), nortriptyline (Pamelor);	Useful in treating emotional lability, neurogenic pain, and associated sleep disorders to enhance willingness to be more active.
Anticonvulsants; e.g., carbamazepine (Tegretol), gabapentin (Neurontin), lamotrigine (Lamictal);	Used to treat neurogenic pain and sudden intermittent spasms related to spinal cord irritation.
Steroids; e.g., prednisone (Deltasone), dexamethasone (Decadron), methylprednisolone (Solu-Medrol);	May be used during acute exacerbations to reduce/prevent edema formation at the sclerotic plaques; however, long-term therapy seems to have little effect on progression of symptoms.
Antineoplastic agents; e.g. mitoxantrone (Novantrone);	May be given to reduce neurologic disability and/or frequency of relapses in clients with secondary (chronic) progressive, or worsening relapsing-remitting MS (such as clients whose neurologic status is significantly abnormal between relapses).
Vitamin B;	Supports nerve-cell replication, enhances metabolic functions, and may increase sense of well-being/energy level (although reports are more anecdotal than research based).
Immunomodulating agents; e.g., cyclophosphamide (Cytoxan), azathioprine (Imuran), methotrexate (Mexate); interferon β-1A (Avonex, Rebif), interferon β-1B (Betaseron), glatiramer (Copaxone), mitoxentrone (Novantrone).	May be used to treat acute relapses, reduce the frequency of relapse, and promote remission. Current research indicates early treatment with drugs that reduce inflammation and lesion formation may limit permanent damage. Therapy of choice is the use of "A, B, C" drugs: Avonex, Betaseron, and Copaxone. Therapeutic benefits have been reported in clients at all stages of disability with reduction in both steroid use and hospital days. (Copaxone chemically resembles a component of myelin and may act as a decoy, diverting immune cells away from myelin target.) *Note:* Novantrone may be used if other medications are not effective but is contraindicated in clients with primary progressive MS.
Prepare for plasma exchange treatment as indicated.	Research suggests that individuals experiencing severe, acute exacerbations not responding to standard high-dose steroid therapy may benefit from a course of plasmapheresis.

NURSING DIAGNOSIS: Self-Care Deficit [specify]

May be related to

Neuromuscular/perceptual impairment; intolerance to activity; decreased strength and endurance; motor impairment, tremors
Pain, discomfort, fatigue
Memory loss
Depression

Possibly evidenced by

Frustration, inability to perform tasks of self-care, poor personal hygiene

DESIRED OUTCOMES/EVALUATION CRITERIA—CLIENT WILL:

Self-Care Activities of Daily Living (ADL) (NOC)

Identify individual areas of weakness/needs.
Demonstrate techniques/lifestyle changes to meet self-care needs.
Perform self-care activities within level of own ability.
Identify personal/community resources that provide assistance.

ACTIONS/INTERVENTIONS	RATIONALE
Self-Care Assistance (NIC)	
Independent	
Determine current activity level/physical condition. Assess degree of functional impairment using 0–4 scale.	Provides information to develop plan of care for rehabilitation. *Note:* Motor symptoms are less likely to improve than sensory ones.
Encourage client to perform self-care to the maximum of ability as defined by client. Do not rush client.	Promotes independence and sense of control, may decrease feelings of helplessness.
Assist according to degree of disability, allow as much autonomy as possible.	Participation in own care can ease the frustration over loss of independence.
Encourage client input in planning schedule.	Client's quality of life is enhanced when desires/likes are considered in daily activities.
Note presence of/accommodate for fatigue.	Fatigue experienced by clients with MS can be very debilitating and greatly impact ability to participate in ADLs. The subjective nature of reports of fatigue can be misinterpreted by healthcare providers and family, leading to conflict and the belief that the client is "manipulative" when, in fact, this may not be the case.
Encourage scheduling activities early in the day or during the time when energy level is best.	Clients with MS expend a great deal of energy to complete ADLs, increasing the risk of fatigue, which often progresses through the day.
Allot sufficient time to perform task(s), and display patience when movements are slow.	Decreased motor skills/spasticity may interfere with ability to manage even simple activities.
Anticipate hygienic needs and calmly assist as necessary with care of nails, skin, hair, mouth care, shaving (use electric razor).	Caregiver's example can set a matter-of-fact tone for acceptance of handling mundane needs that may be embarrassing to client/repugnant to SO.
Provide assistive devices/aids as indicated; e.g., shower chair, elevated toilet seat with arm supports.	Reduces fatigue, enhancing participation in self-care.
Reposition frequently when client is immobile (bed/chair-bound). Provide skin care to pressure points, such as sacrum, ankles, and elbows. Position/encourage to sleep prone as tolerated.	Reduces pressure on susceptible areas, prevents skin breakdown. Minimizes flexor spasms at knees and hips.

ACTIONS/INTERVENTIONS	RATIONALE
Provide massage and active/passive ROM and stretching and toning exercises on a regular schedule. Encourage use of medications, cold packs, and splints/footboards as indicated.	Prevents problems associated with muscle pain, dysfunction, and disuse. Helps maintain muscle tone/strength and joint mobility and proper body alignment. Decreases spasticity and its effects, and reduces risk of loss of calcium from bones.
Problem-solve ways to meet nutritional/fluid needs; e.g., wrap fork handle with tape, cut food, and show client how to hold cup with both hands.	Provides for adequate intake and enhances client's feelings of independence/self-esteem.

Collaborative

Consult with physical/occupational therapist.	Useful in identifying/providing treatments, devices, and equipment to relieve spastic muscles, improve motor functioning; prevent/reduce muscular atrophy and contractures, promoting independence and increasing sense of self-worth.
Administer medications as indicated; e.g.:	
Tizanidine (Zanaflex), baclofen (Lioresal), carbamazepine (Tegretol);	Newer drugs used for reducing spasticity, promoting muscle relaxation, and inhibiting reflexes at the spinal nerve root level. Zanaflex may have an additive effect with Lioresal, but must be used with caution because both drugs have similar side effects. Short duration of action requires careful individualizing of dosage to maximize therapeutic effect.
Diazepam (Valium), clonazepam (Klonopin), cylobenzaprine (Flexeril), gabapentin (Neurontin), dantrolene (Dantrium);	A variety of medications are used to manage spasticity. The mechanisms are not well understood, and responses vary in each person. Therefore, it may take a period of medication trials to discover what provides the most effective relief of muscle spasticity and associated pain. *Note:* Adverse effects may be increased muscle weakness, loss of muscle tone, and liver toxicity.
Meclizine (Antivert), scopolamine patches (Transderm-Scop);	Reduces dizziness when present, allowing client to be more mobile.
Prepare for surgical intervention—deep brain stimulation—as appropriate.	Placement of an electrode (similar to a cardiac pacemaker device) in the region of the thalamus provides for small, adjustable electrical impulses to reduce arm tremors and enhance movement without actually destroying brain tissue.

NURSING DIAGNOSIS: low Self-Esteem, (specify situational/chronic)

May be related to

Change in structure/function
Disruption in how client perceives own body
Role reversal; dependence

Possibly evidenced by

Confusion about sense of self, purpose, direction in life
Denial, withdrawal, anger
Negative/self-destructive behavior
Use of ineffective coping methods
Change in self/other's perception of role/physical capacity to resume role

DESIRED OUTCOMES/EVALUATION CRITERIA—CLIENT WILL:

Self-Esteem (NOC)

Verbalize realistic view and acceptance of body as it is.
View self as a capable person.
Participate in and assume responsibility for meeting own needs.
Recognize and incorporate changes in self-concept/role without negating self-esteem.
Develop realistic plans for adapting to role changes.

ACTIONS/INTERVENTIONS	RATIONALE
Self-Esteem Enhancement (NIC)	
Independent	
Establish/maintain a therapeutic nurse-client relationship, discussing fears/concerns.	Conveys an attitude of caring and develops a sense of trust between client and caregiver in which client is free to express fears of rejection, loss of previous functioning/appearance, feelings of helplessness, powerlessness about changes that may occur. Promotes a sense of support and well-being for client.
Note withdrawn behaviors/use of denial or overconcern with body/disease process.	Initially may be a normal protective response, but if prolonged, may prevent dealing appropriately with reality and may lead to ineffective coping.
Support use of defense mechanisms, allowing client to deal with information in own time and way.	Confronting client with reality of situation may result in increased anxiety and lessened ability to cope with changed self-concept/role.
Acknowledge reality of grieving process related to actual/perceived changes. Help client deal realistically with feelings of anger and sadness.	Nature of the disease leads to ongoing losses and changes in all aspects of life, blocking resolution of grieving process.
Review information about course of disease, possibility of remissions, prognosis.	When client learns about disease and becomes aware that own behavior (including feeling hopeful/maintaining a positive attitude) can significantly improve general well-being and daily functioning, client may feel more in control, enhancing sense of self-esteem. *Note:* Some clients may never have a remission.
Provide accurate verbal and written information about what is happening and discuss with client/SO.	Helps client stay in the "here and now," reduces fear of the unknown, provides reference source for future use.
Explain that labile emotions are not unusual. Problem-solve ways to deal with these feelings.	Relieves anxiety and assists with efforts to manage unexpected emotional displays.
Note presence of depression/impaired thought processes, expressions of suicidal ideation (evaluate on a scale of 1–10).	Adapting to a long-term, progressively debilitating incurable condition is a difficult emotional adjustment. In addition, cognitive impairment may affect adaptation to life changes. A depressed individual may believe that suicide is the best way to deal with what is happening.
Assess interaction between client and SO. Note changes in relationship.	SO may unconsciously/consciously reinforce negative attitudes and beliefs of client, or issues of secondary gain may interfere with progress and ability to manage situation.
Provide open environment for client/SO to discuss concerns about sexuality, including management of fatigue, spasticity, arousal, and changes in sensation.	Physical and psychologic changes often create stressors within the relationship, affecting usual roles/expectations, further impairing self-concept.
Discuss use of medications and adjuncts to improve sexual function.	Client and partner may want to explore trial of medications (e.g., papaverine [Pavabid], dinoprostone [Prostin E_2]) or other avenues of improving sexual relationship.

ACTIONS/INTERVENTIONS	RATIONALE
Collaborative	
Consult with occupational therapist/rehabilitation team.	Identifying assistive devices/equipment enhances level of overall function and participation in activities, enhancing sense of well-being and viewing self as a capable individual.
Refer to psychiatric clinical nurse specialist, social worker, psychologist as indicated.	May require more in-depth/supportive counseling to resolve conflicts, deal with life changes.

NURSING DIAGNOSIS: Powerlessness [specify degree]/Hopelessness

May be related to

Illness-related regimen, unpredictability of disease
Lifestyle of helplessness

Possibly evidenced by

Verbal expressions of having no control or influence over situation
Depression over physical deterioration that occurs despite client compliance with regimen
Nonparticipation in care or decision-making when opportunities are provided
Passivity, decreased verbalization/affect
Verbal cues (despondent content, "I can't," sighing)
Lack of involvement in care/passively allowing care
Isolating behaviors/social withdrawal

DESIRED OUTCOMES/EVALUATION CRITERIA—CLIENT WILL:

Hope (NOC)

Identify and verbalize feelings.
Use coping mechanisms to counteract feelings of hopelessness.
Identify areas over which individual has control.
Participate/monitor and control own self-care and ADLs within limits of the individual situation.

ACTIONS/INTERVENTIONS	RATIONALE
Hope Instillation (NIC)	
Independent	
Note behaviors indicative of powerlessness/hopelessness; e.g., statements of despair, "They don't care," "It won't make any difference."	The degree to which client believes own situation is hopeless, that he or she is powerless to change what is happening, affects how client handles life situation.
Acknowledge reality of situation, at the same time expressing hope for client.	Although the prognosis may be discouraging, remissions may occur, and because the future cannot be predicted, hope for some quality of life should be encouraged. Additionally, research is ongoing and new treatment options are being initiated.
Encourage/assist client to identify activities he or she would like to be involved in (e.g., volunteer work) within the limits of his or her abilities.	Staying active and interacting with others helps counteract feelings of helplessness.

ACTIONS/INTERVENTIONS	RATIONALE
Discuss plans for the future. Suggest visiting alternative care facilities, taking a look at the possibilities for care as condition changes.	When options are considered and plans are made for any eventuality, client has a sense of control over own circumstances.

Self-Responsibility Facilitation (NIC)

ACTIONS/INTERVENTIONS	RATIONALE
Determine degree of mastery client has exhibited in life to the present. Note locus of control; i.e., internal/external.	Client who has assumed responsibility in life previously tends to do the same during difficult times of exacerbation of illness. However, if locus of control has been focused outward, client may blame others and not take control over own circumstances.
Assist client to identify factors that are under own control; e.g., list things that can or cannot be controlled.	Knowing and accepting what is beyond individual control can reduce helpless/acting out behaviors, promote focusing on areas individual can control.
Encourage client to assume control over as much of own care as possible.	Even when unable to do much physical care, individual can help plan and supervise own care, having a voice in what is/is not desired.
Discuss needs openly with client/SO, setting up agreed-on routines for meeting identified needs.	Helps deal with manipulative behavior, when client feels powerless and not listened to.
Incorporate client's daily routine into home care schedule/hospital stay as possible.	Maintains sense of control/self-determination and independence.

Collaborative

ACTIONS/INTERVENTIONS	RATIONALE
Refer to vocational rehabilitation as indicated.	Can assist client to develop and implement a vocational plan incorporating specific interests/abilities.
Identify community resources; e.g., adult day enrichment program.	Participation in structured activities can reduce sense of isolation and may enhance feeling of self-worth.

NURSING DIAGNOSIS: risk for ineffective Coping

Risk factors may include

Physiologic changes (cerebral and spinal lesions)
Psychologic conflicts, anxiety; fear
Impaired judgment, short-term memory loss, confusion, unrealistic perceptions/expectations, emotional lability
Personal vulnerability; inadequate support systems
Multiple life changes
Inadequate coping methods

Possibly evidenced by

[Not applicable; presence of signs and symptoms establishes an *actual* diagnosis.]

DESIRED OUTCOMES/EVALUATION CRITERIA—CLIENT WILL:

Coping (NOC)

Recognize relationship between disease process (cerebral lesions) and emotional responses, changes in thinking/behavior.
Verbalize awareness of own capabilities/strengths.
Display effective problem-solving skills.
Demonstrate behaviors/lifestyle changes to prevent/minimize changes in mentation and maintain reality orientation.

ACTIONS/INTERVENTIONS	RATIONALE
Coping Enhancement (NIC)	
Independent	
Assess current functional capacity/limitations; note presence of distorted thinking processes, labile emotions, cognitive dissonance. Determine how these affect the individual's coping abilities.	Organic or psychologic effects may cause client to be easily distracted, to display difficulties with concentration, problem-solving, dealing with what is happening, being responsible for own care.
Determine client's understanding of current situation and previous methods of dealing with life's problems.	Provides a clue as to how client may deal with what is currently happening, and helps identify individual resources and need for assistance.
Discuss ability to make decisions, care for children/dependent adults, handle finances. Identify options available to individuals involved.	Impaired judgment, confusion, inadequate support systems may interfere with ability to meet own needs/needs of others. Conservatorship, guardianship, or adult protective services may be required until (if ever) client is able to manage own affairs.
Maintain an honest, reality-oriented relationship.	Reduces confusion and minimizes painful, frustrating struggles associated with adaptation to altered environment/lifestyle.
Encourage verbalization of feelings/fears, accepting what client says in a nonjudgmental manner. Note statements reflecting powerlessness, inability to cope. (Refer to ND: Powerlessness/Hopelessness.)	May diminish client's fear, establish trust, and provide an opportunity to identify problems/begin the problem-solving process.
Observe nonverbal communication; e.g., posture, eye contact, movements, gestures, and use of touch. Compare with verbal content and verify meaning with client as appropriate.	May provide significant information about what client is feeling; however, verification is important to ensure accuracy of communication. Discrepancy between feelings and what is being verbalized can interfere with ability to cope, problem-solve.
Provide clues for orientation; e.g., calendars, clocks, notecards, organizers/date book.	These serve as tangible reminders to aid recognition and permeate memory gaps and enable client to cope with situation.
Encourage client to tape record important information and listen to the recording periodically.	Repetition puts information in long-term memory, where it is more easily retrieved and can support decision-making/problem-solving process.
Collaborative	
Refer to cognitive retraining program.	Improving cognitive abilities can enhance basic thinking skills when attention span is short, ability to process information is impaired, client is unable to learn new tasks, or insight, judgment, and problem-solving skills are impaired.
Refer to counseling, psychiatric clinical nurse specialist/psychiatrist as indicated.	May need additional help to resolve issues of self-esteem and regain effective coping skills.
Administer medications as appropriate e.g., amitriptyline (Elavil), bupropion (Wellbutrin), imipramine (Tofranil), trazadone (Desyrel)	Medications to improve mood and restful sleep may be useful in combating depression and relieving degree of fatigue interfering with function.

NURSING DIAGNOSIS: compromised/disabled family Coping

May be related to

Situational crisis; temporary family disorganization and role changes
Highly ambivalent family relationship
Prolonged disease/disability progression that exhausts the supportive capacity of SO
Client providing little support in turn for SO
SO with chronically unexpressed feelings of guilt, anxiety, hostility, despair

Possibly evidenced by

Client expresses/confirms concern or complaint about SO response to client's illness.
SO withdraws or has limited personal communication with client or displays protective behavior disproportionate to client's abilities or need for autonomy.
SO preoccupied with own personal reactions
Intolerance, abandonment
Neglectful care of client
Distortion of reality regarding client's illness

DESIRED OUTCOMES/EVALUATION CRITERIA—FAMILY WILL:

Family Coping (NOC)

Identify/verbalize resources within themselves to deal with the situation.
Express more realistic understanding and expectations of client.
Interact appropriately with client/healthcare providers providing support and assistance as indicated.
Verbalize knowledge and understanding of disability/disease and community resources.

ACTIONS/INTERVENTIONS	RATIONALE
Family Involvement Promotion (NIC)	
Independent	
Note length/severity of illness. Determine client's role in family and how illness has changed the family organization.	Chronic/unresolved illness, accompanied by changes in role performance/responsibility, often exhausts supportive capacity and coping abilities of SO/family.
Determine SO's understanding of disease process and expectations for the future.	Inadequate information/misconception regarding disease process and/or unrealistic expectations affect ability to cope with current situation. *Note:* A particular area of misconception is the fatigue experienced by clients with MS. Family members may view client's inability to perform activities as manipulative behavior rather than an actual physiologic deficit.
Discuss with SO/family members their willingness to be involved in care. Identify other responsibilities/factors impacting participation.	Individuals may not have desire/time to assume responsibility for care. If several family members are available, they may be able to share tasks.
Assess other factors that are affecting abilities of family members to provide needed support; e.g., own emotional problems, work concerns.	Individual members' preoccupation with own needs/concerns can interfere with providing needed care/support for stresses of long-term illness. Additionally, caregiver(s) may incur decrease or loss of income/risk losing own health insurance if they alter their work hours.
Discuss underlying reasons for client's behaviors.	Helps SO understand and accept/deal with behaviors that may be triggered by emotional or physical effects of MS.
Encourage client/SO to develop and strengthen problem-solving skills to deal with situation.	Family may/may not have handled conflict well before illness, and stress of long-term debilitating condition can create additional problems (including unresolved anger).
Encourage free expression of feelings, including frustration, anger, hostility, and hopelessness.	Individual members may be afraid to express "negative" feelings, believing it will discourage client. Free expression promotes awareness and can help with resolution of feelings and problems (especially when done in a caring manner).

ACTIONS/INTERVENTIONS	RATIONALE
Collaborative	
Identify community resources; e.g., local MS organization, support groups, home care agencies, respite programs.	Provides information, opportunities to share with others who are experiencing similar difficulties, and sources of assistance when needed.
Refer to social worker, financial adviser, psychiatric clinical nurse specialist/psychiatrist as appropriate.	May need more in-depth assistance from professional sources.

NURSING DIAGNOSIS: impaired Urinary Elimination

May be related to

Neuromuscular impairment (spinal cord lesions/neurogenic bladder)

Possibly evidenced by

Incontinence, nocturia, frequency
Retention with overflow
Recurrent UTIs

DESIRED OUTCOMES/EVALUATION CRITERIA—CLIENT WILL:

Urine Continence (NOC)

Verbalize understanding of condition.
Demonstrate behaviors/techniques to prevent/minimize infection.
Empty bladder completely and regularly (voluntarily or by catheter as appropriate).
Be free of urine leakage between voidings.

ACTIONS/INTERVENTIONS	RATIONALE
Urinary Elimination Management (NIC)	
Independent	
Note reports of urinary frequency, urgency, burning, incontinence, nocturia, and size/force of urinary stream. Palpate bladder after voiding.	Provides information about degree of interference with elimination or may indicate bladder infection. Fullness over bladder after voiding is indicative of inadequate emptying/retention and requires further evaluation and intervention.
Review drug regimen, including prescribed, OTC, and street drug use.	A number of medications (e.g., some antispasmodics, antidepressants, and narcotic analgesics; OTC medications with anticholinergic or α-agonist properties, or recreational drugs such as cannabis) may interfere with bladder emptying.
Institute bladder training program or timed voidings as appropriate.	Helps restore adequate bladder functioning, lessens occurrence of incontinence and bladder infection.
Encourage adequate fluid intake, avoiding caffeine and use of aspartame, and limiting intake during late evening and at bedtime. Recommend use of cranberry juice and vitamin C.	Sufficient hydration promotes urinary output and aids in preventing infection. *Note:* When client is taking sulfa drugs, sufficient fluids are necessary to ensure adequate excretion of drug, reducing risk of cumulative effects. *Note:* Aspartame, a sugar substitute (e.g., NutraSweet), may cause bladder irritation leading to bladder dysfunction.
Promote continued mobility.	Decreases risk of developing UTI.

ACTIONS/INTERVENTIONS	RATIONALE
Recommend good hand-washing/perineal care.	Reduces skin irritation and risk of ascending infection.
Encourage client to observe for sediment/blood in urine, foul odor, fever, or unexplained increase in MS symptoms (e.g., spasticity, dysarthria).	Indicative of infection requiring further evaluation/ treatment.

Collaborative

Refer to urinary continence specialist as indicated.	Helpful for developing individual plan of care to meet client's specific needs using the latest techniques, continence products.
Administer medications as indicated; e.g., Tolterodine (Detrol), oxybutynin (Ditropan), propantheline (Pro-Banthine), hyoscyamine sulfate (Cytospaz-M), flavoxate(Urispaz)	Reduce bladder spasticity and associated symptoms of frequency, urgency, incontinence, and nocturia.
Catheterize as indicated.	May be necessary as a treatment and for evaluation purposes if client is unable to empty bladder or retains urine.
Teach self-catheterization/instruct in use and care of indwelling catheter.	Helps client maintain autonomy and encourages self-care. Indwelling catheter may be required, depending on client's abilities and degree of urinary problem.
Obtain periodic urinalysis/urine culture and sensitivity as indicated.	Monitors bladder and kidney status. Colony count over 100,000 indicates presence of infection requiring treatment.
Administer anti-infective agents as necessary; e.g., nitrofurantoin macrocrystals (Macrodantin), co-trimoxazole (Bactrim, Septra), ciprofloxacin (Cipro), norfloxacin (Noroxin).	Bacteriostatic agents inhibit bacterial growth and destroy susceptible bacteria. Prompt treatment of infection is necessary to prevent serious complications of sepsis/shock.

NURSING DIAGNOSIS: risk for Caregiver Role Strain

Risk factors may include

Severity of illness of the care receiver, duration of caregiving required, complexity/amount of caregiving task
Caregiver is female, spouse
Care receiver exhibits deviant, bizarre behavior
Family/caregiver isolation, lack of respite and recreation

Possibly evidenced by

[Not applicable; presence of signs/symptoms establishes an *actual* diagnosis.]

DESIRED OUTCOME/EVALUATION CRITERIA—CAREGIVER WILL:

CAREGIVER PERFORMANCE: Direct Care (NOC)

Identify individual risk factors and appropriate interventions.
Demonstrate/initiate behaviors or lifestyle changes to prevent development of impaired function.

CAREGIVER PERFORMANCE: Indirect Care (NOC)

Use available resources appropriately.
Report satisfaction with plan and support available.

ACTIONS/INTERVENTIONS	RATIONALE
Caregiver Support (NIC)	
Independent	
Note physical/mental condition, therapeutic regimen of care receiver.	Determines individual needs for planning care. Identifies strengths and how much responsibility client may be expected to assume, as well as disabilities requiring accommodation.
Determine caregiver's level of commitment, responsibility, involvement in and anticipated length of care. Use assessment tool, such as Burden Interview, to further determine caregiver's abilities when appropriate.	Progressive debilitation taxes caregiver and may alter ability to meet client/own needs. (Refer to ND: compromised/disabled family Coping.)
Discuss caregiver's view of and about situation.	Allows ventilation and clarification of concerns, promoting understanding.
Determine available supports and resources currently used.	Organizations (e.g., National MS Society, local support groups) can provide information regarding adequacy of supports and identify needs/possible options.
Facilitate family conference to share information and develop plan for involvement in care activities as appropriate.	When others are involved in care, the risk of one person becoming overloaded is lessened.
Identify additional resources to include financial, legal assistance.	These areas of concern can add to burden of caregiving if not adequately resolved.
Identify adaptive equipment needs/resources for the home and vehicles.	Enhances independence and safety of both caregiver and client.
Provide information and/or demonstrate techniques for dealing with acting-out/violent or disoriented behavior.	Helps caregiver maintain sense of control and competency. Enhances safety for care receiver and caregiver.
Stress importance of self-nurturing; e.g., pursuing self-development interests, personal needs, hobbies, and social activities.	Taking time for self can lessen risk of "burnout"/being overwhelmed by situation.
Identify alternate care sources (such as sitter/day care facility), senior care services; e.g., Meals on Wheels, respite care, home care agency.	As client's condition worsens, SO may need additional help from several sources to maintain client at home even on a part-time basis.
Assist caregiver to plan for changes that may be necessary for the care receiver (e.g., eventual placement in extended care facility).	Planning for this eventually is important for the time when burden of care becomes too great.
Collaborative	
Refer to supportive services as need indicates.	Medical case manager or social services consultant may be needed to develop ongoing plan to meet changing needs of client and SO/family.

NURSING DIAGNOSIS: deficient Knowledge [Learning Need] regarding condition, prognosis, complications, treatment, and needs

May be related to

Lack of exposure, information misinterpretation
Unfamiliarity with information resources
Cognitive limitation, lack of recall

Possibly evidenced by

Statement of misconception
Request for information
Inaccurate follow-through of instruction; development of preventable complications
Inappropriate or exaggerated behaviors (e.g., hysterical, hostile, agitated, apathetic)

DESIRED OUTCOMES/EVALUATION CRITERIA—CLIENT/CAREGIVER WILL:

KNOWLEDGE: Disease Process (NOC)

Participate in learning process.
Assume responsibility for own learning and begin to look for information and to ask questions.
Verbalize understanding of condition/disease process and treatment.
Initiate necessary lifestyle changes.
Participate in prescribed treatment regimen.

ACTIONS/INTERVENTIONS	RATIONALE
Learning Facilitation (NIC)	
Independent	
Evaluate desire/readiness of client and SO/caregiver to learn.	Determines amount/level of information to provide at any given moment.
Note signs of emotional lability or whether client is in dissociative state (loss of affect, inappropriate emotional responses).	Client will not process/retain information and will have difficulty learning during this time.
Provide information in varied formats depending on client's cognitive/perceptual abilities and considering client's locus of control.	Changes in cognitive, visual, auditory function impact choice of teaching modalities; e.g., verbal instruction, books, pamphlets, audiovisuals, computer programs. Whether locus of control is internal or external affects client's attitude toward helpfulness of learning.
Encourage active participation of client/SO in learning process, including use of self-paced instruction as appropriate.	Enhances sense of independence and control and may strengthen commitment to therapeutic regimen.
TEACHING: Disease Process (NIC)	
Review disease process/prognosis, effects of climate, emotional stress, overexertion, fatigue.	Clarifies client/SO understanding of individual situation.
Identify signs/symptoms requiring further evaluation.	Prompt intervention may help limit severity of exacerbation/complications.
Discuss importance of daily routine of rest, exercise, activity, and eating, focusing on current capabilities. Instruct in use of appropriate devices to assist with ADLs; e.g., eating utensils, walking aids.	Helps client maintain current level of physical independence and may limit fatigue.
Stress necessity of weight control.	Excess weight can interfere with balance and motor abilities and make care more difficult.
Review possible problems that may arise, such as decreased perception of heat and pain, susceptibility to skin breakdown and infections, especially UTI.	These effects of demyelination and associated complications may compromise client's safety and/or precipitate an exacerbation of symptoms.
Identify actions that can be taken to avoid injury; e.g., avoid hot baths, inspect skin regularly, take care with transfers and wheelchair/walker mobility, practice scooter safety, force fluids, and get adequate nutrition. Encourage avoidance of persons with upper respiratory infection.	Review of risk factors can help client take measures to maintain physical state at optimal level/prevent complications.
Discuss increased risk of osteoporosis and review preventive measures; e.g., regular exercise, increased intake of calcium and vitamin D, reduced intake of caffeine, cessation of smoking, hormone replacement therapy (HRT) or alternatives (e.g., bisphosphonates—Fosamax), and fall prevention measures such as wearing low-heeled shoes with nonskid soles, use of handrails/grab bars in bathroom and along stairwells, removal of small area rugs.	Decreased mobility, vitamin D deficiency (possibly a result of decreased exposure to sunlight, which can exacerbate MS symptoms), and decreased likelihood of engaging in preventive measures increase bone mass loss and the risk of fractures.

ACTIONS/INTERVENTIONS	RATIONALE
Identify bowel elimination concerns. Recommend adequate hydration and intake of fiber; use of stool softeners, bulking agents, suppositories, or possibly mild laxatives; bowel training program.	Constipation is common, and bowel urgency and/or accidents may occur as a result of dietary deficiencies or impaction.
Review specifics of individual medications. Recommend avoidance of OTC drugs.	Reduces likelihood of drug interactions/adverse effects, and enhances cooperation with treatment regimen.
Discuss concerns regarding sexual relationships, contraception/reproduction, effects of pregnancy on affected woman. Identify alternative ways to meet individual needs; counsel regarding use of artificial lubrication (females), genitourinary (GU) referral for males regarding available medication/sexual aids.	Pregnancy may be an issue for the young client relative to issues of genetic predisposition and/or ability to manage pregnancy or parent offspring. Increased libido is not uncommon and may require adjustments within the existing relationship or in the absence of an acceptable partner. Information about different positions and techniques and/or other options for sexual fulfillment (e.g., fondling, cuddling) may enhance personal relationship and feelings of self-worth.
Encourage client to set goals for the future while focusing on the "here and now," what can be done today.	Having a plan for the future helps retain hope and provides opportunity for client to see that although today is to be lived, one can plan for tomorrow even in the worst of circumstances.
Identify financial concerns.	Loss or change of employment (for client and/or SO) impacts income, insurance benefits, and level of independence, requiring additional family/social support.
Refer for vocational rehabilitation as appropriate.	May need assessment of capabilities/job retraining as indicated by individual limitations/disease progression.
Recommend contacting local and national MS organizations, relevant support groups.	Ongoing contact (e.g., mailings) informs client of programs/services available, and can update client's knowledge base. Support groups can provide role modeling, sharing of information and enhance problem-solving ability.

POTENTIAL CONSIDERATIONS following acute hospitalization (dependent on client's age, physical condition/presence of complications, personal resources, and life responsibilities)

risk for Trauma—weakness, poor vision, balancing difficulties, reduced temperature/tactile sensation, reduced muscle and hand/eye coordination, cognitive or emotional difficulties, insufficient finances to purchase necessary equipment.

impaired Home Maintenance—insufficient finances, unfamiliarity with neighborhood resources, inadequate support systems.

risk for/[actual] Disuse Syndrome—paralysis/immobilization, severe pain.

ineffective Therapeutic Regimen Management—economic difficulties, family conflict, social support deficits.

7

CHAPTER

Gastrointestinal Disorders

UPPER GASTROINTESTINAL/ESOPHAGEAL BLEEDING

Bleeding duodenal ulcer is the most frequent cause of massive upper gastrointestinal bleed (UGIB), but bleeding may also occur because of gastric ulcers, gastritis, and esophageal varices. Severe vomiting can precipitate gastric bleeding as a result of a tear in the mucosa at the gastroesophageal junction (Mallory-Weiss syndrome). Stress ulcers are often associated with severe burns, major trauma/surgery, or severe systemic disease. Esophagitis, esophageal/gastric carcinoma, hiatal hernia, hemophilia, leukemia, and disseminated intravascular coagulation (DIC) are less common causes of UGIB. *Note:* Eighty to 90% of elderly clients with ulcers have been found to have *Helicobactor pylori* as an underlying cause. Because this organism is easily treated with anti-infectives, complications such as perforation and gastrointestinal (GI) bleeding have dropped dramatically. If *H. pylori* bacteria are not eliminated, ulcers recur in 50%–90% of clients after 1 year when the antiulcer medications are discontinued following ulcer healing. The presence of *H. pylori* increases the risk of peptic ulcer disease 5- to 7-fold, but with the use of nonsteroidal anti-inflammatory drugs (NSAID)s, the risk increases 5- to 20-fold.

CARE SETTING

Generally, a client with severe, active bleeding is admitted directly to a critical care unit; however, a client may develop GI bleeding on the medical-surgical unit or be admitted there for evaluation/treatment of subacute bleeding.

RELATED CONCERNS

Cirrhosis of the liver, page 453
Fluid and electrolyte imbalances, page 919
Psychosocial aspects of care, page 770
Renal failure: acute, page 541
Subtotal gastrectomy/gastric resection, page 320

Client Assessment Database

ACTIVITY/REST

May report: Weakness, fatigue
May exhibit: Tachycardia, tachypnea/hyperventilation (response to activity)

CIRCULATION

May report: Palpitations
Dizziness with position change
May exhibit: Hypotension (including postural)
Tachycardia, dysrhythmias (hypovolemia/hypoxemia)
Weak/thready peripheral pulse
Capillary refill slow/delayed (vasoconstriction)
Skin color: Pallor, cyanosis (depending on the amount of blood loss)
Skin/mucous membrane moisture: Diaphoresis (reflecting shock state, acute pain, psychologic response)

EGO INTEGRITY

May report: Acute or chronic stress factors (financial, relationships, job related)
Feelings of helplessness
May exhibit: Signs of anxiety; e.g., restlessness, pallor, diaphoresis, narrowed focus, trembling, quivering voice

ELIMINATION

May report: Change in usual bowel patterns/characteristics of stool

May exhibit: Abdominal tenderness, distention

Bowel sounds often hyperactive during bleeding, hypoactive after bleeding subsides

Character of stool: Diarrhea; dark bloody, tarry, or occasionally bright red stools; frothy, foul-smelling (steatorrhea); constipation may occur (changes in diet, antacid use)

Urine output may be decreased, concentrated

FOOD/FLUID

May report: Anorexia, nausea, vomiting (protracted vomiting suggests pyloric outlet obstruction associated with duodenal ulcer)

Problems with swallowing, belching, hiccups

Heartburn, indigestion, burping with sour taste

Bloating/distention, flatulence

Food intolerances; e.g., spicy food, chocolate; special diet for preexisting ulcer disease

Weight loss

May exhibit: Vomitus: Coffee-ground or bright red, with or without clots

Mucous membranes dry, decreased mucus production, poor skin turgor (chronic bleeding)

Urine specific gravity may be elevated

NEUROSENSORY

May report: Fainting, dizziness/lightheadedness, weakness

May exhibit: Mental status: Level of consciousness (LOC) may be altered, ranging from slight drowsiness, disorientation/confusion, to stupor and coma (depending on circulating volume/oxygenation)

PAIN/DISCOMFORT

May report: Pain described as sharp, dull, burning, gnawing, sudden, excruciating (can accompany perforation)

Vague sensation of discomfort/distress following large meals and relieved by food (acute gastritis)

Left to midepigastric pain and/or pain radiating to back, often accompanied by vomiting after eating and relieved by antacids (gastric ulcer)

Localized right to midepigastric pain, gnawing, burning, occurring about 2–3 hr after meals when stomach is empty, and relieved by food or antacids (duodenal ulcers)

Midepigastric pain and burning with regurgitation (chronic gastroesophageal reflux disease [GERD])

Absence of pain (esophageal varices or gastritis)

Precipitating factors may be foods (e.g., milk, chocolate, caffeine), smoking, alcohol, certain drugs (salicylates, reserpine, antibiotics, ibuprofen), psychological stressors

May exhibit: Facial grimacing, guarding of affected area, pallor, diaphoresis, narrowed focus

SAFETY

May report: Drug allergies/sensitivities; e.g., acetylsalicylic acid (ASA)

May exhibit: Temperature elevation

Spider angiomas, palmar erythema (reflecting cirrhosis/portal hypertension)

TEACHING/LEARNING

May report: Recent use of prescription/OTC drugs containing acetylsalicylic acid (ASA), alcohol/recreational drugs, steroids, or NSAIDs—leading cause of drug-induced GI bleeding

Current complaint may reveal admission for related (e.g., anemia) or unrelated (e.g., head trauma) diagnosis, intestinal flu, or severe vomiting episode; long-standing health problems; e.g., cirrhosis, alcoholism, hepatitis, eating disorders

History of previous hospitalizations for GI bleeding or related GI problems; e.g., peptic/gastric ulcer, gastritis, gastric surgery, irradiation of gastric area

Discharge plan considerations: May require changes in therapeutic/medication regimen.

Refer to section at end of plan for postdischarge considerations.

DIAGNOSTIC STUDIES

Esophagogastroduodenoscopy (EGD) and colonoscopies: Key diagnostic tests for upper and lower GI bleeding, done to visualize site of bleeding/ degree of tissue ulceration/injury. Capsule endoscopy is a novel diagnostic procedure that has high diagnostic yield in obscure GI bleeding of suspected small-bowel origin. Endoscopy allows estimation of the rate of bleeding and enables various therapeutic options.

Gastrointestinal nuclear scan: Radionuclide uptake at sites of bleeding identifies site (not cause) of bleeding. Test is considered to be more sensitive than EGD, upper GI studies with barium, or angiography in detecting sites of lower GI bleeding or persistent bleeding anywhere in GI tract.

Helicobacter pylori *breath test:* Client drinks a carbon-enriched urea solution. If *H. pylori* is present, it breaks down the compound and releases CO_2. *H. pylori* can also be detected by blood or tissue tests, with blood test now being more common.

Barium swallow with x-ray: May be done after bleeding has ceased for differential diagnosis of cause/site of lesion and presence of structural defects such as strictures.

Gastric aspirate analysis: May be done in suspected peptic ulcer disease as indicated by low to normal pH and/or presence of blood; also in suspected gastric cancer (abnormal acidity, blood and/or abnormal cells on cytologic examination).

Gastric biopsies: Obtained during EGD to help determine presence of *H. pylori* (gram-negative urease-producing bacteria), currently accepted as organism responsible in the elderly for 90% of duodenal and 70%–80% of gastric ulcers.

Angiography: GI vasculature may be reviewed if endoscopy is inconclusive or impractical. Demonstrates collateral circulation and possibly bleeding site.

Stools: Testing for blood will be positive.

Complete blood count (CBC), hemoglobin (Hb)/hematocrit (Hct): Decreased levels occur 6–24 hr after acute bleeding begins. Red blood cells (RBCs) and platelets may also be decreased. White blood cell (WBC) count may be elevated, reflecting body's response to injury.

Prothrombin time (PT) and activated partial thromboplastin time (aPTT); coagulation profile: Prolonged in active bleeding. May indicate need for replacement of coagulation factors (fresh frozen plasma [FFP]). Increased platelets with decreased clotting times may be the body's attempt to restore hemostasis. Severe abnormalities may reveal coagulopathy (e.g., DIC) as cause of bleeding.

Blood urea nitrogen (BUN): Elevated within 24–48 hr as blood proteins are broken down in the GI tract and kidney filtration is decreased.

Creatinine (Cr): Usually not elevated if renal perfusion is maintained.

Ammonia: May be elevated when severe liver dysfunction disrupts the metabolism and proper excretion of urea or when massive whole blood transfusions have been given.

Arterial blood gases (ABGs): May reveal initial respiratory alkalosis (compensating for diminished blood flow through lungs). Later, metabolic acidosis develops in response to sluggish liver flow/accumulation of metabolic waste products.

Sodium: May be elevated as a hormonal compensation to conserve body fluid.

Potassium: May initially be depleted because of massive gastric emptying/vomiting or bloody diarrhea. Elevated potassium levels may occur after multiple transfusions of stored blood or with acute renal impairment.

Serum gastrin analysis: Elevated level suggests Zollinger-Ellison syndrome or possible presence of multiple poorly healed ulcers. Normal or low in type B gastritis.

Serum amylase: Elevated with posterior penetration of duodenal ulcer.

Pepsinogen level: Increased by duodenal ulcer; low level suggestive of gastritis.

Serum parietal cell antibodies: Presence suggestive of chronic gastritis.

NURSING PRIORITIES

1. Control hemorrhage.
2. Achieve/maintain hemodynamic stability.
3. Promote stress reduction.
4. Provide information about disease process/prognosis, treatment needs, and potential complications.

DISCHARGE GOALS

1. Hemorrhage curtailed.
2. Hemodynamically stable.
3. Anxiety/fear reduced to manageable level.
4. Disease process/prognosis, therapeutic regimen, and potential complications understood.
5. Plan in place to meet needs after discharge.

NURSING DIAGNOSIS: deficient Fluid Volume [isotonic]

May be related to

Active fluid volume loss (hemorrhage)

Possibly evidenced by

Hypotension, tachycardia, delayed capillary refill
Changes in mentation, restlessness
Concentrated/decreased urine
Pallor, diaphoresis
Hemoconcentration

DESIRED OUTCOMES/EVALUATION CRITERIA—CLIENT WILL:

Blood Loss Severity (NOC)

Be free of signs of bleeding in GI aspirate/stools, stablization of Hb/Hct.

Hydration (NOC)

Demonstrate improved fluid balance as evidenced by individually adequate urinary output with normal specific gravity, stable vital signs, moist mucous membranes, good skin turgor, prompt capillary refill.

ACTIONS/INTERVENTIONS	RATIONALE
BLEEDING REDUCTION: Gastrointestinal (NIC)	
Independent	
Note color and characteristics of vomitus, nasogastric tube drainage, and/or stools.	The first step in managing bleeding is to determine its location. Bright red blood that does not clear signals recent or acute arterial bleeding, perhaps caused by gastric ulceration; dark red blood may be old blood (retained in intestine) or venous bleeding from varices. Coffee-grounds appearance is suggestive of partially digested blood from slowly oozing area. Undigested food indicates obstruction or gastric tumor. In a rapid upper GI bleed, stool color may be red or maroon because of rapid transit time through the GI tract.
Monitor vital signs; compare with client's normal/previous readings. Take blood pressure (BP) in lying, sitting, standing positions when possible.	Changes in blood pressure (BP) and pulse may be used for rough estimate of blood loss (e.g., BP less than 90 mm Hg and pulse greater than 110 suggest a 25% decrease in volume, or approximately 1000 mL). Postural hypotension reflects a decrease in circulating volume. *Note:* Heart rate may not rise above normal until up to 30% of total blood volume is lost.
Note client's individual physiologic response to bleeding; e.g., changes in mentation, weakness, restlessness, anxiety, pallor, diaphoresis, tachypnea, temperature elevation.	Symptomatology is useful in gauging severity/length of bleeding episode. Worsening of symptoms may reflect continued bleeding, inadequate fluid replacement, and/or shock.
Measure central venous pressure (CVP) if available.	Reflects circulating volume and cardiac response to bleeding and fluid replacement; e.g., CVP values between 5 and 20 cm H_2O usually reflect adequate volume.
Monitor intake and output (I&O) and correlate with weight changes. Measure blood/fluid losses via emesis, gastric suction/lavage, and stools.	Provides guidelines for fluid replacement.

ACTIONS/INTERVENTIONS	RATIONALE
Keep accurate record of subtotals of solutions/blood products during replacement therapy.	Potential exists for overtransfusion of fluids, especially when volume expanders are given before blood transfusions.
Maintain bedrest; prevent vomiting and straining at stool. Schedule activities to provide undisturbed rest periods. Eliminate noxious stimuli.	Activity/vomiting increases intra-abdominal pressure and can predispose to further bleeding.
Elevate head of bed during antacid gavage.	Prevents gastric reflux and aspiration of antacids, which can cause serious pulmonary complications.
Note signs of renewed bleeding after cessation of initial bleed.	Increased abdominal fullness/distention, nausea or renewed vomiting, and bloody diarrhea may indicate rebleeding.
Observe for secondary bleeding; e.g., nose/gums, oozing from puncture sites, appearance of ecchymotic areas following minimal trauma.	Loss of/inadequate replacement of clotting factors may precipitate development of DIC.
Provide clear/bland fluids when intake is resumed. Avoid caffeinated and carbonated beverages.	More easily digested and reduce risk of added irritation to inflamed tissues. Caffeine and carbonated beverages stimulate hydrochloric acid (HCl) production, possibly potentiating rebleeding.

Collaborative

Prepare for urgent endoscopy.	Indicated within 24 hr of acute UGIB for diagnosis and intervention when client presents with hematemesis, melena, or postural changes in blood pressure.
Administer IV fluids/volume expanders as indicated; e.g.:	
0.9% sodium chloride, lactated Ringer's solution;	Fluid replacement with isotonic crystalloid solutions depends on degree of hypovolemia and duration of bleeding (acute or chronic). Other volume expanders, such as albumin, may be infused until type and cross-matching can be completed and blood transfusions begun. Approximately 80%–90% of gastric bleeding is controlled by fluid resuscitation and medical management without transfusion of blood products. *Note:* Use of lactated Ringer's solution may be contraindicated in presence of hepatic failure because metabolism of lactate is impaired, and lactic acidosis may develop.
Fresh whole blood/packed RBCs;	Fresh whole blood is indicated only for acute bleeding with severe volume and RBC depletion because stored blood may be deficient in clotting factors. Packed red blood cells (PRCs) are adequate for stable clients with subacute/chronic bleeding to increase oxygen-carrying capability. *Note:* PRCs are preferred for clients with heart failure (HF) to prevent fluid overload.
Platelets;	Transfused more often than any other blood component, platelets are given to correct deficits in platelet number and clotting function. Clotting factors/components are depleted by two mechanisms: hemorrhagic loss and the clotting process at the site of bleeding.
Fresh frozen plasma.	FFP is an excellent source for clotting factors. Administered to clients with coagulation deficiencies who are bleeding or about to undergo an invasive procedure.
Insert/maintain large-bore nasogastric (NG) tube in acute bleeding.	Provides avenue for removing irritating gastric secretions, blood, and clots; reduces nausea/vomiting; and facilitates diagnostic endoscopy. *Note:* Blood remaining in the stomach/intestines will be broken down into ammonia, which can produce a toxic central nervous system (CNS) effect; e.g., encephalopathy.

ACTIONS/INTERVENTIONS	RATIONALE
Perform gastric lavage with cool or room-temperature saline until aspirate is light pink or clear and free of clots. Simultaneous low-pressure gastric suctioning and continuous saline infusion through the air port of a Salem sump tube may also be used.	Flushes out/breaks up clots and may reduce bleeding by local vasoconstriction. Facilitates visualization by endoscopy to locate bleeding source. *Note:* Research suggests that iced saline is no more effective than room temperature solution in controlling bleeding, and it may actually damage gastric mucosa and lower client's core temperature, which could prolong bleeding by inhibiting platelet function. Controversy also exists as to whether benefit is obtained from any gastric lavage, whether iced or room temperature.
Administer medications as indicated; e.g.:	
Proton pump inhibitor (PPI) (e.g.: omeprazole [Prilosec], lansoprazole [Prevacid], robeprazole [Aciphex], pantoprazole [Protonix]), esomeprasole [Nexium]);	PPIs have been shown in studies to be most effective after GI bleed to reduce occurrence of rebleeding. PPIs (administered orally, by tube, endoscope, or IV) can completely inhibit acid secretion, and have a long duration of action. Used for peptic ulcer disease (PUD) and GERD, or short-term therapy for duodenal ulcers (healing duodenal ulcers in 2–4 wk once severe bleeding is controlled). Typically given with antibiotics when *H. pylori* infection is present. *Note:* Pantoprazole (Protonix) is the only PPI available for IV administration.
Sucralfate (Carafate);	Antiulcer agent that coats the stomach, adheres to the ulcer surface, and reinforces the mucosal barrier. *Note:* Impairs absorption of some drugs; e.g., theophylline, digoxin, phenytoin, tetracycline, amitriptyline.
Cisapride (Propulsid);	Serotonin-4-receptor agonist used to treat PUD, reflux esophagitis.
Misoprostol (Cytotec);	Aids in mucus production and inhibits acid secretions. Used to prevent gastric ulcers associated with NSAID use.
Antacids: e.g., aluminum-based (Amphojel, Basaljel), magnesium-based (e.g., Mylanta, Riopan);	Antacids (administered orally or by gavage) may be used to reduce total acid load within the gastric lumen. Effectiveness is greatest for duodenal ulcers. Antacids maintain gastric pH level at 4.5 or higher and reduce risk of rebleeding. *Note:* Antacids block the gastric absorption of oral histamine antagonists and therefore should not be administered within 1 hr after oral administration of histamine blockers.
Belladonna, atropine;	Anticholinergics may be used to decrease gastric motility, particularly in PUD after acute bleeding has subsided.
Octreotide (Sandostatin);	An analogue of the hormone somatostatin thought to help control esophageal bleeding by decreasing blood flow to the gut, thereby lowering pressure to the portal system. *Note:* Current guidelines do not recommend use of this drug for nonvariceal GI bleeding.
Vasopressin (Pitressin);	Administration of intra-arterial vasoconstrictors may be needed in severe, prolonged bleeding (varices). *Note:* Effects of Pitressin are systemic, whereas octreotide is more regional.
Vitamin K_1 (AquaMEPHYTON);	Promotes hepatic synthesis of coagulation factors to support clotting. *Note:* Use of sucralfate may decrease absorption of vitamin K.
Antiemetics; e.g., metoclopramide (Reglan), prochlorperazine (Compazine);	Alleviate nausea and prevent vomiting.
Supplemental vitamin B_{12};	In diffuse atrophic gastritis, the intrinsic factor necessary for vitamin B_{12} absorption from the GI tract is not secreted, and individual may develop pernicious anemia.

ACTIONS/INTERVENTIONS	RATIONALE
Anti-infectives; e.g., tetracycline (Achromycin), metronidazole (Flagyl), amoxicillin (Amoxil), clarithromycin (Biaxin).	Oral agents may be combined with antacids or histamine blockers to treat infections causing chronic gastritis or peptic ulcers (*H. pylori*). *Note:* Some studies indicate that *H. pylori* is developing widespread resistance to metronidazole (Flagyl).
Monitor laboratory studies; e.g.:	
Hb, Hct, RBC count;	Aids in establishing blood replacement needs and monitoring effectiveness of therapy; e.g., 1 unit of whole blood should raise Hct two to three points. Levels may initially remain stable because of loss of both plasma and RBCs. *Note:* Levels may not accurately reflect early/sudden blood loss, and low baseline levels may indicate preexisting anemia.
BUN/Cr levels.	BUN greater than 40 with normal creatinine level indicates major bleeding. BUN should return to client's normal level approximately 12 hr after bleeding has ceased.
Assist with/prepare for:	
Sclerotherapy; e.g., ethanolamine, polidocanol, or combination of sodium tetradecyl, alcohol, and sodium chloride;	Performed during endoscopy, injection of an irritating (sclerosing) agent into esophageal varices (to create thrombosis) is used to stop bleeding and/or prevent recurrence after initial bleeding is controlled. The percentage of rebleeding is still significant (50%–60%) following this therapy in clients with varices.
Endoscopic variceal ligation (EVL);	Performed during endoscopy, this banding technique is increasingly being used as an effective alternative to sclerotherapy. Active hemorrhage is controlled in a high percentage of clients with fewer complications than with sclerotherapy.
Balloon tamponade;	Short-term intervention technique using Sengstaken-Blakemore tubes when medication or sclerotherapy fails to control esophageal bleed.
Electrocoagulation or photocoagulation (laser) therapy;	Provides direct coagulation of bleeding sites; e.g., gastritis, duodenal ulcer, tumor, esophageal (Mallory-Weiss) tear.
Surgical Intervention.	Total/partial gastrectomy, pyloroplasty, and/or vagotomy may be required to control/prevent future gastric bleeding. Shunt procedures (portacaval, splenorenal, mesocaval, or distal splenorenal) may be done to divert blood flow and reduce pressure within esophageal vessels when other measures fail.

NURSING DIAGNOSIS: risk for ineffective Tissue Perfusion

Risk factors may include

Hypovolemia

Possibly evidenced by

[Not applicable; presence of signs and symptoms establishes an *actual* diagnosis.]

DESIRED OUTCOMES/EVALUATION CRITERIA—CLIENT WILL:

Circulation Status (NOC)

Maintain/improve tissue perfusion as evidenced by stabilized vital signs, warm skin, palpable peripheral pulses, ABGs within client norms, adequate urine output.

ACTIONS/INTERVENTIONS	RATIONALE
Shock Prevention (NIC)	
Independent	
Investigate changes in level of consciousness, reports of dizziness/headache.	Changes may reflect inadequate cerebral perfusion as a result of reduced arterial blood pressure. *Note:* Changes in sensorium may also reflect elevated ammonia levels/hepatic encephalopathy in client with liver disease.
Investigate reports of chest pain. Note location, quality, duration, and what relieves pain.	May reflect cardiac ischemia related to decreased perfusion. *Note:* Impaired oxygenation status resulting from blood loss can bring on myocardial infarction (MI) in client with cardiac disease.
Auscultate apical pulse. Monitor cardiac rate/rhythm if continuous electrocardiogram (ECG) available/indicated.	Dysrhythmias and ischemic changes can occur as a result of hypotension, hypoxia, acidosis, electrolyte imbalance, or cooling near the heart if cold saline lavage is used to control bleeding.
Assess skin for coolness, pallor, diaphoresis, delayed capillary refill, and weak, thready peripheral pulses.	Vasoconstriction is a sympathetic response to lowered circulating volume and/or may occur as a side effect of vasopressin administration.
Note urinary output and specific gravity.	Decreased systemic perfusion may cause kidney ischemia/failure manifested by decreased urine output. Acute tubular necrosis (ATN) may develop if hypovolemic state is prolonged.
Note reports of abdominal pain, especially sudden, severe pain or pain radiating to shoulder.	Pain caused by gastric ulcer is often relieved after acute bleeding because of buffering effects of blood. Continued severe or sudden pain may reflect ischemia due to vasoconstrictive therapy, bleeding into biliary tract (hematobilia), or perforation/onset of peritonitis.
Observe skin for pallor, redness. Massage gently with lotion. Change position frequently.	Compromised peripheral circulation increases risk of skin breakdown.
Collaborative	
Monitor ABGs/pulse oximetry.	Identifies hypoxemia, effectiveness of/need for therapy
Provide supplemental oxygen if indicated.	Treats hypoxemia and lactic acidosis during acute bleed.
Administer IV fluids as indicated.	Maintains circulating volume and perfusion. (Refer to ND: deficient Fluid Volume, [isotonic].)

NURSING DIAGNOSIS: Fear/Anxiety [specify level]

May be related to

Change in health status, threat of death

Possibly evidenced by

Increased tension, restlessness, irritability, fearfulness
Trembling, tachycardia, diaphoresis
Lack of eye contact, focus on self
Verbalization of specific concern
Withdrawal, panic, or attack behavior

DESIRED OUTCOMES/EVALUATION CRITERIA—CLIENT WILL:

Anxiety Self-Control (NOC)

Discuss fears/concerns recognizing healthy versus unhealthy fears.
Verbalize appropriate range of feelings.
Appear relaxed and report anxiety is reduced to a manageable level.
Demonstrate problem solving and effective use of resources.

ACTIONS/INTERVENTIONS	RATIONALE
Anxiety Reduction (NIC)	
Independent	
Monitor physiologic responses, (e.g., tachypnea, palpitations, dizziness, headache, tingling sensations) and behavioral cues, (e.g., restlessness, irritability, lack of eye contact, combativeness/attack behavior).	May be indicative of the degree of fear client is experiencing (e.g., client may feel out of control of the situation or reach a state of panic), but may also be related to physical condition/shock state.
Encourage verbalization of concerns. Assist client in expressing feelings by active listening.	Establishes a therapeutic relationship. Assists client in dealing with feelings, and provides opportunity to clarify misconceptions.
Acknowledge that this is a fearful situation and that others have expressed similar fears.	When client is expressing own fear, the validation that these feelings are normal can help client to feel less isolated.
Provide accurate, concrete information about what is being done; e.g., sensations to expect, usual procedures undertaken.	Involves client in plan of care and decreases unnecessary anxiety about unknowns.
Provide a calm, restful environment.	Removing client from outside stressors promotes relaxation, may enhance coping skills.
Encourage significant other (SO) to stay with client as able. Respond to call signal promptly. Use touch and eye contact as appropriate.	Helps reduce fear of going through a frightening experience alone.
Provide opportunity for SO to express feelings/concerns. Encourage SO to project positive, realistic attitude.	Helps SO to deal with own anxiety/fears that can be transmitted to client. Promotes a supportive attitude that can facilitate recovery.
Demonstrate/encourage relaxation techniques; e.g., visualization, deep-breathing exercises, guided imagery.	Learning ways to relax can be helpful in reducing fear and anxiety. Because client with GI bleeding may be a person who has difficulty relaxing, learning these skills can be important to recovery and prevention of recurrence.
Help client identify and initiate positive coping behaviors used successfully in the past.	Successful behaviors can be fostered in dealing with current fear, enhancing client's sense of self-control and providing reassurance.
Encourage and support client in evaluation of lifestyle.	Changes may be necessary to avoid recurrence of ulcer condition.
Collaborative	
Administer medications as indicated; e.g., diazepam (Valium), clorazepate (Tranxene), alprazolam (Xanax).	Sedatives/antianxiety agents may be used on occasion to reduce anxiety and promote rest, particularly in client with an ulcer.
Refer to psychiatric clinical nurse specialist, social services, spiritual advisor.	May need additional assistance during recovery to deal with consequences of emergency situation/adjustments to required/desired changes in lifestyle.

NURSING DIAGNOSIS: acute/chronic Pain

May be related to

Chemical burn of gastric mucosa, oral cavity
Physical response; e.g., reflex muscle spasm in the stomach wall

Possibly evidenced by

Communication of pain descriptors
Abdominal guarding, rigid body posture, facial grimacing
Autonomic responses; e.g., changes in vital signs (acute pain)

DESIRED OUTCOMES/EVALUATION CRITERIA—CLIENT WILL:

Pain Level (NOC)

Verbalize relief of pain.
Demonstrate relaxed body posture and be able to sleep/rest appropriately.

ACTIONS/INTERVENTIONS	RATIONALE
Pain Management (NIC)	
Independent	
Note reports of pain, including location, duration, intensity (0–10 scale).	Pain is not always present, but if present should be compared with client's previous pain symptoms. This comparison may assist in diagnosis of etiology of bleeding and development of complications.
Review factors that aggravate or alleviate pain.	Helpful in establishing diagnosis and treatment needs.
Note nonverbal pain cues; e.g., restlessness, reluctance to move, abdominal guarding, tachycardia, diaphoresis. Investigate discrepancies between verbal and nonverbal cues.	Nonverbal cues may be both physiologic and psychologic and may be used in conjunction with verbal cues to evaluate extent/severity of the problem.
Provide small, frequent meals as indicated for individual client.	Food has an acid-neutralizing effect and dilutes the gastric contents. Small meals prevent distention and the release of gastrin.
Identify and limit foods that create discomfort.	Specific foods that cause distress vary among individuals. Studies indicate pepper is harmful, and coffee (including decaffeinated) can precipitate dyspepsia.
Assist with active/passive range of motion (ROM) exercises.	Reduces joint stiffness, minimizing pain/discomfort.
Provide frequent oral care and comfort measures; e.g., back rub, position change.	Halitosis from stagnant oral secretions is unappetizing and can aggravate nausea. Gingivitis and dental problems may arise.
Collaborative	
Provide and implement prescribed dietary modifications.	Client may receive nothing by mouth (NPO) initially. When oral intake is allowed, food choices depend on the diagnosis and etiology of the bleeding.
Use regular rather than skim milk if milk is allowed.	Fat in regular milk may decrease gastric secretions; however, the calcium and protein content (especially in skim milk) increases secretions.
Administer medications, as indicated; e.g.:	
Analgesics; e.g., morphine sulfate;	May be narcotic of choice to relieve acute/severe pain and reduce peristaltic activity. *Note:* Meperidine (Demerol) has been associated with increased incidence of nausea/vomiting.
Acetaminophen (Tylenol);	Promotes general comfort and rest.
Antacids;	Decrease gastric acidity by absorption or by chemical neutralization. Evaluate choice of antacid in regard to total health picture; e.g., sodium restriction.
Anticholinergics; e.g., belladonna, atropine.	May be given at bedtime to decrease gastric motility, suppress acid production, delay gastric emptying, and alleviate nocturnal pain associated with gastric ulcer.

NURSING DIAGNOSIS: deficient Knowledge [Learning Need] regarding disease process, prognosis, treatment, self-care, and discharge needs

May be related to

Lack of information/recall
Unfamiliarity with information resources
Information misinterpretation

Possibly evidenced by

Verbalization of the problem, request for information, statement of misconceptions
Inaccurate follow-through of instructions
Development of preventable complications

DESIRED OUTCOMES/EVALUATION CRITERIA—CLIENT WILL:

KNOWLEDGE: Disease Process (NOC)

Verbalize understanding of cause of own bleeding episode (if known) and treatment modalities used.
Begin to discuss own role in preventing recurrence.

KNOWLEDGE: Treatment Regimen (NOC)

Identify/implement necessary lifestyle changes.
Participate in treatment regimen.

ACTIONS/INTERVENTIONS	RATIONALE
TEACHING: Disease Process (NIC)	
Independent	
Determine client perception of cause of bleeding.	Establishes knowledge base and provides some insight into how the teaching plan needs to be constructed for this individual.
Provide/review information regarding etiology of bleeding, cause/effect, relationship of lifestyle behaviors, and ways to reduce risk/contributing factors. Encourage questions.	Provides knowledge base from which client can make informed choices/decisions about future and control of health problems.
Assist client to identify relationship of food intake and precipitation of/relief from epigastric pain, including avoidance of gastric irritants; e.g., pepper, caffeine, alcohol, fruit juices, carbonated beverages, and extremely hot, cold, fatty, or spicy foods.	Caffeine stimulates gastric acidity. Alcohol contributes to erosion of gastric mucosa. Although current research indicates that diet does not contribute to the development of PUD, individuals may find that certain foods/fluids increase gastric secretion and pain.
Recommend small, frequent meals/snacks, chewing food slowly, eating at regular time, and avoiding "skipping" meals.	Frequent eating keeps HCl neutralized, dilutes stomach contents to minimize action of acid on gastric mucosa. Small meals prevent gastric overdistention.
Stress importance of reading labels on OTC drugs and either avoiding products containing aspirin or switching to enteric-coated aspirin. Recommend client discuss alternatives to NSAID use for pain relief.	Aspirin damages the protective mucosa, permitting gastric erosion, ulceration, and bleeding to occur. NSAID use increases the risk of peptic ulcer disease 5–20 times.
Review significance of signs/symptoms such as coffee-grounds emesis, tarry stools, abdominal distention, severe epigastric/abdominal pain radiating to shoulder/back.	Prompt medical evaluation/intervention is required to prevent more serious complications; e.g., perforation, Zollinger-Ellison syndrome.
Support use of stress-management techniques, avoidance of emotional stress.	Decreases extrinsic stimulation of HCl, reducing risk of recurrence of bleeding.

ACTIONS/INTERVENTIONS	RATIONALE
Review drug regimen, possible side effects, and interaction with other drugs as appropriate.	Helpful to client's understanding of reason for taking drugs and what symptoms are important to report to healthcare provider. *Note:* Aluminum-containing antacids inhibit the intestinal absorption of some drugs and affect scheduling of drug intake. Some men may incur impotence when using prescription-strength cimetidine (Tagamet). Alternative drug choices are famotidine (Pepcid) and ranitidine (Zantac).
Encourage client to inform all healthcare providers of bleeding history.	May affect drug choices and/or concomitant prescriptions; e.g., misoprostol (Cytotec) can be given with NSAIDs to inhibit gastric acid secretion and reduce risk of gastric irritability/lesions resulting from NSAID therapy.
Discuss importance of cessation of smoking.	Ulcer healing may be delayed in people who smoke, particularly in those who use cimetidine (Tagamet). Smoking stimulates gastric acidity and is associated with increased risk of peptic ulcer development/recurrence.
Refer to support groups/counseling for lifestyle/behavior changes, reduction of associated risk factors; e.g., substance abuse/stop-smoking clinics.	Alcohol users have a higher incidence of gastritis/esophageal varices, and cigarette smoking is associated with peptic ulcers and delayed healing.

POTENTIAL CONSIDERATIONS following acute hospitalization (dependent on client's age, physical condition/presence of complications, personal resources, and life responsibilities)

ineffective Therapeutic Regimen Management—decisional conflicts (e.g., use of NSAIDs for arthritic/chronic pain condition), perceived benefits (e.g., cessation of smoking), economic difficulties (cost of medication).

SUBTOTAL GASTRECTOMY/GASTRIC RESECTION

Subtotal gastrectomy or *gastric resection* is a surgical treatment indicated for gastric hemorrhage that may be due to perforated or chronic ulcers, pyloric obstruction, or gastric cancer.

RELATED CONCERNS

Cancer, page 857
Pancreatitis, page 467
Peritonitis, page 355
Psychosocial aspects of care, page 770
Surgical intervention, page 788
Total nutritional support: parenteral/enteral feeding, page 488
Upper gastrointestinal/esophageal bleeding, page 309

CARE SETTING

Inpatient or same day outpatient surgical unit. The procedure may be done as an open procedure or via laparoscope.

Client Assessment Database

Data depend on the underlying condition necessitating surgery. (Refer to CP: Upper gastrointestinal/esophageal bleeding.)

TEACHING/LEARNING

Discharge plan considerations: Assistance with administration of enteral feedings/total parenteral nutrition (TPN) if required, and acquisition of supplies

Refer to section at end of plan for postdischarge considerations.

NURSING PRIORITIES

1. Promote healing and adequate nutritional intake.
2. Prevent complications.
3. Provide information about surgical procedure/prognosis, treatment needs, and concerns.

DISCHARGE GOALS

1. Nutritional intake adequate for individual needs.
2. Complications prevented/minimized.
3. Surgical procedure/prognosis, therapeutic regimen, and long-term needs understood.
4. Plan in place to meet needs after discharge.

(In addition to nursing diagnoses identified in this CP, refer to CP: Surgical Intervention.)

NURSING DIAGNOSIS: risk for imbalanced Nutrition: less than body requirements

Risk factors may include

Restriction of fluids and food
Change in digestive process/absorption of nutrients

Possibly evidenced by

[Not applicable; presence of signs and symptoms establishes an *actual* diagnosis.]

DESIRED OUTCOMES/EVALUATION CRITERIA—CLIENT WILL:

Nutritional Status (NOC)

Maintain stable weight/demonstrate progressive weight gain toward goal with normalization of laboratory values.
Be free of signs of malnutrition.

ACTIONS/INTERVENTIONS	RATIONALE
Nutrition Therapy (NIC)	
Independent	
Maintain patency of nasogastric (NG), orogastric (OG) or nasointestinal (NI) tube when used. Be aware of feeding tube placement (e.g. enterostomal/jejunostomal). Notify physician if tube becomes dislodged.	Intestinal tubes are inserted to provide rest for GI tract during acute postoperative phase until return of normal GI function. These are attached to suction. Feeding tubes (e.g., Dobhoff) may be inserted at time of surgery or later, and are used to provide enteral feedings once gut is functional. *Note:* Although several methods have been used to identify tube placement at the bedside (e.g., aspiration of gastric contents, measurement of trypsin, pH, and pepsin levels), abdominal radiographs may be necessary to confirm location of tube, and the physician/surgeon may need to reposition the tube endoscopically to prevent injury to the operative area.
Note character and amount of gastric drainage.	Drainage may be bloody for first 12 hr, and then should clear/turn greenish gold. Continued/recurrent bleeding suggests complications and should be reported to physician. Decline in output may reflect return of GI function.
Caution client to limit the intake of ice chips.	Excessive intake of ice produces nausea and can wash out electrolytes via the NG tube.
Provide oral hygiene on a regular, frequent basis, including petroleum jelly for lips.	Prevents discomfort of dry mouth and cracked lips caused by fluid restriction and the NG tube.
Auscultate for resumption of bowel sounds and note passage of flatus.	Peristalsis can be expected to return about the third postoperative day, signaling readiness to resume oral intake.

ACTIONS/INTERVENTIONS	RATIONALE
Monitor tolerance to fluid and food intake (when resumed), noting abdominal distention, reports of increased pain/cramping, nausea/vomiting.	Complications of paralytic ileus, obstruction, delayed gastric emptying, and gastric dilation may occur, possibly requiring reinsertion of NG tube. Even if the above complications do not occur, "dumping syndrome" is a fairly common after effect of stomach surgery. Symptoms include bloating, nausea, diarrhea, weakness, sweating, and rapid heartbeat 30–60 min after a meal. (Refer to ND: deficient Knowledge [Learning Need], following.)
Note admission weight and compare with subsequent readings.	Provides information about adequacy of dietary intake/determination of nutritional needs.

Collaborative

Administer IV fluids, parenteral or enteral nutrition, as indicated.	Meets fluid/nutritional needs until oral intake can be resumed. *Note:* Early enteral feedings have been found to stimulate gut immunologic function and can assist in maintaining gut structure and function. TPN is usually reserved for clients who are critically ill at the time of surgery. (Refer to CP: Total Nutritional Support: Parenteral/Enteral Feeding, page 478 for additional interventions.)
Monitor laboratory studies; e.g., Hb/Hct, electrolytes, and total protein/prealbumin.	Indicates fluid/nutritional needs and effectiveness of therapy, and detects developing complications.
Progress diet as tolerated, advancing from clear liquid to bland diet with several small feedings.	After NG tube is removed, intake is advanced gradually to prevent gastric irritation/distention.
Administer medications as indicated:	
Anticholinergics/antispasmodics; e.g., atropine, propantheline (Pro-Banthine);	May be given to manage dumping syndrome, enhancing digestion and absorption of nutrients.
Fat-soluble vitamin supplements, including vitamin B_{12} and calcium;	Depending on the type and extent of gastric surgery performed, poor absorption of nutrients, vitamins, and minerals may occur to a significant degree. For example, removal of the stomach prevents absorption of vitamin B_{12} (owing to loss of intrinsic factor) and can lead to pernicious anemia. Rapid emptying of the stomach reduces absorption of calcium.
Iron preparations;	Correct/prevent iron deficiency anemia.
Protein supplements;	Additional protein may be helpful for tissue repair and healing.
Pancreatic enzymes, bile salts;	Enhance digestive process.
Medium-chain triglycerides (MCT).	Promote absorption of fats and fat-soluble vitamins to prevent malabsorption problems.

NURSING DIAGNOSIS: deficient Knowledge [Learning Need] regarding procedure, prognosis, treatment, self-care, and discharge needs

May be related to

Lack of exposure/recall
Information misinterpretation
Unfamiliarity with information resources

Possibly evidenced by

Questions, statement of misconception
Inaccurate follow-through of instruction
Development of preventable complications

DESIRED OUTCOMES/EVALUATION CRITERIA—CLIENT WILL:

KNOWLEDGE: Disease Process (NOC)

Verbalize understanding of procedure, disease process/prognosis.
Verbalize understanding of functional changes.

KNOWLEDGE: Treatment Regimen (NOC)

Identify necessary interventions/behaviors to maintain appropriate weight.
Correctly perform necessary procedures, explaining reasons for actions.

ACTIONS/INTERVENTIONS	RATIONALE
TEACHING: Disease Process (NIC)	
Independent	
Review surgical procedure and long-term expectations.	Provides knowledge base from which informed choices can be made. Recovery following gastric surgery is often slower than may be anticipated with similar types of surgery. Improved strength and partial normalization of dietary pattern may not be evident for at least 3 months, and full return to usual intake (three "normal" meals/day) may take up to 12 months. This prolonged convalescence may be difficult for the client/SO to deal with, especially if he or she has not been adequately prepared.
Discuss and identify stress situations and how to avoid them. Investigate job-related issues.	Stress and stress reactions can alter gastric motility, interfering with optimal digestion, especially if client has been very ill in conjunction with the surgery. *Note:* Client may require vocational counseling if change in employment is indicated.
Review dietary needs/regimen (e.g., low-carbohydrate, low-fat, high-protein) and importance of maintaining vitamin supplementation.	May prevent deficiencies, enhance healing, and promote cooperation with therapy. *Note:* Low-fat diet may be required to reduce risk of alkaline reflux gastritis.
Discuss the importance of eating small, frequent meals slowly and in a relaxed atmosphere; resting after meals; avoiding extremely hot or cold food; restricting high-fiber foods, caffeine, milk products and alcohol, excess sugars and salt; and taking fluids between meals rather than with food.	These measures can be helpful in avoiding gastric distention/irritation and/or stress on surgical repair, dumping syndrome, and reactive hypoglycemia. *Note:* Ice-cold fluids/foods can cause gastric spasms.
Instruct in avoiding certain fibrous foods, and discuss the necessity of chewing food well.	Remaining gastric tissue may have reduced ability to digest such foods as citrus skin/seeds, which can collect, forming a mass (phytobezoar formation) that is not excreted.
Recommend foods containing pectin; e.g., citrus fruits, bananas, apples, yellow vegetables, and beans.	Increased intake of these foods may reduce incidence of dumping syndrome.
Identify foods that can cause gastric irritation and increase gastric acid; e.g., chocolate, spicy foods, whole grains, raw vegetables.	Limiting/avoiding these foods reduces risk of gastric bleeding/ulceration in some individuals. *Note:* Ingesting fresh fruits to reduce risk of dumping syndrome should be tempered with adverse effect of gastric irritation.
Identify symptoms that may indicate dumping syndrome; e.g., weakness, profuse perspiration, epigastric fullness, nausea/vomiting, abdominal cramping, faintness, flushing, explosive diarrhea, and palpitations occurring within 15 min to 1 hr after eating.	Can cause severe discomfort or even shock, and reduces absorption of nutrients. Usually self-limiting (1–3 wk after surgery) but can become chronic.
Discuss signs of hypoglycemia and corrective interventions; e.g., ingesting cheese and crackers, orange/grape juice.	Awareness helps clients take actions to prevent progression of symptoms.

ACTIONS/INTERVENTIONS	RATIONALE
Suggest client weigh self on a regular basis.	Change in dietary pattern, early satiety, and efforts to avoid dumping syndrome may limit intake, causing weight loss.
Review medication purpose, dosage, and schedule and possible side effects.	Understanding Rationale/therapeutic needs can reduce risk of complications; e.g., anticholinergics/pectin powder may be given to reduce incidence of dumping syndrome; antacids/histamine antagonists reduce gastric irritation.
Caution client to read labels and avoid products containing ASA, ibuprofen.	Can cause gastric irritation/bleeding.
Discuss reasons and importance of cessation of smoking.	Smoking stimulates gastric acid production, relaxes lower esophageal sphincter, and may cause vasoconstriction, compromising mucous membranes and increasing risk of gastric and esophageal irritation/ulceration.
Identify signs/symptoms requiring medical evaluation; e.g., persistent nausea/vomiting or abdominal fullness, weight loss, diarrhea, foul-smelling fatty or tarry stools, bloody or coffee-grounds vomitus/presence of bile, fever. Instruct client to report changes in pain characteristics.	Prompt recognition and intervention may prevent serious consequences or potential complications such as pancreatitis, peritonitis, and afferent loop syndrome.
Emphasize importance of regular checkups with healthcare provider.	Necessary to detect developing complications; e.g., anemia, problems with nutrition, and/or recurrence of disease.

POTENTIAL CONSIDERATIONS following acute hospitalization (dependent on client's age, physical condition/presence of complications, personal resources, and life responsibilities)

risk for imbalanced Nutrition: less than body requirements—change in digestive process/absorption of nutrients, early satiety, gastric irritation.

Fatigue—decreased energy production, states of discomfort, increased energy requirements to perform activities of daily living (ADLs).

INFLAMMATORY BOWEL DISEASE: ULCERATIVE COLITIS, REGIONAL ENTERITIS (CROHN'S DISEASE, ILEOCOLITIS)

Inflammatory bowel disease (IBD): *Inflammatory bowel disease* is a general term used for two different diseases, ulcerative colitis and Crohn's disease. Researchers believe that IBD may result from a complex interplay between genetic and environmental factors. Similarities involve (1) chronic inflammation of the alimentary tract and (2) periods of remission interspersed with episodes of acute inflammation, and (3) systemic inflammation affecting most of the body's organ systems; that is, internal organs, the eyes, blood, skin, and musculoskeletal systems (known as extraintestinal manifestations [EMs]). IBD affects both men and women between the ages of 20 and 50 years; however, Crohn's disease has a higher incidence of occurring in late adolescence and the early adult years (15–30). Common symptoms between the two disorders include frequent diarrhea, abdominal pain, fever, and weight loss.

Ulcerative colitis (UC): A chronic condition of unknown cause usually starting in the rectum and distal portions of the colon and possibly spreading upward to involve the sigmoid and descending colon or the entire colon. It is usually intermittent (acute exacerbation with long remissions), but some individuals (30%–40%) have continuous symptoms. Cure is affected only by total removal of colon and rectum/rectal mucosa.

Regional enteritis (Crohn's disease, ileocolitis): May be found in any portion of the alimentary tract from the mouth to the anus, but is most commonly found in the small intestine (terminal ileum). It is a slowly progressive chronic disease of unknown cause with intermittent acute episodes and no known cure. UC and regional enteritis share common symptoms but differ in the segment and layer of intestine involved and the degree of severity and complications. Therefore, separate databases are provided.

CARE SETTING

Usually handled at the community level; however, severe exacerbations (with severe dehydration, anemia, intestinal blockage or perforation) requiring surgical intervention, advanced pain control, nutrition, rehydration necessitating a stay in acute care medical unit.

RELATED CONCERNS

Fecal diversions: postoperative care of ileostomy and colostomy, page 338
Fluid and electrolyte imbalances, page 919
Peritonitis, page 355
Psychosocial aspects of care, page 770
Total nutritional support: parenteral/enteral feeding, page 478

Client Assessment Database—Ulcerative Colitis

ACTIVITY/REST

May report: Weakness, fatigue, malaise, exhaustion
Insomnia, not sleeping through the night because of diarrhea
Feeling restless
Restriction of activities/work due to effects of disease process

CIRCULATION

May exhibit: Tachycardia (response to fever, dehydration, inflammatory process, and pain)
Bruising, ecchymotic areas (insufficient vitamin K)
BP: Hypotension, including postural changes

EGO INTEGRITY

May report: Anxiety, apprehension, emotional upsets; e.g., feelings of helplessness/hopelessness
Acute/chronic stress factors; e.g., family/job-related, expense of treatment
Cultural factor—increased prevalence in Jewish population

May exhibit: Withdrawal, narrowed focus, depression

ELIMINATION

May report: Stool texture varying from soft-formed to mush or watery
Unpredictable, intermittent, frequent, uncontrollable episodes of bloody diarrhea (as many as 20–30 stools/day); sense of urgency/cramping (tenesmus); passing blood/pus/mucus with or without passing feces
Rectal bleeding
Intermittent constipation

May exhibit: Diminished or hyperactive bowel sounds, absence of peristalsis or presence of visible peristaltic waves

FOOD/FLUID

May report: Anorexia; nausea/vomiting
Weight loss (not common, but can occur as a result of decreased intake)
Dietary intolerances/sensitivities; e.g., raw fruits/vegetables, dairy products, fatty foods

May exhibit: Decreased subcutaneous fat/muscle mass
Weakness, poor muscle tone and skin turgor
Mucous membranes pale; sore, inflamed buccal cavity; dry, cracking of tongue (dehydration/malnutrition)

HYGIENE

May report: Inability to maintain self-care

May exhibit: Stomatitis reflecting vitamin deficiency

PAIN/DISCOMFORT

May report: Mild abdominal cramping to severe pain/tenderness in lower-left quadrant (may be relieved with defecation)
Migratory joint pain, tenderness (arthritis)
Eye pain, photophobia (iritis)

May exhibit: Abdominal tenderness, distention, rigidity

SAFETY

May report: History of lupus erythematosus, hemolytic anemia, vasculitis
Arthritis (worsening of symptoms with exacerbations in bowel disease)

Temperature elevation 104°F–105°F (acute exacerbation)
Blurred vision
Allergies to foods/milk products (release of histamine into bowel has an inflammatory effect)

May exhibit: Skin/mucosal lesions may be present; e.g., erythema nodosum (raised, tender, red, and swollen) on arms, face; aphthous ulcerations of mouth; pyoderma gangrenosum (purulent pinpoint lesion/boil with a purple border) on trunk, legs, ankles
Ankylosing spondylitis; osteoporosis
Uveitis, conjunctivitis/iritis

SEXUALITY

May report: Reduced frequency/avoidance of sexual activity

SOCIAL INTERACTION

May report: Relationship/role problems related to condition
Inability to be active socially

TEACHING/LEARNING

May report: Family history of IBD, immune disorders
Use of multiple medications, OTC medications for bowel health; and/or use of herbal remedies (e.g., peppermint, psyllium, chamomile)

Discharge plan considerations: Assistance with dietary requirements, medication regimen, psychological support

Refer to section at end of plan for postdischarge considerations.

DIAGNOSTIC STUDIES

Stool specimens (examinations are used in initial diagnosis and in following disease progression): Mainly composed of mucus, blood, pus, and intestinal organisms, especially *Entamoeba histolytica* (active stage). Fecal leukocytes and RBCs indicate inflammation of GI tract. Stool positive for bacterial pathogens, ova and parasites or clostridia indicates infections. Stool positive for fat indicates malabsorption.

Endoscopic examinations; e.g., sigmoidoscopy, esophagogastroduodenoscopy, or colonoscopy: Gold standard for diagnosis, especially when biopsy included. Identifies inflamed and lacerated tissues, deep ulcerations, adhesions, changes in luminal wall (narrowing/irregularity); rules out bowel obstruction.

Proctosigmoidoscopy: Visualizes ulcerations, edema, hyperemia, and inflammation (result of secondary infection of the mucosa and submucosa). Friability and hemorrhagic areas caused by necrosis and ulceration occur in 85% of these clients.

Cytology and rectal biopsy: Differentiates between infectious process and carcinoma (occurs 10–20 times more often than in general population). Neoplastic changes can be detected, as well as characteristic inflammatory infiltrates called crypt abscesses.

Barium enema: Rarely done during acute, relapsing stage, because it can exacerbate condition.

Abdominal magnetic resonance imaging (MRI)/computed tomography (CT) scan, ultrasound: Detects abscesses, masses, strictures, or fistulas.

CBC: May show hyperchromic anemia (active disease generally present because of blood loss and iron deficiency); leukocytosis may occur, especially in fulminating or complicated cases and in clients on steroid therapy.

Erythrocyte sedimentation rate (ESR and C-reactive protein [CRP]): Elevated in acute inflammation according to severity of disease.

Serum iron levels: Lowered because of blood loss or poor dietary intake.

PT: Prolonged in severe cases from altered factors VII and X caused by vitamin K deficiency.

Thrombocytosis: May occur as a result of inflammatory disease process.

Electrolytes: Decreased potassium, magnesium, and zinc are common in severe disease.

Prealbumin/albumin level: Decreased because of loss of plasma proteins/disturbed liver function, decreased dietary intake.

Alkaline phosphatase: Increased, along with serum cholesterol and hypoproteinemia, indicating disturbed liver function (e.g., cholangitis, cirrhosis).

Disease-specific antibodies: periantineutrophil cytoplasmic antibodies (pANCA), and anti-Saccharomyces cerevisiae antibodies (ASCA): May be positive, but negative results do not rule out diagnosis.

Bone marrow: A generalized depression is common in fulminating types/after a long inflammatory process.

Client Assessment Database—Regional Enteritis (Crohn's Disease, Ileocolitis)

ACTIVITY/REST

May report: Weakness, fatigue, malaise, exhaustion
Feeling restless
Restriction of activities/work due to effects of disease process

EGO INTEGRITY

May report: Anxiety, apprehension, emotional upsets, feelings of helplessness/hopelessness
Acute/chronic stress factors; e.g., family/job-related expense of treatment
Cultural factor—increased prevalence in Jewish population, frequency increasing in individuals of Northern European and Anglo-Saxon derivation

May exhibit: Withdrawal, narrowed focus, depression

ELIMINATION

May report: Unpredictable, intermittent, frequent, uncontrollable episodes of bloody or nonbloody diarrhea, soft or semi-liquid with flatus; foul-smelling and fatty stools (steatorrhea)
History of renal stones (increased oxalates in the urine)

May exhibit: Hyperactive bowel sounds with gurgling, splashing sound (borborygmus)
Visible peristalsis

FOOD/FLUID

May report: Anorexia; nausea/vomiting
Weight loss; failure to grow
Dietary intolerance/sensitivity; e.g., dairy products, fatty foods

May exhibit: Decreased subcutaneous fat/muscle mass
Weakness, poor muscle tone and skin turgor
Mucous membranes pale

HYGIENE

May report: Inability to maintain self-care

May exhibit: Unkempt appearance; body odor

PAIN/DISCOMFORT

May report: Tender abdomen with cramping pain in lower right quadrant (inflammation involving all layers of bowel wall and possibly the mesentery); pain in midlower abdomen (jejunal involvement)
Referred tenderness to periumbilical region
Perineal tenderness/pain
Migratory joint pain, tenderness (arthritis)
Eye pain, photophobia (iritis)

May exhibit: Abdominal tenderness/distention

SAFETY

May report: History of arthritis, systemic lupus erythematosus (SLE), hemolytic anemia, vasculitis
Temperature elevation (low-grade fever)
Blurred vision

May exhibit: Skin/mucosal lesions may present: erythema nodosum (raised tender, red swelling) on face, arms; aphthous ulcerations of mouth; pyoderma gangrenosum (purulent pinpoint lesion/boil with a purple border) on trunk, legs, ankles; perineal lesions/anorectal fistulas (with purulent drainage)
Ankylosing spondylitis, osteoporosis
Uveitis, conjunctivitis/iritis
Clotting disorders

SOCIAL INTERACTION

May report: Relationship/role problems related to condition; inability to be active socially

TEACHING/LEARNING

May report: Family history of IBD, immune disorders
Use of multiple medications, OTC medications for bowel health; and/or use of herbal remedies (e.g., aloe, chamomile, flax, garlic, bosweilia, echinacea, goldenseal)

Discharge plan considerations: Assistance with dietary requirements, medication regimen, psychological support

Refer to section at end of plan for postdischarge considerations.

DIAGNOSTIC STUDIES

Stool examination: Occult blood may be positive (mucosal erosion); white blood cells may be found, indicating infection; steatorrhea and bile salts may be noted.
Endoscopic examination; e.g., sigmoidoscopy, esophagogastroduodenoscopy, or colonoscopy: Gold standard for diagnosis, especially when biopsy included. Identifies inflamed and lacerated tissues, deep ulcerations, adhesions, changes in luminal wall (narrowing/irregularity); rules out bowel obstruction. Any granuloma in the biopsy confirms Crohn's disease.
Radiographic scans: Barium swallow may demonstrate luminal narrowing in the terminal ileum, stiffening of the bowel wall, mucosal irritability or ulceration.
Barium enema: Small bowel is nearly always involved, but the rectal area is affected only 50% of the time. Fistulas are common and are usually found in the terminal ileum but may be present in segments throughout the GI tract.
Abdominal MRI/CT scan, ultrasound: Detects infections/inflammatory conditions.
CBC: Anemia (hypochromic, occasionally macrocytic) may occur because of malnutrition or malabsorption or depressed bone marrow function (chronic inflammatory process); increased white blood cells (WBCs).
ESR and CRP: Increased, reflecting inflammation.
Prealbumin/albumin/total protein: Decreased.
Cholesterol: Elevated (may have gallstones).
Serum iron-binding folic acid capacity/transferrin levels: Decreased because of chronic infection or secondary to blood loss.
Clotting studies: Alterations may occur because of poor vitamin B_{12} absorption.
Electrolytes: Decreased potassium, calcium, and magnesium, with increased sodium.
Urine: Hyperoxaluria (can cause kidney stones).
Urine culture: If *Escherichia coli* organisms are present, suspect fistula formation into the bladder.
Disease-specific antibodies (pANCA), and (ASCA): May be positive, but negative results do not rule out diagnosis.

NURSING PRIORITIES

1. Control diarrhea/promote optimal bowel function.
2. Minimize/prevent complications.
3. Promote optimal nutrition.
4. Minimize mental/emotional stress.
5. Provide information about disease process, treatment needs, and long-term aspects/potential complications of recurrent disease.

DISCHARGE GOALS

1. Bowel function stabilized.
2. Complications prevented/controlled.
3. Dealing positively with condition.
4. Disease process/prognosis, therapeutic regimen, and potential complications are understood.
5. Plan in place to meet needs after discharge.

NURSING DIAGNOSIS: Diarrhea

May be related to

Inflammation, irritation, or malabsorption of the bowel
Presence of toxins
Segmental narrowing of the lumen

Possibly evidenced by

Increased bowel sounds/peristalsis
Frequent, and often severe, watery stools (acute phase)
Changes in stool color
Abdominal pain; urgency (sudden painful need to defecate), cramping

DESIRED OUTCOMES/EVALUATION CRITERIA—CLIENT WILL:

Bowel Elimination (NOC)

Report reduction in frequency of stools, return to more normal stool consistency.
Identify/avoid contributing factors.

ACTIONS/INTERVENTIONS	RATIONALE
Diarrhea Management (NIC)	
Independent	
Observe and record stool frequency, characteristics, amount, and precipitating factors.	Helps differentiate individual disease and assesses severity of episode.
Promote bedrest, provide bedside commode.	Rest decreases intestinal motility and reduces the metabolic rate when infection or hemorrhage is a complication. Urge to defecate may occur without warning and be uncontrollable, increasing risk of incontinence/falls if facilities are not close at hand.
Remove stool promptly. Provide room deodorizers.	Reduces noxious odors to avoid undue client embarrassment.
Identify foods and fluids that precipitate diarrhea; e.g., raw vegetables and fruits, whole-grain cereals, condiments, carbonated drinks, milk products.	Avoiding intestinal irritants promotes intestinal rest.
Restart oral fluid intake gradually. Offer clear liquids hourly; avoid cold fluids.	Provides colon rest by omitting or decreasing the stimulus of foods/fluids. Gradual resumption of liquids may prevent cramping and recurrence of diarrhea; however, cold fluids can increase intestinal motility.
Provide opportunity to vent frustrations related to disease process.	Presence of disease with unknown cause that is difficult to cure and that may require surgical intervention can lead to stress reactions that may aggravate condition.
Observe for fever, tachycardia, lethargy, leukocytosis, decreased serum protein, anxiety, and prostration.	May signify that toxic megacolon or perforation and peritonitis are imminent/have occurred, necessitating immediate medical intervention.
Collaborative	
Administer medications as indicated:	
Anti-inflammatories; e.g., sulfasalazine (Azulfidine), 5-aminosalicylic acids, olsalazine (Dipentum), mesalamine (Pentasa, Asacol, Rowasa), balazide (Colazol);	Useful in treating mild/moderate exacerbations because of both anti-inflammatory and antimicrobial properties. Long-term use may prolong remission. *Note:* Available in oral/time-release and pH-dependent forms. Rowasa may be given as an enema in lieu of sulfasalazine (Azulfidine) for clients who are sensitive to oral sulfa drugs.
Steroids; e.g., hydrocortisone (Cortenema, Cortifoam), prednisolone (Medrol, Deltasone, Cortef), prednisone (Deltasone), butesonide (Entocort EC);	Used to decrease acute inflammatory process when symptoms are refractory to sulfasalasine and 5-aminosalicylic acids, or for sudden flare-ups of the disease process. Steroid enemas (Cortenema) may be given in mild/moderate disease to aid absorption of the drug (possibly with atropine sulfate or belladonna suppository). Current research suggests an 8-wk course of time-release steroids may effect remission in Crohn's disease; however, steroids are contraindicated if intra-abdominal abscesses are suspected.
Immune-modulating agents e.g., azathioprine (Imuran), 6-mercaptopurine (Purinethol), methotrexate (Mexate), cyclosporine (Sandimmune);	Immunosuppressant may be given to block inflammatory response, decrease steroid requirements, promote healing of fistulas.

ACTIONS/INTERVENTIONS	RATIONALE
Biologic response modifiers; e.g., monoclonal antibodies such as IV infliximab (Remicade);	Used for treatment and maintenance of moderate to severe refractory or fistulizing CD. Drug blocks the inflammatory agent's activity, leading to decreased inflammation and promoting intestinal healing.
Anti-infectives; e.g., metronidazole (Flagyl), ciprofloxacin (Cipro);	Used when exacerbation is caused by or accompanied by infection, or may be part of a long-term treatment regimen.
Antidiarrheals; e.g., diphenoxylate (Lomotil), loperamide (Imodium), anodyne suppositories;	Decreases GI motility/propulsion (peristalsis) and diminishes digestive secretions to relieve cramping and diarrhea. *Note:* Used with caution in UC because they may precipitate toxic megacolon and are contraindicated in presence of infection.
Antispasmodics; e.g., L-hyoscyamine (Levsin), dicyclomine (Bentyl), hyoscyamine/atropine/scopolamine/phenobarbital (Donnatal).	May be useful for clients who do not respond to standard interventions.
Assist with/prepare for surgical intervention; e.g., ileostomy, total colostomy, percutaneous abscess drainage.	May be necessary if perforation or bowel obstruction occurs or disease is unresponsive to medical treatment. Total colectomy is considered curative for UC (which affects only the colon). However, it may not resolve extraintestinal manifestations. In Crohn's disease, surgery may be performed to remove a diseased section of bowel, but is not curative, as inflammation can occur anywhere in the GI tract. The client may require a temporary or permanent colostomy. (Refer to CP: Fecal Diversion, p 338.)

NURSING DIAGNOSIS: risk for deficient Fluid Volume

Risk factors may include

Excessive losses through normal routes (severe frequent diarrhea, vomiting)
Hypermetabolic state (inflammation, fever)
Restricted intake (nausea/anorexia)

Possibly evidenced by

[Not applicable; presence of signs and symptoms establishes an *actual* diagnosis.]

DESIRED OUTCOMES/EVALUATION CRITERIA—CLIENT WILL:

Hydration (NOC)

Maintain adequate fluid volume as evidenced by moist mucous membranes, good skin turgor, and capillary refill; stable vital signs; balanced I&O with urine of normal concentration/amount.

ACTIONS/INTERVENTIONS	RATIONALE
Fluid/Electrolyte Management (NIC)	
Independent	
Monitor I&O. Note number, character, and amount of stools. Estimate insensible fluid losses; e.g., diaphoresis. Measure urine specific gravity; observe for oliguria.	Provides information about overall fluid balance, renal function, and bowel disease control, as well as guidelines for fluid replacement.
Assess vital signs (BP, pulse, temperature).	Hypotension (including postural), tachycardia, fever can indicate response to and/or effect of fluid loss.

ACTIONS/INTERVENTIONS	RATIONALE
Observe for excessively dry skin and mucous membranes, decreased skin turgor, slowed capillary refill.	Indicates excessive fluid loss/resultant dehydration.
Weigh daily.	Indicator of overall fluid and nutritional status.
Maintain oral restrictions, bedrest; avoid exertion.	Colon is placed at rest for healing and to decrease intestinal fluid losses.
Observe for overt bleeding and test stool daily for occult blood.	Inadequate diet and decreased absorption may lead to vitamin K deficiency and defects in coagulation, potentiating risk of hemorrhage.
Note generalized muscle weakness or cardiac dysrhythmias.	Excessive intestinal loss may lead to electrolyte imbalance; e.g., potassium, which is necessary for proper skeletal and cardiac muscle function. Minor alterations in serum levels can result in profound and/or life-threatening symptoms.

Collaborative

ACTIONS/INTERVENTIONS	RATIONALE
Administer parenteral fluids, blood transfusions as indicated.	Maintenance of bowel rest requires alternative fluid replacement to correct losses/anemia. *Note:* Fluids containing sodium may be restricted in presence of regional enteritis.
Monitor laboratory studies; e.g., electrolytes (especially potassium, magnesium) and ABGs (acid-base balance).	Determines replacement needs and effectiveness of therapy.
Administer medications as indicated:	
Antidiarrheals (Refer to ND: Diarrhea);	Reduce fluid losses from intestines.
Antiemetics; e.g., trimethobenzamide (Tigan), hydroxyzine (Vistaril), prochlorperazine (Compazine);	Control nausea/vomiting in acute exacerbations.
Antipyretics; e.g., acetaminophen (Tylenol);	Control fever, helping to reduce insensible losses.
Electrolytes; e.g., potassium supplement (KCl-IV; K-Lyte, Slow-K);	Electrolytes are lost in large amounts, especially in bowel with denuded, ulcerated areas, and diarrhea can also lead to metabolic acidosis through loss of bicarbonate (HCO_3).
Vitamin K (Mephyton).	Stimulates hepatic formation of prothrombin, stabilizing coagulation and reducing risk of hemorrhage.

NURSING DIAGNOSIS: imbalanced Nutrition: less than body requirements

May be related to

Altered absorption of nutrients
Hypermetabolic state
Medically restricted intake; fear that eating may cause diarrhea

Possibly evidenced by

Weight loss, decreased subcutaneous fat/muscle mass, poor muscle tone
Hyperactive bowel sounds, steatorrhea
Pale conjunctiva and mucous membranes
Aversion to eating

DESIRED OUTCOMES/EVALUATION CRITERIA—CLIENT WILL:

Nutritional Status (NOC)

Demonstrate stable weight or progressive gain toward goal with normalization of laboratory values and absence of signs of malnutrition.

ACTIONS/INTERVENTIONS	RATIONALE
Nutrition Therapy (NIC)	
Independent	
Assess weight, age, body mass, strength, activity/rest level; ascertain stage of disease process and its effects on client's nutritional status	Provides comparative baseline.
Inspect oral mucosa.	May reveal ulcerations and/or provide information about the integrity of the entire GI tract, affecting ability to eat and absorb nutrients.
Evaluate client's appetite.	Appetite may be suppressed because of altered taste, early satiety, meal-related cramping, diarrhea, or a combination of these factors.
Weigh frequently.	Provides information about dietary needs/effectiveness of therapy.
Encourage bedrest and/or limited activity during acute phase of illness.	Decreasing metabolic needs aids in preventing caloric depletion and conserves energy.
Recommend rest before meals.	Quiets peristalsis and increases available energy for eating.
Provide oral hygiene.	A clean mouth can enhance the taste of food.
Serve foods in well-ventilated, pleasant surroundings, with unhurried atmosphere, congenial company.	Pleasant environment aids in reducing stress and is more conducive to eating.
Avoid/limit foods that might cause/exacerbate abdominal cramping, flatulence (e.g., milk products, foods high in fiber or fat, alcohol, caffeinated beverages, chocolate, peppermint, tomatoes, orange juice).	Individual tolerance varies, depending on stage of disease and area of bowel affected.
Record intake and changes in symptomatology.	Useful in identifying specific deficiencies and determining GI response to foods.
Promote client participation in dietary planning as able.	Provides sense of control for client and opportunity to select foods desired/enjoyed, which may increase intake.
Encourage client to verbalize feelings concerning resumption of diet.	Hesitation to eat may be result of fear that food will cause exacerbation of symptoms.
Collaborative	
Keep client NPO as indicated.	Resting the bowel decreases peristalsis and diarrhea, limiting malabsorption/loss of nutrients.
Resume/advance diet as indicated; e.g., clear liquids progressing to bland, low residue, and then high-protein, high-calorie, caffeine-free, nonspicy, and low-fiber as indicated.	Allows the intestinal tract to readjust to the digestive process. Protein is necessary for tissue healing. Low bulk decreases peristaltic response to meal. *Note:* Dietary measures depend on client's condition; e.g., if disease is mild, client may do well on low-residue, low-fat diet high in protein and calories with lactose restriction. In moderate disease, elemental enteral products may be given to provide nutrition without overstimulating the bowel. Client with toxic colitis is NPO and placed on parenteral nutrition.
Provide nutritional support; e.g.:	
Enteral feedings; e.g., Ultra Clear Plus via NG, percutaneous endoscopic gastrostomy (PEG), or J-tube;	Many clinical studies have shown early enteral feeding is beneficial in reducing the effects of malabsorption and providing essential nutrients. An elemental formula (hypoallergenic, low in fat, protein, and carbohydrates) is easily absorbed and tolerated. Although elemental enteral solutions cannot provide all needed nutrients, they can prevent gut atrophy.
TPN.	This regimen rests the GI tract completely while providing essential nutrients. Short-term TPN is indicated during periods of disease exacerbation when bowel rest is needed. (Refer to CP: Total Nutritional Support: Parenteral/Enteral Feeding, p. 478.)

ACTIONS/INTERVENTIONS	RATIONALE
Administer medications as indicated; e.g.:	
Belladonna alkaloids (Donnatal), butabarbital sodium with belladonna (Butibel), propantheline bromide (Pro-Banthine);	Anticholinergics given 15–30 min before eating provide relief from cramping pain and diarrhea, decreasing gastric motility and enhancing time for absorption of nutrients.
Iron (ImFeD/injectable);	Prevents/treats anemia. Oral route for iron supplement is ineffective because of intestinal alterations that severely reduce absorption.
Vitamin B_{12} (Crystamine, Rubesol);	Malabsorption of vitamin B_{12} results from significant loss of functional ileum. Replacement of vitamin B_{12} reverses bone marrow depression caused by prolonged inflammatory process, promoting RBC production/correction of anemia.
Folic acid (Folvite);	Folate deficiency is common in presence of Crohn's disease because of decreased intake/absorption, effect of drug therapy sulfasalazine (Azulfidine).
Vitamin C (Ascorbicap).	Promotes tissue healing/regeneration.

NURSING DIAGNOSIS: Anxiety [specify level]

May be related to

Physiologic factors/sympathetic stimulation (inflammatory process)
Threat to self-concept (perceived or actual)
Threat to/change in health status, socioeconomic status, role functioning, interaction patterns

Possibly evidenced by

Exacerbation of acute stage of disease
Increased tension, distress, apprehension
Expressed concern regarding changes in life
Somatic complaints
Focus on self

DESIRED OUTCOMES/EVALUATION CRITERIA—CLIENT WILL:

Anxiety Self-Control (NOC)

Appear relaxed and report anxiety reduced to a manageable level.
Verbalize awareness of feelings of anxiety and healthy ways to deal with them.

ACTIONS/INTERVENTIONS	RATIONALE
Anxiety Reduction (NIC)	
Independent	
Note behavioral clues; e.g., restlessness, irritability, withdrawal, lack of eye contact, demanding behavior.	Indicators of degree of anxiety/stress; e.g., client may feel out of control at home/work managing personal problems. Stress may develop as a result of physical symptoms of condition and the reaction of others.
Encourage verbalization of feelings. Provide feedback.	Establishes a therapeutic relationship. Assists client/SO in identifying problems causing stress. Client with severe diarrhea may hesitate to ask for help for fear of becoming a burden to the staff.

ACTIONS/INTERVENTIONS	RATIONALE
Acknowledge that the anxiety and problems are similar to those expressed by others. Active-listen client's concerns.	Validation that feelings are normal can help reduce stress/isolation and belief that "I am the only one."
Provide accurate, concrete information about what is being done; e.g., reason for bed rest, restriction of oral intake, and procedures.	Involving client in plan of care provides sense of control and helps decrease anxiety.
Provide a calm, restful environment.	Removing client from outside stressors promotes relaxation; helps reduce anxiety.
Encourage staff/SO to project caring, concerned attitude.	A supportive manner can help client feel less stressed, allowing energy to be directed toward healing/recovery.
Help client identify/initiate positive coping behaviors used in the past.	Successful behaviors can be fostered in dealing with current problems/stress, enhancing client's sense of self-control.
Assist client to learn new coping mechanisms; e.g., stress management techniques, organizational skills as appropriate.	Learning new ways to cope can be helpful in reducing stress and anxiety, enhancing disease control.

Collaborative

Administer medications as indicated:	
Sedatives; e.g., barbiturates, phenobarbital (Luminal); antianxiety agents; e.g., diazepam (Valium).	May be used to reduce anxiety and to facilitate rest, particularly in the client with UC.
Refer to psychiatric clinical nurse specialist, social services, spiritual advisor.	May require additional assistance in regaining control and coping with acute episodes/exacerbations, as well as learning to deal with the chronicity and consequences of the disease and the therapeutic regimen.

NURSING DIAGNOSIS: acute Pain

May be related to

Hyperperistalsis, prolonged diarrhea, skin/tissue irritation, perirectal excoriation, fissures, fistulas

Possibly evidenced by

Reports of colicky/cramping abdominal pain/referred pain
Guarding/distraction behaviors, restlessness
Facial mask of pain; self-focusing

DESIRED OUTCOMES/EVALUATION CRITERIA—CLIENT WILL:

Pain Level (NOC)

Report pain is relieved/controlled.
Appear relaxed and able to sleep/rest appropriately.

ACTIONS/INTERVENTIONS — RATIONALE

Pain Management (NIC)

Independent

ACTIONS/INTERVENTIONS	RATIONALE
Encourage client to report pain.	May try to tolerate pain rather than request analgesics.
Assess reports of abdominal cramping or pain, noting location, duration, intensity (0–10 scale). Investigate and report changes in pain characteristics.	Colicky intermittent pain occurs with Crohn's disease. Predefecation pain frequently occurs in UC with urgency, which may be severe and continuous. Changes in pain characteristics may indicate spread of disease/developing complications; e.g., bladder fistula, perforation, toxic megacolon.

ACTIONS/INTERVENTIONS	RATIONALE
Note nonverbal cues; e.g., restlessness, reluctance to move, abdominal guarding, withdrawal, and depression. Investigate discrepancies between verbal and nonverbal cues.	Body language/nonverbal cues may be both physiologic and psychologic and may be used in conjunction with verbal cues to determine extent/severity of the problem.
Review factors that aggravate or alleviate pain.	May pinpoint precipitating or aggravating factors (such as stressful events, food intolerance) or identify developing complications.
Encourage client to assume position of comfort; e.g., knees flexed.	Reduces abdominal tension and promotes sense of control.
Provide comfort measures (e.g., back rub, reposition) and diversional activities.	Promotes relaxation, refocuses attention, and may enhance coping abilities.
Cleanse rectal area with mild soap and water/wipes after each stool and provide skin care; e.g., A&D ointment, Sween ointment, karaya gel, Desitin, petroleum jelly.	Protects skin from bowel acids, preventing excoriation.
Provide sitz bath as appropriate.	Enhances cleanliness and comfort in the presence of perianal irritation/fissures.
Observe for ischiorectal and perianal fistulas.	Fistulas may develop from erosion and weakening of intestinal bowel wall.
Observe/record abdominal distention, increased temperature, decreased BP.	May indicate developing intestinal obstruction from inflammation, edema, and scarring.

Collaborative

Implement prescribed dietary modifications; e.g., commence with liquids and increase to solid foods as tolerated.	Complete bowel rest can reduce pain, cramping.
Administer medications as indicated; e.g.:	
Analgesics;	Pain varies from mild to severe and necessitates management to facilitate adequate rest and recovery. *Note:* Opiates should be used with caution because they may precipitate toxic megacolon.
Anticholinergics;	Relieve spasms of GI tract and resultant colicky pain.
Anodyne suppositories.	Relax rectal muscle, decreasing painful spasms.

NURSING DIAGNOSIS: ineffective Coping

May be related to

Multiple stressors, repeated over period of time; situational crisis
Unpredictable nature of disease process
Personal vulnerability, inadequate coping method, lack of support systems
Severe pain
Lack of sleep, rest

Possibly evidenced by

Verbalization of inability to cope, discouragement, anxiety
Preoccupation with physical self, chronic worry, emotional tension, poor self-esteem
Depression and dependency

DESIRED OUTCOMES/EVALUATION CRITERIA—CLIENT WILL:

Coping (NOC)

Assess the current situation accurately.
Identify ineffective coping behaviors and consequences.
Acknowledge own coping abilities.
Demonstrate necessary lifestyle changes to limit/prevent recurrent episodes.

ACTIONS/INTERVENTIONS	RATIONALE
Coping Enhancement (NIC)	
Independent	
Assess client's/SO's understanding and previous methods of dealing with disease process.	Enables the nurse to deal more realistically with current problems. Anxiety and other problems may have interfered with previous health teaching/client learning.
Determine outside stressors; e.g., family, relationships, social or work environment.	Stress can alter autonomic nervous response, affecting the immune system and contributing to exacerbation of disease. Even the goal of independence in the dependent client can be an added stressor.
Provide opportunity for client to discuss how illness has affected relationship, including sexual concerns.	Stressors of illness affect all areas of life, and client may have difficulty coping with feelings of fatigue/pain in relation to relationship/sexual needs.
Help client identify individually effective coping skills.	Use of previously successful behaviors can help client deal with current situation/plan for future.
Provide emotional support:	
Active-listen in a nonjudgmental manner;	Aids in communication and understanding client's viewpoint. Adds to client's feelings of self-worth.
Maintain nonjudgmental body language when caring for client;	Prevents reinforcing client's feelings of being a burden; e.g., frequent need to empty bedpan/commode.
Assign same staff as much as possible.	Provides a more therapeutic environment and lessens the stress of constant adjustments.
Provide uninterrupted sleep/rest periods.	Exhaustion brought on by the disease tends to magnify problems, interfering with ability to cope.
Encourage use of stress management skills; e.g., relaxation techniques, visualization, guided imagery, deep-breathing exercises.	Refocuses attention, promotes relaxation, and enhances coping abilities.
Collaborative	
Include client/SO in team conferences to develop individualized program.	Promotes continuity of care and enables client/SO to feel a part of the plan, imparting a sense of control and increasing cooperation with therapeutic regimen.
Administer medications as indicated: antianxiety agents; e.g., lorazepam (Ativan), alprazolam (Xanax).	Aids in psychologic/physical rest. Conserves energy and may strengthen coping abilities.
Refer to resources as indicated; e.g., local support group, social worker, psychiatric clinical nurse specialist, spiritual advisor.	Additional support and counseling can assist client/SO in dealing with specific stress/problem areas.

NURSING DIAGNOSIS: deficient Knowledge [Learning Need] regarding condition, prognosis, treatment, self-care, and discharge needs

May be related to

Information misinterpretation, lack of recall
Unfamiliarity with resources

Possibly evidenced by

Questions, request for information, statements of misconceptions
Inaccurate follow-through of instructions
Development of preventable complications/exacerbations

DESIRED OUTCOMES/EVALUATION CRITERIA—CLIENT WILL:

KNOWLEDGE: Disease Process (NOC)

Verbalize understanding of disease processes, possible complications.
Identify stress situations and specific action(s) to deal with them.

KNOWLEDGE: Treatment Regimen (NOC)

Verbalize understanding of therapeutic regimen.
Participate in treatment regimen.
Initiate necessary lifestyle changes.

ACTIONS/INTERVENTIONS	RATIONALE
TEACHING: Disease Process (NIC)	
Independent	
Determine client's perception of disease process.	Establishes knowledge base and provides some insight into individual learning needs.
Review disease process, cause/effect relationship of factors that precipitate symptoms, and identify ways to reduce contributing factors. Encourage questions.	Precipitating/aggravating factors are individual; therefore, client needs to be aware of what foods, fluids, and lifestyle factors can precipitate symptoms. Accurate knowledge base provides opportunity for client to make informed decisions/choices about future and control of chronic disease. Although most clients know about their own disease process, they may have outdated information or misconceptions.
Review medications, purpose, frequency, dosage, and possible side effects.	Promotes understanding and may enhance cooperation with regimen.
Remind client to observe for side effects if steroids are given on a long-term basis; e.g., ulcers, facial edema, muscle weakness.	Steroids may be used to control inflammation and to effect a remission of the disease; however, drug may lower resistance to infection and cause fluid retention.
Stress importance of good skin care; e.g., proper handwashing techniques and perineal skin care.	Reduces spread of bacteria and risk of skin irritation/breakdown, infection.
Recommend cessation of smoking.	Can increase intestinal motility, aggravating symptoms.
Emphasize need for long-term follow-up and periodic reevaluation.	Clients with IBD are at increased risk for colon/rectal cancer, and regular diagnostic evaluations may be required.
Identify appropriate community resources; e.g., Crohn's and Colitis Foundation of America (CCFA), United Ostomy Association, home healthcare providers/visiting nurse services, dietitian, and social services.	Client may benefit from the services of these agencies in coping with chronicity of the disease and evaluating treatment options.

POTENTIAL CONSIDERATIONS following acute hospitalization (dependent on client's age, physical condition/presence of complications, personal resources, and life responsibilities)

acute Pain—hyperperistalsis, prolonged diarrhea, skin/tissue irritation, perirectal excoriation, fissures, fistulas.

ineffective Coping—multiple stressors repeated over period of time, unpredictable nature of disease process, personal vulnerability, severe pain, situational crisis.

risk for Infection—traumatized tissue, change in pH of secretions, altered peristalsis, suppressed inflammatory response, chronic disease, malnutrition.

ineffective Therapeutic Regimen Management—complexity of therapeutic regimen, perceived benefit, powerlessness.

FECAL DIVERSIONS: POSTOPERATIVE CARE OF ILEOSTOMY AND COLOSTOMY

An *ileostomy* is an opening constructed in the ileum to treat regional and ulcerative colitis and to divert intestinal contents in cases of colon cancer, polyps, and trauma. It is usually done when the entire colon, rectum, and anus must be removed, in which case the ileostomy is permanent. A temporary ileostomy is done to provide complete bowel rest in conditions such as chronic colitis and in some trauma cases.

A *colostomy* is a diversion of the effluent of the colon and may be temporary or permanent. Ascending, transverse, descending, and sigmoid colostomies may be performed. A transverse colostomy is usually temporary. A sigmoid colostomy is the most common permanent stoma, usually performed for cancer treatment.

Within the past 50 years major advances have occurred in ostomy surgery, including continent diversions such as the Kock pouch and the ileoanal reservoir. However, each year in the United States, 100,000 people still undergo surgery to create ostomies. These incontinent diversions are the primary focus of this plan of care.

CARE SETTINGS

Inpatient acute care surgical unit.

RELATED CONCERNS

Cancer, page 857
Fluid and electrolyte imbalances, page 919
Inflammatory bowel disease: ulcerative colitis, regional enteritis, page 324
Psychosocial aspects of care, page 770
Surgical intervention, page 788
Total nutritional support: parenteral/enteral feeding, page 478

Client Assessment Database

Data depend on the underlying problem, duration, and severity (e.g., obstruction, perforation, inflammation, congenital defects).

TEACHING/LEARNING

Discharge plan considerations: Assistance with dietary concerns, management of ostomy, and acquisition of supplies may be required

Refer to section at end of plan for postdischarge considerations.

NURSING PRIORITIES

1. Assist client/SO in psychosocial adjustment.
2. Prevent complications.
3. Support independence in self-care.
4. Provide information about procedure/prognosis, treatment needs, potential complications, and community resources.

DISCHARGE GOALS

1. Adjusting to perceived/actual changes.
2. Complications prevented/minimized.
3. Self-care needs met by self/with assistance depending on specific situation.
4. Procedure/prognosis, therapeutic regimen, potential complications understood and sources of support identified.
5. Plan in place to meet needs after discharge.

NURSING DIAGNOSIS: risk for impaired Skin Integrity

Risk factors may include

Absence of sphincter at stoma
Character/flow of effluent and flatus from stoma
Reaction to product/chemicals; improper fitting/care of appliance/skin

Possibly evidenced by

[Not applicable; presence of signs and symptoms establishes an *actual* diagnosis.]

DESIRED OUTCOMES/EVALUATION CRITERIA—CLIENT WILL:

Ostomy Self-Care (NOC)

Maintain skin integrity around stoma.
Identify individual risk factors.
Demonstrate behaviors/techniques to promote healing/prevent skin breakdown.

ACTIONS/INTERVENTIONS	RATIONALE
Ostomy Care (NIC)	
Independent	
Inspect stoma/peristomal skin area with each pouch change. Note irritation, bruises (dark, bluish color), rashes.	Monitors healing process/effectiveness of appliances and identifies areas of concern, need for further evaluation/intervention. Early identification of stomal necrosis/ischemia or fungal infection (from changes in normal bowel flora) provides for timely interventions to prevent serious complications. Stoma should be red and moist. Ulcerated areas on stoma may be from a pouch opening that is too small or a faceplate that cuts into stoma. In clients with an ileostomy, the effluent is rich in enzymes, increasing the likelihood of skin irritation. In client with a colostomy, skin care is not as great a concern because the enzymes are no longer present in the effluent.
Clean with warm water and pat dry. Use soap only if area is covered with sticky stool. If paste has collected on the skin, let it dry, and then peel it off.	Maintaining a clean/dry area helps prevent skin breakdown, and increases adherence of appliances.
Measure stoma periodically; e.g., at least weekly for first 6 weeks, then once a month for 6 months. Measure both width and length of stoma.	As postoperative edema resolves (during first 6 wk), the stoma shrinks and size of appliance must be altered to ensure proper fit so that effluent is collected as it flows from the ostomy and contact with the skin is prevented.
Verify that opening on adhesive backing of pouch is at least 1/16 to 1/8 inch (2–3 mm) larger than the base of the stoma, with adequate adhesiveness left to apply pouch.	Prevents trauma to the stoma tissue and protects the peristomal skin. Adequate adhesive area prevents the skin barrier wafer from being too tight. *Note:* Too tight a fit may cause stomal edema or stenosis.
Use a transparent, odor-proof drainable pouch.	A transparent appliance during first 4–6 weeks allows easy observation of stoma without necessity of removing pouch/irritating skin.
Apply appropriate skin barrier; e.g., hydrocolloid wafer, karaya gum, extended-wear skin barrier, or similar products.	Protects skin from pouch adhesive, enhances adhesiveness of pouch, and facilitates removal of pouch when necessary. *Note:* Sigmoid colostomy may not require an appliance if elimination is regulated through irrigation.
Empty, rinse, and cleanse ostomy pouch on a routine basis, using appropriate equipment.	Frequent pouch changes are irritating to the skin and should be avoided. Emptying and rinsing the pouch with the proper solution removes bacteria and odor-causing stool and flatus.
Support surrounding skin when gently removing appliance. Apply adhesive removers as indicated, and then wash thoroughly.	Prevents tissue irritation/destruction associated with "pulling" pouch off.
Investigate reports of burning/itching/blistering around stoma.	Indicative of effluent leakage with peristomal irritation, or possibly *Candida* infection, requiring intervention.
Evaluate adhesive product and appliance fit on ongoing basis.	Provides opportunity for problem-solving. Determines need for further intervention.

ACTIONS/INTERVENTIONS	RATIONALE
Collaborative	
Consult with certified wound, ostomy, continence nurse.	Helpful in choosing products appropriate for client's particular rehabilitation needs, including type of ostomy, physical/mental status, abilities to handle self-care, and financial resources.
Apply corticosteroid aerosol spray and prescribed antifungal powder as indicated.	Assists in healing if peristomal irritation persists/fungal infection develops. *Note:* These products can have potent side effects and should be used sparingly.

NURSING DIAGNOSIS: disturbed Body Image

May be related to

Biophysical: presence of stoma, loss of control of bowel elimination
Psychosocial: altered body structure
Disease process and associated treatment regimen; e.g., cancer, colitis

Possibly evidenced by

Verbalization of change in body image, fear of rejection/reaction of others, and negative feelings about body
Actual change in structure and/or function (ostomy)
Not touching/looking at stoma, refusal to participate in care

DESIRED OUTCOMES/EVALUATION CRITERIA—CLIENT WILL:

Body Image (NOC)

Verbalize acceptance of self in situation, incorporating change into self-concept without negating self-esteem.
Demonstrate beginning acceptance by viewing/touching stoma and participating in self-care.
Verbalize feelings about stoma/illness; begin to deal constructively with situation.

ACTIONS/INTERVENTIONS	RATIONALE
Body Image Enhancement (NIC)	
Independent	
Ascertain whether support and counseling were initiated when the possibility and/or necessity of ostomy was first discussed.	Provides information about client's/SO's level of knowledge and anxiety about individual situation.
Encourage client/SO to verbalize feelings regarding the ostomy. Acknowledge normality of feelings of anger, depression, and grief over loss. Discuss daily "ups and downs" that can occur.	Helps client realize that feelings are not unusual and that feeling guilty about them is not necessary/helpful. Client needs to recognize feelings before they can be dealt with effectively.
Review reason for surgery and future expectations.	Client may find it easier to accept/deal with an ostomy done to correct chronic/long-term disease than for traumatic injury even if ostomy is only temporary. Also, client who will be undergoing a second procedure (to convert ostomy to a continent or anal reservoir) may possibly encounter less severe self-image problems because body function eventually will be "more normal."

ACTIONS/INTERVENTIONS	RATIONALE
Note behaviors of withdrawal, increased dependency, manipulation, or noninvolvement in care.	Suggestive of problems in adjustment that may require further evaluation and more extensive therapy.
Provide opportunities for client/SO to view and touch stoma, using the moment to point out positive signs of healing, normal appearance, and so forth. Remind client that it will take time to adjust, both physically and emotionally.	Although integration of stoma into body image can take months or even years, looking at the stoma and hearing comments (made in a normal, matter-of-fact manner) can help client with this acceptance. Touching stoma reassures client/SO that it is not fragile and that slight movements of stoma actually reflect normal peristalsis.
Provide opportunity for client to deal with ostomy through participation in self-care.	Independence in self-care helps improve self-confidence and acceptance of situation.
Plan/schedule care activities with client.	Promotes sense of control and gives message that client can handle situation, enhancing self-concept.
Maintain positive approach during care activities, avoiding expressions of disdain or revulsion. Do not take angry expressions of client/SO personally.	Assists client/SO to accept body changes and feel all right about self. Anger is most often directed at the situation and lack of control individual has over what has happened (powerlessness), not with the individual caregiver.
Ascertain client's desire to visit with a person with an ostomy. Make arrangements for visit if desired.	A person who is living with an ostomy can be a good support system/role model. Helps reinforce teaching (shared experiences) and facilitates acceptance of change as client realizes "life does go on" and can be relatively normal.

NURSING DIAGNOSIS: acute Pain

May be related to

Physical factors; e.g., disruption of skin/tissues (incisions/drains)
Biologic: activity of disease process (cancer, trauma)
Psychologic factors; e.g., fear, anxiety

Possibly evidenced by

Reports of pain, self-focusing
Guarding/distraction behaviors, restlessness
Autonomic responses; e.g., changes in vital signs

DESIRED OUTCOMES/EVALUATION CRITERIA—CLIENT WILL:

Pain Level (NOC)

Verbalize that pain is relieved/controlled.
Appear relaxed, able to sleep/rest appropriately.

Pain Control (NOC)

Demonstrate use of relaxation skills and general comfort measures as indicated for individual situation.

ACTIONS/INTERVENTIONS	RATIONALE
Pain Management (NIC)	
Independent	
Assess pain, noting location, characteristics, intensity (0–10 scale).	Helps evaluate degree of discomfort and effectiveness of analgesia or may reveal developing complications. Because abdominal pain usually subsides gradually by the third or fourth postoperative day, continued or increasing pain may reflect delayed healing or peristomal skin irritation. *Note:* Pain in anal area associated with abdominal-perineal resection may persist for months.

ACTIONS/INTERVENTIONS	RATIONALE
Encourage client to verbalize concerns. Active-listen these concerns, and provide support by acceptance, remaining with client, and giving appropriate information.	Reduction of anxiety/fear can promote relaxation/comfort.
Provide comfort measures; e.g., mouth care, back rub, repositioning (use proper support measures as needed). Assure client that position change will not injure stoma.	Prevents drying of oral mucosa and associated discomfort. Reduces muscle tension, promotes relaxation, and may enhance coping abilities.
Encourage use of relaxation techniques; e.g., guided imagery, visualization. Provide diversional activities.	Helps client rest more effectively and refocuses attention, thereby reducing pain and discomfort.
Assist with ROM exercises and encourage early ambulation. Avoid prolonged sitting position.	Reduces muscle/joint stiffness. Ambulation returns organs to normal position and promotes return of usual level of functioning. *Note:* Presence of edema, packing, and drains (if perineal resection has been done) increases discomfort and creates a sense of needing to defecate. Ambulation and frequent position changes reduce perineal pressure.
Investigate and report abdominal muscle rigidity, involuntary guarding, and rebound tenderness.	Suggestive of peritoneal inflammation, which requires prompt medical intervention.

Collaborative

Administer medication as indicated; e.g., narcotics, analgesics, client-controlled analgesia (PCA).	Relieves pain, enhances comfort, and promotes rest. PCA may be more beneficial, especially following anal-perineal repair.
Provide sitz baths.	Relieves local discomfort, reduces edema, and promotes healing of perineal wound.
Apply/monitor effects of transcutaneous electrical nerve stimulator (TENS) unit.	Cutaneous stimulation may be used to block transmission of pain stimulus.

NURSING DIAGNOSIS: impaired Skin/Tissue Integrity

May be related to

Invasion of body structure (e.g., perineal resection)
Stasis of secretions/drainage
Altered circulation, edema; malnutrition

Possibly evidenced by

Disruption of skin/tissue: presence of incision and sutures, drains

DESIRED OUTCOMES/EVALUATION CRITERIA—CLIENT WILL:

WOUND HEALING: Primary Intention (NOC)

Achieve timely wound healing free of signs of infection.

ACTIONS/INTERVENTIONS	RATIONALE
Wound Care (NIC)	
Independent	
Observe wounds, note characteristics of drainage.	Postoperative hemorrhage is most likely to occur during first 48 hr, whereas infection may develop at any time. Depending on type of wound closure (e.g., first or second intention), complete healing may take 6–8 months.

ACTIONS/INTERVENTIONS	RATIONALE
Change dressings as needed.	Large amounts of serous drainage require that dressings be changed frequently to reduce skin irritation and potential for infection.
Encourage side-lying position with head elevated. Avoid prolonged sitting.	Promotes drainage from perineal wound/drains, reducing risk of pooling. Prolonged sitting increases perineal pressure, reducing circulation to wound, and may delay healing.

Collaborative

Irrigate wound as indicated, using normal saline (NS), diluted hydrogen peroxide, or antibiotic solution.	May be required to treat preoperative inflammation/infection or intraoperative contamination.
Provide sitz baths.	Promotes cleanliness and facilitates healing, especially after packing is removed (usually day 3–5).

NURSING DIAGNOSIS: risk for deficient Fluid Volume

Risk factors may include

Excessive losses through normal routes; e.g., preoperative emesis and diarrhea; high-volume ileostomy output
Losses through abnormal routes; e.g., NG/intestinal tube, perineal wound drainage tubes
Medically restricted intake
Altered absorption of fluid; e.g., loss of colon function
Hypermetabolic states; e.g., inflammation, healing process

Possibly evidenced by

[Not applicable; presence of signs and symptoms establishes an *actual* diagnosis.]

DESIRED OUTCOMES/EVALUATION CRITERIA—CLIENT WILL:

Hydration (NOC)

Maintain adequate hydration as evidenced by moist mucous membranes, good skin turgor and capillary refill, stable vital signs, and individually appropriate urinary output.

ACTIONS/INTERVENTIONS	RATIONALE
Fluid/Electrolyte Management (NIC)	
Independent	
Monitor intake and output (I&O) carefully, measure liquid stool. Weigh regularly.	Provides direct indicators of fluid balance. Greatest fluid losses occur with ileostomy, but they generally do not exceed 500–800 mL/day.
Monitor vital signs, noting postural hypotension, tachycardia. Evaluate skin turgor, capillary refill, and mucous membranes.	Reflects hydration status/possible need for increased fluid replacement.
Limit intake of ice chips during period of gastric intubation.	Ice chips can stimulate gastric secretions and wash out electrolytes.

ACTIONS/INTERVENTIONS	RATIONALE
Collaborative	
Monitor laboratory results; e.g., Hct and electrolytes.	Detects homeostasis or imbalance, and aids in determining replacement needs.
Administer IV fluid and electrolytes as indicated.	May be necessary to maintain adequate tissue perfusion/organ function.

NURSING DIAGNOSIS: risk for imbalanced Nutrition: less than body requirements

Risk factors may include

Prolonged anorexia/altered intake preoperatively
Hypermetabolic state (preoperative inflammatory disease; healing process)
Presence of diarrhea/altered absorption
Restriction of bulk and residue-containing foods

Possibly evidenced by

[Not applicable; presence of signs and symptoms establishes an *actual* diagnosis.]

DESIRED OUTCOMES/EVALUATION CRITERIA—CLIENT WILL:

Nutritional Status (NOC)

Maintain weight/demonstrate progressive weight gain toward goal with normalization of laboratory values and be free of signs of malnutrition.
Plan diet to meet nutritional needs/limit GI disturbances.

ACTIONS/INTERVENTIONS	RATIONALE
Nutrition Therapy (NIC)	
Independent	
Obtain a thorough nutritional assessment.	Identifies deficiencies/needs to aid in choice of interventions.
Auscultate bowel sounds.	Return of intestinal function indicates readiness to resume oral intake.
Resume solid foods slowly.	Reduces incidence of abdominal cramps, nausea.
Identify odor-causing foods (e.g., cabbage, fish, beans) and temporarily restrict from diet. Gradually reintroduce one food at a time.	Sensitivity to certain foods is not uncommon following intestinal surgery. Client can experiment with food several times before determining whether it is creating a problem.
Recommend client increase use of yogurt, buttermilk, and acidophilus preparations.	May help prevent gas and decrease odor formation.
Suggest client with ileostomy limit prunes, dates, stewed apricots, strawberries, grapes, bananas, cabbage family, beans, and avoid foods high in cellulose; e.g., peanuts.	These products increase ileal effluent. Digestion of cellulose requires colonic bacteria that are no longer present.
Discuss mechanics of swallowed air as a factor in the formation of flatus and some ways client can exercise control.	Drinking through a straw, snoring, anxiety, smoking, ill-fitting dentures, and gulping down food increase the production of flatus. Too much flatus not only necessitates frequent emptying, but also can cause leakage from too much pressure within the pouch.

ACTIONS/INTERVENTIONS	RATIONALE
Collaborative	
Consult with dietitian.	Helpful in assessing client's nutritional needs in light of changes in digestion and intestinal function, including absorption of vitamins/minerals.
Advance diet from liquids to low-residue food when oral intake is resumed.	Low-residue diet may be maintained during first 6–8 weeks to provide adequate time for intestinal healing.
Administer enteral/parenteral feedings when indicated.	In the presence of severe debilitation/intolerance of oral intake, parenteral or enteral feedings may be given to supply needed components for healing and prevention of catabolic state. (Refer to CP: Total Nutritional Support: Parenteral/Enteral Feeding, p. 478.)

NURSING DIAGNOSIS: disturbed Sleep Pattern

May be related to

External factors: necessity of ostomy care, excessive flatus/ostomy effluent
Internal factors: psychologic stress, fear of leakage of pouch/injury to stoma

Possibly evidenced by

Verbalizations of interrupted sleep, not feeling well rested
Changes in behavior; e.g., irritability, listlessness/lethargy

DESIRED OUTCOMES/EVALUATION CRITERIA—CLIENT WILL:

Sleep (NOC)

Sleep/rest between disturbances.
Report increased sense of well-being and feeling rested.

ACTIONS/INTERVENTIONS	RATIONALE
Sleep Enhancement (NIC)	
Independent	
Explain necessity to monitor intestinal function in early postoperative period.	Client is more apt to be tolerant of disturbances by staff if he or she understands the reasons for/importance of care.
Provide adequate pouching system. Empty pouch before retiring and, if necessary, on a preagreed schedule.	Excessive flatus/effluent can occur despite interventions. Emptying on a regular schedule minimizes threat of leakage.
Let client know that stoma will not be injured when sleeping.	Client will be able to rest better if feeling secure about stoma and ostomy function.
Restrict intake of caffeine-containing foods/fluids.	Caffeine may delay client's falling asleep and interfere with REM (rapid eye movement) sleep, resulting in client not feeling well rested.
Support continuation of usual bedtime rituals.	Promotes relaxation and readiness for sleep.
Collaborative	
Determine cause of excessive flatus or effluent and possible actions; e.g., confer with dietitian regarding restriction of foods if diet related.	Identification of cause enables institution of corrective measures that may promote sleep/rest.

ACTIONS/INTERVENTIONS	RATIONALE
Administer analgesics, sedatives at bedtime as indicated.	Pain can interfere with client's ability to fall/remain asleep. Timely medication can enhance rest/sleep during initial postoperative period. *Note:* Pain pathways in the brain lie near the sleep center and may contribute to wakefulness.

NURSING DIAGNOSIS: risk for Constipation/Diarrhea

Risk factors may include

Placement of ostomy in descending or sigmoid colon
Inadequate diet/fluid intake

Possibly evidenced by

[Not applicable; presence of signs and symptoms establishes an *actual* diagnosis.]

DESIRED OUTCOMES/EVALUATION CRITERIA—CLIENT WILL:

Bowel Elimination (NOC)

Establish an elimination pattern suitable to physical needs and lifestyle with effluent of appropriate amount and consistency.

ACTIONS/INTERVENTIONS	RATIONALE
Bowel Management (NIC)	
Independent	
Investigate delayed onset/absence of effluent. Auscultate bowel sounds.	Postoperative paralytic/adynamic ileus usually resolves within 48–72 hr, and ileostomy should begin draining within 12–24 hr. Delay may indicate persistent ileus or stomal obstruction, which may occur postoperatively because of edema, improperly fitting pouch (too tight), prolapse, or stenosis of the stoma.
Inform client with an ileostomy that initially the effluent is liquid. If constipation occurs, it should be reported to enterostomal nurse or physician.	Although the small intestine eventually begins to take on water-absorbing functions to permit a more semisolid, pasty discharge, constipation may indicate an obstruction. Absence of stool requires emergency medical attention.
Review dietary pattern and amount/type of fluid intake.	Adequate intake of fiber and roughage provides bulk, and fluid is an important factor in determining the consistency of the stool.
Review physiology of the colon and discuss irrigation management of sigmoid ostomy if indicated.	This knowledge helps client understand individual care needs.
Ascertain client's previous bowel habits and lifestyle.	Assists in formulation of a timely/effective irrigation schedule for client with a colostomy if appropriate.
Demonstrate use of irrigation equipment per institution policy or under guidance of physician or certified wound, ostomy, continence nurse.	Irrigations may be done on a daily basis if appropriate, although there are differing views on this practice. Many believe cleaning the bowel on a regular basis is helpful. Others believe that this interferes with normal functioning. (Most authorities agree that occasional irrigation is useful for emptying the bowel to avoid leakage when special events are planned.)

ACTIONS/INTERVENTIONS	RATIONALE
Instruct client in the use of closed-end pouch or a patch, dressing/Band-Aid when irrigation is successful and the sigmoid colostomy effluent becomes more manageable, with stool expelled every 24 hr.	Enables client to feel more comfortable socially and is less expensive than regular ostomy pouches.
Involve client in care of the ostomy on an increasing basis.	Rehabilitation can be facilitated by encouraging client independence and control.

Collaborative

Instruct in use of TENS unit if indicated.	Electrical stimulation has been used in some clients to stimulate peristalsis and relieve postoperative ileus.

NURSING DIAGNOSIS: risk for Sexual Dysfunction

Risk factors may include

Altered body structure/function; radical resection/treatment procedures
Vulnerability/psychological concern about response of SO
Disruption of sexual response pattern; e.g., erectile difficulty

Possibly evidenced by

[Not applicable; presence of signs and symptoms establishes an *actual* diagnosis.]

DESIRED OUTCOMES/EVALUATION CRITERIA—CLIENT WILL:

Sexual Functioning (NOC)

Verbalize understanding of relationship of physical condition to sexual problems.
Identify satisfying/acceptable sexual practices and explore alternative methods.
Resume sexual relationship as appropriate.

ACTIONS/INTERVENTIONS — RATIONALE

Sexual Counseling (NIC)

Independent

ACTIONS/INTERVENTIONS	RATIONALE
Determine client's/SO's sexual relationship before the disease and/or surgery and whether they anticipate problems related to presence of ostomy.	Identifies future expectations and desires. Mutilation and loss of privacy/control of a bodily function can affect client's view of personal sexuality. When coupled with the fear of rejection by SO, the desired level of intimacy can be greatly impaired. Sexual needs are very basic, and client will be rehabilitated more successfully when a satisfying sexual relationship is continued/developed as desired.
Review with client/SO sexual functioning in relation to own situation.	Understanding if nerve damage has altered normal sexual functioning (e.g., erection) helps client/SO to understand the need for exploring alternative methods of satisfaction.
Reinforce information given by the physician. Encourage questions. Provide additional information as needed.	Reiteration of data previously given assists client/SO to hear and process the knowledge again, moving toward acceptance of individual limitations/restrictions and prognosis (e.g., that it may take up to 2 years to regain potency after a radical procedure or that a penile prosthesis may be necessary).

ACTIONS/INTERVENTIONS	RATIONALE
Discuss likelihood of resumption of sexual activity in approximately 6 weeks after discharge, beginning slowly and progressing (e.g., cuddling/caressing until both partners are comfortable with body image/function changes). Include alternative methods of stimulation as appropriate.	Knowing what to expect in progress of recovery helps client avoid performance anxiety/reduce risk of "failure." If the couple is willing to try new ideas, this can assist with adjustment and may help to achieve sexual fulfillment.
Encourage dialogue between partners. Suggest wearing pouch cover, T-shirt, short nightgown, or underwear specifically designed for sexual contact.	Disguising ostomy appliance may aid in reducing feelings of self-consciousness, embarrassment during sexual activity.
Stress awareness of factors that might be distracting (e.g., unpleasant odors and pouch leakage). Encourage use of sense of humor.	Promotes resolution of solvable problems. Laughter can help individuals deal more effectively with difficult situation, promote positive sexual experience.
Problem-solve alternative positions for coitus.	Minimizing awkwardness of appliance and physical discomfort can enhance satisfaction.
Discuss/role play possible interactions or approaches when dealing with new sexual partners.	Rehearsal is helpful in dealing with actual situations when they arise, preventing self-consciousness about "different" body image.
Provide birth control information as appropriate and stress that impotence does not necessarily mean client is sterile.	Confusion may exist that can lead to an unwanted pregnancy.

Collaborative

Arrange meeting with an ostomy visitor if appropriate.	Sharing of how these problems have been resolved by others can be helpful and reduce sense of isolation.
Refer to counseling/sex therapy as indicated.	If problems persist longer than several months after surgery, a trained therapist may be required to facilitate communication between client and SO.

NURSING DIAGNOSIS: deficient Knowledge [Learning Need] regarding condition, prognosis, treatment, self-care, and discharge needs

May be related to

Lack of exposure/recall, information misinterpretation
Unfamiliarity with information resources

Possibly evidenced by

Questions; statement of misconception/misinformation
Inaccurate follow-through of instruction/performance of ostomy care
Inappropriate or exaggerated behaviors (e.g., hostile, agitated, apathetic, withdrawal)

DESIRED OUTCOMES/EVALUATION CRITERIA—CLIENT WILL:

KNOWLEDGE: Ostomy Care (NOC)

Verbalize understanding of condition/disease process, prognosis, and potential complications.
Verbalize understanding of therapeutic needs.
Correctly perform necessary procedures, explain reasons for the action.
Initiate necessary lifestyle changes.

ACTIONS/INTERVENTIONS	RATIONALE
Learning Facilitation (NIC)	
Independent	
Evaluate client's emotional, cognitive, and physical capabilities.	These factors affect client's ability to master care tasks and willingness to assume responsibility for ostomy care.
Include written/picture (photo, video, Internet) learning resources.	Provides references for obtaining support, equipment, and additional information after discharge to support client efforts for independence in self-care.
TEACHING: Disease Process (NIC)	
Review anatomy, physiology, and implications of surgical intervention. Discuss future expectations, including anticipated changes in character of effluent.	Provides knowledge base from which client can make informed choices, and offers an opportunity to clarify misconceptions regarding individual situation. (Temporary ileostomy may be converted to ileoanal reservoir at a future date; ileostomy and ascending colostomy cannot be regulated by diet, irrigations, or medications.)
Instruct client/SO in stomal care. Allot time for return demonstrations and provide positive feedback for efforts.	Promotes positive management and reduces risk of improper ostomy care/development of complications.
Recommend increased fluid intake during warm weather months.	Loss of normal colon function of conserving water and electrolytes can lead to dehydration and constipation.
Discuss possible need to decrease salt intake.	Salt can increase ileal output, potentiating risk of dehydration and increasing frequency of ostomy care needs/client's inconvenience.
Identify symptoms of electrolyte depletion; e.g., anorexia, abdominal muscle cramps, feelings of faintness or "cold" in arms/legs, general fatigue/weakness, bloating, decreased sensations in arms/legs.	Loss of colon function altering fluid/electrolyte absorption may result in sodium/potassium deficits requiring dietary correction with foods/fluids high in sodium (e.g., bouillon, Gatorade) or potassium (e.g., orange juice, prunes, tomatoes, bananas, Gatorade).
Discuss need for periodic evaluation/ administration of supplemental vitamins and minerals, as appropriate.	Depending on portion and amount of bowel resected, lack of absorption may cause deficiencies.
Stress importance of chewing food well, adequate intake of fluids with/following meals, only moderate use of high-fiber foods, avoidance of cellulose.	Reduces risk of bowel obstruction in client with ileostomy.
Review foods that are/may be a source of flatus (e.g., carbonated drinks, beer, beans, cabbage family, onions, fish, and highly seasoned foods) or odor (e.g., onions, cabbage family, eggs, fish, and beans).	These foods may be restricted or eliminated, based on individual reaction, for better ostomy control, or it may be necessary to empty the pouch more frequently if they are ingested.
Identify foods associated with diarrhea, such as green beans, broccoli, highly seasoned foods.	Promotes more even effluent and better control of evacuations.
Recommend foods used to manage constipation (e.g., bran, celery, raw fruits), and discuss importance of increased fluid intake.	Proper management can prevent/minimize problems of constipation.
Discuss resumption of presurgery level of activity. Suggest emptying the ostomy appliance before leaving home and carrying fresh supplies. Recommend resources for obtaining attractive appliances and decorative cummerbunds as appropriate.	With a little planning, client should be able to manage same degree of activity as previously enjoyed and in some cases increase activity level. A cummerbund can provide both physical and psychologic support when client is involved in activities such as tennis and swimming.
Talk about the possibility of sleep disturbance, anorexia, loss of interest in usual activities.	"Homecoming depression" may occur, lasting for months after surgery, requiring patience/support and ongoing evaluation as client adjusts to living with a stoma.
Explain necessity of notifying healthcare providers and pharmacists of type of ostomy and avoidance of sustained-release medications (for client with ileostomy).	Presence of ostomy may alter rate/extent of absorption of oral medications and increase risk of drug-related complications; e.g., diarrhea/constipation or peristomal excoriation. Liquid, chewable, or injectable forms of medication are preferred for clients with ileostomy to maximize absorption of drug.

ACTIONS/INTERVENTIONS	RATIONALE
Counsel client concerning medication use and problems associated with altered bowel function. Refer to pharmacist for teaching/advice as appropriate.	Client with an ostomy has two key problems: altered disintegration and absorption of oral drugs and unusual or pronounced adverse effects. Some of the medications that client may respond to differently include laxatives, salicylates, H_2-receptor antagonists, antibiotics, and diuretics.
Discuss effect of medications on effluent; that is, changes in color, odor, consistency of stool, and need to observe for drug residue indicating incomplete absorption.	Understanding decreases anxiety regarding intestinal function and enhances independence in self-care.
Stress necessity of close monitoring of chronic health conditions requiring routine oral medications.	Monitoring of clinical symptoms and serum blood levels is indicated because of altered drug absorption, requiring periodic dosage adjustments.
Identify community resources; e.g. United Ostomy Association, the Crohn's and Colitis Foundation of America, Ostomy rehabilitation program, local ostomy support group; certified Wound, Ostomy, Continence (WOC) nurse; visiting nurse, pharmacy/medical supply house.	Continued support after discharge is essential to facilitate the recovery process and client's independence in care. WOC nurse can be very helpful in solving appliance problems, identifying alternatives to meet individual client needs.

POTENTIAL CONSIDERATIONS following acute hospitalization (dependent on client's age, physical condition/presence of complications, personal resources, and life responsibilities)

risk for Impaired Skin Integrity—absence of sphincter at stoma, character/flow of effluent and flatus from stoma.

ineffective Coping—situational crises, vulnerability.

Impaired Social Interaction—self-concept disturbance, concern for loss of control of bodily functions

APPENDECTOMY

An inflamed appendix may be removed using a laparoscopic approach with laser. However, the presence of multiple adhesions, retroperitoneal positioning of the appendix, or the likelihood of rupture necessitates an open (traditional) procedure. Studies indicate that *laparoscopic appendectomy* results in significantly less postoperative pain, earlier resumption of solid foods, a shorter hospital/same day surgery stay, lower wound infection rate, and a faster return to normal activities than *open appendectomy*.

CARE SETTING

Although many of the interventions included here are appropriate for the short-stay client, this plan of care addresses the traditional appendectomy care provided on a surgical unit, after being diagnosed in the Emergency Department (ED).

RELATED CONCERNS

Peritonitis, page 355
Psychosocial aspects of care, page 770
Surgical intervention, page 788

Client Assessment Database (Preoperative)

ACTIVITY/REST

May report: Malaise

CIRCULATION

May exhibit: Tachycardia

ELIMINATION

May report: Constipation of recent onset
Diarrhea (occasional)

May exhibit: Abdominal distention, tenderness/rebound tenderness, rigidity
Decreased or absent bowel sounds

FOOD/FLUID

May report: Anorexia
Nausea/vomiting (nearly always follows onset of pain)

PAIN/DISCOMFORT

May report: Abdominal pain around the epigastrium and umbilicus, which may have an insidious onset and become increasingly severe; pain may localize in right lower quarter (RLQ), at McBurney's point (halfway between umbilicus and crest of right ileum); pain may be aggravated by walking, sneezing, coughing, or deep respiration
Increasingly severe, generalized pain or the sudden cessation of severe pain (suggests perforation or infarction of the appendix)
Varied reports of pain/vague symptoms (due to location of appendix; e.g., retrocecally or next to ureter) or due to onset of peritonitis

May exhibit: Guarding behavior; lying on side or back with knees flexed; increased RLQ pain with extension of right leg/upright position
Rebound tenderness on left side (suggests peritoneal inflammation)

RESPIRATION

May exhibit: Tachypnea; shallow respirations

SAFETY

May exhibit: Fever (usually low-grade)

TEACHING/LEARNING

May report: History of other conditions associated with abdominal pain; e.g., acute pyelitis, ureteral stone, acute salpingitis, regional ileitis
May occur at any age

Discharge plan considerations: May need brief assistance with transportation, homemaker tasks

Refer to section at end of plan for postdischarge considerations.

DIAGNOSTIC STUDIES

CBC: White blood cells (WBCs) are often elevated above 12,000/mm^3; neutrophil count often elevated to greater than 75%.

Imaging Studies:

Abdominal CT scan: Gold standard test for differentiation of appendicitis from other causes of abdominal pain (e.g., perforating ulcer, cholecystitis, reproductive organ infections) or to localize drainable abscesses.

Ultrasonography: Noninvasive method for quickly scanning abdomen. May be done as screening test, as a normal appendix does not visualize.

Abdominal radiographs: May reveal hardened bit of fecal material in appendix (fecalith), localized ileus. Test is insensitive and nonspecific in diagnosing appendicitis.

NURSING PRIORITIES

1. Prevent complications.
2. Promote comfort.
3. Provide information about surgical procedure/prognosis, treatment needs, and potential complications.

DISCHARGE GOALS

1. Complications prevented/minimized.
2. Pain alleviated/controlled.
3. Surgical procedure/prognosis, therapeutic regimen, and possible complications understood.
4. Plan in place to meet needs after discharge.

NURSING DIAGNOSIS: risk for Infection

Risk factors may include

Inadequate primary defenses; perforation/rupture of the appendix; peritonitis; abscess formation
Invasive procedures, surgical incision

Possibly evidenced by

[Not applicable; presence of signs and symptoms establishes an *actual* diagnosis.]

DESIRED OUTCOMES/EVALUATION CRITERIA—CLIENT WILL:

WOUND HEALING: Primary Intention (NOC)

Achieve timely wound healing; free of signs of infection/inflammation, purulent drainage, erythema, and fever.

ACTIONS/INTERVENTIONS	RATIONALE
Infection Control (NIC)	
Independent	
Practice/instruct in good hand washing and aseptic wound care. Encourage/provide perineal care.	Reduces risk of spread of bacteria.
Inspect incision and dressings. Note characteristics of drainage from wound/drains (if inserted), presence of erythema.	Provides for early detection of developing infectious process, and/or monitors resolution of preexisting peritonitis.
Monitor vital signs. Note onset of fever, chills, diaphoresis, changes in mentation, reports of increasing abdominal pain.	Suggestive of presence of infection/developing sepsis, abscess, peritonitis.
Obtain drainage specimens if indicated.	Gram's stain, culture, and sensitivity testing is useful in identifying causative organism and choice of therapy.
Collaborative	
Administer antibiotics as appropriate; e.g., metronidazole (Flagyl), gentamycin (Garamycin, Gentacidin), cefotetan (Cefotan), meropenem (Merrem).	Antibiotics given before appendectomy are primarily for prophylaxis of wound infection and are not usually continued postoperatively. Therapeutic antibiotics are administered if the appendix is ruptured/abscessed or peritonitis has developed.
Prepare for/assist with incision and drainage (I&D) if indicated.	May be necessary to drain contents of localized abscess.

NURSING DIAGNOSIS: risk for deficient Fluid Volume

Risk factors may include

Preoperative vomiting, postoperative restrictions (e.g., NPO)
Hypermetabolic state (e.g., fever, healing process)
Inflammation of peritoneum with sequestration of fluid

Possibly evidenced by

[Not applicable; presence of signs and symptoms establishes an *actual* diagnosis.]

DESIRED OUTCOMES/EVALUATION CRITERIA—CLIENT WILL:

Hydration (NOC)

Maintain adequate fluid balance as evidenced by moist mucous membranes, good skin turgor, stable vital signs, and individually adequate urinary output.

ACTIONS/INTERVENTIONS	RATIONALE
Fluid Monitoring (NIC)	
Independent	
Monitor BP and pulse.	Variations help identify fluctuating intravascular volumes, or changes in vital signs associated with immune response to inflammation.
Inspect mucous membranes; assess skin turgor and capillary refill.	Indicators of adequacy of peripheral circulation and cellular hydration.
Monitor I&O; note urine color/concentration, specific gravity.	Decreasing output of concentrated urine with increasing specific gravity suggests dehydration/need for increased fluids.
Auscultate bowel sounds. Note passing of flatus, bowel movement.	Indicators of return of peristalsis, readiness to begin oral intake. *Note:* This may not occur in the hospital if client has had a laparoscopic procedure and been discharged in less than 24 hr.
Provide clear liquids in small amounts when oral intake is resumed, and progress diet as tolerated.	Reduces risk of gastric irritation/vomiting to minimize fluid loss.
Give frequent mouth care with special attention to protection of the lips.	Dehydration results in drying and painful cracking of the lips and mouth.
Collaborative	
Maintain gastric/intestinal suction as indicated.	Although not frequently needed, An NG tube may be inserted preoperatively and maintained in immediate postoperative phase to decompress the bowel, promote intestinal rest, and prevent vomiting.
Administer IV fluids and electrolytes.	The peritoneum reacts to irritation/infection by producing large amounts of intestinal fluid, possibly reducing the circulating blood volume, resulting in dehydration and relative electrolyte imbalances.

NURSING DIAGNOSIS: acute Pain

May be related to

Distention of intestinal tissues by inflammation
Presence of surgical incision

Possibly evidenced by

Reports of pain
Facial grimacing, muscle guarding; distraction behaviors
Autonomic responses

DESIRED OUTCOMES/EVALUATION CRITERIA—CLIENT WILL:

Pain Level (NOC)

Report pain is relieved/controlled.
Appear relaxed, able to sleep/rest appropriately.

ACTIONS/INTERVENTIONS	RATIONALE
Pain Management (NIC)	
Independent	
Assess pain, noting location, characteristics, severity (0–10 scale). Investigate and report changes in pain as appropriate.	Useful in monitoring effectiveness of medication, progression of healing. Changes in characteristics of pain may indicate developing abscess/peritonitis, requiring prompt medical evaluation and intervention.
Provide accurate, honest information to client/SO.	Being informed about progress of situation provides emotional support, helping to decrease anxiety
Keep at rest in semi-Fowler's position.	Gravity localizes inflammatory exudate into lower abdomen or pelvis, relieving abdominal tension, which is accentuated by supine position.
Encourage early ambulation.	Promotes normalization of organ function; e.g., stimulates peristalsis and passing of flatus, reducing abdominal discomfort.
Provide diversional activities.	Refocuses attention, promotes relaxation, and may enhance coping abilities.
Collaborative	
Keep NPO/maintain NG suction initially.	Decreases discomfort of early intestinal peristalsis and gastric irritation/vomiting.
Administer analgesics as indicated.	Relief of pain facilitates cooperation with other therapeutic interventions; e.g., ambulation, pulmonary toilet.
Place ice bag on abdomen periodically during initial 24–48 hr as appropriate.	Soothes and relieves pain through desensitization of nerve endings. *Note*: Do not use heat because it may cause tissue congestion/increase edema formation.

NURSING DIAGNOSIS: deficient Knowledge [Learning Need] regarding condition, prognosis, treatment, self-care, and discharge needs

May be related to

Lack of exposure/recall; information misinterpretation
Unfamiliarity with information resources

Possibly evidenced by

Questions, request for information, verbalization of problem/concerns
Statement of misconception
Inaccurate follow-through of instruction
Development of preventable complications

DESIRED OUTCOMES/EVALUATION CRITERIA—CLIENT WILL:

KNOWLEDGE: Illness Care (NOC)

Verbalize understanding of disease process and potential complications.
Verbalize understanding of therapeutic needs.
Participate in treatment regimen.

ACTIONS/INTERVENTIONS	RATIONALE
TEACHING: Disease Process (NIC)	
Independent	
Identify symptoms requiring medical evaluation; e.g., increasing pain, edema/erythema of wound, presence of drainage, fever.	Prompt intervention reduces risk of serious complications; e.g., delayed wound healing, peritonitis.
Review postoperative activity restrictions; e.g., heavy lifting, exercise, sex, sports, driving.	Provides information for client to plan for return to usual routines without untoward incidents.
Encourage progressive activities as tolerated with periodic rest periods.	Prevents fatigue, promotes healing and feeling of well-being, and facilitates resumption of normal activities.
Recommend use of mild laxative/stool softeners as necessary and avoidance of enemas.	Assists with return to usual bowel function; prevents undue straining for defecation.
Discuss care of incision, including dressing changes, bathing restrictions, and return to physician for suture/staple removal.	Understanding promotes cooperation with therapeutic regimen, enhancing healing and recovery process.

POTENTIAL CONSIDERATIONS following acute hospitalization (dependent on client's age, physical condition/presence of complications, personal resources, and life responsibilities)

risk for Ineffective Therapeutic Regimen Management—perceived seriousness/susceptibility, perceived benefit, demands made on individual (family, work).

PERITONITIS

Peritonitis is defined as inflammation of the serosal membrane that lines the abdominal cavity and the organs contained therein. Peritonitis is often the result of the introduction of an infection (e.g., bacteria) or sterile (e.g., chemical irritating material). It is categorized as primary, secondary, or tertiary and can be acute or chronic in nature.

Primary peritonitis is a rare condition in which the peritoneum is spontaneously infected via the blood/lymphatic circulation. Chronic liver disease is the most common etiology of primary peritonitis. *Secondary peritonitis* is related to a pathologic processes in a visceral organ, with sources of inflammation being the GI tract (e.g., ruptured appendix, perforated gastric or duodenal ulcer, perforated colon caused by diverticulitis or cancer, pancreatitis, ulcerative colitis, and Crohn's disease), ovaries/uterus (e.g., pelvic inflammatory disease, ovarian cyst), traumatic injuries (e.g., blunt and penetrating trauma), or surgical contaminants. *Tertiary peritonitis* is a persistent or recurrent infection after adequate initial therapy.

The intra-abdominal infection may be localized or generalized, with or without abscess formation. The most common pathogens include gram-negative organisms (e.g., *Escherichia coli* [40%]) and gram-positive organisms (e.g., *Streptococcus*). Resistant and unusual organisms (e.g., *Enterococcus, Candida, Enterobacter*) are found in a significant proportion of tertiary cases.

Surgical intervention may be curative in localized peritonitis, as occurs with appendicitis/appendectomy, ulcer plication, and bowel resection. If peritonitis is diffuse, medical management is necessary before or in place of surgical treatment.

CARE SETTING

Inpatient acute medical or surgical unit

RELATED CONCERNS

Appendectomy, page 350
Inflammatory bowel disease: ulcerative colitis, regional enteritis (Crohn's disease, ileocolitis), page 324
Pancreatitis, page 467
Psychosocial aspects of care, page 770
Renal dialysis: peritoneal, page 575
Sepsis/septicemia, page 701
Surgical intervention, page 788
Total nutritional support: parenteral/enteral feeding, page 478
Upper gastrointestinal/esophageal bleeding, page 309

Client Assessment Database

ACTIVITY/REST

May report: Weakness
May exhibit: Difficulty ambulating

CIRCULATION

May exhibit: Tachycardia, diaphoresis, pallor, hypotension (signs of shock)
Tissue edema

ELIMINATION

May report: Inability to pass stool or flatus
Diarrhea (occasionally)

May exhibit: Hiccups; abdominal distention; quiet abdomen
Decreased urinary output, dark color
Decreased/absent bowel sounds (ileus); intermittent loud, rushing bowel sounds (obstruction); abdominal rigidity, distention, rebound tenderness; hyperresonance/tympani (ileus); loss of dullness over liver (free air in abdomen)

FOOD/FLUID

May report: Anorexia, nausea/vomiting, thirst
May exhibit: Hypoactive bowel sounds (generalized ileus)
Projectile vomiting
Dry mucous membranes, swollen tongue, poor skin turgor

PAIN/DISCOMFORT

May report: Sudden, severe, or persistent severe abdominal pain.
Pain may be generalized, localized, referred to shoulder, intensified by movement

May exhibit: Abdominal distention, rigidity, rebound tenderness
Distraction behaviors; restlessness; self-focus
Muscle guarding (abdomen); flexion of knees

RESPIRATION

May exhibit: Shallow respirations, tachypnea

SAFETY

May report: Fever (usually greater than 38°C {101°F], although hypothermia may be present with severe sepsis), chills

SEXUALITY

May report: History of pelvic organ inflammation (salpingitis), puerperal infection, septic abortion, retroperitoneal abscess

TEACHING/LEARNING

May report: History of recent trauma with abdominal penetration; e.g., gunshot/stab wound or blunt trauma to the abdomen, bladder perforation/ruptured gallbladder, perforated carcinoma of the stomach, perforated gastric/duodenal ulcer, gangrenous obstruction of the bowel, perforation of diverticulum, UC, regional ileitis, strangulated hernia

Discharge plan considerations: Assistance with homemaker/maintenance tasks

Refer to section at end of plan for postdischarge considerations.

DIAGNOSTIC STUDIES

CBC: WBCs elevated, sometimes more than 20,000, except in client with immunocompromise or certain infections (e.g., fungal, cytomegalovirus), who may demonstrate leukopenia. RBC count may be increased, indicating hemoconcentration.
Serum protein/albumin: May be decreased because of fluid shifts.
Serum amylase and lipase: Usually elevated when pancreatitis is cause.
Serum electrolytes: Hypokalemia may be present.
ABGs: Respiratory alkalosis and metabolic acidosis may be noted.
Cultures: Causative organism (often *E. coli,* streptococci, staphylococcus, or rarely, pneumococcus) may be identified from blood, exudate/secretions, ascitic fluid, cloudy peritoneal dialysate.
CT scan (abdominal and pelvic): Gold standard for diagnosis of peritonitis, peritoneal abscess and related visceral pathology.
MRI: Emerging imaging modality for the diagnosis of intra-abdominal abscesses.
Abdominal radiographs: May reveal gas distention of bowel/ileus. When perforated viscera is the cause, free air will be found in the abdomen.
Chest x-ray: May reveal elevation of diaphragm.
Abdominal and/or pelvic ultrasound: Can often diagnose peritonitis cause (e.g., cholecystitis, perihepatic abscess, pancreatitis, ruptured appendix, ovarian abscess, or diverticulitis). Ultrasonography can also detect increased amounts of peritoneal fluid (ascites).
Paracentesis: Peritoneal fluid samples generally demonstrate low pH and glucose, elevated protein and lactate dehydrogenase (LDH) levels, and may contain blood, pus/exudate, amylase, bile, and creatinine.

NURSING PRIORITIES

1. Control infection.
2. Restore/maintain circulating volume.
3. Promote comfort.
4. Maintain nutrition.
5. Provide information about disease process, possible complications, and treatment needs.

DISCHARGE GOALS

1. Infection resolved.
2. Complications presented/minimized.
3. Pain relieved.
4. Disease process, potential complications, and therapeutic regimen understood.
5. Plan in place to meet needs after discharge.

NURSING DIAGNOSIS: risk for Infection, [septicemia]

Risk factors may include

Inadequate primary defenses (broken skin, traumatized tissue, altered peristalsis)
Inadequate secondary defenses (immunosuppression)
Invasive procedures

Possibly evidenced by

[Not applicable; presence of signs and symptoms establishes an *actual* diagnosis.]

DESIRED OUTCOMES/EVALUATION CRITERIA—CLIENT WILL:

Infection Status (NOC)

Achieve timely healing, be free of purulent drainage or erythema, be afebrile.

Risk Control (NOC)

Verbalize understanding of the individual causative/risk factor(s).

ACTIONS/INTERVENTIONS	RATIONALE
Infection Control (NIC)	
Independent	
Note individual risk factors; e.g., abdominal trauma, acute appendicitis, peritoneal dialysis.	Influences choice of interventions.
Assess vital signs frequently, noting unresolved or progressing hypotension, decreased pulse pressure, tachycardia, fever, tachypnea.	Signs of impending septic shock. Circulating endotoxins eventually produce vasodilation, shift of fluid from circulation, and a low cardiac output state. Note: These clients frequently are critically ill and medical or postsurgical intensive care is required. (Refer to CP: Sepsis/septicemia, p. 701.)
Note changes in mental status (e.g., confusion, stupor).	Hypoxemia, hypotension, and acidosis can cause deteriorating mental status.
Note skin color, temperature, moisture.	Warm, flushed, dry skin is early sign of septicemia. Later manifestations include cool, clammy, pale skin and cyanosis as shock becomes refractory.
Monitor urine output.	Oliguria develops as a result of decreased renal perfusion, circulating toxins, effects of antibiotics.
Maintain strict aseptic technique in caring for abdominal drains, incisions/open wounds, dressings, and invasive sites. Cleanse with appropriate solution.	Prevents access or limits spread of infecting organisms/cross-contamination.
Perform/model good hand-washing technique. Monitor staff/client compliance.	Reduces risk of cross-contamination/spread of infection.
Observe drainage from wounds/drains.	Provides information about status of infection.
Maintain sterile technique when catheterizing client, and provide catheter care/encourage perineal cleansing on a routine basis.	Prevents access, limits bacterial growth in urinary tract.
Monitor/restrict visitors and staff as appropriate. Provide protective isolation if indicated.	Reduces risk of exposure to/acquisition of secondary infection in immunosuppressed client.
Collaborative	
Obtain specimens/monitor results of serial blood, urine, wound cultures.	Identifies causative microorganisms and helps in assessing effectiveness of antimicrobial regimen.
Assist with peritoneal aspiration if indicated.	May be done to remove fluid and to identify infecting organisms so appropriate antibiotic therapy can be instituted.
Administer antimicrobials; e.g., second- and third-generation cephalosporins (e.g., cefamandole [Mandole], cefotetan [Cefotan]; cefotaxime [Claforan], ceftriaxone [Rocephin]), extended spectrim penicillins (e.g., piperacillin/tazobactam [Zosyn]), fluoroquinolones (e.g., ciprofloxacin [Cipro], alatrovafloxacin [Trovan]), antifungals (e.g., metronidazole [Flagyl]), aminoglycosides (e.g., gentamicin [Garamycin, amikacin [Amikin]).	Therapy is systemic and directed at the particular identified organism(s) (e.g., anaerobic bacteria, fungus, gram-negative bacilli). Optimal duration of antimicrobial therapy depends on the underlying pathology, severity of infection, and speed/effectiveness of source control. Antimicrobials may be administered by IV and/or by intraoperative lavage (IOPL).
Prepare for surgical intervention (e.g., open incision, or laparoscopic débridement and lavage) if indicated.	Surgery may be treatment of choice (curative) in acute, localized peritonitis; e.g., to drain localized abscess; remove peritoneal exudates, ruptured appendix/gallbladder; plicate perforated ulcer; or resect bowel. Intraoperative lavage may be used to remove necrotic debris and treat inflammation that is poorly localized/diffuse. Multiple reoperations may be needed to control source of infection, drain abscesses, or clean out necrotic material. In this instance, the abdominal closure is temporary using various dressings, mesh coverings, and Velcro-like skin-closure devices, providing ready access to affected area while preventing contamination from the outside. Later surgical procedures may also be required for permanent closure/repair of abdominal wall. Temporary colostomy procedure may be performed during this time (if the colon is source of infection; e.g., ruptured diverticulum) to facilitate treatment of the infection and bowel healing.

NURSING DIAGNOSIS: deficient Fluid Volume, [mixed]

May be related to

Fluid shifts from extracellular, intravascular, and interstitial compartments into intestines and/or peritoneal space
Vomiting; medically restricted intake; NG/intestinal aspiration
Fever/hypermetabolic state

Possibly evidenced by

Dry mucous membranes, poor skin turgor, delayed capillary refill, weak peripheral pulses
Diminished urinary output, dark/concentrated urine
Hypotension, tachycardia

DESIRED OUTCOMES/EVALUATION CRITERIA—CLIENT WILL:

Fluid Balance (NOC)

Demonstrate improved fluid balance as evidenced by adequate urinary output with normal specific gravity, stable vital signs, moist mucous membranes, good skin turgor, prompt capillary refill, and weight within acceptable range.

ACTIONS/INTERVENTIONS	RATIONALE
Fluid/Electrolyte Management (NIC)	
Independent	
Monitor vital signs, noting presence of hypotension (including postural changes), tachycardia, tachypnea, fever. Measure central venous pressure (CVP) if available.	Aids in evaluating degree of fluid deficit/effectiveness of fluid replacement therapy and response to medications.
Maintain accurate I&O and correlate with daily weights. Include measured/estimated losses; e.g., gastric suction, drains, dressings, Hemovacs, diaphoresis, and abdominal girth for third spacing of fluid.	Reflects overall hydration status. Urine output may be diminished because of hypovolemia and decreased renal perfusion, but weight may still increase, reflecting tissue edema/ascites accumulation. Gastric suction losses may be large, and a great deal of fluid can be sequestered in the bowel and peritoneal space (ascites).
Measure urine specific gravity.	Reflects hydration status and changes in renal function, which may warn of developing acute renal failure in response to hypovolemia and effect of toxins. *Note:* Many antibiotics also have nephrotoxic effects that may further affect kidney function/urine output.
Observe skin/mucous membrane dryness, turgor. Note peripheral/sacral edema.	Hypovolemia, fluid shifts, and nutritional deficits contribute to poor skin turgor, taut edematous tissues.
Eliminate noxious sights/smells from environment. Limit intake of ice chips.	Reduces gastric stimulation and vomiting response. *Note:* Excessive use of ice chips during gastric aspiration can increase gastric washout of electrolytes.
Change position frequently, provide frequent skin care, and maintain dry/wrinkle-free bedding.	Edematous tissue with compromised circulation is prone to breakdown.
Collaborative	
Monitor laboratory studies; e.g., Hb/Hct, electrolytes, protein, albumin, BUN, Cr.	Provides information about hydration and organ function. Varied alterations with significant consequences to systemic function are possible as a result of fluid shifts, hypovolemia, hypoxemia, circulating toxins, and necrotic tissue products.

ACTIONS/INTERVENTIONS	RATIONALE
Administer plasma/blood, fluids, electrolytes, diuretics as indicated.	Replenishes/maintains circulating volume and electrolyte balance. Colloids (plasma, blood) help move water back into intravascular compartment by increasing osmotic pressure gradient. Diuretics may be used to assist in excretion of toxins and to enhance renal function.
Maintain NPO status with nasogastric/intestinal aspiration.	Reduces vomiting caused by hyperactivity of bowel, manages stomach and intestinal fluids.

NURSING DIAGNOSIS: acute Pain

May be related to

Chemical irritation of the parietal peritoneum (toxins)
Trauma to tissues
Accumulation of fluid in abdominal/peritoneal cavity (abdominal distention)

Possibly evidenced by

Verbalizations of pain
Muscle guarding, rebound tenderness
Facial mask of pain, self-focus
Distraction behavior, autonomic/emotional responses (anxiety)

DESIRED OUTCOMES/EVALUATION CRITERIA—CLIENT WILL:

Pain Control (NOC)

Report pain is relieved/controlled.
Demonstrate use of relaxation skills, other methods to promote comfort.

ACTIONS/INTERVENTIONS	RATIONALE
Pain Management (NIC)	
Independent	
Investigate pain reports, noting location, duration, intensity (0–10 scale), and characteristics (e.g., dull, sharp, constant).	Changes in location/intensity are not uncommon but may reflect developing complications. Pain tends to become constant, more intense, and diffuse over the entire abdomen as inflammatory process accelerates; pain may localize if an abscess develops.
Maintain semi-Fowler's position as indicated.	Facilitates fluid/wound drainage by gravity, reducing diaphragmatic irritation and abdominal tension, thereby reducing pain.
Move client slowly and deliberately, splinting painful area.	Reduces muscle tension/guarding, which may help minimize pain of movement.
Provide comfort measures; e.g., massage, back rubs, deep breathing. Instruct in relaxation/visualization exercises. Provide diversional activities.	Promotes relaxation and may enhance client's coping abilities by refocusing attention.
Provide frequent oral care. Remove noxious environmental stimuli.	Reduces nausea/vomiting, which can increase intra-abdominal pressure/pain.

ACTIONS/INTERVENTIONS	RATIONALE
Collaborative	
Administer medications as indicated:	
Analgesics, narcotics;	Reduces metabolic rate and intestinal irritation from circulating/local toxins, which aid in pain relief and promote healing. *Note:* Pain is usually severe and may require narcotic pain control. Analgesics may be withheld during initial diagnostic process because they can mask signs/symptoms.
Antiemetics; e.g., hydroxyzine (Vistaril);	Reduces nausea and vomiting, which can increase abdominal pain.
Antipyretics; e.g., acetaminophen (Tylenol).	Reduces discomfort associated with fever/chills.

NURSING DIAGNOSIS: risk for imbalanced Nutrition: less than body requirements

Risk factors may include

Nausea/vomiting, intestinal dysfunction
Metabolic abnormalities, increased metabolic needs

Possibly evidenced by

[Not applicable; presence of signs and symptoms establishes an *actual* diagnosis.]

DESIRED OUTCOMES/EVALUATION CRITERIA—CLIENT WILL:

Nutritional Status (NOC)

Maintain usual weight and positive nitrogen balance.

ACTIONS/INTERVENTIONS	RATIONALE
Nutrition Management (NIC)	
Independent	
Auscultate bowel sounds, noting absent/hyperactive sounds.	Although bowel sounds are frequently absent, inflammation/irritation of the intestine may be accompanied by intestinal hyperactivity, diminished water absorption, and diarrhea.
Monitor NG tube output. Note presence of vomiting, diarrhea.	Large amounts of gastric aspirant, or severe vomiting and diarrhea suggest bowel obstruction, requiring further evaluation.
Measure abdominal girth.	Provides quantitative evidence of changes in gastric/intestinal distention and/or accumulation of ascites.
Assess abdomen frequently for return to softness, reappearance of normal bowel sounds, and passage of flatus.	Indicates return of normal bowel function and ability to resume oral intake.
Weigh regularly.	Initial losses/gains reflect changes in hydration, but sustained losses suggest nutritional deficit.
Collaborative	
Monitor BUN, protein, prealbumin/albumin, glucose, nitrogen balance as indicated.	Reflects organ function and nutritional status/needs.

ACTIONS/INTERVENTIONS	RATIONALE
Administer enteral/parenteral feedings as indicated.	Enteral feedings, even at low volumes, have been shown to maintain gut mucosal integrity and to reduce the incidence of infectious complications, making the choice of enteral feedings preferable over parenteral solutions whenever possible. (Refer to CP: Total Nutritional Support: Enteral/Parenteral Feedings, page 478)
Advance diet as tolerated; e.g., clear liquids to soft food.	Client may have some degree of gut dysfunction for quite some time, making it necessary for careful progression of diet when oral intake is resumed.

NURSING DIAGNOSIS: Anxiety [specify level]/Fear

May be related to

Situational crisis
Threat of death/change in health status
Physiologic factors, hypermetabolic state

Possibly evidenced by

Increased tension/helplessness
Apprehension, uncertainty, worry, sense of impending doom
Sympathetic stimulation; restlessness, focus on self

DESIRED OUTCOMES/EVALUATION CRITERIA—CLIENT WILL:

Anxiety Self-Control (NOC)

Verbalize awareness of feelings and healthy ways to deal with them.
Report anxiety is reduced to a manageable level.
Appear relaxed.

ACTIONS/INTERVENTIONS — RATIONALE

Anxiety Reduction (NIC)

Independent

ACTIONS/INTERVENTIONS	RATIONALE
Evaluate anxiety level, noting client's perception of situation, verbal and nonverbal responses. Encourage free expression of emotions.	Apprehension may be escalated by severe pain, increasingly ill feeling, urgency of diagnostic procedures, and possibility of surgery.
Review physiologic factors present (e.g., sepsis/toxins related to infection, medications, and metabolic imbalances).	These factors are present in seriously ill client and cause/contribute to anxiety.
Provide ongoing information regarding disease process and anticipated treatment.	Knowing what to expect can reduce anxiety for both client/SO. Also, ongoing review helps to identify those factors adding to anxiety that could be changed; e.g., client getting more uninterrupted sleep or adding or deleting medications.
Provide presence. Acknowledge anxiety/fear. Do not deny or reassure client that everything will be all right. Be accurate and factual in providing information. Correct misconceptions about disease process and possible treatments.	Affirms client's value as a human being in need of assistance in dealing with a serious health threat; helps client/SO identify and deal with reality.
Schedule adequate rest and uninterrupted periods for sleep.	Limits fatigue, conserves energy, and can enhance coping ability.
Provide comfort measures; e.g., family presence, quiet environment, soft music, back rub, therapeutic touch (TT).	Promotes relaxation and enhances ability to deal with situation.

Refer to CP: Psychosocial Aspects for Care, for additional interventions.

NURSING DIAGNOSIS: deficient Knowledge [Learning Need] regarding condition, prognosis, treatment, self-care, and discharge needs

May be related to

Lack of exposure/recall
Information misinterpretation
Unfamiliarity with information resources

Possibly evidenced by

Questions, request for information
Statement of misconception
Inaccurate follow-through of instruction

DESIRED OUTCOMES/EVALUATION CRITERIA—CLIENT WILL:

KNOWLEDGE: Disease Process (NOC)

Verbalize understanding of disease process and potential complications.
Identify relationship of signs/symptoms to the disease process and correlate symptoms with causative factors.

KNOWLEDGE: Treatment Regimen (NOC)

Verbalize understanding of therapeutic needs.
Correctly perform necessary procedures and explain reasons for actions.

ACTIONS/INTERVENTIONS	RATIONALE
TEACHING: Disease Process (NIC)	
Independent	
Review underlying disease process and recovery expectations.	Provides knowledge base from which client can make informed choices.
Identify signs/symptoms requiring medical evaluation; e.g., recurrent abdominal pain/distention, vomiting, fever, chills, or presence of purulent drainage, swelling/erythema of surgical incision (if present).	Early recognition and treatment of developing complications may prevent more serious illness/injury.
Discuss medication regimen, schedule, and possible side effects.	Antibiotics may be continued for varying periods of time after discharge depending on extent of the infection and length of stay in acute care facility.
Recommend gradual resumption of usual activities, allowing for adequate rest.	Prevents fatigue, enhances feeling of well-being.
Review activity restrictions/limitations; e.g., avoid heavy lifting, constipation.	Avoids unnecessary increase of intra-abdominal pressure and muscle tension.
Demonstrate sterile or clean dressing change—colostomy or wound care—as appropriate. Have client/SO demonstrate ability to manage these procedures.	Client/SO may have a long period of home management of surgical wound(s) depending on extent of infection and treatment, as slow recovery time is often associated with such a complex condition.
Emphasize importance of medical follow-up	Necessary to monitor resolution of infection and resumption of usual activities.
Refer to community resources, as needed/desired; e.g., visiting nurse, home healthcare, durable medical equipment suppliers.	Supports transition to home, promotes self-care, and increases likelihood of successful outcome.

POTENTIAL CONSIDERATIONS following acute hospitalization (dependent on client's age, physical condition/presence of complications, personal resources, and life responsibilities)

Fatigue—decreased metabolic energy production, increased energy requirements to perform ADLs, states of discomfort.

acute Pain—chemical irritation of the peritoneum, prolonged healing process.

CHOLECYSTITIS WITH CHOLELITHIASIS

Cholecystitis with cholelithiasis is an acute or chronic inflammation of the gallbladder associated with obstruction by gallstone(s) of the cystic or common bile ducts. Common bile duct stones are either *primary* (formed in the bile ducts) or *secondary* (formed in and transported from the gallbladder). Although stones most often develop in (and obstruct) the common bile duct or the cystic duct, they have also been found in the hepatic, small bile, and pancreatic ducts. Stones (calculi) are made up of cholesterol, calcium bilirubinate, or a mixture caused by changes in the bile composition. Crystals can also form in the submucosa of the gallbladder causing widespread inflammation. Infection is thought to be a consequence rather than cause of cholecystitis.

Acute cholecystitis with cholelithiasis is usually treated by surgery, although several other treatment methods (fragmentation and dissolution of stones) are also used.

CARE SETTING

Severe acute attacks may require brief hospitalization on a medical unit. This plan of care deals with the acutely ill, hospitalized client.

RELATED CONCERNS

Cholecystectomy, page 371
Fluid and electrolyte imbalances, page 919
Psychosocial aspects of care, page 770
Total nutritional support: parenteral/enteral feeding, page 478

Client Assessment Database

ACTIVITY/REST

May report: Fatigue
May exhibit: Restlessness

CIRCULATION

May exhibit: Tachycardia, diaphoresis

ELIMINATION

May report: Change in color of urine and stools
May exhibit: Abdominal distention
Palpable mass in right upper quadrant (RUQ)
Dark, concentrated urine
Clay-colored stool, steatorrhea

FOOD/FLUID

May report: Anorexia, nausea/vomiting
Intolerance of fatty and "gas-forming" foods, recurrent regurgitation, heartburn, indigestion, flatulence, bloating (dyspepsia)
Belching (eructation)
May exhibit: Obesity, recent weight loss
Normal to hypoactive bowel sounds

PAIN/DISCOMFORT

May report: Severe epigastric and right upper abdominal pain, may radiate to mid-back, right shoulder/scapula, or to front of chest; often increases with movement
Midepigastric colicky pain associated with eating, especially after meals rich in fats
Episodes of pain severe/ongoing, starting suddenly, sometimes at night, with episodes of constant pain typically lasting 1–5 hr
Recurring episodes of similar pain

May exhibit: Rebound tenderness, muscle guarding, or abdominal rigidity when RUQ is palpated; positive Murphy's sign

RESPIRATION

May exhibit: Increased respiratory rate
Splinted respiration marked by short, shallow breathing

SAFETY

May exhibit: Low-grade fever, high-grade fever and chills (septic complications)
Jaundice (not common), with dry, itching skin (pruritus)
Bleeding tendencies (vitamin K deficiency)

TEACHING/LEARNING

May report: Familial tendency for gallstones
Recent pregnancy/delivery; history of diabetes mellitus (DM), IBD, blood dyscrasias

Discharge plan considerations: May require support with dietary changes/weight reduction

Refer to section at end of plan for postdischarge considerations.

DIAGNOSTIC STUDIES

Biliary ultrasound: Most common screening test, ultrasound is 90%–95% sensitive for cholecystitis and 98% sensitive and specific for simple cholelithiasis. Sonographic Murphy's sign (pain when the probe is pushed directly on the gallbladder) is 86%–92% sensitive. Ultrasound also identifies abnormalities of surrounding tissues (e.g., dilated common bile duct or dilated intrahepatic ducts).

Oral cholecystography (OCG): Preferred method of visualizing general appearance and function of gallbladder, including presence of filling defects, structural defects, and/or stone in ducts/biliary tree. Can be done IV (IVC) when nausea/vomiting prevent oral intake, when the gallbladder cannot be visualized during OCG, or when symptoms persist following cholecystectomy. IVC may also be done perioperatively to assess structure and function of ducts, detect remaining stones after lithotripsy or cholecystectomy, and/or to detect surgical complications. Dye can also be injected via T-tube drain postoperatively.

Endoscopic retrograde cholangiopancreatography (ERCP): Visualizes biliary tree by cannulation of the common bile duct through the duodenum.

Percutaneous transhepatic cholangiography (PTC): Fluoroscopic imaging distinguishes between gallbladder disease and cancer of the pancreas (when jaundice is present); supports the diagnosis of obstructive jaundice and reveals calculi in ducts.

Cholecystograms (for chronic cholecystitis): Reveals stones in the biliary system. *Note:* Contraindicated in acute cholecystitis because client is too ill to take the dye by mouth.

CT Hepatobiliary (HIDA, PIPIDA) scan: May be done to confirm diagnosis of cholecystitis, especially when barium studies are contraindicated. Scan may be combined with cholecystokinin injection to demonstrate abnormal gallbladder ejection.

Abdominal radiographs (multipositional): Radiopaque (calcified) gallstones present in 10%–15% of cases; calcification of the wall or enlargement of the gallbladder.

CBC: Moderate leukocytosis may be present (acute cholecystitis), but a normal WBC count does not rule out cholecystitis.

Serum bilirubin and amylase: Elevation may indicate common bile duct stone or presence of pancreatitis complicating cholelithiasis.

Serum liver enzymes—AST; ALT; ALP; LDH: Slight elevation; alkaline phosphatase and 5-nucleotidase are markedly elevated in biliary obstruction.

Prothrombin levels: Reduced when obstruction to the flow of bile into the intestine decreases absorption of vitamin K.

NURSING PRIORITIES

1. Relieve pain and promote rest.
2. Maintain fluid and electrolyte balance.
3. Prevent complications.
4. Provide information about disease process, prognosis, and treatment needs.

DISCHARGE GOALS

1. Pain relieved.
2. Homeostasis achieved.
3. Complications prevented/minimized.
4. Disease process, prognosis, and therapeutic regimen understood.
5. Plan in place to meet needs after discharge.

NURSING DIAGNOSIS: acute Pain

May be related to

Biologic injuring agents: obstruction/ductal spasm, inflammatory process, tissue ischemia/necrosis

Possibly evidenced by

Reports of pain, biliary colic (waves of pain)
Facial mask of pain; guarding behavior
Autonomic responses (changes in BP, pulse)
Self-focusing; narrowed focus

DESIRED OUTCOMES/EVALUATION CRITERIA—CLIENT WILL:

Pain Control (NOC)

Report pain is relieved/controlled.
Demonstrate use of relaxation skills and diversional activities as indicated for individual situation.

ACTIONS/INTERVENTIONS	RATIONALE
Pain Management (NIC)	
Independent	
Observe and document location, severity (0–10 scale), and character of pain (e.g., steady, intermittent, colicky).	Assists in differentiating cause of pain, and provides information about disease progression/resolution, development of complications, and effectiveness of interventions.
Note response to medication, and report to physician if pain is not being relieved.	Severe pain not relieved by routine measures may indicate developing complications/need for further intervention.
Promote bed rest, allowing client to assume position of comfort.	Bed rest in low-Fowler's position reduces intra-abdominal pressure; however, client will naturally assume least painful position.
Use soft/cotton linens, calamine lotion, oil (Alpha Keri) bath, cool/moist compresses as indicated.	Reduces irritation/dryness of the skin and itching sensation.
Control environmental temperature.	Cool surroundings aid in minimizing dermal discomfort.
Encourage use of relaxation techniques; e.g., guided imagery, visualization, deep-breathing exercises. Provide diversional activities.	Promotes rest, redirects attention, may enhance coping.
Make time to listen to and maintain frequent contact with client.	Helpful in alleviating anxiety and refocusing attention, which can relieve pain.
Collaborative	
Maintain NPO status; insert/maintain NG suction as indicated.	Removes gastric secretions that stimulate release of cholecystokinin and gallbladder contractions.
Administer medications as indicated:	
Anticholinergics; e.g., dicyclomine (Bentyl), clycopyrrolate (Robinul), propantheline (Pro-Banthine);	Antispasmodics and anticholinergics are thought to decrease gallbladder and biliary tree tone, which decreases pain.
Sedatives; e.g., phenobarbital;	Promote rest and relax smooth muscle, relieving pain.
Narcotics; e.g., meperidine hydrochloride (Demerol);	When pain is unrelieved by medications such as dicylomine (Bentyl), narcotics may be given to reduce severe pain. The narcotic of choice is Demerol owing to potential problems of increased tone of the sphincter of Oddi with morphine use.

ACTIONS/INTERVENTIONS	RATIONALE
Antibiotics, either single agent (e.g., penicillin [Ampicillin], tazobactam [Zosyn], and clavulanate [Augmentin] or combinations (e.g., piperacillin/tazobactam [Pipracil], a penicillin and metronidazole [Flagyl], imipenem/cilastatin [Primaxin], or many other anti-infective combinations);	To treat infectious process, reducing inflammation, and potential for systemic complications. Treatment for acute cholecystitis usually requires single-agent therapy, but for more serious infections, combination drug treatment has increased broad-spectrum coverage.
Oral dissolution therapy; e.g., chenodeoxycholic acid (Chenix), ursodeoxycholic acid (Urso, Actigall).	Although a rarely chosen option for mainstream treatment of cholecystitis with cholelithiasis, oral dissolution is possible (e.g., dissolves some stones <5 mm in size). The therapy takes 6–12 months and stones usually recur.
Prepare for procedures; e.g.:	
Endoscopic sphincterotomy plus extraction or chemical dissolution (e.g., monoctanoin [Moctanin]);	Procedure done to widen the mouth of the common bile duct where it empties into the duodenum. The procedure may also be done to retrieve stones from the common duct by means of a tiny basket or balloon on the end of the endoscope. Stones must be smaller than 15 mm. Moctanin may be used for retained stones or for newly formed large stones in the bile duct. It is a lengthy treatment (1–3 weeks) and is administered via a nasobiliary tube. A cholangiogram is done periodically to monitor stone dissolution.
Extracorporeal shock wave lithotripsy (ESWL);	Shock wave treatment is an exciting technologic invention, but is a little-used therapy owing due to high recurrence of stones. It may be indicated in a client with mild to moderate symptoms, a single cholesterol stone (0.5 mm or larger), without biliary tract obstruction. *Note:* This procedure is contraindicated in clients with pacemakers or implantable defibrillators.
Laparoscopic or open surgical intervention.	Cholecystectomy may be indicated because of the size of stones and degree of tissue involvement/presence of necrosis. (Refer to CP: Cholecystectomy, page 371.)

NURSING DIAGNOSIS: risk for deficient Fluid Volume

Risk factors may include

Excessive losses through gastric suction; vomiting, distention, and gastric hypermotility
Medically restricted intake
Altered clotting process

Possibly evidenced by

[Not applicable; presence of signs and symptoms and establishes an *actual* diagnosis.]

DESIRED OUTCOMES/EVALUATION CRITERIA—CLIENT WILL:

Hydration (NOC)

Demonstrate adequate fluid balance evidenced by stable vital signs, moist mucous membranes, good skin turgor, capillary refill, individually appropriate urinary output, absence of vomiting.

ACTIONS/INTERVENTIONS	RATIONALE
Fluid/Electrolyte Management (NIC)	
Independent	
Maintain accurate record of I&O, noting output less than intake, increased urine specific gravity. Assess skin/mucous membranes, peripheral pulses, and capillary refill.	Provides information about fluid status/circulating volume and replacement needs.
Monitor for signs/symptoms of increased/continued nausea or vomiting, abdominal cramps, weakness, twitching, seizures, irregular heart rate, paresthesia, hypoactive or absent bowel sounds, depressed respirations.	Prolonged vomiting, gastric aspiration, and restricted oral intake can lead to deficits in sodium, potassium, and chloride.
Eliminate noxious sights/smells from environment.	Reduces stimulation of vomiting center.
Perform frequent oral hygiene with alcohol-free mouthwash, apply lubricants.	Decreases dryness of oral mucous membranes, reduces risk of oral bleeding.
Use small-gauge needles for injections and apply firm pressure for longer than usual after venipuncture.	Reduces trauma, risk of bleeding/hematoma formation.
Assess for unusual bleeding; e.g., oozing from injection sites, epistaxis, bleeding gums, ecchymosis, petechiae, hematemesis/melena.	Prothrombin is reduced and coagulation time prolonged when bile flow is obstructed, increasing risk of bleeding/hemorrhage.
Collaborative	
Keep client NPO as necessary.	Decreases GI secretions and hypermotility.
Insert NG tube, connect to suction, and maintain patency as indicated.	Provides rest for GI tract and relief of vomiting.
Administer antiemetics; e.g., promethazine (Phenergan, Prorex), prochlorperazine (Compazine).	Helpful in reducing nausea and vomiting often associated with cholecystitis and particularly, common bile duct obstruction.
Review laboratory studies; e.g., Hb/Hct, electrolytes, ABGs (pH), clotting times.	Aids in evaluating circulating volume, identifies deficits, and influences choice of intervention for replacement/correction.
Administer IV fluids, electrolytes, and vitamin K.	Maintains circulating volume and corrects imbalances.

NURSING DIAGNOSIS: risk for imbalanced Nutrition: less than body requirements

Risk factors may include

Self-imposed or prescribed dietary restrictions, nausea/vomiting, dyspepsia, pain
Loss of nutrients; impaired fat digestion due to obstruction of bile flow

Possibly evidenced by

[Not applicable; presence of signs and symptoms establishes an *actual* diagnosis.]

DESIRED OUTCOMES/EVALUATION CRITERIA—CLIENT WILL:

Nutritional Status (NOC)

Report relief of nausea/vomiting.
Demonstrate progression toward desired weight gain or maintain weight as individually appropriate.

ACTIONS/INTERVENTIONS	RATIONALE
Nutrition Management (NIC)	
Independent	
Estimate/calculate caloric intake. Keep comments about appetite to a minimum.	Identifies nutritional deficiencies/needs. Focusing on problem creates a negative atmosphere and may interfere with intake.
Weigh as indicated.	Monitors effectiveness of dietary plan.
Consult with client about likes/dislikes, foods that cause distress, and preferred meal schedule.	Involving client in planning enables client to have a sense of control and encourages eating.
Provide a pleasant atmosphere at mealtime; remove noxious stimuli.	Useful in promoting appetite/reducing nausea.
Provide oral hygiene before meals.	A clean mouth enhances appetite.
Offer effervescent drinks with meals if tolerated.	May lessen nausea and relieve gas. *Note:* May be contraindicated if beverage causes gas formation/gastric discomfort.
Assess for abdominal distention, frequent belching, guarding, reluctance to move.	Nonverbal signs of discomfort associated with impaired digestion, gas pain.
Ambulate and increase activity as tolerated.	Helpful in expulsion of flatus, reduction of abdominal distention. Contributes to overall recovery and sense of well-being and decreases possibility of secondary problems related to immobility (e.g., pneumonia, thrombophlebitis).
Collaborative	
Consult with dietitian/nutritional support team as indicated.	Useful in establishing individual nutritional needs and most appropriate route.
Begin low-fat liquid diet after NG tube is removed.	Limiting fat content reduces stimulation of gallbladder and pain associated with incomplete fat digestion and is helpful in preventing recurrence.
Advance diet as tolerated, usually low-fat, nonspicy, high-fiber. Restrict gas-producing foods (e.g., onions, cabbage, popcorn) and foods/fluids high in fats (e.g., butter, fried foods, nuts).	Meets nutritional requirements while minimizing stimulation of the gallbladder.
Monitor laboratory studies; e.g., BUN, prealbumin, albumin, total protein, transferrin levels.	Provides information about nutritional deficits/effectiveness of therapy.
Provide parenteral/enteral feedings as needed.	Alternative feeding may be required depending on degree of disability/gallbladder involvement and need for prolonged gastric rest.

NURSING DIAGNOSIS: deficient Knowledge [Learning Need] regarding condition, prognosis, treatment, self-care, and discharge needs

May be related to

Lack of knowledge/recall
Information misinterpretation
Unfamiliarity with information resources

Possibly evidenced by

Questions; request for information
Statement of misconception
Inaccurate follow-through of instruction
Development of preventable complications

DESIRED OUTCOMES/EVALUATION CRITERIA—CLIENT WILL:

KNOWLEDGE: Illness Care (NOC)

Verbalize understanding of disease process, prognosis, potential complications.
Verbalize understanding of therapeutic needs.
Initiate necessary lifestyle changes and participate in treatment regimen.

ACTIONS/INTERVENTIONS	RATIONALE
TEACHING: Disease Process (NIC)	
Independent	
Provide explanations of/reasons for test procedures and preparation needed.	Information can decrease anxiety, thereby reducing sympathetic stimulation.
Review disease process/prognosis. Discuss hospitalization and prospective treatment as indicated. Encourage questions, expression of concern.	Provides knowledge base from which client can make informed choices. Effective communication and support at this time can diminish anxiety and promote healing.
Review drug regimen, possible side effects.	Gallstones often recur, necessitating long-term therapy. Development of diarrhea/cramps during chenodiol (Chenix) therapy may be dose-related/correctable. *Note:* Women of childbearing age should be counseled regarding birth control to prevent pregnancy and risk of fetal hepatic damage.
Discuss weight reduction programs if indicated.	Obesity is a risk factor associated with cholecystitis, and weight loss is beneficial in medical management of chronic condition.
Instruct client to avoid food/fluids high in fats (e.g., whole milk, ice cream, butter, fried foods, nuts, gravies, pork), gas producers (e.g., cabbage, beans, onions, carbonated beverages), or gastric irritants (e.g., spicy foods, caffeine, citrus).	May prevent recurrence of/limit severity of gallbladder attacks.
Review signs/symptoms requiring medical intervention; e.g., recurrent fever; persistent nausea/vomiting, pain; jaundice of skin or eyes; itching; dark urine; clay-colored stools; blood in urine, stools, vomitus; or bleeding from mucous membranes.	Indicative of progression of disease process/development of complications requiring further intervention.
Recommend resting in semi-Fowler's position after meals.	Promotes flow of bile and general relaxation during initial digestive process.
Suggest client limit gum chewing, sucking on drinking straw/hard candy, or smoking.	Promotes gas formation, which can increase gastric distention/discomfort.
Discuss avoidance of aspirin-containing products, forceful blowing of nose, straining for bowel movement, contact sports. Recommend use of soft toothbrush, electric razor.	Reduces risk of bleeding related to changes in coagulation time, mucosal irritation, and trauma.

POTENTIAL CONSIDERATIONS following acute hospitalization (dependent on client's age, physical condition/presence of complications, personal resources, and life responsibilities)

acute Pain—recurrence of obstruction/ductal spasm; inflammation, tissue ischemia.

CHOLECYSTECTOMY

Cholecystectomy is performed most frequently through laparoscopic incisions using a laser. However, traditional open cholecystectomy is the treatment of choice for many clients with multiple/large gallstones either because of acute symptomatology or to prevent recurrence of stones.

CARE SETTING

This procedure is usually done on a short-stay basis; however, in the presence of suspected complications, e.g., empyema, gangrene, or perforation, an inpatient stay on a surgical unit is indicated.

RELATED CONCERNS

Cholecystitis with cholelithiasis, page 364
Pancreatitis, page 467
Peritonitis, page 355
Psychosocial aspects of care, page 770
Surgical intervention, page 788

Client Assessment Database/Diagnostic Studies

Refer to CP: Cholecystitis with Cholelithiasis.

TEACHING/LEARNING

Discharge plan considerations: May require assistance with wound care/supplies, homemaker tasks

Refer to section at end of plan for postdischarge considerations.

NURSING PRIORITIES

1. Promote respiratory function.
2. Prevent complications.
3. Provide information about disease, procedure(s), prognosis, and treatment needs.

DISCHARGE GOALS

1. Ventilation/oxygenation adequate for individual needs.
2. Complications prevented/minimized.
3. Disease process, surgical procedure, prognosis, and therapeutic regimen understood.
4. Plan in place to meet needs after discharge.

NURSING DIAGNOSIS: ineffective Breathing Pattern

May be related to

Pain
Muscular impairment
Decreased energy/fatigue

Possibly evidenced by

Tachypnea,respiratory depth changes, reduced vital capacity
Holding breath, reluctance to cough

DESIRED OUTCOMES/EVALUATION CRITERIA—CLIENT WILL:

Respiratory Status: Ventilation (NOC)

Establish effective breathing pattern.
Experience no signs of respiratory compromise/complications.

ACTIONS/INTERVENTIONS	RATIONALE
Respiratory Monitoring (NIC)	
Independent	
Observe respiratory rate/depth.	Shallow breathing, splinting with respirations, holding breath may result in hypoventilation/atelectasis.
Auscultate breath sounds.	Areas of decreased/absent breath sounds suggest atelectasis, whereas adventitious sounds (wheezes, rhonchi) reflect congestion.
Assist client to turn, cough, and deep breathe periodically. Demonstrate how to splint incision. Instruct in effective breathing techniques.	Promotes ventilation of all lung segments and mobilization and expectoration of secretions.
Elevate head of bed; maintain low-Fowler's position. Support abdomen when coughing, ambulating.	Facilitates lung expansion. Splinting provides incisional support/decreases muscle tension to promote cooperation with therapeutic regimen.
Collaborative	
Assist with respiratory treatments; e.g., incentive spirometer.	Maximizes expansion of lungs to prevent/resolve atelectasis.
Administer analgesics regularly/continuously (PCA), or before treatments; e.g. incentive spirometry, deep-breathing exercises.	Facilitates more effective coughing, deep breathing, and activity.

NURSING DIAGNOSIS: risk for deficient Fluid Volume

Risk factors may include

Losses from NG aspiration, vomiting
Medically restricted intake
Altered coagulation; e.g., reduced prothrombin, prolonged coagulation time

Possibly evidenced by

[Not applicable; presence of signs and symptoms establishes an *actual* diagnosis.]

DESIRED OUTCOMES/EVALUATION CRITERIA—CLIENT WILL:

Hydration (NOC)

Display adequate fluid balance as evidenced by stable vital signs, moist mucous membranes, good skin turgor/capillary refill, and individually appropriate urinary output.

ACTIONS/INTERVENTIONS	RATIONALE
Fluid/Electrolyte Management (NIC)	
Independent	
Monitor I&O, including drainage from NG tube, T-tube, and wound. Weigh client periodically.	Provides information about replacement needs and organ function. Initially, 200–500 mL of bile drainage may be expected via the T-tube, decreasing as more bile enters the intestine. Continuing large amounts of bile drainage may be an indication of unresolved obstruction or, occasionally, a biliary fistula.

ACTIONS/INTERVENTIONS	RATIONALE
Monitor vital signs. Assess mucous membranes, skin turgor, peripheral pulses, and capillary refill.	Indicators of adequacy of circulating volume/perfusion.
Observe for signs of bleeding; e.g., hematemesis, melena, petechiae, ecchymosis.	Prothrombin is reduced and coagulation time prolonged when bile flow is obstructed, increasing risk of bleeding/hemorrhage.
Use small-gauge needles for injections, and apply firm pressure for longer than usual after venipuncture.	Reduces trauma, risk of bleeding/hematoma formation.
Have client use soft toothbrush or cotton/sponge swabs and alcohol-free mouthwash instead of a toothbrush if bleeding is a problem.	Avoids trauma and bleeding of the gums. Alcohol can be drying and cause irritation to mucosa.

Collaborative

Monitor laboratory studies; e.g., Hb/Hct, electrolytes, prothrombin level/clotting time.	Provides information about circulating volume, electrolyte balance, and adequacy of clotting factors.
Administer IV fluids, blood products, as indicated:	Maintain adequate circulating volume and aid in replacement of clotting factors.
Electrolytes;	Correct imbalances resulting from excessive gastric/wound losses.
Vitamin K.	Provides replacement of factors necessary for clotting process.

NURSING DIAGNOSIS: impaired Skin/Tissue Integrity

May be related to

Chemical substance (bile), stasis of secretions
Altered nutritional state (obesity)/metabolic state
Invasion of body structure (T-tube)

Possibly evidenced by

Disruption of skin/subcutaneous tissues

DESIRED OUTCOMES/EVALUATION CRITERIA—CLIENT WILL:

WOUND HEALING: Primary/Secondary Intention (NOC)

Achieve timely wound healing without complications.
Demonstrate behaviors to promote healing/prevent skin breakdown.

ACTIONS/INTERVENTIONS — RATIONALE

Wound Care (NIC)

Independent

ACTIONS/INTERVENTIONS	RATIONALE
Observe the color and character of NG, T-tube drainage.	Initially, drainage may contain blood and bloodstained fluid, normally changing to greenish brown (bile color) after the first several hours.
Change dressings as often as necessary. Clean the skin with soap and water. Use sterile petroleum jelly gauze, zinc oxide, or karaya powder around the incision.	Keeps the skin around the incision clean and provides a barrier to protect skin from excoriation.
Apply Montgomery straps.	Facilitates frequent dressing changes and minimizes skin trauma.

ACTIONS/INTERVENTIONS	RATIONALE
Use a disposable ostomy bag over a stab wound drain.	Ostomy appliance may be used to collect heavy drainage for more accurate measurement of output and protection of the skin.
Place client in low- or semi-Fowler's position.	Facilitates drainage of bile.
Monitor puncture sites (three to five) if endoscopic procedure is done.	These areas may bleed, or staples and Steri-Strips may loosen at puncture wound sites.
Check the T-tube and incisional drains; make sure they are free flowing.	T-tube may remain in common bile duct for 7–10 days to remove retained tiny stones/gravel. Incision site drains are used to remove any accumulated fluid and bile. Correct positioning prevents backup of the bile in the operative area.
Maintain T-tube in closed collection system.	Prevents skin irritation and facilitates measurement of output. Reduces risk of contamination.
Anchor drainage tube, allowing sufficient tubing to permit free turning and avoid kinks and twists.	Avoids dislodging tube and/or occlusion of the lumen.
Observe for hiccups, abdominal distention, or signs of peritonitis, pancreatitis.	Dislodgment of the T-tube can result in diaphragmatic irritation or more serious complications if bile drains into abdomen or pancreatic duct is obstructed.
Observe skin, sclera, urine for change in color.	Developing jaundice may indicate obstruction of bile flow.
Note color and consistency of stools.	Clay-colored stools result when bile is not present in the intestines.
Investigate reports of increased/unrelenting RUQ pain; development of fever, tachycardia; leakage of bile drainage around tube/from wound.	Signs suggestive of abscess or fistula formation, requiring medical intervention.

Collaborative

Administer antibiotics as indicated.	Necessary for treatment of abscess/infection.
Clamp the T-tube per schedule.	Tests the patency of the common bile duct before tube is removed.
Prepare for surgical interventions as indicated.	Drainage of blocked duct or fistulectomy may be required to treat abscess or repair fistula.
Monitor laboratory studies; e.g., WBC.	Leukocytosis reflects inflammatory process; e.g., abscess formation or development of peritonitis/pancreatitis.

NURSING DIAGNOSIS: deficient Knowledge [Learning Need] regarding condition, prognosis, treatment, self-care, and discharge needs

May be related to

Lack of exposure; information misinterpretation
Unfamiliarity with information resources
Lack of recall

Possibly evidenced by

Questions; statement of misconception
Request for information
Inaccurate follow-through of instructions

DESIRED OUTCOMES/EVALUATION CRITERIA—CLIENT WILL:

KNOWLEDGE: Illness Care (NOC)

Verbalize understanding of disease process, surgical procedure/prognosis, and potential complications.
Verbalize understanding of therapeutic needs.
Correctly perform necessary procedures and explain reasons for the actions.
Initiate necessary lifestyle changes and participate in therapeutic regimen.

ACTIONS/INTERVENTIONS	RATIONALE
TEACHING: Disease Process (NIC)	
Independent	
Review disease process, surgical procedure/prognosis.	Provides knowledge base on which client can make informed choices.
Demonstrate care of incisions/dressings and drains.	Promotes independence in care and reduces risk of complications (e.g., infection, biliary obstruction).
Recommend periodic drainage of T-tube collection bag and recording of output.	Reduces risk of reflux, strain on tube/appliance seal. Provides information about resolution of ductal edema/return of ductal function for appropriate timing of T-tube removal.
Emphasize importance of maintaining low-fat diet, eating frequent small meals, gradual reintroduction of foods/fluids containing fats over a 4- to 6-month period.	During initial 6 months after surgery, low-fat diet limits need for bile and reduces discomfort associated with inadequate digestion of fats.
Discuss use of medication such as florantyrone (Sancho) or dehydrocholic acid (Decholin).	Oral replacement of bile salts may be required in certain clients, to facilitate digestion/treat malabsorption of fats.
Discuss avoiding/limiting use of alcoholic beverages.	Minimizes risk of pancreatic involvement.
Inform client that loose stools may occur for several months.	Intestines require time to adjust to stimulus of continuous output of bile.
Advise client to note and avoid foods that seem to aggravate the diarrhea.	Although radical dietary changes are not usually necessary, certain restrictions may be helpful; e.g., fats in small amounts are usually tolerated. After a period of adjustment, client usually will not have problems with most foods.
Identify signs/symptoms requiring notification of healthcare provider; e.g., dark urine, jaundiced color of eyes/skin, clay-colored stools, excessive stools, or recurrent heartburn, bloating.	Indicators of obstruction of bile flow/altered digestion, requiring further evaluation and intervention.
Review activity limitations, depending on individual situation.	Resumption of usual activities is normally accomplished within 4–6 weeks.

POTENTIAL CONSIDERATIONS following acute hospitalization (dependent on client's age, physical condition/presence of complications, personal resources, and life responsibilities)

Diarrhea—continuous excretion of bile into bowel, changes in digestive process.

risk for Infection—invasive procedure (discharge with T-tube in place).

8 CHAPTER

Metabolic and Endocrine Disorders

EATING DISORDERS: ANOREXIA NERVOSA/BULIMIA NERVOSA

Anorexia nervosa (AN) is a serious, chronic illness of starvation associated with a severe disturbance of body image and a morbid fear of obesity. The disorder can be divided into early/mild or established stages. AN is more common in girls and women, although approximately 15% of cases occur in boys and men. AN is found mainly in the white (>95%) adolescent (>75%) population, although it can occur in either sex and in people of any race, age, or social stratum. Only about 50% of those affected recover, with best results occurring if treatment is begun within the first 6 months of onset and supportive parents/family are present. Mortality rates range from 10% to 20%, and is often related to length of illness.

Bulimia nervosa (BN) is an eating disorder (binge-purge syndrome) characterized by normal weight, but may be seen in overweight clients, without anorexia or extreme overeating followed by self-induced vomiting and/or abuse of laxatives, enemas, and diuretics. Fear of gaining weight motivates the purging behavior. BN affects primarily adolescent girls (6%) and college-age women (5%). Lifetime prevalence is about 3%.

Both disorders can be present in the same individual. Occurrence of these disorders has increased over the past 30 years due in part to earlier recognition and better diagnosis. The best treatment is behavioral therapy with operant conditioning plus reinforcement and privileges.

CARE SETTING

Acute care is provided through inpatient stay on medical or behavioral unit and for correction of severe nutritional deficits/electrolyte imbalances or initial psychiatric stabilization. Long-term care is provided in outpatient/day treatment program (partial hospitalization) or in the community.

RELATED CONCERNS

Dysrhythmias, page 85
Fluid and electrolyte imbalances, page 919
Metabolic alkalosis (primary base bicarbonate excess), page 495
Total nutritional support: parenteral/enteral feeding, page 478
Psychosocial aspects of care, page 770

Client Assessment Database

ACTIVITY/REST

May report:
Disturbed sleep patterns; e.g., early-morning insomnia; fatigue
Feeling "hyper" and/or anxious
Increased activity/avid exerciser, participation in high-energy sports
Employment in positions/professions that stress/require weight control (e.g., athletics such as gymnasts, swimmers, jockeys, models, flight attendants)

May exhibit:
Periods of hyperactivity, constant vigorous exercising

CIRCULATION

May report:
Feeling cold even when room is warm

May exhibit:
Low blood pressure (BP), orthostatic changes in BP or HR
Cold hands and feet
Tachycardia, bradycardia, dysrhythmias

EGO INTEGRITY

May report:

Powerlessness/helplessness lack of control over eating (e.g., cannot stop eating/control what or how much is eaten [bulimia]); feeling disgusted with self, depressed or very guilty because of overeating
Distorted (unrealistic) body image, reports self as fat regardless of weight (denial), and sees thin body as fat; persistent overconcern with body shape and weight (fears gaining weight)
High self-expectations
Stress factors; e.g., family move/divorce, onset of puberty
Suppression of anger

May exhibit:

Emotional states of depression, withdrawal, anger, anxiety, pessimistic outlook

ELIMINATION

May report:

Diarrhea/constipation
Vague abdominal pain and distress, bloating
Laxative/diuretic abuse

FOOD/FLUID

May report:

Constant hunger or denial of hunger; normal or exaggerated appetite that rarely vanishes until late in the disorder (anorexia)
Intense fear of gaining weight (females); may have prior history of being overweight (particularly males)
Preoccupation with food; e.g., calorie counting, gourmet cooking
An unrealistic pleasure in weight loss, while denying self pleasure in other areas
Refusal to maintain body weight over minimal norm for age/height (anorexia)
Recurrent episodes of binge eating, a feeling of lack of control over behavior during eating binges, a minimum average of two binge-eating episodes a week for at least 3 months (bulimia)
Regularly engages in self-induced vomiting (binge-purge syndrome, bulimia) either independently or as a complication of anorexia, or strict dieting or fasting

May exhibit:

Weight loss/maintenance of body weight 15% or more below that expected (anorexia), or weight may be normal or slightly above or below normal (bulimia)
No medical illness evident to account for weight loss
Cachectic appearance, skin may be dry, yellowish/pale with poor turgor (anorexia)
Preoccupation with food (e.g., calorie counting, hiding food, cutting food into small pieces, rearranging food on plate)
Irrational thinking about eating, food, and weight
Peripheral edema
Swollen salivary glands; sore, inflamed buccal cavity; continuous sore throat (bulimia)
Vomiting, bloody vomitus (may indicate esophageal tearing [Mallory-Weiss syndrome])
Excessive gum chewing

HYGIENE

May exhibit:

Increased hair growth on body (lanugo), hair loss (axillary/pubic), hair is dull/not shiny
Brittle nails
Signs of erosion of tooth enamel, gums in poor condition, ulcerations of mucosa

NEUROSENSORY

May exhibit:

Appropriate affect (except in regard to body and eating) or depressive affect
Mental changes: Apathy, confusion, memory impairment (brought on by malnutrition/starvation)
Hysterical or obsessive personality style, absence of other psychiatric illness or evidence of a psychiatric thought disorder present (although a significant number may show evidence of an affective disorder)

PAIN/DISCOMFORT

May report:

Headaches, sore throat/mouth, generalized vague complaints

SAFETY

May exhibit:

Body temperature below normal

Recurrent infectious processes (indicative of depressed immune system)
Eczema/other skin problems, abrasions/calluses may be noted on back of hands from sticking finger down throat to induce vomiting

SEXUALITY

May report:

Absence of at least three consecutive menstrual cycles (decreased levels of estrogen in response to malnutrition) (anorexia)
Promiscuity or denial/loss of sexual interest
History of sexual abuse
Homosexual/bisexual orientation (higher percentage in male clients than in general population)

May exhibit:

Breast atrophy, amenorrhea related to hypothalamic function

SOCIAL INTERACTION

May report:

Middle-class or upper-class family background
History of being a quiet, cooperative child
Problems of control issues in relationships, difficult communications with others/authority figures, poor communication within family of origin
Engagement in power struggles
An emotional crisis of some sort, such as the onset of puberty or a family move
Altered relationships or problems with relationships (not married/divorced), withdrawal from friends/social contacts
Abusive family relationships
Sense of helplessness
History of legal difficulties (e.g., shoplifting)

May exhibit:

Passive father/dominant mother, family members closely fused, togetherness prized, personal boundaries not respected

TEACHING/LEARNING

May report:

Family history of higher than normal incidence of depression, other family members with eating disorders (genetic predisposition)
Onset of the illness usually between the ages of 10 and 22
Health beliefs/practice (e.g., certain foods have "too many" calories, use of "health" foods)
High academic achievement
Substance abuse
Use of herbal or over-the-counter (OTC) preparations to control weight gain; e.g., bitter orange, green tea extract, guarana rodiola, laxatives (e.g., bisacodyl, cascara, senna), high- fiber supplements
Use of prescription diet medications; e.g., Meridia, phentolamine, Xenical (often obtained without prescription via Internet)

Discharge plan considerations:

Assistance with maintenance of treatment plan

Refer to section at end of plan for postdischarge considerations.

DIAGNOSTIC STUDIES

Complete blood count (CBC) with differential: Determines presence of anemia, leukopenia, lymphocytosis. Platelets show significantly less than normal activity by the enzyme monoamine oxidase (thought to be a marker for depression).

Electrolytes: Imbalances may include decreased potassium, sodium, chloride, and magnesium. Hypokalemia, hyochloremic metabolic alkalosis are observed with vomiting, acidosis is present in cases of laxative abuse.

Endocrine studies:

Thyroid function: Thyroxine (T_4) levels usually normal; however, circulating triiodothyronine (T_3) levels may be low.

Pituitary function: Thyroid-stimulating hormone (TSH) response to thyrotropin-releasing hormone (TRH) is abnormal in anorexia nervosa. Propranolol-glucagon stimulation test studies the response of human growth hormone (hGH), which is depressed in anorexia. Gonadotropic hypofunction is noted.

Cortisol metabolism: May be elevated.

Dexamethasone suppression test (*DST*): Evaluates hypothalamic-pituitary function. Dexamethasone resistance indicates cortisol suppression, suggesting malnutrition and/or depression.

Luteinizing hormone (LH) secretions test: Pattern often resembles those of prepubertal girls.
Estrogen: Decreased.
MHP 6 levels: Decreased, suggestive of malnutrition/depression.

Serum glucose and basal metabolic rate (BMR): May be low.

Other chemistries: Liver function studies (e.g., aspartate transaminase [AST]) may be minimally elevated. Dramatic elevations may be noted in cholesterol levels (in starvation). Serum protein and albumin are often normal in AN because although the amount of food is restricted, it often contains high-quality proteins.

Urinalysis and renal function: Blood urea nitrogen (BUN) may be normal or elevated, ketones present reflecting starvation, decreased urinary 17-ketosteroids, increased specific gravity/dehydration.

Electrocardiogram (ECG): Abnormal tracing with low-voltage, T-wave inversion, dysrhythmias.

Genetic testing: Gene for agouti-related protein has been found to be higher in anorexic clients than in the general population.

NURSING PRIORITIES

1. Obtain client's cooperation in treatment.
2. Reestablish adequate/appropriate nutritional intake.
3. Correct fluid and electrolyte imbalance.
4. Assist client to develop realistic body image/improve self-esteem.
5. Provide support/involve significant other (SO), if available, in treatment program.
6. Coordinate total treatment program with other disciplines.
7. Provide information about disease, prognosis, and treatment to client/SO.

DISCHARGE GOALS

1. Adequate nutrition and fluid intake maintained.
2. Maladaptive coping behaviors and stressors that precipitate anxiety recognized.
3. Adaptive coping strategies and techniques for anxiety reduction and self-control implemented.
4. Self-esteem increased.
5. Disease process, prognosis, and treatment regimen understood.
6. Plan in place to meet needs after discharge.

NURSING DIAGNOSIS: imbalanced Nutrition: less than body requirements

May be related to

Inadequate food intake, self-induced vomiting
Chronic/excessive laxative use

Possibly evidenced by

Body weight 15% (or more) below expected, or may be within normal range/ overweight (bulimia)
Pale conjunctiva and mucous membranes, poor skin turgor/muscle tone, edema
Excessive loss of hair, increased growth of hair on body (lanugo)
Amenorrhea
Hypothermia
Bradycardia, cardiac irregularities, hypotension

DESIRED OUTCOMES/EVALUATION CRITERIA—CLIENT WILL:

KNOWLEDGE: Diet (NOC)

Verbalize understanding of nutritional needs.

Nutritional Status (NOC)

Establish a dietary pattern with caloric intake adequate to regain/maintain appropriate weight.
Demonstrate weight gain toward individually expected range.

ACTIONS/INTERVENTIONS	RATIONALE
Eating Disorders Management (NIC)	
Independent	
Establish a minimum weight goal and daily nutritional requirements.	Provides comparative baseline for effectiveness of therapy. *Note:* Malnutrition is a mood-altering condition, leading to depression and affecting cognitive function and decision making. Improved nutritional status enhances thinking ability, allowing initiation of psychologic work.
Contract with client regarding commitment to therapeutic program and meeting specific dietary needs and goals.	When client agrees to a contract, individual success is enhanced.
Use a consistent approach. Sit with client while eating; present and remove food without persuasion and/or comment. Promote pleasant environment and record intake.	Client detects urgency and may react to pressure. Any comment that might be seen as coercion provides focus on food. When staff responds in a consistent manner, client can begin to trust staff responses. The single area in which client has exercised power and control is food/eating, and she or he may experience guilt or rebellion if forced to eat. Structuring meals and decreasing discussions about food will decrease power struggles with client and avoid manipulative games.
Provide small, frequent, and nutritionally dense meals and supplemental snacks as appropriate.	Gastric dilation may occur if refeeding is too rapid following a period of starvation dieting. *Note:* Refeeding syndrome (e.g., excessive bloating, edema, and [rarely] congestive heart failure) can occur because of too rapid an increase in oral intake. In any event, client may feel bloated for weeks while body adjusts to increased food intake.
Make selective menu available, and allow client to control choices as much as possible.	Client who gains confidence in self and feels in control of environment is more likely to eat preferred foods.
Be alert to choices of low-calorie foods/beverages, hoarding food, disposing of food in various places, such as pockets or wastebaskets.	Client will try to avoid taking in what is viewed as excessive calories and may go to great lengths to avoid eating.
Maintain a regular weighing schedule, such as Monday/Friday before breakfast in same attire, and graph results.	Provides accurate ongoing record of weight loss/gain. Also diminishes obsessing about changes in weight.
Weigh with back to scale (depending on program protocols).	Although some programs prefer that client does not see the results of the weighing, this can force the issue of trust in client who usually does not trust others.
Avoid room checks and other control devices whenever possible.	External control reinforces feelings of powerlessness and therefore is usually not helpful.
Provide one-to-one supervision and have client with bulimia remain in the day room area/in sight with no bathroom privileges for a specified period (e.g., 2–3 hours) following eating if contracting is unsuccessful.	Prevents vomiting during or immediately after eating. Client may desire food and eating, but use a binge-purge syndrome to control weight. *Note:* Some clients purge for the first time in response to establishment of a weight-gain program.
Monitor exercise program and set limits on physical activities. Chart activity/level of work (pacing and so on).	Moderate exercise helps in maintaining muscle tone/weight and combating depression; however, client may exercise excessively to burn calories.
Maintain matter-of-fact, nonjudgmental attitude if giving tube feedings, parenteral fluids, and so on.	Perception of punishment is counterproductive to client's self-confidence and faith in own ability to control destiny.
Be alert to possibility of client disconnecting feeding tube and emptying enteral/parenteral fluids if used. Check measurements, and tape tubing snugly.	Sabotage behavior is common in attempt to prevent weight gain.
Collaborative	
Provide nutritional therapy within a hospital treatment program as indicated when condition is life threatening.	Cure of the underlying problem cannot happen without improved nutritional status. Hospitalization provides a controlled environment in which food intake, vomiting, elimination, medications, and activities can be monitored. It also separates client from SO (who may be contributing factor) and provides exposure to others with the same problem, creating an atmosphere for sharing.

ACTIONS/INTERVENTIONS	RATIONALE
Involve client in setting up/carrying out program of behavior modification. Provide reward for weight gain as individually determined; ignore loss.	Provides structured eating situation while allowing client some control in choices. Behavior modification may be effective in mild cases or for short-term weight gain.
Provide diet and snacks with substitutions of preferred foods when available.	Having a variety of foods available enables client to have a choice of potentially enjoyable foods.
Administer nutritional diet by prescripted means; e.g., regular food with supplements, high-calorie liquid diet, tube feedings if needed.	When caloric intake is insufficient to sustain metabolic needs, nutritional support can be used to prevent malnutrition/death while therapy is continuing. High-calorie liquid feedings may be given as medication, at preset times separate from meals, as an alternative means of increasing caloric intake.
Blenderize and tube-feed anything left on the tray after a given period of time if indicated.	This method of feeding may be used as part of behavior modification program to provide total intake of needed calories.
Administer enteral or parenteral nutrition as appropriate.	Total parenteral nutrition (also known as TPN or hyperalimentation) may be required for life-threatening situations; however, enteral feedings are preferred because they preserve gastrointestinal (GI) function and reduce atrophy of the gut.
Avoid giving laxatives.	Use is counterproductive because they may be used by client to rid body of food/calories.
Administer medication as indicated:	In anorexia nervosa, medication is usually limited to use in managing medical complications; e.g., calcium and vitamin D for osteopenia (which can be severe); potassium, magnesium, and phosphorus.
Serotonin and histamine antagonist; e.g., cyproheptadine (Periactin),	May be used for client with severe anorexia and no bingeing/purging. A serotonin and histamine antagonist that may be used in high doses to stimulate the appetite, decrease preoccupation with food, and combat depression. Does not appear to have serious side effects, although decreased mental alertness may occur.
Selective serotonin reuptake inhibitors (SSRIs); e.g., fluoxetine (Prozac), other antidepressants (e.g., tricyclic antidepressants [e.g., amitriptyline (Elavil), imipramine (Tofranil)]), dopamine reuptake blocker (e.g., bupropion [Wellbutrin]), 5-HT2 blockers (e.g., trazadone [Desryel]);	Various antidepressant class drugs may be used to lift depression, stimulate appetite, and stabilize AN. Many of these same drugs are also found to be useful in reducing binge-purge cycles in BN, *Note:* Use must be closely monitored because of potential side effects, although side effects from SSRIs are less significant than those associated with tricyclics.
Monoamine oxidase inhibitors (MAOIs); e.g., phenelzine (Nardil), tranylcypromine sulfate (Parnate);	May be used to treat depression when other drug therapy is ineffective; decreases urge to binge in bulimia.
Antipsychotic drugs; e.g., risperadone (Risperdal), olanzapine (Zyprexa), chlorpromazine (Thorazine), lithium (Eskalith, Lithane, Lithobid).	Newer antipsychotic drugs (e.g., Risperdal, Zyprexa) are being used to manage eating disorders, especially in presence of dual disorder; e.g., bulimia and bipolar disorder. These drugs can reduce tension, anxiety, and nervousness and increase cooperation with psychotherapeutic program. However, some antipsychotic drugs are used only when absolutely necessary for severely delusional/overactive/hospitalized client as a last resort (e.g., Thorazine). Possibility of extrapyramidal side effects is a concern.
Perform AIMS (Abnormal Involuntary Movement Scale) after initiation of, and periodically during, treatment with antipsychotic medications.	Used to provide baseline and monitor for the development of extrapyramidal side effects indicating need for change in therapy.
Prepare for/assist with electroconvulsive therapy (ECT) if indicated. Discuss reasons for use and help client understand this is not punishment.	In rare and difficult cases in which malnutrition is severe/life threatening, a short-term ECT series may enable client to begin eating and become accessible to psychotherapy.

NURSING DIAGNOSIS: actual or risk for deficient Fluid Volume

May be related to

Inadequate intake of food and liquids
Consistent self-induced vomiting
Chronic/excessive laxative/diuretic use

Possibly evidenced by (actual)

Dry skin and mucous membranes, decreased skin turgor
Increased pulse rate, body temperature, decreased BP
Output greater than input (diuretic use); concentrated urine/decreased urine output (dehydration)
Weakness
Change in mental state
Hemoconcentration, altered electrolyte balance

DESIRED OUTCOMES/EVALUATION CRITERIA—CLIENT WILL:

Hydration (NOC)

Maintain/demonstrate improved fluid balance, as evidenced by adequate urine output, stable vital signs, moist mucous membranes, good skin turgor.

Risk Control (NOC)

Verbalize understanding of causative factors and behaviors necessary to correct fluid deficit.

ACTIONS/INTERVENTIONS	RATIONALE
Fluid/Electrolyte Management (NIC)	
Independent	
Monitor vital signs, capillary refill, status of mucous membranes, skin turgor.	Indicators of adequacy of circulating volume. Orthostatic hypotension may occur with risk of falls/injury following sudden changes in position.
Monitor amount and types of fluid intake. Measure urine output accurately.	Client may abstain from all intake, with resulting dehydration, or substitute fluids for caloric intake, disturbing electrolyte balance.
Discuss strategies to stop vomiting and laxative/diuretic use.	Helping client deal with the feelings that lead to vomiting and/or laxative/diuretic use will prevent continued fluid loss. *Note:* Client with bulimia has learned that vomiting provides a release of anxiety.
Identify actions necessary to regain/maintain optimal fluid balance; e.g., specific fluid intake schedule.	Involving client in plan to correct fluid imbalances improves chances for success.
Collaborative	
Review electrolyte/renal function test results.	Fluid/electrolyte shifts, decreased renal function can adversely affect client's recovery/prognosis and may require additional intervention.
Administer/monitor IV fluids and electrolytes, as indicated.	Used to correct fluid/electrolyte imbalances and prevent cardiac dysrhythmias.

NURSING DIAGNOSIS: disturbed Thought Processes

May be related to

Severe malnutrition/electrolyte imbalance
Psychologic conflicts; e.g., sense of low self-worth, perceived lack of control

Possibly evidenced by

Impaired ability to make decisions, problem-solve
Non–reality-based verbalizations
Ideas of reference
Altered sleep patterns; e.g., may go to bed late (stay up to binge/purge) and get up early
Altered attention span/distractibility
Perceptual disturbances with failure to recognize hunger, fatigue, anxiety, and depression

DESIRED OUTCOMES/EVALUATION CRITERIA—CLIENT WILL:

Distorted Thought Control (NOC)

Verbalize understanding of causative factors and awareness of impairment.
Demonstrate behaviors to change/prevent malnutrition.
Display improved ability to make decisions, problem-solve.

ACTIONS/INTERVENTIONS	RATIONALE
Delusion Management (NIC)	
Independent	
Be aware of client's distorted thinking ability.	Allows caregiver to have more realistic expectations of client and provide appropriate information and support.
Listen to/avoid challenging irrational, illogical thinking. Present reality concisely and briefly.	It is difficult to respond logically when thinking ability is physiologically impaired. Client needs to hear reality, but challenging client leads to distrust and frustration. *Note:* Even though client may gain weight, she or he may continue to struggle with attitudes/behaviors typical of eating disorders, major depression, and/or alcohol dependence for a number of years.
Adhere strictly to nutritional regimen.	Improved nutrition is essential to improved brain functioning. (Refer to ND: imbalanced Nutrition: less than body requirements.)
Collaborative	
Review electrolyte/renal function tests.	Imbalances negatively affect cerebral functioning, and require correction before therapeutic interventions can begin.

NURSING DIAGNOSIS: disturbed Body Image/ chronic low Self-Esteem

May be related to

Morbid fear of obesity, perceived loss of control in some aspect of life
Personal vulnerability; unmet dependency needs
Dysfunctional family system
Continual negative evaluation of self

Possibly evidenced by

Distorted body image (views self as fat even in the presence of normal body weight or severe emaciation)
Expresses little concern, uses denial as a defense mechanism, and feels powerless to prevent/make changes
Expressions of shame/guilt
Overly conforming, dependent on others' opinions

DESIRED OUTCOMES/EVALUATION CRITERIA—CLIENT WILL:

Body Image (NOC)

Establish a more realistic body image.

Self-Esteem (NOC)

Acknowledge self as an individual.
Accept responsibility for own actions.

ACTIONS/INTERVENTIONS	RATIONALE
Body Image Enhancement (NIC)	
Independent	
Have client draw picture of self.	Provides opportunity to discuss client's perception of self/body image and realities of individual situation.
Involve in personal development program, preferably in a group setting. Provide information about proper application of makeup and grooming.	Learning about methods to enhance personal appearance may be helpful to long-range sense of self-esteem/image. Feedback from others can promote feelings of self-worth.
Recommend consultation with an image consultant.	Positive image enhances sense of self-esteem.
Suggest disposing of "thin" clothes as weight gain occurs.	Provides incentive to at least maintain and not lose weight. Not seeing "thin" clothes removes visual reminder of thinner self.
Assist client to confront changes associated with puberty/sexual fears. Provide sex education as necessary.	Major physical/psychologic changes in adolescence can contribute to development of eating disorders. Feelings of powerlessness and loss of control of feelings (in particular sexual sensations) can lead to an unconscious desire to desexualize self. Client often believes that these fears can be overcome by taking control of bodily appearance/development/function.
Self-Esteem Enhancement (NIC)	
Establish a therapeutic nurse/client relationship.	Within a helping relationship, client can begin to trust and try out new thinking and behaviors.
Promote self-concept without moral judgment.	Client sees self as weak willed even though part of person may feel sense of power and control (e.g., dieting/weight loss).
State rules clearly regarding weighing schedule, remaining in sight during medication and eating times, and consequences of not following the rules. Without undue comment, be consistent in carrying out rules.	Consistency is important in establishing trust. As part of the behavior modification program, client knows risks involved in not following established rules (e.g., decrease in privileges). Failure to follow rules is viewed as client's choice and accepted by staff in matter-of-fact manner so as not to provide reinforcement for the undesirable behavior.

ACTIONS/INTERVENTIONS	RATIONALE
Respond (confront) with reality when client makes unrealistic statements such as "I'm gaining weight, so there's nothing really wrong with me."	Client may be denying the psychologic aspects of own situation and is often expressing a sense of inadequacy and depression.
Be aware of own reaction to client's behavior. Avoid arguing.	Feelings of disgust, hostility, and infuriation are not uncommon when caring for these clients. Prognosis often remains poor even with a gain in weight because other problems may remain. Many clients continue to see themselves as fat, and there is also a high incidence of affective disorders, social phobias, obsessive-compulsive symptoms, drug abuse, and psychosexual dysfunction. Nurse needs to deal with own response/feelings so they do not interfere with care of client.
Assist client to assume control in areas other than dieting/weight loss; e.g., management of own daily activities, work/leisure choices.	Feelings of personal ineffectiveness, low self-esteem, and perfectionism are often part of the problem. Client feels helpless to change and requires assistance to problem-solve methods of control in life situations.
Help client formulate goals for self (not related to eating) and create a manageable plan for reaching those goals, one at a time, progressing from simple to more complex.	Client needs to recognize ability to control other areas in life and may need to learn problem-solving skills to achieve this control. Setting realistic goals fosters success.
Note client's withdrawal from and/or discomfort in social settings.	May indicate feelings of isolation and fear of rejection/judgment by others. Avoidance of social situations and contact with others can compound feelings of worthlessness.
Encourage client to take charge of own life in a more healthful way by making own decisions and accepting self as she or he is at this moment (including inadequacies and strengths).	Client often does not know what she or he may want for self. Parents (mother) often make decisions for client. Client may also believe she or he has to be the best in everything and holds self responsible for being perfect.
Let client know that it is acceptable to be different from family, particularly mother.	Developing a sense of identity separate from family and maintaining sense of control in other ways besides dieting and weight loss is a desirable goal of therapy/program.
Encourage client to express anger and acknowledge when it is verbalized.	Important to know that anger is part of self and as such is acceptable. Expressing anger may need to be taught to client because anger is generally considered unacceptable in the family, and therefore client does not express it.
Assist client to learn strategies other than eating for dealing with feelings. Have client keep a diary of feelings, particularly when thinking about food.	Feelings are the underlying issue, and client often uses food instead of dealing with feelings appropriately. Client needs to learn to recognize feelings and how to express them clearly.
Assess feelings of helplessness/hopelessness.	Lack of control is a common/underlying problem for this client and may be accompanied by more serious emotional disorders. *Note:* Fifty-four percent of clients with anorexia have a history of major affective disorder, and 33% have a history of minor affective disorder.
Be alert to suicidal ideation/behavior.	Intense anxiety/panic about weight gain, depression, and hopeless feelings may lead to suicidal attempts, particularly if client is impulsive.

Collaborative

Use cognitive-behavioral or interpersonal psychotherapy approach rather than interpretive therapy.	Although both therapies have similar results, cognitive-behavioral seems to work more quickly. Interaction between individuals is more helpful for client to discover feelings/impulses/needs from within own self. Client has not learned this internal control as a child and may not be able to interpret or attach meaning to behavior.
Involve in group therapy.	Provides an opportunity to talk about feelings and try out new behaviors.

ACTIONS/INTERVENTIONS	RATIONALE
Refer to occupational/recreational therapy.	Can develop interest and skills to fill time that has been occupied by obsession with eating. Involvement in recreational activities encourages social interactions with others and promotes fun and relaxation.
Encourage participation in directed activities; e.g., group hiking, bicycle tours, and wilderness adventures, such as Outward Bound Program.	Although exercise is often used negatively by these clients, participation in these directed activities provides an opportunity to learn self-reliance, enhance self-esteem, and realize that food is the fuel required by the body to do its work.
Refer to therapist trained in dealing with sexuality as indicated.	May need professional assistance to deal with sexuality issues and accept self as a sexual adult.

NURSING DIAGNOSIS: impaired Parenting

May be related to

Issues of control in family
Situational/maturational crises
History of inadequate coping methods

Possibly evidenced by

Dissonance among family members
Family developmental tasks not being met
Focus on "identified client" (IP)
Family needs not being met
Family member(s) acting as enablers for IP
Ill-defined family rules, function, and roles

DESIRED OUTCOMES/EVALUATION CRITERIA—FAMILY WILL:

Parenting (NOC)

Demonstrate individual involvement in problem-solving process directed at encouraging client toward independence.
Express feelings freely and appropriately.
Demonstrate more autonomous coping behaviors with individual family boundaries more clearly defined.
Recognize and resolve conflict appropriately with the individuals involved.

ACTIONS/INTERVENTIONS	RATIONALE
Family Therapy (NIC)	
Independent	
Identify patterns of interaction. Encourage each family member to speak for self. Do not allow two members to discuss a third without that member's participation.	Helpful information for planning interventions. The enmeshed, overinvolved family members often speak for each other and need to learn to be responsible for their own words and actions.
Discourage members from asking for approval from each other. Be alert to verbal or nonverbal checking with others for approval. Acknowledge competent actions of client.	Each individual needs to develop own internal sense of self-esteem. Individual often is living up to others' (family's) expectations rather than making own choices. Acknowledgment provides recognition of self in positive ways.

ACTIONS/INTERVENTIONS	RATIONALE
Listen with regard when client speaks.	Sets an example and provides a sense of competence and self-worth in that client has been heard and attended to.
Encourage individuals not to answer to everything.	Reinforces individualization and return to privacy.
Communicate message of separation—that it is acceptable for family members to be different from each other.	Individuation needs reinforcement. Such a message confronts rigidity and opens options for different behaviors.
Encourage and allow expression of feelings (e.g., crying, anger) by individuals.	Often these families have not allowed free expression of feelings and need help and permission to learn and accept this.
Prevent intrusion in dyads by other members of the family.	Inappropriate interventions in family subsystems prevent individuals from working out problems successfully.
Reinforce importance of parents as a couple who have rights of their own.	The focus on the child with anorexia is very intense and often is the only area around which the couple interacts. The couple needs to explore their own relationship and restore the balance within relationship to help prevent its disintegration.
Prevent client from intervening in conflicts between parents. Assist parents in identifying and solving their marital differences.	Triangulation occurs in which a parent-child coalition exists. Sometimes the child is openly pressed to ally self with one parent against the other. The symptom (anorexia) is the regulator in the family system, and the parents deny their own conflicts.
Be aware and confront sabotage behavior on the part of family members.	Feelings of blame, shame, and helplessness may lead to unconscious behavior designed to maintain the status quo.

Collaborative

Refer to community resources such as family therapy groups, parents' groups, and parent effectiveness classes as indicated.	May help reduce overprotectiveness, support/facilitate the process of dealing with unresolved conflicts and change.

NURSING DIAGNOSIS: risk for impaired Skin Integrity

Risk factors may include

Altered nutritional/metabolic state; edema
Dehydration/cachectic changes (skeletal prominence)

Possibly evidenced by

[Not applicable; presence of signs and symptoms establishes an *actual* diagnosis.]

DESIRED OUTCOMES/EVALUATION CRITERIA—CLIENT WILL:

Risk Control (NOC)

Verbalize understanding of causative factors and absence of itching.
Identify and demonstrate behaviors to maintain soft, supple, intact skin.

ACTIONS/INTERVENTIONS	RATIONALE
Skin Surveillance (NIC)	
Independent	
Observe for reddened, blanched, excoriated areas.	Indicators of increased risk of breakdown, requiring more intensive treatment.

ACTIONS/INTERVENTIONS	RATIONALE
Encourage bathing every other day instead of daily if this is an area of concern.	Frequent baths contribute to dryness of the skin.
Use skin cream twice a day and after bathing.	Lubricates skin and decreases itching.
Massage skin gently, especially over bony prominences.	Improves circulation to the skin, enhances skin tone.
Discuss importance of frequent position changes, need for remaining active.	Enhances circulation and perfusion to skin by preventing prolonged pressure on tissues.
Emphasize importance of adequate nutrition/fluid intake. (Refer to ND: imbalanced Nutrition: less than body requirements.)	Improved nutrition and hydration will improve skin condition.

NURSING DIAGNOSIS: deficient Knowledge [Learning Need] regarding condition, prognosis, treatment, self-care, and discharge needs

May be related to

Lack of exposure to/unfamiliarity with information about condition
Learned maladaptive coping skills

Possibly evidenced by

Verbalization of misconception of relationship of current situation and behaviors
Preoccupation with extreme fear of obesity and distortion of own body image
Refusal to eat, binging and purging, abuse of laxatives and diuretics, excessive exercising
Verbalization of need for new information
Expressions of desire to learn more adaptive ways of coping with stressors

DESIRED OUTCOMES/EVALUATION CRITERIA—CLIENT WILL:

KNOWLEDGE: Illness Care (NOC)

Verbalize awareness of and plan for lifestyle changes to maintain normal weight.
Identify relationship of signs/symptoms (weight loss, tooth decay) to behaviors of not eating/bingeing-purging.
Assume responsibility for own learning.
Seek out sources/resources to assist with making identified changes.

ACTIONS/INTERVENTIONS — RATIONALE

Learning Facilitation (NIC)

Independent

ACTIONS/INTERVENTIONS	RATIONALE
Determine level of knowledge and readiness to learn.	Learning is easier when it begins where the learner is.
Note blocks to learning; e.g., physical/intellectual/emotional.	Malnutrition, family problems, drug abuse, affective disorders, and obsessive-compulsive symptoms can be blocks to learning requiring resolution before effective learning can occur.

ACTIONS/INTERVENTIONS	RATIONALE
TEACHING: Disease Process (NIC)	
Independent	
Discuss familial tendencies and/or genetic risk for eating disorder.	Recent research supports the findings suggesting that anorexia and bulimia are disorders that occur in families; e.g., this client is more likely to have an immediate family member (or even a more distant relative) with either disorder. There also may be a genetic risk
Provide written information for client/SOs.	Helpful as reminder of and reinforcement for learning.
Discuss consequences of behavior and potential for recovery and relapse.	Sudden death can occur because of electrolyte imbalances, suppression of the immune system and liver damage may result from protein deficiency, or gastric rupture may follow binge eating/vomiting.
Review dietary needs, answering questions as indicated. Encourage inclusion of high-fiber foods and adequate fluid intake.	Client/family may need assistance with planning for new way of eating. Constipation may occur when laxative use is curtailed.
Encourage the use of relaxation and other stress-management techniques; e.g., visualization, guided imagery, biofeedback.	New ways of coping with feelings of anxiety and fear help client manage these feelings in more effective ways, assisting in giving up maladaptive behaviors of not eating/bingeing-purging.
Assist with establishing a sensible exercise program. Caution regarding overexercise.	Exercise can assist with developing a positive body image and combats depression (release of endorphins in the brain enhances sense of well-being). However, client may use excessive exercise as a way to control weight.
Discuss need for information about sex and sexuality.	Because avoidance of own sexuality is an issue for this client, realistic information can be helpful in beginning to deal with self as a sexual being.
Refer to National Association of Anorexia Nervosa and Associated Disorders, Overeaters Anonymous, and other local resources as appropriate.	May be a helpful source of support and information for client/SO.

POTENTIAL CONSIDERATIONS following acute hospitalization (dependent on client's age, physical condition/presence of complications, personal resources, and life responsibilities)

risk for imbalanced Nutrition: less than body requirements—inadequate food intake, self-induced vomiting, history of chronic laxative use.

ineffective Therapeutic Regimen Management—complexity of therapeutic regimen, perceived seriousness/benefits, mistrust of regimen and/or healthcare personnel, excessive demands made on individual, family conflict.

Sample CP: Eating Disorders Program. ELOS: 28 Days Behavioral Unit

ND and Categories of Care	Time Dimension	Goals/Actions	Time Dimension	Goals/Actions	Time Dimension	Goals/Actions
Imbalanced nutrition: less than body requirements R/T inadequate intake, self-induced vomiting, laxative use	Ongoing	Gain 3 lb/wk as indicated	Day 2–28	Consume at least 75% of food provided at each meal	Day 15–28	Demonstrate ability to select foods to meet at least 80% of nutritional needs
Risk for deficient fluid volume R/T inadequate intake, self-induced vomiting, laxative use	Ongoing	Be free of S/S of dehydration	Day 2–28	Ingest at least 1500 mL fluid/day	Day 22–28	Refrain from self-induced vomiting
	Ongoing	Display balanced I & O	Day 3	Vital signs WNL	Day 28	Be free of S/S of malnutrition with all laboratory results WNL
Referral	Day 1 & prn	Dietitian				
Diagnostic Studies	Day 1	Electrolytes, CBC, BUN/Cr, Thyroid function UA ECG as indicated	Day 14	Repeat selected studies		
Additional assessments	Day 1–2	Vital signs/I & O q shift	Day 3–7	q AM	Day 8–28	As indicated
	Day 1	Weight	Day 7, 14	7:30 AM/same clothes		
	Day 1–28	Types of amount of food/fluid intake Behavior/purging following meals Level of activity				
Medications Allergies:	Day 1–28	Periactin Tricyclic antidepressant Vitamin supplement				
Client education	Day 1 & prn	Orient to unit and schedule Behavior modification program Minimum weight goal and initial nutritional needs	Day 7–14	Principles of nutrition; foods for maintenance of wellness	Day 21–28	Incorporating nutritional plan into lifestyle and home setting
Additional nursing actions	Day 1–3	Assist client with formulation of behavioral contract and monitoring of cooperation	Day 7–28	Involve mother/SO as appropriate in nutritional counseling and planning for future		
	Day 1–7	Administer tube feeding/ blenderized food as indicated				
	Day 1–21	Bathroom locked for 1 hr following meals				
	Day 1–28	Provide social setting for meals				

Ineffective denial R/T presence of overwhelming anxiety-producing feelings, learned response pattern, personal/family value system	Ongoing	Participate in behavior modification program and adhere to unit policies	Day 8–28	Attend and contribute to group sessions	Day 18–28	Verbalize acceptance of reality that eating behaviors are maladaptive Demonstrate ability to cope more adaptively
			Day 14	Develop trusting relationship with at least one staff member on each shift		
	Day 2–28	Cooperate with therapy to restore nutritional well-being			Day 28	Identify ways to gain control in life situation Refrain from use of manipulation of others to achieve control Plan in place to meet needs after discharge
Referrals	Day 5 (or when physical condition stable)	Psychologist Social worker Psychodramatist	Day 8–28	Group psychotherapy sessions	Day 25	Community resource contact person(s)
Additional assessments	Day 1/ongoing	Degree and stage of denial Perception of situation	Day 5–7	Readiness to participate in group sessions		
	Day 1–17	Ability to trust Use of manipulation to achieve control	Day 7–28	Congruence between verbalizations and behaviors (insight)		
			Day 8–28	Degree/quality of involvement in group sessions		
Client education	Day 1 and prn	Privileges and responsibilities of behavior modification Consequences of behaviors	Day 3/ongoing	Eating disorder and consequences of eating behavior	Day 21	Role of support group/community resources
Additional nursing actions	Day 1/ongoing	Encourage expression of feelings Avoid agreeing with inaccurate statements/perceptions	Day 5–28	Promote involvement in unit activities Support interactions with family members	Day 21–28	Involve family (as appropriate in long-range planning for meeting individual needs)
		Provide positive feedback for desired insight/behaviors Set limits on maladaptive behavior	Day 8–28	Encourage interactions in group sessions		
Disturbed body image/chronic low self-esteem R/T perceived loss of control, unmet dependency needs, personal vulnerability, negative evaluation of self	Day 7	Acknowledge that attention will not be given to discussion of body image and food	Day 21	Acknowledge misperception of body image as fat Verbalize positive self-attributes	Day 28	Demonstrate realistic body image and self-awareness Verbalize acceptance of self including "imperfections" Acknowledge self as sexual being

(Continued on the following page)

Sample CP: Eating Disorders Program. ELOS: 28 Days Behavioral Unit *(continued)*

ND and Categories of Care	Time Dimension	Goals/Actions	Time Dimension	Goals/Actions	Time Dimension	Goals/Actions
Referrals	Day 1 (or when physical condition stable)	Therapists: occupational, recreational, music, art	Day 14	Image consultant	Day 28	Therapist to address issue of sexuality postdischarge as indicated
Additional assessments	Day 1–7	Suicidal ideation/behaviors	Day 8	Individual strengths/weaknesses		
	Day 3	Sexual history including abuse	Day 8–28	Congruency of feelings/perceptions with actions		
	Day 3–28	Perception of body image Family patterns of interaction				
Client education	Day 1–28	Responsibility for self in family setting	Day 8–10	General wellness needs	Day 21–28	Sex education reflecting individual sexuality and needs
	Day 7–28	Clarify misconceptions of body image	Day 8–28	Human behavior and interactions with family/others—transactional analysis (TA)		
			Day 14	Personal appearance and grooming		
			Day 14–28	Alternative coping strategies for dealing with feelings		
Additional nursing actions	Day 1	Develop therapeutic relationship	Day 7	Compare actual measurement of client's body with client's perceptions	Day 14–28	Have client keep diary of feelings, especially when thinking of food Role-play new behaviors for dealing with feelings and conflicts
	Day 1–28	Provide positive feedback for participation and independent decision making Confront sabotage behavior by family members	Day 7–9	Assist with planning to meet individual goals		
			Day 8–28	Involve in physical activity/exercise program		
	Day 3–5	Encourage control in areas other than diet				
	Day 4–6	Support development of goals not related to eating				

EATING DISORDERS: OBESITY

Obesity is chronic condition, defined as an excess accumulation of body fat (at least 20% over average desired weight for age, sex, and height, or a body mass index [BMI—measured in kilograms/height in square meters] greater than 30% for persons of either sex).

The causes of obesity are multiple and complex and cannot be attributed simply to a disorder of willpower or the result of insufficient exercise. Variations in metabolism, body fat distribution, and appetite regulation can be attributed to genetic factors. Environmental influences and behavioral and societal issues are also involved in obesity in Americans (e.g., availability of high fat, calorie-dense convenience foods, large portions, and sedentary lifestyle). Obesity negatively impacts all body systems and increases client risk of multiple physical and psychologic pathologies, including hypertension, heart disease, diabetes, arthritis, depression and anxiety disorders, difficulty maintaining personal relationships, prejudice and discrimination, and limited access to public conveniences.

The general prognosis for achieving and maintaining weight loss is poor; however, the desire for a healthier lifestyle and reduction of risk factors associated with life-threatening illnesses motivate many people toward diets and weight-loss programs.

CARE SETTING

Community level unless morbid obesity requires brief inpatient stay.

RELATED CONCERNS

Cerebrovascular accident (CVA)/stroke, page 236
Cholecystitis with cholelithiasis, page 364
Cirrhosis of the liver, page 453
Diabetes mellitus/diabetic ketoacidosis, page 412
Heart failure: chronic, page 47
Hypertension: severe, page 35
Myocardial infarction, page 72
Obesity: surgical interventions (gastric partitioning/gastroplasty, gastric bypass), page 402
Psychosocial aspects of care, page 770
Thrombophlebitis: deep vein thrombosis, page 108

Client Assessment Database

ACTIVITY/REST

May report: Fatigue, constant drowsiness
Inability/lack of desire to be active or engage in regular exercise, sedentary lifestyle
Dyspnea with exertion

May exhibit: Increased heart rate/respirations with activity

CIRCULATION

May exhibit: Hypertension, edema

EGO INTEGRITY

May report: History of cultural/lifestyle factors affecting food choices
Weight may/may not be perceived as a problem
Eating relieves unpleasant feelings; e.g., loneliness, frustration, boredom
Perception of body image as undesirable
SO's resistance to weight loss (may sabotage client's efforts)

FOOD/FLUID

May report: Normal/excessive ingestion of food
Experimentation with numerous types of diets ("yo-yo" dieting) with varied/short-lived results
History of recurrent weight loss and gain

May exhibit: Weight disproportionate to height
Endomorphic body type (soft/round)
Failure to adjust food intake to diminishing requirements (e.g., change in lifestyle from active to sedentary, aging)

PAIN/DISCOMFORT

May report: Pain/discomfort on weight-bearing joints or spine

RESPIRATION

May report: Dyspnea
May exhibit: Cyanosis, respiratory distress (pickwickian syndrome)

SEXUALITY

May report: Menstrual disturbances, amenorrhea

TEACHING/LEARNING

May report: Problem may be lifelong or related to life event
Family history of obesity
Concomitant health problems may include hypertension, diabetes, gallbladder and cardiovascular disease, hypothyroidism

Discharge plan considerations: May require support with therapeutic regimen; home modifications, assistive devices/equipment.

Refer to section at end of plan for postdischarge considerations.

DIAGNOSTIC STUDIES

Metabolic/endocrine studies: May reveal abnormalities; e.g., hypothyroidism, hypopituitarism, hypogonadism, Cushing's syndrome (increased insulin levels), hyperglycemia, hyperlipidemia, hyperuricemia, hyperbilirubinemia. It is also suggested that the cause of these disorders may arise from neuroendocrine abnormalities within the hypothalamus, which result in various chemical disturbances.
Anthropometric measurements: Measures fat-to-muscle ratio.

NURSING PRIORITIES

1. Assist client to identify a workable method of weight control incorporating healthful foods and activity.
2. Promote improved self-concept, including body image, self esteem.
3. Encourage health practices to provide for weight control throughout life.

DISCHARGE GOALS

1. Healthy patterns for eating and weight control identified.
2. Weight loss toward desired goal established.
3. Positive perception of self verbalized.
4. Plans developed for future weight control.
5. Plan in place to meet needs after discharge.

NURSING DIAGNOSIS: imbalanced Nutrition: more than body requirements

May be related to

Food intake that exceeds body needs
Psychosocial factors
Socioeconomic status

Possibly evidenced by

Weight of 20% or more over optimum body weight; excess body fat by skinfold/other measurements
Reported/observed dysfunctional eating patterns, intake more than body requirements

DESIRED OUTCOMES/EVALUATION CRITERIA—CLIENT WILL:

KNOWLEDGE: Diet (NOC)

Identify inappropriate behaviors and consequences associated with overeating or weight gain.

Demonstrate appropriate change in lifestyle and behaviors, including eating patterns, food quantity/quality; and involvement in individual exercise program.

Nutritional Status (NOC)

Display weight loss with optimal maintenance of health.

ACTIONS/INTERVENTIONS	RATIONALE
Weight Reduction Assistance (NIC)	
Independent	
Review individual cause for obesity; e.g., organic or nonorganic.	Identifies/influences choice of some interventions.
Ascertain previous dieting history. Determine which diets and strategies have been used, results, individual frustrations/factors interfering with success.	Client may have tried multiple diets, with little lasting change in body weight and feel negatively about embarking on another plan.
Implement/review daily food diary; e.g., total caloric intake, types and amounts of food, eating habits and associated feelings.	Provides the opportunity for the individual to focus on/internalize a realistic picture of the amount of food ingested and corresponding eating habits/feelings. Identifies patterns requiring change and/or a base on which to tailor the dietary program.
Determine client's motivation for weight loss (e.g., health issues, own satisfaction, to gain approval from others). Discuss client/SO's view of self, including what being fat does for the client. Notice occurrence of negative feedback from SO(s).	Helps to clarify client's motivation and potential for success in weight reduction. Client's family and cultural practices greatly influence client's self-view regarding food and body image. Feedback from family may reveal control issues impacting motivation for change.
Formulate an eating plan with the client, using knowledge of individual's height, body build, age, gender, and individual patterns of eating, as well as energy, and nutrient requirements.	An important factor in the success of any weight loss program is good adherence to a sensible nutritional plan. Although there is little basis for recommending one commercial diet plan over another, a good reducing diet should contain foods from all basic food groups with a focus on low-fat intake and adequate protein intake to prevent loss of lean muscle mass. It is helpful to keep the plan as similar to client's usual eating pattern as possible. A plan developed with and agreed to by the client is more likely to be successful.
Emphasize the importance of avoiding fad diets.	Elimination of needed components can lead to metabolic imbalances; e.g., excessive reduction of carbohydrates can lead to fatigue, headache, instability/weakness, and metabolic acidosis (ketosis), interfering with effectiveness of weight loss program.
Discuss need to give self permission to include desired/craved food items in dietary plan.	Denying self by excluding desired/favorite foods results in a sense of deprivation and feelings of guilt/failure when individual "succumbs to temptation." These feelings can sabotage weight loss.
Be alert to binge eating and develop strategies for dealing with these episodes; e.g., substituting other actions for eating.	The client who binges experiences guilt about it, which is also counterproductive because negative feelings may sabotage further weight loss efforts.
Identify realistic incremental goals for weekly weight loss.	Reasonable weight loss (1–2 lb/wk) results in more lasting effects. Excessive/rapid loss may result in fatigue and irritability and ultimately lead to failure in meeting goals for weight loss. Motivation is more easily sustained by meeting "stair-step" goals.

ACTIONS/INTERVENTIONS	RATIONALE
Weigh periodically as individually indicated, and obtain appropriate body measurements.	Provides information about effectiveness of therapeutic regimen and visual evidence of success of client's efforts. (During hospitalization for controlled fasting, daily weighing may be required. Weekly weighing is more appropriate after discharge.)
Determine current activity level and exercise program. Factor in caloric needs.	Exercise furthers weight loss by reducing appetite, sense of well-being, and accomplishment.
Develop an appetite reeducation plan with client.	Signals of hunger and fullness often are not recognized, have become distorted, or are ignored.
Emphasize the importance of avoiding tension at mealtimes and not eating too quickly.	Reducing tension provides a more relaxed eating atmosphere and encourages more leisurely eating patterns. This is important because a period of time is required for the appestat mechanism to know the stomach is full.
Encourage client to eat only at a table or designated eating place and to avoid standing while eating.	Techniques that modify behavior may be helpful in avoiding diet failure.
Discuss restriction of salt intake and diuretic drugs if used.	Water retention may be a problem because of increased fluid intake and fat metabolism.
Reassess caloric requirements every 2–4 weeks; provide additional support when plateaus occur.	Changes in weight and exercise necessitate changes in plan. As weight is lost, changes in metabolism occur, resulting in plateaus when weight remains stable for periods of time. This can create distrust and lead to accusations of "cheating" on caloric intake, which are not helpful. Client may need additional support at this time.

Collaborative

ACTIONS/INTERVENTIONS	RATIONALE
Perform comprehensive nutritional assessment to determine calorie, nutrient, and vitamin/supplement requirements for individual	Intake can be calculated by several different formulas, but weight reduction is based on the basal caloric requirement for 24 hr depending on client's sex, age, current/desired weight, and length of time estimated to achieve desired weight. *Note:* Standard tables are subject to error when applied to individual situations, and circadian rhythms/lifestyle patterns need to be considered.
Provide medications as indicated:	
Appetite-suppressant drugs; e.g., diethylpropion (Tenuate), mazindol (Sanorex), sibutramine (Meridia);	May be used with caution/supervision at the beginning of a weight-loss program to support client during stress of behavioral/lifestyle changes. They are effective for only a few weeks and may cause problems of dependence in some people.
Hormonal therapy; e.g., thyroid (Euthroid), levothyroxine (Synthroid);	May be necessary when hypothyroidism is present. When no deficiency is present, replacement therapy is not helpful and may actually be harmful. *Note:* Other hormonal treatments, such as human chorionic gonadrotropin (hCG), although widely publicized, have no documented evidence of value.
Orlistat (Xenical);	Lipase inhibitor blocks absorption of approximately 30% of dietary fat. Facilitates weight loss/maintenance when used in conjunction with a reduced-calorie diet. Also reduces risk of regaining after weight loss.
Vitamin, mineral supplements.	Obese individuals have large fuel reserves but are often deficient in vitamins and minerals. *Note:* Use of Xenical inhibits absorption of water-soluble vitamins and β-carotene. Vitamin supplement should be given at least 2 hr before or after Xenical.
Hospitalize for fasting regimen and/or stabilization of medical problems when indicated.	Aggressive therapy/support may be necessary to initiate weight loss, although fasting is not generally a treatment of choice. Client can be monitored more effectively in a controlled setting to minimize complications such as postural hypotension, anemia, cardiac irregularities, and decreased uric acid excretion with hyperuricemia.

ACTIONS/INTERVENTIONS	RATIONALE
Prepare for surgical interventions; e.g., gastric partitioning/bypass as indicated.	These interventions may be necessary to help the client lose weight when obesity is life-threatening. (Refer to CP: Obesity: Surgical Interventions.)

NURSING DIAGNOSIS: sedentary Lifestyle

May be related to

Lack of interest/motivation, resources
Lack of training or knowledge of specific exercise needs
Safety concerns/fear of injury

Possibly evidenced by

Demonstrates physical deconditioning
Chooses a daily routine lacking physical exercise

DESIRED OUTCOMES/EVALUATION CRITERIA—CLIENT WILL:

KNOWLEDGE: Prescribed Activity (NOC)

Verbalize understanding of importance of regular exercise to weight loss/general well-being.
Identify necessary precautions/safety concerns and self-monitoring techniques.
Formulate realistic exercise program with gradual increase in activity.

ACTIONS/INTERVENTIONS	RATIONALE
Exercise Promotion (NIC)	
Independent	
Review necessity for/benefits of regular exercise.	Exercise furthers weight loss by reducing appetite, increasing energy, toning muscles, enhancing cardiac fitness, sense of well-being, and accomplishment.
Determine current activity level and plan progressive exercise program (e.g., walking) tailored to the individual's goals and choice.	Commitment on the part of the client enables the setting of more realistic goals and adherence to the plan.
Identify barriers (perceived and actual) to exercise.	Lack of resources for proper apparel (e.g., supportive shoes, comfortable clothing), safe place to walk, facility/membership for water aerobics decreases likelihood of individual adhering to specific program. In addition, fear of discrimination or ridicule by others may limit client's willingness to exercise in public.
Discuss appropriate warm-up exercises, cool-down activities, and specific techniques to avoid injury.	Preventing muscle injuries allows client to stay active. Time spent recuperating from exercise-induced injuries may result in relapse to sedentary habits.
Determine optimal exercise heart rate. Demonstrate proper technique to monitor pulse and signs/symptoms requiring modification of activity.	Promotes safety as client exercises to tolerance, not peer pressure.
Identify alternatives to chosen activity program to accommodate weather, travel, and so on.	Promotes continuation of program.

ACTIONS/INTERVENTIONS	RATIONALE
Discuss use of mechanical devices/equipment for weight reduction.	Fat loss occurs on a generalized overall basis, and there is no evidence that spot reducing or mechanical devices aid in weight loss in specific areas; however, specific types of exercise or equipment may be useful in toning specific body parts.
Recommend keeping a graph of activity as exercise program advances.	Provides visual record of progress and positive reinforcement for efforts.
Suggest client identify an exercise "buddy."	Provides support and companionship, increasing likelihood of adherence to program.
Encourage involvement in social activities that are not centered on food; e.g., bike ride/nature hike, attending musical event, group sporting activities.	Activities/exercise use calories to help maintain desired weight. Also provides opportunity for pleasure and relaxation without "temptation."

Collaborative

Involve physical therapist/exercise physiologist in developing progressive program.	Facilitates development of an appropriate program of activities that are geared to obese individual, considers impact of client's weight on ability to perform specific activities and safety concerns.

NURSING DIAGNOSIS: disturbed Body Image/chronic low Self-Esteem

May be related to

Biophysical/psychosocial factors such as client's view of self (slimness is valued in this society, and mixed messages are received when thinness is stressed); changes in health status/body image, personal identity
Family/subculture encouragement of overeating
Perceived failure at ability to control weight
Control, sex, and love issues

Possibly evidenced by

Verbalization of negative feelings about body (mental image often does not match physical reality)
Fear of rejection/reaction by others
Feelings of hopelessness/powerlessness
Preoccupation with change (attempts to lose weight)
Lack of follow-through with diet plan
Verbalization of powerlessness to change eating habits

DESIRED OUTCOMES/EVALUATION CRITERIA—CLIENT WILL:

Body Image (NOC)

Verbalize a more realistic self-image.
Demonstrate some acceptance of self as is rather than an idealized image.

Self-Esteem (NOC)

Seek information and actively pursue appropriate weight loss.
Acknowledge self as an individual who has responsibility for self.

ACTIONS/INTERVENTIONS	RATIONALE
Body Image Enhancement (NIC)	
Independent	
Determine client's view of being fat and what it does for the individual.	Mental image includes our ideal and is usually not up-to-date. Fat and compulsive eating behaviors may have deep-rooted psychologic implications (e.g., compensation for lack of love and nurturing or a defense against intimacy). In addition, chronically obese client may report long-term discrimination in family, social and professional settings. She/he may experience mixed feelings of fear and shame, or compensate for psychologic trauma by developing a strong (big) personality.
Promote open communication avoiding criticism/judgment about client's behavior.	Supports client's own responsibility for weight loss, enhances sense of control, and promotes willingness to discuss difficulties/setbacks and problem-solve. *Note:* Distrust and accusations of "cheating" on caloric intake are not helpful.
Outline and clearly state responsibilities of client and nurse.	It is helpful for each individual to understand area of own responsibility in the program so that misunderstandings do not arise.
Graph weight on a weekly basis.	Provides ongoing visual evidence of weight changes (reality orientation).
Ensure availability of properly sized equipment (e.g., gowns; blood pressure cuff; wide/strong wheelchair, bed, commode; transfer devices) when providing inpatient care.	Healthcare providers have a moral and legal obligation to meet the client's needs for comfort and safety.
Encourage client to use imagery to visualize self at desired weight and to practice handling of new behaviors.	Mental rehearsal is very useful in helping the client plan for and deal with anticipated change in self-image or occasions that may arise (family gatherings, special dinners) where constant decisions about eating many foods will occur.
Provide information about the use of makeup, hairstyles, and ways of dressing to maximize figure assets.	Enhances feelings of self-esteem, promotes improved body image.
Encourage buying clothes instead of food treats as a reward for weight loss, life successes.	Properly fitting clothes enhance the body image as small losses are made and the individual feels more positive. Waiting until the desired weight loss is reached can become discouraging.
Suggest the client dispose of "fat clothes" as weight loss occurs.	Removes the "safety valve" of having clothes available "in case" the weight is regained. Retaining fat clothes can convey the message that the weight loss will not occur/be maintained.
Be alert to myths the client/SO may have about weight and weight loss.	Beliefs about what an ideal body looks like or unconscious motivations can sabotage efforts to lose weight. Some of these include the feminine thought of "If I become thin, men will view me as a sexual object"; the masculine counterpart, "I don't trust myself to stay in control of my sexual feelings"; as well as issues of strength, power, or the "good cook" image.
Help staff be aware of and deal with own feelings when caring for client.	Judgmental attitudes, feelings of disgust, anger, and weariness can interfere with care/be transmitted to client, reinforcing negative self-concept/image.
Self-Esteem Enhancement (NIC)	
Identify basic sense of self-esteem, image client has of existential, physical, psychologic self. Determine locus of control.	Provides insight into view of self as fat and own ability to control weight. Information necessary to determine individual needs and treatment plan.

ACTIONS/INTERVENTIONS	RATIONALE
Determine client perception of threat to self.	Client's perception of problem weight poses is more important than what the threat really is and needs to be dealt with before reality can be addressed.
Provide privacy during care activities.	Individual knows size makes it hard to care for her or him and usually is sensitive/self-conscious about body.
Have client recall coping patterns related to food in family of origin and explore how these may affect current situation.	Parents act as role models for the child. Maladaptive coping patterns (overeating) are learned within the family system and are supported through positive reinforcement. Food may be substituted by the parent for affection and love, and eating is associated with a feeling of satisfaction, becoming the primary defense.
Determine relationship history and possibility of sexual abuse.	May contribute to current issues of self-esteem/patterns of coping.
Identify client's motivation for weight loss and assist with goal setting.	The individual may harbor repressed feeling of hostility, which may be expressed inward on the self. Because of a poor self-concept, the person often has difficulty with relationships. *Note:* When losing weight for someone else, the client is less likely to be successful/maintain weight loss.
Assist client to identify feelings that lead to compulsive eating. Encourage journaling.	Awareness of emotions that lead to overeating can be the first step in behavior change (e.g., people often eat because of depression, anger, and guilt).
Develop strategies for doing something besides eating for dealing with these feelings; e.g., talking with a friend.	Replacing eating with other activities helps retrain old patterns and establish new ways to deal with feelings.

Collaborative

Refer to community support and/or therapy group.	Support groups can provide companionship, enhance motivation, decrease loneliness and social ostracism, and give practical solutions to common problems. Group therapy can be helpful in dealing with underlying psychologic concerns.

NURSING DIAGNOSIS: impaired Social Interaction

May be related to

Verbalized or observed discomfort in social situations
Self-concept disturbance

Possibly evidenced by

Reluctance to participate in social gatherings
Verbalization of a sense of discomfort with others

DESIRED OUTCOMES/EVALUATIONS CRITERIA—CLIENT WILL:

Social Involvement (NOC)

Verbalize awareness of feelings that lead to poor social interactions.
Become involved in achieving positive changes in social behaviors and interpersonal relationships.

ACTIONS/INTERVENTIONS	RATIONALE
Socialization Enhancement (NIC)	
Independent	
Review family patterns of relating and social behaviors.	Social interaction is primarily learned within the family of origin. When inadequate patterns are identified, actions for change can be instituted.
Encourage client to express feelings and perceptions of problems.	Helps identify and clarify reasons for difficulties in interacting with others; e.g., may feel unloved/unlovable or insecure about sexuality.
Assess client's use of coping skills and defense mechanisms.	May have coping skills that will be useful in the process of weight loss. Defense mechanisms used to protect the individual may contribute to feelings of aloneness/isolation.
Have client list behaviors that cause discomfort.	Identifies specific concerns and suggests actions that can be taken to effect change.
Involve in role playing new ways to deal with identified behaviors/situations.	Practicing these new behaviors enables the individual to become comfortable with them in a safe situation.
Discuss negative self-concepts and self-talk; e.g., "No one wants to be with a fat person," "Who would be interested in talking to me?"	May be impeding positive social interactions.
Encourage use of positive self-talk such as telling one-self "I am OK," or "I can enjoy social activities and do not need to be controlled by what others think or say."	Positive strategies enhance feelings of comfort and support efforts for change.
Collaborative	
Refer for ongoing family or individual therapy as indicated.	Client benefits from involvement of SO to provide support and encouragement.

NURSING DIAGNOSIS: deficient Knowledge [Learning Need] regarding condition, prognosis, treatment, self care, and discharge needs

May be related to

Lack of/misinterpretation of information
Lack of interest in learning, lack of recall
Inaccurate/incomplete information presented

Possibly evidenced by

Statements of lack of/request for information about obesity and nutritional requirements
Verbalization of problem with weight reduction
Inadequate follow-through with previous diet and exercise instructions

DESIRED OUTCOMES/EVALUATION CRITERIA—CLIENT WILL:

KNOWLEDGE: Diet (NOC)

Verbalize understanding of need for lifestyle changes to maintain/control weight.
Establish individual goal and plan for attaining that goal.
Begin to look for information about nutrition and ways to control weight.

ACTIONS/INTERVENTIONS	RATIONALE
TEACHING: Prescribed Diet (NIC)	
Independent	
Determine level of nutritional knowledge and what client believes is most urgent need.	Necessary to know what additional information to provide. When client's views are listened to, trust is enhanced.
Identify individual holistic long-term goals for health (e.g., lowering blood pressure, controlling serum lipid and glucose levels).	A high relapse rate at 5-year follow-up suggests obesity cannot be reliably reversed/cured. Shifting the focus from initial weight loss/percentage of body fat to overall wellness may enhance rehabilitation.
Provide information about ways to maintain satisfactory food intake in settings away from home.	"Smart" eating when dining out or when traveling helps individual manage weight while still enjoying social outlets.
Identify other sources of information; e.g., books, tapes, community classes, groups.	Using different avenues of accessing information furthers client's learning. Involvement with others who are also losing weight can provide support.
Emphasize necessity of continued follow-up care/counseling, especially when plateaus occur.	As weight is lost, changes in metabolism occur, interfering with further loss by creating a plateau as the body activates a survival mechanism, attempting to prevent "starvation." This requires new strategies and aggressive support to continue weight loss.
Discuss use of medications; advise client to discuss with physician/pharmacist any additions to regimen (e.g., OTC medications, antibiotics, herbal supplements).	Obesity can alter the pharmacokinetic properties of medications. Changes in dosages may be needed based on the degree to which drugs are absorbed (drugs can be subtherapeutic or toxic) or dangerous side effects/interactions that might occur.
Instruct client about risk of deep vein thrombosis (DVT) and self-care (e.g., ankle exercises, walking to limit of ability, reporting any unusual discomfort in legs).	Very obese client is at higher risk for DVT and pulmonary embolism than general population because of immobility, stasis, and polycythemia related to chronic respiratory insufficiency.
Discuss necessity of good skin care, especially in skin folds (e.g., abdomen, breasts, groin, perineal areas) during hot weather and times of immobility or following exercise.	Client is at risk for developing pressure ulcers and can be prone to yeast infections Frequent skin care (e.g., cleansing and drying the tissues, using antifungal creams in skin folds) can prevent skin breakdown.
Identify alternative ways to "reward" self/family for accomplishments or to provide solace.	Reduces likelihood of relying on food to deal with feelings.

POTENTIAL CONSIDERATIONS following acute hospitalization (dependent on client's age, physical condition/presence of complications, personal resources, and life responsibilities) in addition to above nursing diagnoses

ineffective Therapeutic Regimen Management—complexity of therapeutic regimen, perceived seriousness/benefits, mistrust of regimen and/or health care personnel, excessive demands made on individual, family conflict.

OBESITY: SURGICAL INTERVENTIONS (GASTRIC PARTITIONING/GASTROPLASTY, GASTRIC BYPASS)

Weight-reduction (bariatric) surgery has been reported to improve several comorbid conditions associated with morbid obesity, such as sleep apnea, glucose intolerance and diabetes, hypertension, and hyperlipidemia. A number of surgical treatments have been tried and discarded because of ineffectiveness or complications. The procedures of choice are *gastric restriction* (by means of stapling or banding) or *gastric restriction and malabsorption* (gastric bypass or roux-en-Y gastric bypass). Procedures may be performed via open abdominal incision or laparoscopy.

Gastroplasty (gastric stapling/banding): A small pouch with a restricted outlet is created across the stomach just distal to the gastroesophageal junction. A small opening remains through which food passes into stomach. *Vertical banded gastroplasty* (VBG) is accomplished by placing rows of staples vertically in the strongest sidewall of the stomach and insertion of a polypropylene band around the outlet of the resulting pouch. Postoperatively, food is digested normally and the risk of anemia or vitamin deficiencies is lower than with gastric bypass.

Gastric bypass (roux-en-Y): Anastomosis of a segment of the small intestine to the upper portion of the stomach creates a small stomach pouch that has been partitioned by a horizontal staple line or banding. Postoperatively, food bypasses 90% of the stomach, the duodenum, and a portion of the jejunum, so fewer calories are absorbed.

CARE SETTING

Inpatient acute surgical unit

RELATED CONCERNS

Eating disorders: obesity, page 393
Peritonitis, page 355
Psychosocial aspects of care, page 770
Surgical intervention, page 788
Thrombophlebitis: deep vein thrombosis, page 108

(Refer to Endocrine Disorders: Obesity Database for additional assessment information.)

Client Assessment Database

ACTIVITY/REST

May report: Difficulty sleeping
Exertional discomfort, inability to participate in desired activity/sports

EGO INTEGRITY

May report: Motivated to lose weight for oneself (or for gratification of others)
History of psychiatric illness/treatment

May exhibit: Anxiety, depression

ELIMINATION

May report: Urinary stress incontinence

FOOD/FLUID

May report: "Yo-yo" dieting, years of failed dieting
Weight fluctuations
Dysfunctional eating patterns

May exhibit: Weight exceeding ideal body weight by 100 lb or more, or a body mass index (BMI) of more than 40% (morbid obesity)

HYGIENE

May report: Difficulty dressing, bathing

TEACHING/LEARNING

May report: Presence of chronic conditions (hypertension, diabetes, heart failure, arthritis, sleep apnea, pickwickian syndrome, infertility)
Adequate trials and failure of other treatment approaches
Desire to lose weight

Discharge plan considerations: May require support with therapeutic regimen/weight loss, assistance with self-care, homemaker/maintenance tasks

Refer to section at end of plan for postdischarge considerations.

DIAGNOSTIC STUDIES

Studies depend on individual situation and are used to rule out underlying disease and provide a preoperative workup, including psychiatric evaluation.

NURSING PRIORITIES

1. Support respiratory function.
2. Prevent/minimize complications.
3. Provide appropriate nutritional intake.
4. Provide information regarding surgical procedure, postoperative expectations, and treatment needs.

DISCHARGE GOALS

1. Ventilation and oxygenation adequate for individual needs.
2. Complications prevented/controlled.
3. Nutritional intake modified for specific procedure.
4. Procedure, prognosis, and therapeutic regimen understood.
5. Plan in place to meet needs after discharge.

NURSING DIAGNOSIS: ineffective Breathing Pattern

May be related to

Decreased lung expansion
Pain, anxiety
Decreased energy, fatigue
Tracheobronchial obstruction

Possibly evidenced by

Shortness of breath, dyspnea
Tachypnea, respiratory depth changes, reduced vital capacity
Wheezes, rhonchi
Abnormal arterial blood gases (ABGs)

DESIRED OUTCOMES/EVALUATION CRITERIA—CLIENT WILL:

RESPIRATORY STATUS: Ventilation (NOC)

Maintain adequate ventilation.
Experience no cyanosis or other signs of hypoxia, with ABGs within acceptable range.

ACTIONS/INTERVENTIONS	RATIONALE
Ventilation Assistance (NIC)	
Independent	
Monitor respiratory rate/depth. Auscultate breath sounds. Investigate presence of pallor/cyanosis, increased restlessness, or confusion.	Respirations may be shallow because of incisional pain, analgesia, immobility, and obesity itself, causing hypoventilation and potentiating risk of atelectasis and hypoxia. *Note:* Many anesthetic agents are fat soluble, so that postoperative "resedation" and the potential for respiratory complications are increased.
Elevate head of bed 30–45 degrees.	Encourages optimal diaphragmatic excursion/lung expansion and minimizes pressure of abdominal contents on the thoracic cavity. *Note:* When kept recumbent, obese clients are at high risk for severe hypoventilation postoperatively.
Encourage deep-breathing exercises. Assist with coughing and splint incision.	Promotes maximal lung expansion and aids in clearing airways, thus reducing risk of atelectasis, pneumonia. *Note*: Use of abdominal binder (properly fitted and placed at least 2 inches below the xiphoid process) can encourage deep breathing.
Turn periodically and ambulate as early as possible.	Promotes aeration of all segments of the lung, mobilizing and aiding movement of secretions. *Note*: If client was a good candidate for bariatric surgery, she or he was probably relatively healthy before operation, and is usually able to turn self, walk, and transfer to chair within 8 hr of surgery.

ACTIONS/INTERVENTIONS	RATIONALE
Pad side rails and teach client to use them as armrests.	Using the side rail as an armrest allows for greater chest expansion.
Use small pillow under head when indicated.	Many obese clients have large, thick necks, and use of large, fluffy pillows may obstruct the airway.

Collaborative

ACTIONS/INTERVENTIONS	RATIONALE
Administer supplemental oxygen.	Maximizes available O_2 for exchange and reduces work of breathing.
Assist in use of intermittent positive-pressure breathing (IPPB) and/or respiratory adjuncts; e.g., incentive spirometer.	Enhances lung expansion; reduces potential for atelectasis.
Monitor/graph serial ABGs/pulse oximetry when indicated.	Reflects ventilation/oxygenation and acid-base status. Used as a basis for evaluating need for/effectiveness of respiratory therapies.
Monitor client-controlled analgesia (PCA)/administer analgesics as appropriate.	Maintenance of comfort level enhances participation in respiratory therapy and promotes increased lung expansion.

NURSING DIAGNOSIS: risk for ineffective peripheral Tissue Perfusion

Risk factors may include

Diminished blood flow, hypovolemia
Immobility/bedrest
Interruption of venous blood flow (thrombosis)

Possibly evidenced by

[Not applicable; presence of signs and symptoms establishes an *actual* diagnosis.]

DESIRED OUTCOMES/EVALUATION CRITERIA—CLIENT WILL:

Circulation Status (NOC)

Maintain perfusion as individually appropriate; e.g., skin warm/dry, peripheral pulses present/strong, vital signs within acceptable range.

Risk Control (NOC)

Identify causative/risk factors.
Demonstrate behaviors to improve/maintain circulation.

ACTIONS/INTERVENTIONS — RATIONALE

Surveillance (NIC)

Independent

ACTIONS/INTERVENTIONS	RATIONALE
Monitor vital signs, palpate peripheral pulses routinely, evaluate capillary refill and changes in mentation. Note 24-hr fluid balance.	Indicators of circulatory adequacy. (Refer to ND: risk for deficient Fluid Volume, following.)
Encourage frequent range-of-motion (ROM) exercises for legs and ankles. Maintain schedule of sequential compression devices (SCD) on lower extremities when used.	Stimulates circulation in the lower extremities, reduces high risk complications associated with venous stasis (e.g., DVT and PE).
Assess for redness, edema, and discomfort in calf.	Indicators of thrombus formation, but warning signs may not always be present in obese individuals.

ACTIONS/INTERVENTIONS	RATIONALE
Encourage early ambulation, discourage sitting and/or dangling legs at the bedside.	Sitting constricts venous flow, whereas walking encourages venous return.
Provide adequate/appropriate equipment (e.g., trapeze for turning, transfer device, walker, wheelchair) and sufficient staff for handling client.	Helpful in dealing with obese client for moving and ambulating. Reduces risk of traumatic injury to both client and caregivers.
Evaluate for complications; e.g., rigid abdomen, nonincisional abdominal pain, fever, tachycardia, low blood pressure.	Although rare, client can develop abdominal complications, (e.g., abdominal compartment syndrome, sepsis/septic shock secondary to anastomotic leak or wound infection) requiring intensive interventions/return to surgery.

Collaborative

Administer heparin therapy as indicated.	May be used prophylactically to reduce risk of thrombus formation or to treat thromboemboli.
Monitor hemoglobin (Hb)/hematocrit (Hct) and coagulation studies.	Provides information about circulatory volume/alterations in coagulation and indicates therapy needs/effectiveness.

NURSING DIAGNOSIS: risk for deficient Fluid Volume

Risk factors may include

Excessive gastric losses: nasogastric suction, diarrhea
Reduced intake

Possibly evidenced by

[Not applicable; presence of signs and symptoms establishes an *actual* diagnosis.]

DESIRED OUTCOMES/EVALUATION CRITERIA—CLIENT WILL:

Hydration (NOC)

Maintain adequate fluid volume with balanced intake and output (I&O) and be free of signs reflecting dehydration.

ACTIONS/INTERVENTIONS	RATIONALE
Fluid/Electrolyte Management (NIC)	
Independent	
Assess vital signs, noting changes in BP (postural), tachycardia, fever. Assess skin turgor, capillary refill, and moisture of mucous membranes.	Indicators of dehydration/hypovolemia, adequacy of current fluid replacement. *Note:* Adequately-sized cuff must be used to ensure factual measurement of BP. If cuff is too small, reading will be falsely elevated.
Monitor I&O, measuring nasogastric (NG) suction losses.	Changes in gastric capacity/intestinal motility and nausea greatly influence intake and fluid needs, increasing risk of dehydration.
Evaluate muscle strength/tone. Observe for muscle tremors.	Large gastric losses may result in decreased magnesium and calcium, leading to neuromuscular weakness/tetany.
Establish individual needs/replacement schedule.	Determined by amount of measured losses/estimated insensible losses and dependent on gastric capacity.
Encourage increased oral intake when able.	Permits discontinuation of invasive fluid support measures and contributes to return of normal bowel functioning.

ACTIONS/INTERVENTIONS	RATIONALE
Collaborative	
Administer IV fluids as indicated.	Replaces fluid losses and restores fluid balance in immediate postoperative phase and/or until client is able to take sufficient oral fluids.
Monitor electrolyte levels and replace as indicated.	Use of NG tube and/or vomiting, onset of diarrhea can deplete electrolytes, affecting organ function.

NURSING DIAGNOSIS: risk for imbalanced Nutrition: less than body requirements

Risk factors may include

Decreased intake, dietary restrictions, early satiety
Increased metabolic rate/healing
Malabsorption of nutrients/impaired absorption of vitamins

Possibly evidenced by

[Not applicable; presence of signs and symptoms establishes an *actual* diagnosis.]

DESIRED OUTCOMES/EVALUATION CRITERIA—CLIENT WILL:

KNOWLEDGE: Diet (NOC)

Identify individual nutritional needs.

Nutritional Status (NOC)

Display behaviors to maintain adequate nutritional intake.
Demonstrate appropriate weight loss with normalization of laboratory values.

ACTIONS/INTERVENTIONS	RATIONALE
Weight Reduction Assistance (NIC)	
Independent	
Establish hourly intake schedule. Measure/provide food and fluids in amount specified.	After gastric restriction procedures, stomach capacity is reduced to approximately 50 mL, necessitating frequent/small feedings. Ultimately, management of optimal nutrition depends on reducing the amount of food/fluid (e.g., 1 oz of fluid or 300 calories) passing through the gastrointestinal (GI) system at one time.
Instruct in how to sip and eat slowly.	Increases satiety and reduces risk of dehydration.
Stress importance of being aware of satiety and stopping intake.	Overeating may cause nausea/vomiting or damage partitioning.
Require that client sit up to drink/eat.	Reduces possibility of aspiration.
Determine foods that are gas forming and eliminate them from diet.	May cause nausea and interfere with appetite/digestion, restricting nutritional intake.
Discuss food preferences with client and include those foods in pureed diet when possible.	May enhance intake, promote sense of participation/control.
Weigh on regular schedule.	Monitors losses and aids in assessing nutritional needs/effectiveness of therapy.

ACTIONS/INTERVENTIONS	RATIONALE
Collaborative	
Provide liquid diet, advancing intake as prescribed.	Provides nutrients without exceeding calorie limits *Note:* Liquid diet is usually maintained for 8 wk after partitioning procedure.
Refer to dietitian/multidisciplinary team.	Provides assistance in planning a diet that meets nutritional needs, as well as offering individualized treatment and support.
Administer vitamin supplements and vitamin B_{12} injections, folate, and calcium as indicated.	Supplements may be needed for life to prevent anemia because absorption is impaired. Increased intestinal motility following bypass procedure lowers calcium level and increases absorption of oxalates, which can lead to urinary stone formation.

NURSING DIAGNOSIS: actual and risk for impaired Skin Integrity

May be related to

Trauma/surgery, difficulty in approximation of suture line of fatty tissue
Reduced vascularity, altered circulation
Altered nutritional state: obesity

Possibly evidenced by (actual)

Disruption of skin surface, altered healing

DESIRED OUTCOMES/EVALUATION CRITERA—CLIENT WILL:

WOUND HEALING: Primary Intention (NOC)

Display timely wound healing without complication.
Demonstrate behaviors to reduce tension on suture line.

ACTIONS/INTERVENTIONS	RATIONALE
Wound Care (NIC)	
Independent	
Support and instruct client in incisional support when turning, coughing, deep breathing, and ambulating.	Reduces possibility of dehiscence and incisional hernia.
Observe incisions periodically, noting approximation of wound edges, hematoma formation and resolution, presence of bleeding/drainage.	Verifies status of healing, provides for early detection of developing complications requiring prompt evaluation and influencing choice of interventions.
Provide routine incisional care, being careful to keep dressing dry and sterile. Assess/maintain patency of drains.	Promotes healing. Accumulation of serosanguineous drainage in subcutaneous layers increases tension on suture line, may delay wound healing, and serves as a medium for bacterial growth.
Skin Surveillance (NIC)	
Encourage frequent positional change, inspect pressure points, and massage gently as indicated. Apply transparent skin barrier to elbows/heels.	Reduces pressure on skin, promoting peripheral circulation and reducing risk of skin breakdown. Skin barrier reduces risk of shearing injury.
Provide meticulous skin care, pay particular attention to skin folds.	Moisture or excoriation enhances growth of bacteria that can lead to postoperative infection.

ACTIONS/INTERVENTIONS	RATIONALE
Collaborative	
Provide foam/air mattress or kinetic therapy as indicated.	Reduces skin pressure and enhances circulation.

NURSING DIAGNOSIS: risk for Infection

Risk factors may include

Inadequate primary defenses: broken/traumatized tissues, decreased ciliary action, stasis of body fluids

Invasive procedures

Possibly evidenced by

[Not applicable; presence of signs and symptoms establishes an *actual* diagnosis.]

DESIRED OUTCOMES/EVALUATION CRITERIA—CLIENT WILL:

IMMOBILITY CONSEQUENCES: Physiological (NOC)

Be free of nosocomial infection.

WOUND HEALING: Primary Intention (NOC)

Achieve timely wound healing free of signs of local or generalized infectious process.

ACTIONS/INTERVENTIONS	RATIONALE
Infection Protection (NIC)	
Independent	
Emphasize/model proper hand-washing technique.	Prevents spread of bacteria, cross-contamination.
Maintain aseptic technique in dressing changes, invasive procedures.	Reduces risk of nosocomial infection.
Inspect surgical incisions/invasive sites for erythema, purulent drainage.	Early detection of developing infection provides for prevention of more serious complications.
Encourage frequent position changes, deep breathing, coughing, use of respiratory adjuncts; e.g., incentive spirometer.	Promotes mobilization of secretions, reducing risk of pneumonia.
Provide routine catheter care/encourage good perineal care.	Prevents ascending bladder infections.
Encourage client to drink acid-ash juices, such as cranberry.	Maintains urine acidity to retard bacterial growth.
Observe for reports of abdominal pain (especially after third postoperative day), elevated temperature, increased white blood cell (WBC) count.	Suggests possibility of developing peritonitis.
Collaborative	
Apply topical antimicrobials/antibiotics as indicated.	Reduces bacterial or fungal colonization on skin, prevents infection in wound.
Administer IV antibiotics as indicated.	A prophylactic antibiotic regimen is usually standard in these clients to reduce risk of perioperative contamination and/or peritonitis.

ACTIONS/INTERVENTIONS	RATIONALE
Obtain specimen of purulent drainage/sputum for culture and sensitivity.	Identifies infectious agent, aids in choice of appropriate therapy.

NURSING DIAGNOSIS: Diarrhea

May be related to

Rapid transit of food through shortened small intestine
Changes in dietary fiber and bulk
Inflammation, irritation, and malabsorption of bowel

Possibly evidenced by

Loose, liquid stools, increased frequency
Increased/hyperactive bowel sounds

DESIRED OUTCOMES/EVALUATION CRITERIA—CLIENT WILL:

TREATMENT BEHAVIOR: Illness or Injury (NOC)

Verbalize understanding of causative factors and rationale of treatment regimen.
Follow through with treatment recommendations.

Bowel Elimination (NOC)

Regain near-normal bowel function.

ACTIONS/INTERVENTIONS — RATIONALE

Diarrhea Management (NIC)

Independent

ACTIONS/INTERVENTIONS	RATIONALE
Observe/record stool frequency, characteristics, and amount.	Diarrhea often develops after resumption of diet because of shortened transit time through the GI tract and/or dumping syndrome. This condition is usually self-limiting, but can cause discomfort and social difficulties when persistent.
Encourage diet high in fiber/bulk within dietary limitations, with moderate fluid intake as diet resumes.	Increases consistency of the effluent. Although fluid is necessary for optimal body function, excessive amounts contribute to diarrhea.
Restrict fat intake as indicated.	Low-fat diet reduces risk of steatorrhea and limits laxative effect of decreased fat absorption.
Observe for signs of dumping syndrome; e.g., instant diarrhea, sweating, nausea, and weakness after eating.	Rapid emptying of food from the stomach may result in gastric distress and alter bowel function.
Assist with frequent perianal care, using ointments as indicated. Provide whirlpool bath.	Anal irritation, excoriation, and pruritus occur because of diarrhea. The client often cannot reach the area for proper cleansing and may be embarrassed to ask for help.

Collaborative

ACTIONS/INTERVENTIONS	RATIONALE
Administer medications as indicated; e.g., diphenoxylate with atropine [Lomotil]).	Antidiarrheals may be necessary to control frequency of stools until body adjusts to changes in function brought about by surgery.
Monitor serum electrolytes.	Large gastric losses potentiate the risk of electrolyte imbalance, which can lead to more serious/life-threatening complications.

NURSING DIAGNOSIS: deficient Knowledge [Learning Need] regarding condition, prognosis, treatment, self-care, and discharge needs

May be related to

Lack of exposure, unfamiliarity with resources
Information misinterpretation
Lack of recall

Possibly evidenced by

Questions, request for information
Statement of misconceptions
Inaccurate follow-through of instructions
Development of preventable complications

DESIRED OUTCOMES/EVALUATION CRITERIA—CLIENT WILL:

KNOWLEDGE: Disease Process (NOC)

Verbalize understanding of surgical procedure, potential complications, and postoperative expectations.

KNOWLEDGE: Treatment Regimen (NOC)

Verbalize understanding of therapeutic needs and rationale for actions.
Initiate necessary lifestyle changes and participate in treatment regimen.

ACTIONS/INTERVENTIONS	RATIONALE
TEACHING: Disease Process (NIC)	
Independent	
Review specific surgical procedure and postoperative expectations.	Provides knowledge base from which informed choices can be made and goals formulated. Initial weight loss is rapid, with client often losing half of the total weight loss during the first 6 months. Weight loss then gradually stabilizes over a 2-year period.
Address concerns about altered body size/image.	Anticipation of problems can be helpful in dealing with situations that arise. (Refer to CP: Eating Disorders: Obesity, ND: disturbed Body Image/ chronic low Self-Esteem.) *Note:* Feelings that often occur during more conventional weight loss therapies generally are not encountered in the surgically treated client.
Review medication regimen, dosage, and side effects.	Knowledge may enhance cooperation with therapeutic regimen and maintenance of schedule.
Recommend avoidance of alcohol.	May contribute to liver/pancreatic dysfunction.
Discuss responsibility for self-care with client/SO.	Full cooperation is important for successful outcome after procedure.
Stress importance of regular medical follow-up, including laboratory studies, and discuss possible health problems.	Periodic assessment/evaluation (e.g., over 3–12 months) promotes early recognition/prevention of such complications as liver dysfunction, malnutrition, electrolyte imbalances, and kidney stones, which may develop following bypass procedure.
Encourage progressive exercise/activity program balanced with adequate rest periods.	Promotes weight loss, enhances muscle tone, and minimizes postoperative complications while preventing undue fatigue.

ACTIONS/INTERVENTIONS	RATIONALE
Review proper eating habits; e.g., eat small amounts of food slowly and chew well, sit at table in calm/relaxed environment, eat only at prescribed times, avoid between-meal snacking, do not "make up" skipped feedings.	Focuses attention on eating, increasing awareness of intake and feelings of satiety.
Avoid fluid intake 30 min before/after meals and use of carbonated beverages.	May cause gastric fullness/gaseous distention, limiting intake of food.
Identify signs of hypokalemia; e.g., diarrhea, muscle cramps/weakness of lower extremities, weak/irregular pulse, dizziness with position changes.	Increasing dietary intake of potassium (e.g., milk, coffee, potatoes, carrots, bananas, oranges) may correct deficit, preventing serious respiratory/cardiac complications.
Discuss symptoms that may indicate dumping syndrome; e.g., weakness, profuse perspiration, nausea, vomiting, faintness, flushing, and epigastric discomfort or palpitations occurring during or immediately following meals. Problem-solve solutions.	Generally occurring in early postoperative period (1–3 weeks), syndrome is usually self-limiting but may become chronic and require medical intervention.
Review symptoms requiring medical evaluation; e.g., persistent nausea/vomiting, abdominal distention/tenderness, change in pattern of bowel elimination, fever, purulent wound drainage, excessive weight loss or plateauing/weight gain.	Early recognition of developing complications allows for prompt intervention, preventing serious outcome.
Refer to community support groups.	Involvement with others who have dealt with same problems enhances coping; may promote cooperation with therapeutic regimen and long-term positive recovery.

POTENTIAL CONSIDERATIONS following acute hospitalization (dependent on client's age, physical condition/presence of complications, personal resources, and life responsibilities)

risk for imbalanced Nutrition: more than body requirements—dysfunctional eating patterns, observed use of food as reward/comfort measure, history of morbid obesity.

Refer to Potential Considerations in Surgical Intervention plan of care.

DIABETES MELLITUS/DIABETIC KETOACIDOSIS

There are more than 14 million Americans diagnosed with *diabetes mellitus* (DM). It affects 20% of people over the age of 65 years, and approximately 625,000 new cases of diabetes are diagnosed annually in the general population. Conditions or situations known to exacerbate glucose/insulin imbalance include (1) previously undiagnosed or newly diagnosed type I diabetes, (2) food intake in excess of available insulin, (3) adolescence and puberty, (4) exercise in uncontrolled diabetes, and (5) stress associated with illness, infection, trauma, or emotional distress. Type I diabetes can be complicated by instability and *diabetic ketoacidosis* (DKA). DKA is a life-threatening emergency caused by a relative or absolute deficiency of insulin.

CARE SETTINGS

Although DKA may be encountered in any setting and mild DKA may be managed at the community level, severe metabolic imbalance requires inpatient acute care on a medical unit.

RELATED CONCERNS

Amputation, page 657
Fluid and electrolyte imbalances, page 919
Metabolic acidosis (primary base bicarbonate deficiency), page 492
Psychosocial aspects of care, page 770

Client Assessment Database

Data depend on the severity and duration of metabolic imbalance, length/stage of diabetic process, and effects on other organ function.

ACTIVITY/REST

May report: Sleep/rest disturbances
Weakness, fatigue, difficulty walking/moving
Muscle cramps, decreased muscle strength

May exhibit: Tachycardia and tachypnea at rest or with activity
Lethargy/disorientation, coma
Decreased muscle strength/tone

CIRCULATION

May report: History of hypertension; acute myocardial infarction (MI)
Claudication, numbness, tingling of extremities (long-term effects)
Leg ulcers, slow healing

May exhibit: Tachycardia
Postural BP changes; hypertension
Decreased/absent pulses
Dysrhythmias
Crackles; jugular venous distention (JVD) (if heart failure present)
Hot, dry, flushed skin; sunken eyeballs

EGO INTEGRITY

May report: Stress; dependence on others
Life stressors including financial concerns related to condition

May exhibit: Anxiety, irritability

ELIMINATION

May report: Change in usual voiding pattern (polyuria), nocturia
Pain/burning, difficulty voiding (infection or neurogenic bladder), recent/recurrent urinary tract infection (UTI)
Abdominal tenderness, bloating
Diarrhea

May exhibit: Pale, yellow, dilute urine; polyuria (may progress to oliguria/anuria if severe hypovolemia occurs)
Cloudy, odorous urine (infection)
Abdomen firm, distended
Bowel sounds diminished or hyperactive (diarrhea)

FOOD/FLUID

May report: Loss of appetite, nausea/vomiting
Not following prescribed diet, increased intake of glucose/carbohydrates
Weight loss over a period of days/weeks
Thirst
Use of medications exacerbating dehydration, such as diuretics

May exhibit: Dry/cracked skin, poor skin turgor
Abdominal rigidity/distention
Thyroid may be enlarged (increased metabolic needs with increased blood sugar)
Halitosis/sweet, fruity odor (acetone breath)

NEUROSENSORY

May report: Fainting spells/dizziness
Headaches
Tingling, numbness, weakness in muscles
Visual disturbances

May exhibit: Confusion/disorientation; drowsiness, lethargy, stupor/coma (later stages)
Memory impairment (recent, remote)
Deep tendon reflexes (DTRs) decreased (coma)
Seizure activity (late stages of DKA or hypoglycemia)

PAIN/DISCOMFORT

May report: Abdominal bloating/pain (mild/severe)

May exhibit: Facial grimacing with palpation; guarding

RESPIRATION

May report: Air hunger (late stages of DKA)
Cough, with/without purulent sputum (infection)

May exhibit: Increased respiratory rate (tachypnea), deep, rapid (Kussmaul's) respirations (metabolic acidosis)
Rhonchi, wheezes
Yellow or green sputum (infection)

SAFETY

May report: Dry, itching skin, skin ulcerations
Paresthesia (diabetic neuropathy)

May exhibit: Fever, diaphoresis
Skin breakdown, lesions/ulcerations
Decreased general strength/ROM
Weakness/paralysis of muscles, including respiratory musculature (if potassium levels are markedly decreased)

SEXUALITY

May report: Vaginal discharge (prone to infection)
Problems with impotence (men); orgasmic difficulty (women)

TEACHING/LEARNING

May report: Familial risk factors: diabetes mellitus, heart disease, strokes, hypertension
Slow/delayed healing
Use of drugs; e.g., steroids, thiazide diuretics, phenytoin (Dilantin), and phenobarbital (can increase glucose levels)
May/may not be taking diabetic medications as ordered

Discharge plan considerations: May need assistance with dietary regimen, medication administration/supplies, self-care, glucose monitoring

Refer to section at end of plan for postdischarge considerations.

DIAGNOSTIC STUDIES

Serum glucose: DKA is defined as glucose greater than 250 mg/dL in association with an arterial pH of less than 7.30 or serum bicarbonate of less than 15 mEq/L and ketonemia (serum ketones).
Fatty acids: Lipids, triglycerides, and cholesterol levels elevated.
Serum osmolality: Elevated but usually less than 330 mOsm/L.
Glucagon: Elevated level is associated with conditions that produce (1) actual hypoglycemia, (2) relative lack of glucose (e.g., trauma, infection), or (3) lack of insulin. Therefore, glucagon may be elevated with severe DKA despite hyperglycemia.
A_{1C} (glycosylated hemoglobin/HbA1c): Currently, the gold standard for measuring glycemic control, the A_{1c} reflects client's overall blood glucose during past 8–12 wk, with the previous 2 wk most heavily weighted. Useful in differentiating inadequate control versus incident-related DKA (e.g., current upper respiratory infection [URI]). A result greater than 8% represents average blood glucose of 200+ mg/dL and signals a need for changes in treatment.
Serum insulin: May be decreased/absent (type I) or normal to high (type II), indicating insulin insufficiency/improper utilization (endogenous/exogenous). Insulin resistance may develop secondary to formation of antibodies.
Electrolytes:
Sodium: May be normal, elevated, or decreased.
Potassium: Normal or falsely elevated (cellular shifts), then markedly decreased.
Phosphorus: Frequently decreased.
Arterial blood gases (ABGs): Usually reflect low pH and decreased HCO_3 (metabolic acidosis) with compensatory respiratory alkalosis.
CBC: Hct may be elevated (dehydration); leukocytosis suggests hemoconcentration, response to stress or infection.
BUN: May be normal or elevated (dehydration/decreased renal perfusion).
Serum amylase: May be elevated, indicating acute pancreatitis as cause of DKA.
Thyroid function tests: Increased thyroid activity can increase blood glucose and insulin needs.
Urine: Urine glucose correlates poorly with blood glucose, being dependent on renal glucose threshold (150–300 mg/dL) and should be used only if measuring of blood glucose is not possible (or as a confirmatory test). Ketones should be self-monitored during febrile illness or when DKA symptoms are present (e.g., nausea, vomiting, abdominal pain). In DKA, urine tests are positive for glucose and ketones; specific gravity and osmolality may be elevated.
Cultures and sensitivities: Possible UTI, respiratory or wound infections.

NURSING PRIORITIES

1. Restore fluid/electrolyte and acid-base balance.
2. Correct/reverse metabolic abnormalities.
3. Identify/assist with management of underlying cause/disease process.
4. Prevent complications.
5. Provide information about disease process/prognosis, self-care, and treatment needs.

DISCHARGE GOALS

1. Homeostasis achieved.
2. Causative/precipitating factors corrected/controlled.
3. Complications prevented/minimized.
4. Disease process/prognosis, self-care needs, and therapeutic regimen understood.
5. Plan in place to meet needs after discharge.

NURSING DIAGNOSIS: deficient Fluid Volume [specify]

May be related to

Osmotic diuresis (from hyperglycemia)
Excessive gastric losses: diarrhea, vomiting
Restricted intake: nausea, confusion

Possibly evidenced by

Increased urinary output, dilute urine
Weakness; thirst, sudden weight loss
Dry skin/mucous membranes, poor skin turgor
Hypotension, tachycardia, delayed capillary refill

DESIRED OUTCOMES/EVALUATION CRITERIA—CLIENT WILL:

Fluid Balance (NOC)

Demonstrate adequate hydration as evidenced by stable vital signs, palpable peripheral pulses, good skin turgor and capillary refill, individually appropriate urinary output, and electrolyte levels within normal range.

ACTIONS/INTERVENTIONS	RATIONALE
Fluid/Electrolyte Management (NIC)	
Independent	
Obtain history from client/SO related to duration/intensity of symptoms such as vomiting, excessive urination.	Assists in estimation of total volume depletion. Symptoms may have been present for varying amounts of time (hours to days). Presence of infectious process results in fever and hypermetabolic state, increasing insensible fluid losses.
Monitor vital signs:	
Note orthostatic BP changes;	Hypovolemia may be manifested by hypotension and tachycardia. Estimates of severity of hypovolemia may be made when client's systolic BP drops more than 10 mm Hg from a recumbent to a sitting/standing position. *Note:* Cardiac neuropathy may block reflexes that normally increase heart rate.

ACTIONS/INTERVENTIONS	RATIONALE
Respiratory pattern; e.g., Kussmaul's respirations, acetone breath;	Lungs remove carbonic acid through respirations, producing a compensatory respiratory alkalosis for ketoacidosis. Acetone breath is due to breakdown of acetoacetic acid and should diminish as ketosis is corrected. Although fever is a common precipitating factor for DKA, clients may be normothermic or hypothermic because of peripheral vasodilation.
Respiratory rate and quality; use of accessory muscles, periods of apnea, and appearance of cyanosis;	Correction of hyperglycemia and acidosis will cause the respiratory rate and pattern to approach normal. In contrast, increased work of breathing; shallow, rapid respirations; and presence of cyanosis may indicate respiratory fatigue and/or that client is losing ability to compensate for acidosis.
Temperature, skin color/moisture.	Although fever, chills, and diaphoresis are common with infectious process, fever with flushed, dry skin may reflect dehydration.
Assess peripheral pulses, capillary refill, skin turgor, and mucous membranes.	Indicators of level of hydration, adequacy of circulating volume.
Monitor I&O, note urine specific gravity.	Provides ongoing estimate of volume replacement needs, kidney function, and effectiveness of therapy.
Weigh daily.	Provides the best assessment of current fluid status and adequacy of fluid replacement.
Maintain fluid intake of at least 2500 mL/day within cardiac tolerance when oral intake is resumed.	Maintains hydration/circulating volume.
Promote comfortable environment. Cover client with light sheets.	Avoids overheating, which could promote further fluid loss.
Investigate changes in mentation/sensorium.	Changes in mentation can be due to abnormally high or low glucose, electrolyte abnormalities, acidosis, decreased cerebral perfusion, or developing hypoxia. Regardless of the cause, impaired consciousness can predispose client to aspiration.

Collaborative

ACTIONS/INTERVENTIONS	RATIONALE
Administer fluids as indicated:	
Isotonic (0.9%) or lactated Ringer's solution without additives;	Type and amount of fluid depend on degree of deficit and individual client response. *Note:* Client with DKA is often severely dehydrated, and commonly needs 5–10 L of isotonic saline (2–3 L within first 2 hr of treatment).
Albumin, plasma, dextran.	Plasma expanders may occasionally be needed if the deficit is life threatening/BP does not normalize with rehydration efforts.
Insert/maintain indwelling urinary catheter.	Provides for accurate/ongoing measurement of urinary output, especially if autonomic neuropathies result in neurogenic bladder (urinary retention/overflow incontinence). May be removed when client is stable to reduce risk of infection.
Monitor laboratory studies; e.g.:	
Hct;	Assesses level of hydration and is often elevated because of hemoconcentration associated with osmotic diuresis.
BUN/creatinine (Cr);	Elevated values may reflect cellular breakdown from dehydration or signal the onset of renal failure.
Serum osmolality;	Elevated because of hyperglycemia and dehydration.
Sodium;	May be decreased, reflecting shift of fluids from the intracellular compartment (osmotic diuresis). High sodium values reflect severe fluid loss/dehydration or sodium reabsorption in response to aldosterone secretion.

ACTIONS/INTERVENTIONS	RATIONALE
Potassium.	Initially, hyperkalemia occurs in response to metabolic acidosis, but as this potassium is lost in the urine, the absolute potassium level in the body is depleted. As insulin is replaced and acidosis is corrected, serum potassium deficit becomes apparent.
Administer potassium and other electrolytes via IV and/or by oral route as indicated.	Potassium should be added to the IV (as soon as urinary flow is adequate) to prevent hypokalemia. *Note:* Potassium phosphate may be drug of choice when IV fluids contain sodium chloride in order to prevent chloride overload. Phosphate concentrations tend to decrease with insulin therapy.
Administer bicarbonate if indicated (e.g., if pH is less than 7.1).	Not routinely necessary, and given with caution to help correct acidosis in the presence of hypotension or shock, lactic acidosis, or severe hyperkalemia.
Insert NG tube and attach to suction as indicated.	Decompresses stomach and may relieve vomiting.

NURSING DIAGNOSIS: imbalanced Nutrition: less than body requirements

May be related to

Insulin deficiency: decreased uptake/utilization of glucose by the tissues (resulting in increased protein/fat metabolism), omitting insulin (especially with young people in an effort to decrease weight)
Decreased oral intake: anorexia, nausea, gastric fullness, abdominal pain; eating disorders, altered consciousness
Hypermetabolic state: release of stress hormones (e.g., epinephrine, cortisol, and growth hormone), infectious process

Possibly evidenced by

Increased urinary output, dilute urine
Reported inadequate food intake, lack of interest in food
Recent weight loss, weakness, fatigue, poor muscle tone
Diarrhea
Increased ketones (endproduct of fat metabolism)

DESIRED OUTCOMES/EVALUATION CRITERIA—CLIENT WILL:

Nutritional Status (NOC)

Ingest appropriate amounts of calories/nutrients.
Display usual energy level.
Demonstrate stabilized weight or gain toward usual/desired range with normal laboratory values.

ACTIONS/INTERVENTIONS	RATIONALE
Hyperglycemia Management (NIC)	
Independent	
Weigh daily or as indicated.	Assesses adequacy of nutritional intake (absorption and utilization). *Note*: Eating disorders are a contributing factor in 20% of recurrent DKA in young clients.
Ascertain client's dietary program and usual pattern; compare with recent intake.	Identifies deficits and deviations from therapeutic needs.

ACTIONS/INTERVENTIONS	RATIONALE
Auscultate bowel sounds. Note reports of abdominal pain/bloating, nausea, vomiting of undigested food. Maintain nothing by mouth (NPO) status as indicated.	Hyperglycemia and fluid and electrolyte disturbances can decrease gastric motility/function (distension or ileus), affecting choice of interventions. *Note:* Long-term difficulties with decreased gastric emptying and poor intestinal motility suggest autonomic neuropathies affecting the GI tract and requiring symptomatic treatment.
Provide liquids containing nutrients and electrolytes as soon as client can tolerate oral fluids; progress to more solid food as tolerated.	Oral route is preferred when client is alert and bowel function is restored.
Identify food preferences, including ethnic/cultural needs.	Incorporating as many of the client's food preferences into the meal plan as possible increases cooperation with dietary guidelines after discharge.
Include SO in meal planning as indicated.	Promotes sense of involvement; provides information for SO to understand nutritional needs of client. *Note:* Various methods available for dietary planning include carbohydrate counting, exchange list, point system, or preselected menus.
Observe for signs of hypoglycemia; e.g., changes in level of consciousness, cool/clammy skin, rapid pulse, hunger, irritability, anxiety, headache, lightheadedness, shakiness.	Once carbohydrate metabolism resumes (blood glucose level reduced) and as insulin is being adjusted, hypoglycemia can occur. If client is comatose, hypoglycemia may occur without notable change in level of consciousness (LOC). This potentially life-threatening emergency should be assessed and treated quickly per protocol. *Note:* Type I diabetics of long standing may not display usual signs of hypoglycemia because normal response to low blood sugar may be diminished.

Collaborative

ACTIONS/INTERVENTIONS	RATIONALE
Perform fingerstick glucose testing.	Bedside analysis of serum glucose is more accurate (displays current levels) than monitoring urine sugar, which is not sensitive enough to detect fluctuations in serum levels and can be affected by client's individual renal threshold or the presence of urinary retention/renal failure. *Note:* Some studies have found that urine glucose of 20% may be correlated to blood glucose of 140–360 mg/dL.
Monitor laboratory studies; e.g., serum glucose, acetone, pH, HCO_3.	Blood glucose will decrease slowly with controlled fluid replacement and insulin therapy. With the administration of optimal insulin dosages, glucose can then enter the cells and be used for energy. When this happens, acetone levels decrease and acidosis is corrected.
Administer rapid-acting insulins (e.g., regular [Humulin R], lispro [Humalog], aspart [Novalog]) by intermittent or continuous IV method; e.g., IV bolus followed by a continuous drip via pump of approximately 5–10 U/hr so that glucose is reduced by 50–75 mg/dL/hr.	Rapid-acting insulins are used in hyperglycemic crisis. The IV route is the initial route of choice because absorption from subcutaneous tissues may be erratic. Many believe the continuous method is the optimal way to facilitate transition to carbohydrate metabolism and reduce incidence of hypoglycemia. *Note:* Intermediate (NPH, Humulin N, Lente) and long-acting insulins (e.g., Ultralente, protamine zinc insulin [PZI], glargine) may be part of the client's usual or added insulin, but are not part of crisis hyperglycemic treatment.
Administer glucose solutions; e.g., 5% dextrose and half-normal saline.	Glucose solutions may be added after insulin and fluids have brought the blood glucose to approximately 400 mg/dL. As carbohydrate metabolism approaches normal, care must be taken to avoid hypoglycemia.
Consult with dietitian for resumption of oral intake.	Useful in calculating and adjusting diet to meet client's needs; answer questions and assist client/SO in developing meal plans.

ACTIONS/INTERVENTIONS	RATIONALE
Provide diet of approximately 60% carbohydrates, 20% proteins, 20% fats in designated number of meals/snacks.	Complex carbohydrates (e.g., corn, peas, carrots, broccoli, dried beans, oats, apples) decrease glucose levels/insulin needs, reduce serum cholesterol levels, and promote satiation. Food intake is scheduled according to specific insulin characteristics (e.g., peak effect) and individual client response. *Note:* A snack at bedtime (HS) of complex carbohydrates is especially important (if insulin is given in divided doses) to prevent hypoglycemia during sleep and potential Somogyi response.
Administer other medications as indicated; e.g., metoclopramide (Reglan), erythromycin.	May be useful in treating symptoms related to autonomic neuropathies affecting GI tract, thus enhancing oral intake and absorption of nutrients.

NURSING DIAGNOSIS: risk for Infection, [sepsis]

Risk factors may include

High glucose levels, decreased leukocyte function, alterations in circulation
Preexisting respiratory infection, or UTI

Possibly evidenced by

[Not applicable; presence of signs and symptoms establishes an *actual* diagnosis.]

DESIRED OUTCOMES/EVALUATION CRITERIA—CLIENT WILL:

KNOWLEDGE: Infection Control (NOC)

Identify interventions to prevent/reduce risk of infection.
Demonstrate techniques, lifestyle changes to prevent development of infection.

Infection Control (NIC)

Independent

ACTIONS/INTERVENTIONS	RATIONALE
Observe for signs of infection and inflammation; e.g., fever, flushed appearance, wound drainage, purulent sputum, cloudy urine.	Client may be admitted with infection, which could have precipitated the ketoacidotic state, or may develop a nosocomial infection.
Promote good hand washing by staff and client.	Reduces risk of cross-contamination.
Maintain aseptic technique for IV insertion procedure, administration of medications, and providing site care. Rotate IV sites as indicated.	High glucose in the blood creates an excellent medium for bacterial growth.
Provide catheter/perineal care. Teach the female client to clean from front to back after elimination.	Minimizes risk of UTI. Comatose client may be at particular risk if urinary retention occurred before hospitalization. *Note:* Elderly female diabetic clients are especially prone to urinary tract/vaginal yeast infections. Many UTIs are asymptomatic, possibly related to neurogenic bladder.
Provide conscientious skin care, gently massage bony areas, keep the skin dry, keep linens dry and wrinkle-free.	Peripheral circulation may be impaired, placing client at increased risk for skin irritation/breakdown and infection.
Auscultate breath sounds.	Rhonchi indicate accumulation of secretions possibly related to pneumonia/bronchitis (may have precipitated the DKA). Pulmonary congestion/edema (crackles) may result from rapid fluid replacement/HF.

ACTIONS/INTERVENTIONS	RATIONALE
Place in semi-Fowler's position.	Facilitates lung expansion, reduces risk of aspiration.
Reposition and encourage coughing/deep breathing if client is alert and cooperative. Otherwise, suction airway, using sterile technique, as needed.	Aids in ventilating all lung areas and mobilizing secretions. Prevents stasis of secretions with increased risk of infection.
Provide tissues and trash bag in a convenient location for sputum and other secretions. Instruct client in proper handling of secretions.	Minimizes spread of infection.
Encourage/assist with oral hygiene.	Reduces risk of oral/gum disease.
Encourage adequate dietary and fluid intake (at least 2500 mL/day if not contraindicated by cardiac or renal dysfunction), including 8 oz of cranberry juice per day as appropriate.	Decreases susceptibility to infection. Increased urinary flow prevents stasis and aids in maintaining urine pH/acidity, reducing bacteria growth and flushing organisms out of system. *Note:* Use of cranberry juice can help prevent bacteria from adhering to the bladder wall, reducing the risk of recurrent UTI.

Collaborative

Obtain specimens for culture and sensitivities as indicated.	Identifies organism(s) so that most appropriate drug therapy can be instituted.
Administer antibiotics as appropriate.	Early treatment may help prevent sepsis.

NURSING DIAGNOSIS: risk for disturbed Sensory Perception, (specify)

Risk factors may include

Endogenous chemical alteration: glucose/insulin and/or electrolyte imbalance

Possibly evidenced by

[Not applicable; presence of signs and symptoms establishes an *actual* diagnosis.]

DESIRED OUTCOMES/EVALUATION CRITERIA—CLIENT WILL:

Neurologic Status (NOC)

Maintain usual level of mentation.
Recognize and compensate for existing sensory impairments.

ACTIONS/INTERVENTIONS — RATIONALE

Neurologic Monitoring (NIC)

Independent

ACTIONS/INTERVENTIONS	RATIONALE
Monitor vital signs and mental status.	Provides a baseline from which to compare abnormal findings; e.g., fever may affect mentation.
Address client by name; reorient as needed to place, person, time, and situation. Give short explanations, speaking slowly and enunciating clearly.	Decreases confusion and helps maintain contact with reality.
Schedule nursing time to provide for uninterrupted rest periods.	Promotes restful sleep, reduces fatigue, and may improve cognition.
Keep client's routine as consistent as possible. Encourage participation in activities of daily living (ADLs) as able.	Helps keep client in touch with reality and maintain orientation to the environment.

ACTIONS/INTERVENTIONS	RATIONALE
Protect client from injury (avoid/limit use of restraints as able, place bed in low position) when cognition is impaired. Pad bed rails if client is prone to seizures.	Disoriented client is prone to injury, especially at night, and precautions need to be taken as indicated. Seizure precautions reduce risk of physical injury.
Evaluate visual acuity as indicated.	Retinal edema/detachment, hemorrhage, presence of cataracts or temporary paralysis of extraocular muscles may impair vision, requiring corrective therapy and/or supportive care.
Investigate reports of hyperesthesia, pain, or sensory loss in the feet/legs. Look for ulcers, reddened areas, pressure points, loss of pedal pulses.	Peripheral neuropathies may result in severe discomfort, lack of/distortion of tactile sensation, potentiating risk of dermal injury and impaired balance. *Note:* Mononeuropathy affects a single nerve (most often femoral or cranial), causing sudden pain and loss of motor/sensory function along affected nerve path.
Provide bed cradle. Keep hands/feet warm, avoiding exposure to cool drafts/hot water or use of heating pad.	Reduces discomfort and potential for dermal injury. *Note:* Sudden development of cold hands/feet may reflect hypoglycemia, suggesting need to evaluate serum glucose level.
Assist with ambulation/position changes.	Promotes client safety, especially when sense of balance is affected.

Collaborative

Carry out prescribed regimen for correcting DKA as indicated.	Alteration in thought processes/potential for seizure activity is usually alleviated once hyperosmolar state is corrected.
Monitor laboratory values; e.g., blood glucose, serum osmolality, Hb/Hct, BUN/Cr.	Imbalances can impair mentation. *Note:* If fluid is replaced too quickly, excess water may enter brain cells and cause alteration in the level of consciousness (water intoxication).

NURSING DIAGNOSIS: Fatigue

May be related to

Decreased metabolic energy production
Altered body chemistry: insufficient insulin
Increased energy demands: hypermetabolic state/infection

Possibly evidenced by

Overwhelming lack of energy, inability to maintain usual routines, decreased performance, accident-prone
Impaired ability to concentrate, listlessness, disinterest in surroundings

DESIRED OUTCOMES/EVALUATION CRITERIA—CLIENT WILL:

Endurance (NOC)

Verbalize increase in energy level.
Display improved ability to participate in desired activities.

ACTIONS/INTERVENTIONS — RATIONALE

Energy Management (NIC)

Independent

ACTIONS/INTERVENTIONS	RATIONALE
Discuss with client the need for activity. Plan schedule with client and identify activities that lead to fatigue.	Education may provide motivation to increase activity level even though client may feel too weak initially.
Alternate activity with periods of rest/uninterrupted sleep.	Prevents excessive fatigue.

ACTIONS/INTERVENTIONS	RATIONALE
Monitor pulse, respiratory rate, and BP before/after activity.	Indicates physiologic levels of tolerance.
Discuss ways of conserving energy while bathing, transferring, and so on.	Client will be able to accomplish more with a decreased expenditure of energy.
Increase client participation in ADLs as tolerated.	Increases confidence level/self-esteem and tolerance level. *Note:* Elderly clients may experience a "lag effect" in which exercise may precipitate hypoglycemia as late as 24 hr after exercising, leading to extensive fatigue and muscle tremors.

NURSING DIAGNOSIS: Powerlessness

May be related to

Long-term/progressive illness that is not curable
Dependence on others

Possibly evidenced by

Reluctance to express true feelings, expressions of having no control/influence over situation
Apathy, withdrawal, anger
Does not monitor progress, nonparticipation in care/decision making
Depression over physical deterioration/complications despite client cooperation with regimen

DESIRED OUTCOMES/EVALUATION CRITERIA—CLIENT WILL:

HEALTH BELIEFS: Perceived Control (NOC)

Acknowledge feelings of helplessness.
Identify healthy ways to deal with feelings.
Assist in planning own care and independently take responsibility for self-care activities.

ACTIONS/INTERVENTIONS	RATIONALE
Self-Responsibility Facilitation (NIC)	
Independent	
Encourage client/SO to express feelings about hospitalization and disease in general.	Identifies concerns and facilitates problem-solving.
Acknowledge normality of feelings.	Recognition that reactions are normal can help client problem-solve and seek help as needed. Diabetic control is a full-time job that serves as a constant reminder of both presence of condition and threat to client's health/life.
Assess how client has handled problems in the past, identify locus of control.	Knowledge of individual's style helps determine needs for treatment goals. Client whose locus of control is internal usually looks at ways to gain control over own treatment program. Client who operates with an external locus of control wants to be cared for by others and may project blame for circumstances onto external factors.
Provide opportunity for SO to express concerns and discuss ways in which he or she can be helpful to client.	Enhances sense of being involved and gives SO a chance to problem-solve solutions to help client prevent recurrence.

ACTIONS/INTERVENTIONS	RATIONALE
Ascertain expectations/goals of client and SO.	Unrealistic expectations/pressure from others or self may result in feelings of frustration/loss of control and may impair coping abilities. *Note:* Even with rigid adherence to medical regimen, complications/setbacks may occur.
Determine whether a change in relationship with SO has occurred.	Constant energy and thought required for diabetic control often shifts the focus of a relationship. Development of psychologic concerns/visceral neuropathies affecting self-concept (especially sexual role function) may add further stress.
Encourage client to make decisions related to care; e.g., ambulation, time for activities, and so forth.	Communicates to client that some control can be exercised over care.
Support participation in self-care and give positive feedback for efforts.	Promotes feeling of control over situation.

NURSING DIAGNOSIS: deficient Knowledge [Learning Need] regarding disease, prognosis, treatment, self-care, and discharge needs

May be related to

Lack of exposure/recall, information misinterpretation
Unfamiliarity with information resources

Possibly evidenced by

Questions/request for information, verbalization of the problem
Inaccurate follow-through of instructions, development of preventable complications

DESIRED OUTCOMES/EVALUATION CRITERIA—CLIENT WILL:

KNOWLEDGE: Diabetes Management (NOC)

Verbalize understanding of disease process, potential complications.
Identify relationship of signs/symptoms to the disease process and correlate symptoms with causative factors.
Correctly perform necessary procedures and explain reasons for the actions.
Initiate necessary lifestyle changes and participate in treatment regimen.

ACTIONS/INTERVENTIONS	RATIONALE
Learning Facilitation (NIC)	
Independent	
Create an environment of trust by listening to concerns, being available.	Rapport and respect need to be established before client will be willing to take part in the learning process.
Work with client in setting mutual goals for learning.	Participation in the planning promotes enthusiasm and cooperation with the principles learned.
Select a variety of teaching strategies; e.g., demonstrate needed skills and have client do return demonstration, incorporate new skills into the hospital routine.	Use of different means of accessing information promotes learner retention.

ACTIONS/INTERVENTIONS	RATIONALE
TEACHING: Disease Process (NIC)	
Discuss essential elements; e.g.:	
What the normal blood glucose range is and how it compares with client's level, the type of diabetes the client has, the relationship between insulin deficiency and a high glucose level;	Provides knowledge base from which client can make informed lifestyle choices.
Reasons for the ketoacidotic episode;	Knowledge of the precipitating factors may help avoid recurrences.
Acute and chronic complications of the disease, including visual disturbances, neurosensory and cardiovascular changes, renal impairment, hypertension.	Awareness helps client be more consistent with care and may prevent/delay onset of complications.
Demonstrate fingerstick testing, or similar (e.g., palm or armstick, or continuous glucose monitoring system [Glucowatch]), and have client/SO return demonstration until proficient. Instruct client to check urine ketones if glucose is higher than 250 mg/dL.	Self-monitoring of blood glucose four or more times a day allows flexibility in self-care, promotes tighter control of serum levels (e.g., 60–150 mg/dL), and may prevent/delay development of long-term complications. *Note:* Various new devices have been released or are in testing. Some use a laser perforator instead of a sharp lancet, others are bloodless. In addition to glucose levels, several devices can measure glycosylated albumin (fructosamine) in the home, providing a measure of blood glucose control over the past 7–10 days.
Discuss dietary plan, limiting intake of sugar, fat, salt, and alcohol; eating complex carbohydrates, especially those high in fiber (fruits, vegetables, whole grains); and ways to deal with meals outside the home.	Medical nutrition therapy for diabetes encourages client to make meal choices based on individual unique needs and preferences. Awareness of importance of dietary control aids client in planning meals/sticking to regimen. Fiber can slow glucose absorption, decreasing fluctuations in serum levels, but may cause GI discomfort, increase flatus, and affect vitamin/mineral absorption.
Review medication regimen, including onset, peak, and duration of prescribed insulin, as applicable, with client/SO.	Understanding all aspects of drug usage promotes proper use. Dose algorithms are created, taking into account drug dosages established during inpatient evaluation, usual amount and schedule of physical activity, and meal plan. Including SO provides additional support/resource for client.
Review client's type of basal insulin (e.g., lente, NPH, ultralente, glargine [Lantus]) and bolus insulin (e.g., regular, lispro, aspart [Novolog]) as indicated. Review self-administration of insulin (e.g., injection or pump) and care of equipment. Have client demonstrate procedure (e.g., drawing up and injecting insulin, insulin pen technique, or use of continuous pump).	Verifies understanding and correctness of procedure. Identifies potential problems (e.g., vision, memory, and so on) so that alternative solutions can be found for insulin administration. *Note:* If multiple daily injections are required, combinations of rapid acting plus short acting, intermediate, and new long-acting insulin Lantus are used. Lantus has a minimal peak and is used as basal insulin with rapid action at meal. If the pump method is used, client programs his or her own basal and bolus settings. Only rapid-acting insulin, Humalog or Novolog, is administered, with a basal dose throughout the day and bolus doses before meals and as needed. An insulin pump more closely mimics normal pancreatic activity because the basal rate may be changed relative to client's activity level, presence of stressors/infection or menstrual cycle.
Discuss timing of insulin injection and mealtime.	One of the many inconveniences people with diabetes cope with is having to decide at least 30–60 min in advance when they are going to have a meal for the timely administration of regular human injections. A newer product, insulin lispro (Humalog), or aspart (Novolog) may be helpful because it works best when taken within 15 min of eating. With the onset twice as fast as regular human insulin and a duration approximately half as long, Humalog/ Novolog closely mimics pancreatic activity. However, hypoglycemia may develop more rapidly and be more severe than with use of regular insulin. A blood glucose level below 80 mg/dL indicates that insulin should be injected after eating rather than before the meal.

ACTIONS/INTERVENTIONS	RATIONALE
Review individual's target blood glucose levels.	Although this range varies per person, the ideal range for the adult diabetic is considered to be 80–120 mg/dL. *Note:* Clients with an insulin pump may maintain blood glucose levels between 120 mg/dL and 200 mg/dL with no urinary ketones.
Stress importance and necessity of maintaining diary of glucose testing, medication dose/time, dietary intake, activity, feelings/sensations, life events.	Aids in creating overall picture of client situation to achieve better disease control, and promotes self-care/independence.
Discuss factors that play a part in diabetic control; e.g., exercise (aerobic versus isometric), stress, surgery, and illness. Review "sick day" rules.	This information promotes diabetic control and can greatly reduce the occurrence of ketoacidosis. *Note:* Aerobic exercise (e.g., walking, swimming) promotes effective use of insulin, lowering glucose levels, and strengthens the cardiovascular system. A "sick day" management plan helps maintain equilibrium during illness, minor surgery, severe emotional stress, exogenous steroids (e.g., as with spinal or joint injections or any oral treatment for asthma, arthritis) or any condition that might send glucose spiraling upward.
Review effects of smoking on insulin use. Encourage cessation of smoking.	Nicotine constricts the small blood vessels, and insulin absorption is delayed for as long as these vessels remain constricted. *Note:* Insulin absorption may be reduced by as much as 30% below normal in the first 30 min after smoking.
Establish regular exercise/activity schedule and identify corresponding insulin concerns.	Exercise times should not coincide with the peak action of insulin. A snack should be ingested before or during exercise as needed, and rotation of injection sites should avoid the muscle group that will be used in the activity (e.g., abdominal site is preferred over thigh/arm before jogging or swimming) to prevent accelerated uptake of insulin.
Identify the symptoms of hypoglycemia (e.g., weakness, dizziness, lethargy, hunger, irritability, diaphoresis, pallor, tachycardia, tremors, headache, changes in mentation) and explain causes.	May promote early detection and treatment, preventing/limiting occurrence. (However, approximately 30% of insulin-dependent clients are asymptomatic when hypoglycemic.) *Note:* Early-morning hyperglycemia may reflect the "dawn phenomenon" (indicating need for additional insulin) or a rebound response to hypoglycemia during sleep (Somogyi effect), requiring a decrease in insulin dosage/change in diet (e.g., HS snack). Testing serum levels at 3 AM aids in identifying the specific problem.
Instruct SO in emergency use of glucagon.	Given for treatment of severe hypoglycemia when client is unable to take oral carbohydrates. Prompt intervention may prevent more serious complications.
Instruct in importance of routine daily examination of the feet and proper foot care. Demonstrate ways to examine feet, inspect shoes for fit, and care for toenails, calluses, and corns. Encourage use of natural fiber stockings.	Prevents/delays complications associated with peripheral neuropathies and/or circulatory impairment, especially cellulitis, gangrene, and amputation. *Note:* Studies show that approximately 15% of all clients with diabetes will develop a foot or leg ulcer during the course of the disease. Also 50% of all nontraumatic lower extremity amputations occur in people with diabetes. Prevention is therefore critical.
Demonstrate/discuss proper use of transcutaneous electrical nerve stimulator (TENS) unit. Identify safety concerns following local nerve block.	May provide relief of discomfort associated with neuropathies.
Stress importance of regular eye examinations, especially for clients who have had type I diabetes for 5 yr or more.	Changes in vision may be gradual and are more pronounced in persons with poorly controlled DM and BP. Problems include changes in visual acuity and may progress to retinopathy and blindness. Note: Retinopathy is the most frequent cause of new blindness among adults 20 to 74 years of age. During the first 2 decades of disease, nearly *all* clients with type I diabetes will have retinopathy.

ACTIONS/INTERVENTIONS	RATIONALE
Arrange for vision aids when needed; e.g., magnifying sleeve for insulin syringe, prefilled insulin pens, large-print instructions, one-touch/talking glucose meters.	Adaptive aids have been developed in recent years to help the visually impaired manage their own DM more effectively.
Discuss sexual functioning and answer questions client/SO may have.	Impotence may be first symptom of onset of DM. *Note:* Counseling and/or use of penile prosthesis may be of benefit.
Stress importance of use of identification bracelet.	Can promote quick entry into the health system and appropriate care with fewer resultant complications in the event of an emergency.
Recommend reading product labels/avoidance of OTC drugs without prior approval of healthcare provider.	These products may contain sugars/interact with prescribed medications.
Discuss importance of follow-up care.	Helps maintain tighter control of disease process and may prevent exacerbations of DM, retarding development of systemic complications.
Review signs/symptoms requiring medical evaluation; e.g., fever, cold, or flu symptoms; cloudy, odorous urine; painful urination; delayed healing of cuts/sores; sensory changes (pain or tingling) of lower extremities; changes in blood sugar level, presence of ketones in urine.	Prompt intervention may prevent development of more serious/life-threatening complications.
Identify community resources; e.g., American Diabetic Association, Internet resources/online diabetes bulletin boards, visiting nurse, weight-loss/stop-smoking clinics, contact person/diabetic instructor.	Continued support is usually necessary to sustain lifestyle changes and promote well-being.

POTENTIAL CONSIDERATIONS following acute hospitalization (dependent on client's age, physical condition/presence of complications, personal resources, and life responsibilities)

ineffective Therapeutic Regimen Management—complexity of therapeutic regimen, economic concerns, perceived susceptibility (recurrence of problem).

disturbed peripheral/visual Sensory Perception—endogenous chemical alternations (elevated glucose level).

HYPERTHYROIDISM (THYROTOXICOSIS, GRAVES' DISEASE)

Hyperthyroidism is a metabolic imbalance that results from overproduction of the thyroid hormones triiodothyronine (T_3) and thyroxine (T_4). The most common form is *Graves' disease*, but other forms of hyperthyroidism include toxic adenoma, thyroid-stimulating hormone (TSH)–secreting pituitary tumor, subacute or silent thyroiditis, and some forms of thyroid cancer.

Thyroid storm (also called *thyrotoxicosis*) is a rarely encountered manifestation of hyperthyroidism that can be precipitated by such events as thyroid ablation (surgical or radioiodine), medication overdosage, and trauma. This condition constitutes a medical emergency.

CARE SETTING

Most people with classic hyperthyroidism rarely need hospitalization. Critically ill clients, those with extreme manifestations of thyrotoxicosis plus a significant concurrent illness, require inpatient acute care on a medical unit.

RELATED CONCERNS

Heart failure: chronic, page 47
Psychosocial aspects of care, page 770
Thyroidectomy, page 437

Client Assessment Database

Data depend on the severity/duration of hormone imbalance and involvement of other organs.

ACTIVITY/REST

May report:	Nervousness, increased irritability, insomnia Muscle weakness, incoordination Extreme fatigue
May exhibit:	Muscle atrophy

CIRCULATION

May report: Palpitations
Chest pain (angina)

May exhibit: Dysrhythmias (atrial fibrillation), gallop rhythm, murmurs
Elevated BP with widened pulse pressure
Tachycardia at rest
Circulatory collapse, shock (thyrotoxic crisis)

ELIMINATION

May report: Urinating in large amounts
Stool changes; diarrhea

EGO INTEGRITY

May report: Recent stressful experience (emotional/physical)

May exhibit: Emotional lability (mild euphoria to delirium); anxiety/depression

FOOD/FLUID

May report: Recent/sudden weight loss
Increased appetite, large meals, frequent meals, thirst
Nausea/vomiting

May exhibit: Enlarged thyroid, goiter
Nonpitting edema, especially in pretibial area

NEUROSENSORY

May exhibit: Rapid and hoarse speech
Mental status and behavior alterations; e.g., confusion, disorientation, nervousness, irritability, delirium, frank psychosis, stupor, coma
Fine tremor in hands; purposeless, quick, jerky movements of body parts
Hyperactive deep tendon reflexes (DTRs)
Paralysis (thyrotoxic hypokalemia)

PAIN/DISCOMFORT

May report: Orbital pain, photophobia (eye movement)

RESPIRATION

May report: Difficulty breathing

May exhibit: Increased respiratory rate, tachypnea
Breath sounds: crackles, wheezes (pulmonary edema associated with thyrotoxic crisis)

SAFETY

May report: Heat intolerance, excessive sweating
Allergy to iodine (may be used in testing)

May exhibit: Elevated temperature (above 100°F), diaphoresis
Skin smooth, warm, and flushed; hair fine, silky, straight
Exophthalmos, lid retraction, conjunctival irritation, tearing
Pruritic, erythematous lesions (often in pretibial area) that become brawny

SEXUALITY

May report: Decreased libido
Hypomenorrhea, amenorrhea
Impotence

TEACHING/LEARNING

May report: Family history of thyroid problems
History of hypothyroidism, thyroid hormone replacement therapy or antithyroid therapy, premature withdrawal of antithyroid drugs, recent partial thyroidectomy
History of insulin-induced hypoglycemia, cardiac disorders or surgery, recent illness (pneumonia), trauma; x-ray contrast studies

Discharge plan considerations: May require assistance with treatment regimen, self-care activities, homemaker/maintenance tasks

Refer to section at end of plan for postdischarge considerations.

DIAGNOSTIC STUDIES

Thyroid hormone blood tests:

Thyroid-stimulating hormone (*TSH*): Test first done to evaluate thyroid function and considered a reliable method of detecting a thyroid problem. TSH is suppressed in hyperthyroidism to < 0.1 μU/mL (except when etiology is a TSH-secreting pituitary tumor or pituitary resistant to thyroid hormone). Hyperthyroidism is indicated if TSH fails to rise after administration of thyrotropin-releasing hormone (TRH). (Normal TSH is 0.4–4.5 milli-international units/liter.)

Tyyroxine (T_4): Produced by the thyroid gland when the pituitary gland releases TSH. Free T_4 can be measured directly (FT_4) or calculated by index (FTI). Total T_4 measures both bound and free T_4. Free T_4 affects tissue function, bound T_4 does not. (Normal total T_4 is 5–12 micrograms per deciliter.) Total T_4, FT_4, and free thyroxine index (FTI) are values used to monitor treatment for hyperthyroidism.

Triiodothyronine (T_3): Small amount produced directly by thyroid gland. Most T_3 is made by other tissues that convert T_4 into T_3. T_4 has a greater effect on metabolism than T_3 even though T_3 is normally present in lower amounts than T_4. Total T_3 measures both bound and free T_3 (FT_3). (Normal total T_3 is 70–195 [nanograms per deciliter].) Both T_3 and T_4 are increased in hyperthyroidism; however, T_3 appears to be the more accurate diagnostic indicator of hyperthyroidism than T_4. T_3 levels become abnormal earlier than T_4 levels, and return to normal later that T_4 in hyperthyroidism.

Triiodothyronine uptake (T_3U): An indirect measurement of the amount of the protein thyroxine-binding globulin (TBG) that can bind T_3 and T_4. A high T_4 value combined with a high T_3U value usually confirms the presence of hyperthyroidism.

Thyroid scan: Differentiates between Graves' disease and Plummer's disease, both of which result in hyperthyroidism.

Radioactive iodine (RAI) uptake test: Used in differential diagnoses; e.g., high in Graves' disease and toxic nodular goiter, low in thyroiditis.

Needle or open biopsy: May be done to determine cause of hyperthyroidism, differentiate cysts or tumors, diagnose enlargement of thyroid gland.

ECG: Atrial fibrillations, shorter systole time, cardiomegaly, heart enlarged with fibrosis and necrosis (late signs or in elderly with masked hyperthyroidism).

Serum glucose: Elevated (related to adrenal involvement).

Plasma cortisol: Low levels (less adrenal reserve).

Alkaline phosphatase and serum calcium: Increased.

Liver function tests: Abnormal.

Electrolytes: Hyponatremia may reflect adrenal response or dilutional effect in fluid replacement therapy. Hypokalemia occurs because of GI losses and diuresis.

Serum catecholamines: Decreased.

Urine creatinine: Increased.

NURSING PRIORITIES

1. Reduce metabolic demands and support cardiovascular function.
2. Provide psychological support.
3. Prevent complications.
4. Provide information about disease process/prognosis and therapy needs.

DISCHARGE GOALS

1. Homeostasis achieved.
2. Client effectively dealing with current situation.
3. Complications prevented/minimized.
4. Disease process/prognosis and therapeutic regimen understood.
5. Plan in place to meet needs after discharge.

NURSING DIAGNOSIS: risk for decreased Cardiac Output

Risk factors may include

Uncontrolled hyperthyroidism, hypermetabolic state
Increasing cardiac workload
Changes in venous return and systemic vascular resistance
Alterations in rate, rhythm, conduction

Possibly evidenced by

[Not applicable; presence of signs and symptoms establishes an *actual* diagnosis.]

DESIRED OUTCOMES/EVALUATION CRITERIA—CLIENT WILL:

Circulatory Status (NOC)

Maintain adequate cardiac output for tissue needs as evidenced by stable vital signs, palpable peripheral pulses, good capillary refill, usual mentation, and absence of dysrhythmias.

ACTIONS/INTERVENTIONS	RATIONALE
Hemodynamic Regulation (NIC)	
Independent	
Monitor BP lying, sitting, and standing, if able. Note widened pulse pressure.	General/orthostatic hypotension may occur as a result of excessive peripheral vasodilation and decreased circulating volume. Widened pulse pressure reflects compensatory increase in stroke volume and decreased systemic vascular resistance (SVR).
Monitor central venous pressure (CVP) if available.	Provides more direct measure of circulating volume and cardiac function.
Investigate reports of chest pain/angina.	May reflect increased myocardial oxygen demands/ ischemia.
Assess pulse/heart rate while client is sleeping.	Provides a more accurate assessment of tachycardia.
Auscultate heart sounds, noting extra heart sounds, development of gallops and systolic murmurs.	Prominent S_1 and murmurs are associated with forceful cardiac output of hypermetabolic state; development of S_3 may warn of impending cardiac failure.
Monitor electrocardiogram (ECG), noting rate/rhythm. Document dysrhythmias.	Tachycardia (greater than normally expected with fever/ increased circulatory demand) may reflect direct myocardial stimulation by thyroid hormone. Dysrhythmias often occur and may compromise cardiac function/output.
Auscultate breath sounds, noting adventitious sounds (e.g., crackles).	Early sign of pulmonary congestion, reflecting developing cardiac failure.
Monitor temperature, provide cool environment, limit bed linens/clothes, administer tepid sponge baths.	Fever (may exceed 104°F) can occur as a result of excessive hormone levels increasing diuresis/dehydration, causing increased peripheral vasodilation, venous pooling, and hypotension.
Observe signs/symptoms of severe thirst, dry mucous membranes, weak/thready pulse, poor capillary refill, decreased urinary output, and hypotension.	Rapid dehydration can occur, which reduces circulating volume and compromises cardiac output.
Record I&O. Note urine specific gravity.	Significant fluid losses (through vomiting, diarrhea, diuresis, diaphoresis) can lead to profound dehydration, concentrated urine, and weight loss.
Weigh daily. Encourage chair rest/bedrest; limit nonessential activity.	Activity increases metabolic/circulatory demands, which may potentiate cardiac failure.
Note history of asthma/bronchoconstrictive disease, sinus bradycardia/heart blocks, advanced HF, or current pregnancy.	Presence/potential recurrence of these conditions affects choice of therapy; e.g., use of β-adrenergic blocking agents is contraindicated.
Observe for adverse side effects of adrenergic antagonists; e.g., severe decrease in pulse, BP; signs of vascular congestion/HF; cardiac arrest.	Indicates need for reduction/discontinuation of therapy.

ACTIONS/INTERVENTIONS	RATIONALE
Collaborative	
Administer IV fluids as indicated.	Rapid fluid replacement may be necessary to improve circulating volume but must be balanced against signs of cardiac failure/need for inotropic support.
Administer medications as indicated:	
β-blockers; e.g., propranolol (Inderal), atenolol (Tenormin), nadolol (Corgard), pindolol (Visken);	Given to control thyrotoxic effects of tachycardia, tremors, and nervousness and is first drug of choice for acute storm. Decreases heart rate/cardiac work by blocking β-adrenergic receptor sites and blocking conversion of T_4 to T_3. *Note:* If severe bradycardia develops, atropine may be required.
Thyroid hormone antagonists; e.g., propylthiouracil (PTU), methimazole (Tapazole);	Antithryroid drugs block thyroid hormone synthesis and inhibit conversion of T_4 to T_3. May be definitive long-term treatment or used to prepare client for surgery; but effect is slow, and will not relieve thyroid storm. *Note:* Once PTU therapy is begun, abrupt withdrawal may precipitate thyroid crisis.
Strong iodine solution (Lugol's solution) or supersaturated potassium iodide (SSKI) orally;	Acts to prevent release of thyroid hormone into circulation by increasing the amount of thyroid hormone stored within the gland. May interfere with RAI treatment and may exacerbate the disease in some people. May be used as surgical preparation to decrease size and vascularity of the gland or to treat thyroid storm. *Note:* Should be started 1–3 hr after initiation of antithyroid drug therapy to minimize hormone formation from the iodine.
RAI ($Na^{131}I$ or $Na^{125}I$) following NRC regulations for radiopharmaceutical;	Radioactive iodine therapy is the treatment of choice for almost all clients with Graves' disease because it destroys abnormally functioning gland tissue. Peak results take 6–12 wk (several treatments may be necessary); however, a single dose controls hyperthyroidism in about 90% of clients. *Note:* This therapy is contraindicated during pregnancy. Also, people preparing or administering the dose must have their own thyroid burden measured, and contaminated supplies and equipment must be monitored and stored until decayed.
Corticosteroids; e.g., dexamethasone (Decadron);	Provides glucocorticol support, decreases hyperthermia, relieves relative adrenal insufficiency, inhibits calcium absorption, and reduces peripheral conversion of T_4 to T_3. *Note:* May be given before thyroidectomy and discontinued after surgery.
Digoxin (Lanoxin);	Digitalization may be required in clients with HF before β-adrenergic blocking therapy can be considered/safely initiated.
Furosemide (Lasix);	Diuresis may be necessary if heart failure (HF) occurs. *Note:* It also may be effective in reducing calcium level if neuromuscular function is impaired.
Potassium (KCl, K-Lyte);	Increased losses of K^+ through intestinal/renal routes may result in dysrhythmias if not corrected.
Acetaminophen (Tylenol);	Drug of choice to reduce temperature and associated metabolic demands. Aspirin is contraindicated because it actually increases level of circulating thyroid hormones by blocking binding of T_3 and T_4 with thyroid-binding proteins.
Sedatives, barbiturates;	Promotes rest, thereby reducing metabolic demands/cardiac workload.
Muscle relaxants.	Reduces shivering associated with hyperthermia, which can further increase metabolic demands.

ACTIONS/INTERVENTIONS	RATIONALE
Monitor laboratory/diagnostic studies as indicated; e.g.:	
Serum potassium;	Hypokalemia resulting from intestinal losses, altered intake, or diuretic therapy may cause dysrhythmias and compromise cardiac function/output. *Note:* In the presence of thyrotoxic paralysis (primarily occurring in Asian men), close monitoring and cautious replacement are indicated because rebound hyperkalemia can occur as condition abates, releasing potassium from the cells.
Serum calcium;	Elevation may alter cardiac contractility.
Sputum culture;	Pulmonary infection is most frequent precipitating factor of crisis.
Serial ECGs;	May demonstrate effects of electrolyte imbalance or ischemic changes reflecting inadequate myocardial oxygen supply in presence of increased metabolic demands.
Chest x-rays.	Cardiac enlargement may occur in response to increased circulatory demands. Pulmonary congestion may be noted with cardiac decompensation.
Provide supplemental O_2 as indicated.	May be necessary to support increased metabolic demands/O_2 consumption.
Provide hypothermia blanket as indicated.	Occasionally used to lower uncontrolled hyperthermia (104°F and higher) to reduce metabolic demands/O_2 consumption and cardiac workload.
Administer transfusions, assist with plasmapheresis, hemoperfusion, dialysis.	May be done to achieve rapid depletion of extrathyroidal hormone pool in desperately ill/comatose client.
Prepare for surgery.	Subtotal thyroidectomy (removal of five-sixths of the gland) may be treatment of choice for hyperthyroidism once euthyroid state is achieved.

NURSING DIAGNOSIS: Fatigue

May be related to

Hypermetabolic state with increased energy requirements
Irritability of central nervous system (CNS), altered body chemistry

Possibly evidenced by

Verbalization of overwhelming lack of energy to maintain usual routine, decreased performance
Emotional lability/irritability; nervousness, tension
Jittery behavior
Impaired ability to concentrate

DESIRED OUTCOMES/EVALUATION CRITERIA—CLIENT WILL:

Endurance (NOC)

Verbalize increase in level of energy.
Display improved ability to participate in desired activities.

ACTIONS/INTERVENTIONS	RATIONALE
Energy Management (NIC)	
Independent	
Monitor vital signs, noting pulse rate at rest and when active.	Pulse is typically elevated and, even at rest, tachycardia (up to 160 beats/min) may be noted.
Note development of tachypnea, dyspnea, pallor, and cyanosis.	O_2 demand and consumption are increased in hypermetabolic state, potentiating risk of hypoxia with activity.
Provide quiet environment, cool room, decreased sensory stimuli, soothing colors, quiet music.	Reduces stimuli that may aggravate agitation, hyperactivity, and insomnia.
Encourage client to restrict activity and rest in bed as much as possible.	Helps counteract effects of increased metabolism.
Provide comfort measures; e.g., judicious touch/massage, cool showers.	May decrease nervous energy, promoting relaxation.
Provide for diversional activities that are calming; e.g., reading, radio, television.	Allows for use of nervous energy in a constructive manner, serves as a distraction, and may reduce anxiety.
Avoid topics that irritate or upset client. Discuss ways to respond to these feelings.	Increased irritability of the CNS may cause client to be easily excited, agitated, and prone to emotional outbursts.
Discuss with SO reasons for fatigue and emotional lability.	Understanding that the behavior is physically based may enhance coping with current situation and encourage SO to respond positively and provide support for client.
Collaborative	
Administer medications as indicated:	
Sedatives (e.g., phenobarbital [Luminal]), antianxiety agents (e.g., chlordiazepoxide [Librium]).	Combats nervousness, hyperactivity, and insomnia.

NURSING DIAGNOSIS: risk for imbalanced Nutrition: less than body requirements

Risk factors may include

Increased metabolism (increased appetite/intake with loss of weight)
Nausea/vomiting, diarrhea
Relative insulin insufficiency, hyperglycemia

Possibly evidenced by

[Not applicable; presence of signs and symptoms establishes an *actual* diagnosis.]

DESIRED OUTCOMES/EVALUATION CRITERIA—CLIENT WILL:

Nutritional Status (NOC)

Demonstrate stable weight with normal laboratory values and be free of signs of malnutrition.

ACTIONS/INTERVENTIONS	RATIONALE
Nutrition Therapy (NIC)	
Independent	
Monitor daily food intake. Weigh daily and report losses.	Continued weight loss in face of adequate caloric intake may indicate failure of antithyroid therapy.

ACTIONS/INTERVENTIONS	RATIONALE
Encourage client to eat and increase number of meals and snacks, using high-calorie foods that are easily digested.	Aids in keeping caloric intake high enough to keep up with rapid expenditure of calories caused by hypermetabolic state.
Avoid foods that increase peristalsis (e.g., tea, coffee, fibrous and highly seasoned foods) and fluids that cause diarrhea (e.g., apple/prune juice).	Increased motility of GI tract may result in diarrhea and impair absorption of needed nutrients.

Collaborative

Consult with dietitian to provide diet high in calories, protein, carbohydrates, and vitamins.	May need assistance to ensure adequate intake of nutrients, identify appropriate supplements.
Administer medications as indicated:	
Glucose, vitamin B complex;	Given to meet energy requirements and prevent or correct hypoglycemia.
Insulin (small doses).	Aids in controlling serum glucose if elevated.

NURSING DIAGNOSIS: Anxiety [specify level]

May be related to

Physiologic factors: hypermetabolic state (CNS stimulation), pseudocatecholamine effect of thyroid hormones

Possibly evidenced by

Increased feelings of apprehension, shakiness, loss of control, panic
Changes in cognition, distortion of environmental stimuli
Extraneous movements, restlessness, tremors

DESIRED OUTCOMES/EVALUATION CRITERIA—CLIENT WILL:

Anxiety Self-Control (NOC)

Appear relaxed.
Report anxiety reduced to a manageable level.
Identify healthy ways to deal with feelings.

ACTIONS/INTERVENTIONS | RATIONALE

Anxiety Reduction (NIC)

Independent

ACTIONS/INTERVENTIONS	RATIONALE
Observe behavior indicative of level of anxiety.	Mild anxiety may be displayed by irritability and insomnia. Severe anxiety progressing to panic state may produce feelings of impending doom, terror, inability to speak or move, shouting/swearing.
Monitor physical responses, noting palpitations, repetitive movements, hyperventilation, insomnia.	Increased number of β-adrenergic receptor sites, coupled with effects of excess thyroid hormones, produces clinical manifestations of catecholamine excess even when normal levels of norepinephrine/epinephrine exist.
Stay with client, maintaining calm manner. Acknowledge fear and allow client's behavior to belong to client.	Affirms to client/SO that although client feels out of control, environment is safe. Avoiding personal responses to inappropriate remarks or actions prevents conflicts/overreaction to stressful situation/client behavior.

ACTIONS/INTERVENTIONS	RATIONALE
Describe/explain procedures, surrounding environment, or sounds that may be heard by client.	Provides accurate information, which reduces distortions/misinterpretations that can contribute to anxiety/fear reactions.
Speak in brief statements, using simple words.	Attention span may be shortened, concentration reduced, limiting ability to assimilate information.
Reduce external stimuli: Place in quiet room; provide soft, soothing music; reduce bright lights; reduce number of persons interacting with client.	Creates a therapeutic environment, shows recognition that unit activity/personnel may increase client's anxiety.
Discuss with client/SO reasons for emotional lability/psychotic reaction. (Refer to ND: risk for disturbed Thought Processes, following.)	Understanding that behavior is physically based enhances acceptance of situation and encourages different responses/approaches.
Reinforce expectation that emotional control should return as drug therapy progresses.	Provides information and reassures client that the situation is temporary and will improve with treatment.

Collaborative

Administer antianxiety agents or sedatives and monitor effects.	May be used in conjunction with medical regimen to reduce effects of hyperthyroid secretion.
Refer to support systems as needed; e.g., counseling, social services, pastoral care.	Ongoing therapy support may be desired/required by client/SO if crisis precipitates lifestyle alterations.

NURSING DIAGNOSIS: risk for disturbed Thought Processes

Risk factors may include

Physiologic changes: increased CNS stimulation/accelerated mental activity
Altered sleep patterns

Possibly evidenced by

[Not applicable; presence of signs and symptoms establishes an *actual* diagnosis.]

DESIRED OUTCOMES/EVALUATION CRITERIA—CLIENT WILL:

Distorted Thought Self-Control (NOC)

Maintain usual reality orientation.
Recognize changes in thinking/behavior and causative factors.

ACTIONS/INTERVENTIONS | RATIONALE

Delirium Management (NIC)

Independent

ACTIONS/INTERVENTIONS	RATIONALE
Assess thinking processes; e.g., memory, attention span, orientation to person/place/time/situation.	Determines extent of interference with sensory processing.
Note changes in behavior.	May be hypervigilant, restless, extremely sensitive, or crying, or may develop frank psychosis.
Assess level of anxiety. (Refer to ND: Anxiety)	Anxiety may alter thought processes, ability to think clearly.
Provide quiet environment; decreased stimuli, cool room, dim lights. Limit procedures/personnel.	Reduction of external stimuli may decrease hyperactivity/hyperreflexia, CNS irritability, auditory/visual hallucinations.

ACTIONS/INTERVENTIONS	RATIONALE
Reorient to person/place/time/situation as indicated.	Helps establish and maintain awareness of reality/environment.
Present reality concisely and briefly without challenging illogical thinking.	Limits defensive reaction.
Provide clock, calendar, and room with outside window; alter level of lighting to simulate day/night.	Promotes continual orientation cues to assist client in maintaining sense of normalcy.
Encourage visits by family/SO. Provide support as needed.	Aids in maintaining socialization and orientation. *Note:* Client's agitation/psychotic behavior may precipitate family quarrels/conflicts.
Provide safety measures; e.g., padded side rails, close supervision, or soft restraints as last resort as necessary.	Prevents injury to client who may be hallucinating/disoriented.

Collaborative

Administer medication as indicated; e.g., sedatives/antianxiety agents/antipsychotic drugs.	Promotes relaxation, reduces CNS hyperactivity/agitation to enhance thinking ability.

NURSING DIAGNOSIS: risk for impaired Tissue Integrity

Risk factors may include

Alterations of protective mechanisms of eye: impaired closure of eyelid (exophthalmos)

Possibly evidenced by

[Not applicable; presence of signs and symptoms establishes an *actual* diagnosis.]

DESIRED OUTCOMES/EVALUATION CRITERIA—CLIENT WILL:

TISSUE INTEGRITY: Skin & Mucous Membranes (NOC)

Maintain moist eye membranes, free of ulcerations.

Risk Control (NOC)

Identify measures to provide protection for eyes and prevent complications.

Surveillance (NIC)

Independent

ACTIONS/INTERVENTIONS	RATIONALE
Encourage use of dark glasses when awake and taping the eyelids shut during sleep as needed.	Protects exposed cornea if client is unable to close eyelids completely because of edema/fibrosis of fat pads.
Elevate the head of the bed and restrict salt intake if indicated.	Decreases tissue edema when appropriate; e.g., HF, which can aggravate existing exophthalmos.
Instruct client in extraocular muscle exercises if appropriate.	Improves circulation and maintains mobility of the eyelids.
Provide opportunity for client to discuss feelings about altered appearance and measures to enhance self-image.	Protruding eyes may be viewed as unattractive. Appearance can be enhanced with proper use of makeup, overall grooming, and use of shaded glasses.

ACTIONS/INTERVENTIONS	RATIONALE
Collaborative	
Administer medications as indicated:	
Methylcellulose drops;	Lubricates the eyes, reducing risk of lesion formation.
Adrenocorticotropic hormone (ACTH), prednisone;	Given to decrease rapidly progressive and marked inflammation.
Antithyroid drugs;	May decrease signs/symptoms or prevent worsening of the condition.
Diuretics.	Can decrease edema in mild involvement.
Prepare for surgery as indicated.	Eyelids may need to be sutured shut temporarily to protect the corneas until edema resolves (rare), or increasing space within sinus cavity and adjusting musculature may return eye to a more normal position.

NURSING DIAGNOSIS: deficient Knowledge [Learning Need] regarding condition, prognosis, treatment, self-care, and discharge needs

May be related to

Lack of exposure/recall
Information misinterpretation
Unfamiliarity with information resources

Possibly evidenced by

Questions, request for information, statement of misconception
Inaccurate follow-through of instructions/development of preventable complications

DESIRED OUTCOMES/EVALUATION CRITERIA—CLIENT WILL:

KNOWLEDGE: Illness Care (NOC)

Verbalize understanding of disease process and potential complications.
Identify relationship of signs/symptoms to the disease process and correlate symptoms with causative factors.
Verbalize understanding of therapeutic needs.
Initiate necessary lifestyle changes and participate in treatment regimen.

ACTIONS/INTERVENTIONS	RATIONALE
TEACHING: Disease Process (NIC)	
Independent	
Review disease process and future expectations.	Provides knowledge base from which client can make informed choices.
Provide information appropriate to individual situation.	Severity of condition, cause, age, and concurrent complications determine course of treatment.
Identify stressors and discuss precipitators to thyroid crises; e.g., personal/social and job concerns, infection, pregnancy.	Psychogenic factors are often of prime importance in the occurrence/exacerbation of this disease.
Provide information about signs/symptoms of hypothyroidism and the need for continuing follow-up care.	Client who has been treated for hyperthyroidism needs to be aware of possible development of hypothyroidism, which can occur immediately after treatment or as long as 5 yr later.

ACTIONS/INTERVENTIONS	RATIONALE
Discuss drug therapy, including need for adhering to regimen, and expected therapeutic and side effects.	Antithyroid medication (either as primary therapy or in preparation for thyroidectomy) requires adherence to a medical regimen over an extended period to inhibit hormone production. Agranulocytosis is the most serious side effect that can occur, and alternative drugs may be given if problems arise.
Identify signs/symptoms requiring medical evaluation; e.g., fever, sore throat, and skin eruptions.	Early identification of toxic reactions (thiourea therapy) and prompt intervention are important in preventing development of agranulocytosis.
Explain need to check with physician/pharmacist before taking other prescribed or OTC drugs.	Antithyroid medications can affect or be affected by numerous other medications, requiring monitoring of medication levels, side effects, and interactions.
Emphasize importance of planned rest periods.	Prevents undue fatigue, reduces metabolic demands. As euthyroid state is achieved, stamina and activity level will increase.
Review need for nutritious diet and periodic review of nutrient needs; avoid caffeine, red/yellow food dyes, artificial preservatives.	Provides adequate nutrients to support hypermetabolic state. As hormonal imbalance is corrected, diet will need to be readjusted to prevent excessive weight gain. Irritants and stimulants should be limited to avoid cumulative systemic effects.
Stress necessity of continued medical follow-up.	Required to monitor effectiveness of therapy and for prevention of potentially fatal complications.

POTENTIAL CONSIDERATIONS following acute hospitalization (dependent on client's age, physical condition/presence of complications, personal resources, and life responsibilities)

Fatigue—hypermetabolic state diminishing body energy reserves, prolonged recovery.

risk for imbalanced Nutrition: more than body requirements—change in BMR and metabolic needs.

THYROIDECTOMY

Thyroidectomy, although rare, may be performed in clients with thyroid cancer, hyperthyroidism, drug reactions to antithyroid agents, pregnant women who cannot be managed with drugs, clients who do not want radiation therapy, and clients with large goiters who do not respond to antithyroid drugs. Surgery may be done as an open or endoscopic procedure. The three types of thyroidectomy include:

Total thyroidectomy: The entire gland and surrounding lymph nodes are removed. This is done in the case of malignancy, or when there is a high risk of developing multiple sites of thyroid cancer, when there are many separate nodules, or when an enlarged thyroid makes breathing and swallowing difficult. Thyroid replacement therapy is necessary for life.

Lobectomy: A lobe is removed (with or without the isthmus between the lobes). Done to remove single nodule or multiple nodules in a single lobe.

Subtotal thyroidectomy: Up to five-sixths of the gland is removed when antithyroid drugs do not correct hyperthyroidism or RAI therapy is contraindicated. This is the procedure used for hyperthyroidism and is 95% curative.

CARE SETTING

Inpatient acute surgical unit

RELATED CONCERNS

Cancer, page 857
Hyperthyroidism (thyrotoxicosis, Graves' disease), page 426
Psychosocial aspects of care, page 770
Surgical intervention, page 788

Client Assessment Database

Refer to CP: Hyperthyroidism (Thyrotoxicosis, Graves' disease), for assessment information.

Discharge plan considerations: Assistance with self-care and other ADLs, transportation.

Refer to section at end of plan for postdischarge considerations.

NURSING PRIORITIES

1. Reverse/manage hyperthyroid state preoperatively.
2. Prevent complications.
3. Relieve pain.
4. Provide information about surgical procedure, prognosis, and treatment needs.

DISCHARGE GOALS

1. Complications prevented/minimized.
2. Pain alleviated.
3. Surgical procedure/prognosis and therapeutic regimen understood.
4. Plan in place to meet needs after discharge.

NURSING DIAGNOSIS: risk for ineffective Airway Clearance

Risk factors may include

Tracheal obstruction; swelling, bleeding, laryngeal spasms

Possibly evidenced by

[Not applicable; presence of signs and symptoms establishes an *actual* diagnosis.]

DESIRED OUTCOMES/EVALUATION CRITERIA—CLIENT WILL:

RESPIRATORY STATUS: Airway Patency (NOC)

Maintain patent airway, with aspiration prevented.

ACTIONS/INTERVENTIONS	RATIONALE
Airway Management (NIC)	
Independent	
Monitor respiratory rate, depth, and work of breathing.	Respirations may remain somewhat rapid because of hyperthyroid state, but development of respiratory distress is indicative of tracheal compression from edema or hemorrhage.
Auscultate breath sounds, noting presence of rhonchi.	Rhonchi may indicate airway obstruction/accumulation of copious thick secretions.
Assess for dyspnea, stridor, "crowing," and cyanosis. Note quality of voice.	Indicators of tracheal obstruction/laryngeal spasm, requiring prompt evaluation and intervention.
Keep head of bed elevated 30–45 degrees. Caution client to avoid bending neck; support head with pillows in the immediate postoperative period.	Enhances breathing and reduces likelihood of tension on surgical wound.
Assist with repositioning, deep breathing exercises, and/or coughing as indicated.	Maintains clear airway and ventilation. Although "routine" coughing is not encouraged and may be painful, it may be necessary to clear secretions.
Suction mouth and trachea as indicated, noting color and characteristics of sputum.	Edema/pain may impair client's ability to clear own airway.
Check dressing frequently, especially posterior portion.	If bleeding occurs, anterior dressing may appear dry because blood pools dependently. *Note*: Highest risk of bleeding is first 2 hr postoperative, but risk continues up to 24 hr.

ACTIONS/INTERVENTIONS	RATIONALE
Investigate reports of difficulty swallowing, drooling of oral secretions.	May indicate edema/sequestered bleeding in tissues surrounding operative site.
Keep tracheostomy tray at bedside.	Compromised airway may create a life-threatening situation requiring emergency procedure.

Collaborative

ACTIONS/INTERVENTIONS	RATIONALE
Provide steam inhalation; humidify room air.	Reduces discomfort of sore throat and tissue edema and promotes expectoration of secretions.
Assist with/prepare for procedures; e.g.:	
Tracheostomy;	Although rare, tracheostomy may be necessary to obtain airway if obstructed by edema of glottis or hemorrhage.
Return to surgery.	May require ligation of bleeding vessels.

NURSING DIAGNOSIS: impaired verbal Communication

May be related to

Vocal cord injury/laryngeal nerve damage
Tissue edema; pain/discomfort

Possibly evidenced by

Impaired articulation, does not/cannot speak; use of nonverbal cues such as gestures

DESIRED OUTCOMES/EVALUATION CRITERIA—CLIENT WILL:

Communication (NOC)

Establish method of communication in which needs can be understood.

COMMUNICATION ENHANCEMENT: Speech Deficit (NIC)

Independent

ACTIONS/INTERVENTIONS	RATIONALE
Assess speech periodically, encourage voice rest.	Hoarseness and sore throat may occur secondary to tissue edema or surgical damage to recurrent laryngeal nerve and may last several days. Permanent nerve damage can occur (rare) that causes paralysis of vocal cords and/or compression of the trachea.
Keep communication simple, ask yes/no questions.	Reduces demand for response; promotes voice rest.
Provide alternative methods of communication as appropriate; e.g., slate board, letter/picture board. Place IV line to minimize interference with written communication.	Facilitates expression of needs.
Anticipate needs as possible. Visit client frequently.	Reduces anxiety and client's need to communicate.
Post notice of client's voice limitations at central station and answer call light promptly.	Prevents client from straining voice to make needs known/summon assistance.
Maintain quiet environment.	Enhances ability to hear whispered communication and reduces necessity for client to raise/strain voice to be heard.

NURSING DIAGNOSIS: risk for Injury, [tetany]

Risk factors may include

Chemical imbalance: excessive CNS stimulation

Possibly evidenced by

[Not applicable; presence of signs and symptoms establishes an *actual* diagnosis.]

DESIRED OUTCOMES/EVALUATION CRITERIA—CLIENT WILL:

Physical Injury Severity (NOC)

Demonstrate absence of injury with complications minimized/controlled.

ACTIONS/INTERVENTIONS	RATIONALE
Surveillance (NIC)	
Independent	
Monitor vital signs noting elevating temperature, tachycardia (140–200 beats/min), dysrhythmias, respiratory distress, cyanosis (developing pulmonary edema/HF).	Manipulation of gland during subtotal thyroidectomy may result in increased hormone release, causing thyroid storm.
Evaluate reflexes periodically. Observe for neuromuscular irritability; e.g., twitching, numbness, paresthesias, positive Chvostek's and Trousseau's signs, seizure activity.	Hypocalcemia with tetany (usually transient) may occur 1–7 days postoperatively and indicates hypoparathyroidism, which can occur as a result of inadvertent trauma to/partial to total removal of parathyroid gland(s) during surgery.
Keep side rails raised/padded, bed in low position, and airway at bedside. Avoid use of restraints.	Reduces potential for injury if seizures occur. (Refer to CP: Seizure Disorders, ND: risk for Trauma/Suffocation.)
Collaborative	
Monitor serum calcium levels.	Clients with levels less than 7.5 mg/100 mL generally require replacement therapy.
Administer medications as indicated:	
Calcium (gluconate, lactate);	Corrects deficiency, which is usually temporary but may be permanent. *Note:* Use with caution in clients taking digitalis because calcium increases cardiac sensitivity to digitalis, potentiating risk of toxicity.
Phosphate-binding agents;	Helpful in lowering elevated phosphorus levels associated with hypocalcemia.
Sedatives;	Promotes rest, reducing exogenous stimulation.
Anticonvulsants.	Controls seizure activity until corrective therapy is successful.

NURSING DIAGNOSIS: acute Pain

May be related to

Surgical interruption/manipulation of tissues/muscles
Postoperative edema

Possibly evidenced by

Reports of pain
Narrowed focus, guarding behavior; restlessness
Autonomic responses

DESIRED OUTCOMES/EVALUATION CRITERIA—CLIENT WILL:

Pain Control (NOC)

Report pain is relieved/controlled.
Demonstrate use of relaxation skills and diversional activities appropriate to situation.

ACTIONS/INTERVENTIONS	RATIONALE
Pain Management (NIC)	
Independent	
Assess verbal/nonverbal reports of pain, noting location, intensity (0–10 scale), and duration.	Useful in evaluating pain, choice of interventions, effectiveness of therapy.
Place in semi-Fowler's position and support head/neck in neutral position with sandbags or small pillows as required in immediate postoperative phase. Instruct client to use hands to support neck during movement and to avoid hyperextension of neck.	Prevents hyperextension of the neck and protects integrity of the suture line. Movement restriction is imposed for only a few hours postoperatively to prevent stress on the suture line and reduce muscle tension. Gentle flexing and stretching is then permitted according to pain tolerance to help prevent neck soreness.
Keep call light and frequently needed items within easy reach.	Limits stretching, muscle strain in operative area.
Give cool liquids or soft foods, such as ice cream or popsicles.	Although both may be soothing to sore throat, soft foods may be tolerated better than liquids if client experiences difficulty swallowing.
Encourage client to use relaxation techniques; e.g., guided imagery, soft music, progressive relaxation.	Helps refocus attention and assists client to manage pain/discomfort more effectively.
Collaborative	
Administer analgesics and throat sprays/lozenges as necessary.	Reduces pain and discomfort, enhances rest.
Provide ice collar if indicated.	Reduces tissue edema and decreases perception of pain.

NURSING DIAGNOSIS: deficient Knowledge [Learning Need] regarding condition, prognosis, treatment, self-care, and discharge needs

May be related to

Lack of exposure/recall, misinterpretation
Unfamiliarity with information resources

Possibly evidenced by

Questions; request for information; statement of misconception
Inaccurate follow-through of instructions/development of preventable complications

DESIRED OUTCOMES/EVALUATION CRITERIA—CLIENT WILL:

KNOWLEDGE: Disease Process (NOC)

Verbalize understanding of surgical procedure and prognosis and potential complications.

KNOWLEDGE: Treatment Regimen (NOC)

Verbalize understanding of therapeutic needs.
Participate in treatment regimen.
Initiate necessary lifestyle changes.

ACTIONS/INTERVENTIONS	RATIONALE
TEACHING: Disease Process (NIC)	
Independent	
Review surgical procedure and future expectations.	Provides knowledge base from which client can make informed decisions.
Discuss need for well-balanced, nutritious diet and, when appropriate, inclusion of iodized salt.	Promotes healing and helps client regain/maintain appropriate weight. Use of iodized salt is often sufficient to meet iodine needs unless salt is restricted for other healthcare problems; e.g., HF.
Recommend avoidance of goitrogenic foods; e.g., excessive ingestion of seafood, soybeans, turnips.	Contraindicated after partial thyroidectomy because these foods inhibit thyroid activity.
Identify foods high in calcium (e.g., dairy products) and vitamin D (e.g., fortified dairy products, egg yolks, liver).	Maximizes supply and absorption of calcium if parathyroid function is impaired.
Encourage progressive general exercise program.	In clients with subtotal thyroidectomy, exercise can stimulate the thyroid gland and production of hormones, facilitating recovery of general well-being.
Review postoperative exercises to be instituted after incision heals; e.g., flexion, extension, rotation, and lateral movement of head and neck.	Regular ROM exercises strengthen neck muscles, enhance circulation and healing process.
Review importance of rest and relaxation, avoiding stressful situations and emotional outbursts.	Effects of hyperthyroidism usually subside completely, but it takes some time for the body to recover.
Instruct in incisional care; e.g., cleansing, dressing application.	Enables client to provide competent self-care. *Note*: Neck incisions heal rapidly and are watertight within 24–36 hr.
Recommend the use of loose-fitting scarves to cover scar, avoiding the use of jewelry.	Covers the incision without aggravating healing or precipitating infections of suture line.
Apply moisturizers/vitamin E after sutures have been removed.	Softens tissues and may help minimize scarring.
Discuss possibility of change in voice.	Normal surgical area swelling and/or alteration in vocal cord function may cause changes in pitch and quality of voice, which may be temporary or permanent.
Review drug therapy and the necessity of continuing even when feeling well.	If thyroid hormone replacement is needed because of surgical removal of gland, client needs to understand rationale for replacement therapy and consequences of failure to routinely take medication.
Identify signs/symptoms requiring medical evaluation; e.g., fever, chills, continued/purulent wound drainage, erythema, gaps in wound edges, sudden weight loss, intolerance to heat, nausea/vomiting, diarrhea, insomnia, weight gain, fatigue, intolerance to cold, constipation, drowsiness.	Early recognition of developing complications such as infection, hyperthyroidism, or hypothyroidism may prevent progression to life-threatening situation. *Note:* As many as 43% of clients with subtotal thyroidectomy will develop hypothyroidism in time.
Stress necessity of continued medical follow-up.	Provides opportunity for evaluating effectiveness of therapy and prevention of complications.

POTENTIAL CONSIDERATIONS following acute hospitalization (dependent on client's age, physical condition/presence of complications, personal resources, and life responsibilities)

Fatigue—decreased metabolic energy production, altered body chemistry (hypothyroidism)

Refer to Potential Considerations in Surgical Intervention plan of care.

HEPATITIS

Hepatitis is an umbrella term for a variety of viral, bacterial, and noninfectious causes of widespread inflammation that results in necrosis and scarring of liver cells. Inflammation of the liver can be due to viral or bacterial invasion. Noninfectious causes include physical or toxic chemical agents (e.g., drugs, alcohol, industrial chemicals) and nonalcoholic or autoimmune hepatitis.

Viral infections can be transmitted by blood and body fluids and/or food. These viruses are designated by letters of the alphabet, (A, B, C, D, E, G) and variously used (e.g., B is known as HBV, or HepB). HCV is responsible for about 30% of viral hepatitis cases. Other causes of hepatitis include cytomegalovirus (CMV), Epstein-Barr virus (EBV), *Mycobacterium avium* complex (MAC), toxoplasmosis, and histoplasmosis. Studies have shown that almost 25% of persons with human immunodeficiency virus (HIV) infection also have hepatitis.

Hepatitis can be acute or chronic. Although most cases of hepatitis are self-limiting, approximately 5%–10% of clients with hepatitis B and 80%–85% of clients with hepatitis C progress to a chronic state. Chronic inflammation can lead to fibrotic scarring (cirrhosis) and can be fatal.

CARE SETTING

Care can frequently be provided in the outpatient setting or at the community level. In states of acute hepatic inflammation, brief inpatient acute care on a medical unit may be required to monitor/treat hepatic failure or hepatic encephalopathy.

RELATED CONCERNS

Alcohol: acute withdrawal, page 831
Cirrhosis of the liver, page 453
Psychosocial aspects of care, page 770
Renal dialysis, page 564
Substance dependence/abuse rehabilitation, page 843
Total nutritional support: parenteral/enteral feeding, page 478

Client Assessment Database

Data depend on the cause (type of hepatitis) and severity of liver involvement/damage.

ACTIVITY/REST

May report: Fatigue, weakness, general malaise, muscle aches

CIRCULATION

May exhibit: Bradycardia (severe hyperbilirubinemia)
Jaundiced sclera, skin, mucous membranes

ELIMINATION

May report: Dark urine
Diarrhea/constipation, clay-colored stools
Current/recent hemodialysis

FOOD/FLUID

May report: Loss of appetite (anorexia), weight loss or gain (edema)
Nausea/vomiting

May exhibit: Ascites

NEUROSENSORY

May exhibit: Irritability, drowsiness, lethargy, asterixis, headache

PAIN/DISCOMFORT

May report: Abdominal cramping, right upper quadrant (RUQ) tenderness
Myalgias, arthralgias; headache
Itching (pruritus)

May exhibit: Muscle guarding, restlessness

RESPIRATION

May report: Distaste for/aversion to cigarettes (smokers)
Recent flu-like URI signs and symptoms

SAFETY

May report: Transfusion of blood/blood products in the past

May exhibit: Fever
Urticaria, maculopapular lesions, irregular patches of erythema
Exacerbation of acne
Spider angiomas, palmar erythema, gynecomastia in men (sometimes present in alcoholic hepatitis)
Splenomegaly, posterior cervical node enlargement

SEXUALITY

May report: Lifestyle/behaviors increasing risk of exposure (e.g., sexual promiscuity, sexually active homosexual/bisexual male)

TEACHING/LEARNING

May report: History of known/possible exposure to virus, bacteria, or toxins (contaminated food, water, needles, surgical equipment or blood), carriers (symptomatic or asymptomatic), recent surgical procedure with halothane anesthesia, exposure to toxic chemicals (e.g., carbon tetrachloride, vinyl chloride)
History of known/possible exposure to hepatotoxic prescription (e.g., sulfonamides, phenothiazines, isoniazid) or OTC drug use (e.g., acetaminophen)
Use of herbal supplements associated with hepatotoxicity, (e.g., chaparral, JinBuHuan, germander, comfrey, mistletoe, skullcap, margosa oil, pennyroral)
Use of street injection drugs or alcohol
Travel to/immigration from China, Africa, Southeast Asia, Middle East (hepatitis B [HBV] and C [HVC] are endemic in these areas)
Concurrent diabetes, HF, malignancy, or renal disease

Discharge plan considerations: May require assistance with home making, maintenance tasks, shopping, transportation

Refer to section at end of plan for postdischarge considerations.

DIAGNOSTIC STUDIES

Liver enzymes/isoenzymes: Abnormal (4–10 times normal values). However, of limited value in differentiating viral from nonviral hepatitis.
AST/ALT: Initially elevated. May rise 1–2 weeks before jaundice is apparent, then decline.
Alkaline phosphatase (ALP): Slight elevation (unless severe cholestasis present).
Hepatitis A, B, C, D, E panels (antibody/antigen tests): Specify type and stage of disease and determine possible carriers.
CBC: Red blood cells (RBCs) decreased because of shortened lifespan of RBCs (liver enzyme alterations) or hemorrhage.
WBC count and differential: Leukopenia, leukocytosis, monocytosis, atypical lymphocytes, and plasma cells may be present.
Serum albumin: Decreased.
Blood glucose: Transient hyperglycemia/hypoglycemia (altered liver function).
Prothrombin time: May be prolonged (liver dysfunction).
Serum bilirubin: Above 2.5 mg/100 mL. (If above 200 mg/100 mL, poor prognosis is probable because of increased cellular necrosis.)
Stools: Clay-colored, steatorrhea (decreased hepatic function).
Bromsulphalein (BSP) excretion test: Blood level elevated.
Liver biopsy: Usually not needed, but should be considered if diagnosis is uncertain, or if clinical course is atypical or unduly prolonged.
Liver scan: Aids in estimation of severity of parenchymal damage.
Urinalysis: Elevated bilirubin levels; protein/hematuria may occur.

NURSING PRIORITIES

1. Reduce demands on liver while promoting physical well-being.
2. Prevent complications.

3. Enhance self-concept, acceptance of situation.
4. Provide information about disease process, prognosis, and treatment needs.

DISCHARGE GOALS

1. Meeting basic self-care needs.
2. Complications prevented/minimized.
3. Dealing with reality of current situation.
4. Disease process, prognosis, transmission, and therapeutic regimen understood.
5. Plan in place to meet needs after discharge.

NURSING DIAGNOSIS: Fatigue

May be related to

Decreased metabolic energy production
States of discomfort
Altered body chemistry (e.g., changes in liver function, effect on target organs)

Possibly evidenced by

Reports of lack of energy/inability to maintain usual routines
Decreased performance
Increase in physical complaints

DESIRED OUTCOMES/EVALUATION CRITERIA—CLIENT WILL:

Endurance (NOC)

Report improved sense of energy.
Perform ADLs and participate in desired activities at level of ability.

ACTIONS/INTERVENTIONS	RATIONALE
Energy Management (NIC)	
Independent	
Encourage bedrest/chair (recliner) rest during toxic state. Provide quiet environment; limit visitors as needed.	Promotes rest and relaxation. Available energy is used for healing. Activity and an upright position are believed to decrease hepatic blood flow, which prevents optimal circulation to the liver cells.
Recommend changing position frequently. Provide/instruct caregiver in good skin care.	Promotes optimal respiratory function and minimizes pressure areas to reduce risk of tissue breakdown.
Do necessary tasks quickly and at one time as tolerated.	Allows for extended periods of uninterrupted rest.
Determine and prioritize role responsibilities and alternative providers/possible community resources available; e.g., Meals on Wheels, homemaker/housekeeper services.	Promotes problem-solving of most pressing needs of individual/family.
Identify energy-conserving techniques; e.g., sitting to shower and brush teeth, planning steps of activity so that all needed materials are at hand, scheduling rest periods.	Helps minimize fatigue, allowing client to accomplish more and feel better about self.
Increase activity as tolerated, demonstrate passive/active ROM exercises.	Prolonged bedrest can be debilitating. This can be offset by limited activity alternating with rest periods.
Encourage use of stress management techniques; e.g., progressive relaxation, visualization, guided imagery. Discuss appropriate diversional activities; e.g., radio, TV, reading.	Promotes relaxation and conserves energy, redirects attention, and may enhance coping.
Monitor for recurrence of anorexia and liver tenderness/enlargement.	Indicates lack of resolution/exacerbation of the disease, requiring further rest, change in therapeutic regimen.

ACTIONS/INTERVENTIONS	RATIONALE
Collaborative	
Administer medications as indicted: sedatives, antianxiety agents; e.g., diazepam (Valium), lorazepam (Ativan).	Assists in managing required rest. *Note:* Use of certain medications (e.g., prochlorperazine [Compazine] and chlorpromazine [Thorazine]}, is contraindicated because of hepatotoxic effects.
Monitor serial liver enzyme levels.	Aids in determining appropriate levels of activity because premature increase in activity potentiates risk of relapse.
Administer antidote or assist with procedures as indicated (e.g., lavage, catharsis, hyperventilation) depending on route of exposure.	Removal of causative agent in toxic hepatitis may limit degree of tissue involvement/damage.

NURSING DIAGNOSIS: imbalanced Nutrition: less than body requirements

May be related to

Insufficient intake to meet metabolic demands: anorexia, nausea/vomiting
Altered absorption and metabolism of ingested foods: reduced peristalsis (visceral reflexes), bile stasis
Increased caloric needs/hypermetabolic state

Possibly evidenced by

Aversion to eating/lack of interest in food; altered taste sensation
Abdominal pain/cramping
Loss of weight; poor muscle tone

DESIRED OUTCOMES/EVALUATION CRITERIA—CLIENT WILL:

TREATMENT BEHAVIOR: Illness or Injury (NOC)

Initiate behaviors, lifestyle changes to regain/maintain appropriate weight.

Nutritional Status (NOC)

Demonstrate progressive weight gain toward goal with normalization of laboratory values and no signs of malnutrition.

ACTIONS/INTERVENTIONS	RATIONALE
Weight Gain Assistance (NIC)	
Independent	
Monitor dietary intake/calorie count. Suggest several small feedings and offer "largest" meal at breakfast.	Large meals are difficult to manage when client is anorexic. Anorexia may also worsen during the day, making intake of food difficult later in the day.
Encourage mouth care before meals.	Eliminating unpleasant taste may enhance appetite.
Recommend eating in upright position.	Reduces sensation of abdominal fullness and may enhance intake.
Encourage intake of fruit juices, carbonated beverages, and hard candy throughout the day.	These supply extra calories and may be more easily digested/tolerated than other foods.

ACTIONS/INTERVENTIONS	RATIONALE
Collaborative	
Consult with dietitian, nutritional support team to provide diet according to client's needs, with fat and protein intake as tolerated.	Useful in formulating dietary program to meet individual needs. Fat metabolism varies according to bile production and excretion and may necessitate restriction of fat intake if diarrhea develops. If tolerated, a normal or increased protein intake helps with liver regeneration. Protein restriction may be indicated in severe disease (e.g., fulminating hepatitis) because the accumulation of the endproducts of protein metabolism can potentiate hepatic encephalopathy.
Monitor serum glucose as indicated.	Hyperglycemia/hypoglycemia may develop, necessitating dietary changes/insulin administration. Fingerstick monitoring may be done by client on a regular schedule to determine therapy needs.
Administer medications as indicated:	
Antiemetics; e.g., metoclopramide (Reglan), trimethobenzamide (Tigan);	Given 30 min before meals, may reduce nausea and increase food tolerance. *Note:* Prochlorperazine (Compazine) is contraindicated in hepatic disease.
Antiulcer agents/antacids; e.g., lansoprazole (Prevacid), esomeprazole [Nexium], magnesium hydroxide/aluminum hydroxide [Maalox, Mylanta];	Counteracts gastric acidity, reducing irritation/risk of bleeding.
Vitamins; e.g., B complex, C, other dietary supplements as indicated;	Corrects deficiencies and aids in the healing process.
Steroid therapy; e.g., prednisone (Deltasone), alone or in combination with azathioprine (Imuran).	Steroids may be contraindicated because they can increase risk of relapse/development of chronic hepatitis in clients with viral hepatitis; however, anti-inflammatory effect may be useful in chronic active hepatitis (especially idiopathic) to reduce nausea/vomiting and enable client to retain food and fluids. Steroids may decrease serum aminotransferase and bilirubin levels, but they do not affect liver necrosis or regeneration. Combination therapy has fewer steroid-related side effects.
Provide supplemental feedings, enteral/parenteral nutrition if needed.	May be necessary to meet caloric requirements if marked deficits are present/symptoms are prolonged.

NURSING DIAGNOSIS: risk for deficient Fluid Volume

Risk factors may include

Excessive losses through vomiting and diarrhea, third-space shift
Altered clotting process

Possibly evidenced by

[Not applicable; presence of signs and symptoms establishes an *actual* diagnosis.]

DESIRED OUTCOMES/EVALUATION CRITERIA—CLIENT WILL:

Hydration (NOC)

Maintain adequate hydration, as evidenced by stable vital signs, good skin turgor, capillary refill, strong peripheral pulses, and individually appropriate urinary output.

Coagulation Status (NOC)

Be free of signs of hemorrhage with clotting times WNL.

ACTIONS/INTERVENTIONS	RATIONALE
Fluid/Electrolyte Management (NIC)	
Independent	
Monitor I&O, compare with periodic weight. Note enteric losses; e.g., vomiting and diarrhea.	Provides information about replacement needs/effects of therapy. *Note:* Diarrhea may be due to transient flu-like response to viral infection or may represent a more serious problem of obstructed portal blood flow with vascular congestion in the GI tract, or it may be the intended result of medication use (neomycin, lactulose) to decrease serum ammonia levels in the presence of hepatic encephalopathy.
Assess vital signs, peripheral pulses, capillary refill, skin turgor, and mucous membranes.	Indicators of circulating volume/perfusion.
Bleeding Precautions (NIC)	
Check for ascites for edema formation. Measure abdominal girth as indicated.	Useful in monitoring progression/resolution of fluid shifts (edema/ascites).
Use small-gauge needles for injections, applying pressure for longer than usual after venipuncture.	Reduces possibility of bleeding into tissues.
Have client use cotton/sponge swabs and alcohol-free mouthwash instead of toothbrush.	Avoids trauma and bleeding of the gums. *Note:* Alcohol-based mouthwash may be irritating/dry mucosa.
Observe for signs of bleeding; e.g., hematuria/melena, ecchymosis, oozing from gums/puncture sites.	Prothrombin levels are reduced and coagulation times prolonged when vitamin K absorption is altered in GI tract and synthesis of prothrombin is decreased in affected liver.
Fluid/Electrolyte Management (NIC)	
Collaborative	
Monitor periodic laboratory values; e.g., Hgb/Hct, Na, albumin, and clotting times.	Reflects hydration and identifies sodium retention/protein deficits, which may lead to edema formation. Deficits in clotting potentiate risk of bleeding/hemorrhage.
Administer antidiarrheal agents; e.g., diphenoxylate with atropine (Lomotil).	Reduces fluid/electrolyte loss from GI tract.
Provide IV fluids (usually glucose), electrolytes:	Provides fluid and electrolyte replacement in acute toxic state.
Protein hydrolysates.	Correction of albumin/protein deficits can aid in return of fluid from tissues to the circulatory system. May follow albumin administration with an IV diuretic to pull fluids from interstitial space into intravascular space to reduce ascites.
Bleeding Precautions (NIC)	
Administer medications as indicated; e.g.:	
Vitamin K;	Because absorption is altered, supplementation may prevent coagulation problems, which may occur if clotting factors/prothrombin time (PT) is depressed.
Antacids or H_2-receptor antagonists; e.g., lansoprazole (Prevacid), cimetidine (Tagamet).	Neutralize/reduce gastric secretions to lower risk of gastric irritation/bleeding.
Infuse fresh frozen plasma, as indicated.	May be required to replace clotting factors in the presence of coagulation defects.

NURSING DIAGNOSIS: situational low Self-Esteem

May be related to

Annoying/debilitating symptoms, confinement/isolation, length of illness/recovery period

Possibly evidenced by

Verbalization of change in lifestyle, fear of rejection/reaction of others, negative feelings about body, feelings of helplessness
Depression, lack of follow-through, self-destructive behavior

DESIRED OUTCOMES/EVALUATION CRITERIA—CLIENT WILL:

Self-Esteem (NOC)

Verbalize feelings.
Identify methods for coping with negative perception of self.
Verbalize acceptance of self in situation, including length of recovery/need for isolation.
Acknowledge self as worthwhile; be responsible for self.

ACTIONS/INTERVENTIONS	RATIONALE
Self-Esteem Enhancement (NIC)	
Independent	
Contract with client regarding time for listening. Encourage discussion of feelings/concerns.	Establishing time enhances trusting relationship. Providing opportunity to express feelings allows client to feel more in control of the situation. Verbalization can decrease anxiety and depression and facilitate positive coping behaviors. Client may need to express feelings about being ill, length and cost of illness, possibility of infecting others, and (in severe illness) fear of death. May have concerns regarding the stigma of the disease.
Avoid making moral judgments regarding lifestyle (e.g., alcohol use, drug abuse, sexual practices).	Client may already feel upset/angry and condemn self; judgments from others will further damage self-esteem.
Discuss recovery expectations.	Recovery period may be prolonged (months), potentiating family/situational stress and necessitating need for planning, support, and follow-up.
Assess effect of illness on economic factors of client/SO.	Financial problems may exist because of loss of client's role functioning in the family/prolonged recovery.
Offer diversional activities based on energy level.	Enables client to use time and energy in constructive ways that enhance self-esteem and minimize anxiety and depression.
Suggest client wear bright reds or blues/blacks instead of yellows or greens.	Enhances appearance because yellow skin tones are intensified by yellow/green colors. *Note:* Jaundice usually peaks within 1–2 weeks, then gradually resolves over 2–4 weeks.
Collaborative	
Make appropriate referrals for help as needed; e.g., case manager/discharge planner, social services, and/or other community agencies.	Can facilitate problem solving and help involved individuals cope more effectively with situation.

NURSING DIAGNOSIS: risk for Infection

Risk factors may include

Inadequate secondary defenses (e.g., leukopenia, suppressed inflammatory response) and immunosuppression
Malnutrition
Insufficient knowledge to avoid exposure to pathogens

Possibly evidenced by

[Not applicable; presence of signs and symptoms establishes an *actual* diagnosis.]

DESIRED OUTCOMES/EVALUATION CRITERIA—CLIENT WILL:

Risk Control (NOC)

Verbalize understanding of individual causative/risk factor(s).
Demonstrate techniques; initiate lifestyle changes to avoid reinfection/transmission to others.

ACTIONS/INTERVENTIONS	RATIONALE
Infection Control (NIC)	
Independent	
Establish isolation techniques for enteric and respiratory infections according to infection guidelines/policy. Encourage/model effective hand washing.	Prevents transmission of viral disease to others. Thorough hand washing is effective in preventing virus transmission. Types A and E are transmitted by oral-fecal route, contaminated water, milk, and food (especially inadequately cooked shellfish). Types A, B, C, and D are transmitted by contaminated blood/blood products, needle punctures, open wounds, and contact with saliva, urine, stool, and semen. Incidence of both HBV and HCV has increased among healthcare providers and high-risk clients. *Note:* Toxic and alcoholic types of hepatitis are not communicable and do not require special measures/isolation.
Stress need to monitor/restrict visitors as indicated.	Client exposure to infectious processes (especially respiratory) potentiates risk of secondary complications.
Explain isolation procedures to client/SO.	Understanding reasons for safeguarding themselves and others can lessen feelings of isolation and stigmatization. Isolation may last 2–3 weeks from onset of illness depending on type/duration of symptoms.
Collaborative	
Administer medications as indicated:	The particular (or combination) medication used depends on the type of infection.
Antiviral drugs: e.g., vidarabine (Vira-A), acyclovir (Zovirax), lamivudine (Epivir), adefovir dipivoxil (Hepsera);	Useful in reducing viral load/treating chronic active HAV and HBV.
Interferon alfa-2a (Roferon A), interferon alfa-2b (Intron A);	Biologic response modifiers (BMRs) used to reduce viral load/treat symptoms of HCV and may lead to temporary improvement in liver function.
Pegylated interferons; e.g., peginterferon alfa-2a, (Pegasys), peginterferon alfa-2b (Peg-Intron);	These BMRs have largely replaced standard interferons in the treatment of HCV.

ACTIONS/INTERVENTIONS	RATIONALE
Ribavirin (Rebetol, Copegus);	Used in conjunction with interferon and peginterferon to improve the effectiveness of that drug. *Note:* These treatments lead to improvement, not cure of the disease.
Antinfectives appropriate to causative agents (e.g., gram-negative, anaerobic bacteria, fungus) or secondary infectious process.	Used to treat bacterial hepatitis or to prevent/limit secondary infections.

NURSING DIAGNOSIS: risk for impaired Skin/Tissue Integrity

Risk factors may include

Chemical substance: bile salt accumulation in the tissues

Possibly evidenced by

[Not applicable; presence of signs and symptoms establishes an *actual* diagnosis.]

DESIRED OUTCOMES/EVALUATION CRITERIA—CLIENT WILL:

TISSUE INTEGRITY: Skin and Mucous Membranes (NOC)

Display intact skin/tissues free of excoriation.
Report absence/decrease of pruritus/scratching.

ACTIONS/INTERVENTIONS	RATIONALE
Skin Surveillance (NIC)	
Independent	
Encourage use of cool showers and baking soda or starch baths. Avoid use of alkaline soaps. Apply calamine lotion as indicated.	Prevents excessive dryness of skin. Provides relief from itching.
Provide diversional activities.	Aids in refocusing attention, reducing tendency to scratch.
Suggest use of knuckles if desire to scratch is uncontrollable. Keep fingernails cut short, apply gloves on comatose client or during hours of sleep. Recommend loose-fitting clothing. Provide soft cotton linens.	Reduces potential for dermal injury.
Provide a soothing massage at bedtime.	May be helpful in promoting sleep by reducing skin irritation.
Observe skin for areas of redness, breakdown.	Early detection of problem areas allows for additional intervention to prevent complications/promote healing.
Avoid comments regarding client's appearance.	Minimizes psychologic stress associated with skin changes.
Collaborative	
Administer medications as indicated:	
Antihistamines; e.g., diphenhydramine (Benadryl), azatadine (Optimine);	Relieves itching. *Note:* Use cautiously in severe hepatic disease.
Antilipemics; e.g., cholestyramine (Questran).	May be used to bind bile acids in the intestine and prevent their absorption. Note side effects of nausea and constipation.

NURSING DIAGNOSIS: deficient Knowledge [Learning Need] regarding condition, prognosis, treatment, self-care, and discharge needs

May be related to

Lack of exposure/recall; information misinterpretation
Unfamiliarity with resources

Possibly evidenced by

Questions or statements of misconception, request for information
Inaccurate follow-through of instructions, development of preventable complications

DESIRED OUTCOMES/EVALUATION CRITERIA—CLIENT WILL:

KNOWLEDGE: Illness Care (NOC)

Verbalize understanding of disease process, prognosis, and potential complications.
Identify relationship of signs/symptoms to the disease and correlate symptoms with causative factors.
Verbalize understanding of therapeutic needs.
Initiate necessary lifestyle changes and participate in treatment regimen.

ACTIONS/INTERVENTIONS	RATIONALE
TEACHING: Disease Process (NIC)	
Independent	
Assess level of understanding of the disease process, expectations/prognosis, possible treatment options.	Identifies areas of lack of knowledge/misinformation and provides opportunity to give additional information as necessary. *Note:* Liver transplantation may be needed in the presence of fulminating disease with liver failure.
Provide specific information regarding prevention/transmission of disease; e.g., contacts may require γ-globulin, personal items should not be shared, observe strict hand washing and sanitizing of clothes, dishes, and toilet facilities while liver enzymes are elevated. Avoid intimate contact, such as kissing and sexual contact, and exposure to infections, especially respiratory infections.	Needs/recommendations vary with type of hepatitis (causative agent) and individual situation.
Plan resumption of activity as tolerated with adequate periods of rest. Discuss restriction of heavy lifting, strenuous exercise/contact sports.	It is not necessary to wait until serum bilirubin levels return to normal to resume activity (may take as long as 2 months), but strenuous activity needs to be limited until the liver returns to normal size. When client begins to feel better, he or she needs to understand the importance of continued adequate rest in preventing relapse or recurrence. (Relapse occurs in 5%–25% of adults.) *Note:* Energy level may take up to 3–6 months to return to normal.
Help client identify appropriate diversional activities.	Enjoyable activities promote rest and help client avoid focusing on prolonged convalescence.
Encourage continuation of balanced diet.	Promotes general well-being and enhances energy for healing process/tissue regeneration.
Identify ways to maintain usual bowel function; e.g., adequate intake of fluids/dietary roughage, moderate activity/exercise to tolerance.	Decreased level of activity, changes in food/fluid intake, and slowed bowel motility may result in constipation.

ACTIONS/INTERVENTIONS	RATIONALE
Discuss the side effects and dangers of taking OTC/certain prescribed drugs that are known to have adverse effects on the liver. Advise client to notify pharmacists and all future healthcare providers of diagnosis.	Some drugs are toxic to the liver; many others are metabolized by the liver and should be avoided in severe liver diseases because they may cause cumulative toxic effects/chronic hepatitis.
Discuss restrictions on donating blood.	Prevents spread of infectious disease. Most state laws prevent accepting as donors those who have a history of any type of hepatitis.
Emphasize importance of follow-up physical examination and laboratory evaluation.	Disease process may take several months to resolve. If symptoms persist longer than 6 months, liver biopsy may be required to verify presence of chronic hepatitis.
Discuss need for immunizations.	Recovery from hepatitis A and B results in protective antibodies in the client, so he or she will not get those strains again. There is currently no vaccine available against HepC. However, people should be vaccinated against HepA and HepB. Guidelines include: everyone under the age of 18 years, individuals exposed to blood and body fluids, or sharing a household with an infected person; people traveling to areas where infection rates are known to be high; men who have sex with men; illicit IV drug users; persons receiving hemodialysis; or who have clotting disorders or liver disease.
Give information regarding availability of γ-globulin, ISG, H-BIG, HB vaccine (Recombivax HB, Engerix-B) through health department or family physician.	Immune globulins may be effective in preventing viral hepatitis in those who have been exposed depending on type of hepatitis and period of incubation.
Review necessity of avoidance of alcohol, illicit drugs, and tobacco.	These substances increase hepatic irritation, and may interfere with recovery.
Refer to community resources, drug/alcohol treatment program as indicated.	May need additional assistance to withdraw from substance and maintain abstinence to avoid further liver damage.

POTENTIAL CONSIDERATIONS following acute hospitalization (dependent on client's age, physical condition/presence of complications, personal resources, and life responsibilities)

Fatigue—generalized weakness, decreased strength/endurance, pain, imposed activity restrictions, depression.

impaired Home Maintenance—prolonged recovery/chronic condition, insufficient finances, inadequate support systems, unfamiliarity with neighborhood resources.

imbalanced Nutrition: less than body requirements—insufficient intake to meet metabolic demands: anorexia, nausea/vomiting; altered absorption and metabolism of ingested foods; increased calorie needs/hypermetabolic state.

risk for Infection—inadequate secondary defenses; malnutrition; insufficient knowledge to avoid exposure to pathogens.

CIRRHOSIS OF THE LIVER

Cirrhosis is a chronic disease of the liver characterized by alteration in structure, degenerative changes, and widespread destruction of hepatic cells, impairing cellular function and impeding blood flow through the liver. The damage to the liver is usually irreversible. In the United States, over 60% of cases of cirrhosis are the result of hepatitis C, alcoholic liver disease, or a combination of the two. In 2002, cirrhosis was listed as the twelfth leading cause of death in the United States.

Cirrhosis is associated with multiple causes including (1) various liver diseases (e.g., Wilson's disease, α_1-antitrypsin deficiency, hemochromatosis), (2) hepatitis (viral, bacterial, autoimmune, alcohol-induced or other drug-induced cirrhosis), (3) obesity, and (4) cholestatic diseases (e.g., biliary atresia, primary biliary cirrhosis, cystic fibrosis, and primary sclerosing cholangitis).

The goals of treatment are to slow the progression of the disease and to alleviate the symptoms such as pruritus, nutritional deficits, and variceal bleeding. Liver transplantation appears to be the only life-saving procedure for end-stage disease.

CARE SETTING

May be hospitalized on a medical unit during initial or recurrent acute episodes with potentially life-threatening complications. Otherwise, this condition is managed at the community, outpatient level.

RELATED CONCERNS

Alcohol: acute withdrawal, page 831
Substance dependence/abuse rehabilitation, page 843
Fluid and electrolyte imbalances, page 919
Psychosocial aspects of care, page 770
Renal dialysis, page 564
Renal failure: acute, page 541
Total nutritional support: parenteral/enteral feeding, page 478
Upper gastrointestinal/esophageal bleeding, page 309

Client Assessment Database

Data depend on underlying cause of the condition.

ACTIVITY/REST

May report: Weakness, fatigue, exhaustion

May exhibit: Lethargy
Decreased muscle mass/tone

CIRCULATION

May report: History of/recent onset of HF, pericarditis, rheumatic heart disease, or cancer (causing liver impairment leading to failure)
Easy bruising, nosebleeds, bleeding gums

May exhibit: Hypertension or hypotension (fluid shifts)
Dysrhythmias, extra heart sounds (S_3, S_4)
Jugular venous distention (JVD), distended abdominal veins, spider angiomas/collateral circulation
Ecchymosis, petechiae
Anemia, leukopenia, thromboctyopenia, coagulation disorders, splenomegaly

ELIMINATION

May report: Flatulence
Diarrhea or constipation; gradual abdominal enlargement

May exhibit: Abdominal distention (hepatomegaly, splenomegaly, ascites)
Decreased/absent bowel sounds
Clay-colored stools, melena
Hemorrhoidal varices
Dark, concentrated urine; oliguria (hepatorenal syndrome/failure)

FOOD/FLUID

May report: Anorexia, food intolerance/ingestion
Nausea/vomiting, hematemesis

May exhibit: Weight loss or gain (fluid)
Tissue wasting, delayed wound healing
Edema generalized in tissues
Dry skin, poor turgor
Halitosis/fetor hepaticus, bleeding gums
Hypoalbuminemia

NEUROSENSORY

May report: SO(s) may report personality changes, depressed mentation

May exhibit: Changes in mentation, confusion, hallucinations, coma
Slowed/slurred speech
Asterixis (involuntary jerking movements of hands/tongue/feet associated with hepatic encephalopathy)

PAIN/DISCOMFORT

May report: Abdominal tenderness/RUQ pain
Severe itching
Pins/needles sensation, burning pain in extremities (peripheral neuropathy)

May exhibit: Guarding/distraction behaviors
Self-focus

RESPIRATION

May report: Dyspnea

May exhibit: Tachypnea, shallow respiration, adventitious breath sounds
Limited thoracic expansion (ascites)
Hypoxia

SAFETY

May report: Itching/dryness of the skin

May exhibit: Fever (more common in alcoholic cirrhosis)
Jaundiced skin and sclera, pruritus
Spider angiomas/telangiectasis, palmar erythema
Confusion progressing to delirium and coma (hepatic encephalopathy)
Unsteady or shaky/jerking movements

SEXUALITY

May report: Menstrual disorders (women), impotence (men)

May exhibit: Testicular atrophy, gynecomastia, loss of hair (chest, underarm, pubic)

TEACHING/LEARNING

May report: History of long-term alcohol or IV drug use/abuse, alcoholic liver disease, use of drugs affecting liver function
History of biliary disease, hepatitis, exposure to toxins, liver trauma, complications of portal hypertension (e.g., episodes of bleeding esophageal varices and hepatorenal syndrome)

Discharge plan considerations: May need assistance with self-care and other activities of daily living (ADLs), homemaker/maintenance

Refer to section at end of plan for postdischarge considerations.

DIAGNOSTIC STUDIES

Laparoscopic liver scan/biopsy: Detects fatty infiltrates, fibrosis, destruction of hepatic tissues, tumors (primary or metastatic), associated ascites.

Percutaneous transhepatic cholangiography (PTHC): May be done to rule out/differentiate causes of jaundice or to perform liver biopsy.

Esophagogastroduodenoscopy (EGD): May demonstrate presence of esophageal varices, stomach irritation or ulceration, duodenal ulceration or bleeding.

Percutaneous transhepatic portal angiography (PTPA): Visualizes portal venous system circulation.

Hepatobiliary iminodiacetic acid (HIDA) scan: Assists in the evaluation of the function of the gallbladder and bile ducts. The client is given a radioactive tracer (IV) that is excreted by the liver into bile ducts.

Serum bilirubin: Elevated because of cellular disruption, inability of liver to conjugate, or biliary obstruction.

Liver enzymes:

AST/ALT, LDH, and isoenzymes (LDH_5): Increased because of cellular damage and release of enzymes.

Alkaline phosphatase (ALP) and isoenzyme (LAP_1): Elevated because of reduced excretion.

Gamma glutamyl transpeptidase (GTT): Elevated.

Serum albumin: Decreased because of depressed synthesis.

Immunoglobulin (IgA, IgG, and IgM): Increased synthesis.

CBC: Hb/Hct and RBCs may be decreased because of bleeding. RBC destruction and anemia is seen with hypersplenism and iron deficiency. Leukopenia may be present as a result of hypersplenism.

PT/activated partial thromboplastin time (aPTT): Prolonged (decreased synthesis of prothrombin).

Fibrinogen: Decreased.

BUN: Elevation indicates breakdown of blood/protein.

Serum ammonia: Elevated because of inability to convert ammonia to urea.

Serum glucose: Hypoglycemia suggests impaired glycogenesis.

Electrolytes: Hypokalemia may reflect increased aldosterone, although various imbalances may occur. Hypocalcemia may occur because of impaired absorption of vitamin D.

Nutrient studies: Deficiency of vitamins A, B_{12}, C, K; folic acid; and iron may be noted.

Urine urobilinogen: May/may not be present. Serves as guide for differentiating liver disease, hemolytic disease, and biliary obstruction.

Fecal urobilinogen: Decreased.

NURSING PRIORITIES

1. Maintain adequate nutrition.
2. Prevent complications.
3. Enhance self-concept, acceptance of situation.
4. Provide information about disease process/prognosis, potential complications, and treatment needs.

DISCHARGE GOALS

1. Nutritional intake adequate for individual needs.
2. Complications prevented/minimized.
3. Dealing effectively with current reality.
4. Disease process, prognosis, potential complications, and therapeutic regimen understood.
5. Plan in place to meet needs after discharge.

NURSING DIAGNOSIS: imbalanced Nutrition: less than body requirements

May be related to

Inadequate diet; inability to process/digest nutrients
Anorexia, nausea/vomiting, indigestion, early satiety (ascites)
Abnormal bowel function

Possibly evidenced by

Weight loss
Changes in bowel sounds and function
Poor muscle tone/wasting; [fatigue]
Imbalances in nutritional studies

DESIRED OUTCOMES/EVALUATION CRITERIA—CLIENT WILL:

Nutritional Status (NOC)

Demonstrate progressive weight gain toward goal with client-appropriate normalization of laboratory values.
Experience no further signs of malnutrition.

ACTIONS/INTERVENTIONS	RATIONALE
Nutrition Therapy (NIC)	
Independent	
Evaluate client's risk for malnutrition.	Eighty-five percent to 90% of the blood that leaves the stomach and intestines carries nutrients to the liver where they are converted into substances the body can use. The client with liver dysfunction often has malnutrition because of inadequate dietary intake (e.g., poor food choices, preference for alcohol rather than food) and/or may currently have malabsorption syndrome (e.g., inability to process/digest nutrients, anorexia, nausea/vomiting, indigestion, early satiety [ascites]).

ACTIONS/INTERVENTIONS	RATIONALE
Determine interest in eating and ability to chew, swallow, and taste. Discuss eating habits, including food preferences, intolerances/aversions. Note availability/use of support systems.	Factors that affect ingestion and/or digestion of nutrients.
Determine dietary intake/perform calorie count if client is eating.	Provides information about intake, needs/deficiencies. Client with cirrhosis requires a balanced protein diet providing 2000–3000 calories/day to permit liver cell regeneration.
Weigh as indicated. Compare changes in fluid status, recent weight history.	It may be difficult to use weight as a direct indicator of nutritional status in view of edema/ascites.
Assist/encourage client to eat; explain reasons for the types of diet. Feed client if tiring easily, or have SO assist client. Consider preferences in food choices.	Improved nutrition/diet is vital to recovery. Client may eat better if family is involved and preferred foods are included as much as possible. Client and family must understand protein intake limitations and how best to meet needs/desires within limitations.
Encourage client to eat all meals/supplementary feedings.	Client may demonstrate loss of interest in food because of nausea, fatigue (often first reported symptom), generalized weakness, malaise.
Recommend/provide small, frequent meals.	Poor tolerance to larger meals may be due to increased intra-abdominal pressure/ascites.
Limit high-salt foods (e.g., canned soups and vegetables, processed meats, condiments). Provide salt substitutes if allowed; avoid those containing ammonium.	Salt limitations can help manage fluid complications in cirrhosis (e.g., ascites or tissue edema). Salt substitutes enhance the flavor of food and aid in increasing appetite; ammonia potentiates risk of encephalopathy.
Restrict intake of caffeine, gas-producing or spicy and excessively hot or cold foods.	Aids in reducing gastric irritation/diarrhea and abdominal discomfort that may impair oral intake/digestion.
Encourage/provide frequent mouth care, especially before meals.	Client is prone to sore and/or bleeding gums and bad taste in mouth, which contributes to anorexia.
Provide assistance with activities as needed. Promote undisturbed rest periods, especially before meals.	Conserving energy reduces metabolic demands on the liver and promotes cellular regeneration.
Recommend cessation of smoking.	Reduces excessive gastric stimulation and risk of irritation/bleeding.

Collaborative

Monitor nutritional laboratory studies; e.g., serum glucose, prealbumin/albumin, total protein, ammonia.	Glucose may be decreased because of impaired glycogenesis, depleted glycogen stores, or inadequate intake. Protein may be low because of impaired metabolism, decreased hepatic synthesis, or loss into peritoneal cavity (ascites). Protein-calorie malnutrition contributes to further development of fatty liver and deterioration of function. Elevation of ammonia level may require restriction of protein intake to prevent serious complications.
Maintain NPO status when indicated.	Gastrointestinal rest may be required in acutely ill clients to reduce demands on the liver and production of ammonia/urea in the GI tract. When this is the case, nutrition must be supplied by another method; e.g., enteral/parenteral feedings.
Determine nutritional/caloric needs, using appropriate method (e.g., total energy expenditure [TEE], body mass index [BMI], Harris-Benedict equation, indirect calorimetry test) as indicated.	Identifies energy requirements and deficits. Skinfold measurements and/or indirect calorimetry are useful in assessing changes in muscle mass, energy expenditure, and subcutaneous fat reserves.

ACTIONS/INTERVENTIONS	RATIONALE
Consult with dietitian/nutritionist to provide diet that is high in calories and simple carbohydrates, low in fat (or using fat substitutes), and low to moderate in protein. Limit sodium as necessary. Provide liquid supplements as indicated.	High-calorie foods are desired inasmuch as client intake is usually limited. Carbohydrates supply readily available energy. Fats are poorly absorbed because of liver dysfunction and may contribute to abdominal discomfort. Proteins are needed to improve serum protein levels (reduces edema) and to promote liver cell regeneration. However, protein can also elevate ammonia levels, and must be restricted if ammonia level is elevated, or if client has clinical signs of hepatic encephalopathy. In addition, these individuals may tolerate vegetable protein better than meat protein.
Provide enteral tube feedings, TPN, lipids if indicated.	May be required to supplement diet or to provide nutrients when client is too nauseated or anorexic to eat or when esophageal varices interfere with oral intake. (Refer to CP: Total nutritional support: Enteral/parenteral feedings.)
Administer medications as indicated; e.g.:	
Vitamin supplements (especially fat-soluble vitamins A, D, E, K) and B vitamins (e.g., thiamine, iron, folic acid);	Client may be vitamin deficient because of previous poor dietary habits. Also, the injured liver is unable to utilize vitamins, and anemia (due to iron and folic acid deficiencies) may exist.
Digestive enzymes; e.g., pancrelipase (Viokase); lactulose;	May be tried to promote digestion of fats, and reduce incidence of steatorrhea and diarrhea.
Antiemetics; e.g., trimethobenzamide (Tigan).	Used with caution to reduce nausea/vomiting and increase oral intake.

NURSING DIAGNOSIS: excess Fluid Volume

May be related to

Compromised regulatory mechanism (e.g., syndrome of inappropriate antidiuretic hormone [SIADH], decreased plasma proteins, malnutrition)
Excess sodium/fluid intake

Possibly evidenced by

Edema, anasarca, weight gain
Intake greater than output, oliguria, changes in urine specific gravity
Dyspnea, adventitious breath sounds, pleural effusion
BP changes, altered CVP
JVD, positive hepatojugular reflex
Altered electrolyte levels
Change in mental status

DESIRED OUTCOMES/EVALUATION CRITERIA—CLIENT WILL:

Fluid Balance (NOC)

Demonstrate stabilized fluid volume, with balanced I&O, stable weight, vital signs within client's normal range, and absence of edema.

ACTIONS/INTERVENTIONS	RATIONALE
Fluid/Electrolyte Management (NIC)	
Independent	
Measure I&O, noting positive balance (intake in excess of output). Weigh daily, and note gain more than 0.5 kg/day.	Reflects circulating volume status, developing/resolution of fluid shifts, and response to therapy. Positive balance/weight gain often reflects continuing fluid retention. *Note:* Decreased circulating volume (fluid shifts) may directly affect renal function/urine output, resulting in hepatorenal syndrome.
Monitor BP (and CVP if available). Note JVD/abdominal vein distention.	BP elevations are usually associated with fluid volume excess but may not occur because of fluid shifts out of the vascular space. Distention of external jugular and abdominal veins is associated with vascular congestion.
Assess respiratory status, noting increased respiratory rate, dyspnea.	Indicative of pulmonary congestion/edema.
Auscultate lungs, noting diminished/absent breath sounds and developing adventitious sounds (e.g., crackles).	Increasing pulmonary congestion may result in consolidation, impaired gas exchange, and complications; e.g., pulmonary edema.
Monitor for cardiac dysrhythmias. Auscultate heart sounds, noting development of S_3/S_4 gallop rhythm.	May be caused by heart failure, decreased coronary arterial perfusion, or electrolyte imbalance.
Assess degree of peripheral/dependent edema.	Fluids shift into tissues as a result of sodium and water retention, decreased albumin, and increased antidiuretic hormone (ADH).
Measure abdominal girth.	Reflects accumulation of fluid (ascites) resulting from loss of plasma proteins/fluid into peritoneal space. *Note:* Excessive fluid accumulation can reduce circulating volume, resulting in a deficit (signs of dehydration).
Encourage bedrest when ascites is present.	May promote recumbency-induced diuresis.
Provide frequent mouth care; occasional ice chips (particularly if NPO), schedule fluid intake around the clock.	Decreases sensation of thirst, especially when fluid intake restricted.
Collaborative	
Monitor serum albumin and electrolytes (particularly potassium and sodium).	Decreased serum albumin affects plasma colloid osmotic pressure, resulting in edema formation. Reduced renal blood flow accompanied by elevated ADH and aldosterone levels and the use of diuretics (to reduce total body water) may cause various electrolyte shifts/imbalances.
Monitor serial chest x-rays.	Vascular congestion, pulmonary edema, and pleural effusions frequently occur.
Restrict sodium and fluids as indicated.	Sodium may be restricted to minimize fluid retention in extravascular spaces. Fluid restriction may be necessary to correct/prevent dilutional hyponatremia.
Administer salt-free albumin/plasma expanders as indicated.	Albumin may be used to increase the colloid osmotic pressure in the vascular compartment (pulling fluid into vascular space), thereby increasing effective circulating volume and decreasing formation of ascites.
Administer medications as indicated:	
Diuretics; e.g., spironolactone (Aldactone), furosemide (Lasix);	Used with caution to control edema and ascites, block effect of aldosterone, and increase water excretion while sparing potassium when conservative therapy with bedrest and sodium restriction does not alleviate problem. Diuretic given in coordination with albumin administration may enhance fluid removal.
Potassium;	Serum and cellular potassium are usually depleted because of liver disease and urinary losses.
Positive inotropic drugs and arterial vasodilators.	Given to increase cardiac output/improve renal blood flow and function, thereby reducing excess fluid.

NURSING DIAGNOSIS: risk for impaired Skin Integrity

Risk factors may include

Altered circulation/metabolic state
Accumulation of bile salts in skin
Poor skin turgor, skeletal prominence, presence of edema, ascites

Possibly evidenced by

[Not applicable; presence of signs and symptoms establishes an *actual* diagnosis.]

DESIRED OUTCOMES/EVALUATION CRITERIA—CLIENT WILL:

Risk Control (NOC)

Maintain skin integrity.
Identify individual risk factors and demonstrate behaviors/techniques to prevent skin breakdown.

ACTIONS/INTERVENTIONS	RATIONALE
Skin Surveillance (NIC)	
Independent	
Inspect skin surfaces/pressure points routinely. Gently massage bony prominences or areas of continued stress. Use emollient lotions, limit use of soap for bathing.	Edematous tissues are more prone to breakdown and to the formation of decubitus ulcers. Ascites may stretch the skin to the point of tearing in severe cirrhosis.
Encourage/assist with repositioning on a regular schedule, while in bed/chair, and active/passive ROM exercises as appropriate.	Repositioning reduces pressure on edematous tissues to improve circulation. Exercises enhance circulation and improve/maintain joint mobility.
Recommend elevating lower extremities.	Enhances venous return and reduces edema formation in extremities.
Keep linens dry and free of wrinkles.	Moisture aggravates pruritus and increases risk of skin breakdown.
Suggest clipping fingernails short, provide mittens/gloves if indicated.	Prevents client from inadvertently injuring the skin, especially while sleeping.
Encourage/provide perineal care following urination and bowel movement.	Prevents skin excoriation breakdown from bile salts.
Collaborative	
Use alternating pressure mattress, egg-crate mattress, waterbed, sheepskins, as indicated.	Reduces dermal pressure, increases circulation, and diminishes risk of tissue ischemia/breakdown.
Apply calamine lotion, provide baking soda baths.	May be soothing/provide relief of itching (pruritus).
Administer medications such as hydroxyzine (Vistaril, Atarax), cholestyramine (Questran), colestipol (Colestid), hydroxyzine (Atarax), dronabinol (Marinol) if indicated.	Although the cause of pruritus is unknown, it may be associated with jaundice or bile salts in skin, and may respond to these treatments.

NURSING DIAGNOSIS: risk for ineffective Breathing Pattern

Risk factors may include

Intra-abdominal fluid collection (ascites)
Decreased lung expansion, accumulated secretions
Decreased energy, fatigue

Possibly evidenced by

[Not applicable; presence of signs and symptoms establishes an *actual* diagnosis.]

DESIRED OUTCOMES/EVALUATION CRITERIA—CLIENT WILL:

RESPIRATORY STATUS: Ventilation (NOC)

Maintain effective respiratory pattern; be free of dyspnea and cyanosis, with ABGs and vital capacity within acceptable range.

ACTIONS/INTERVENTIONS	RATIONALE
Ventilation Assistance (NIC)	
Independent	
Monitor respiratory rate, depth, and effort.	Rapid shallow respirations/dyspnea may be present because of hypoxia and/or fluid accumulation in abdomen.
Auscultate breath sounds, noting crackles, wheezes, rhonchi.	Indicates developing complications (e.g., presence of adventitious sounds reflects accumulation of fluid/secretions; absent/diminished sounds suggest atelectasis), increasing risk of infection.
Investigate changes in level of consciousness.	Changes in mentation may reflect hypoxemia and respiratory failure, which often accompany hepatic coma.
Keep head of bed elevated. Position on sides.	Facilitates breathing by reducing pressure on the diaphragm, and minimizes risk of aspiration of secretions.
Encourage frequent repositioning and deep-breathing exercises/coughing as appropriate.	Aids in lung expansion and mobilizing secretions.
Monitor temperature. Note presence of chills, increased coughing, changes in color/character of sputum.	Indicative of onset of infection; e.g., pneumonia.
Collaborative	
Monitor serial ABGs, pulse oximetry, vital capacity measurements, chest x-rays.	Reveals changes in respiratory status, developing pulmonary complications.
Provide supplemental O_2 as indicated.	May be necessary to treat/prevent hypoxia. If respirations/oxygenation inadequate, mechanical ventilation may be required.
Demonstrate/assist with respiratory adjuncts; e.g., incentive spirometer.	Reduces incidence of atelectasis, enhances mobilization of secretions.
Prepare for/assist with acute care procedures; e.g.:	
Paracentesis;	Occasionally done to remove ascites fluid to relieve abdominal pressure when respiratory embarrassment is not corrected by other measures.
Peritoneovenous shunt.	Surgical implant of a catheter to return accumulated fluid in the abdominal cavity to systemic circulation via the vena cava; provides long-term relief of ascites and improvement in respiratory function.

NURSING DIAGNOSIS: risk for Injury [hemorrhage]

Risk factors may include

Abnormal blood profile; altered clotting factors (decreased production of prothrombin, fibrinogen, and factors VIII, IX, and X; impaired vitamin K absorption; and release of thromboplastin)
Portal hypertension, development of esophageal varices

Possibly evidenced by

[Not applicable; presence of signs and symptoms establishes an *actual* diagnosis.]

DESIRED OUTCOMES/EVALUATION CRITERIA—CLIENT WILL:

Coagulation Status (NOC)

Maintain homeostasis with absence of bleeding.

Risk Control (NOC)

Demonstrate behaviors to reduce risk of bleeding.

ACTIONS/INTERVENTIONS	RATIONALE
Bleeding Precautions (NIC)	
Independent	
Assess for signs/symptoms of GI bleeding; e.g., check all secretions for frank or occult blood. Observe color and consistency of stools, NG drainage, or vomitus.	The GI tract (esophagus and rectum) is the most usual source of bleeding because of its mucosal fragility and alterations in homeostasis associated with cirrhosis.
Observe for presence of petechiae, ecchymosis, bleeding from one or more sites.	Subacute disseminated intravascular coagulation (DIC) may develop secondary to altered clotting factors.
Monitor pulse, BP (and CVP if available).	An increased pulse with decreased BP and CVP can indicate loss of circulating blood volume, requiring further evaluation.
Note changes in mentation/level of consciousness.	Changes may indicate decreased cerebral perfusion secondary to hypovolemia, hypoxemia.
Avoid rectal temperature, be gentle with GI tube insertions.	Rectal and esophageal vessels are most vulnerable to rupture.
Encourage use of soft toothbrush, electric razor, avoiding straining for stool, forceful nose blowing, and so forth.	In the presence of clotting factor disturbances, minimal trauma can cause mucosal bleeding.
Use small needles for injections. Apply pressure to small bleeding/venipuncture sites for longer than usual.	Minimizes damage to tissues, reducing risk of bleeding/hematoma.
Recommend avoidance of aspirin-containing products.	Prolongs coagulation, potentiating risk of hemorrhage.
Collaborative	
Monitor Hb/Hct, platelets, and clotting factors.	Indicators of anemia, active bleeding, or impending complications (e.g., DIC).
Administer medications as indicated:	
Supplemental vitamins (e.g., vitamins K, D, and C);	Promotes prothrombin synthesis and coagulation if liver is functional. Vitamin C deficiencies increase susceptibility of GI system to irritation/bleeding.

ACTIONS/INTERVENTIONS	RATIONALE
Stool softeners.	Prevents straining for stool with resultant increase in intra-abdominal pressure and risk of vascular rupture/hemorrhage.
Provide gastric lavage with room temperature/cool saline solution or water as indicated.	In presence of acute bleeding, evacuation of blood from GI tract may reduce ammonia production and risk of hepatic encephalopathy. (Refer to CP: Upper gastrointestinal/esophageal bleeding.)
Assist with insertion/maintenance of GI/esophageal tube (e.g., Sengstaken-Blakemore tube).	Temporarily controls bleeding of esophageal varices when control by other means (e.g., lavage) and hemodynamic stability cannot be achieved.
Prepare for procedures; e.g., direct ligation (banding) of varices, esophagogastric resection, transjugular intrahepatic portosystemic shunt (TIPS), splenorenal-portacaval anastomosis.	May be needed to control active hemorrhage or to decrease portal and collateral blood vessel pressure to minimize risk of recurrence of bleeding. TIPS is a nonsurgical procedure to relieve portal hypertension and decompress varices by creating a shunt between the systemic and portal venous systems to redirect portal blood flow.

NURSING DIAGNOSIS: risk for acute Confusion

Risk factors may include

Alcohol abuse
Inability of liver to detoxify certain enzymes/drugs

Possibly evidenced by

[Not applicable; presence of signs and symptoms establishes an *actual* diagnosis.]

DESIRED OUTCOMES/EVALUATION CRITERIA—CLIENT WILL:

Cognition (NOC)

Maintain usual level of mentation/reality orientation.
Initiate behaviors/lifestyle changes to prevent or minimize recurrence of problem.

ACTIONS/INTERVENTIONS	RATIONALE
Reality Orientation (NIC)	
Independent	
Observe for changes in behavior and mentation; e.g., lethargy, confusion, drowsiness, slowing/slurring of speech, and irritability (may be intermittent). Arouse client at intervals as indicated.	Ongoing assessment of behavior and mental status is important because of fluctuating nature of impending hepatic coma.
Review current medication regimen/schedules.	Adverse drug reactions or interactions (e.g., cimetidine plus antacids) may potentiate/exacerbate confusion.
Evaluate sleep/rest schedule.	Difficulty falling/staying asleep leads to sleep deprivation, resulting in diminished cognition and lethargy.
Note development/presence of asterixis, fetor hepaticus, seizure activity.	Suggests elevating serum ammonia levels; increased risk of progression to encephalopathy.
Consult with SO about client's usual behavior and mentation.	Provides baseline for comparison of current status.
Have client write name periodically and keep this record for comparison. Report deterioration of ability. Have client do simple arithmetic computations.	Easy test of neurologic status and muscle coordination.

ACTIONS/INTERVENTIONS	RATIONALE
Reorient to time, place, person, situation as needed.	Assists in maintaining reality orientation, reducing confusion/anxiety.
Maintain a pleasant, quiet environment and approach in a slow, calm manner. Encourage uninterrupted rest periods.	Reduces excessive stimulation/sensory overload, promotes relaxation, and may enhance coping.
Provide continuity of care. If possible, assign same nurse over a period of time.	Familiarity provides reassurance, aids in reducing anxiety, and provides a more accurate documentation of subtle changes.
Reduce provocative stimuli, confrontation. Refrain from forcing activities. Assess potential for violent behavior.	Avoids triggering agitated, violent responses; promotes client safety.
Discuss current situation, future expectation.	Client/SO may be reassured that intellectual (as well as emotional) function may improve as liver involvement resolves.
Maintain bedrest, assist with self-care activities.	Reduces metabolic demands on liver, prevents fatigue, and promotes healing, lowering risk of ammonia buildup.
Identify/provide safety needs; e.g., supervision during smoking, bed in low position, side rails up and pad if necessary. Provide close supervision.	Reduces risk of injury when confusion, seizures, or violent behavior occurs.
Investigate temperature elevations. Monitor for signs of infection.	Infection may precipitate hepatic encephalopathy caused by tissue catabolism and release of nitrogen.
Recommend avoidance of narcotics or sedatives, antianxiety agents, and limiting/restricting use of medications metabolized by the liver.	Certain drugs are toxic to the liver, whereas other drugs may not be metabolized because of cirrhosis, causing cumulative effects that affect mentation, mask signs of developing encephalopathy, or precipitate coma.

Collaborative

ACTIONS/INTERVENTIONS	RATIONALE
Monitor laboratory studies; e.g., ammonia, electrolytes, pH, BUN, glucose, CBC with differential.	Elevated ammonia levels, hypokalemia, metabolic alkalosis, hypoglycemia, anemia, and infection can precipitate or potentiate development of hepatic coma.
Eliminate or restrict protein in diet. Provide glucose supplements, adequate hydration.	Ammonia (product of the breakdown of protein in the GI tract) is responsible for mental changes in hepatic encephalopathy. Dietary changes may result in constipation, which also increases bacterial action and formation of ammonia. Glucose provides a source of energy, reducing need for protein catabolism. *Note:* Vegetable protein may be better tolerated than meat protein.
Administer medications as indicated:	
Ursodeoxycholic acid (UDCA; urosodiol [Actigal]);	Major medication used to slow the progression of the disease; may delay need for transplantation.
Immunosuppressive agents (e.g., corticosteroids (Prednisolone, DeltaCortef), methotrexate (Rheumatrex/Folex), cycolsporine (Sandimmune/Neoral), anti-inflammatory agents; e.g., colchicines;	These agents may inhibit immune reactions that mediate inflammatory processes/progression of the disease.
Electrolytes;	Corrects imbalances and may improve cerebral function/metabolism of ammonia.
Stool softeners, colonic purges (e.g., magnesium sulfate), enemas, lactulose;	Removes protein and blood from intestines. Acidifying the intestine produces diarrhea and decreases production of nitrogenous substances, reducing risk/severity of encephalopathy. *Note:* Long-term use of lactulose may be required for clients with hepatic encephalopathy to reduce ammonia on a daily/regular basis.
Bactericidal agents; e.g., neomycin (Mycifradin), kanamycin (Kantrex).	Destroys intestinal bacteria, reducing production of ammonia, to prevent encephalopathy.
Administer supplemental O_2.	Mentation is affected by O_2 concentration and utilization in the brain.
Assist with procedures as indicated; e.g., dialysis, plasmapheresis, or extracorporeal liver perfusion.	May be used to reduce serum ammonia levels if encephalopathy develops/other measures are not successful.

NURSING DIAGNOSIS: Self-Esteem [specify]/disturbed Body Image

May be related to

Biophysical changes/altered physical appearance
Uncertainty of prognosis, changes in role function
Personal vulnerability
Self-destructive behavior (alcohol-induced disease)

Possibly evidenced by

Verbalization of change/restriction in lifestyle
Fear of rejection or reaction by others
Negative feelings about body/abilities
Feelings of helplessness, hopelessness, or powerlessness

DESIRED OUTCOMES/EVALUATION CRITERIA—CLIENT WILL:

Self-Esteem (NOC)

Verbalize understanding of changes and acceptance of self in the present situation.
Identify feelings and methods for coping with negative perception of self.

ACTIONS/INTERVENTIONS	RATIONALE
Self-Esteem Enhancement (NIC)	
Independent	
Discuss situation/encourage verbalization of fears and concerns. Explain relationship between nature of disease and symptoms.	Client is very sensitive to body changes and may also experience feelings of guilt when cause is related to alcohol (70%) or other drug use.
Support and encourage client, provide care with a positive, friendly attitude.	Caregivers sometimes allow judgmental feelings to affect the care of client and need to make every effort to help client feel valued as a person.
Encourage family/SO to verbalize feelings, visit freely/participate in care.	Family members may feel guilty about client's condition and may be fearful of impending death. They need nonjudgmental emotional support and free access to client. Participation in care helps them feel useful and promotes trust between staff, client, and SO.
Assist client/SO to cope with change in appearance; suggest clothing that does not emphasize altered appearance; e.g., use of red, blue, or black clothing.	Client may present unattractive appearance as a result of jaundice, ascites, ecchymotic areas. Providing support can enhance self-esteem and promote client sense of control.
Collaborative	
Refer to support services; e.g., counselors, psychiatric resources, social service, clergy, and/or alcohol treatment program.	Increased vulnerability/concerns associated with this illness may require services of additional professional resources.

NURSING DIAGNOSIS: deficient Knowledge [Learning Need] regarding condition, prognosis, treatment, self-care, and discharge needs

May be related to

Lack of exposure/recall; information misinterpretation
Unfamiliarity with information resources

Possibly evidenced by

Questions; request for information, statement of misconception
Inaccurate follow-through of instructions/development of preventable complications

DESIRED OUTCOMES/EVALUATION CRITERIA—CLIENT WILL:

KNOWLEDGE: Illness Care (NOC)

Verbalize understanding of disease process/prognosis, potential complications.
Correlate symptoms with causative factors.

KNOWLEDGE: Health Behaviors (NOC)

Identify/initiate necessary lifestyle changes and participate in care.

ACTIONS/INTERVENTIONS	RATIONALE
TEACHING: Disease Process (NIC)	
Independent	
Review disease process/prognosis and future expectations.	Provides knowledge base from which client can make informed choices.
Stress importance of avoiding alcohol. Give information about community services available to aid in alcohol rehabilitation if indicated.	Alcohol is one of the leading causes in the development of cirrhosis.
Inform client of altered effects of medications with cirrhosis and the importance of using only drugs prescribed or cleared by a healthcare provider who is familiar with client's history.	Some drugs are hepatotoxic (especially narcotics, sedatives, and hypnotics). In addition, the damaged liver has a decreased ability to metabolize all drugs, potentiating cumulative effect and/or aggravation of bleeding tendencies.
Review procedure for maintaining function of peritoneovenous shunt when present.	Insertion of a Denver shunt requires client to periodically pump the chamber to maintain patency of the device. Clients with a LeVeen shunt may wear an abdominal binder and/or engage in a Valsalva maneuver to maintain shunt function.
Assist client identifying support person(s).	Because of length of recovery, potential for relapses, and slow convalescence, support systems are extremely important in maintaining behavior modifications.
Emphasize the importance of good nutrition. Recommend avoidance of high-protein/salty foods, onions, and strong cheeses. Provide written dietary instructions.	Proper dietary maintenance and avoidance of foods high in sodium and protein aid in remission of symptoms and help prevent ammonia buildup and further liver damage. Written instructions are helpful for client to refer to at home.
Stress necessity of follow-up care and adherence to therapeutic regimen.	Chronic nature of disease has potential for life-threatening complications. Provides opportunity for evaluation of effectiveness of regimen, including patency of shunt if used.
Discuss sodium and salt substitute restrictions and necessity of reading labels on food, OTC drugs, and herbal agents.	Minimizes ascites and edema formation. Overuse of substitutes may result in other electrolyte imbalances. Food, OTC medications and personal care products (e.g., antacids, some mouthwashes) may contain sodium or alcohol and may be toxic to the liver and/or be primarily metabolized by the liver.
Encourage scheduling activities with adequate rest periods.	Adequate rest decreases metabolic demands on the body and increases energy available for tissue regeneration.
Promote diversional activities that are enjoyable to client.	Prevents boredom, facilitates rest, and minimizes anxiety and depression.

ACTIONS/INTERVENTIONS	RATIONALE
Recommend avoidance of persons with infections, especially URI.	Decreased resistance, altered nutritional status, and immune response (e.g., leukopenia may occur with splenomegaly) potentiate risk of infection.
Identify environmental dangers; e.g., carbon tetrachloride–type cleaning agents, exposure to hepatitis.	Can precipitate recurrence.
Instruct client/SO of signs/symptoms that warrant notification of healthcare provider; e.g., increased abdominal girth, rapid weight loss/gain, increased peripheral edema, increased dyspnea, fever, blood in stool or urine, excess bleeding of any kind, jaundice.	Prompt reporting of symptoms reduces risk of further hepatic damage and provides opportunity to treat complications before they become life-threatening. *Note*: Client may be evaluated for additional medical or surgical interventions, including liver transplantation.
Instruct SO to notify healthcare providers of any confusion, untidiness, night wandering, tremors, or personality change.	Changes (reflecting deterioration) may be more apparent to SO, although insidious changes may be noted by others with less frequent contact with client.

POTENTIAL CONSIDERATIONS following acute hospitalization (dependent on client's age, physical condition/presence of complications, personal resources, and life responsibilities)

Fatigue—decreased metabolic energy production, states of discomfort, altered body chemistry (e.g., changes in liver function, effect on target organs, alcohol withdrawal).

imbalanced Nutrition: less than body requirements—inadequate diet, inability to process/digest nutrients, anorexia, nausea/vomiting, indigestion, early satiety (ascites), abnormal bowel function.

risk for ineffective Therapeutic Regimen Management—perceived benefit, social support deficit, economic difficulties.

dysfunctional Family Processes: alcoholism—abuse of alcohol, resistance to treatment, inadequate coping/lack of problem-solving skills, addictive personality/codependency.

risk for Caregiver Role Strain—addiction or codependency, family dysfunction before caregiving situation, presence of situational stressors, such as economic vulnerability, hospitalization, changes in employment.

PANCREATITIS

Pancreatitis is a painful inflammatory condition in which the pancreatic enzymes are prematurely activated resulting in autodigestion of the pancreas. An estimated 80,000 individuals are diagnosed with pancreatitis annually in the United States. The most common causes of acute pancreatitis are (1) biliary tract disease (e.g., gallstones) and (2) alcoholism; however, it can also be the result of (3) trauma (e.g., blunt/penetrating), (4) procedures (e.g., endoscopic or surgical), (5) viral infections (e.g., mumps, mononucleosis, varicella), (6) bacterial infections (e.g., *Mycoplasma pneumoniae*, salmonellosis, tuberculosis), (7) genetic mutations (e.g., cystic fibrosis transmembrane regulator [CFTR] or pancreatic secretory protease inhibitor), and (8) drugs (e.g., sulfonamides, glucocorticoids, thiazide diuretics, nonsteroidal anti-inflammatory drugs).

Pancreatitis may be acute or chronic, with symptoms ranging from mild to severe. Acute pancreatitis can be life threatening.

CARE SETTING

Inpatient acute medical unit and/or intensive care unit for initial incident or exacerbations with serious complications; otherwise condition is managed at the community level.

RELATED CONCERNS

Alcohol: acute withdrawal, page 831
Substance dependence/abuse rehabilitation, page 843
Diabetes mellitus/diabetic ketoacidosis, page 412
Peritonitis, page 355
Psychosocial aspects of care, page 770
Renal failure: acute, page 541
Sepsis/septicemia, page 701
Total nutritional support; parenteral/enteral feeding, page 478

Client Assessment Database

ACTIVITY/REST

May report: Malaise, fatigue
May exhibit: Agitation, restlessness, distress, apprehension

CIRCULATION

May exhibit: Hypertension (acute pain), hypotension and tachycardia (hypovolemic shock or sepsis/systemic inflammatory response syndrome [SIRS])
Edema, ascites
Skin pale, mottled areas with diaphoresis (vasoconstriction/fluid shifts); flushing may be present in acute stage from systemic inflammation; jaundiced (inflammation/obstruction of common duct); blue-green-brown discoloration around umbilicus (Cullen's sign) from accumulation of blood (hemorrhagic pancreatitis)

ELIMINATION

May report: Diarrhea or no elimination
May exhibit: Bowel sounds decreased/absent (reduced peristalsis/ileus)
Dark amber or brown, foamy urine (bile)
Frothy, foul-smelling, grayish, greasy, nonformed stool (steatorrhea)
Oliguria progressing to anuria (hypovolemic compensatory response)

FOOD/FLUID

May report: Food intolerance, anorexia; frequent/persistent vomiting, retching, dry heaves
Weight loss
May exhibit: Diffuse epigastric/abdominal tenderness to palpation, abdominal rigidity, distention
Hypoactive bowel sounds
Hyperglycemia and urine positive for glucose

NEUROSENSORY

May exhibit: Confusion, agitation
Coarse tremors of extremities (hypocalcemia)

PAIN/DISCOMFORT

May report: Unrelenting severe deep abdominal pain, usually located in the epigastrium and periumbilical regions but may radiate to the back; onset may be sudden and may be associated with heavy drinking or a large meal
Radiation to chest and back; may increase in supine position
May exhibit: Abdominal guarding; may curl up on left side with both arms over abdomen and knees/hips flexed
Abdominal rigidity

RESPIRATION

May exhibit: Tachypnea with/without dyspnea
Decreased depth of respiration with splinting/guarding actions
Bibasilar crackles (pleural effusion/infiltration)

SAFETY

May exhibit: Fever (76%)
Agitation, confusion (hypovolemia and septic shock)

SEXUALITY

May exhibit: Current pregnancy (third trimester) with shifting of abdominal contents and compression of biliary tract

TEACHING/LEARNING

May report: Family history of pancreatitis
Signs and symptoms of hyperglycemic crisis
History of cholelithiasis with partial or complete common bile duct obstruction, gastritis, duodenal ulcer, duodenitis, diverticulitis, Crohn's disease, recent abdominal surgery (e.g., procedures on the pancreas, biliary tract, stomach, or duodenum), external abdominal trauma

Excessive alcohol intake (90% of cases)
Uses of medications; e.g., salicylates, pentamidine, antihypertensives, opiates, thiazides, steroids, some antibiotics, estrogens
Infectious diseases; e.g., mumps, hepatitis B, Coxsackie viral infection

Discharge plan considerations: May require assistance with dietary program and ADLs at home

Refer to section at end of plan for postdischarge considerations

DIAGNOSTIC STUDIES

Ultrasound of abdomen: Most useful initial test for determining etiology of pancreatitis, to identify pancreatic inflammation, abscess, pseudocysts, carcinoma, or obstruction of biliary tract by gallstones.
CT scan: Shows an enlarged pancreas and pancreatic cysts and determines extent of edema and necrosis.
Magnetic resonance cholangiopancreatography (MRCP): Emerging role in diagnosis of suspected biliary and pancreatic duct obstruction in the presence of pancreatitis.
Endoscopic retrograde cholangiopancreatography (ERCP): Useful to diagnose fistulas, obstructive biliary disease, and pancreatic duct strictures/anomalies (procedure is contraindicated in acute phase).
Endoscopic ultrasonography (EUS): Allows a more detailed image to be obtained than with ERCP because the high-frequency transducer can be introduced adjacent to the pancreas.
CT-guided needle aspiration: Done to determine whether infection is present or if pseudocyst develops that requires aspiration.
Abdominal radiographs: May demonstrate dilated loop of small bowel adjacent to pancreas or other intra-abdominal precipitator of pancreatitis, presence of free intraperitoneal air caused by perforation or abscess formation, pancreatic calcification.
Chest radiograph: May demonstrate diffuse, pulmonary infiltrates. Client may demonstrate signs and symptoms of hypoxemia requiring mechanical ventilation/support.
Upper GI series: Frequently exhibits evidence of pancreatic enlargement/inflammation.
Serum amylase: Increased because of obstruction of normal outflow of pancreatic enzymes (normal level does not rule out disease). May be five or more times normal level in acute pancreatitis, and then fall back within normal ranges as pancreatitis resolves.
Serum lipase: Elevates along with amylase, but stays elevated longer.
Serum bilirubin: Elevation is common (may be caused by alcoholic liver disease or compression of common bile duct).
Alkaline phosphatase: Usually elevated if pancreatitis is accompanied by biliary disease.
C-reactive protein (CRP): An acute-phase reactant not specific for pancreatitis: however, when elevated >10mg/dL, is suggestive of severe pancreatitis.
Serum albumin and protein: May be decreased (increased capillary permeability and transudation of fluid into extracellular space).
Serum calcium: Hypocalcemia may appear 2–3 days after onset of illness (usually indicates fat necrosis and may accompany pancreatic necrosis).
Potassium: Hypokalemia may occur because of gastric losses; hyperkalemia may develop secondary to tissue necrosis, acidosis, renal insufficiency.
Triglycerides: Levels may exceed 1700 mg/dL and may be causative agent in acute pancreatitis.
LDH/AST: May be elevated up to 15 times normal because of biliary and liver involvement.
CBC: WBC count of 10,000–25,000 is present in 80% of clients. Hgb may be lower because of bleeding. Hct may be elevated (hemoconcentration associated with vomiting, hypovolemia, or from effusion of fluid into pancreas or retroperitoneal area).
Serum glucose: Transient elevations of more than 200 mg/dL are common, especially during initial/acute attacks. Sustained hyperglycemia reflects widespread cell damage and pancreatic necrosis and is a poor prognostic sign.
Partial thromboplastin time (PTT): Prolonged if coagulopathy develops because of liver involvement and fat necrosis.
Urinalysis: Glucose, myoglobin, blood, and protein may be present.
Urine amylase: Can increase dramatically within 2–3 days after onset of attack.
Stool: Increased fat content (steatorrhea) indicative of insufficient digestion of fats and protein.

NURSING PRIORITIES

1. Control pain and promote comfort.
2. Prevent/treat fluid and electrolyte imbalance.
3. Reduce pancreatic stimulation while maintaining adequate nutrition.
4. Prevent complications.
5. Provide information about disease process/prognosis and treatment needs.

DISCHARGE GOALS

1. Pain relieved/controlled.
2. Hemodynamically stable.
3. Complications prevented/minimized.
4. Disease process/prognosis, potential complications, and therapeutic regimen understood.
5. Plan in place to meet needs after discharge.

NURSING DIAGNOSIS: acute Pain

May be related to

Obstruction of pancreatic, biliary ducts
Chemical contamination of peritoneal surfaces by pancreatic exudate/autodigestion of pancreas
Extension of inflammation to the retroperitoneal nerve plexus

Possibly evidenced by

Reports of pain
Self-focusing, grimacing, distraction/guarding behaviors
Autonomic responses, alteration in muscle tone

DESIRED OUTCOMES/EVALUATION CRITERIA—CLIENT WILL:

Pain Control (NOC)

Report pain is relieved/controlled.
Follow prescribed therapeutic regimen.
Demonstrate use of methods that provide relief.

ACTIONS/INTERVENTIONS	RATIONALE
Pain Management (NIC)	
Independent	
Investigate verbal reports of pain, noting specific location and intensity (0–10 scale). Note factors that aggravate and relieve pain.	Pain is often diffuse, severe, and unrelenting in acute or hemorrhagic pancreatitis. Severe pain is often the major symptom in client with chronic pancreatitis. Isolated pain in the right upper quadrant (RUQ) reflects involvement of the head of the pancreas. Pain in the left upper quadrant (LUQ) suggests involvement of the pancreatic tail. Localized pain may indicate development of pseudocysts or abscesses.
Maintain bedrest during acute attack, provide quiet, restful environment.	Decreases metabolic rate and GI stimulation/secretions, thereby reducing pancreatic activity.
Promote position of comfort; e.g., on one side with knees flexed, sitting up and leaning forward.	Reduces abdominal pressure/tension, providing some measure of comfort and pain relief. *Note:* Supine position often increases pain.
Provide alternative comfort measures (e.g., back rub), encourage relaxation techniques (e.g., guided imagery, visualization), quiet diversional activities (e.g., TV, radio).	Promotes relaxation and enables client to refocus attention; may enhance coping.
Keep environment free of food odors.	Sensory stimulation can activate pancreatic enzymes, increasing pain.
Administer IV analgesics in timely manner, smaller, more frequent doses, during acute episode. Consider use of patient-controlled analgesia (PCA) if appropriate.	Severe/prolonged pain can aggravate shock and is more difficult to relieve, requiring larger doses of medication, which can mask underlying problems/complications and may contribute to respiratory depression.

ACTIONS/INTERVENTIONS	RATIONALE
Maintain meticulous skin care, especially in presence of draining abdominal wall fistulas.	Pancreatic enzymes can digest the skin and tissues of the abdominal wall, creating a chemical burn.

Collaborative

ACTIONS/INTERVENTIONS	RATIONALE
Administer medication as indicated:	
Narcotic analgesics; e.g., meperidine (Demerol), morphine sulfate; fentanyl (Sublimaze), pentazocine (Talwin);	Meperidine is usually effective in relieving pain and may be preferred over morphine, which may have a side effect of biliary-pancreatic spasms. Paravertebral block has been used to achieve prolonged pain control. *Note:* Pain in clients who have recurrent or chronic pancreatitis episodes may be more difficult to manage because they may develop tolerance to normal doses of the narcotics given for pain control.
Sedatives; e.g., diazepam (Valium), antispasmodics; e.g., atropine;	Potentiates action of narcotic to promote rest and to reduce muscular/ductal spasm, thereby reducing metabolic needs, enzyme secretions.
Antacids; e.g., Mylanta, Maalox, Amphojel, Riopan;	Neutralizes gastric acid to reduce production of pancreatic enzymes and to reduce incidence of upper GI bleeding.
Lansoprazole (Prevacid), cimetidine (Tagamet), ranitidine (Zantac), famotidine (Pepcid).	Decreasing secretion of HCl reduces stimulation of the pancreas and associated pain.
Withhold food and fluid as indicated.	Client should be kept NPO until pain and nausea subside to limit/reduce release of pancreatic enzymes and resultant pain.
Maintain gastric suction when used.	NG tube may be used for client with ileus or protracted vomiting to prevent accumulation of gastric secretions and pancreatic enzyme activity.
Prepare for surgical intervention if indicated.	Surgical exploration may be required in presence of intractable pain/complications involving the biliary tract, such as pancreatic abscess or pseudocyst.

NURSING DIAGNOSIS: risk for deficient Fluid Volume

Risk factors may include

Excessive losses: vomiting, gastric suctioning
Increase in size of vascular bed (vasodilation, effects of kinins)
Third-space fluid transudation, ascites formation
Alteration of clotting process, hemorrhage

Possibly evidenced by

[Not applicable; presence of signs and symptoms establishes an *actual* diagnosis.]

DESIRED OUTCOMES/EVALUATION CRITERIA—CLIENT WILL:

Hydration (NOC)

Maintain adequate hydration as evidenced by stable vital signs, good skin turgor, prompt capillary refill, strong peripheral pulses, and individually appropriate urinary output.

ACTIONS/INTERVENTIONS	RATIONALE
Fluid/Electrolyte Management (NIC)	
Independent	
Auscultate heart sounds; note rate and rhythm. Monitor/document rhythm, changes.	Cardiac changes/dysrhythmias may reflect hypovolemia and/or electrolyte imbalance, commonly hypokalemia/hypocalcemia. Hyperkalemia may occur related to tissue necrosis, acidosis, and renal insufficiency and may precipitate lethal dysrhythmias if uncorrected. S_3 gallop in conjunction with JVD and crackles suggest HF/pulmonary edema. *Note:* Cardiovascular complications are common and include MI, pericarditis, and pericardial effusion with/without tamponade.
Monitor blood pressure, noting trends. Measure CVP if available.	Fluid sequestration (shifts into third space), bleeding, and release of vasodilators (kinins) and cardiac depressant factor triggered by pancreatic ischemia may result in profound hypotension. Reduced cardiac output/poor organ perfusion secondary to a hypotensive episode can precipitate widespread systemic complications. Systemic infection (septic shock) is also possible exacerbating hypovolemic status.
Investigate changes in sensorium; e.g., confusion, slowed responses.	Changes may be related to hypovolemia, hypoxia, electrolyte imbalance, or impending delirium tremens (in client with acute pancreatitis secondary to excessive alcohol intake). Severe pancreatic disease may cause toxic psychosis.
Measure I&O including vomiting/gastric aspirate, diarrhea. Calculate 24-hr fluid balance.	Indicators of replacement needs/effectiveness of therapy.
Note decrease in urine output (less than 400 mL/24 hr).	Oliguria may occur, signaling renal impairment/acute tubular necrosis (ATN), related to increase in renal vascular resistance or reduced/altered renal blood flow.
Record color and character of gastric drainage, measure pH, and note presence of occult blood.	Risk of gastric bleeding/hemorrhage is high.
Weigh as indicated; correlate with calculated fluid balance.	Weight loss may suggest hypovolemia; however, edema, fluid retention, and ascites may be reflected by increased or stable weight, even in the presence of muscle wasting.
Note poor skin turgor, dry skin/mucous membranes, reports of thirst.	Further physiologic indicators of dehydration.
Observe/record peripheral and dependent edema. Measure abdominal girth if ascites present.	Edema/fluid shifts occur as a result of increased vascular permeability, sodium retention, and decreased colloid osmotic pressure in the intravascular compartment. *Note:* Fluid loss (sequestration) of more than 6 L/48 hr is considered a poor prognostic sign.
Inspect skin for petechiae, hematomas, and unusual wound or venipuncture bleeding. Note hematuria, mucous membrane bleeding, and bloody gastric contents.	Disseminated intravascular coagulapathy (DIC) may be initiated by release of active pancreatic proteases into the circulation. The most frequently affected organs are the kidneys, skin, and lungs.
Observe/report coarse muscle tremors, twitching, positive Chvostek's or Trousseau's sign.	Symptoms of calcium imbalance. Calcium binds with free fats in the intestine and is lost by excretion in the stool.
Collaborative	
Administer fluid replacement as indicated; e.g., saline solutions, albumin, blood/blood products, dextran.	Choice of replacement solution may be less important than rapidity and adequacy of volume restoration. Saline solutions and albumin may be used to promote mobilization of fluid back into vascular space. Low-molecular-weight dextran is sometimes used to reduce risk of renal dysfunction and pulmonary edema associated with pancreatitis.

ACTIONS/INTERVENTIONS	RATIONALE
Monitor laboratory studies; e.g., Hgb/Hct, protein, albumin, electrolytes, BUN, creatinine, urine osmolality, and sodium/potassium, coagulation studies.	Identifies deficits/replacement needs and developing complications, (e.g., ATN, DIC, septic shock, acute respiratory distress syndrome [ARDS]).
Replace electrolytes; e.g., sodium, potassium, chloride, calcium as indicated.	Decreased oral intake and excessive losses greatly affect electrolyte/acid-base balance, which is necessary to maintain optimal cellular/organ function.
Prepare for/assist with peritoneal lavage, hemoperitoneal dialysis.	Removes toxic chemicals/pancreatic enzymes and may allow for more rapid correction of metabolic abnormalities in severe/unresponsive cases of acute pancreatitis.

NURSING DIAGNOSIS: imbalanced Nutrition: less than body requirements

May be related to

Vomiting, decreased oral intake; prescribed dietary restrictions
Loss of digestive enzymes and insulin (related to pancreatic outflow obstruction or necrosis/autodigestion)

Possibly evidenced by

Reported inadequate food intake
Aversion to eating, reported altered taste sensation, lack of interest in food
Weight loss
Poor muscle tone

DESIRED OUTCOMES/EVALUATION CRITERIA—CLIENT WILL:

Nutritional Status (NOC)

Demonstrate progressive weight gain toward goal with normalization of laboratory values
Experience no signs of malnutrition.

KNOWLEDGE: Diet (NOC)

Demonstrate behaviors, lifestyle changes to regain and/or maintain appropriate weight.

ACTIONS/INTERVENTIONS — RATIONALE

Nutrition Management (NIC)

Independent

ACTIONS/INTERVENTIONS	RATIONALE
Assess abdomen, noting presence/character of bowel sounds, abdominal distention, and reports of nausea.	Gastric distention and intestinal atony are frequently present, resulting in reduced/absent bowel sounds. Return of bowel sounds and relief of symptoms signal readiness for discontinuation of gastric aspiration (NG tube).
Provide frequent oral care.	Decreases vomiting stimulus and inflammation/irritation of dry mucous membranes associated with dehydration and mouth breathing when NG tube is in place.
Assist client in selecting food/fluids that meet nutritional needs and restrictions when diet is resumed.	Previous dietary habits may be unsatisfactory in meeting current needs for tissue regeneration and healing. Use of gastric stimulants; e.g., caffeine, alcohol, cigarettes, gas-producing foods, or ingestion of large meals may result in excessive stimulation of the pancreas/recurrence of symptoms.

ACTIONS/INTERVENTIONS	RATIONALE
Observe color/consistency/amount of stools. Note frothy consistency/foul odor.	Steatorrhea may develop from incomplete digestion of fats.

Hyperglycemia Management (NIC)

ACTIONS/INTERVENTIONS	RATIONALE
Note signs of increased thirst and urination or changes in mentation and visual acuity.	May warn of developing hyperglycemia associated with increased release of glucagon (damage to α cells) or decreased release of insulin (damage to β cells).
Perform/monitor results of bedside fingerstick glucose testing and dipstick testing of urine for sugar and acetone (ketones).	Early detection of inadequate glucose utilization may prevent development of hyperglycemic crisis. IV insulin may be required to control serum glucose within normal ranges.
Maintain NPO status and gastric suctioning during acute phase.	Prevents stimulation and release of pancreatic enzymes (secretin) when chyme and HCl enter the duodenum.
Administer enteral/parenteral feedings (hyperalimentation and lipids) if indicated.	Enteral feedings may be preferred to prevent gut atrophy when tolerated, However, IV administration of calories, lipids, and amino acids should be instituted before nutrition/nitrogen depletion is advanced. (Refer to CP: Total nutritional support: Enteral/parenteral feedings.)
Resume oral intake with clear liquids and advance diet slowly to provide high-protein, high-carbohydrate diet, when indicated.	Oral feedings given too early in the course of illness may exacerbate symptoms. Loss of pancreatic function/reduced insulin production may require initiation of a diabetic diet.

Nutrition Management (NIC)

Collaborative

ACTIONS/INTERVENTIONS	RATIONALE
Provide medium-chain triglycerides (MCTs) (e.g., MCT, Portagen).	MCTs are elements of enteral feedings (NG or J-tube) that provide supplemental calories/nutrients that do not require pancreatic enzymes for digestion/absorption.
Administer medications as indicated:	
Vitamins; e.g., A, D, E, K;	Replacement required because fat metabolism is altered, reducing absorption/storage of fat-soluble vitamins.
Replacement enzymes; e.g., pancreatin (Dizymes), pancrelipase (Viokase, Cotazym).	Used in chronic pancreatitis to correct deficiencies to promote digestion and absorption of nutrients.

Hyperglycemia Management (NIC)

ACTIONS/INTERVENTIONS	RATIONALE
Monitor serum glucose.	Indicator of insulin needs because hyperglycemia is frequently present, although not usually in levels high enough to produce ketoacidosis.
Provide insulin as appropriate.	Corrects persistent hyperglycemia caused by injury to cells and increased release of glucocorticoids. Insulin therapy is usually short-term unless permanent damage to pancreas occurs. Aggressive insulin therapy during acute exacerbations has been associated with better outcomes.

NURSING DIAGNOSIS: risk for Infection, [sepsis]

Risk factors may include

Inadequate primary defenses: stasis of body fluids, altered peristalsis, change in pH of secretions
Immunosuppression
Nutritional deficiencies
Tissue destruction, chronic disease

Possibly evidenced by:

[Not applicable; presence of signs and symptoms establishes an *actual* diagnosis.]

DESIRED OUTCOMES/EVALUATION CRITERIA—CLIENT WILL:

Immune Status (NOC)

Achieve timely healing; be free of signs of infection.
Be afebrile.

Risk Control (NOC)

Participate in activities to reduce risk of infection.

ACTIONS/INTERVENTIONS	RATIONALE
Infection Protection (NIC)	
Independent	
Use strict aseptic technique when changing surgical dressings or working with IV lines, indwelling catheters/tubes, drains. Change soiled dressings promptly.	Limits sources of infection, which can lead to sepsis in a compromised client. *Note:* Studies indicate that infectious complications are responsible for about 80% of deaths associated with pancreatitis.
Stress importance of good hand washing.	Reduces risk of cross-contamination.
Observe rate and characteristics of respirations, breath sounds. Note occurrence of cough and sputum production.	Pulmonary complications of pancreatitis include atelectasis, pleural effusion, pneumonia, and ARDS. Fluid accumulation and limited mobility predispose to respiratory infections and atelectasis. Accumulation of ascites fluid may cause elevated diaphragm and shallow abdominal breathing.
Encourage frequent position changes, deep breathing, and coughing. Assist with ambulation as soon as stable.	Enhances ventilation of all lung segments and promotes mobilization of secretions.
Observe for signs of infection; e.g.:	
Fever and respiratory distress in conjunction with jaundice;	Cholestatic jaundice and decreased pulmonary function may be first sign of sepsis/ARDS.
Increased abdominal pain, rigidity/rebound tenderness, diminished/absent bowel sounds;	Suggestive of peritonitis.
Increased abdominal pain/tenderness, recurrent fever (higher than 101°F), leukocytosis, hypotension, tachycardia, and chills.	Abscesses can occur 2 weeks or more after the onset of pancreatitis (mortality can exceed 50%) and should be suspected whenever client is deteriorating despite supportive measures.
Collaborative	
Obtain culture specimens; e.g., blood, wound, urine, sputum, or pancreatic aspirate.	Identifies presence of infection and causative organism.
Administer anti-infective therapies as indicated; e.g., imipenem/cilastatin (Primaxin), metronidazole (Flagyl), levofloxan (Levoquin), cephalosporins, cefoxitin sodium (Mefoxin), plus aminoglycosides; e.g., gentamicin (Garamycin), tobramycin (Nebcin).	Broad-spectrum anti-infectives are generally recommended for pancreatitis sepsis; however, therapy will be based on the specific organisms cultured.
Prepare for surgical intervention as necessary.	Abscesses may be surgically drained with resection of necrotic tissue. Sump tubes may be inserted for antibiotic irrigation and drainage of pancreatic debris. Pseudocysts (persisting for several weeks) may be drained because of the risk and incidence of infection/rupture.

NURSING DIAGNOSIS: risk for ineffective Breathing Pattern/impaired Gas Exchange

May be related to

Pain/splinting of respirations, upper abdominal distention/elevated diaphragm, pleural effusion
Alveolar/capillary membrane changes: interstitial edema, pulmonary congestion

Possibly evidenced by

[Not applicable; presence of signs and symptoms establishes an *actual* diagnosis.]

DESIRED OUTCOMES/EVALUATION CRITERIA—CLIENT WILL:

RESPIRATORY STATUS: Ventilation (NOC)

Maintain adequate ventilation with respiratory rate/rhythm normal for client, breath sounds clear, and free of dyspnea/shortness of breath.

RESPIRATORY STATUS: Gas Exchange (NOC)

Display ABGs within client's normal range.

ACTIONS/INTERVENTIONS	RATIONALE
Respiratory Monitoring (NIC)	
Independent	
Evaluate respiratory rate and depth. Note respiratory effort; e.g., presence of dyspnea, use of accessory muscles, nasal flaring.	Client responses are variable. Rate and effort may be increased by pain, accumulation of secretions, or abdominal distention (elevation of diaphragm). Respiratory suppression (decreased rate) can occur with use of narcotic analgesics. Early recognition and treatment of abnormal ventilation may prevent complications.
Auscultate breath sounds. Note areas of diminished/absent breath sounds and presence of adventitious sounds; e.g., rhonchi, or crackles.	Loss of active breath sounds in an area of previous ventilation may reflect atelectasis. Crackles or rhonchi may be indicative of fluid accumulation (interstitial edema, pulmonary congestion, or infection).
Encourage client participation/responsibility for deep-breathing exercises, use of adjuncts, and coughing as indicated. Reposition frequently.	Stimulates respiratory function/lung expansion. Effective in preventing and resolving pulmonary congestion. Coughing is not necessary unless wheezes/rhonchi are present, indicating retention of secretions.
Reinforce splinting of abdomen with pillows during deep breathing/coughing.	May enhance effectiveness of cough effort.
Note increasing restlessness, confusion, lethargy.	May indicate impaired gas exchange, possible ARDS requiring prompt evaluation and intervention.
Collaborative	
Monitor/graph serial ABGs, pulse oximetry, review chest x-ray reports.	Decreasing PaO_2/SaO_2 and increasing $PaCO_2$ (impaired gas exchange) and changes in chest x-rays suggest developing complications requiring further evaluation/treatment.
Administer supplemental oxygen if indicated.	Increases available O_2 for optimal oxygenation. (Inability to maintain adequate oxygenation indicates need for more aggressive therapy/mechanical ventilation. (Refer to CP: Ventilation assistance [mechinical], p. 170.)

NURSING DIAGNOSIS: deficient Knowledge [Learning Need] regarding condition, prognosis, treatment, self-care, and discharge needs

May be related to

Lack of exposure/recall
Information misinterpretation, unfamiliarity with information resources

Possibly evidenced by

Questions, request for information, statement of misconception
Inaccurate follow-through of instructions/development of preventable complications

DESIRED OUTCOMES/EVALUATION CRITERIA—CLIENT WILL:

KNOWLEDGE: Illness Care (NOC)

Verbalize understanding of condition/disease process and potential complications.
Verbalize understanding of therapeutic needs.
Correctly perform necessary procedures and explain reasons for the actions.
Initiate necessary lifestyle changes and participate in treatment regimen.

ACTIONS/INTERVENTIONS	RATIONALE
TEACHING: Disease Process (NIC)	
Independent	
Review specific cause of current episode and prognosis. Discuss other causative/associated factors; e.g., excessive alcohol intake, gallbladder disease, duodenal ulcer, hyperlipoproteinemias, some drugs (e.g., oral contraceptives, thiazides, furosemide [Lasix], isoniazid [INH], glucocorticoids, sulfonamides).	Provides knowledge base on which client can make informed choices. Avoidance may help limit damage and prevent development of a chronic condition.
Explore availability of treatment programs/rehabilitation of chemical dependency if indicated.	Alcohol abuse is currently the most common cause of recurrence of chronic pancreatitis. Usage of other drugs, whether prescribed or illicit, is increasing as a factor. *Note:* Pain of pancreatitis can be severe and prolonged and may lead to narcotic tolerance/dependence, possibly benefiting from referral to a pain clinic.
Stress the importance of follow-up care, and review symptoms that need to be reported immediately to physician; e.g., recurrence of pain, persistent fever, nausea/vomiting, abdominal distention, frothy/foul-smelling stools, general intolerance of food.	Prolonged recovery period requires close monitoring to prevent recurrence/complications; e.g., infection, pancreatic pseudocysts.
Review importance of initially continuing bland, low-fat diet with frequent small feedings and restricted caffeine, with gradual resumption of a normal diet within individual tolerance.	Understanding the purpose of the diet in maximizing the use of available enzymes while avoiding overstimulation of the pancreas may enhance client involvement in self-monitoring of dietary needs and responses to foods.
Instruct in use of pancreatic enzyme replacements and bile salt therapy as indicated, avoiding concomitant ingestion of hot foods/fluids.	If permanent damage to the pancreas has occurred, exocrine deficiencies will occur, requiring long-term replacement. Hot foods/fluids can inactivate enzymes.
Recommend cessation of smoking.	Nicotine stimulates gastric secretions and unnecessary pancreatic activity.
Discuss signs/symptoms of diabetes mellitus; i.e., polydipsia, polyuria, weakness, weight loss.	Damage to the β cells may result in a temporary or permanent alteration of insulin production.

POTENTIAL CONSIDERATIONS following acute hospitalization (dependent on client's age, physical condition/presence of complications, personal resources, and life responsibilities)

imbalanced Nutrition: less than body requirements—preexisting malnutrition, prescribed dietary restrictions, persistent nausea/vomiting, imbalances in digestive enzymes.

acute/chronic Pain—chemical irritation of peritoneal surfaces by pancreatic enzymes, spasms of biliary ducts, general inflammatory process.

dysfunctional Family Processes: alcoholism—abuse of alcohol, resistance to treatment, inadequate coping/lack of problem-solving skills, addictive personality/codependency.

ineffective Therapeutic Regimen Management—complexity of therapeutic regimen, economic difficulties, mistrust of regimen, perceived benefit, social support deficits

TOTAL NUTRITIONAL SUPPORT: PARENTERAL/ENTERAL FEEDING

Nutritional status is a key factor in client's overall immune function and ability to mount a stress response. Underfeeding a client may lead to increased nosocomial infections, poor wound healing, respiratory muscle dysfunction, and respiratory failure. Overfeeding clients, in contrast, may increase physiologic stress and lead to problems such as hyperglycemia, fluid overload, azotemia, and hepatic dysfunction. Therefore, measuring energy expenditure and determining the client's caloric requirements and feeding status should be included in a thorough nutritional assessment. Specifically designed nutritional therapy can be administered via a parenteral or enteral route to prevent/correct protein-calorie malnutrition when oral intake is inadequate or not possible.

Enteral nutrition is preferred for the client who has a functional GI tract but is unable to consume an adequate nutritional intake or for whom oral intake is contraindicated/impossible. Feeding may be done via flexible catheter (e.g., nasogastric, orogastric tube) or enterostomal (e.g., gastrostomy, duodenostomy, or jejunostomy tube). A feeding tube may be inserted short-term for supplementation of oral intake or long-term to provide all of the client's nutrition.

Parenteral nutrition may be chosen because of altered metabolic states or when mechanical or functional abnormalities of the GI tract prevent enteral feeding. Amino acids, fat, carbohydrates, trace elements, vitamins, and electrolytes may be infused via a central or peripheral vein.

CARE SETTING

May be any setting, including community/home care

RELATED CONCERNS

Burns: thermal/chemical/electrical (acute and convalescent phases), page 680
Cancer, page 857
Chronic obstructive pulmonary disease (COPD) and asthma, page 117
Fluid and electrolyte imbalances, page 919
Inflammatory bowel disease, page 324
Pancreatitis, page 467
Psychosocial aspects of care, page 770
Renal failure: chronic, page 553
Surgical intervention, page 788

Client Assessment Database

Clinical signs listed here depend on the degree and duration of malnutrition and include observations indicative of vitamin, mineral, and protein/calorie deficiencies.

ACTIVITY/REST

May exhibit: Muscle wasting (temporal, intercostal, gastrocnemius, dorsum of hand), thin extremities, flaccid muscles, decreased activity tolerance

CIRCULATION

May exhibit: Tachycardia, bradycardia
Diaphoresis, cyanosis

ELIMINATION

May report: Diarrhea or constipation, flatulence associated with food intake

May exhibit: Abdominal distention/increased girth, ascites, tenderness on palpation
Stools may be loose, hard-formed, fatty, or clay-colored

FOOD/FLUID

May report: Recent weight loss/weight loss of 10% or more of body weight within previous 6 months
Problems with chewing, swallowing, choking, or saliva production
Changes in the taste of food, anorexia, nausea/vomiting, inadequate oral intake (NPO) status for 7–10 days, long-term use of 5% dextrose intravenously

May exhibit: Actual weight (measured) as compared with usual or preillness weight is less than 90% of ideal body weight for height, sex, and age or equal to or greater than 120% of ideal or usual body weight (client risk in obesity is a tendency to overlook protein and caloric requirements). A distorted actual weight may occur because of the presence of edema, ascites, organomegaly, tumor bulk, anasarca, amputation
Edentulous or ill-fitting dentures
Bowel sounds diminished, hyperactive, or absent
Thyroid, parotid enlargement
Lips dry, cracked, red, swollen; angular stomatitis
Tongue may be smooth, pale, slick, coated; color often magenta, beefy red; lingual papillae atrophy/swelling
Gums swollen/bleeding, multiple caries
Mucous membranes dry, pale, red, swollen

NEUROSENSORY

May exhibit: Lethargy, apathy, listlessness, irritability, disorientation, coma
Gag/swallow reflex may be decreased/absent; e.g., cerebrovascular accident (CVA), head trauma, nerve injury
Loss of balance and coordination

RESPIRATION

May exhibit: Increased respiratory rate; respiratory distress
Dyspnea, increased sputum production
Breath sounds, crackles (protein deficiency/related fluid shifts)

SAFETY

May report: Recent course of radiation therapy (radiation enteritis)

May exhibit: Hair may be fragile, coarse, lackluster, falling out (alopecia); decreased pigmentation may be present
Skin dry, scaly, tented; "flaky paint" dermatosis; edema; draining or unhealed wounds; pressure sores; ecchymoses; perifollicular petechiae; subcutaneous fat loss
Eyes sunken, dull, dry, with pale conjunctiva; Bitot's spots (triangular, shiny, gray spots on the conjunctiva seen in vitamin A deficiency) or scleral icterus
Nails may be brittle, thin, flattened, ridged, spoon shaped

SEXUALITY

May report: Loss of libido
Amenorrhea

TEACHING/LEARNING

May report: History/presence of conditions causing protracted protein/caloric losses; e.g., malabsorption or short-gut syndrome, diarrhea, acute pancreatitis, renal dialysis, fistulas, draining wounds, thermal injuries, problems with chewing/swallowing (e.g., CVA or Parkinson's disease)
Presence of factors known to alter nutritional requirements/increase energy demands; e.g., single or multiorgan failure, sepsis, fever, AIDS, cancer, trauma, extensive burns, use of steroids, antitumor agents, immunosuppressants
Use of treatments that greatly alter intake and medications that cause untoward drug/nutrient interactions; e.g., laxatives, anticonvulsants, diuretics, antacids, narcotics, immunosuppresants, radiation, high-dose chemotherapy
Illness of psychiatric origin; e.g., anorexia nervosa/bulimia
Educational/social factors; e.g., lack of nutrition knowledge and/or kitchen facilities, reduced/limited financial resources

Discharge plan considerations: May require assistance with solution preparation, therapy supplies, and maintenance of feeding device for home nutritional care

Refer to section at end of plan for postdischarge considerations.

DIAGNOSTIC STUDIES

Weight: Ideal body weight (IBW): Men—106 lb for first 5 feet plus 6 lb for each additional inch of height. Women—100 lb for first 5 feet plus 5 lb for each additional inch of height. Obesity defined as 120% of IBW; 70%–79% of IBW is moderately underweight. Weight may be inaccurate as a result of factors such as edema, ascites.

Anthropometrics: Includes measurement of weight-to-height ratio, osteometry, and ratios of lean-to-fat weight:

Triceps skin-fold measurement: Estimates subcutaneous fat stores; fat reserves less than 10th percentile suggest advanced depletion; levels less than the 30th percentile suggest mild-to-moderate depletion.

Midarm muscle circumference: Measures somatic muscle mass and is used in combination with triceps skinfold measurement; a decrease of 15–20 percentiles from the expected value suggests a significant reduction.

Visceral proteins: (*Note:* Recent research questions the reliability of serum albumin and transferrin as markers for malnutrition.)

Serum albumin (the classic marker measured): Values of 2.7–3.4 g/dL indicate mild depletion; 2.1–2.7 g/dL, moderate depletion; and less than 2.1 g/dL, severe depletion. Decreased levels are due to poor protein intake, nephrotic syndrome, sepsis, burns, HF, cirrhosis, eclampsia, protein-losing enteropathy; above-normal values (more than 4.5 g/dL) are seen in dehydration. (Serum prealbumin has a shorter half-life than albumin, so body stores turn over quickly, theoretically making it a more sensitive indicator of improvement/change in protein status.)

Serum transferrin: More sensitive to changes in visceral protein stores than albumin; levels of 150–200 mg/dL reflect mild depletion; 100–150 mg/dL, moderate depletion; and 100 mg/dL, severe depletion. Elevated values are seen with iron deficiency, pregnancy, hypoxia, and chronic blood loss. Decreased values are seen with pernicious anemia, chronic infection, liver disease, iron overload, and protein-losing enteropathy.

Thyroxine-binding prealbumin: Reflects rapid changes in hepatic protein synthesis and thus is a more sensitive indicator of visceral protein depletion. Decreased levels less than 200 mEq/mL are noted with cirrhosis, inflammation, and surgical trauma.

Amino acid profile: Alterations reflect an imbalance of plasma proteins with depressed levels of branched-chain amino acids (common with hepatic encephalopathy or sepsis).

Tests of immune system:

Total lymphocyte count: Less than 1500 cells/mm^3 indicates leukopenia and results from decreased generation of T cells, which are very sensitive to malnutrition. Less than 800 cells/mm^3 indicates severe depletion. Levels are also altered by severe stress, renal failure, cancer, infection, and administration of corticosteroids.

Tests of micronutrients:

Potassium: Deficiency occurs with inadequate intake and with loss of potassium-containing fluids (e.g., urine, diarrhea, vomiting, fistula drainage, continuous NG suctioning). Potassium is also lost from cells during muscle wasting and is excreted by the kidneys.

Sodium: Levels depend on state of hydration/presence of active loss as may exist in excessive diuresis, GI suctioning, burns.

Phosphorus: May be decreased, reflecting inadequate intake or increased cellular uptake; may be elevated in renal failure.

Magnesium: Deficiency is common in alcoholics, chronic vomiting, diarrhea; may be elevated in renal failure.

Calcium: Levels are decreased with conditions associated with hypoalbuminemia; e.g., renal failure (majority of calcium is bound to albumin). Absorption is decreased by fat malabsorption and low-protein diet.

Zinc: Deficiency is seen in alcoholic cirrhosis, or may be secondary to hypoalbuminemia and GI losses (diarrhea).

Tests reflecting protein (nitrogen) loss:

Nitrogen balance studies: Nitrogen (protein) excretion via urine, stool, and insensible losses often exceeds nitrogen intake in the acutely ill, reflecting catabolic response to stress and use of endogenous protein stores for energy production (gluconeogenesis). BUN may be severely decreased as a result of chronic malnutrition and depletion of skeletal protein stores.

24-Hr creatinine excretion: Because Cr is concentrated in muscle mass, there is a correlation between lean body mass and 24-hr Cr excretion. Actual values are compared with ideal values (based on height and weight) times 100, known as the Cr height index: 60%–80% indicates moderate depletion; less than 60%, severe depletion.

Tests of GI function (include Schilling test, D-xylose test, 72-hr stool fat, GI series): Determine malabsorption.

Chest x-ray: May be normal or show evidence of pleural effusion; small heart silhouette.

ECG: May be normal or demonstrate low voltage, dysrhythmias/patterns reflective of electrolyte imbalances.

NURSING PRIORITIES

1. Promote consistent intake of adequate calorie and protein requirements.
2. Prevent complications.
3. Minimize energy losses/needs.
4. Provide information about condition, prognosis, and treatment needs.

DISCHARGE GOALS

1. Nutritional intake adequate for individual needs.
2. Complications prevented/minimized.
3. Fatigue alleviated.
4. Condition, prognosis, and therapeutic regimen understood.
5. Plan in place to meet needs after discharge.

NURSING DIAGNOSIS: imbalanced Nutrition: less than body requirements

May be related to

Conditions that interfere with nutrient intake or increase nutrient need/metabolic demand; e.g., cancer and associated treatments, anorexia, surgical procedures, dysphagia/difficulty swallowing, depressed mental status/level of consciousness

Possibly evidenced by

Body weight 10% or more under ideal
Decreased subcutaneous fat/muscle mass, poor muscle tone
Changes in gastric motility and stool characteristics

DESIRED OUTCOMES/EVALUATION CRITERIA—CLIENT WILL:

Nutritional Status (NOC)

Demonstrate stable weight or progressive weight gain toward goal with normalization of laboratory values and no signs of malnutrition.

ACTIONS/INTERVENTIONS	RATIONALE
Nutrition Therapy (NIC)	
Independent	
General	
Assess nutritional status continually, during daily nursing care, noting energy level; condition of skin, nails, hair, oral cavity; desire to eat/anorexia.	Provides the opportunity to observe deviations from normal client baseline, and influences choice of interventions.
Weigh daily and compare with admission weight.	Establishes baseline, aids in monitoring effectiveness of therapeutic regimen, and alerts nurse to inappropriate trends in weight loss/gain.
Document oral intake by use of 24-hour recall, food history, calorie counts as appropriate.	Identifies imbalance between estimated nutritional requirements and actual intake.
Ensure accurate collection of specimens (urine and stool) for nitrogen balance studies.	Inaccurate collection can alter test results, leading to improper interpretation of client's current status and needs.
Administer nutritional solutions at prescribed rate via infusion control device as needed. Adjust rate to deliver prescribed hourly intake. Do not increase rate to "catch up" if infusion slows.	Nutritional support prescriptions are based on individually estimated caloric and protein requirements. A consistent rate of nutrient administration ensures proper utilization with fewer side effects, such as hyperglycemia or dumping syndrome. *Note:* Continuous and cyclic infusions of enteral formulas are generally better tolerated than bolus feedings and result in improved absorption.
Be familiar with electrolyte content of nutritional solutions.	Metabolic complications of nutritional support often result from a lack of appreciation of changes that can occur as a result of refeeding; e.g., hyperglycemic, hyperosmolar nonketotic coma (HHNC), electrolyte imbalances.

ACTIONS/INTERVENTIONS	RATIONALE
Schedule activities with adequate rest periods. Promote relaxation techniques.	Conserves energy/reduces calorie needs. (Refer to ND: Fatigue.)

Total Parenteral Nutrition (TPN)

Administration (NIC)

Observe appropriate "hang" time of parenteral solutions per protocol.	Effectiveness of IV vitamins diminishes and solution degrades after 24 hr.
Monitor fingerstick glucose per protocol (e.g., qid during initiation of therapy).	High glucose content of solutions may lead to pancreatic fatigue, requiring use of supplemental insulin to prevent hyperglycemic complications. *Note:* Fingerstick determination of glucose level is more accurate than urine testing because of variations in renal glucose threshold.

Enteral Tube Feeding (NIC)

Assess GI function and tolerance to enteral feedings—knowing type of tube used (e.g., NG, small bowel): note bowel sounds, reports of nausea, abdominal discomfort; presence of diarrhea/constipation, development of weakness, lightheadedness, diaphoresis, tachycardia, abdominal cramping.	Because protein turnover of the GI mucosa occurs approximately every 3 days, the GI tract is at great risk for early dysfunction and atrophy from disease and malnutrition. Intolerance of formula/presence of dumping syndrome may require alteration of rate of administration/concentration or type of formula, or possibly change to parenteral administration. *Note*: Use of post–pyloric feeding tube eliminates need for active bowel sounds as a criterion for tolerance.
Check gastric residuals if bolus feedings are done and as otherwise indicated. Hold feeding/return aspirate per protocol for type/rate of feeding used if residual is greater than predetermined level.	Delayed gastric emptying can be caused by a specific disease process; e.g., paralytic ileus/surgery, shock; by drug therapy (especially narcotics); or the protein/fat content of the individual formula. *Note:* Replacement of gastric aspirate reduces loss of gastric acid/electrolytes.
Maintain patency of enteral feeding tubes by flushing with warm water before and after feeding and as indicated; e.g., between multiple doses of medications or when checking gastric residuals.	Enteral formulas contain protein that can clog feeding tubes (more likely with small-bore or silicone than with polyurethane tubes), necessitating removal/replacement of tube. *Note:* Cranberry juice or colas are not recommended because they may actually cause an obstruction by promoting formula coagulation. Pancrelipase (a pancreatic enzyme) may be effective in clearing tubing of persistent clog.
Transitional	
Emphasize importance of transition to oral feedings as appropriate.	Although client may have little interest in food or desire to eat, transition to oral feedings is preferred in view of potential side effects/complications of nutritional support therapy.
Assess gag reflex, ability to chew/swallow, and motor skills when progressing to transitional feedings.	May require additional interventions; e.g., retraining by dysphagia expert (speech therapist) or long-term nutritional support.
Provide self-help utensils as indicated; e.g., plate guard, utensils with built-up handles, lidded cups.	Clients with neuromuscular deficits, e.g., post-CVA, brain injury, may require use of special aids developed to facilitate feeding.
Create optimal environment; e.g., remove noxious stimuli, bedpans, soiled linens. Provide cheerful, attractive tray/table, soft music, companionship.	Encourages client's attempts to eat, reduces anorexia, and introduces some of the social pleasures usually associated with mealtime.
Allow adequate time for chewing, swallowing, savoring food; provide socialization and feeding assistance as indicated.	Clients need encouragement/assistance to overcome underlying problems such as anorexia, fatigue, muscular weakness.
Offer small, frequent feedings; incorporate client likes/dislikes in meal planning as much as possible, and include "home foods," as appropriate.	May enhance client's desire for food and amount of intake.

ACTIONS/INTERVENTIONS	RATIONALE
Provide calorie-containing beverages when oral intake is possible; e.g., juices/Jell-O water, dietary supplements (Sustacal, Ensure); add Polycase to beverages/water.	Maximizes calorie intake when oral intake is limited/restricted.

Collaborative

ACTIONS/INTERVENTIONS	RATIONALE
Refer to nutritional team/registered dietitian.	Aids in identification of nutrient deficits and specific need for parenteral/enteral nutritional intervention.
Determine nutritional/caloric needs, using appropriate method (e.g., TEE, BMI, Harris-Benedict equation, indirect calorimetry test) as indicated.	Several methods are available to provide an estimation of calorie and protein needs. TEE is based on resting and activity energy expenditure, and thermic effect of food. BMI estimates caloric needs according to energy requirements per kilogram of body weight. Harris-Benedict provides a reasonable estimate of resting energy expenditure in kcal/day. Indirect calorimetry test measures O_2 consumption at basal or resting metabolic rate to aid in estimating calorie/protein requirements. *Note:* Although any of these tests may accurately determine individual needs, a standard formula for projecting energy requirements in the ill client is to provide 30 Kcal/kg for weight maintenance, 25 Kcal/kg for weight loss, or 35 Kcal/kg for weight gain.

Enteral Tube Feeding (NIC)/TPN Administration (NIC)

ACTIONS/INTERVENTIONS	RATIONALE
Assist with insertion and confirm proper placement of infusion/feeding line (e.g., chest x-ray for central venous catheter, or aspiration of gastric [green] or small bowel [golden] contents from feeding tube) before administration of solutions.	Reduces risk of feeding-induced complications, including pneumothorax/hemothorax, hydrothorax, air embolus, arterial puncture (central venous line), or aspiration (NG tube).
Administer dextrose-electrolyte or dextrose–amino acid and lipid emulsions (3-in-1) solutions as indicated.	Solutions provide calories, essential amino acids, and micronutrients, usually combined with lipids for complete nutrition known as total nutrient admixtures (TNA). Solutions are modified to meet specific needs; e.g., renal and liver failure (lower protein), respiratory failure (higher fat). *Note:* 3-in-1 solution bags are larger (2–3 L) and can infuse over a 24-hr period, eliminating the need for frequent bag changes and reducing line manipulation/risk of contamination.
Co-infuse lipid emulsions if 3-in-1 solutions are not used.	Useful in meeting excessive caloric requirements (e.g., burns) or as a source of essential fatty acids during long-term hyperalimentation. *Note:* Lipid solutions may be contraindicated in clients with alterations in fat metabolism or in the presence of pancreatitis, liver damage, anemia, coagulation disorders, pulmonary disease.
Administer medications, as indicated; e.g.:	
Multivitamin preparations;	Water-soluble vitamins are added to parenteral solutions. Other vitamins may be given for identified deficiencies.
Insulin;	High glucose content of solutions may require exogenous insulin for metabolism, especially in presence of pancreatic insufficiency or disease. *Note:* Insulin is usually now added directly to parenteral solution.
Diphenoxylate with atropine (Lomotil), camphorated tincture of opium (paregoric), and metoclopramide (Reglan).	GI side effects of enteral feeding may need to be controlled with antidiarrheal agents (Lomotil/paregoric) or peristaltic stimulants (Reglan) if more conservative measures such as alteration of rate/strength or type of formula are not successful.

ACTIONS/INTERVENTIONS	RATIONALE
Monitor laboratory studies; e.g., serum glucose, electrolytes, transferrin, prealbumin/albumin, total protein, phosphate, BUN/Cr, liver enzymes, CBC, ABGs.	Serum chemistries, blood counts, and lipid profiles are performed before initiation of therapy, providing a baseline for comparison with repeat (monitoring) studies to determine therapy needs/complications. Untoward metabolic effects of TPN include hypokalemia, hyponatremia and fluid retention, hyperglycemia, hypophosphatemia, increased CO_2 production resulting in respiratory compromise, elevation of liver function tests, renal dysfunction.

NURSING DIAGNOSIS: risk for Infection

Risk factors may include

Invasive procedures: insertion of venous catheter; surgically placed gastrostomy/jejunostomy feeding tube

Malnutrition; chronic disease

Environmental exposure: access devices in place for extended periods, improper preparation/handling/contamination of the feeding solution

Possibly evidenced by

[Not applicable; presence of signs and symptoms establishes an *actual* diagnosis.]

DESIRED OUTCOMES/EVALUATION CRITERIA—CLIENT WILL:

Immune Status (NOC)

Experience no fever or chills.

Demonstrate clean catheter insertion sites, free of drainage and erythema/edema.

ACTIONS/INTERVENTIONS — RATIONALE

Infection Protection (NIC)

Independent

ACTIONS/INTERVENTIONS	RATIONALE
Stress/model proper hand washing technique.	Reduces risk of cross-contamination.
Maintain sterile technique for invasive procedures. Provide routine site care as appropriate.	Prevents entry of bacteria, reducing risk of nosocomial infections.
Encourage frequent position changes and out of bed/ambulation as tolerated.	Limits stasis of body fluids, promotes optimal functioning of organ systems, GI tract.
Screen visitors/care providers for infectious processes, especially URI.	Reduces risk of transmission of viruses that are difficult to treat.
Monitor/assist with respiratory exercises, use of adjuncts; e.g., incentive spirometer. Auscultate lungs for adventitious sounds.	Promotes deep breathing to clear airways and reduce risk of pneumonia. Presence of wheezes suggests retained secretions, potential complications requiring intervention.
Assess vital signs, including temperature per protocol.	A rise in pulse and temperature may provide warning of infectious process unless client's immune system is too compromised to respond.

Total Parenteral Nutrition (TPN) Administration (NIC)

ACTIONS/INTERVENTIONS	RATIONALE
Maintain an optimal aseptic environment during bedside insertion of central venous catheters and during changes of TPN bottles and administration tubing.	Catheter-related sepsis may result from entry of pathogenic microorganisms through skin insertion tract or from touch contamination during manipulations of TPN system.

ACTIONS/INTERVENTIONS	RATIONALE
Secure external portion of catheter/administration tubing to dressing with tape. Note intactness of skin suture.	Manipulation of catheter in/out of insertion site can result in tissue trauma (coring) and potentiate entry of skin organisms into catheter tract.
Maintain a sterile occlusive dressing over catheter insertion site. Perform central/peripheral venous catheter dressing care per protocol.	Protects catheter insertion sites from potential sources of contamination. *Note:* Central venous catheter sites can easily become contaminated from tracheostomy/endotracheal secretions or from wounds of the head, neck, and chest.
Inspect insertion site of catheter for erythema, induration, drainage, tenderness.	The catheter is a potential irritant to the surrounding skin and subcutaneous skin tract, and extended use may result in insertion site irritation and infection.
Refrigerate premixed solutions before use; observe a 24-hr hang time for amino acid or total nutrient admixtures solutions and a 12-hr hang time for IV fat emulsions.	TPN solutions and fat emulsions have been shown to support the growth of a variety of pathogenic organisms once contaminated.
Monitor urinary output and serum glucose levels.	A rise in temperature or loss of glucose tolerance (glycosuria, hyperglycemia) are early indications of possible catheter-related sepsis.

Enteral Tube Feeding (NIC)

ACTIONS/INTERVENTIONS	RATIONALE
Keep manipulations of enteral feeding system to a minimum and wash hands before opening system. Handle the system as little as possible.	Touch contamination of formula is caused by caregiver administration technique.
Alternate nares for tube placement in long-term NG feedings.	Reduces risk of trauma/infection of paranasal tissue (especially important in facial trauma/burns).
Provide daily/prn site care to abdominally placed feeding tubes.	GI secretions leaking through or around gastrostomy/jejunostomy tube tracts can cause skin breakdown severe enough to require removal of the feeding tube.
Refrigerate reconstituted enteral formulas before use; observe a hang time of 4–8 hr; discard unused formula after 24 hr.	Enteral formulas easily support bacterial growth (due to high concentration of glucose and lipids) and can be contaminated from several sources (e.g., when preparation is mixed or poured, or via frequent aspiration of gastric/small bowel contents, use of open system, use of blue dye).

Infection Protection (NIC)

Collaborative

ACTIONS/INTERVENTIONS	RATIONALE
Aseptically prepare parenteral solutions/enteral formulas for administration. When possible, use prepackaged sterile enteral feeding formula.	TPN solutions should be prepared under a laminar flow hood in the pharmacy. Enteral formulas should be mixed in a clean environment in the dietary or pharmacy department. *Note:* Additives to TPN solutions, as a rule, should not be made on the unit because of the potential for contamination and drug incompatibilities.
Notify physician if signs of infection present. Follow protocol for obtaining appropriate culture specimens; e.g., blood, solutions, and change bottle/tubing as indicated.	Necessary to identify source of infection and initiate appropriate therapy. May require removal of TPN line and culture of catheter tip.
Administer antibiotics as indicated.	May be given prophylactically or for specifically identified organism.

NURSING DIAGNOSIS: risk for Injury, [multifactor]

Risk factors may include

External environment: catheter-related complications (air emboli and septic thrombophlebitis)
Internal factors: aspiration; effects of therapy/drug interactions

Possibly evidenced by

[Not applicable; presence of signs and symptoms establishes an *actual* diagnosis.]

DESIRED OUTCOMES/EVALUATION CRITERIA—CLIENT WILL:

Risk Control (NOC)

Be free of complications associated with nutritional support.
Modify environment/correct hazards to enhance safety for in-home therapy.

ACTIONS/INTERVENTIONS	RATIONALE
Surveillance (NIC)	
Independent	
Parenteral	
Maintain a closed central IV system using Luer-Lok connections/taping of all connections.	Inadvertent disconnection of central IV system can result in lethal air emboli.
Administer appropriate TPN solution via peripheral or central venous route (including peripherally inserted central catheter [PICC] lines and tunneled catheters).	Solutions containing high concentrations of dextrose (more than 10%) must be delivered via a central vein because they result in chemical phlebitis when delivered through small peripheral veins.
Monitor for potential drug/nutrient interactions.	Various interactions are possible; e.g., digoxin (in conjunction with diuretic therapy) can cause hypomagnesemia; hypokalemia may result from chronic use of laxatives, mineralocorticosteroids, diuretics, or amphotericin.
Assess catheter for signs of displacement out of central venous position; i.e., extended length of catheter on skin surface, leaking of IV solution onto dressing, client complaints of neck/arm pain, tenderness at catheter site, or swelling of extremity on side of catheter insertion.	Central venous catheter tip may slip out of superior vena cava and migrate into smaller innominate and jugular veins, causing a chemical thrombophlebitis. Incidence of subclavian or superior vena cava thrombosis is increased with extended use of central venous catheters.
Inspect peripheral TPN catheter site routinely and change sites at least every other day, or per protocol.	Peripheral TPN solutions (although less hyperosmolar) can still irritate small veins and cause phlebitis. Peripheral venous access is often limited in malnourished clients, but site should still be changed if signs of irritation develop.
Investigate reports of severe chest pain/coughing in clients with central line. Turn client to left side in Trendelenburg's position if indicated and notify physician.	Suggests presence of air embolus requiring immediate intervention to displace air into apex of heart away from the pulmonary artery.
Maintain an occlusive dressing on catheter insertion sites for 24 hr after subclavian catheter is removed.	Extended catheter use may result in development of catheter skin tract. Once the catheter is removed, air embolus is still a potential risk until skin tract has sealed.
Enteral	
Assess gastrostomy or jejunostomy tube sites for evidence of malposition.	Indwelling and mushroom catheters are still used for feeding tubes inserted via the abdomen. Migration of the catheter balloon can result in duodenal or jejunal obstruction. Improperly sutured gastrostomy tubes may easily fall out.
Collaborative	
Review chest x-ray as indicated.	Central parenteral line placement is routinely confirmed by x-ray.

ACTIONS/INTERVENTIONS	RATIONALE
Consult with pharmacist in regard to site/time of delivery of drugs that might have action adversely affected by enteral formula.	Absorption of vitamin D is impaired by administration of mineral oil (inhibits micelle formation of bile salts) and by neomycin (inactivates bile salts). Aluminum-containing antacids bind with the phosphorus in the feeding solution, potentiating hypophosphatemia.

NURSING DIAGNOSIS: risk for Aspiration

Risk factors may include

Presence of GI tube, bolus tube feedings, medication administration
Increased intragastric pressure, delayed gastric emptying

Possibly evidenced by

[Not applicable; presence of signs and symptoms establishes an *actual* diagnosis.]

DESIRED OUTCOMES/EVALUATION CRITERIA—CLIENT WILL:

RESPIRATORY STATUS: Ventilation (NOC)

Maintain clear airway, be free of signs of aspiration.

ACTIONS/INTERVENTIONS	RATIONALE
Aspiration Precautions (NIC)	
Independent	
Confirm placement of nasoenteral feeding tubes. Determine feeding tube position in stomach by x-ray, confirmation of pH of 0–5 of the gastric fluid withdrawn through tube, or auscultation of injected air before intermittent feedings. Observe for ability to speak/cough.	Malplacement of nasoenteral feeding tubes may result in aspiration of enteral formula. Clients at particular risk include those who are intubated or obtunded and those who have had a CVA or surgery of the head/neck and upper GI system. *Note:* The reliability of the pH method is reduced if antacids or certain other medications have been given po/NG in the past 4 hr. Also when using auscultatory method to assess tube placement, air sounds can be transmitted to the epigastrium even if the tube is malpositioned (i.e., in lung or proximal jejunum).
Maintain aspiration precautions during enteral feedings; e.g.:	
Keep head of bed elevated at 30–45 degrees during feeding and at least 1 hr after feeding;	Reduces risk of regurgitation/gastric reflux.
Inflate tracheostomy cuff during and for 1 hr after intermittent feeding. Interrupt continuous feeding when client is in prone position;	Aspiration of enteral formulas is highly irritating to the lung parenchyma and may result in pneumonia and respiratory compromise.
Add blue food coloring to enteral formula as indicated.	Helps identify aspiration of enteral formula and/or tracheal esophageal fistula, if discovered in sputum/lung secretions. *Note:* Avoid use of methylene blue dye, which may cause false-positive guaiac test when assessing for GI bleeding.
Monitor gastric residuals between/before bolus feedings (as previously noted in ND: imbalanced Nutrition: less than body requirements).	Presence of large gastric residuals may potentiate an incompetent esophageal sphincter, leading to vomiting and aspiration.

ACTIONS/INTERVENTIONS	RATIONALE
Note characteristics of sputum/tracheal aspirate. Investigate development of dyspnea, cough, tachypnea, cyanosis. Auscultate breath sounds.	Presence of formula in tracheal secretions or signs/symptoms reflecting respiratory distress suggests aspiration.
Note indicators of NG tube intolerance; e.g., absence of gag reflex, high risk of aspiration, frequent removal of NG feeding tubes.	May require consideration of surgically placed feeding tube/percutaneous endoscopic gastrostomy (PEG), or jejunostomy for client safety and consistency of enteral formula delivery.

Collaborative

Review abdominal x-ray if done.	Confirmation of placement of gastric feeding tube may be obtained by x-ray.

NURSING DIAGNOSIS: risk for imbalance Fluid Volume

Risk factors may include

Active loss and/or failure of regulatory mechanisms (specific to underlying disease process/trauma); complications of nutrition therapy; e.g., high-glucose solutions, hyperglycemia (hyperosmolar nonketotic coma and severe dehydration)
Inability to obtain/ingest fluids

Possibly evidenced by

[Not applicable; presence of signs and symptoms establishes an *actual* diagnosis.]

DESIRED OUTCOMES/EVALUATION CRITERIA—CLIENT WILL:

Fluid Balance (NOC)

Display moist skin/mucous membranes, stable vital signs, individually adequate urinary output; be free of edema and excessive weight loss/inappropriate gain.

ACTIONS/INTERVENTIONS | RATIONALE

Fluid Management (NIC)

Independent

ACTIONS/INTERVENTIONS	RATIONALE
Assess for clinical signs of dehydration (e.g., thirst, dry skin/mucous membranes, hypotension) or fluid excess (e.g., peripheral edema, tachycardia, adventitious breath sounds).	Early detection and intervention may prevent occurrence of excessive fluctuation in fluid balance. *Note:* Severely malnourished clients have an increased risk of developing refeeding syndrome; e.g., life-threatening fluid overload, intracellular electrolyte shifts, and cardiac strain occurring during initial 3–5 days of therapy.
Incorporate knowledge of caloric density of enteral formulas into assessment of fluid balance.	Enteric solutions are usually concentrated and do not meet free water needs.
Provide additional water/flush tubing as indicated.	With higher calorie formula, additional water is needed to prevent dehydration/hyperglycemic complications.
Record I&O, calculate fluid balance, measure urine specific gravity.	Excessive urinary losses may reflect developing HHNC. Specific gravity is an indicator of hydration and renal function.
Weigh daily or as indicated; evaluate changes.	Rapid weight gain (reflecting fluid retention) can predispose/potentiate HF or pulmonary edema. Gain of more than 0.5 lb/day indicates fluid retention and not deposition of lean body mass.

ACTIONS/INTERVENTIONS	RATIONALE
Collaborative	
Monitor laboratory studies; e.g.:	
Serum potassium/phosphorus;	Hypokalemia/phosphatemia can occur because of intracellular shifts during initial refeeding and may compromise cardiac function if not corrected.
Hct;	Reflects hydration/circulating volume.
Serum albumin.	Hypoalbuminemia/decreased colloidal osmotic pressure leads to third spacing of fluid (edema).
Dilute formula or change from hypertonic to isotonic formula as indicated.	May decrease gastric intolerance, reducing occurrence of diarrhea and associated fluid losses.

NURSING DIAGNOSIS: Fatigue

May be related to

Decreased metabolic energy production; increased energy requirements (hypermetabolic states, healing process)
Altered body chemistry: medications, chemotherapy

Possibly evidenced by

Overwhelming lack of energy, inability to maintain usual routines/accomplish routine tasks
Lethargy, impaired ability to concentrate

DESIRED OUTCOMES/EVALUATION CRITERIA—CLIENT WILL:

Endurance (NOC)

Report increased sense of well-being/energy level.
Demonstrate measurable increase in physical activity.

ACTIONS/INTERVENTIONS	RATIONALE
Energy Management (NIC)	
Independent	
Monitor physiologic response to activity; e.g., changes in BP, or heart/respiratory rate.	Tolerance varies greatly, depending on the stage of the disease process, nutritional state, and fluid balance.
Establish realistic activity goals with client.	Provides for a sense of control and feelings of accomplishment.
Plan care to allow for rest periods. Schedule activities for periods when client has most energy. Involve client/SO in schedule planning.	Frequent rest periods are needed to restore/conserve energy. Planning allows client to be active during times when energy level is higher, which may restore a feeling of well-being and a sense of control.
Encourage client to do whatever possible; e.g., self-care, sitting up in chair, walking. Increase activity level as indicated.	Increases strength/stamina and enables client to become more active without undue fatigue.
Provide passive/active ROM exercises to bedridden clients.	The development of healthy lean muscle mass depends on the provision of both isotonic and isometric exercises.
Keep bed in low position, pathways clear of furniture; assist with ambulation.	Protects client from injury during activities.
Assist with self-care needs as necessary.	Generalized weakness may make ADLs almost impossible for client to complete.

ACTIONS/INTERVENTIONS	RATIONALE
Collaborative	
Provide supplemental O_2 as indicated.	Presence of anemia/hypoxemia reduces O_2 available for cellular uptake and contributes to fatigue.
Refer to physical/occupational therapy.	Programmed daily exercises and activities help client maintain/increase strength and muscle tone and enhance sense of well-being.

NURSING DIAGNOSIS: deficient Knowledge [Learning Need] regarding condition, prognosis, treatment, self-care, and discharge needs

May be related to

Lack of exposure/recall, information misinterpretation
Cognitive limitation

Possibly evidenced by

Request for information, questions/statement of misconception
Inaccurate follow-through of instructions/development of preventable complications

DESIRED OUTCOMES/EVALUATION CRITERIA—CLIENT WILL:

KNOWLEDGE: Disease Process (NOC)

Verbalize understanding of condition/disease process and individual nutritional needs.

KNOWLEDGE: Treatment Procedure (NOC)

Correctly perform necessary procedures and explain reasons for the actions.

ACTIONS/INTERVENTIONS	RATIONALE
TEACHING: Prescribed Diet (NIC)	
Independent	
Assess client's/SO's knowledge of nutritional state. Review individual situation, signs/symptoms of malnutrition, future expectations, transitional feeding needs.	Provides information from which client/SO can make informed choices. Knowledge of the interaction between malnutrition and illness is helpful in understanding need for special therapy.
Discuss reasons for use of parenteral/enteral nutrition support.	May experience anxiety regarding inability to eat and may not comprehend the nutritional value of the prescribed TPN/tube feedings.
Provide adequate time for teaching client/SO when client is going home on enteral/parenteral feedings. Document client's/SO's understanding and ability/competence to deliver safe home therapy.	Generally, 3–4 days is sufficient for client/SO to become proficient with tube feedings. Parenteral therapy is more complex, and client/SO may require a week or longer to feel ready for home management; follow-up in the home is required.
Discuss proper handling, storage, preparation of nutritional solutions or blenderized feedings; also discuss aseptic or clean techniques for care of insertion sites and use of dressings.	Reduces risk of formula-/solution-related problems, metabolic complications, and infection.

ACTIONS/INTERVENTIONS	RATIONALE
Review use/care of nutritional support devices.	Client understanding and cooperation are key to the safe insertion and maintenance of nutritional support access devices and prevention of complications.
Review specific precautions depending on type of feeding; e.g., checking placement of tube, sitting upright for enteral feeding, maintaining patency of tube, anchoring of tubing and adequate length of tubing for nighttime feeding.	Promotes safe self-care and reduces risk of complications.
Discuss/demonstrate reinsertion of enterostomal feeding tube if appropriate.	Tube may be changed routinely or inserted only for feedings. Intermittent feedings enhance client mobility and aid in transition to regular feeding pattern.
Identify signs/symptoms requiring medical evaluation; e.g., nausea/vomiting, abdominal cramping or bloating, diarrhea, rapid weight changes, erythema, drainage, foul odor at tube insertion site, fever/chills, coughing/choking, or difficulty breathing during enteral feeding.	Early evaluation and treatment of problems (e.g., feeding intolerance, infection, aspiration) may prevent progression to more serious complications.
Instruct client/SO in glucose monitoring if indicated.	Timely recognition of changes in blood glucose levels reduces risk of hyperglycemic or hypoglycemic reactions in client on hyperalimentation.
Discuss signs/symptoms and treatment of hyperglycemia/hypoglycemia.	Hyperglycemia is more common for clients receiving parenteral feedings and those who have pancreas or liver disease or are taking large doses of corticosteroids. Rebound hypoglycemia can occur when feedings are intentionally/accidentally discontinued.
Encourage use of diary for recording test results, physical feelings/reactions, activity level, oral intake if any, I&O, weekly weight.	Provides resource for review by healthcare providers for optimal management of individual situation.
Recommend daily exercise/activity to tolerance, scheduling of adequate rest periods.	Enhances gastric motility for enteral/transition feedings, promotes feelings of general well-being, and prevents undue fatigue.
Ascertain that all supplies are in place in the home before discharge, make arrangements as needed with suppliers; e.g., hospital, pharmacy, medical equipment company, laboratory.	Provides for successful and competent home therapy.
Refer to nutritional support team, home healthcare agency, and counseling resources. Provide with immediate access phone numbers.	Client/SO needs readily available support persons to assist with nutrition therapy, equipment problems, and emotional adjustments in long-term/home-based therapy.

POTENTIAL CONSIDERATIONS following acute hospitalization (dependent on client's age, physical condition/presence of complications, personal resources, and life responsibilities)

Fatigue—decreased metabolic energy production, increased energy requirements (hypermetabolic states, healing process), altered body chemistry; e.g., medications, chemotherapy.

risk for Injury—catheter-related complications (catheter breaks, dislodgement, occlusion), effects of therapy (e.g., electrolyte/fluid shifts, diarrhea)/drug interactions, aspiration.

risk for Infection—invasive tubes, environmental exposure, malnutrition, chronic disease.

interrupted Family Processes—situational crises.

METABOLIC ACID-BASE IMBALANCES

The body has the remarkable ability to maintain plasma pH within the narrow range of 7.35–7.45. It does so by means of chemical buffering mechanisms by the kidneys and the lungs. Although single acid-base (e.g., metabolic acidosis) imbalances do occur, mixed acid-base imbalances are more common (e.g., metabolic acidosis/respiratory acidosis as occurs with cardiac arrest).

METABOLIC ACIDOSIS (PRIMARY BASE BICARBONATE [HCO_3] DEFICIENCY)

Metabolic acidosis (primary base bicarbonate [HCO_3] deficiency) reflects an excess of acid (hydrogen) and a deficit of base (bicarbonate) resulting from acid overproduction, loss of intestinal bicarbonate, inadequate conservation of bicarbonate, and excretion of acid, or anaerobic metabolism.

Metabolic acidosis is characterized by normal or high anion gap situations. If the primary problem is direct loss of bicarbonate, gain of chloride, or decreased ammonia production, the anion gap is within normal limits. If the primary problem is the accumulation of organic anions (such as ketones or lactic acid), the condition is known as *high anion gap acidosis.* Compensatory mechanisms to correct this imbalance include an increase in respirations to blow off excess CO_2, an increase in ammonia formation, and acid excretion (H^+) by the kidneys, with retention of bicarbonate and sodium.

High anion gap acidosis occurs in diabetic ketoacidosis, severe malnutrition or starvation, alcoholic lactic acidosis, renal failure, high-fat, low-carbohydrate diets/lipid administration, poisoning (e.g., salicylate intoxication [after initial stage]), paraldehyde intoxication, and drug therapy (e.g., acetazolamide [Diamox], NH_4Cl).

Normal anion gap acidosis is associated with loss of bicarbonate from the body, as may occur in renal tubular acidosis, hyperalimentation, vomiting/diarrhea, small-bowel/pancreatic fistulas, and ileostomy and use of IV sodium chloride in presence of preexisting kidney dysfunction, acidifying drugs (e.g., ammonium chloride).

CARE SETTING

This condition does not occur in isolation but rather is a complication of a broader problem that may require inpatient care in a medical-surgical or subacute unit.

RELATED CONCERNS

Plans of care specific to predisposing factors
Fluid and electrolyte imbalances, page 919
Renal dialysis, page 564
Respiratory acidosis (primary carbonic acid excess), page 194
Respiratory alkalosis (primary carbonic acid deficit), page 198

Client Assessment Database (Dependent on Underlying Cause)

ACTIVITY/REST

May report: Lethargy, fatigue; muscle weakness

CIRCULATION

May exhibit: Hypotension, wide pulse pressure
Pulse may be weak, irregular (dysrhythmias)
Jaundiced sclera, skin, mucous membranes (liver failure)

ELIMINATION

May report: Diarrhea
May exhibit: Dark/concentrated urine

FOOD/FLUID

May report: Anorexia, nausea/vomiting
May exhibit: Poor skin turgor, dry mucous membranes

NEUROSENSORY

May report: Headache, drowsiness, decreased mental function
May exhibit: Changes in sensorium; e.g., stupor, confusion, lethargy, depression, delirium, coma
Decreased deep-tendon reflexes, muscle weakness

RESPIRATION

May report: Dyspnea on exertion
May exhibit: Hyperventilation, Kussmaul's respirations (deep, rapid breathing is best recognized sign of metabolic acidosis)

SAFETY

May report: Transfusion of blood/blood products
Exposure to hepatitis virus
May exhibit: Fever, signs of sepsis

TEACHING/LEARNING

May report: History of diabetes, alcohol abuse or prolonged starvation
Use of carbonic anhydrase inhibitors or anion-exchange resins; e.g., cholestyramine (Questran)
Ingestion of drugs or toxins (e.g., salicylates, acetazolamide, cyclosporine, ethylene glycol, methanol)

Discharge plan considerations: May require change in therapies for underlying disease process/condition

Refer to section at end of plan for postdischarge considerations

DIAGNOSTIC STUDIES

Arterial pH: Decreased, below 7.35.
Bicarbonate (HCO_3): Decreased, less than 22 mEq/L.
$PaCO_2$: Below 35 mm Hg.
Base excess: Negative.
Anion gap: Above 14 mEq/L (high anion gap) or range of 10–14 mEq/L (normal anion gap).
Serum potassium: Increased (except in diarrhea, renal tubular acidosis).
Serum chloride: Increased.
Serum glucose: May be decreased or increased depending on etiology.
Serum ketones: Increased in DM, starvation, alcohol intoxication.
Plasma lactic acid: Elevated in lactic acidosis.
Urine pH: Decreased, less than 4.5 (in absence of renal disease).
ECG: Cardiac dysrhythmias (bradycardia) and pattern changes associated with hyperkalemia; e.g., tall T wave.

NURSING PRIORITIES

1. Achieve homeostasis.
2. Prevent/minimize complications.
3. Provide information about condition/prognosis and treatment needs as appropriate.

DISCHARGE GOALS

1. Physiological balance restored.
2. Free of complications.
3. Condition, prognosis, and treatment needs understood.
4. Plan in place to meet needs after discharge.

Because no current nursing diagnosis speaks clearly to metabolic imbalances, the following interventions are presented in a general format for inclusion in the primary plan of care.

DESIRED OUTCOMES/EVALUATION CRITERIA—CLIENT WILL:

Electrolyte & Acid/Base Balance (NOC)

Display serum bicarbonate and electrolytes within normal limits (WNL).
Be free of symptoms of imbalance; e.g., absence of neurological impairment, vital signs WNL.

ACTIONS/INTERVENTIONS	RATIONALE
ACID-BASE MANAGEMENT: Metabolic Acidosis (NIC)	
Independent	
Monitor BP.	Arteriolar dilation/decreased cardiac contractility (e.g., sepsis) and hypovolemia (e.g., ketoacidosis) occur, resulting in systemic shock, evidenced by hypotension and tissue hypoxia.

ACTIONS/INTERVENTIONS	RATIONALE
Assess LOC and note progressive changes in neuromuscular status; e.g., strength, tone, movement.	Decreased mental function, confusion, seizures, weakness, flaccid paralysis can occur because of hypoxia, hyperkalemia, and decreased pH of CNS fluid.
Provide seizure/coma precautions; e.g., bed in low position, use of padded side rails, frequent observation.	Protects client from injury resulting from decreased mentation/convulsions.
Monitor heart rate/rhythm.	Acidemia may be manifested by changes in ECG configuration and presence of bradydysrhydythmias as well as increased ventricular irritability such as fibrillation (signs of hyperkalemia). Life-threatening cardiovascular collapse may also occur because of vasodilation and decreased cardiac contractility. *Note:* Hypokalemia can occur as acidosis is corrected, resulting in premature ventricular contractions (PVCs)/ventricular tachycardia.
Observe for altered respiratory excursion, rate, and depth.	Deep, rapid respirations (Kussmaul's) may be noted as a compensatory mechanism to eliminate excess acid; however, as potassium shifts out of cell in an attempt to correct acidosis, respirations may become depressed. Transient respiratory depression may be the result of overcorrection of metabolic acidosis with sodium bicarbonate.
Assess skin temperature, color, capillary refill.	Evaluates circulatory status, tissue perfusion, effects of hypotension.
Auscultate bowel sounds; measure abdominal girth as indicated.	In the presence of coexisting hyperkalemia, GI distress (e.g., distention, diarrhea, and colic) may occur.
Monitor I&O closely and weigh daily.	Marked dehydration may be present because of vomiting, diarrhea. Therapy needs are based on underlying cause and fluid balance.
Test/monitor urine pH.	Kidneys attempt to compensate for acidosis by excreting excess hydrogen in the form of weak acids and ammonia. Maximum urine acidity is pH of 4.
Provide oral hygiene with sodium bicarbonate washes, lemon/glycerine swabs.	Neutralizes mouth acids and provides protective lubrication.

Collaborative

ACTIONS/INTERVENTIONS	RATIONALE
Assist with identification/treatment of underlying cause.	Treatment of disorder is directed at mild correction of acidosis until organ(s) function is improved. Addressing the primary condition (e.g., DKA, liver/renal failure, drug poisoning, sepsis) promotes correction of the acid-base disorder.
Monitor/graph serial ABGs.	Evaluates therapy needs/effectiveness. Blood bicarbonate and pH should slowly increase toward normal levels.
Monitor serum electrolytes; e.g., potassium.	As acidosis is corrected, serum potassium deficit may occur as potassium shifts back into the cells.
Replace fluids, as indicated depending on underlying etiology; e.g., D_5W/saline solutions.	Choice of solution varies with cause of acidosis; e.g., DKA. *Note:* Lactate-containing solutions may be contraindicated in the presence of lactic acidosis.
Administer medications as indicated; e.g.:	
Sodium bicarbonate/lactate or saline IV;	Corrects bicarbonate deficit, but is used cautiously to correct severe acidosis (pH less than 7.2) because sodium bicarbonate can cause rebound metabolic alkalosis.
Potassium chloride;	May be required as potassium re-enters the cell, causing a serum deficit.
Phosphate;	May be administered to enhance acid excretion in presence of chronic acidosis with hypophosphatemia.
Calcium.	May be given to improve neuromuscular conduction/function.

ACTIONS/INTERVENTIONS	RATIONALE
Modify diet as indicated; e.g., low-protein, high-carbohydrate diet in presence of renal failure, or adjust medical nutritional therapy for the person with diabetes.	Restriction of protein may be necessary to decrease production of acid waste products, whereas addition of complex carbohydrates will correct acid production from the metabolism of fats.
Administer exchange resins and/or assist with dialysis as indicated.	May be desired to reduce acidosis by decreasing excess potassium and acid waste products if pH less than 7.1 and other therapies are ineffective or HF develops.

POTENTIAL CONSIDERATIONS: Refer to Potential Considerations relative to underlying cause of acid-base disorder.

METABOLIC ALKALOSIS (PRIMARY BASE BICARBONATE EXCESS)

Metabolic alkalosis is characterized by a high pH (loss of hydrogen ions) and high plasma bicarbonate caused by excessive intake of sodium bicarbonate, loss of gastric/intestinal acid, renal excretion of hydrogen and chloride, prolonged hypercalcemia, hypokalemia, and hyperaldosteronism. Compensatory mechanisms include slow, shallow respirations to increase CO_2 level and an increase of bicarbonate excretion and hydrogen reabsorption by the kidneys.

CARE SETTING

This condition does not occur in isolation but rather is a complication of a broader problem that may require inpatient care in a medical-surgical or subacute unit.

RELATED CONCERNS

Plans of care specific to predisposing factors
Fluid and electrolyte imbalances, page 919
Renal dialysis, page 564
Respiratory acidosis (primary carbonic acid excess), page 194
Respiratory alkalosis (primary carbonic acid deficit), page 198

Client Assessment Database (Dependent on Underlying Cause)

CIRCULATION

May exhibit: Tachycardia, irregularities/dysrhythmias
Hypotension
Cyanosis

ELIMINATION

May report: Diarrhea (with high chloride content)
Use of potassium-losing diuretics (Diuril, Hygroton, Lasix, Edecrin)
Laxative abuse

FOOD/FLUID

May report: Anorexia, nausea/prolonged vomiting
High salt intake; excessive ingestion of licorice
Recurrent indigestion/heartburn with frequent use of antacids/baking soda

NEUROSENSORY

May report: Tingling of fingers and toes; circumoral paresthesia
Muscle twitching, weakness
Dizziness

May exhibit: Hypertonicity of muscles, tetany, tremors, convulsions, loss of reflexes
Confusion, irritability, restlessness, belligerence, apathy, coma
Picking at bedclothes

SAFETY

May report: Recent blood transfusions (citrated blood)

RESPIRATION

May exhibit: Hypoventilation (increases P_{CO_2} and conserves carbonic acid), periods of apnea

TEACHING/LEARNING

May report: History of primary aldosteronism, Cushing's syndrome, primary reninism, Bartter's syndrome, milk-alkali syndrome, corticosteroid therapy; pyloric stenosis or ulcers, self-induced vomiting (bulimia), long-term use of diuretics

Discharge plan considerations: May require change in therapy for underlying disease process/condition.

Refer to section at end of plan for postdischarge considerations.

DIAGNOSTIC STUDIES

Arterial pH: Increased, higher than 7.45.
Bicarbonate (HCO_3): Increased, higher than 26 mEq/L (primary).
$PaCO_2$: Slightly increased, above 45 mm Hg (compensatory).
Base excess: Increased.
Serum chloride: Decreased, less than 98 mEq/L, disproportionately to serum sodium decreases (if alkalosis is hypochloremic).
Serum sodium and potassium: Decreased.
Serum calcium: Usually decreased. Prolonged hypercalcemia (nonparathyroid) may be a predisposing factor.
Urine pH: Increased, higher than 7.0.
Urine chloride: Less than 10 mEq/L suggests chloride-responsive alkalosis, whereas levels above 20 mEq/L suggest chloride resistance.
ECG: May show hypokalemic changes including peaked P waves, flat T waves, depressed ST segment, low T wave merging to P wave, and elevated U waves.

NURSING PRIORITIES

1. Achieve homeostasis.
2. Prevent/minimize complications.
3. Provide information about condition/prognosis and treatment needs as appropriate.

DISCHARGE GOALS

1. Physiologic balance restored.
2. Free of complications.
3. Condition, prognosis, and treatment needs understood.
4. Plan in place to meet needs after discharge.

Because no current nursing diagnosis speaks clearly to metabolic imbalances, the following interventions are presented in a general format for inclusion in the primary plan of care.

DESIRED OUTCOMES/EVALUATION CRITERIA—CLIENT WILL:

Electrolyte & Acid/Base Balance (NOC)

Display serum bicarbonate and electrolytes WNL.
Be free of symptoms of imbalance; e.g., absence of neurologic impairment/irritability.

ACTIONS/INTERVENTIONS	RATIONALE
Metabolic Alkalosis Management (NIC)	
Independent	
Monitor respiratory rate, rhythm, and depth.	Hypoventilation is a compensatory mechanism to conserve carbonic acid and represents definite risks to the individual; e.g., hypoxemia and respiratory failure.

ACTIONS/INTERVENTIONS	RATIONALE
Assess level of consciousness and neuromuscular status; e.g., strength, tone, movement; note presence of Chvostek's/Trousseau's signs.	The CNS may be hyperirritable (increased pH of CNS fluid), resulting in tingling, numbness, dizziness, restlessness, or apathy and confusion. Hypocalcemia may contribute to tetany (although occurrence is rare).
Monitor heart rate/rhythm.	Atrial/ventricular ectopic beats and tachydysrhythmias may develop.
Record amount and source of output.	Helpful in identifying source of ion loss; e.g., potassium and HCl are lost in vomiting and GI suctioning.
Monitor intake and daily weight.	Useful in monitoring fluid status.
Restrict oral intake and reduce noxious environmental stimuli; use intermittent/low suction during NG suctioning; irrigate gastric tube with isotonic solutions rather than water.	Limits gastric losses of HCl, potassium, and calcium.
Provide seizure/safety precautions as indicated; e.g., padded side rails, airway protection, bed in low position, frequent observation.	Changes in mentation and CNS/neuromuscular hyperirritability may result in client harm, especially if tetany/convulsions occur.
Encourage intake of foods and fluids high in potassium and possibly calcium (dependent on blood level); e.g., canned grapefruit and apple juices, bananas, cauliflower, dried peaches, figs, and wheat germ.	Useful in replacing potassium losses when oral intake permitted.
Review medication regimen for use of diuretics, such as thiazides (Diuril, Hygroton), furosemide (Lasix), and ethacrynic acid (Edecrin).	Discontinuation of these potassium-wasting drugs may prevent recurrence of imbalance.
Instruct client to avoid use of excessive amounts of sodium bicarbonate.	Ulcer clients can cause alkalosis by taking baking soda and milk of magnesia in addition to prescribed alkaline antacids.

Collaborative

ACTIONS/INTERVENTIONS	RATIONALE
Assist with identification/treatment of underlying disorder.	Addressing the primary condition (e.g., prolonged vomiting/diarrhea, hyperaldosteronism, Cushing's syndrome) promotes correction of the acid-base disorder.
Monitor laboratory studies as indicated; e.g., ABGs/pH, serum electrolytes (especially potassium), and BUN.	Evaluates therapy needs/effectiveness and monitors renal function.
Administer medications as indicated:	
chloride solutions; e.g., sodium chloride PO/Ringer's solution IV unless contraindicated;	Correcting sodium, water, and chloride defects may be all that is needed to permit kidneys to excrete bicarbonate and correct alkalosis, but must be used with caution in clients with HF or renal insufficiency.
Potassium chloride;	Hypokalemia is frequently present. Chloride is needed so kidney can absorb sodium with chloride, enhancing excretion of bicarbonate.
Ammonium chloride or arginine hydrochloride;	Although used only in severe cases, ammonium chloride may be given to increase amount of circulating hydrogen ions. Monitor administration closely to prevent too rapid a decrease in pH, hemolysis of RBCs. *Note:* May cause rebound metabolic acidosis and is usually contraindicated in clients with renal/hepatic failure.
Carbonic anhydrase inhibitors: e.g., acetazolamide (Diamox); spironolactone (Aldactone).	Blocks HCO_3 reabsorption in the proximal renal tubules, promoting renal excretion of bicarbonate. Effective in treating chloride-resistant alkalosis and its excess fluid volume effects.
Avoid/limit use of sedatives or hypnotics.	If respirations are depressed, may cause hypoxia/respiratory failure.
Encourage fluids IV/PO.	Replaces extracellular fluid losses, and adequate hydration facilitates removal of pulmonary secretions to improve ventilation.

ACTIONS/INTERVENTIONS	RATIONALE
Administer supplemental O_2 as indicated and respiratory treatments to improve ventilation.	Respiratory compensation for metabolic alkalosis is hypoventilation, which may cause decreased PaO_2 levels/hypoxia.
Prepare client for/assist with dialysis as needed.	Useful when renal dysfunction prevents clearance of bicarbonate.

POTENTIAL CONSIDERATIONS: Refer to Potential Considerations relative to underlying cause of acid/base disorder.

9

CHAPTER

Diseases of The Blood/ Blood-Forming Organs

ANEMIAS (IRON DEFICIENCY, PERNICIOUS, APLASTIC, HEMOLYTIC)

Anemia is a symptom of an underlying condition, such as loss of blood components, inadequate elements, or lack of required nutrients for the formation of blood cells that result in decreased oxygen-carrying capacity of the blood. In most grading systems, adult anemia is defined as a hemoglobin (Hb) level lower than 11 g/dL, with severe anemia (Hb $<$ 8 g/dL) being associated with many physiologic complications, including dyspnea; fatigue; dizziness; decreased cognitive, sleep, and sexual function; and significant debilitation.

Clients at risk for anemias include those with family history of hematologic problems; client history of chronic illness, recent infection, inflammatory conditions, surgery (e.g., partial or total gastrectomy); social history of alcohol consumption, endurance exercise; occupational history of lead exposure; inadequate or inappropriate dietary intake; medication use (e.g., prescription/nonprescription, aspirin, nonsteroidal anti-inflammatory drugs [NSAIDs], cancer drugs, herbal supplements).

There are numerous types of anemias with various causes. The following types of anemia are discussed here: (1) *iron deficiency anemia* (ID), the result of inadequate absorption or excessive loss of iron, and the most common form of anemia seen in primary care; (2) *pernicious anemia* (PA), the result of a lack of the intrinsic factor essential for the absorption of vitamin B_{12}; (3) *aplastic anemia*, due to failure of bone marrow; and (4) *hemolytic anemia*, due to red blood cell (RBC) destruction.

The most frequent cause of ID is physiologic iron loss secondary to blood loss; e.g., menstruating women. Pathologic iron loss occurs most often from gastrointestinal tract bleeding (e.g., gastric or duodenal ulcers, diverticula, hemorrhoids, ulcerative colitis). Inadequate nutrition, malabsorption syndromes, and lead exposure can also cause ID.

PA is an autoimmune disorder characterized by the production of autoantibodies to gastric parietal cells and their secretory product, intrinsic factor, which is needed for vitamin B_{12} absorption. Conditions that interfere with the body's absorption and use of B_{12} include Crohn's and Whipple's diseases, gastrectomy/gastric bypass, and the use of chemotherapeutic medications.

Bone marrow failure can be associated with conditions such as certain cancers, lymphoma, and renal, hepatic, or endocrine disorders that affect erythropoietin production and/or secretion. Hemolytic anemia is marked by an accelerated destruction of red blood cells associated with various causes such as hereditary factors (e.g., sickle cell trait or disease), blood transfusion reactions, acute viral or infectious agents, drugs (e.g., quinidine, penicillins, methyldopa), and toxins (e.g., chemicals, venoms).

Nursing care for the anemic client has a common theme (e.g., physical symptoms and quality-of-life issues) even though the medical treatments vary widely.

CARE SETTING

Treated at the community level except in the presence of severe cardiovascular/immune compromise.

RELATED CONCERNS

Acquired immunodeficiency syndrome (AIDS), page 726
Burns: thermal/chemical/electrical (acute and convalescent phases), page 680
Cancer, page 857
Cirrhosis of the liver, page 453
Heart failure: chronic, page 47
Psychosocial aspects of care, page 770
Renal failure: acute, page 541
Renal failure: chronic, page 553
Rheumatoid arthritis, page 750
Pulmonary tuberculosis (TB), page 184
Upper gastrointestinal/esophageal bleeding, page 309

Client Assessment Database

ACTIVITY/REST

May report:
Fatigue, weakness, general malaise
Loss of productivity; diminished enthusiasm for work
Low exercise tolerance
Greater need for rest and sleep

May exhibit:
Tachycardia/tachypnea; dyspnea on exertion or at rest (severe or aplastic anemia)
Lethargy, withdrawal, apathy, lassitude, and lack of interest in surroundings
Muscle weakness and decreased strength
Ataxia, unsteady gait
Slumping of shoulders, drooping posture, slow walk, and other cues indicative of fatigue

CIRCULATION

May report:
History of chronic blood loss; e.g., chronic gastrointestinal bleeding, heavy menses (ID), angina, heart failure (due to increased cardiac workload)
History of chronic infective endocarditis
Palpitations (compensatory tachycardia)

May exhibit:
Blood pressure (BP): Increased systolic with stable diastolic and a widened pulse pressure, postural hypotension
Dysrhythmias, electrocardiogram abnormalities; e.g., ST-segment depression and flattening or depression of the T wave, tachycardia
Throbbing carotid pulsations (reflects increased cardiac output as a compensatory mechanism to provide oxygen/nutrients to cells)
Systolic murmur (ID)
Extremities (color): Pallor of the skin and mucous membranes (conjunctiva, mouth, pharynx, lips) and nailbeds, or grayish cast in black client; waxy, pale skin (aplastic, PA) or bright lemon yellow (PA)
Sclera blue or pearl white (ID), jaundice (PA)
Capillary refill delayed (diminished blood flow to the periphery and compensatory vasoconstriction)
Nails brittle, spoon shaped (koilonychia) (ID)

EGO INTEGRITY

May report:
Negative feelings about self, ability to handle situation/events

May exhibit:
Depression

ELIMINATION

May report:
History of pyelonephritis, renal failure
Flatulence, malabsorption syndrome (ID)
Hematemesis, fresh blood in stool, melena
Diarrhea or constipation
Diminished urine output

May exhibit:
Abdominal distention

FOOD/FLUID

May report:
Decreased dietary intake, low intake of animal protein/high intake of cereal products (ID)
Mouth or tongue pain, difficulty swallowing (ulcerations in pharynx)
Nausea/vomiting, dyspepsia, anorexia
Recent weight loss
Insatiable craving, or pica, for unnatural food such as ice, dirt, cornstarch, paint, clay, and others

May exhibit:
Beefy red/smooth appearance of tongue (PA, folic acid and vitamin B_{12} deficiencies)
Dry, pale mucous membranes
Skin turgor poor with dry, shriveled appearance/loss of elasticity (ID)
Stomatitis and glossitis (deficiency states)
Lips: Cheilitis; i.e., inflammation of the lips with cracking at the corners of the mouth (ID)

HYGIENE

May report:
Difficulty maintaining activities of daily living (ADLs)

May exhibit: Unkempt appearance, poor personal hygiene
Hair dry, brittle, thinning; premature graying (PA)

NEUROSENSORY

May report: Headaches, fainting, dizziness, vertigo, tinnitus, inability to concentrate
Insomnia, dimness of vision, and spots before eyes
Weakness, poor balance, wobbly legs, paresthesias of hands/feet (PA), claudication
Sensation of being cold

May exhibit: Irritability, restlessness, depression, drowsiness, apathy
Mentation: Notable slowing and dullness in response
Ophthalmic: Retinal hemorrhages (aplastic, PA)
Epistaxis, bleeding from other orifices (aplastic)
Disturbed coordination, ataxia, decreased vibratory and position sense, positive Romberg's sign, paralysis (PA)

PAIN/DISCOMFORT

May report: Vague abdominal pains, headache (ID)
Oral pain

RESPIRATION

May report: History of TB, lung abscesses
Shortness of breath at rest and with activity

May exhibit: Tachypnea, orthopnea, and dyspnea

SAFETY

May report: History of occupational exposure to chemicals; e.g., benzene, lead, insecticides, phenylbutazone, naphthalene
History of exposure to radiation either as a treatment modality or by accident
History of cancer, cancer therapies
Cold and/or heat intolerance
Previous blood transfusions
Impaired vision
Poor wound healing, frequent infections

May exhibit: Low-grade fever, chills, night sweats
Generalized lymphadenopathy
Petechiae and ecchymosis (aplastic)

SEXUALITY

May report: Changes in menstrual flow; e.g., menorrhagia or amenorrhea in women (ID)
Loss of libido (men and women)
Impotence in men

May exhibit: Pale cervix and vaginal walls

TEACHING/LEARNING

May report: Family tendency for anemia (ID, PA)
Past/present use of anticonvulsants, antibiotics, chemotherapeutic agents (bone marrow failure), aspirin, anti-inflammatory drugs, or anticoagulants
Chronic use of alcohol
Religious/cultural beliefs affecting treatment choices; e.g., refusal of blood transfusions
Recent/current episode of active bleeding (ID)
History of liver, renal disease; hematologic problems; celiac or other malabsorption disease; regional enteritis; tapeworm manifestations; polyendocrinopathies; autoimmune problem (e.g., antibodies to parietal cells, intrinsic factor, thyroid and T-cell antibodies)
Prior surgeries; e.g., splenectomy; tumor excision; prosthetic valve replacement; surgical excision of duodenum or gastric resection, partial/total gastrectomy (ID, PA)
History of problems with wound healing or bleeding; chronic infections, chronic granulomatous disease, or cancer (secondary anemias)

Discharge plan considerations: May require assistance with treatment (injections); self-care activities and/or homemaker/maintenance tasks; changes in dietary plan

Refer to section at end of plan for postdischarge considerations.

DIAGNOSTIC STUDIES

Complete blood count (CBC):

Hemoglobin (Hb) and hematocrit (Hct): Decreased in anemias and overhydration caused by excessive IV fluids, bleeding problems, bone marrow suppression.

Erythrocyte (RBC) count: Decreased (PA), severely decreased (aplastic) mean corpuscular volume (MCV) and mean corpuscular hemoglobin (MCH) decreased and microcytic with hypochromic erythrocytes (ID), elevated (PA), pancytopenia (aplastic).

Stained RBC examination: Detects changes in color and shape (may indicate particular type of anemia).

Reticulocyte count: Varies; helps assess bone marrow function; e.g., decreased (PA, cirrhosis, folic acid deficiency, bone marrow failure, radiation therapy), elevated (blood loss/hemolysis, leukemias, compensated anemias).

White blood cells (WBCs): Total cell count and specific WBCs (differential) may be increased (hemolytic) or decreased (aplastic).

Platelet count: Decreased (aplastic), elevated (ID), normal or high (hemolytic).

Erythrocyte sedimentation rate (ESR): Elevation indicates presence of inflammatory reaction; e.g., increased RBC destruction or malignant disease.

RBC survival time: Useful in the differential diagnosis of anemias because RBCs have shortened life spans in pernicious and hemolytic anemias.

Erythrocyte fragility test: Decreased (ID), increased fragility confirms hemolytic and autoimmune anemias.

Hemoglobin electrophoresis: Identifies type of hemoglobin structure, aids in determining source of hemolytic anemia.

Serum folate and vitamin B_{12}: Aids in diagnosing anemias related to deficiencies in dietary intake/malabsorption.

Serum iron: Absent (ID), elevated (hemolytic, aplastic).

Serum total iron-binding capacity (TIBC): Increased (ID), normal or slightly reduced (AP).

Serum ferritin: Decreased (ID).

Serum bilirubin (unconjugated): Elevated (PA, hemolytic).

Serum lactate dehydrogenase (LDH): May be elevated (PA).

Bleeding time: Prolonged (aplastic).

Schilling's test: Decreased urinary excretion of vitamin B_{12} (PA).

Guaiac: May be positive for occult blood in urine, stools, and gastric contents, reflecting acute/chronic bleeding (ID).

Gastric analysis: Decreased secretions with elevated pH and absence of free HCl (PA).

Bone marrow aspiration/biopsy examination: Cells may show changes in number, size, and shape, helping to differentiate type of anemia; e.g., increased megaloblasts (PA), fatty marrow with diminished or absence of blood cells at several sites (aplastic).

Endoscopic and radiographic studies: Checks for bleeding sites; e.g., acute/chronic gastrointestinal (GI) bleeding.

NURSING PRIORITIES

1. Enhance tissue perfusion.
2. Provide nutritional/fluid needs.
3. Prevent complications.
4. Provide information about disease process, prognosis, and treatment regimen.

DISCHARGE GOALS

1. ADLs met by self or with assistance of others.
2. Complications prevented/minimized.
3. Disease process/prognosis and therapeutic regimen understood.
4. Plan in place to meet needs after discharge.

NURSING DIAGNOSIS: Activity Intolerance

May be related to

Imbalance between oxygen supply (delivery) and demand

Possibly evidenced by

Weakness and fatigue
Reports of decreased exercise/activity tolerance
Greater need for sleep/rest
Palpitations, tachycardia, increased BP/respiratory response with minor exertion

DESIRED OUTCOMES/EVALUATION CRITERIA—CLIENT WILL:

Endurance (NOC)

Report an increase in activity tolerance (including ADLs).
Demonstrate a decrease in physiological signs of intolerance; e.g., pulse, respirations, and BP remain within client's normal range.
Display laboratory values, e.g., Hb/Hct, within acceptable range.

ACTIONS/INTERVENTIONS	RATIONALE
Energy Management (NIC)	
Independent	
Assess client's ability to perform normal tasks/ADLs, noting reports of weakness, fatigue, and difficulty accomplishing tasks.	Influences choice of interventions/needed assistance.
Note changes in balance/gait disturbance, muscle weakness.	May indicate neurologic changes associated with vitamin B_{12} deficiency, affecting client safety/risk of injury.
Monitor BP, pulse, respirations during and after activity. Note adverse responses to increased levels of activity (e.g., increased heart rate [HR]/BP, dysrhythmias, dizziness, dyspnea, tachypnea, cyanosis of mucous membranes/nailbeds).	Cardiopulmonary manifestations result from attempts by the heart and lungs to supply adequate amounts of oxygen to the tissues.
Recommend quiet atmosphere; bedrest if indicated. Stress need to monitor and limit visitors, phone calls, and repeated unplanned interruptions.	Enhances rest to lower body's oxygen requirements, and reduces strain on the heart and lungs.
Elevate head of bed as tolerated.	Enhances lung expansion to maximize oxygenation for cellular uptake. *Note:* May be contraindicated if hypotension is present.
Suggest client change position slowly, monitor for dizziness.	Postural hypotension or cerebral hypoxia may cause dizziness, fainting, and increased risk of injury.
Assist client to prioritize ADLs/desired activities. Alternate rest periods with activity periods. Write out schedule for client to refer to.	Promotes adequate rest, maintains energy level, and alleviates strain on the cardiac and respiratory systems.
Provide/recommend assistance with activities/ambulation as necessary, allowing client to do as much as possible.	Although help may be necessary, self-esteem is enhanced when client does some things for self.
Plan activity progression with client, including activities that client views as essential. Increase activity levels as tolerated.	Promotes gradual return to normal activity level and improved muscle tone/stamina without undue fatigue. Increases self-esteem and sense of control.
Identify/implement energy-saving techniques; e.g., shower chair, sitting to perform tasks.	Encourages client to do as much as possible, while conserving limited energy and preventing fatigue.
Instruct client to stop activity if palpitations, chest pain, shortness of breath, weakness, or dizziness occur.	Cellular ischemia potentiates risk of infarction and excessive cardiopulmonary strain/stress may lead to decompensation and failure.
Discuss importance of maintaining environmental temperature and body warmth as indicated.	Vasoconstriction (shunting of blood to vital organs) decreases peripheral circulation, impairing tissue perfusion. Client's comfort/need for warmth must be balanced with need to avoid excessive heat with resultant vasodilation (reduces organ perfusion).
Collaborative	
Monitor laboratory studies; e.g., Hb/Hct and RBC count, arterial blood gases (ABGs).	Identifies deficiencies in RBC components affecting oxygen transport and treatment needs/response to therapy.

ACTIONS/INTERVENTIONS	RATIONALE
Provide supplemental oxygen as indicated.	Maximizing oxygen transport to tissues improves ability to function.
Administer as indicated:	
Colony-stimulating factors (CSFs); e.g., aldesleukin (Interleukin-2);	CSFs may be given to stimulate growth of specific blood elements.
Erythropoiesis-stimulating therapies; e.g., epoietin-Alpha (Procrit, EPO);	Large-scale clinical studies have shown the effectiveness of EPO in increasing erythrocyte and hemoglobin levels relieving clinical and quality-of-life manifestations associated with anemia.
Whole blood/packed RBCs (PRCs), blood products as indicated. Monitor closely for transfusion reactions.	Increases number of oxygen-carrying cells; corrects deficiencies to reduce risk of hemorrhage in acutely compromised individuals. *Note:* Transfusions are reserved for severe blood loss anemias with cardiovascular compromise; used after other therapies have failed to restore homeostasis.
Prepare for surgical intervention if indicated.	Surgery is useful to control bleeding in patients who are anemic because of bleeding (e.g., ulcers, uterine bleeding); or to remove spleen as treatment of autoimmune hemolytic anemia. Bone marrow and stem cell transplantation may be done in presence of bone marrow failure/aplastic anemia.

NURSING DIAGNOSIS: imbalanced Nutrition: less than body requirements

May be related to

Failure to ingest or inability to digest food/absorb nutrients necessary for formation of normal RBCs

Possibly evidenced by

Weight loss/weight below normal for age, height, and build
Decreased triceps skin fold measurement
Changes in gums, oral mucous membranes
Decreased tolerance for activity, weakness, and loss of muscle tone

DESIRED OUTCOMES/EVALUATION CRITERIA—CLIENT WILL:

Nutritional Status (NOC)

Demonstrate progressive weight gain or stable weight, with normalization of laboratory values.
Experience no signs of malnutrition.
Demonstrate behaviors, lifestyle changes to regain and/or maintain appropriate weight.

ACTIONS/INTERVENTIONS	RATIONALE
Nutrition Therapy (NIC)	
Independent	
Review nutritional history, including food preferences.	Identifies deficiencies, suggests possible interventions. *Note*: Daily meal diary over period of time may be necessary to identify anemia related to nutrient deficiencies; e.g., no meat in diet (iron and vitamin B_{12}), few leafy vegetables in diet (folic acid deficiency).

ACTIONS/INTERVENTIONS	RATIONALE
Observe and record client's food intake.	Monitors caloric intake or insufficient quality of food consumption.
Weigh periodically as appropriate (e.g., weekly).	Monitors weight loss and effectiveness of nutritional interventions.
Recommend small, frequent meals and/or between meal nourishment.	May reduce fatigue and thus enhance intake while preventing gastric distention. Use of Ensure/Isomil or similar product provides additional protein and calories.
Suggest bland diet, low in roughage, avoiding hot, spicy, or very acidic foods as indicated.	When oral lesions are present, pain may restrict type of foods client can tolerate.
Have client record and report occurrence of nausea/vomiting, flatus, and other related symptoms such as irritability or impaired memory.	May reflect effects of anemias (hypoxia, vitamin B_{12} deficiency) on organs.
Encourage/assist with good oral hygiene before and after meals, use soft-bristled toothbrush for gentle brushing. Provide dilute, alcohol-free mouthwash if oral mucosa is ulcerated.	Enhances appetite and oral intake. Diminishes bacterial growth, minimizing possibility of infection. Special mouth-care techniques may be needed if tissue is fragile/ulcerated/bleeding and pain is severe.

Collaborative

Consult with dietitian.	Aids in establishing dietary plan to meet individual needs.
Monitor laboratory studies; e.g., Hb/Hct, blood urea nitrogen (BUN), prealbumin/albumin, protein, transferrin, serum iron, vitamin B_{12}, folic acid, total iron-binding capacity (TIBC), serum electrolytes.	Evaluates effectiveness of treatment regimen, including dietary sources of needed nutrients.
Administer medications as indicated, e.g.:	
Vitamin and mineral supplements; e.g., cyanocobalamin (vitamin B_{12}), folic acid (Folvite), ascorbic acid (vitamin C);	Replacements needed depend on type of anemia and/or presence of poor oral intake and identified deficiencies.
Oral iron supplements; e.g., ferrous sulfate (Feosol, Mol-Iron, Fer-In-Sol), ferrous gluconate (Fergon), ferrous fumarate (Ircon, Femiron);	May be useful in some types of iron deficiency anemias. Oral preparations are taken between meals to enhance absorption and usually correct anemia and replace iron stores over a period of several months.
Iron dextran (InFeD) IM/IV;	Administered until estimated deficit is corrected. Reserved for those who cannot absorb or comply with oral iron therapy or when blood loss is too rapid for oral replacement to be effective.
Antifungal or anesthetic mouthwash if indicated.	May be needed in the presence of stomatitis/glossitis to promote oral tissue healing and facilitate intake.

NURSING DIAGNOSIS: Constipation/Diarrhea

May be related to

Decreased dietary intake, changes in digestive processes
Drug therapy side effects

Possibly evidenced by

Changes in frequency, characteristics, and amount of stool
Nausea/vomiting, decreased appetite
Reports of abdominal pain, urgency, cramping
Altered bowel sounds

DESIRED OUTCOMES/EVALUATION CRITERIA—CLIENT WILL:

Bowel Elimination (NOC)

Establish/return to normal patterns of bowel functioning.
Demonstrate changes in behaviors/lifestyle, as necessitated by causative, contributing factors.

ACTIONS/INTERVENTIONS	RATIONALE
Bowel Management (NIC)	
Independent	
Determine stool color, consistency, frequency, and amount.	Assists in identifying causative/contributing factors and appropriate interventions.
Auscultate bowel sounds.	Bowel sounds are generally increased in diarrhea and decreased in constipation.
Monitor intake and output (I&O) with specific attention to food/fluid intake.	May identify dehydration, excessive loss of fluids or aid in identifying dietary deficiencies.
Encourage fluid intake of 2500–3000 mL/day within cardiac tolerance.	Assists in improving stool consistency if constipated. Helps maintain hydration status if diarrhea is present.
Recommend avoiding gas-forming foods.	Decreases gastric distress and abdominal distention.
Assess perianal skin condition frequently, noting changes or beginning breakdown. Encourage/assist with perineal care after each bowel movement (BM) if diarrhea is present.	Prevents skin excoriation and breakdown.
Discuss use of stool softeners, mild stimulants, bulk-forming laxatives, or enemas as indicated. Monitor effectiveness.	Facilitates defecation when constipation is present.
Collaborative	
Consult with dietitian to provide well-balanced diet high in fiber and bulk.	Fiber resists enzymatic digestion and absorbs liquids in its passage along the intestinal tract and thereby produces bulk, which acts as a stimulant to defecation.
Administer antidiarrheal medications; e.g., diphenoxylate hydrochloride with atropine (Lomotil), and water-absorbing drugs; e.g., Metamucil.	Decreases intestinal motility when diarrhea is present.

NURSING DIAGNOSIS: risk for Infection

Risk factors may include

Inadequate secondary defenses; e.g., decreased hemoglobin, leukopenia, or decreased granulocytes (suppressed inflammatory response)
Inadequate primary defenses; e.g., broken skin, stasis of body fluids, invasive procedures, chronic disease, malnutrition

Possibly evidenced by

[Not applicable; presence of signs and symptoms establishes an *actual* diagnosis.]

DESIRED OUTCOMES/EVALUATION CRITERIA—CLIENT WILL:

Risk Control (NOC)

Identify behaviors to prevent/reduce risk of infection.

Immune Status (NOC)

Be free of signs of infection, achieve timely wound healing (if present).

ACTIONS/INTERVENTIONS	RATIONALE
Infection Protection (NIC)	
Independent	
Perform/promote meticulous hand washing by caregivers and client.	Prevents cross-contamination/bacterial colonization. *Note:* Client with severe/aplastic anemia may be at risk from normal skin flora.
Maintain strict aseptic techniques with procedures/wound care.	Reduces risk of bacterial colonization/infection.
Provide meticulous skin, oral, and perianal care.	Reduces risk of skin/tissue breakdown and infection.
Encourage frequent position changes/ambulation, coughing, and deep-breathing exercises.	Promotes ventilation of all lung segments and aids in mobilizing secretions to prevent pneumonia.
Promote adequate fluid intake.	Assists in liquefying respiratory secretions to facilitate expectoration and prevent stasis of body fluids (e.g., respiratory and renal).
Emphasize need to monitor/limit visitors. Provide protective isolation if appropriate. Restrict live plants/cut flowers.	Limits exposure to bacteria/infections. Protective isolation may be required in aplastic anemia, when immune response is most compromised.
Monitor temperature. Note presence of chills and tachycardia with/without fever.	Reflective of inflammatory process/infection, requiring evaluation and treatment. *Note:* With bone marrow suppression, leukocytic failure may lead to fulminating infections.
Observe for wound erythema/drainage.	Indicators of local infection. *Note:* Pus formation may be absent if granulocytes are depressed.
Collaborative	
Obtain specimens for culture/sensitivity as indicated.	Verifies presence of infection, identifies specific pathogen, and influences choice of treatment.
Administer topical antiseptics; systemic antibiotics.	May be used prophylactically to reduce colonization or used to treat specific infectious process.

NURSING DIAGNOSIS: deficient Knowledge [Learning Need] regarding condition, prognosis, treatment, self-care, and discharge needs

May be related to

Lack of exposure/recall
Information misinterpretation
Unfamiliarity with information resources

Possibly evidenced by

Questions; request for information; statement of misconception
Inaccurate follow-through of instructions, development of preventable complications

DESIRED OUTCOMES/EVALUATION CRITERIA—CLIENT WILL:

KNOWLEDGE: Illness Care (NOC)

Verbalize understanding of the nature of the disease process, diagnostic procedures, and potential complications.
Identify causative factors.
Verbalize understanding of therapeutic needs.
Initiate necessary behaviors/lifestyle changes.

ACTIONS/INTERVENTIONS	RATIONALE
TEACHING: Disease Process (NIC)	
Independent	
Provide information about specific anemia and explain that therapy depends on the type and severity of the anemia.	Provides knowledge base from which client can make informed choices. Allays anxiety and may promote cooperation with therapeutic regimen.
Discuss effects of anemias on preexisting conditions.	Anemias aggravate heart, lung, and cerebrovascular disease.
Review purpose and preparations for diagnostic studies.	Anxiety/fear of the unknown increases stress level, which in turn increases the cardiac workload. Knowledge of what to expect can diminish anxiety.
Explain that blood taken for laboratory studies will not worsen anemia.	This is often an unspoken concern that can potentiate client's anxiety.
Review required diet alterations to meet specific dietary needs (determined by type of anemia/deficiency).	Red meat, liver, seafood, green leafy vegetables, whole wheat bread, and dried fruits are sources of iron. Green vegetables, whole grains, liver, and citrus fruits are sources of folic acid and vitamin C (enhances absorption of iron).
Discuss foods to avoid (e.g., coffee, tea, egg yolks, milk, fiber, and soy protein) at the time when client is eating high-iron foods.	These foods block absorption of iron and should be taken at a different meal. For example, red meat and milk taken at the same time can block absorption of the iron from the meat.
Assess resources (e.g., financial) and ability to obtain/prepare food).	Inadequate resources may affect ability to purchase/prepare appropriate food items.
Encourage cessation of smoking.	Smoking decreases available oxygen and causes vasonstriction.
Provide information about purpose, dosage, schedule, precautions, and potential side effects, interactions, and adverse reactions to all prescribed medications.	Information enhances cooperation with regimen. Recovery from anemias can be slow, requiring lengthy treatment and prevention of secondary complications.
Stress importance of reporting signs of fatigue, weakness, paresthesias, irritability, impaired memory.	Indicates that anemia is progressing or failing to resolve, necessitating further evaluation/treatment changes.
Instruct and demonstrate self-administration of oral iron preparations:	Iron replacement usually takes 3–6 months, whereas vitamin B_{12} injections may be necessary for the rest of client's life.
Discuss importance of taking only prescribed dosages;	Overdose of iron medication can be toxic.
Advise taking with meals or immediately after meals;	Iron is best absorbed on an empty stomach. However, iron salts are gastric irritants and may cause dyspepsia, diarrhea, and abdominal discomfort if taken on an empty stomach.
Dilute liquid preparations (preferably with orange juice) and administer through a straw.	Undiluted liquid iron preparations may stain the teeth. Ascorbic acid promotes iron absorption.

ACTIONS/INTERVENTIONS	RATIONALE
Suggest use of protective devices; e.g., sheepskin, egg-crate, alternating air pressure/water mattress, heel/elbow protectors, and pillows as indicated.	Avoids skin breakdown by preventing/reducing pressure against skin surfaces.
Review good oral hygiene, necessity for regular dental care.	Effects of anemia (oral lesions) and/or iron supplements increase risk of infection/bacteremia.
Instruct to avoid use of aspirin products.	Increases bleeding tendencies.
Refer to appropriate community resources when indicated; e.g., social services for food stamps, Meals on Wheels.	May need assistance with groceries/meal preparation.

POTENTIAL CONSIDERATIONS following acute hospitalization (dependent on client's age, physical condition/presence of complications, personal resources, and life responsibilities)

Activity Intolerance—imbalance between oxygen supply (delivery) and demand.

imbalanced Nutrition: less than body requirements—failure to ingest or inability to digest food/absorb nutrients necessary for formation of normal RBCs.

risk for Infection—inadequate secondary defenses; e.g., decreased hemoglobin, leukopenia, or decreased granulocytes (suppressed inflammatory response); inadequate primary defenses; e.g., broken skin, stasis of body fluids; invasive procedures; chronic disease; malnutrition.

ineffective Therapeutic Regimen Management—economic difficulties, perceived benefits.

SICKLE CELL CRISIS

The term *sickle cell disease* (sickle hemoglobinopathies) comprises a group of genetic diseases, with the most common forms being homozygous hemoglobin SS disease (sickle cell anemia), hemoglobin SC disease, and sickle β-thalassemia.

Sickle cell disease primarily affects black populations of African descent (1 in 600 African-Americans has inherited sickle cell hemoglobin from both parents and therefore has the disease); it also affects people of South/Central American, Caribbean, Mediterranean, Arabian, and East Indian descent. It renders the individual vulnerable to repeated painful crises that can progressively destroy vital organs. These crises are:

Vaso-occlusive/thrombocytic crisis: Related to infection, dehydration, fever, hypoxia, and characterized by multiple infarcts of bones, joints, and other target organs, with tissue pain and necrosis caused by plugs of sickled cells in the microcirculation.

Hypoplastic/aplastic crisis: May be secondary to severe (usually viral) infection or folic acid deficiency, resulting in cessation of production of RBCs and bone marrow.

Hyperhemolytic crisis: Reticulocytes are increased in peripheral blood, and bone marrow is hyperplastic. Characterized by anemia and jaundice (effects of hemolysis).

Sequestration crisis (more commonly occurs in infants): Massive, sudden erythrostasis with pooling of blood in the viscera (splenomegaly), resulting in hypovolemic shock/possible death. This crisis occurs in clients with intact splenic function.

CARE SETTING

Sickle cell disease is generally managed at the community level, with many of the interventions included here being appropriate for this focus; however, this plan of care addresses sickle cell crisis, which usually requires hospitalization during the acute phase to address oxygenation and severe pain.

RELATED CONCERNS

Cerebrovascular accident (CVA)/stroke, page 236
Cholecystitis with cholelithiasis, page 364
Chronic obstructive pulmonary disease (COPD) and asthma, page 117
Cirrhosis of the liver, page 453
Heart failure: chronic, page 47
Pneumonia, page 128
Psychosocial aspects of care, page 770
Seizure disorders, page 208
Sepsis/septicemia, page 701

Client Assessment Database

Depends on severity of condition, presence of complications.

ACTIVITY/REST

May report: Lethargy, fatigue, weakness, general malaise
Loss of productivity; decreased exercise tolerance; greater need for sleep and rest

May exhibit: Listlessness, severe weakness and increasing pallor (aplastic crisis)
Gait disturbances (pain, kyphosis, lordosis), inability to walk (pain)
Poor body posture (slumping of shoulders indicative of fatigue)
Decreased range-of-motion (ROM) (swollen, inflamed joints), joint, bone deformities
Generalized retarded growth, tower-shaped skull with frontal bossing, disproportionately long arms and legs, short trunk, narrowed shoulders/hips, and long, tapered fingers

CIRCULATION

May report: Palpitations or anginal chest pain (concomitant coronary artery disease [CAD]/myocardial ischemia, acute chest syndrome)
Intermittent claudication

May exhibit: Apical pulse: Point of maximal impulse (PMI) may be displaced to the left (cardiomegaly)
Tachycardia, dysrhythmias (hypoxia), systolic murmurs
BP: Widened pulse pressure
Generalized symptoms of shock; e.g., hypotension, rapid thready pulse, and shallow respirations (sequestration crisis)
Peripheral pulses throbbing on palpation
Bruits (reflects compensatory mechanisms of anemia, may also be auscultated over the spleen because of multiple splenic infarcts)
Capillary refill delayed (anemia or hypovolemia)
Skin color: Pallor or cyanosis of skin, mucous membranes, and conjunctiva. (*Note:* Pallor may appear as yellowish brown color in brown-skinned clients and as ashen gray in black-skinned clients).
Jaundice: Scleral icterus, generalized icteric coloring (excessive RBC hemolysis)
Dry skin/mucous membranes
Diaphoresis (either sequestration or vaso-occlusive crisis, acute pain or shock)

ELIMINATION

May report: Frequent voiding, voiding in large amounts, nocturia

May exhibit: Right upper quadrant (RUQ) abdominal tenderness, enlargement/distention (hepatomegaly), ascites
Left upper quadrant (LUQ) abdominal fullness (spleen may be enlarged or may be atrophic and nonfunctional from repeated splenic infarcts and fibrosis)
Dilute, pale, straw-colored urine, hematuria or smoky appearance (multiple renal infarcts)
Inability to concentrate urine
Urine specific gravity decreased (may be fixed with progressive renal disease)

EGO INTEGRITY

May report: Resentment and frustration with disease, fear of rejection from others
Negative feelings about self, ability to deal with life/situation.
Concern regarding being a burden to significant others (SOs), financial concerns, possible loss of insurance/benefits, lost time at work/school, fear of genetic transmission of disease

May exhibit: Anxiety, restlessness, irritability, apprehension, withdrawal, narrowed focus, self-focusing, unresponsiveness to questions, regression, depression, decreased self-concept
Dependent relationship with whomever can offer security and protection

FOOD/FLUID

May report: Thirst
Anorexia, nausea/vomiting

May exhibit: Height/weight usually in the lower percentiles
Poor skin turgor with visible tenting (crisis, infection, and dehydration)
Dry skin/mucous membranes
Jugular venous distention (JVD) and general peripheral edema (concomitant HF)

HYGIENE

May report: Difficulty maintaining ADLs (pain or severe anemia)
May exhibit: Unkempt appearance, poor personal hygiene

NEUROSENSORY

May report: Headaches or dizziness
Visual disturbances (e.g., hemianopsia, retinopathy, nystagmus)
Tingling in the extremities
Disturbances in pain and position sense
May exhibit: Mental status usually unaffected except in cases of severe sickling (cerebral infarction/intracranial hemorrhage)
Weakness of the mouth, tongue, and facial muscles; aphasia (in cerebral infarction of dominant hemisphere)
Abnormal reflexes, decreased muscle strength/tone, abnormal involuntary movements, hemiplegia or sudden hemiparesis, quadriplegia
Ataxia, seizures
Meningeal irritation (intracranial hemorrhage); e.g., decreasing level of consciousness (LOC), nuchal rigidity, focal neurologic deficits, vomiting, severe headache

PAIN/DISCOMFORT

May report: Pain as severe, throbbing, gnawing of varied location [localized, migratory, or generalized—common sites extremities, abdomen, back, chest])
Recurrent, sharp, transient headaches
Back pain (changes in vertebral column from recurrent infarctions); joint/bone pain accompanied by warmth, tenderness, erythema, and occasional effusions (vaso-occlusive crisis); deep bone infarctions may have no apparent signs of irritation
Gallbladder tenderness and pain (excessive accumulation of bilirubin as a result of increased erythrocyte destruction)
May exhibit: Sensitivity to palpation over affected areas
Guarding/holding joints in position of comfort, decreased ROM (result of joint pain and swelling)
Maladaptive pain behaviors; e.g., guilt for being ill, denial of any aspect of disease, indulgence in precipitating factors (overwork, strenuous exercise)

RESPIRATION

May report: Dyspnea on exertion or at rest
History of repeated pulmonary infections/infarctions, pulmonary fibrosis, pulmonary hypertension or cor pulmonale
May exhibit: Acute respiratory distress; e.g., dyspnea, chest pain, and cyanosis (especially in crisis)
Bronchial/bronchovesicular sounds in lung periphery, diminished breath sounds (pulmonary fibrosis)
Crackles, rhonchi, wheezes, diminished breath sounds (HF)
Increased anteroposterior (AP) diameter of the chest (barrel chest)

SAFETY

May report: History of repeated/frequent transfusions
May exhibit: Low-grade fever
Impaired vision (sickle retinopathy), decreased visual acuity (temporary/permanent blindness)
Leg ulcers (common in adult clients, especially found on the internal and external malleoli and the medial aspect of the tibia)
Lymphadenopathy

SEXUALITY

May report: Loss of libido, amenorrhea, priapism, impotence
May exhibit: Delayed sexual maturity
Pale cervix and vaginal walls (anemia)

TEACHING/LEARNING

May report: History of HF (chronic anemic state); pulmonary hypertension or cor pulmonale (multiple pulmonary infections/infarctions); chronic leg ulcers, delayed healing
Discharge plan considerations: May need assistance with shopping, transportation, self-care, homemaker/maintenance tasks

Refer to section at end of plan for postdischarge considerations.

DIAGNOSTIC STUDIES

CBC: Hb (5–10 g/dL) and total RBCs are decreased. Reticulocytes elevated (count may vary from 30% to 50%); leukocytes elevated (especially in vaso-occlusive crisis), with counts over 20,000; platelets increased and a normal-to-elevated MCV.

Stained RBC examination: Demonstrates partially or completely sickled, crescent-shaped cells, anisocytosis, poikilocytosis, polychromasia, target cells, Howell-Jolly bodies, basophilic stippling, occasional nucleated RBCs (normoblasts).

Sickle-turbidity tube test (Sickledex): Routine screening test that determines the presence of hemoglobin S (HbS) but does not differentiate between sickle cell anemia and trait.

Hemoglobin electrophoresis: Identifies any abnormal hemoglobin types and differentiates between sickle cell trait and sickle cell anemia. Results may be inaccurate if client has received a blood transfusion within 3–4 months before testing.

ESR: Elevated.

Erythrocyte fragility: Decreased (osmotic fragility or RBC fragility), RBC survival time decreased (accelerated breakdown).

ABGs: May reflect decreased PO_2 (defects in gas exchange at the alveolar capillary level), acidosis (hypoxemia and acidic states in vaso-occlusive crisis).

Serum bilirubin (total and indirect): Elevated (increased RBC hemolysis).

Acid phosphatase (ACP): Elevated (release of erythrocytic ACP into the serum).

Alkaline phosphatase: Elevated during vaso-occlusive crisis (bone and liver damage).

LDH: Elevated (RBC hemolysis).

Serum potassium and uric acid: Elevated during vaso-occlusive crisis (RBC hemolysis).

Serum iron: May be elevated or normal (increased iron absorption due to excessive RBC destruction).

Total iron-binding capacity (TIBC): Normal or decreased.

Urine/fecal urobilinogen: Increased (more sensitive indicators of RBC destruction than serum levels).

Intravenous pyelogram (IVP): May be done to evaluate kidney damage.

Bone radiographs: May demonstrate skeletal changes; e.g., bone thinning, osteoporosis, osteosclerosis, osteomyelitis, or avascular necrosis.

NURSING PRIORITIES

1. Promote adequate cellular oxygenation/perfusion.
2. Alleviate pain.
3. Prevent complications.
4. Provide information about disease process/prognosis, and treatment needs.

DISCHARGE GOALS

1. Oxygenation/perfusion adequate to meet cellular needs.
2. Pain relieved/controlled.
3. Complications prevented/minimized.
4. Disease process, future expectations, potential complications, and therapeutic regimen understood.
5. Plan in place to meet needs after discharge.

NURSING DIAGNOSIS: impaired Gas Exchange

May be related to

Decreased oxygen-carrying capacity of the blood, reduced RBC life span/premature destruction, abnormal RBC structure, sensitivity to low oxygen tension (strenuous exercise, increase in altitude)

Increased blood viscosity (occlusions created by sickled cells packing together within the capillaries) and pulmonary congestion (impairment of surface phagocytosis)

Predisposition to bacterial pneumonia, pulmonary infarcts

Possibly evidenced by

Dyspnea, use of accessory muscles

Restlessness, confusion

Tachycardia

Cyanosis (hypoxia)

DESIRED OUTCOMES/EVALUATION CRITERIA—CLIENT WILL:

RESPIRATORY STATUS: Gas Exchange (NOC)

Demonstrate improved ventilation/oxygenation as evidenced by respiratory rate within normal limits, absence of cyanosis and use of accessory muscles, clear breath sounds.
Participate in ADLs without weakness and fatigue.
Display improved/normal pulmonary function tests.

ACTIONS/INTERVENTIONS	RATIONALE
Respiratory Monitoring (NIC)	
Independent	
Monitor respiratory rate/depth, use of accessory muscles, areas of cyanosis.	Indicators of adequacy of respiratory function or degree of compromise and therapy needs/effectiveness.
Auscultate breath sounds, noting presence/absence, and adventitious sounds.	Development of atelectasis and stasis of secretions can impair gas exchange.
Monitor vital signs, note changes in cardiac rhythm.	Compensatory changes in vital signs and development of dysrhythmias reflect effects of hypoxia on cardiovascular system.
Investigate reports of chest pain and increasing fatigue. Observe for signs of increased fever, cough, adventitious breath sounds.	Reflective of developing acute chest syndrome (i.e., chest pain, dyspnea, fever, and leukocytosis), which increases the workload of the heart and oxygen demand.
Assess level of consciousness/mentation regularly.	Brain tissue is very sensitive to decreases in oxygen and changes in mentation may be an early indicator of developing hypoxia.
Ventilation Assistance (NIC)	
Assist in turning, coughing, and deep-breathing exercises.	Promotes optimal chest expansion, mobilization of secretions, and aeration of all lung fields; reduces risk of stasis of secretions/pneumonia.
Evaluate activity tolerance; limit activities to those within client tolerance or place client on bedrest. Assist with ADLs and mobility as needed.	Reduction of the metabolic requirements of the body reduces the oxygen requirements/degree of hypoxia.
Encourage client to alternate periods of rest and activity. Schedule rest periods as indicated.	Protects from excessive fatigue, reduces oxygen demands/degree of hypoxia.
Demonstrate and encourage use of relaxation techniques; e.g., guided imagery and visualization.	Relaxation decreases muscle tension and anxiety and hence the metabolic demand for oxygen.
Promote adequate fluid intake; e.g., 2–3 L/day within cardiac tolerance.	Sufficient intake is necessary to provide for mobilization of secretions and to prevent hyperviscosity of blood/capillary occlusion.
Screen health status of visitors/staff.	Protects from potential sources of respiratory infection.
Collaborative	
Administer supplemental humidified oxygen as indicated.	Maximizes oxygen transport to tissues, particularly in presence of pulmonary insults/pneumonia. *Note:* Oxygen should be given only in the presence of confirmed hypoxemia because oxygen can suppress erythropoietin levels, further reducing the production of RBCs.
Monitor laboratory studies; e.g., CBC, cultures, ABGs/pulse oximetry, chest x-ray, pulmonary function tests.	Client is particularly prone to pneumonia, which is potentially fatal because of its hypoxemic effect of increasing sickling.
Perform/assist with chest physiotherapy, intermittent positive-pressure breathing (IPPB), and incentive spirometer.	Mobilizes secretions and increases aeration of lung fields.

ACTIONS/INTERVENTIONS	RATIONALE
Administer packed RBCs (PRCs) or exchange transfusions as indicated.	Increases number of oxygen-carrying cells, dilutes the percentage of HbS to prevent sickling, improves circulation, and removes/decreases number of sickled cells. PRCs are used because they are less likely to create circulatory overload. *Note:* Partial transfusions are sometimes used prophylactically in high-risk situations; e.g., chronic, severe leg ulcers, preparation for general anesthesia, third trimester of pregnancy.
Administer medications as indicated:	
Antipyretics; e.g., acetaminophen (Tylenol);	Maintains normothermia to reduce metabolic oxygen demands without affecting serum pH, which may occur with aspirin.
Antibiotics.	A broad-spectrum antibiotic is started immediately pending culture results of suspected infections then may be changed when the specific pathogen is identified.

NURSING DIAGNOSIS: acute/chronic Pain

May be related to

Intravascular sickling with localized stasis, occlusion, and infarction/necrosis
Activation of pain fibers due to deprivation of oxygen and nutrients, accumulation of noxious metabolites

Possibly evidenced by

Localized, migratory, or more generalized pain, described as throbbing, gnawing, or severe and incapacitating; affecting peripheral extremities, bones, joints, back, abdomen, or head (headaches recurrent/transient)
Decreased ROM, guarding of the affected areas
Facial grimacing, narrowed/self-focus

DESIRED OUTCOMES/EVALUATION CRITERIA—CLIENT WILL:

Pain Level (NOC)

Verbalize relief/control of pain.
Demonstrate relaxed body posture, freedom of movement, ability to sleep/rest appropriately.

ACTIONS/INTERVENTIONS	RATIONALE
Pain Management (NIC)	
Independent	
Assess reports of pain, including location, duration, and intensity (scale of 0–10). Have client help differentiate current pain from typical/usual pain problems.	Vaso-occlusive pain crises are the most common manifestation of sickle cell disease, where sickling potentiates cellular hypoxia, resulting in severe pain. Typically, pain occurs deep in the bones and muscles of back, ribs, and limbs and lasts 5–7 days. However, client may also have acute pain from another cause (e.g., ulcers, appendicitis), chronic pain from sickle cell damage (e.g., usually bone pain that is present daily), chronic pain from other causes (e.g., old injuries, arthritis), and/or chronic nerve pain caused by damage from sickle cell blockage or other conditions, like diabetes.

ACTIONS/INTERVENTIONS	RATIONALE
Observe nonverbal pain cues; e.g., gait disturbances, body positioning, reluctance to move, facial expressions, and physiologic manifestations of acute pain (e.g., elevated BP, tachycardia, increased respiratory rate). Explore discrepancies between verbal and nonverbal cues.	Pain is unique to each client; therefore, one may encounter varying descriptions because of individualized perceptions. Nonverbal cues may aid in evaluation of pain and effectiveness of therapy.
Discuss with the client/SO what pain relief measures were effective in the past.	Involves client/SO in care and allows for identification of remedies that have already been found to relieve pain. Helpful in establishing individualized treatment needs.
Explore alternative pain relief measures; e.g., relaxation techniques, biofeedback, yoga, meditation, progressive relaxation techniques, distraction (e.g., visual, auditory, tactile, kinesthetic, guided imagery, and breathing techniques).	Cognitive-behavioral interventions may reduce reliance on pharmacologic therapy and enhance client's sense of control.
Provide support for and carefully position affected extremities.	Reduces edema, discomfort, and risk of injury, especially if osteomyelitis is present.
Apply local massage gently to affected areas.	Helps reduce muscle tension.
Encourage ROM exercises.	Prevents joint stiffness and possible contracture formation.
Plan activities during peak analgesic effect.	Maximizes movement of joints, enhancing mobility.
Maintain adequate fluid intake.	Dehydration increases sickling/vaso-occlusion and corresponding pain.

Collaborative

Apply warm, moist compresses to affected joints or other painful areas. Avoid use of ice or cold compresses.	Warmth causes vasodilation and increases circulation to hypoxic areas. Cold causes vasoconstriction and compounds the crisis.
Administer medications as indicated: narcotics; e.g., continuous infusion or around-the-clock morphine (Astramorph, Duramorph), hydromorphone (Dilaudid), nalbuphine (Nubain); long-acting opiate combinations; e.g., morphine (MS Contin), oxycodone (Oxycontin); non-narcotic analgesics; e.g., acetaminophen (Tylenol); oral opiate combination analgesics; e.g., acetaminophen with codeine (Tylenol #3), hydrocodone (Vicodin). Antiseizure medications, e.g. gabapentin (Neurontin).	Various types of analgesics are needed to manage different types of pain. Narcotics are the mainstay of pain control during crisis, and are usually administered via patient-controlled analgesia (PCA). Acetaminophen (Tylenol) can be used for control of headache, pain, and fever. Aspirin should be avoided because it alters blood pH and can make cells sickle more easily. *Note*: Meperidine (Demerol) should not be used because its metabolite, normeperidine, can cause CNS excitation; e.g., anxiety, tremors, seizures.
Consult with/refer to physical therapy.	Determine/provide appropriate therapies (e.g., massage, heat therapies, transcutaneous electrical nerve stimulation [TENS]).
Administer/monitor RBC transfusion.	Although transfusion does not halt the pain in an acute crisis, frequency of painful crises may be reduced by regular partial exchange transfusions to maintain population of normal RBCs.

NURSING DIAGNOSIS: ineffective Tissue Perfusion, (specify)

May be related to

Vaso-occlusive nature of sickling, inflammatory response
Arteriovenous (AV) shunts in both pulmonary and peripheral circulation
Myocardial damage from small infarcts, iron deposits, and fibrosis

Possibly evidenced by

Changes in vital signs, diminished peripheral pulses/capillary refill, general pallor
Decreased mentation, restlessness
Angina, palpitations

Tingling in extremities, intermittent claudication, bone pain
Transient visual disturbances
Ulcerations of lower extremities, delayed healing

DESIRED OUTCOMES/EVALUATION CRITERIA—CLIENT WILL:

Circulation Status (NOC)

Demonstrate improved tissue perfusion as evidenced by stabilized vital signs, strong/palpable peripheral pulses, adequate urine output, absence of pain; usual mentation; normal capillary refill; skin warm/dry; nailbeds and lips of natural pale, pink color; absence of paresthesias.

ACTIONS/INTERVENTIONS	RATIONALE
CIRCULATORY CARE: Arterial [or] Venous Insufficiency (NIC)	
Independent	
Monitor vital signs carefully. Assess pulses for rate, rhythm, and volume. Note hypotension; rapid, weak, thready pulse; and increased/shallow respirations.	Sludging and sickling in peripheral vessels may lead to complete or partial obliteration of a vessel with diminished perfusion to surrounding tissues. Sudden massive splenic sequestration of cells can lead to shock.
Assess skin for coolness, pallor, cyanosis, diaphoresis, delayed capillary refill.	Changes reflect diminished circulation/hypoxia potentiating capillary occlusion. (Refer to ND: impaired Gas Exchange.)
Note changes in level of consciousness; reports of headaches, dizziness; development of sensory/motor deficits (e.g., hemiparesis or paralysis); seizure activity.	Changes may reflect diminished perfusion to the central nervous system (CNS) due to ischemia or infarction. Stagnant cells must be mobilized immediately to reduce further ischemia/infarction.
Maintain adequate fluid intake. (Refer to ND: risk for deficient Fluid Volume, following.) Monitor urine output.	Dehydration not only causes hypovolemia but increases sickling and occlusion of capillaries. Decreased renal perfusion/failure may occur because of vascular occlusion.
Assess lower extremities for skin texture, edema, ulcerations (especially of internal and external malleoli).	Reduced peripheral circulation often leads to dermal changes and delayed healing.
Investigate reports of change in character of pain, or development of bone pain, angina, tingling of extremities, eye pain/vision disturbances.	Changes may reflect increased sickling of cells/diminished circulation with further involvement of organs; e.g., myocardial infarction (MI) or pulmonary infarction, occlusion of vasculature of the eye.
Maintain environmental temperature and body warmth without overheating. Avoid hypothermia.	Prevents vasoconstriction, aids in maintaining circulation and perfusion. Excessive body heat may cause diaphoresis, adding to insensible fluid losses and risk of dehydration. Hypothermia may exacerbate cardiovascular compromise with severe anemia.
Evaluate for developing edema (including genitals in men).	Vaso-occlusion/circulatory stasis may lead to edema of extremities (and priapism in men), potentiating risk of tissue ischemia/necrosis.
Collaborative	
Monitor laboratory studies, e.g.:	
ABGs, CBC, LDH, AST/ALT, CPK, BUN;	Decreased tissue perfusion may lead to gradual infarction of organ tissues, such as the brain, liver, spleen, kidney, skeletal muscle, and so forth, with consequent release of intracellular enzymes.

ACTIONS/INTERVENTIONS	RATIONALE
Serum electrolytes. Provide replacements as indicated.	Electrolyte losses (especially sodium) are increased during crisis because of fever, diarrhea, vomiting, diaphoresis.
Administer hypo-osmolar solutions (e.g., 0.45 normal saline) via an infusion pump.	Hydration lowers the HbS concentration within the RBCs, which decreases the sickling tendency and also reduces blood viscosity, which helps to maintain perfusion. Infusion pump may prevent circulatory overload. *Note:* Lactated Ringer's solution or D_5W may cause RBC hemolysis and potentiate thrombus formation.
Administer hydroxyurea (Droxia), or experimental antisickling agents (e.g., sodium cyanate) carefully. Observe for possible lethal side effects;	Hydroxyurea, a cytotoxic agent, dramatically decreases the number of sickle cell episodes by as much as 50% and reduces the severity of complications such as fever and severe chest pain by increasing the level of fetal hemoglobin (hemoglobin F). Levels greater than 20% may prolong life. Antisickling agents (currently under investigational use) are aimed at prolonging erythrocyte survival and preventing sickling by affecting cell membrane changes. *Note:* Use of anticoagulants, plasma expanders, nitrates, vasodilators, and alkylating agents has proved essentially unsuccessful in the management of the vaso-occlusive crisis.
Deferoxamine (Desferal), vitamin C.	Chelation therapy may be indicated to correct iron overload (serum ferritin levels of 1500–2000 mEq/L) associated with intermittent transfusions. Vitamin C may enhance excretion especially in clients who are vitamin deficient. *Note*: Phlebotomy and exchange transfusions may be used in conjunction with chelation therapy.
Assist with/prepare for surgical diathermy or photocoagulation.	Direct coagulation of bleeding sites in the eye (resulting from vascular stasis/edema) may prevent progression of proliferative changes if initiated early.
Assist with/prepare for needle aspiration of blood from corpora cavernosa;	Sickling within the penis can cause sustained erection (priapism) and edema. Removal of sludged sickled cells can improve circulation, decreasing psychological trauma and risk of necrosis/infection.
Surgical intervention.	Direct incision and ligation of the dorsal arteries of the penis and saphenocavernous shunting may be necessary in severe cases of priapism to prevent tissue necrosis.

NURSING DIAGNOSIS: risk for deficient Fluid Volume

Risk factors may include

Increased fluid needs; e.g., hypermetabolic state/fever, inflammatory processes
Renal parenchymal damage/infarctions limiting the kidney's ability to concentrate urine (hyposthenuria)

Possibly evidenced by

[Not applicable; presence of signs and symptoms establishes an *actual* diagnosis.]

DESIRED OUTCOMES/EVALUATION CRITERIA—CLIENT WILL:

Hydration (NOC)

Maintain adequate fluid balance as evidenced by individually appropriate urine output with a near-normal specific gravity, stable vital signs, moist mucous membranes, good skin turgor, and prompt capillary refill.

ACTIONS/INTERVENTIONS	RATIONALE
Fluid Monitoring (NIC)	
Independent	
Maintain accurate I&O. Weigh daily.	Client may reduce fluid intake during periods of crisis because of malaise, anorexia, and so on. Dehydration from vomiting, diarrhea, fever may reduce urine output and precipitate a vaso-occlusive crisis.
Note urine characteristics and specific gravity.	Kidney can lose its ability to concentrate urine, resulting in excessive losses of dilute urine and fixation of the specific gravity.
Monitor vital signs, comparing with client's usual/previous readings. Take BP in lying, sitting, and standing positions if possible.	Reduction of circulating blood volume can occur from increased fluid loss, resulting in hypotension and tachycardia.
Observe for fever, changes in level of consciousness, poor skin turgor, dryness of skin and mucous membranes, pain.	Symptoms reflective of dehydration/hemoconcentration with consequent vaso-occlusive state.
Monitor vital signs closely during blood transfusions and note presence of dyspnea, crackles, rhonchi, wheezes, JVD, diminished breath sounds, cough, frothy sputum, and cyanosis.	Client's heart may already be weakened and prone to failure because of chronic demands placed on it by the anemic state. Heart may be unable to tolerate the added fluid volume from transfusions or rapid IV fluid administered to treat crisis/shock.
Collaborative	
Administer IV fluids as indicated.	Replaces losses/deficits; may reverse renal concentration of RBCs/presence of failure. Fluids must be given immediately (especially in CNS involvement) to decrease hemoconcentration and prevent further infarction.
Monitor laboratory studies; e.g., Hb/Hct;	Elevations may indicate hemoconcentration. Post-transfusion hemoglobin level of 8–9 g/dL is generally recommended to avoid the risk of hyperviscosity that may occur several days after transfusion when RBCs sequestered in the spleen may return to the circulation and increase the hemoglobin levels.
Serum and urine electrolytes.	Kidneys' loss of ability to concentrate urine may result in serum depletions of Na^+, K^-, and Cl^-, necessitating replacement.

NURSING DIAGNOSIS: impaired physical Mobility

May be related to

Multiple/recurrent bone infarctions or infections (weight-bearing bones)
Pain/discomfort: kyphosis of upper back/lordosis of lower back, possible joint effusions
Osteoporosis with fragmentation/collapse of femoral head or vertebra (compression deformities)
Bacterial infections (osteomyelitis)

Possibly evidenced by

Reports of pain
Limited joint ROM, reluctance to move, inability to walk/perform ADLs, guarding of joints, gait disturbances
Generalized weakness, therapeutic restrictions (e.g., bed rest)

DESIRED OUTCOMES/EVALUATION CRITERIA—CLIENT WILL:

Mobility (NOC)

Maintain/increase strength and function of affected body parts.
Participate in activities with absence of or improvement in gait disturbances, increased joint ROM, and absence of inflammatory signs.

Refer to CP: Extended Care, ND: impaired physical Mobility for appropriate actions/interventions.

NURSING DIAGNOSIS: risk for impaired Skin integrity

Risk factors may include

Impaired circulation (venous stasis and vaso-occlusion); altered sensation
Decreased mobility/bedrest

Possibly evidenced by

[Not applicable; presence of signs and symptoms establishes an *actual* diagnosis.]

DESIRED OUTCOMES/EVALUATION CRITERIA—CLIENT WILL:

TISSUE INTEGRITY: Skin and Mucous Membranes (NOC)

Prevent dermal ischemic injury.
Display improvement in wound/lesion healing if present.

Risk Control (NOC)

Participate in behaviors to reduce risk factors/skin breakdown.

ACTIONS/INTERVENTIONS	RATIONALE
Skin Surveillance (NIC)	
Independent	
Reposition frequently, even when sitting in chair.	Prevents prolonged tissue pressure where circulation is already compromised, reducing risk of tissue trauma/ischemia.
Inspect skin/pressure points regularly for redness, provide gentle massage.	Poor circulation may predispose to rapid skin breakdown.
Protect bony prominences with sheepskin, heel/elbow protectors, pillows, as indicated.	Decreases pressure on tissues, preventing skin breakdown.
Keep skin surfaces dry and clean and linens dry/wrinkle free.	Moist, contaminated areas provide excellent media for growth of pathogenic organisms.
Monitor ischemic areas, leg bruises, cuts, bumps closely for ulcer formation.	Potential entry sites for pathogenic organisms. In presence of altered immune system, this increases risk of infection/delayed healing.
Elevate lower extremities when sitting.	Enhances venous return, reducing venous stasis/edema formation.

ACTIONS/INTERVENTIONS	RATIONALE
Collaborative	
Provide egg-crate, alternating air pressure, or water mattress.	Reduces tissue pressure and aids in maximizing cellular perfusion to prevent dermal injury.
Cleanse/debride open wounds/ulcers with wet-to-dry/moist occlusive dressings, Unna's boot (zinc oxide–impregnated bandage) as indicated. Monitor distribution, size, depth, character, and drainage.	Improvement or delayed healing reflects status of tissue perfusion and effectiveness of interventions. *Note:* These clients are at increased risk of serious complications because of lowered resistance to infection and decreased nutrients for healing.
Prepare for/assist with hyperbaric oxygenation to ulcer sites.	Maximizes oxygen delivery to tissues, enhancing healing.

NURSING DIAGNOSIS: risk for Infection

Risk factors may include

Chronic disease process, tissue destruction; e.g., infarction, fibrosis, loss of spleen (autosplenectomy)
Inadequate primary defenses (broken skin, stasis of body fluids, decreased ciliary action)

Possibly evidenced by

[Not applicable; presence of signs and symptoms establishes an *actual* diagnosis]

DESIRED OUTCOMES/EVALUATION CRITERIA—CLIENT WILL:

KNOWLEDGE: Infection Control (NOC)

Verbalize understanding of individual causative/risk factors.
Identify interventions to prevent/reduce risk of infection.

Refer to CPs: Pneumonia, Sepsis/Septicemia, Fractures, ND: risk for Infection.

NURSING DIAGNOSIS: deficient Knowledge [Learning Need] regarding condition, prognosis, treatment, self-care, and discharge needs

May be related to

Lack of exposure/recall
Information misinterpretation
Unfamiliarity with resources

Possibly evidenced by

Questions, request for information, statement of misconceptions
Inaccurate follow-through of instructions; development of preventable complications
Verbal/nonverbal cues of anxiety

DESIRED OUTCOMES/EVALUATION CRITERIA—CLIENT WILL:

KNOWLEDGE: Disease Process (NOC)

Verbalize understanding of disease process, including symptoms of crisis, potential complications.

KNOWLEDGE: Treatment Regimen (NOC)

Verbalize understanding of therapeutic needs.
Initiate necessary behaviors/lifestyle changes to prevent complications.
Participate in continued medical follow-up, genetic counseling/family planning services.

ACTIONS/INTERVENTIONS	RATIONALE
TEACHING: Disease Process (NIC)	
Independent	
Review disease process and treatment needs.	Provides knowledge base from which client can make informed choices. *Note:* The median age at death for women is 48 years, and 42 years for men, with death often being due to organ failure. However, significant number of individuals are living much longer.
Review precipitating factors, e.g.:	
Cold environmental temperatures, failure to dress warmly when engaging in winter activities; wearing tight, restrictive clothing; stressful situations;	Causes peripheral vasoconstriction, which may result in sludging of the circulation, increased sickling, and may precipitate a vaso-occlusive crisis.
Strenuous physical activity/contact-type sports, and extremely warm temperatures;	Increases metabolic demand for oxygen and increases insensible fluid losses (evaporation and perspiration) leading to dehydration, which may increase blood viscosity and tendency to sickle.
Travel to places more than 7000 ft above sea level or flying in unpressurized aircraft.	Decreased oxygen tension present at higher altitudes causes hypoxia and potentiates sickling of cells.
Encourage consumption of at least 3–4 L of fluid daily, during a steady state, increasing to 6–8 L during a painful crisis or while engaging in activities that might precipitate dehydration.	Prevents dehydration and consequent hyperviscosity that can potentiate sickling/crisis.
Discuss use of antimetabolites: hydroxyurea (Hydrea).	May reduce frequency of pain episodes in adults.
Encourage ROM exercise and regular physical activity with a balance between rest and activity.	Prevents bone demineralization and may reduce risk of fractures. Aids in maintaining level of resistance and decreases oxygen needs.
Review client's current diet, reinforcing the importance of diet including liver, green leafy vegetables, citrus fruits, and wheat germ. Provide necessary instruction regarding supplementary vitamins such as folic acid.	Sound nutrition is essential because of increased demands placed on bone marrow (e.g., folate and vitamin B_{12} are used in greater quantities than usual). Folic acid supplements are frequently ordered to prevent aplastic crisis.
Discourage smoking and alcohol consumption; identify appropriate community support groups.	Nicotine induces peripheral vasoconstriction and decreases oxygen tension, which may contribute to cellular hypoxia and sickling. Alcohol increases the possibility of dehydration (precipitating sickling). Maintaining these changes in behavior/lifestyle may require prolonged support.
Discuss principles of skin/extremity care and protection from injury. Encourage prompt treatment of cuts, insect bites, sores/lesions.	Because of impaired tissue perfusion, especially in the periphery, distal extremities are especially susceptible to altered skin integrity/infection.
Include instructions on care of leg ulcers that might develop.	Fosters independence and maintenance of self-care at home.
Instruct client to avoid persons with infections such as upper respiratory infections (URIs).	Altered immune response places client at risk for infections, especially bacterial pneumonia.
Recommend client avoid cold remedies and decongestants containing ephedrine and large amounts of caffeine. Stress the importance of reading labels on over-the counter (OTC) drugs and consulting healthcare provider before consuming any drugs/herbal supplements.	Those remedies containing vasoconstrictors may decrease peripheral tissue perfusion and cause sludging of sickled cells.

ACTIONS/INTERVENTIONS	RATIONALE
Discuss conditions for which medical attention should be sought, e.g.:	
Urine that appears blood tinged or smoky;	Symptoms suggestive of sickling in the renal medulla.
Indigestion, persistent vomiting, diarrhea, high fever, excessive thirst;	Dehydration may trigger a vaso-occlusive crisis.
Severe joint or bone pain;	May signify a vaso-occlusive crisis due to sickling in the bones or spleen (ischemia or infarction) or onset of osteomyelitis.
Severe chest pain, with or without cough;	May reflect acute chest syndrome, with pulmonary infiltrates/pneumonia.
Abdominal pain; gastric distress following meals;	Cholelithiasis, primarily with bilirubin stones, is present in more than 50% of adults.
Priaprism episode persisting over 3–4 hours with no resolution;	Suggestive of sickling in the penis.
Persistent fever (greater than 100°F/38°C), increasing fatigue/pallor, dizziness, drowsiness, nonhealing leg ulcers;	Suggestive of infections that may precipitate a vaso-occlusive crisis if dehydration develops. *Note:* Severe infections are the most frequent cause of aplastic crisis.
Any neurologic symptom or sign.	Stroke can occur due to cerebral infarction, although it is more common in children than adults. Without long-term transfusion therapy, approximately one third of clients will experience recurrent strokes.
Review/strengthen coping abilities; e.g., deal appropriately with anxiety, get adequate information, use relaxation techniques.	Promotes client's sense of control, may avert a crisis.
Recommend wearing a medical alert bracelet or carrying a wallet card.	May prevent inappropriate treatment in emergency situation.
Discuss genetic implications of the condition. Encourage SO/family members to seek testing to determine presence of HbS.	Screening may identify other family members with sickle cell trait. Hereditary nature of the disease with the possibility of transmitting the mutation may have a bearing on the reproductive decisions.
Explore concerns regarding childbearing/family planning and refer to community resources and obstetrician knowledgeable about sickle cell disease, as indicated.	Provides opportunity to correct misconceptions/present information necessary to make informed decisions. Pregnancy can precipitate a vaso-occlusive crisis because the placenta's tortuous blood supply and low oxygen tension potentiate sickling, which in turn can lead to fetal hypoxia.
Encourage client to have routine follow-ups, e.g.:	
Periodic laboratory studies; e.g., CBC;	Monitors changes in blood components; identifies need for changes in treatment regimen. When using hydroxyurea, frequent monitoring of CBC is required because of narrow margin between efficacy (acceptable degree of bone marrow suppression) and toxicity (neutropenia, anemia, thrombocytopenia).
Biannual dental examination;	Sound oral hygiene limits opportunity for bacterial invasion/sepsis.
Annual ophthalmologic examination.	Detects development of sickle retinopathy with either proliferative or nonproliferative ocular changes predisposing to retinal hemorrhages/detachments, increased intraocular pressure.
Determine need for vocational/career guidance.	Sedentary career may be necessary because of the decreased oxygen-carrying capacity and diminished exercise tolerance.
Encourage participation in community support groups available to sickle cell clients/SO, such as the Sickle Cell Disease Association of America, March of Dimes, public health/visiting nurse.	Helpful in adjustment to long-term situation; reduces feelings of isolation and enhances problem-solving through sharing of common experiences. *Note:* Failure to resolve concerns/deal with situation may require more intensive therapy/psychological support.

POTENTIAL CONSIDERATIONS following acute hospitalization (dependent on client's age, physical condition/presence of complications, personal resources, and life responsibilities)

acute/chronic Pain—intravascular sickling with localized stasis, occlusion, and infarction/necrosis; activation of pain fibers due to deprivation of oxygen and nutrients, accumulation of noxious metabolites.

risk for deficient Fluid Volume—increased fluid needs; e.g., hypermetabolic state/fever, inflammatory processes; renal parenchymal damage/infarctions limiting the kidneys' ability to concentrate urine (hyposthenuria).

risk for Infection—chronic disease process, tissue destruction; e.g., infarction, fibrosis, loss of spleen (autosplenectomy); inadequate primary defenses (broken skin, stasis of body fluids, decreased ciliary action).

LEUKEMIAS

The term *leukemia* describes a malignant disorder of the blood and lymph-forming tissues of the body. The blood's cellular components originate primarily in the marrow of bones such as the sternum, iliac crest, and cranium. All blood cells begin as immature cells (blasts or stem cells) that differentiate and mature into RBCs, platelets, and various types of WBCs. In leukemia, many immature or ineffective WBCs crowd out the developing normal cells. As the normal cells are replaced by leukemic cells, anemia, neutropenia, and thrombocytopenia occur.

Leukemia is *acute* when WBCs proliferate so rapidly that they lose the ability to regulate cell division and do not differentiate into mature cells. In the *chronic* forms of leukemia, the disease develops gradually. The type of leukemia is based on the predominant cell line that is affected. In adults, the most common of the acute leukemias is *acute myelocytic leukemia*, which affects any type of WBC other than lymphocytes. The most common of the chronic leukemias is *chronic lymphocytic leukemia*, which is characterized by an abnormal increase in lymphocytes.

Current treatments include chemotherapy, biologic therapy (e.g., monoclonal antibodies or interferon), radiation therapy, or transplantation (bone marrow transplant, peripheral stem cell transplant, or umbilical cord blood transplant).

CARE SETTING

Acute inpatient care on medical or oncology unit for initial evaluation and treatment typically 4–6 weeks, and then at the community level.

RELATED CONCERNS

Cancer, page 857
Psychosocial aspects of care, page 770
Transplantation considerations (postoperative and lifelong), page 761

Client Assessment Database

Data depend on degree/duration of the disease and other organ involvement.

ACTIVITY/REST

May report: Fatigue, malaise, weakness, inability to engage in usual activities, flu-like symptoms
May exhibit: Muscle wasting, anemia
Increased need for sleep, somnolence

CIRCULATION

May report: Palpitations
May exhibit: Tachycardia, heart murmurs
Pallor of skin, mucous membranes
Cranial nerve deficits and/or signs of cerebral hemorrhage

EGO INTEGRITY

May report: Feelings of helplessness/hopelessness
May exhibit: Depression, withdrawal, anxiety, fear, anger, irritability
Mood changes, confusion

ELIMINATION

May report: Diarrhea, perianal tenderness, pain
Bright red blood on tissue paper, tarry stools
Blood in urine, decreased urine output
May exhibit: Perianal abscess; hematuria

FOOD/FLUID

May report: Loss of appetite, anorexia, vomiting
Change in taste/taste distortions
Weight loss
Pharyngitis, dysphagia

May exhibit: Abdominal distention, decreased bowel sounds
Splenomegaly, hepatomegaly, jaundice
Stomatitis, oral ulcerations
Gum hypertrophy (gum infiltration may be indicative of acute monocytic leukemia)

NEUROSENSORY

May report: Lack of coordination/decreased coordination
Mood changes, confusion, disorientation, lack of concentration
Dizziness; numbness, tingling, paresthesias

May exhibit: Muscle irritability, seizure activity, uncoordinated movements

PAIN/DISCOMFORT

May report: Abdominal pain, headaches, bone/joint pain, sternal tenderness, muscle cramping

May exhibit: Guarding/distraction behaviors, restlessness; self-focus

RESPIRATION

May report: Shortness of breath with minimal exertion

May exhibit: Dyspnea, tachypnea
Cough
Crackles, rhonchi
Decreased breath sounds

SAFETY

May report: History of recent/recurrent infections, falls
Visual disturbances/impairment
Nosebleeds or other hemorrhages, spontaneous uncontrollable bleeding with minimal trauma

May exhibit: Fever, infections
Bruises, purpura, retinal hemorrhages, gum bleeding, or epistaxis
Enlarged lymph nodes, spleen, or liver (due to tissue invasion)
Papilledema and exophthalmos
Leukemic infiltrates in the dermis

SEXUALITY

May report: Changes in libido
Changes in menstrual flow, menorrhagia
Impotence

TEACHING/LEARNING

May report: History of exposure to chemicals; e.g., benzene (commercially used toxic liquid that is also present in lead-free gasoline), excessive levels of ionizing radiation, previous treatment with chemotherapy, especially alkalizing agents
Chromosomal disorder; e.g., Down syndrome or Fanconi's aplastic anemia
Exposure to virus; e.g., human T-cell leukemia/lymphoma virus-I (HTLV-I)

Discharge plan considerations: May need assistance with therapy and treatment needs/supplies, shopping, food preparation, self-care activities, homemaker/maintenance tasks, transportation

Refer to section at end of plan for postdischarge considerations.

DIAGNOSTIC STUDIES

CBC: Usually indicates a normocytic, normochromic anemia.

Hemoglobin: May be less than 10 g/100 mL.

Reticulocytes: Count is usually low. "Teardrop" and nucleated red blood cells may be seen.

Platelet count: May vary from normal to very low (less than 50,000/mm).

WBC: May be more than 50,000/cm with increased immature WBCs ("shift to left"). Leukemic blast cells may be present.
Prothrombin time (PT)/activated partial thromboplastin time (aPTT): May be prolonged. (Disseminated intravascular coagulation [DIC] may occur with acute myelogenous leukemia, but it is especially common in acute promyelocytic leukemia.)
LDH: May be elevated.
Serum/urine uric acid: May be elevated.
Bence Jones protein (urine): May be increased.
Bone marrow biopsy: Abnormal WBCs usually make up 50% or more of the WBCs in the bone marrow. Often 60%–90% of the cells are blast cells, with erythroid precursors, mature cells, and megakaryocytes reduced.
Chest radiograph and lymph node biopsies: May indicate degree of involvement.
Lumbar puncture: May find leukemic cells in cerebrospinal fluid (CSF).
Cytogenetics: Examination of chromosome abnormalities from samples of peripheral blood, bone marrow, or lymph nodes that may indicate prognostic features.

NURSING PRIORITIES

1. Prevent infection during acute phases of disease/treatment.
2. Maintain circulating blood volume.
3. Alleviate pain.
4. Promote optimal physical functioning.
5. Provide psychologic support.
6. Provide information about disease process/prognosis and treatment needs.

DISCHARGE GOALS

1. Complications prevented/minimized.
2. Pain relieved/controlled.
3. ADLs met by self or with assistance.
4. Dealing with disease realistically.
5. Disease process/prognosis and therapeutic regimen understood.
6. Plan in place to meet needs after discharge.

Refer to CP: Cancer, for further discussion/expansion of interventions related to cancer care and for client teaching.

NURSING DIAGNOSIS: risk for Infection

Risk factors may include

Inadequate secondary defenses: alterations in mature WBCs (low granulocyte and abnormal lymphocyte count), increased number of immature lymphocytes; immunosuppression, bone marrow suppression (effects of therapy/transplant)
Inadequate primary defenses (stasis of body fluids, traumatized tissue)
Invasive procedures
Malnutrition; chronic disease

Possibly evidenced by

[Not applicable; presence of signs and symptoms establishes an *actual* diagnosis.]

DESIRED OUTCOMES/EVALUATION CRITERIA—CLIENT WILL:

KNOWLEDGE: Infection Control (NOC)

Identify actions to prevent/reduce risk of infection.
Demonstrate techniques, lifestyle changes to promote safe environment, achieve timely healing.

ACTIONS/INTERVENTIONS	RATIONALE
Infection Protection (NIC)	
Independent	
Place in private room. Screen/limit visitors as indicated. Prohibit use of live plants/cut flowers. Restrict fresh fruits and vegetables or make sure they are washed or peeled.	Protect client from potential sources of pathogens/infection. *Note:* Profound bone marrow suppression, neutropenia, and chemotherapy place client at great risk for infection.
Require good hand-washing protocol for all personnel and visitors.	Prevents cross-contamination/reduces risk of infection.
Monitor temperature. Note correlation between temperature elevations and chemotherapy treatments. Observe for fever associated with tachycardia, hypotension, subtle mental changes.	Although fever may accompany some forms of chemotherapy, progressive hyperthermia occurs in some types of infections, and fever (unrelated to drugs or blood products) occurs in most leukemia clients. *Note:* Septicemia may occur without fever.
Prevent chilling. Force fluids, administer tepid sponge bath.	Helps reduce fever, which contributes to fluid imbalance, discomfort, and CNS complications.
Encourage frequent turning and deep breathing.	Prevents stasis of respiratory secretions, reducing risk of atelectasis/pneumonia.
Auscultate breath sounds, noting crackles, rhonchi; inspect secretions for changes in characteristics; e.g., increased sputum production or change in sputum color. Observe urine for signs of infection; e.g., cloudy, foul-smelling, or presence of urgency or burning with voids.	Early intervention is essential to prevent sepsis/septicemia in immunosuppressed person.
Handle client gently. Keep linens dry/wrinkle free.	Prevents sheet burn/skin excoriation.
Inspect skin for tender, erythematous areas; open wounds. Cleanse skin with antibacterial solutions.	May indicate local infection. *Note:* Open wounds may not produce pus because of insufficient number of granulocytes.
Inspect oral mucous membranes. Provide good oral hygiene. Use a soft toothbrush, sponge, or swabs for frequent mouth care.	The oral cavity is an excellent medium for growth of organisms and is susceptible to ulceration and bleeding.
Promote good perianal hygiene. Examine perianal area at least daily during acute illness. Provide sitz baths, using Betadine or Hibiclens if indicated. Avoid rectal temperatures, use of suppositories.	Promotes cleanliness, reducing risk of perianal abscess; enhances circulation and healing. *Note:* Perianal abscess can contribute to septicemia and death in immunosupressed clients.
Coordinate procedures and tests to allow for uninterrupted rest periods.	Conserves energy for healing, cellular regeneration.
Encourage increased intake of foods high in protein and fluids with adequate fiber.	Promotes healing and prevents dehydration. *Note:* Constipation potentiates retention of toxins and risk of rectal irritation/tissue injury.
Avoid/limit invasive procedures (e.g., venipuncture and injections) as possible.	Break in skin could provide an entry for pathogenic/potentially lethal organisms. Use of central venous lines (e.g., tunneled catheter or implanted port) can effectively reduce need for frequent invasive procedures and risk of infection. *Note:* Myelosuppression may be cumulative in nature, especially when multiple drug therapy (including steroids) is prescribed.
Collaborative	
Monitor laboratory studies, e.g.:	
CBC, noting whether WBC count falls or sudden changes occur in neutrophils;	Decreased numbers of normal/mature WBCs can result from the disease process or chemotherapy, compromising the immune response and increasing risk of infection.
Gram's stain cultures/sensitivity.	Verifies presence of infections; identifies specific organisms and appropriate therapy.
Review serial chest x-rays.	Indicator of development/resolution of respiratory complications.

ACTIONS/INTERVENTIONS	RATIONALE
Prepare for/assist with leukemia-specific treatments such as chemotherapy, radiation, and/or bone marrow transplant.	Leukemia is usually treated with a combination of these agents, each requiring specific safety precautions for client and care providers.
Administer medications as indicated, e.g.: antibiotics;	May be given prophylactically or to treat specific infection.
Colony-stimulating factors (CSFs): e.g., sargramostim (Leukine), filgrastim (Neupogen), pegfilgrastim (Neulasta).	Restores WBCs destroyed by chemotherapy and reduces risk of severe infection and death in certain types of leukemia.
Avoid use of aspirin-containing antipyretics.	Aspirin can cause gastric bleeding and further decrease platelet count.
Provide nutritious diet, high in protein and calories, avoiding raw fruits, vegetables, or uncooked meats.	Proper nutrition enhances immune system. Minimizes potential sources of bacterial contamination.

NURSING DIAGNOSIS: risk for deficient Fluid Volume

Risk factors may include

Excessive losses; e.g., vomiting, hemorrhage, diarrhea
Decreased fluid intake; e.g., nausea, anorexia
Increased fluid need; e.g., hypermetabolic state, fever, predisposition for kidney stone formation/tumor lysis syndrome

Possibly evidenced by

[Not applicable; presence of signs and symptoms establishes an *actual* diagnosis.]

DESIRED OUTCOMES/EVALUATION CRITERIA—CLIENT WILL:

Hydration (NOC)

Demonstrate adequate fluid volume, as evidenced by stable vital signs; palpable pulses; urine output, specific gravity, and pH within normal limits.

Risk Control (NOC)

Identify individual risk factors and appropriate interventions.
Initiate behaviors/lifestyle changes to prevent development of dehydration.

ACTIONS/INTERVENTIONS	RATIONALE
Fluid Management (NIC)	
Independent	
Monitor I&O. Calculate insensible losses and fluid balance. Note decreased urine output in presence of adequate intake. Measure urine specific gravity and pH.	Tumor lysis syndrome occurs when destroyed cancer cells release toxic levels of potassium, phosphorus, and uric acid. Elevated phosphorus and uric acid levels can cause crystal formation in the renal tubules, impairing filtration and leading to renal failure.
Weigh daily.	Measure of adequacy of fluid replacement and kidney function. Continued intake greater than output may indicate renal insult/obstruction.
Monitor BP and HR.	Changes may reflect effects of hypovolemia (bleeding/dehydration).
Evaluate skin turgor, capillary refill, and general condition of mucous membranes.	Indirect indicators of fluid status/hydration.

ACTIONS/INTERVENTIONS	RATIONALE
Note presence of nausea, fever.	Affects intake, fluid needs, and route of replacement.
Encourage fluids of up to 3–4 L/day when oral intake is resumed.	Promotes urine flow, prevents uric acid precipitation, and enhances clearance of antineoplastic drugs.

Bleeding Precautions (NIC)

Inspect skin/mucous membranes for petechiae, ecchymotic areas; note bleeding gums, frank or occult blood in stools and urine, oozing from invasive line sites.	Suppression of bone marrow and platelet production places client at risk for spontaneous/uncontrolled bleeding.
Implement measures to prevent tissue injury/bleeding; e.g., gentle brushing of teeth or gums with soft toothbrush, cotton swab, or sponge-tipped applicator; using electric razor instead of sharp razors when shaving; avoiding forceful nose blowing and needlesticks when possible; using sustained pressure (sandbags or pressure dressings) on oozing puncture/IV sites.	Fragile tissues and altered clotting mechanisms increase the risk of hemorrhage following even minor trauma.
Limit oral care to mouth rinse if indicated (e.g., a mixture of 1/4 tsp baking soda and 1/8 tsp salt in 8 oz water; may use hydrogen peroxide in water or saline for bleeding or infected oral tissue). Avoid mouthwashes with alcohol.	When bleeding is present, even gentle brushing may cause more tissue damage. Alcohol has a drying effect and may be painful to irritated tissues.
Provide soft diet.	May help reduce gum irritation.

Fluid Management (NIC)

Collaborative

Administer IV fluids as indicated.	Maintains fluid/electrolyte balance in the absence of oral intake; prevents or minimizes tumor lysis syndrome, reduces risk of renal complications.
Administer medications as indicated, e.g.:	
Antiemetics: 5-HT_3 receptor antagonist drugs such as ondansetron (Zofran) or granisetron (Kytril);	Relieves nausea/vomiting associated with administration of chemotherapy agents.
Allopurinol (Zyloprim);	Improves renal excretion of toxic byproducts from breakdown of leukemia cells. Reduces the chances of nephropathy as a result of uric acid production.
Potassium acetate or citrate, sodium bicarbonate;	May be used to alkalinize the urine, preventing or minimizing tumor lysis syndrome/kidney stones.
Antiemetics.	Reducing nausea enhances oral intake.

Bleeding Precautions (NIC)

Monitor laboratory studies; e.g., platelets, Hb/Hct, clotting.	When the platelet count is less than 20,000/mm (because of proliferation of WBCs and/or bone marrow suppression secondary to antineoplastic drugs), client is prone to spontaneous life-threatening bleeding. Decreasing Hb/Hct is indicative of bleeding (may be occult).
Administer RBCs, platelets, clotting factors.	Restores/normalizes RBC count and oxygen-carrying capacity to correct anemia. Used to prevent/treat hemorrhage.
Maintain external central vascular access device (subclavian or tunneled catheter or implanted port).	Eliminates peripheral venipuncture as source of bleeding.
Administer medications, e.g.:	
Stool softeners;	Helpful in reducing straining at stool, which can cause trauma to rectal tissues.
Oral contraceptives.	Minimizes blood loss by stopping or slowing menstrual flow.

NURSING DIAGNOSIS: acute Pain

May be related to

Physical agents; e.g., enlarged organs/lymph nodes, bone marrow packed with leukemic cells
Chemical agents; e.g., antileukemic treatments
Psychologic manifestations; e.g., anxiety, fear

Possibly evidenced by

Reports of pain (bone, nerve, headaches, and so forth)
Guarding/distraction behaviors, facial grimacing, alteration in muscle tone
Autonomic responses

DESIRED OUTCOMES/EVALUATION CRITERIA—CLIENT WILL:

Pain Level (NOC)

Report pain is relieved/controlled.
Appear relaxed and able to sleep/rest appropriately.

Pain Control (NOC)

Demonstrate behaviors to manage pain.

ACTIONS/INTERVENTIONS	RATIONALE
Pain Management (NIC)	
Independent	
Investigate reports of pain. Note changes in degree (use scale of 0–10) and site.	Helpful in assessing need for intervention; may indicate developing complications.
Monitor vital signs, note nonverbal cues; e.g., muscle tension, restlessness.	May be useful in evaluating verbal comments and effectiveness of interventions.
Provide quiet environment and reduce stressful stimuli; e.g., noise, lighting, constant interruptions.	Promotes rest and enhances coping abilities.
Place in position of comfort and support joints, extremities with pillows/padding.	May decrease associated bone/joint discomfort.
Reposition periodically and provide/assist with gentle ROM exercises.	Improves tissue circulation and joint mobility.
Provide comfort measures (e.g., massage, cool packs) and psychologic support (e.g., encouragement, presence).	Minimizes need for/enhances effects of medication.
Review/promote client's own comfort interventions; e.g., position, physical activity/nonactivity.	Successful management of pain requires client involvement. Use of effective techniques provides positive reinforcement, promotes sense of control, and prepares client for interventions to be used after discharge.
Evaluate and support client's coping mechanisms.	Using own learned perceptions/behaviors to manage pain can help client cope more effectively.
Encourage use of stress management techniques; e.g., relaxation/deep-breathing exercises, guided imagery, visualization, therapeutic touch.	Facilitates relaxation, augments pharmacologic therapy, and enhances coping abilities.
Assist with/provide diversional activities, relaxation techniques.	Helps with pain management by redirecting attention.

ACTIONS/INTERVENTIONS	RATIONALE
Collaborative	
Monitor uric acid level as appropriate.	Rapid turnover and destruction of leukemic cells during chemotherapy can elevate uric acid, causing swollen painful joints in some clients. *Note:* Massive infiltration of WBCs into joints can also result in intense pain.
Administer medications as indicated:	
Analgesics; e.g., acetaminophen (Tylenol);	Given for mild pain not relieved by comfort measures. *Note:* Avoid aspirin-containing products because they may potentiate hemorrhage.
Opioids; e.g., codeine, morphine, hydromorphone (Dilaudid);	Use around-the-clock, rather than prn, when pain is severe. *Note:* Use of patient-controlled analgesia (PCA) is beneficial in preventing peaks and valleys associated with intermittent drug administration and increases client's sense of control.
Antianxiety agents; e.g., diazepam (Valium), lorazepam (Ativan).	May be given to enhance the action of analgesics/opioids.

NURSING DIAGNOSIS: Activity Intolerance

May be related to

Generalized weakness; reduced energy stores, increased metabolic rate from massive production of leukocytes
Imbalance between oxygen supply and demand (anemia/hypoxia)
Therapeutic restrictions (isolation/bedrest); effect of drug therapy

Possibly evidenced by

Verbal report of fatigue or weakness
Exertional discomfort or dyspnea
Abnormal HR or BP response

DESIRED OUTCOMES/EVALUATION CRITERIA—CLIENT WILL:

Endurance (NOC)

Report a measurable increase in activity tolerance.
Participate in ADLs to level of ability.
Demonstrate a decrease in physiological signs of intolerance; e.g., pulse, respiration, and BP remain within client's normal range.

ACTIONS/INTERVENTIONS	RATIONALE
Energy Management (NIC)	
Independent	
Evaluate reports of fatigue, noting inability to participate in activities or ADLs.	Effects of leukemia, anemia, and chemotherapy may be cumulative (especially during acute and active treatment phase), necessitating assistance.
Encourage client to keep a diary of daily routines and energy levels, noting activities that increase fatigue.	Helps client prioritize activities and arrange them around fatigue pattern.
Provide quiet environment and uninterrupted rest periods. Encourage rest periods before meals.	Restores energy needed for activity and cellular regeneration/tissue healing.

ACTIONS/INTERVENTIONS	RATIONALE
Implement energy-saving techniques; e.g., sitting, rather than standing, use of shower chair. Assist with ambulation/other activities as indicated.	Maximizes available energy for self-care tasks.
Recommend small, nutritious, high-protein meals and snacks throughout the day. Schedule meals around chemotherapy. Give oral hygiene before meals.	Smaller meals require less energy for digestion than larger meals. Increased intake provides fuel for energy. (Refer to CP: Cancer, ND: imbalanced Nutrition: less than body requirements.)
Collaborative	
Provide supplemental oxygen.	Maximizes oxygen available for cellular uptake, improving tolerance of activity.

NURSING DIAGNOSIS: deficient Knowledge [Learning Need] regarding disease, prognosis, treatment, self-care, and discharge needs

May be related to

Lack of exposure to resources
Information misinterpretation/lack of recall

Possibly evidenced by

Verbalization of problem/request for information
Statement of misconception

DESIRED OUTCOMES/EVALUATION CRITERIA—CLIENT WILL:

KNOWLEDGE: Illness Care (NOC)

Verbalize understanding of condition/disease process and potential complications.
Verbalize understanding of therapeutic needs.
Initiate necessary lifestyle changes.
Participate in treatment regimen.

ACTIONS/INTERVENTIONS	RATIONALE
TEACHING: Disease Process (NIC)	
Independent	
Review pathology of specific form of leukemia and various treatment options.	Treatments can include various antineoplastic drugs, transfusions, peripheral progenitor (stem) cell transplant or bone marrow transplant.

For additional interventions refer to CP: Cancer, ND: deficient Knowledge.

POTENTIAL CONSIDERATIONS following acute hospitalization (dependent on client's age, physical condition/presence of complications, personal resources, and life responsibilities)

risk for Infection—inadequate secondary defenses: alterations in mature WBCs (low granulocyte and abnormal lymphocyte count), increased number of immature lymphocytes, immunosuppression, bone marrow suppression (effects of therapy/transplant).

ineffective Role Performance—situational crisis, health alterations, change in physical capacity.

ineffective Therapeutic Regimen Management—complexity of therapeutic regimen, decisional conflicts, economic difficulties, excessive demands made on individual or family, perceived benefits, powerlessness.

interrupted Family Processes—situational crisis (illness, disabling/expensive treatments).

LYMPHOMAS

Malignant lymphomas are cancers of the lymphoid system and include distinct entities defined by clinical, histologic, immunologic, molecular, and genetic characteristics. Based on histologic characteristics, lymphomas are divided into two major categories: *Hodgkin's disease* and *non-Hodgkin's lymphoma* (NHL). There are five subtypes of Hodgkin's disease and about 30 subtypes of NHL. Because there are so many different subtypes of lymphomas, the system used to classify lymphomas is very complicated.

These diseases are staged (I–IV) according to the microscopic appearance of involved lymph nodes and the extent and severity of the disorder. They can be further classified by letters of the alphabet (e.g., A, B) according to symptoms present at the time of diagnosis. And in NHL, subtypes can be called low grade, intermediate, and high grade when discussing clinical behaviors of the disease. **Accurate staging is most important in deciding subsequent treatment regimens and prognosis.**

HODGKIN'S DISEASE

The etiology of *Hodgkin's disease* is unclear, but indirect evidence indicates a viral cause. Signs and symptoms of Hodgkin's disease are distinctive—clients present with a slow, insidious, superficial lymphadenopathy with lymph (cervical, supraclavicular, mediastinal) nodes that are firm, rubbery, and freely movable. The disease spreads in a generally predictable manner to contiguous lymph nodes via lymphatic channels.

Because of many histologic subtypes and ongoing biologic, pathologic, and clinical studies, classifying lymphomas is controversial. However, in 1999, the World Health Organization (WHO) suggested a change in the subtyping of Hodgkin's disease that would assist physicians in selecting treatment protocols.

Treatment for Hodgkin's disease may include radiation, a combination of radiation and chemotherapy, or chemotherapy alone. The cure rate for newly diagnosed cases is higher than 90%, making Hodgkin's disease one of the most treatable forms of cancer. Bone marrow transplant or peripheral progenitor (stem) cell transplants with high-dose chemotherapy are recommended for clients who have relapsed/failed primary chemotherapy regimen.

NON-HODGKIN'S LYMPHOMA

Non-Hodgkin's lymphoma is a malignancy of the B-lymphocyte and T-lymphocyte cell lines. Abnormal lymphocytes accumulate and form masses in lymph tissue such as the lymph nodes, spleen, or other organs. Malignant lymphocytes travel through the circulation to distant sites. Common extranodal sites include the lungs, liver, gastrointestinal tract, meninges, skin, and bones. Most clients with non-Hodgkin's lymphoma fall into two broad categories related to their clinical features: the nodular indolent type, and the diffuse, aggressive lymphomas. Malignant lymphocytes accumulate in lymph nodes. If the normal follicular structure of the nodes remains intact, the lymphoma is called follicular or nodular. When malignant cells destroy the follicles, the lymphoma is considered diffuse. For treatment purposes, they may be separated into two categories: low-grade lymphoma and aggressive lymphoma (which includes intermediate-grade and high-grade lymphomas).

Treatment for non-Hodgkin's lymphomas includes watching and waiting, radiation, chemotherapy (usually multiple combinations of antineoplastic agents), monoclonal antibodies (rituximab [Rituxan]), peripheral progenitor (stem) cell transplant, or bone marrow transplant. With or without treatment, low-grade lymphomas can transform into a more aggressive lymphoma, or the tumor replaces the hematopoietic and lymphoid tissue, which leads to multiple systemic dysfunction and death. Intermediate- and high-grade lymphomas tend to be more responsive to treatment.

CARE SETTING

Acute inpatient care on a medical unit for initial evaluation and treatment, and then at the community level. This plan of care addresses potential complications that may be encountered in acute care or hospice settings.

RELATED CONCERNS

Anemias (iron deficiency, pernicious, aplastic, hemolytic), page 499
Cancer, page 857
Leukemias page 523
Psychosocial aspects of care, page 770
Sepsis/septicemia, page 701
Spinal cord injury (acute rehabilitative phase), page 271
Transplantation considerations (postoperative and lifelong), page 761
Upper gastrointestinal/esophageal bleeding, page 309

CLIENT ASSESSMENT DATABASE

ACTIVITY/REST

May report: Fatigue, weakness, or general malaise
Loss of productivity and decreased exercise tolerance
Excessive sleepiness

May exhibit: Diminished strength, slumping of the shoulders, slow walk, and other cues indicative of fatigue
Night sweats

CIRCULATION

May report: Palpitations, angina/chest pain

May exhibit: Tachycardia, dysrhythmias
Cyanosis and edema of the face and neck or right arm (superior vena cava syndrome—obstruction of venous drainage from enlarged lymph nodes is a rare occurrence)
Scleral icterus and a generalized jaundice related to liver damage and consequent obstruction of bile ducts by enlarged lymph nodes (may be a late sign)
Pallor (anemia), diaphoresis, night sweats

EGO INTEGRITY

May report: Increased stress; e.g., school, job, family
Fear related to diagnosis and possibility of dying
Concerns about diagnostic testing and treatment modalities (chemotherapy, radiation therapy)
Financial concerns: Hospital costs, treatment expenses, fear of losing job-related benefits because of lost time from work
Relationship status: Fear and anxiety related to being a burden on family/SO

May exhibit: Varied behaviors; e.g., angry, withdrawn, passive

ELIMINATION

May report: Changes in characteristics of urine and/or stool, vague abdominal pain
History of intestinal obstruction; e.g., intussusception or malabsorption syndrome (infiltration from retroperitoneal lymph nodes)

May exhibit: Abdomen: RUQ tenderness and enlargement on palpation (hepatomegaly); LUQ tenderness and enlargement on palpation (splenomegaly)
Decreased output, dark/concentrated urine, anuria (ureteral obstruction/renal failure)
Bowel and bladder dysfunction (spinal cord compression occurs late)

FOOD/FLUID

May report: Anorexia/loss of appetite
Dysphagia (pressure on the esophagus)
Recent unexplained weight loss equivalent to 10% or more of body weight in previous 6 months with no attempt at dieting

May exhibit: Edema of the lower extremities (inferior vena cava obstruction from intra-abdominal lymph node enlargement associated with non-Hodgkin's lymphoma)
Ascites (inferior vena cava obstruction related to intra-abdominal lymph node enlargement)

NEUROSENSORY

May report: Nerve pain (neuralgias) reflecting compression of nerve roots by enlarged lymph nodes in the brachial, lumbar, and sacral plexuses
Muscle weakness, paresthesia

May exhibit: Mental status: Lethargy, withdrawal, general lack of interest in surroundings
Paraplegia (tumor involvement/spinal cord compression from collapse of vertebral body, disc involvement with compression/degeneration, or compromised blood supply to the spinal cord)

PAIN/DISCOMFORT

May report: Tenderness/pain over involved lymph nodes; e.g., in or around the mediastinum; chest pain, back pain (vertebral compression); stiff neck; generalized bone pain (lymphomatous bone involvement)
Immediate pain in involved areas following ingestion of alcohol (rare finding in Hodgkin's disease but may give hints to visceral sites of involvement)

May exhibit: Self-focusing; guarding behaviors

RESPIRATION

May report: Dyspnea on exertion or at rest, chest pain

May exhibit: Dyspnea, tachypnea
Dry, nonproductive cough (hilar lymphadenopathy)
Signs of respiratory distress; e.g., increased respiratory rate and depth, use of accessory muscles, stridor, cyanosis
Hoarseness/laryngeal paralysis (pressure from enlarged nodes on the laryngeal nerve)

SAFETY

May report: History of frequent/recurrent infections (abnormalities in cellular immunity predispose client to systemic herpes virus infections, tuberculosis (TB), toxoplasmosis, or bacterial infections), mononucleosis (higher risk of Hodgkin's disease in client with high titers of Epstein-Barr virus), HIV (risk of non-Hodgkin's lymphoma is 60–100 times higher in these clients compared with the general population)
Administration of immunosuppressive drugs after organ transplantation
History/presence of ulcers/perforation, gastric bleeding
Waxing and waning pattern of lymph node size
Cyclical pattern of evening temperature elevations lasting a few days to weeks (Pel-Ebstein fever) followed by alternate afebrile periods; drenching night sweats without chills

May exhibit: Unexplained, persistent fever higher than 100.4°F (38°C) without symptoms of infection
Asymmetric, painless, yet swollen/enlarged lymph nodes (cervical nodes most commonly involved, left side more than right; then axillary and mediastinal nodes)
Nodes may feel rubbery and hard, discrete and movable
Tonsilar enlargement
Generalized pruritus/urticaria (Hodgkin's disease)
Patchy areas of loss of melanin pigmentation (vitiligo)

SEXUALITY

May report: Concern about fertility/pregnancy (although disease does not affect either, treatment does)
Decreased libido

TEACHING/LEARNING

May report: Familial risk factors (higher incidence among families of Hodgkin's clients than in general population)
History of infections (e.g., HIV, human T-lymphocytic virus type 1 [HTLV-1], Epstein-Barr virus [EBV], *Helicobacter pylori* may be associated risk factors)
Occupational exposure to pesticides and herbicides or other chemicals; e.g., benzene, creosote, lead, formaldehyde, paint thinner

Discharge plan considerations: May need assistance with medical therapies/supplies, self-care activities and/or homemaker/maintenance tasks, transportation, shopping

Refer to section at end of plan for post discharge considerations.

DIAGNOSTIC STUDIES

Radiographic studies:

Chest x-ray: May reveal mediastinal or hilar adenopathy, nodular infiltrates, or pleural effusions.

X-rays of thoracic, lumbar vertebrae, proximal extremities, pelvis, or areas of bone tenderness: Determines areas of involvement and assists in staging.

Scanning studies:

Whole lung/ chest computed tomography (CT): Done if hilar adenopathy is present to reveal possible involvement of mediastinal lymph nodes.

Abdominal and pelvic CT scan: May be done to rule out diseased nodes in the abdomen and pelvis and associated organs.

Bone scans: Done to detect bone involvement.

Positron Emission Tomography Scan (PET): Identifies extent of disease and can reveal occult metastases that may not be revealed through other diagnostic studies.

Gallium scan: Not part of routine staging. In client who presents with large mediastinal mass, can distinguish between residual or recurrent disease and persistent scar.

Thoracentesis: May be performed with cytologic studies of pleural fluid.

Abdominal ultrasound: Evaluates extent of involvement of retroperitoneal lymph nodes.

Lymphangiogram: Historically a very important diagnostic tool. Seldom done today because of newer scanning technologies.

Biopsies:

Bone marrow: Determines bone marrow involvement, which is seen in advanced stages.

Lymph node: Establishes the diagnosis of lymphoma and cell type involved.

Other tests:

Blood studies may vary from completely normal to marked abnormalities. In stage I, few clients have abnormal blood findings.

CBC:

WBC: Variable, may be normal, decreased, or markedly elevated.

Differential WBC: Neutrophilia, monocytosis, basophilia, and eosinophilia may be found. Complete lymphopenia (late symptom).

RBC and Hb/Hct: Decreased. Anemia is usually present in chronic disease.

Erythrocytes: Stained RBC examination: May demonstrate mild to moderate normocytic, normochromic anemia (hypersplenism).

Platelets: Decreased or may be elevated.

ESR: Elevated during active stages and indicates inflammatory or malignant disease. Useful to monitor clients in remission and to detect early evidence of recurrence of disease.

Erythrocyte osmotic fragility: Increased.

Gamma globulin: Hypergammaglobulinemia is common; may occur in advanced disease.

Serum cryoglobulins: May be positive with Hodgkin's disease.

Serum haptoglobin: May be elevated in Hodgkin's disease and with cancer of the lung, large intestine, stomach, breast, and liver.

Coombs' test: Positive reaction (hemolytic anemia) may occur; however, a negative result usually occurs in advanced disease.

C-reactive protein (CRP) serum titer: May be positive with Hodgkin's disease.

Serum iron and TIBC: Decreased.

Serum copper: Elevation may be seen in exacerbations.

Serum calcium: May be elevated when bone is involved.

Serum cytokines e.g. (interleukin-6, interleukin-10, IL-2 receptors): Correlates with tumor burden, systemic symptoms, and prognosis.

Liver function tests:

Serum alkaline phosphatase: Elevation may indicate either liver or bone involvement.

Serum LDH: Elevated. Important prognostic indicator in non-Hodgkin's lymphoma, and may indicate a more aggressive cancer.

Kidney function tests:

BUN: May be elevated when kidney involvement is present.

Serum creatinine, bilirubin, antistreptolysin (ASL), creatinine clearance: May be done to detect organ involvement.

Serum uric acid: Elevation related to increased destruction of nucleoproteins and liver and kidney involvement.

Staging laparotomy: Although rarely performed, may be done to obtain specimens of retroperitoneal nodes, of both lobes of the liver, and/or to remove the spleen.

NURSING PRIORITIES

1. Provide physical and psychological support during extensive diagnostic testing and treatment regimen.
2. Prevent complications.
3. Alleviate pain.
4. Provide information about disease process/prognosis and treatment needs.

DISCHARGE GOALS

1. Complications prevented/minimized.
2. Dealing with individual situation realistically.
3. Pain relieved/controlled.
4. Disease process/prognosis, possible complications, and therapeutic regimen understood.
5. Plan in place to meet needs after discharge.

Refer to CPs: Cancer and Leukemias for shared nursing diagnoses such as Fear/Anxiety, Self-Esteem, Grieving, Pain, and Nutrition to accomplish corresponding nursing priorities/discharge goals.

The nurse is referred to other related cancer care plans for nursing interventions related to treatments such as radiation, chemotherapy, and bone marrow transplant.

NURSING DIAGNOSIS: risk for impaired Gas Exchange

Risk factors may include

Altered oxygen-carrying capacity of blood
Tracheobronchial obstruction: enlarged mediastinal nodes and/or airway edema (Hodgkin's and non-Hodgkin's), superior vena cava syndrome (non-Hodgkin's)

Possibly evidenced by

[Not applicable; presence of signs and symptoms establishes an *actual* diagnosis.]

DESIRED OUTCOMES/EVALUATION CRITERIA—CLIENT WILL:

RESPIRATORY STATUS: Ventilation (NOC)

Maintain a normal/effective respiratory pattern, free of dyspnea, cyanosis, or other signs of respiratory distress; and ABGs WNL.

ACTIONS/INTERVENTIONS	RATIONALE
Ventilation Assistance (NIC)	
Independent	
Assess/monitor respiratory rate, depth, rhythm. Note reports of dyspnea and/or use of accessory muscles, nasal flaring, altered chest excursion.	Changes (such as tachypnea, dyspnea, use of accessory muscles) may indicate progression of respiratory involvement/compromise requiring prompt intervention.
Place client in position of comfort, usually with head of bed elevated or sitting upright leaning forward (weight supported on arms), feet dangling.	Maximizes lung expansion, decreases work of breathing, and reduces risk of aspiration.
Reposition and assist with turning periodically.	Promotes aeration of all lung segments and mobilizes secretions.
Instruct in/assist with deep-breathing techniques and/or pursed-lip or abdominal diaphragmatic breathing if indicated.	Helps promote gas diffusion and expansion of small airways. Provides client with some control over respiration, helping to reduce anxiety.
Monitor/evaluate skin color, noting pallor, development of cyanosis (particularly in nailbeds, ear lobes, and lips).	Proliferation of WBCs can reduce oxygen-carrying capacity of the blood, leading to hypoxemia.
Assess respiratory response to activity. Note reports of dyspnea/"air hunger," increased fatigue. Schedule rest periods between activities.	Decreased cellular oxygenation reduces activity tolerance. Rest reduces oxygen demands and minimizes fatigue and dyspnea.
Identify/encourage energy-saving techniques; e.g., rest periods before and after meals, use of shower chair, sitting for care.	Aids in reducing fatigue and dyspnea, and conserves energy for cellular regeneration and respiratory function.
Promote bedrest and provide care as indicated during acute/prolonged exacerbation.	Worsening respiratory involvement/hypoxia may necessitate cessation of activity to prevent more serious respiratory compromise.
Encourage expression of feelings. Acknowledge reality of situation and normality of feelings.	Anxiety increases oxygen demand, and hypoxemia potentiates respiratory distress/cardiac symptoms, which in turn escalates anxiety.
Provide calm, quiet environment.	Promotes relaxation, conserving energy and reducing oxygen demand.
Observe for neck vein distention, headache, dizziness, periorbital/facial edema, dyspnea, and stridor.	Non-Hodgkin's clients are at risk for superior vena cava syndrome, which may result in tracheal deviation and airway obstruction, representing an oncologic emergency.

ACTIONS/INTERVENTIONS	RATIONALE
Provide support to family/caregivers. Encourage open expression of feelings.	Development of this complication is very frightening for client and family because it may indicate end stage of disease process/approaching death, especially in the hospice setting. Keeping family informed may diminish their anxiety and minimize transmission to client.

Collaborative

ACTIONS/INTERVENTIONS	RATIONALE
Provide supplemental oxygen.	Maximizes oxygen available for circulatory uptake, aids in reducing hypoxemia.
Monitor laboratory studies; e.g., ABGs, pulse oximetry.	Measures adequacy of respiratory function and effectiveness of therapy.
Administer analgesics and tranquilizers as indicated.	Reducing physiologic responses to pain/anxiety decreases oxygen demands and may limit respiratory compromise.
Assist with respiratory treatments/adjuncts; e.g., IPPB, incentive spirometer if appropriate.	Promotes maximal aeration of all lung segments, preventing atelectasis.
Assist with intubation and mechanical ventilation.	May be necessary to support respiratory function until airway edema is resolved in acutely ill hospitalized client.
Prepare for emergency radiation therapy when indicated.	Treatment of choice for superior vena cava syndrome.

NURSING DIAGNOSIS: Sexual Dysfunction

May be related to

Altered body structure or function (drugs, surgery, disease process, radiation [loss of sexual desire, disruption of sexual response pattern])

Possibly evidenced by

Verbalization of problem
Actual or perceived limitation imposed by disease and/or therapy
Alteration in relationship with SO

DESIRED OUTCOMES/EVALUATION CRITERIA—CLIENT WILL:

Sexual Functioning (NOC)

Verbalize understanding of individual reasons for sexual problems.
Identify stressors in lifestyle that may contribute to the dysfunction.
Discuss concerns about body image, sex role, desirability as a sexual partner with partner/SO.

Sexual Counseling (NIC)

Independent

ACTIONS/INTERVENTIONS	RATIONALE
Have client describe problem in own words.	Provides more accurate picture of client experience with which to develop plan.
Determine importance of sex to individual/partner and client's motivation for change.	Because lymphomas often affect the relatively young who are in their productive years, these people may be affected more by these problems and may be less knowledgeable about the possibilities of change.

ACTIONS/INTERVENTIONS	RATIONALE
Assess knowledge of client/SO regarding sexual function and effects of current situation/condition.	Helps identify areas of concern, misconception, and actual problems related to therapy side effects.
Identify preexisting and current stress factors that may be affecting the relationship.	Client may be concerned about other issues, such as job, financial, and illness-related problems.
Determine specific pathophysiology, illness/surgery/trauma involved and impact on (perception of) individual.	Client's perception of the individual effects of this illness is crucial to planning interventions that will be appropriate to those affected (client and family).
Assist with treatment of underlying condition.	As illness is treated and client can see improvement, hope is restored and client can begin to look to the future.
Provide factual information.	Promotes trust in caregivers.
Encourage and accept expressions of concern, anger, grief, fear.	Helps client identify feelings and begin to deal with them.
Encourage client to share thoughts/concerns with partner and to clarify values/impact of condition on relationship.	Helps couple begin to deal with issues that can strengthen or weaken relationship.

Collaborative

Refer to appropriate community resources/support groups; e.g., American Cancer Society.	Provides information about resources that are available to help with individual needs. Meeting with others who are dealing with the effects of devastating illness can help client/family.
Provide written material, Internet sites, and other resources appropriate to age/situation.	Reinforces information client has received.
Refer to psychiatric clinical nurse specialist/professional sexual therapist as indicated.	May need additional in-depth assistance to resolve existing problems.

NURSING DIAGNOSIS: deficient Knowledge [Learning Need] regarding disease process, prognosis, treatment regimen, self-care, and discharge needs

May be related to

Lack of exposure/recall
Information misinterpretation
Unfamiliarity with information resources
Cognitive limitations

Possibly evidenced by

Request for information, verbalization of problem, statements reflecting misconceptions
Inaccurate follow-through of instruction, development of preventable complications

DESIRED OUTCOMES/EVALUATION CRITERIA—CLIENT WILL:

KNOWLEDGE: Illness Care (NOC)

Verbalize understanding of condition, prognosis, and potential complications.
Identify relationship of signs/symptoms to disease process.
Initiate necessary lifestyle changes.

TEACHING: Disease Process (NIC)

Independent

ACTIONS/INTERVENTIONS	RATIONALE
Review with client/SO their understanding of client's diagnosis and outlook.	Although lymhomas are complex and have intensive treatment regimens, the outlook has improved in recent years. The 5-year survival rate after treatment in both categories of lymphomas has improved significantly, and many people live with lymphoma in remission.
Review potential treatments client may be considering (e.g., radiation therapy, chemotherapy, biologic therapy, hematopoietic stem call transplantation [HSCT]; combinations of therapies).	May assist client/SO in making informed choices. Although medical treatments are fairly standardized, different doctors have different philosophies and practices. In general, the goal of therapy is remission of the lymphoma, and treatments vary according to the disease process and stage. For example, Hodgkin's disease stages I-A and II-A are usually treated with radiation therapy or a combination of chemotherapy and radiation. When B symptoms are present, chemotherapy is recommended regardless of stage. *Note*: Splenectomy is controversial because it may increase the risk of infection and is currently not usually done unless client has clinical manifestations of stage IV disease.
Discuss potential complications relative to specific therapeutic regimen.	Possible side effects/long-term physical complications of radiation (direct or indirect) and some chemotherapy agents include hypothyroidism, thyroid cancer, coronary artery disease, and valvular heart disease. Following treatment, there is increased risk of secondary malignancies (e.g., lung cancer, breast cancer, thyroid, myeloid leukemia, non-Hodgkin's lymphoma) in addition to other complications listed.
Emphasize need for ongoing medical follow-up.	After completion of primary therapy, appropriate tests will be repeated to determine efficacy of therapy. Also certain monitoring tests are continued; e.g., thyroid-stimulating hormone (TSH) levels should be monitored yearly starting 8–10 years following radiation therapy (XRT). Yearly Pap smears are recommended for female clients because Hodgkin's cells may be found on the cervix. Women receiving XRT are at higher risk of developing breast cancer and should receive yearly mammograms starting 8 years following the completion of treatment.
Identify signs/symptoms requiring further evaluation; e.g., cough, fever, chills, malaise, dyspnea, weight gain, slow pulse, decreased energy level, intolerance to cold, moderate fever, chest pain, dry cough, dyspnea, rapid pulse (pericarditis[rare]); dyspnea, fatigue, chest pain, dizziness/syncope (cardiomyopathy [rare]).	Prompt intervention can identify recurrence, or perhaps limit progression of complications, reduce further debilitating effects.
Recommend regular exercise in moderation, with adequate rest. Discuss energy conservation techniques.	Promotes general well-being. *Note:* Fatigue is associated with disease process and treatment regimen, as well as developing complications. Therefore, balancing activity with rest enhances client's ability to perform ADLs.
Determine financial needs/concerns. Identify community resources, vocational services.	Although survival rates are relatively good, clients often have limitations in physical activities/employment because of dyspnea, chronic fatigue, and difficulties in concentration or memory. Presence of the disease can also impact client's ability to work or qualify for bank loans or obtain insurance.

ACTIONS/INTERVENTIONS	RATIONALE
Recommend/refer to appropriate community resources, e.g., support groups, social worker, counselor, pastor; home health assistance, medical equipment/supplies; hospice; Lymphoma Research Foundation, American Cancer Society.	Client/SO may benefit from many available resources/networks for such help as care assistance, transportation to treatments, sources of financial resources, long-term support/counseling.

POTENTIAL CONSIDERATIONS following acute hospitalization (dependent on client's age, physical condition/presence of complications, personal resources, and life responsibilities)

Fatigue—decreased metabolic energy production, overwhelming psychologic or emotional demands, states of discomfort, altered body chemistry; e.g., chemotherapy.

interrupted Family Processes—situational crisis (illness, disabling/expensive treatments).

10
CHAPTER

Renal and Urinary Tract

RENAL FAILURE: ACUTE

Acute renal failure (ARF) is a sudden loss of kidney function with a buildup of toxic wastes (such as urea and creatinine) in the blood. Although ARF has many causes, ischemia and toxicity are the most common. If the underlying cause is correctable, the nephrons may recover; however, in some cases, damage is permanent and renal failure becomes chronic. ARF has four well-defined stages: onset, oliguric or anuric, diuretic, and convalescent. Treatment depends on stage and severity of renal compromise. ARF can be divided into three major classifications, depending on site:

Prerenal: Prerenal failure (also known as azotemia) is the most common type and is caused by interference with renal perfusion (e.g., blood volume depletion, volume shifts ["third-space" sequestration of fluid], or excessive/too-rapid volume expansion), manifested by decreased glomerular filtration rate (GFR). Disorders that lead to prerenal failure include hemorrhagic, septic, anaphylactic, or cardiogenic shock; heart failure (HF) with renal insufficiency; myocardial infarction (MI); advanced liver disease; burns; trauma; use of certain drugs (e.g., nonsteroidal anti-inflammatory drugs {NSAIDs], cyclooxygenase inhibitors, ACE inhibitors); and renal artery obstruction.

Renal (or intrarenal): Intrarenal causes for renal failure are associated with parenchymal changes caused by ischemia (e.g., renal artery stenosis) or nephrotoxic substances (e.g., radiocontrast media, cyclosporine, heavy metals, aminoglycoside antibiotics). A major cause of intrarenal failure is acute tubular necrosis (ATN)—damage to the renal tubules. Destruction of tubular epithelial cells results from (1) ischemia/hypoperfusion (similar to prerenal hypoperfusion except that correction of the causative factor may be followed by continued oliguria for up to 30 days) and/or (2) direct damage from nephrotoxins.

Postrenal: Postrenal failure occurs as the result of an obstruction in the urinary tract anywhere from the tubules to the urethral meatus. Obstruction most commonly occurs with stones in the ureters, bladder, or urethra; however, trauma, edema associated with infection, prostate enlargement, and strictures also cause postrenal failure.

CARE SETTING

Inpatient acute medical or surgical unit

RELATED CONCERNS

Metabolic acidosis (primary base bicarbonate deficiency), page 492
Fluid and electrolyte imbalances, page 919
Psychosocial aspects of care, page 770
Renal dialysis, page 564
Renal failure: chronic, page 553
Sepsis/septicemia, page 701
Total nutritional support: parenteral/enteral feeding, page 478
Upper gastrointestinal/esophageal bleeding, page 309

Client Assessment Database

ACTIVITY/REST

May report: Fatigue, weakness, malaise
May exhibit: Muscle weakness, loss of tone

CIRCULATION

May exhibit: Hypotension or hypertension (including malignant hypertension, eclampsia/pregnancy-induced hypertension)
Cardiac dysrhythmias
Weak/thready pulses, orthostatic hypotension (hypovolemia)

Jugular venous distention (JVD), full/bounding pulses (hypervolemia); flat neck veins (diuretic phase)
Generalized tissue edema (including periorbital area, ankles, sacrum)
Pallor (anemia); bleeding tendencies

ELIMINATION

May report: Change in usual urination pattern: Increased frequency, polyuria (early failure and early recovery), or decreased frequency/oliguria (later phase)
Dysuria, hesitancy, urgency, and retention (inflammation/obstruction/infection)
Abdominal bloating, diarrhea, or constipation
History of benign prostatic hyperplasia (BPH) or kidney/bladder stones/calculi

May exhibit: Change in urinary color; e.g., absence of color, deep yellow, red, brown, cloudy
Oliguria (may last 12–21 days and occurs in 70% of clients), polyuria (2–6 L/day of urine, lacking concentration and regulation of waste products)

FOOD/FLUID

May report: Weight gain (edema), weight loss (dehydration)
Nausea, anorexia, heartburn, vomiting
Metallic taste
Use of diuretics

May exhibit: Changes in skin turgor/moisture
Edema (generalized, dependent)

NEUROSENSORY

May report: Headache, blurred vision
Muscle cramps/twitching; "restless leg" syndrome, numbness, tingling

May exhibit: Altered mental state; e.g., decreased attention span, inability to concentrate, loss of memory, confusion, decreasing level of consciousness (LOC) (azotemia, electrolyte and acid-base imbalance)
Twitching, muscle fasciculation, seizure activity

PAIN/DISCOMFORT

May report: Flank pain, headache

May exhibit: Guarding/distraction behaviors, restlessness

RESPIRATION

May report: Shortness of breath

May exhibit: Tachypnea, dyspnea, increased rate/depth (Kussmaul's respirations), ammonia breath
Cough productive of pink-tinged sputum (pulmonary edema)

SAFETY

May report: Recent transfusion reaction

May exhibit: Fever (sepsis, dehydration)
Petechiae, ecchymotic areas on skin
Pruritus, dry skin

TEACHING/LEARNING

May report: Family history of polycystic disease, hereditary nephritis, urinary calculus, malignancy
History of exposure to toxins; e.g., drugs (cyclosporine, amphotericin B, cocaine), environmental poisons (e.g., ethyl alcohol, ethylene glycol, mercury vapors, lead, cadmium/other heavy metals), substance abuse
Current/recent use of nephrotoxic drugs; e.g., aminoglycoside antibiotics, amphotericin B; anesthetics; angiotensin-converting enzyme (ACE) inhibitors, vasodilators; NSAIDs
Recent diagnostic testing with radiographic contrast media
Concurrent conditions: Tumors in the urinary tract, gram-negative sepsis, trauma/crush injuries, hemorrhage, disseminated intravascular coagulation (DIC), burns, electrocution injury, autoimmune disorders (e.g., scleroderma, vasculitis), vascular occlusion/surgery, diabetes mellitus (DM), cardiac/liver failure

Discharge plan considerations: May require alteration/assistance with medications, treatments, supplies, transportation, homemaker/maintenance tasks

Refer to section at end of plan for postdischarge considerations.

DIAGNOSTIC STUDIES

Urine:

Volume: Usually less than 400 mL/24 hr (oliguric phase), which occurs within 24–48 hr after renal insult. May be 50 mL/24 or less per/hr (anuric phase) or more than 400 mL/24 hr (nonoliguric) when renal damage is associated with nephrotoxic agents (e.g., contrast media or antibiotics).

Color: Dirty, brown sediment indicates presence of RBCs, hemoglobin, myoglobin, porphyrins.

Specific gravity: Less than 1.020 reflects kidney disease; e.g., glomerulonephritis, pyelonephritis with loss of ability to concentrate; fixed at 1.010 reflects severe renal damage.

pH: Greater than 7 found in urinary tract infections (UTIs), renal tubular necrosis, and chronic renal failure (CRF).

Osmolality: Less than 350 mOsm/kg is indicative of tubular damage, and urine/serum ratio is often 1:1.

Creatinine (Cr) clearance: Renal function may be significantly decreased before blood urea nitrogen (BUN) and serum Cr show significant elevation.

Sodium: Usually increased if ATN is cause for ARF, more than 40 mEq/L if kidney is not able to reabsorb sodium, although it is typically decreased in other causes of prerenal azotemia.

Fractional sodium (FeNa): Ratio of sodium excreted to total sodium filtered by the kidneys reveals inability of tubules to reabsorb sodium. Readings of less than 1% indicate prerenal problems; higher than 1% reflects intrarenal disorders.

Bicarbonate: Elevated if metabolic acidosis is present.

Red blood cells (RBCs): May be present because of infection, stones, trauma, tumor, or altered glomerular filtration (GF).

Protein: High-grade proteinuria (3–4+) strongly indicates glomerular damage when RBCs and casts are also present. Low-grade proteinuria (1–2+) and white blood cells (WBCs) may be indicative of infection or interstitial nephritis. In ATN, proteinuria is usually minimal.

Casts: Usually signal renal disease or infection. Cellular casts with brownish pigments and numerous renal tubular epithelial cells are diagnostic of ATN. Red casts suggest acute glomerular nephritis.

Blood:

BUN/Cr: Elevated and usually rise in proportion with ratio of 10:1 or higher. ARF presents clinically as a rapidly rising Cr over several hours or days.

Complete blood count (CBC): Hemoglobin (Hb) decreased in presence of anemia (which is main hemotolgic effect of ARF). RBCs often decreased because of increased fragility/decreased survival.

Arterial blood gases (ABGs): Metabolic acidosis (pH less than 7.2) may develop because of decreased renal ability to excrete hydrogen and end products of metabolism. Bicarbonate decreased.

Sodium: Usually increased, but may vary.

Potassium: Elevated related to retention and cellular shifts (acidosis) or tissue release (red cell hemolysis).

Chloride, phosphorus, and magnesium: Usually elevated.

Calcium: Decreased.

Serum osmolality: More than 285 mOsm/kg; often equal to urine.

Protein: Decreased serum level may reflect protein loss via urine, fluid shifts, decreased intake, or decreased synthesis because of lack of essential amino acids.

Other tests:

Kidney/abdominal ultrasound: Determines kidney size and presence of masses, cysts, obstruction in upper urinary tract.

Voiding cystoureterogram: Shows bladder size, reflux into ureters, retention.

Kidney, ureter, bladder (KUB) radiograph: Demonstrates size of kidneys/ureters/bladder, presence of cysts, tumors, and kidney displacement or obstruction (stones).

IVP and retrograde pyelogram: Outlines abnormalities of renal pelvis and ureters.

Excretory urography (intravenous urogram or pyelogram): Radiopaque contrast concentrates in urine and facilitates visualization of KUB.

Computed tomography (CT) scan, with/without enhancement: Cross-sectional view of kidney and urinary tract detects presence/extent of disease.

Magnetic resonance imaging (MRI): Provides information about soft tissue damage.

Radionuclide imaging: May reveal calicectasis, hydronephrosis, narrowing, and delayed filling or emptying as a cause of ARF.

Aortorenal angiography: Assesses renal circulation and identifies extravascularities, masses.

Endourology: Direct visualization may be done of urethra, bladder, ureters, and kidney to diagnose problems, biopsy, and remove small lesions and/or calculi.

Electrocardiogram (ECG): May be abnormal, reflecting electrolyte and acid-base imbalances.

NURSING PRIORITIES

1. Reestablish/maintain fluid and electrolyte balance.
2. Prevent complications.

3. Provide emotional support for client/significant other (SO).
4. Provide information about disease process/prognosis and treatment needs.

DISCHARGE GOALS

1. Homeostasis achieved.
2. Complications prevented/minimized.
3. Dealing realistically with current situation.
4. Disease process/prognosis and therapeutic regimen understood.
5. Plan in place to meet needs after discharge.

NURSING DIAGNOSIS: excess Fluid Volume

May be related to

Compromised regulatory mechanism (renal failure)

Possibly evidenced by

Intake greater than output, oliguria; changes in urine specific gravity
Venous distention; blood pressure (BP)/central venous pressure (CVP) changes
Generalized tissue edema, weight gain
Changes in mental status, restlessness
Decreased Hb/hematocrit (Hct), altered electrolytes, pulmonary congestion on x-ray

DESIRED OUTCOMES/EVALUATION CRITERIA—CLIENT WILL:

Fluid Overload Severity (NOC)

Display appropriate urinary output with specific gravity/laboratory studies near normal; stable weight, vital signs within client's normal range; and absence of edema.

ACTIONS/INTERVENTIONS	RATIONALE
Fluid/Electrolyte Management (NIC)	
Independent	
Record accurate intake and output (I&O). Include "hidden" fluids such as IV antibiotic additives, liquid medications, ice chips, frozen treats. Measure gastrointestinal (GI) losses and estimate insensible losses; e.g., diaphoresis.	Low urine output (less than 400 mL/24 hr) may be first indicator of acute failure, especially in a high-risk client. Accurate I&O is necessary for determining renal function and fluid replacement needs and reducing risk of fluid overload. *Note:* Hypervolemia occurs in the anuric phase of ARF.
Monitor urine specific gravity.	Measures the kidney's ability to concentrate urine. In intrarenal failure, specific gravity is usually equal to/less than 1.010, indicating loss of ability to concentrate the urine.
Weigh daily at same time of day, on same scale, with same equipment and clothing.	Daily body weight is best monitor of fluid status. A weight gain of more than 0.5 kg/day suggests fluid retention.
Assess skin, face, and dependent areas for edema. Evaluate degree of edema (on scale of +1 to +4).	Edema occurs primarily in dependent tissues of the body, e.g., hands, feet, lumbosacral area. Client can gain up to 10 lb (4.5 kg) of fluid before pitting edema is detected. Periorbital edema may be a presenting sign of this fluid shift because these fragile tissues are easily distended by even minimal fluid accumulation.

ACTIONS/INTERVENTIONS	RATIONALE
Monitor heart rate (HR), BP, and CVP.	Tachycardia and hypertension can occur because of (1) failure of the kidneys to excrete urine, (2) excessive fluid resuscitation during efforts to treat hypovolemia/hypotension or convert oliguric phase of renal failure, and/or (3) changes in the renin-angiotensin system. *Note:* Invasive monitoring may be needed for assessing intravascular volume, especially in clients with poor cardiac function.
Auscultate lung and heart sounds.	Fluid overload may lead to pulmonary edema and HF evidenced by development of adventitious breath sounds, extra heart sounds. (Refer to ND: risk for decreased Cardiac Output, following.)
Assess level of consciousness; investigate changes in mentation, presence of restlessness.	May reflect fluid shifts, accumulation of toxins, acidosis, electrolyte imbalances, or developing hypoxia.
Plan oral fluid replacement with client, within multiple restrictions. Intersperse desired beverages throughout 24 hr. Vary offerings; e.g., hot, cold, frozen.	Helps avoid periods without fluids, minimizes boredom of limited choices, and reduces sense of deprivation and thirst.

Collaborative

ACTIONS/INTERVENTIONS	RATIONALE
Correct any reversible cause of ARF; e.g., replace blood loss, maximize cardiac output, discontinue nephrotoxic drug, relieve obstruction via surgery.	Kidneys may be able to return to normal functioning, preventing or limiting residual effects.
Insert/maintain indwelling catheter, as indicated.	Catheterization excludes lower tract obstruction and provides means of accurate monitoring of urine output during acute phase; however, indwelling catheterization may be contraindicated because of increased risk of infection.
Monitor laboratory/diagnostic studies; e.g.:	
BUN, Cr;	Assesses progression and management of renal dysfunction/failure. Although both values may be increased, Cr is a better indicator of renal function because it is not affected by hydration, diet, and tissue catabolism. *Note:* Dialysis is indicated if ratio is higher than 10:1 or if therapy fails to correct fluid overload or metabolic acidosis.
Urine sodium and Cr;	In ATN, tubular functional integrity is lost and sodium resorption is impaired, resulting in increased sodium excretion. Urine creatinine is usually decreased as serum creatinine elevates.
Serum sodium;	Hyponatremia may result from fluid overload (dilutional) or kidney's inability to conserve sodium. Hypernatremia indicates total body water deficit.
Serum potassium;	Lack of renal excretion and/or selective retention of potassium to excrete excess hydrogen ions leads to hyperkalemia, requiring prompt intervention.
Hb/Hct;	Decreased values may indicate hemodilution (hypervolemia); however, during prolonged failure, anemia frequently develops as a result of RBC loss/decreased production. Other possible causes (active or occult hemorrhage) should also be evaluated.
Serial chest x-rays.	Increased cardiac size, prominent pulmonary vascular markings, pleural effusion, infiltrates/congestion indicate acute responses to fluid overload or chronic changes associated with renal and heart failure.

ACTIONS/INTERVENTIONS	RATIONALE
Administer/restrict fluids as indicated.	Fluid management is usually calculated to replace output from all sources plus estimated insensible losses (metabolism, diaphoresis). Prerenal failure (azotemia) is treated with volume replacement and/or vasopressors. The oliguric client with adequate circulating volume or fluid overload who is unresponsive to fluid restriction and diuretics requires dialysis. *Note:* During oliguric phase, "push/pull" therapy (push IV fluids and diurese with diuretics) may be tried to stimulate kidney function.
Administer medication as indicated:	
Diuretics; e.g., furosemide (Lasix), bumetanide (Bumex), torsemide (Demadex), mannitol (Osmitrol);	Given early in oliguric phase of ARF in an effort to convert to nonoliguric phase, flush the tubular lumen of debris, reduce hyperkalemia, and promote adequate urine volume.
Antihypertensives; e.g., clonidine (Catapres), methyldopa (Aldomet), prazosin (Minipress);	May be given to treat hypertension by counteracting effects of decreased renal blood flow and/or circulating volume overload.
Vasodilators; e.g., dopamine (Intropin), fenoldapam (Corlopam);	Given in small doses, dopamine causes selective dilation of the renal vasculature, enhancing renal perfusion. Fenoldopam maintains or increases renal perfusion while it lowers blood pressure, which may be particularly beneficial in clients with renal sufficiency who present in hypertensive crisis.
Calcium channel blockers; e.g., nifedipine (Adalat);	Given early in nephrotoxic ATN to reduce influx of calcium into kidney cells, thereby helping to maintain cell integrity and improve GFR.
Prostaglandins.	Vasodilatory effect may improve circulating volume and reestablish renal blood flow to aid in clearing nephrotoxic agents from nephrons.
Prepare for dialysis as indicated; e.g., hemodialysis, peritoneal dialysis, continuous renal replacement therapy (CRRT).	Done to correct volume overload and electrolyte and acid-base imbalances and to remove toxins. The type of dialysis chosen for ARF depends on the degree of hemodynamic compromise and client's ability to withstand the procedure. (Refer to CP: Renal Dialysis.)

NURSING DIAGNOSIS: risk for decreased Cardiac Output

Risk factors may include

Fluid overload (kidney dysfunction/failure, overzealous fluid replacement)
Fluid shifts, fluid deficit (excessive losses)
Electrolyte imbalance (potassium, calcium), severe acidosis
Uremic effects on cardiac muscle/oxygenation

Possibly evidenced by

[Not applicable; presence of signs and symptoms establishes an *actual* diagnosis.]

DESIRED OUTCOMES/EVALUATION CRITERIA—CLIENT WILL:

Circulation Status (NOC)

Maintain cardiac output as evidenced by BP and HR/rhythm within client's normal limits; peripheral pulses strong and equal with adequate capillary refill time.

ACTIONS/INTERVENTIONS	RATIONALE
Hemodynamic Regulation (NIC)	
Independent	
Monitor BP and HR.	Fluid volume excess, combined with hypertension (often occurs in renal failure) and effects of uremia, increases cardiac workload, and can lead to cardiac failure. In ARF, cardiac failure is usually reversible.
Observe electrocardiogram (ECG) or telemetry for changes in rhythm.	Changes in electromechanical function may become evident in response to progressing renal failure/accumulation of toxins and electrolyte imbalance. For example, hyperkalemia is associated with peaked T wave, wide QRS, prolonged PR interval, flattened/absent P wave. Hypokalemia is associated with flat T wave, peaked P wave, and appearance of U waves. Prolonged QT interval may reflect calcium deficit.
Auscultate heart sounds.	Development of S_3/S_4 is indicative of failure. Pericardial friction rub may be only manifestation of uremic pericarditis, requiring prompt intervention/possibly acute dialysis.
Assess color of skin, mucous membranes, and nailbeds. Note capillary refill time.	Pallor may reflect vasoconstriction or anemia (common in ARF, whether associated with actual blood loss or abnormalities in life of RBCs). Cyanosis is a late sign and is related to pulmonary congestion and/or cardiac failure.
Note occurrence of slow pulse, hypotension, flushing, nausea/vomiting, and depressed level of consciousness (central nervous system [CNS] depression).	Using drugs (e.g., antacids) containing magnesium can result in hypermagnesemia, potentiating neuromuscular dysfunction and risk of respiratory/cardiac arrest.
Investigate reports of muscle cramps, numbness/tingling of fingers, with muscle twitching, hyperreflexia.	Neuromuscular indicators of hypocalcemia, which can also affect cardiac contractility and function.
Maintain bedrest or encourage adequate rest and provide assistance with care and desired activities.	Reduces oxygen consumption/cardiac workload.
Collaborative	
Monitor laboratory studies; e.g.:	
Potassium;	During oliguric phase, hyperkalemia is present but often shifts to hypokalemia in diuretic or recovery phase. Any potassium value associated with ECG changes requires intervention. *Note:* A serum level of 6.5 mEq or higher constitutes a medical emergency.
Calcium;	In addition to its own cardiac effects, calcium deficit enhances the toxic effects of potassium.
Phosphorus;	May be abnormal because of reduced renal excretion and/or excess release of cellular phosphate.
Magnesium.	Dialysis or calcium administration may be necessary to combat the CNS-depressive effects of an elevated serum magnesium level.
Administer/restrict fluids as indicated. (Refer to NDs: excess Fluid Volume, and risk for deficient Fluid Volume)	Cardiac output depends on circulating volume (affected by both fluid excess and deficit) and myocardial muscle function.
Provide supplemental oxygen if indicated.	Maximizes available oxygen for myocardial uptake to reduce cardiac workload and cellular hypoxia.
Administer medications as indicated:	
Inotropic agents; e.g., digoxin (Lanoxin);	May be used to improve cardiac output by increasing myocardial contractility and stroke volume. Dosage depends on renal function and potassium balance to obtain therapeutic effect without toxicity.

ACTIONS/INTERVENTIONS	RATIONALE
Calcium gluconate;	Serum calcium is often low but usually does not require specific treatment in ARF. Calcium gluconate may be given to treat hypocalcemia and to offset the effects of hyperkalemia by modifying cardiac irritability.
Aluminum hydroxide gels (Amphojel, Basalgel);	Increased phosphate levels may occur as a result of failure of glomerular filtration and require use of phosphate-binding antacids to limit phosphate absorption from the GI tract.
Glucose/insulin solution;	Temporary measure to lower serum potassium by driving potassium into cells when cardiac rhythm is endangered.
Sodium bicarbonate or sodium citrate;	May be used to correct metabolic acidosis or hyperkalemia (by increasing serum pH) if client is severely acidotic. (Note: Used with caution as it can exacerbate fluid overload and cause tetany by decreasing the ionized calcium concentration.) Acidosis that does not respond to medical therapy is an indication for dialysis.
Sodium polystyrene sulfonate (Kayexalate) with/without sorbitol.	Exchange resin trades sodium for potassium in the GI tract to lower serum potassium level. Sorbitol may be included to cause osmotic diarrhea to help excrete potassium.
Prepare for/assist with dialysis as necessary.	May be indicated for persistent dysrhythmias, progressive HF unresponsive to other therapies.

NURSING DIAGNOSIS: risk for imbalanced Nutrition: less than body requirements

Risk factors may include

Protein catabolism; dietary restrictions to reduce nitrogenous waste products
Increased metabolic needs
Anorexia, nausea/vomiting; ulcerations of oral mucosa

Possibly evidenced by

[Not applicable; presence of signs and symptoms establishes an *actual* diagnosis.]

DESIRED OUTCOMES/EVALUATION CRITERIA—CLIENT WILL:

Nutritional Status (NOC)

Maintain/regain weight as indicated by individual situation, free of edema.

ACTIONS/INTERVENTIONS	RATIONALE
Nutrition Therapy (NIC)	
Independent	
Assess/document dietary intake.	Aids in identifying deficiencies and dietary needs. General physical condition, uremic symptoms (e.g., nausea, anorexia, altered taste), and multiple dietary restrictions affect food intake.
Provide frequent, small feedings.	Minimizes anorexia and nausea associated with uremic state/diminished peristalsis.
Give client/SO a list of permitted foods/fluids and encourage involvement in menu choices.	Provides client with a measure of control within dietary restrictions. Food from home may enhance appetite.

ACTIONS/INTERVENTIONS	RATIONALE
Offer frequent mouth care/rinse with dilute (0.25%) acetic acid solution; provide gum, hard candy, breath mints between meals.	Mucous membranes may become dry and cracked. Mouth care soothes, lubricates, and helps freshen mouth taste, which is often unpleasant because of uremia and restricted oral intake. Rinsing with acetic acid helps neutralize ammonia formed by conversion of urea.
Weigh daily.	The fasting/catabolic client normally loses 0.2–0.5 kg/day. Changes in excess of 0.5 kg may reflect shifts in fluid balance.

Collaborative

ACTIONS/INTERVENTIONS	RATIONALE
Monitor laboratory studies; e.g., BUN, prealbumin/albumin, transferrin, sodium, and potassium.	Indicators of nutritional needs, restrictions, and necessity for/effectiveness of therapy.
Consult with dietitian/nutritional support team.	Determines individual calorie and nutrient needs within the restrictions, and identifies most effective route and product; e.g., oral supplements, enteral or parenteral nutrition.
Provide high-calorie, low-/moderate-protein diet. Include complex carbohydrates and fat sources to meet caloric needs (avoiding concentrated sugar sources) and essential amino acids.	The amount of needed exogenous protein is less than normal unless client is on dialysis. Carbohydrates meet energy needs and limit tissue catabolism, preventing ketoacid formation from protein and fat oxidation. Carbohydrate intolerance mimicking DM may occur in severe renal failure. Essential amino acids improve nitrogen balance and nutritional status, stimulate repair of tubular epithelial cells, and enhance client's ability to fight systemic complications.
Restrict potassium, sodium, and phosphorus intake as indicated.	Restriction of these electrolytes may be needed to prevent further renal damage, especially if dialysis is not part of treatment, and/or during recovery phase of ARF.
Administer medications as indicated:	
Iron preparations;	Iron deficiency may occur if protein is restricted, client is anemic, or GI function is impaired.
Calcium carbonate;	Restores normal serum levels to improve cardiac and neuromuscular function, blood clotting, and bone metabolism. *Note:* Low serum calcium is often corrected as phosphate absorption is decreased in the GI system. Calcium may be substituted as a phosphate binder.
Vitamin D;	Necessary to facilitate absorption of calcium from the GI tract.
B complex and C vitamins, folic acid;	Vital as coenzyme in cell growth and actions. Intake is decreased because of protein restrictions.
Antiemetics; e.g. prochlorperazine (Compazine), trimethobenzamide (Tigan).	Given to relieve nausea/vomiting and may enhance oral intake.

NURSING DIAGNOSIS: risk for Infection

Risk factors may include

Depression of immunologic defenses (secondary to uremia)
Invasive procedures/devices (e.g., urinary catheter)
Changes in dietary intake/malnutrition

Possibly evidenced by

[Not applicable; presence of signs and symptoms establishes an *actual* diagnosis.]

DESIRED OUTCOMES/EVALUATION CRITERIA—CLIENT WILL:

Immune Status (NOC)

Experience no signs/symptoms of infection.

ACTIONS/INTERVENTIONS	RATIONALE
Infection Protection (NIC)	
Independent	
Promote good hand washing by client and staff.	Reduces risk of cross-contamination.
Avoid invasive procedures, instrumentation, and manipulation of indwelling catheters whenever possible. Use aseptic technique when caring for/manipulating IV/invasive lines. Change site/dressings per protocol. Note edema, purulent drainage.	Limits introduction of bacteria into body. Early detection/treatment of developing infection may prevent sepsis.
Provide routine catheter care and promote meticulous perianal care. Keep urinary drainage system closed and remove indwelling catheter as soon as possible.	Reduces bacterial colonization and risk of ascending UTI.
Encourage deep breathing, coughing, frequent position changes.	Prevents atelectasis and mobilizes secretions to reduce risk of pulmonary infections.
Assess skin integrity. (Refer to CP: Renal Failure: Chronic; ND: risk for impaired Skin Integrity.)	Excoriations from scratching may become secondarily infected.
Monitor vital signs.	Fever (higher than 100.4°F) with increased pulse and respirations is typical of increased metabolic rate resulting from inflammatory process, although sepsis can occur without a febrile response.
Collaborative	
Monitor laboratory studies; e.g., WBC count with differential.	Although elevated WBCs may indicate generalized infection, leukocytosis is commonly seen in ARF and may reflect inflammation/injury within the kidney. A shifting of the differential to the left is indicative of infection.
Obtain specimen(s) for culture and sensitivity and administer appropriate antibiotics as indicated.	Verification of infection and identification of specific organism aids in choice of the most effective treatment. *Note:* A number of anti-infective agents require adjustments of dose and/or time while renal clearance is impaired.

NURSING DIAGNOSIS: risk for deficient Fluid Volume

Risk factors may include

Excessive loss of fluid (diuretic phase of ARF, with rising urinary volume and delayed return of tubular reabsorption capabilities)

Possibly evidenced by

[Not applicable; presence of signs and symptoms establishes an *actual* diagnosis.]

DESIRED OUTCOMES/EVALUATION CRITERIA—CLIENT WILL:

Fluid Balance (NOC)

Display I&O near balance, good skin turgor, moist mucous membranes, palpable peripheral pulses, stable weight and vital signs, electrolytes within normal range.

ACTIONS/INTERVENTIONS	RATIONALE
Fluid Monitoring (NIC)	
Independent	
Measure I&O accurately. Weigh daily. Calculate insensible fluid losses.	Helps estimate fluid replacement needs. Fluid intake should approximate losses through urine, nasogastric/wound drainage, and insensible losses (e.g., diaphoresis and metabolism). *Note:* Some sources believe that fluid replacement should not exceed two-thirds of the previous day's output to prevent prolonging the diuresis.
Provide allowed fluids throughout 24-hr period.	Diuretic phase of ARF may revert to oliguric phase if fluid intake is not maintained or nocturnal dehydration occurs.
Monitor BP (noting postural changes) and HR.	Orthostatic hypotension and tachycardia suggest hypovolemia.
Note signs/symptoms of dehydration; e.g., dry mucous membranes, thirst, dulled sensorium, peripheral vasoconstriction.	In diuretic or postobstructive phase of renal failure, urine output can exceed 3 L/day. Extracellular fluid volume depletion activates the thirst center, and sodium depletion causes persistent thirst, unrelieved by drinking water. Continued fluid losses/inadequate replacement may lead to hypovolemic state.
Control environmental temperature; limit bed linens as indicated.	May reduce diaphoresis, which contributes to overall fluid losses.
Collaborative	
Monitor laboratory studies; e.g., sodium.	In nonoliguric ARF or in diuretic phase of ARF, large urine losses may result in sodium wasting while elevated urinary sodium acts osmotically to increase fluid losses. Restriction of sodium may be indicated to break the cycle.

NURSING DIAGNOSIS: deficient Knowledge [Learning Need] regarding condition, prognosis, treatment, self-care, and discharge needs

May be related to

Lack of exposure/recall
Information misinterpretation
Unfamiliarity with information resources

Possibly evidenced by

Questions/request for information, statement of misconception
Inaccurate follow-through of instructions/development of preventable complications

DESIRED OUTCOMES/EVALUATION CRITERIA—CLIENT WILL:

KNOWLEDGE: Disease Process (NOC)

Verbalize understanding of condition/disease process, prognosis, and potential complications.
Identify relationship of signs/symptoms to the disease process and correlate symptoms with causative factors.

KNOWLEDGE: Treatment Regimen (NOC)

Verbalize understanding of therapeutic needs.
Initiate necessary lifestyle changes and participate in treatment regimen.

ACTIONS/INTERVENTIONS	RATIONALE
TEACHING: Disease Process (NIC)	
Independent	
Review disease process, prognosis, and precipitating factors if known.	Provides knowledge base from which client can make informed choices.
Explain level of renal function after acute episode is over.	Client may experience residual defects in kidney function, which may/may not be permanent.
Discuss renal dialysis or transplantation if these are likely options for the future.	Although these options would have been previously presented by the physician, client may now be at a point when options need to be considered/decisions made and may desire additional input.
Review dietary plan/restrictions. Include fact sheet listing food restrictions.	Adequate nutrition is necessary to promote healing/tissue regeneration; adherence to restrictions may prevent complications.
Encourage client to observe characteristics of urine and amount/frequency of output.	Changes may reflect alterations in renal function/need for dialysis.
Establish regular schedule for weighing.	Useful tool for monitoring fluid and dietary status/needs.
Review fluid intake/restriction. Remind client to spread fluids over entire day and to include all fluids (e.g., ice) in daily fluid counts.	Depending on the cause/stage of ARF, client may need to either restrict or increase intake of fluids.
Discuss activity restriction and gradual resumption of desired activity. Encourage use of energy-saving and relaxation techniques, and diversional activities.	Client with severe ARF may need to restrict activity and/or may feel weak for an extended period during lengthy recovery phase, requiring measures to conserve energy and reduce boredom/depression.
Discuss reality of continued presence of fatigue.	Decreased metabolic energy production, presence of anemia, and states of discomfort commonly result in fatigue.
Determine/prioritize ADLs and personal responsibilities. Identify available resources/support systems.	Helps client manage lifestyle changes and meet personal/family needs.
Recommend scheduling activities with adequate rest periods.	Prevents excessive fatigue and conserves energy for healing, tissue regeneration.
Discuss/review medication use. Encourage client to discuss all medications (including over-the-counter [OTC] drugs) and herbal supplements with healthcare provider.	Medications that are concentrated in/excreted by the kidneys can cause toxic cumulative reactions and/or permanent damage to kidneys. Some supplements may interact with prescribed medications/contain electrolytes.
Stress necessity of follow-up care, laboratory studies.	Renal function may be slow to return following acute failure (up to 12 months), and deficits may persist, requiring changes in therapy to avoid recurrence/complications.
Identify symptoms requiring medical intervention; e.g., decreased urinary output, sudden weight gain, presence of edema, lethargy, bleeding, signs of infection, altered mentation.	Prompt evaluation and intervention may prevent serious complications/progression to CRF.

POTENTIAL CONSIDERATIONS following acute hospitalization (dependent on client's age, physical condition/presence of complications, personal resources, and life responsibilities)

deficient Fluid Volume (specify)—dependent on cause, duration, and stage of recovery.

Fatigue—decreased metabolic energy production/dietary restriction, anemia, increased energy requirements; e.g., fever/inflammation, tissue regeneration.

risk for Infection—depression of immunologic defenses (secondary to uremia), changes in dietary intake/malnutrition, increased environmental exposure.

ineffective Therapeutic Regimen Management—complexity of therapeutic regimen, economic difficulties, perceived benefit.

RENAL FAILURE: CHRONIC

Chronic renal failure (CRF) is the end result of a gradual, progressive loss of kidney function. Causes include chronic infections (glomerulonephritis, pyelonephritis), vascular diseases (hypertension, nephrosclerosis), obstructive processes (renal calculi), polycystic kidney disease, collagen diseases (systemic lupus), nephrotoxic agents (drugs, such as aminoglycosides), and endocrine diseases (diabetes, hyperparathyroidism). This syndrome is generally progressive and produces major changes in all body systems. The final stage of renal dysfunction, end-stage renal disease (ESRD), is demonstrated by a glomerular filtration rate (GFR) of 15%–20% of normal or less. Diabetes and hypertension together are responsible for more than 70% of all cases of end-stage kidney disease.

CARE SETTING

Primary focus is at the community level, although inpatient acute hospitalization may be required for life-threatening complications.

RELATED CONCERNS

Anemias (iron deficiency, pernicious, aplastic, hemolytic), page 499
Fluid and electrolyte imbalances, page 919
Heart failure: chronic, page 47
Hypertension: severe, page 35
Metabolic acidosis (primary base bicarbonate deficiency), page 492
Psychosocial aspects of care, page 770
Upper gastrointestinal/esophageal bleeding, page 309

Additional associated nursing diagnoses are found in:

Renal dialysis, page 564
Renal failure: acute, page 541
Seizure disorders/epilepsy, page 208

Client Assessment Database

Clients with chronic renal failure may not have any symptoms at all until normal kidney function declines to 20% or less. At that stage, an array of symptoms such as the following may appear.

ACTIVITY/REST

May report: Extreme fatigue, weakness, malaise
Sleep disturbances (insomnia/restlessness or somnolence)

May exhibit: Muscle weakness, loss of tone, decreased range-of-motion (ROM)

CIRCULATION

May report: History of prolonged or severe hypertension
Palpitations; chest pain (angina)

May exhibit: Hypertension, JVD, full/bounding pulses, generalized tissue and pitting edema of feet, legs, hands
Cardiac dysrhythmias, distant heart sounds
Weak thready pulses, orthostatic hypotension reflects hypovolemia (rare in end-stage disease)
Pericardial friction rub
Pallor, bronze-gray, yellow skin
Bleeding tendencies

EGO INTEGRITY

May report: Stress factors; e.g., financial, relationship
Feelings of helplessness, hopelessness, powerlessness

May exhibit: Denial, anxiety, fear, anger, irritability, personality changes

ELIMINATION

May report: Decreased urinary frequency; oliguria, anuria (advanced failure)
Abdominal bloating, diarrhea, or constipation

May exhibit: Change in urine color; e.g., deep yellow, red, brown, cloudy
Oliguria, may become anuric

FOOD/FLUID

May report: Rapid weight gain (edema), weight loss (malnutrition)
Anorexia, heartburn, nausea/vomiting, unpleasant metallic taste in the mouth (ammonia breath)
Use of diuretics

May exhibit: Abdominal distention/ascites, liver enlargement (end-stage)
Changes in skin turgor/moisture
Edema (generalized, dependent)
Gum ulcerations, bleeding of gums/tongue
Muscle wasting, decreased subcutaneous fat, debilitated appearance

HYGIENE

May report: Difficulty performing ADLs

May exhibit: Unkempt appearance

NEUROSENSORY

May report: Headache, blurred vision
Muscle cramps/twitching, "restless leg" syndrome, burning numbness of soles of feet
Numbness/tingling and weakness, especially of lower extremities (peripheral neuropathy)

May exhibit: Altered mental state; e.g., decreased attention span, inability to concentrate, loss of memory, confusion, decreasing level of consciousness, stupor, coma
Gait abnormalities
Twitching, muscle fasciculation, seizure activity
Thin, dry, brittle nails and hair

PAIN/DISCOMFORT

May report: Flank pain, headache, muscle cramps/leg pain (worse at night)

May exhibit: Guarding/distraction behaviors, restlessness

RESPIRATION

May report: Shortness of breath, paroxysmal nocturnal dyspnea, cough with/without thick, tenacious sputum

May exhibit: Tachypnea, dyspnea, increased rate/depth (Kussmaul's respiration)
Cough productive of pink-tinged sputum (pulmonary edema)

SAFETY

May report: Itching skin, frequent scratching
Recent/recurrent infections

May exhibit: Scratch marks, petechiae, ecchymotic areas on skin
Fever (sepsis, dehydration); normothermia may actually represent an elevation in client who has developed a lower than normal body temperature (effect of CRF/depressed immune response)
Bone fractures; calcium phosphate deposits (metastatic calcifications) in skin, soft tissues, joints; limited joint movement

SEXUALITY

May report: Decreased libido, amenorrhea, infertility

SOCIAL INTERACTION

May report: Difficulties imposed by condition; e.g., unable to work, maintain social contacts or usual role function in family

TEACHING/LEARNING

May report: Family history of polycystic disease, hereditary nephritis, urinary calculus, malignancy
History of poorly controlled hypertension or diabetes (high risk for renal failure), exposure to toxins; e.g., nephrotoxic drugs, drug overdose, environmental poisons
Current/recent use of nephrotoxic antibiotics, ACE inhibitors, chemotherapy agents, heavy metals, NSAIDs, radiocontrast agents

Discharge plan considerations: May require alteration/assistance with medications, treatments, supplies; transportation, homemaker/maintenance tasks

Refer to section at end of plan for postdischarge considerations.

DIAGNOSTIC STUDIES

Urine:

Volume: Usually less than 400 mL/24 hr (oliguria) or urine is absent (anuria).

Color: Abnormally cloudy urine may be caused by pus, bacteria, fat, colloidal particles, phosphates, or urates. Dirty, brown sediment indicates presence of RBCs, hemoglobin, myoglobin, porphyrins.

Specific gravity: Less than 1.015 (fixed at 1.010 reflects severe renal damage).

Protein: High-grade persistent proteinuria (3−4+) strongly indicates glomerular damage, especially when RBCs and casts are also present. This dipstick test is used as a screening tool. When glomerular injury (prevalent in persons with diabetes, hypertension or glomerular disease) causes glomeruli to lose the selective permeability and leak, the amount of protein (particularly albumin) excreted in urine rises.

Total protein-creatinine ratio >200 mg/g or albumin-creatinine ratio >30 mg/g on dipstick testing should be referred for further diagnostic workup.

Osmolality: Less than 350 mOsm/kg is indicative of tubular damage, and urine/serum ratio is often 1:1.

Creatinine clearance: May be significantly decreased (less than 80 mL/min in early failure; less than 10 mL/min in ESRD).

Sodium: More than 40 mEq/L because kidney is not able to reabsorb sodium.

Blood:

BUN/Cr: Elevated, usually in proportion. Creatinine level of 12 mg/dL suggests ESRD. A BUN of >25 mg/dL is indicative of renal damage.

Glomerular filtration rate (GFR): Calculated from serum creatinine levels and adjusted for mean normal body surface area, the GFR is variable, but in general is approximately 90 mL/min in the adult. GFR is used to stage renal failure. Symptoms are typically absent until GFR falls below 60 (stage 2). The person in severe chronic renal failure with GFR between 15 and 29 (stages 4–5) is candidate for dialysis/transplantation.

CBC: Hb decreased because of anemia, usually less than 7–8 g/dL.

RBCs: Life span decreased because of erythropoietin deficiency and azotemia.

ABGs: pH decreased. Metabolic acidosis (less than 7.2) occurs because of loss of renal ability to excrete hydrogen and ammonia or end products of protein catabolism. Bicarbonate and Pco_2 decreased.

Serum sodium: May be low (if kidney "wastes sodium") or normal (reflecting dilutional state of hypernatremia).

Potassium: Elevated related to retention and cellular shifts (acidosis) or tissue release (RBC hemolysis). In ESRD, ECG changes may not occur until potassium is 6.5 mEq or higher. Potassium may also be decreased if client is on potassium-wasting diuretics or when client is receiving dialysis treatment.

Magnesium, phosphorus: Elevated.

Calcium/phosphorus: Decreased.

Proteins (especially albumin): Decreased serum level may reflect protein loss via urine, fluid shifts, decreased intake, or decreased synthesis because of lack of essential amino acids.

Serum osmolality: Higher than 285 mOsm/kg; often equal to urine.

Other tests:

Renal ultrasound: Determines kidney size and presence of masses, cysts, obstruction in upper urinary tract.

Computed tomographic/magnetic resonance imaging (CT/MRI) scan: Demonstrates vessel disorders and kidney mass.

Abdominal (KUB) radiograph: Demonstrates size of kidneys/ureters/bladder and presence of obstruction (stones).

Aortorenal angiography: Assesses renal circulation and identifies extravascularities, masses.

Retrograde pyelogram: Outlines abnormalities of renal pelvis and ureters.

Renal arteriogram: Assesses renal circulation and identifies extravascularities, masses.

Voiding cystourethrogram: Shows bladder size, reflux into ureters, retention.

Renal biopsy: May be done endoscopically to examine tissue cells for histologic diagnosis.

Renal endoscopy, nephroscopy: Done to examine renal pelvis; flush out calculi, hematuria; and remove selected tumors.

ECG: May be abnormal, reflecting electrolyte and acid-base imbalances.

X-ray of feet, skull, spinal column, and hands: May reveal demineralization/calcifications resulting from electrolyte shifts associated with CRF.

NURSING PRIORITIES

1. Maintain homeostasis.
2. Prevent complications.
3. Provide information about disease process/prognosis and treatment needs.
4. Support adjustment to lifestyle changes.

DISCHARGE GOALS

1. Fluid/electrolyte balance stabilized.
2. Complications prevented/minimized.

3. Disease process/prognosis and therapeutic regimen understood.
4. Dealing realistically with situation; initiating necessary lifestyle changes.
5. Plan in place to meet needs after discharge.

NURSING DIAGNOSIS: risk for decreased Cardiac Output

Risk factors may include

Fluid imbalances affecting circulating volume, myocardial workload, and systemic vascular resistance (SVR)
Alterations in rate, rhythm, cardiac conduction (electrolyte imbalances, hypoxia)
Accumulation of toxins (urea), soft-tissue calcification (deposition of calcium phosphate)

Possibly evidenced by

[Not applicable; presence of signs and symptoms establishes an *actual* diagnosis.]

DESIRED OUTCOMES/EVALUATION CRITERIA—CLIENT WILL:

Circulation Status (NOC)

Maintain cardiac output as evidenced by BP and heart rate within client's normal range; peripheral pulses strong and equal with prompt capillary refill time.

(In addition to interventions here, refer to CP: Renal Failure: Acute; ND: risk for decreased Cardiac Output.)

ACTIONS/INTERVENTIONS	RATIONALE
Hemodynamic Regulation (NIC)	
Independent	
Auscultate heart and lung sounds. Evaluate presence of peripheral edema/vascular congestion and reports of dyspnea.	S_3/S_4 heart sounds with muffled tones, tachycardia, irregular heart rate, tachypnea, dyspnea, crackles, wheezes, and edema/jugular distention suggest heart failure (HF).
Assess presence/degree of hypertension: monitor BP; note postural changes; e.g., sitting, lying, standing.	Significant hypertension can occur because of disturbances in the renin-angiotensin-aldosterone system (caused by renal dysfunction). Although hypertension is common, orthostatic hypotension may occur because of intravascular fluid deficit, response to effects of antihypertensive medications, or uremic pericardial tamponade.
Investigate reports of chest pain, noting location, radiation, severity (0–10 scale), and whether or not it is intensified by deep inspiration and supine position.	Although hypertension and chronic HF may cause MI, approximately half of CRF clients on dialysis develop pericarditis, potentiating risk of pericardial effusion/tamponade.
Evaluate heart sounds (note friction rub), BP, peripheral pulses, capillary refill, vascular congestion, temperature, and sensorium/mentation.	Presence of sudden hypotension, paradoxical pulse, narrow pulse pressure, diminished/absent peripheral pulses, marked jugular distention, pallor, and a rapid mental deterioration indicate tamponade, which is a medical emergency.
Assess activity level, response to activity.	Weakness can be attributed to heart failure and anemia.
Collaborative	
Monitor laboratory/diagnostic studies; e.g.:	
Electrolytes (potassium, sodium, calcium, magnesium), BUN/Cr;	Imbalances can alter electrical conduction and cardiac function.

ACTIONS/INTERVENTIONS	RATIONALE
Chest x-rays.	Useful in identifying developing cardiac failure or soft-tissue calcification.
Administer antihypertensive drugs; e.g., prazosin (Minipress), captopril (Capoten), clonidine (Catapres), hydralazine (Apresoline).	Reduces systemic vascular resistance and/or renin release to decrease myocardial workload and aid in prevention of HF and/or MI.
Prepare for renal replacement therapy (e.g., hemodialysis).	Reduction of uremic toxins and correction of electrolyte imbalances and fluid overload may limit/prevent cardiac manifestations, including hypertension and pericardial effusion.
Assist with pericardiocentesis as indicated.	Accumulation of fluid within pericardial sac can compromise cardiac filling and myocardial contractility, impairing cardiac output and potentiating risk of cardiac arrest.

NURSING DIAGNOSIS: risk for ineffective Protection

Risk factors may include

Abnormal blood profile (suppressed erythropoietin production/secretion, decreased RBC production and survival, altered clotting factors, increased capillary fragility)

Possibly evidenced by

[Not applicable; presence of signs and symptoms establishes an *actual* diagnosis.]

DESIRED OUTCOMES/EVALUATION CRITERIA—CLIENT WILL:

Coagulation Status (NOC)

Experience no signs/symptoms of bleeding/hemorrhage.
Maintain/demonstrate improvement in laboratory values.

ACTIONS/INTERVENTIONS	RATIONALE
Energy Management (NIC)	
Independent	
Note reports of increasing fatigue, weakness. Observe for tachycardia, pallor of skin/mucous membranes, dyspnea, and chest pain. Plan client activities to avoid fatigue.	May reflect effects of anemia and cardiac response necessary to keep cells oxygenated.
Monitor level of consciousness and behavior.	Anemia may cause cerebral hypoxia manifested by changes in mentation, orientation, and behavioral responses.
Evaluate response to activity, ability to perform tasks. Assist as needed and develop schedule for rest.	Anemia decreases tissue oxygenation and increases fatigue, which may require intervention, changes in activity, and rest.
Limit vascular sampling, combine laboratory tests when possible.	Recurrent/excessive blood sampling can worsen anemia.
Bleeding Precautions (NIC)	
Observe for oozing from venipuncture sites, bleeding/ecchymotic areas following slight trauma, petechiae, joint swelling or mucous membrane involvement; e.g., bleeding gums, recurrent epistaxis, hematemesis, melena, and hazy/red urine.	Bleeding can occur easily because of capillary fragility/altered clotting functions and may worsen anemia.

ACTIONS/INTERVENTIONS	RATIONALE
Hematest GI secretions/stool for blood.	Mucosal changes and altered platelet function due to uremia may result in gastric mucosal erosion/GI hemorrhage.
Provide soft toothbrush, electric razor; use smallest needle possible and apply prolonged pressure following injections/vascular punctures.	Reduces risk of bleeding/hematoma formation.

Collaborative

ACTIONS/INTERVENTIONS	RATIONALE
Monitor laboratory studies; e.g.:	
RBCs, Hb/Hct;	Uremia (e.g., elevated ammonia, urea, other toxins) decreases production of erythropoietin and depresses RBC production and survival time. In CRF, Hb and Hct are usually low but tolerated; e.g., client may not be symptomatic until Hb is below 7.
Platelet count, clotting factors;	Suppression of platelet formation and inadequate levels of factors III and VIII impair clotting and potentiate risk of bleeding. *Note:* Bleeding may become intractable in ESRD.
Prothrombin time (PT) level.	Abnormal prothrombin consumption lowers serum levels and impairs clotting.
Administer fresh blood, packed RBCs (packed red cells [PRCs]) as indicated.	May be necessary when client is symptomatic with anemia. PRCs are usually given when client is experiencing fluid overload or receiving dialysis treatment. Washed RBCs are used to prevent hyperkalemia associated with stored blood.
Administer medications, as indicated; e.g.:	
Erythropoietin preparations (Epogen, EPO, Procrit);	Corrects many of the symptoms of CRF resulting from anemia by stimulating the production and maintenance of RBCs, thus decreasing the need for transfusion.
Iron preparations: folic acid (Folvite), cyanocobalamin (Rubesol-1000);	Useful in managing symptomatic anemia related to nutritional/dialysis-induced deficits. *Note:* Iron should not be given with phosphate binders because they may decrease iron absorption.
Cimetidine (Tagamet), ranitidine (Zantac); antacids;	May be given prophylactically to reduce/neutralize gastric acid and thereby reduce the risk of GI hemorrhage.
Hemostatics/fibrinolysis inhibitors; e.g., aminocaproic acid (Amicar);	Inhibits bleeding that does not subside spontaneously/respond to usual treatment.
Stool softeners (e.g., Colace); bulk laxative (e.g., Metamucil).	Straining to pass hard-formed stool increases likelihood of mucosal/rectal bleeding.

NURSING DIAGNOSIS: disturbed Thought Processes

May be related to

Physiologic changes: accumulation of toxins (e.g., urea, ammonia), metabolic acidosis, hypoxia; electrolyte imbalances, calcifications in the brain

Possibly evidenced by

Disorientation to person, place, time, situation
Memory deficit; altered attention span, decreased ability to grasp ideas
Impaired ability to make decisions, problem-solve
Changes in sensorium: somnolence, stupor, coma
Changes in behavior: irritability, withdrawal, depression, psychosis

DESIRED OUTCOMES/EVALUATION CRITERIA—CLIENT WILL:

Cognition (NOC)

Regain/maintain optimal level of mentation.
Identify ways to compensate for cognitive impairment/memory deficits.

ACTIONS/INTERVENTIONS	RATIONALE
Reality Orientation (NIC)	
Independent	
Assess extent of impairment in thinking ability, memory, and orientation. Note attention span.	Uremic syndrome's effect can begin with minor confusion/irritability and progress to altered personality or inability to assimilate information and participate in care. Awareness of changes provides opportunity for evaluation and intervention.
Ascertain from SO client's usual level of mentation.	Provides comparison to evaluate progression/resolution of impairment.
Provide SO with information about client's status.	Some improvement in mentation may be expected with restoration of more normal levels of BUN, electrolytes, and serum pH.
Provide quiet/calm environment and judicious use of television, radio, and visitation.	Minimizes environmental stimuli to reduce sensory overload/confusion while preventing sensory deprivation.
Reorient to surroundings, person, and so forth. Provide calendars, clocks, outside window.	Provides clues to aid in recognition of reality.
Present reality concisely, briefly, and do not challenge illogical thinking.	Confrontation potentiates defensive reactions and may lead to client mistrust and heightened denial of reality.
Communicate information/instructions in simple, short sentences. Ask direct, yes/no questions. Repeat explanations as necessary.	May aid in reducing confusion, and increases possibility that communications will be understood/remembered.
Establish a regular schedule for expected activities.	Aids in maintaining reality orientation and may reduce fear/confusion.
Promote adequate rest and undisturbed periods for sleep.	Sleep deprivation may further impair cognitive abilities.
Collaborative	
Monitor laboratory studies; e.g., BUN/Cr, serum electrolytes, glucose level, and ABGs (PO_2, pH).	Correction of elevations/imbalances can have profound effects on cognition/mentation.
Provide supplemental O_2 as indicated.	Correction of hypoxia alone can improve cognition.
Avoid use of barbiturates and opiates.	Drugs normally detoxified in the kidneys will have increased half-life/cumulative effects, worsening confusion.
Prepare for dialysis.	Marked deterioration of thought processes may indicate worsening of azotemia and general condition, requiring prompt intervention to regain homeostasis.

NURSING DIAGNOSIS: risk for impaired Skin Integrity

Risk factors may include

Altered metabolic state, circulation (anemia with tissue ischemia), and sensation (peripheral neuropathy)
Alterations in skin turgor (edema/dehydration)
Reduced activity/immobility
Accumulation of toxins in the skin

Possibly evidenced by

[Not applicable; presence of signs and symptoms establishes an *actual* diagnosis.]

DESIRED OUTCOMES/EVALUATION CRITERIA—CLIENT WILL:

TISSUE INTEGRITY: Skin and Mucous Membranes (NOC)

Maintain intact skin.

Risk Management (NOC)

Demonstrate behaviors/techniques to prevent skin breakdown/injury.

ACTIONS/INTERVENTIONS	RATIONALE
Skin Surveillance (NIC)	
Independent	
Inspect skin for changes in color, turgor, vascularity. Note redness, excoriation. Observe for ecchymosis, purpura.	Indicates areas of poor circulation/breakdown that may lead to decubitus formation/infection.
Monitor fluid intake and hydration of skin and mucous membranes.	Detects presence of dehydration or overhydration that affects circulation and tissue integrity at the cellular level.
Inspect dependent areas for edema. Elevate legs as indicated.	Edematous tissues are more prone to breakdown. Elevation promotes venous return, limiting venous stasis/edema formation.
Change position frequently, move client carefully, pad bony prominences with sheepskin, elbow/heel protectors.	Decreases pressure on edematous, poorly perfused tissues to reduce ischemia.
Provide soothing skin care, restrict use of soaps, apply ointments or creams (e.g., lanolin, Aquaphor).	Baking soda and cornstarch baths decrease itching and are less drying than soaps. Lotions and ointments may be desired to relieve dry, cracked skin.
Keep linens dry, wrinkle free.	Reduces dermal irritation and risk of skin breakdown.
Investigate reports of itching.	Although dialysis has largely eliminated skin problems associated with uremic frost, itching can occur because the skin is an excretory route for waste products; e.g., phosphate crystals (associated with hyperparathyroidism in ESRD).
Recommend client use cool, moist compresses to apply pressure (rather than scratch) pruritic areas. Keep fingernails short; encourage use of gloves during sleep if needed.	Alleviates discomfort and reduces risk of dermal injury.
Suggest wearing loose-fitting cotton garments.	Prevents direct dermal irritation and promotes evaporation of moisture on the skin.
Collaborative	
Provide foam/flotation mattress.	Reduces prolonged pressure on tissues, which can limit cellular perfusion, potentiating ischemia/necrosis.

NURSING DIAGNOSIS: risk for impaired Oral Mucous Membrane

Risk factors may include

Lack of/decreased salivation, fluid restrictions
Chemical irritation, conversion of urea in saliva to ammonia

Possibly evidenced by

[Not applicable; presence of signs and symptoms establishes an *actual* diagnosis.]

DESIRED OUTCOMES/EVALUATION CRITERIA—CLIENT WILL:

Oral Health (NOC)

Maintain integrity of mucous membranes.
Identify/initiate specific interventions to promote healthy oral mucosa.

ACTIONS/INTERVENTIONS	RATIONALE
Oral Health Maintenance (NIC)	
Independent	
Inspect oral cavity; note moistness, character of saliva, presence of inflammation, ulcerations, leukoplakia.	Provides opportunity for prompt intervention and prevention of infection.
Provide fluids throughout 24-hr period within prescribed limit.	Prevents excessive oral dryness from prolonged period without oral intake.
Offer frequent mouth care/rinse with 0.25% acetic acid solution. Provide gum, hard candy, breath mints between meals.	Mucous membranes may become dry and cracked. Mouth care soothes, lubricates, and helps freshen mouth taste, which is often unpleasant because of uremia and restricted oral intake. Rinsing with acetic acid helps neutralize ammonia formed by conversion of urea.
Encourage good dental hygiene after meals and at bedtime. Recommend avoidance of dental floss.	Reduces bacterial growth and potential for infection. Dental floss may cut gums, potentiating bleeding.
Recommend client stop smoking and avoid lemon/glycerin products or mouthwash containing alcohol.	These substances are irritating to the mucosa and have a drying effect, potentiating discomfort.
Provide artificial saliva as needed; e.g., Ora-Lube.	Prevents dryness, buffers acids, and promotes comfort.

NURSING DIAGNOSIS: deficient Knowledge [Learning Need] regarding condition, prognosis, treatment, self-care, and discharge needs

May be related to

Lack of exposure/recall, information misinterpretation
Cognitive limitation

Possibly evidenced by

Questions/request for information, statement of misconception
Inaccurate follow-through of instructions, development of preventable complications

DESIRED OUTCOMES/EVALUATION CRITERIA—CLIENT WILL:

KNOWLEDGE: Disease Process (NOC)

Verbalize understanding of condition/disease process and potential complications.

KNOWLEDGE: Treatment Regimen (NOC)

Verbalize understanding of therapeutic needs.
Correctly perform necessary procedures and explain reasons for the actions.
Demonstrate/initiate necessary lifestyle changes.
Participate in treatment regimen.

(In addition to interventions outlined in CP: Renal Failure: Acute, ND: deficient Knowledge.)

ACTIONS/INTERVENTIONS	RATIONALE
TEACHING: Disease Process (NIC)	
Independent	
Review disease process/prognosis and future expectations.	Provides knowledge base from which client can make informed choices. Kidney failure choices (depending on stage of disease) include doing no treatment, hemodialysis, peritoneal dialysis, and kidney transplantation. No matter which option is chosen, the client faces many lifestyle changes, including a complicated treatment plan involving several medications, diet and exercise modification, and appointments with numerous healthcare providers. Note: Client at stage 4 must be evaluated/prepared for renal replacement therapy (e.g., dialysis, transplantation).
Address client/SO feelings, concerns, methods of dealing with situation. Offer compassionate listening and honest answers to questions. Refer to appropriate support resources.	Common reactions to diagnosis include disbelief, anxiety, anger at self and others, mild to severe depression (including suicidal ideation). (Refer to CP: Psychosocial Aspects of Care, ND: risk for self-/other-directed Violence.)
Review dietary modifications/restrictions, including:	
Phosphorus (e.g., milk, cheese, carbonated drinks, processed foods, poultry, corn, peanuts) and magnesium (e.g., whole grain products, legumes);	Retention of phosphorus stimulates the parathyroid glands to shift calcium from bones (renal osteodystrophy), and accumulation of magnesium can impair neuromuscular function and mentation.
Fluid, potassium and sodium restrictions when indicated.	If fluid retention is a problem, client may need to restrict intake of fluid (e.g., previous day's output plus 500 mL for insensible losses) and restrict dietary potassium and sodium as prescribed. If fluid overload is present, diuretic therapy or dialysis will be part of the regimen. (Refer to CP: Renal Failure, Acute, ND: excess Fluid Volume.)
Discuss other nutritional concerns; e.g., regulating protein intake according to level of renal function (generally 0.6–0.7 g/kg of body weight per day of good quality protein, such as meat, chicken, fish, eggs).	Metabolites that accumulate in blood derive almost entirely from protein catabolism; as renal function declines, proteins may be restricted proportionately. Too little protein can result in malnutrition. *Note:* Client on dialysis may not need to be as vigilant with protein intake.
Encourage adequate calorie intake, especially from carbohydrates in the nondiabetic client.	Spares protein, prevents wasting, and provides energy. *Note:* Use of special glucose polymer powders can add calories to enhance energy level without extra food or fluid intake.
Discuss drug therapy, including use of calcium supplements and phosphate binders; e.g., aluminum hydroxide antacids (Amphojel, Basalgel) and avoidance of magnesium antacids (Mylanta, Maalox, Gelusil); and vitamin D.	Prevents serious complications; e.g., reducing phosphate absorption from the GI tract and supplying calcium to maintain normal serum levels, reducing risk of bone demineralization/fractures, tetany; however, use of aluminum-containing products should be monitored because accumulation in the bones potentiates osteodystrophy. Magnesium products potentiate risk of hypermagnesemia. *Note:* Supplemental vitamin D may be required to facilitate calcium absorption.
Stress importance of reading all product labels (drugs and food) and not taking medications without prior approval of healthcare provider.	It is difficult to maintain electrolyte balance when exogenous intake is not factored into dietary restrictions; e.g., hypercalcemia can result from routine supplement use in combination with increased dietary intake of calcium-fortified foods and medications containing calcium.
Instruct in/review blood pressure or glucose monitoring at home, and provide information on obtaining monitoring equipment, as indicated.	Because hypertension and poor glycemic control are high risk factors in kidney disease progression, self-monitoring and management are important. Also, hypertension is worsened by CRF, often requiring management with antihypertensive drugs, necessitating close observation of treatment effects; e.g., vascular response to medication.

ACTIONS/INTERVENTIONS	RATIONALE
Emphasize need for smoking cessation, when client smokes. Refer for nicotine medications, and/or support resources.	Smoking increases renal vasoconstriction, and exacerbates hypertension.
Review strategies to prevent constipation, including stool softeners (Colace) and bulk laxatives (Metamucil) but avoiding magnesium products (milk of magnesia).	Reduced fluid intake, changes in dietary pattern and use of phosphate-binding products often result in constipation that is not responsive to nonmedical interventions. Use of products containing magnesium increases risk of hypermagnesemia.
Review measures to prevent bleeding/hemorrhage (e.g., use of soft toothbrush, electric razor), avoidance of constipation, forceful blowing of nose, strenuous exercise/contact sports.	Reduces risks related to alteration of clotting factors/decreased platelet count.
Caution against exposure to external temperature extremes; e.g., heating pad/snow.	Peripheral neuropathy may develop, especially in lower extremities (effects of uremia, electrolyte/acid-base imbalances), impairing peripheral sensation and potentiating risk of tissue injury.
Discuss role of fatigue in client's daily/desired activities. Advise establishing a routine exercise program within limits of individual ability and rest periods with activities. Instruct in energy conservation techniques.	Fatigue due to anemia, sleep disturbances, malnutrition, and/or failure of kidneys to clear toxins can greatly reduce client's tolerance for activity. At the same time, exercise is needed to maintain muscle tone and joint flexibility; reduces risks associated with immobility (including bone demineralization).
Address sexual concerns.	Physiologic effects of uremia/antihypertensive therapy may impair sexual desire/performance.
Identify available resources (e.g., nephrologist, nutritionist, other specialists) as indicated. Stress necessity of medical and laboratory follow-up.	Close monitoring of renal function and electrolyte balance is necessary to adjust dietary prescription, treatment and/or make decisions about possible options such as dialysis/transplantation.
Discuss quality of life concerns (e.g., pros and cons of each treatment option), refusing/withdrawing dialysis, medical care advance directives, durable power of attorney.	When kidney failure is chronic or end-stage, client/SO may want to discuss issues with others (e.g., family, social worker, religious counselor), and should have the opportunity to receive information to make informed choices.
Identify signs/symptoms requiring immediate medical evaluation; e.g.:	
Low-grade fever, chills, changes in characteristics of urine/sputum, tissue swelling/drainage, oral ulcerations;	Depressed immune system, anemia, malnutrition all contribute to increased risk of infection.
Numbness/tingling of digits, abdominal/muscle cramps, carpopedal spasms, pain/tenderness in extremities;	Uremia and decreased absorption of calcium may lead to peripheral neuropathies. Note: Client is also at risk for development of thrombophlebitic complications.
Joint swelling/tenderness, decreased ROM, reduced muscle strength;	Hyperphosphatemia with corresponding calcium shifts from the bone may result in deposition of the excess calcium phosphate as calcifications in joints and soft tissues. Symptoms of skeletal involvement are often noted before impairment in organ function is evident.
Headaches, blurred vision, periorbital/sacral edema, "red eyes";	Suggestive of development/poor control of hypertension, and/or changes in eyes caused by calcium.
Provide information resources; e.g. patient/family education books, articles, Internet sites; National Kidney Foundation, American Association of Kidney Patients.	Offers client/SO opportunity to obtain information, support and/or sources of funding.

POTENTIAL CONSIDERATIONS following acute hospitalization (dependent on client's age, physical condition/presence of complications, personal resources, and life responsibilities)

excess Fluid Volume—compromised regulatory mechanism.

Fatigue—decreased metabolic energy production/dietary restriction, anemia, increased energy requirements; e.g., fever/inflammation, tissue regeneration.

ineffective Therapeutic Regimen Management—complexity of therapeutic regimen, decisional conflicts: client value system; health beliefs; cultural influences; powerlessness; economic difficulties; family conflict; lack of/refusal of support systems.

Hopelessness—deteriorating physiologic condition, long-term stress, prolonged activity limitations.

RENAL DIALYSIS (GENERAL CONSIDERATIONS)

Dialysis is a process that substitutes for renal function by removing excess fluid and/or accumulated endogenous or exogenous toxins. Dialysis is most often used for clients with acute renal failure (ARF) and/or chronic (end-stage) renal disease.

Dialysis (also called renal replacement) therapies include intermittent hemodialysis (IHD), continuous arteriovenous hemodialysis (CAVHD), continuous venovenous hemodialysis (CVVHD), and continuous ambulatory peritoneal dialysis (CAPD). The two most common types are IHD and CAPD.

Clients with ARF are sometimes so hemodynamically unstable that they cannot tolerate conventional hemodialysis. These clients may benefit from continuous renal replacement therapy (CRRT), which more slowly removes plasma water and compensates for the loss of intravascular volume. Ultrafiltration methods include continuous arteriovenous hemofiltration (CAVH) and continuous venovenous hemofiltration (CVVH).

The chosen type of fluid and/or solute removal depends on the client's underlying pathophysiology, current hemodynamic status, vascular access, availability of equipment/resources, and healthcare providers' training.

CARE SETTING

Community level/dialysis center, although inpatient acute stay may be required during initiation of therapy.

RELATED CONCERNS

Anemias (iron deficiency, pernicious, aplastic, hemolytic), page 499
Heart failure: chronic, page 47
Peritonitis, page 355
Psychosocial aspects of care, page 770
Sepsis/septicemia, page 701
Total nutritional support: parenteral/enteral feeding, page 478
Transplantation considerations (postoperative and lifelong), page 761

Client Assessment Database

Refer to CPs: Renal Failure: Acute; Renal Failure: Chronic, for assessment information.

Discharge plan considerations: May require assistance with treatment regimen, transportation, activities of daily living (ADLs), homemaker/maintenance tasks

Refer to section at end of plan for postdischarge considerations.

DIAGNOSTIC STUDIES

Studies and results are variable, depending on reason for dialysis (e.g., removal of excess fluid or toxins/drugs), degree of renal involvement, and client considerations (e.g., distance from treatment center, cognition, available support).

NURSING PRIORITIES

1. Promote homeostasis.
2. Maintain comfort.
3. Prevent complications.
4. Support client independence/self-care.
5. Provide information about disease process/prognosis and treatment needs.

DISCHARGE GOALS

1. Fluid and electrolyte balance maximized.
2. Complications prevented/minimized.
3. Discomfort alleviated.
4. Dealing realistically with current situation; independent within limits of condition.
5. Disease process/prognosis and therapeutic regimen understood.
6. Plan in place to meet needs after discharge.

GENERAL CONSIDERATIONS

This section addresses the general nursing management issues of client receiving some form of dialysis.

NURSING DIAGNOSIS: imbalanced Nutrition: less than body requirements

May be related to

GI disturbances (result of uremia/medication side effects): anorexia, nausea/vomiting, and stomatitis
Sensation of feeling full (abdominal distention during continuous ambulatory peritoneal dialysis [CAPD])
Dietary restrictions (bland, tasteless food); lack of interest in food
Loss of peptides and amino acids (building blocks for proteins) during dialysis

Possibly evidenced by

Inadequate food intake, aversion to eating, altered taste sensation
Poor muscle tone/weakness
Sore, inflamed buccal cavity, pale conjunctiva/mucous membranes

DESIRED OUTCOMES/EVALUATION CRITERIA—CLIENT WILL:

Nutritional Status (NOC)

Demonstrate stable weight/gain toward goal with normalization of laboratory values and no signs of malnutrition.

ACTIONS/INTERVENTIONS	RATIONALE
Nutrition Therapy (NIC)	
Independent	
Monitor food/fluid ingested and calculate daily caloric intake.	Identifies nutritional deficits/therapy needs, which are extremely variable, depending on client's age, stage of renal disease, other coexisting conditions, and the type of dialysis being planned.
Recommend client/SO keep a food diary, including estimation of ingested calories, electrolytes of individual concern (e.g., sodium, potassium, chloride, magnesium, phosphorus), and protein.	Helps client realize "big picture" and allows opportunity to alter dietary choices to meet individual desires within identified restriction.
Note presence of nausea/anorexia.	Symptoms accompany accumulation of endogenous toxins that can alter/reduce intake and require intervention.
Encourage client to participate in menu planning.	May enhance oral intake and promote sense of control/responsibility.
Recommend small, frequent meals. Schedule meals according to dialysis needs.	Smaller portions may enhance intake. Type of dialysis influences meal patterns; e.g., clients receiving hemodialysis might not be fed directly before/during procedure because this can alter fluid removal, and clients undergoing peritoneal dialysis may be unable to ingest food while abdomen is distended with dialysate.
Encourage use of herbs/spices; e.g., garlic, onion, pepper, parsley, cilantro, and lemon.	Adds zest to food to help reduce boredom with diet. *Note:* Some salt substitutes are high in K^+, and regular soy sauce is high in Na^+, and therefore are to be avoided.
Suggest socialization during meals.	Provides diversion and promotes social aspects of eating.

ACTIONS/INTERVENTIONS	RATIONALE
Encourage frequent mouth care.	Reduces discomfort of oral stomatitis and undesirable/metallic taste in mouth, which can interfere with food intake.

Collaborative

ACTIONS/INTERVENTIONS	RATIONALE
Refer to nutritionist/dietitian.	Necessary to develop complex and highly individual dietary program to meet cultural/lifestyle needs within specific kilocalories and protein restrictions while controlling phosphorus, sodium, and potassium. Dietary needs may change as kidney function/dialysis therapy changes. From 25% to 40% of chronic dialysis clients suffer protein malnutrition. *Note:* Dietary allowances tend to be somewhat more liberal for clients receiving peritoneal/home dialysis because of the frequency of exchanges.
Perform complete nutrition assessment; e.g. measure muscle mass via triceps skin fold or similar procedure. Determine muscle to fat ratio.	Assesses need and adequacy of nutrient utilization by measuring changes that may suggest presence/absence of tissue catabolism.
Provide a balanced diet usually of 2000–2200 calories/day of complex carbohydrates and ordered amount of high-quality protein and essential amino acids.	Provides sufficient nutrients to improve energy and prevent muscle wasting (catabolism); promotes tissue regeneration/healing, and electrolyte balance. *Note:* Fifty percent of protein intake should be derived from protein sources with high biological value, such as red meat, poultry, fish, eggs.
Restrict sodium/potassium as indicated; e.g., avoid bacon, ham, other processed meats and foods, orange juice, tomato soup.	These electrolytes can quickly accumulate, causing fluid retention, weakness, and potentially lethal cardiac dysrhythmias. *Note:* Peritoneal dialysis is not as effective in lowering elevated Na^+ level, necessitating tighter control of Na^+ intake.
Administer multivitamins, including ascorbic acid (vitamin C), folic acid, vitamins B_6 and D, and iron supplements, as indicated.	Replaces vitamin/mineral deficits resulting from malnutrition/anemia or lost during dialysis.
Administer parenteral supplements as indicated, or intradialytic parenteral nutrition (IDPN) as necessary.	Hyperalimentation may be needed to enhance renal tubular regeneration/resolution of underlying disease process and to provide nutrients if oral/enteral feeding is contraindicated. IDPN may be required when parenteral route is also unavailable/contraindicated. Research suggests IDPN may be more efficient at increasing protein synthesis and decreasing proteolysis resulting in a shift from an essentially catabolic state to a positive nitrogen balance.
Monitor laboratory studies; e.g.:	
Serum protein, prealbumin/albumin levels;	Indicators of protein needs. *Note:* Peritoneal dialysis is associated with significant protein loss. *Note*: Serum albumin levels below 3.4 g/dL suggest need for IDPN infusions.
Hb, RBC, and iron levels.	Anemia is the most pervasive complication affecting energy levels in ESRD.
Administer medications as appropriate:	
Antiemetics; e.g., prochlorperazine (Compazine);	Reduces stimulation of the vomiting center.
Histamine blockers; e.g., famotidine (Pepcid);	Gastric distress is common and may be a neuropathy-induced gastric paresis. Hypersecretion can cause persistent gastric distress and digestive dysfunction.
Hormones and supplements as indicated; e.g., erythropoietin (EPO, Epogen) and iron supplement (Niferex).	Although EPO is given to increase numbers of RBCs, it is not effective without iron supplementation. Niferex is preferred because it can be given once daily and has fewer side effects than many iron preparations.
Insert/maintain nasogastric (NG) or enteral feeding tube if indicated.	May be necessary when persistent vomiting occurs or when enteral feeding is desired.

NURSING DIAGNOSIS: impaired physical Mobility

May be related to

Restrictive therapies; e.g., lengthy dialysis procedure
Fear of/real danger of dislodging dialysis lines/catheter
Decreased strength/endurance; musculoskeletal impairment
Perceptual/cognitive impairment

Possibly evidenced by

Reluctance to attempt movement
Inability to move within physical environment
Decreased muscle mass/tone and strength
Impaired coordination
Pain, discomfort

DESIRED OUTCOMES/EVALUATION CRITERIA—CLIENT WILL:

Mobility (NOC)

Maintain optimal mobility/function.
Display increased strength and be free of associated complications (e.g., contractures, decubitus ulcers).

ACTIONS/INTERVENTIONS	RATIONALE
Bed Rest Care (NIC)	
Independent	
Assess activity limitations, noting presence/degree of restriction/ability.	Influences choice of interventions.
Encourage frequent change of position when on bedrest or chair rest; support affected body parts/joints with pillows, rolls, sheepskin, elbow/heel pads as indicated.	Decreases discomfort, maintains muscle strength/joint mobility, enhances circulation, and prevents skin breakdown.
Provide gentle massage. Keep skin clean and dry. Keep linens dry and wrinkle free.	Stimulates circulation; prevents skin irritation.
Encourage deep breathing and coughing. Elevate head of bed as appropriate.	Mobilizes secretions, improves lung expansion, and reduces risk of respiratory complications; e.g., atelectasis, pneumonia.
Suggest/provide diversion as appropriate to client's condition; e.g., visitors, radio/television, books. Take time to interact with client, showing interest in his or her life.	Decreases boredom; promotes relaxation. *Note:* Recent studies indicate that clients on dialysis do feel bored and that caregivers/dialysis staff do not tend to talk with them, resulting in clients feeling like they are "just part of the scenery."
Instruct in and assist with active/passive ROM exercises.	Maintains joint flexibility, prevents contractures, and aids in reducing muscle tension.
Exercise Promotion (NIC)	
Institute a planned activity/exercise program as appropriate, with client's input.	Increases client's energy and sense of well-being/control. Studies have shown that regular exercise programs have benefited clients with ESRD both physically and emotionally. Stable clients have not been shown to have adverse effects.

ACTIONS/INTERVENTIONS	RATIONALE
Bed Rest Care (NIC)	
Collaborative	
Provide foam/flotation mattress or soft chair cushion.	Reduces tissue pressure and may enhance circulation, thereby reducing risk of dermal ischemia/breakdown.

NURSING DIAGNOSIS: Self-Care Deficit (specify)

May be related to

Intolerance to activity; decreased strength and endurance; pain/discomfort
Perceptual/cognitive impairment (accumulated toxins)

Possibly evidenced by

Reported inability to carry out ADLs
Disheveled/unkempt appearance, strong body odor

DESIRED OUTCOMES/EVALUATION CRITERIA—CLIENT WILL:

SELF-CARE: Activities of Daily Living (ADL) (NOC)

Participate in ADLs within level of own ability/constraints of the illness.

ACTIONS/INTERVENTIONS	RATIONALE
Self-Care Assistance (NIC)	
Independent	
Determine client's ability to participate in self-care activities (scale of 0–4).	Underlying condition dictates level of deficit/needs affecting choice of interventions. *Note:* Psychologic factors (e.g., depression, motivation, and degree of support) also have a major impact on the client's abilities.
Provide assistance with activities as necessary.	Meets needs while supporting client participation and independence.
Encourage/use energy-saving techniques; e.g., sitting, not standing; using shower chair; doing tasks in small increments.	Conserves energy, reduces fatigue, and enhances client's ability to perform tasks.
Recommend scheduling activities to allow client sufficient time to accomplish tasks to fullest extent of ability.	Unhurried approach reduces frustration, promotes client participation, enhancing self-esteem.

NURSING DIAGNOSIS: risk for Constipation

Risk factors may include

Decreased fluid intake, altered dietary pattern
Reduced intestinal motility, compression of bowel (peritoneal dialysate), electrolyte imbalances, decreased mobility

Possibly evidenced by

[Not applicable; presence of signs and symptoms establishes an *actual* diagnosis.]

DESIRED OUTCOMES/EVALUATION CRITERIA—CLIENT WILL:

Bowel Elimination (NOC)

Maintain usual/improved bowel function.

ACTIONS/INTERVENTIONS	RATIONALE
Constipation/Impaction Management (NIC)	
Independent	
Auscultate bowel sounds. Note consistency/frequency of bowel movements (BMs), presence of abdominal distention.	Decreased bowel sounds; passage of hard-formed/dry stools suggests constipation and requires ongoing intervention to manage.
Review current medication regimen.	Side effects of some drugs (e.g., iron products, some antacids) may compound problem.
Ascertain usual dietary pattern/food choices.	Although restrictions may be present, thoughtful consideration of menu choices can aid in controlling problem.
Suggest adding fresh fruits, vegetables, and fiber to diet (within restrictions) when indicated.	Provides bulk, which improves stool consistency.
Encourage/assist with ambulation when able.	Activity may stimulate peristalsis, promoting return to normal bowel activity.
Provide privacy at bedside commode/bathroom.	Promotes psychological comfort needed for elimination.
Collaborative	
Administer stool softeners (e.g., Colace), bulk-forming laxatives (e.g., Metamucil) as appropriate.	Produces a softer/more easily evacuated stool.
Keep client NPO; insert NG tube as indicated.	Decompresses stomach when recurrent episodes of unrelieved vomiting occur. Large gastric output suggests ileus (common early complication of peritoneal dialysis) with accumulation of gas and intestinal fluid that cannot be passed rectally.

NURSING DIAGNOSIS: risk for disturbed Thought Processes

Risk factors may include

Physiologic changes; e.g., presence of uremic toxins, electrolyte imbalances, hypervolemia/fluid shifts; hyperglycemia (infusion of a dialysate with a high glucose concentration)

Possibly evidenced by

[Not applicable; presence of signs and symptoms establishes an *actual* diagnosis.]

DESIRED OUTCOMES/EVALUATION CRITERIA—CLIENT WILL:

Cognition (NOC)

Regain usual/improved level of mentation.
Recognize changes in thinking/behavior and demonstrate behaviors to prevent/minimize changes.

ACTIONS/INTERVENTIONS	RATIONALE
Delirium Management (NIC)	
Independent	
Assess for behavioral change/change in level of consciousness; e.g., disorientation to time/place/person/situation, lethargy, decreased concentration/memory, altered sleep patterns.	May indicate level of uremic toxicity, response to or developing complication of dialysis (e.g., "dialysis dementia"), and requires further assessment/intervention.
Keep explanations simple, reorient frequently as needed. Provide "normal" day/night lighting patterns, clock, calendar.	Improves reality orientation.
Provide a safe environment, restrain as indicated, pad side rails during procedure as appropriate.	Prevents client trauma and/or inadvertent removal of dialysis lines/catheter.
Drain peritoneal dialysate promptly at end of specified equilibration period.	Prompt outflow will decrease risk of hyperglycemia/hyperosmolar fluid shifts affecting cerebral function.
Investigate reports of headache, associated with onset of dizziness, nausea/vomiting, confusion/agitation, hypotension, tremors, or seizure activity.	May reflect development of disequilibrium syndrome, which can occur near completion of/following hemodialysis and is thought to be caused by ultrafiltration or by the too-rapid removal of urea from the bloodstream not accompanied by equivalent removal from brain tissue. The hypertonic cerebrospinal fluid (CSF) causes a fluid shift into the brain, resulting in cerebral edema and increased intracranial pressure.
Monitor changes in speech pattern, development of dementia, myoclonus activity during hemodialysis.	Occasionally, accumulation of aluminum may cause dialysis dementia, progressing to death if untreated.
Collaborative	
Monitor BUN/Cr, serum glucose levels, determine urea reduction ratio (URR).	Follows progression/resolution of azotemia. Pre- and postdialysis BUN levels are used to determine efficacy of procedure. URR greater than 65% is desirable.
Alternate/change dialysate concentrations or add insulin as indicated.	Hyperglycemia may develop secondary to glucose crossing peritoneal membrane and entering circulation. May require initiation of insulin therapy.
Administer normal saline IV as appropriate.	Volume restoration may be sufficient to reverse effects of disequilibrium syndrome.
Administer medication, as indicated; e.g., phenytoin (Dilantin), mannitol (Osmitrol), and barbiturates.	If disequilibrium syndrome occurs during dialysis, medication may be needed to control seizures in addition to a change in dialysis prescription or discontinuation of therapy. Postprocedure, an osmotic diuresis may be required to reduce cerebral edema along with anticonvulsant therapy and barbiturates to slow brain metabolism.
Obtain aluminum level as indicated.	Elevation may warn of impending cerebral involvement/dialysis dementia.

NURSING DIAGNOSIS: Anxiety [specify level]/Fear

May be related to

Situational crisis, threat to self-concept; change in health status/role functioning, socioeconomic status
Threat of death, unknown consequences/outcome

Possibly evidenced by

Increased tension, apprehension, uncertainty, fear
Expressed concerns
Sympathetic stimulation; focus on self

DESIRED OUTCOMES/EVALUATION CRITERIA—CLIENT WILL:

Anxiety [or] Fear Self-Control (NOC)

Verbalize awareness of feelings and reduction of anxiety/fear to a manageable level.
Demonstrate problem-solving skills and effective use of resources.
Appear relaxed, able to rest/sleep appropriately.

ACTIONS/INTERVENTIONS	RATIONALE
Anxiety Reduction (NIC)	
Independent	
Assess level of fear of both client and SO. Note signs of denial, depression, or narrowed focus of attention.	Helps determine the kind of interventions required.
Explain procedures/care as delivered. Repeat explanations frequently/as needed. Provide information in multiple formats, including pamphlets and films.	Fear of unknown is lessened by information/knowledge and may enhance acceptance of permanence of ESRD and necessity for dialysis. Alteration in thought processes and high levels of anxiety/fear may reduce comprehension, requiring repetition of important information. *Note:* Uremia can impair short-term memory, requiring repetition/reinforcement of information provided.
Acknowledge normalcy of feelings in this situation.	Knowing feelings are normal can allay fear that client is losing control.
Provide opportunities for client/SO to ask questions and verbalize concerns.	Creates feeling of openness and cooperation and provides information that will assist in problem identification/solving.
Encourage SO to participate in care, as able/desired.	Involvement promotes sense of sharing, strengthens feelings of usefulness, provides opportunity to acknowledge individual capabilities, and may lessen fear of the unknown.
Acknowledge concerns of client/SO.	Prognosis/possibility of need for long-term dialysis and resultant lifestyle changes are a major concern for this client and those who may be involved in future care.
Point out positive indicators of treatment; e.g., improvement in laboratory values, stable BP, lessened fatigue.	Promotes sense of success/progress in an otherwise chronic process that seems endless while client still is experiencing physical deterioration and depression.
Collaborative	
Arrange for visit to dialysis center/meeting with another dialysis client as appropriate.	Interaction with others who have encountered similar problems may assist client/SO to work toward acceptance of chronic condition/focus on problem-solving activities.
Address financial considerations. Refer to appropriate resources.	Treatment for kidney failure is expensive, although many health insurance programs pay much of the cost.

NURSING DIAGNOSIS: disturbed Body Image/situational low Self-Esteem

May be related to

Situational crisis, chronic illness with changes in usual roles/body image

Possibly evidenced by

Verbalization of changes in lifestyle, focus on past function, negative feelings about body; feelings of helplessness, powerlessness

Continuous physical deterioration, premature aging, disfigurement
Extension of body boundary to incorporate environmental objects (e.g., dialysis equipment)
Change in social involvement
Overdependence on others for care, not taking responsibility for self-care/lack of follow-through, self-destructive behavior

DESIRED OUTCOMES/EVALUATION CRITERIA—CLIENT WILL:

Self-Esteem (NOC)

Identify feelings and methods for coping with negative perception of self.
Verbalize acceptance of self in situation.
Demonstrate adaptation to changes/events that have occurred, as evidenced by setting realistic goals and active participation in care/life.

ACTIONS/INTERVENTIONS	RATIONALE
Body Image [or] Self-Esteem Enhancement (NIC)	
Independent	
Assess level of client's knowledge about condition and treatment and anxiety related to current situation.	Identifies extent of problem/concern and necessary interventions.
Support active information seeking by client/SO.	Concern/belief that sharing of information may be "controlled" by healthcare providers perpetuates sense of a "power differential," potentiating dependence/mistrust.
Discuss meaning of loss/change to client.	Some clients may view situation as a challenge, although many have difficulty dealing with changes in life/role performance and loss of ability to control own body.
Note withdrawn behavior, ineffective use of denial, or behaviors indicative of overconcern with body and its functions. Investigate reports of feelings of depersonalization or the bestowing of humanlike qualities on machinery.	Indicators of developing difficulty handling stress of what is happening. *Note:* Some clients may feel tied to/controlled by technology central to their survival, even to the point of extending body boundary to incorporate dialysis equipment.
Assess for use of addictive substances (e.g., alcohol), self-destructive/suicidal behavior.	May reflect dysfunctional coping and attempt to handle problems in an ineffective manner.
Determine stage of grieving. Note signs of severe/prolonged depression.	Identification of stage client is experiencing provides guide to recognizing and dealing appropriately with behavior as client/SO work to come to terms with loss and limitations associated with condition. Prolonged depression may indicate need for further intervention.
Acknowledge normalcy of feelings.	Recognition that feelings are to be expected helps client accept and deal with them more effectively.
Encourage verbalization of personal and work conflicts that may arise. Active-listen concerns.	Helps client identify problems and problem-solve solutions. *Note*: Home dialysis may provide more flexibility and enhance sense of control for clients who are appropriate candidates for this form of therapy.
Determine client's role in family constellation and client's perception of expectation of self and others.	Long-term/permanent illness and disability alter client's ability to fulfill usual role(s) in family/work setting. Unrealistic expectations can undermine self-esteem and affect outcome of illness.

ACTIONS/INTERVENTIONS	RATIONALE
Recommend SO treat client normally and not as an invalid.	Conveys expectation that client is able to manage situation, and helps maintain sense of self-worth and purpose in life.
Assist client to incorporate disease management into lifestyle.	Necessities of treatment assume a more normal aspect when they are a part of the daily routine.
Identify strengths, past successes, previous methods client has used to deal with life stressors.	Focusing on these reminders of own ability to deal with problems can help client deal with current situation.
Help client identify areas over which he or she has some measure of control. Provide opportunity to participate in decision-making process.	Provides sense of control over seemingly uncontrollable situation, fostering independence.

Collaborative

Recommend participation in local support group.	Reduces sense of isolation as client learns that others have been where client is now. Provides role models for dealing with situation, problem-solving and "getting on with life." Reinforces that therapeutic regimen can be beneficial.
Refer to healthcare/community resources; e.g., social service, vocational counselor, psychiatric clinical nurse specialist.	Provides additional assistance for long-term management of chronic illness/change in lifestyle.

NURSING DIAGNOSIS: deficient Knowledge [Learning Need] regarding condition, prognosis, treatment, self-care, and discharge needs

May be related to

Lack of exposure/recall
Unfamiliarity with information resources
Cognitive limitations

Possibly evidenced by

Questions/request for information; statement of misconception
Inaccurate follow-through of instruction, development of preventable complications

DESIRED OUTCOMES/EVALUATION CRITERIA—CLIENT WILL:

KNOWLEDGE: Disease Process (NOC)

Verbalize understanding of condition and relationship of signs/symptoms of the disease process, and potential complications.

KNOWLEDGE: Treatment Regimen (NOC)

Verbalize understanding of therapeutic needs.
Correctly perform necessary procedures and explain reasons for actions.

ACTIONS/INTERVENTIONS — RATIONALE

TEACHING: Disease Process (NIC)

Independent

ACTIONS/INTERVENTIONS	RATIONALE
Note level of anxiety/fear and alteration of thought processes. Time teaching appropriately.	These factors directly affect ability to participate/access and use knowledge. In addition, studies indicate that during the dialysis procedure, client's cognitive function may be impaired, and clients themselves state that they feel "fuzzy." Therefore, learning may not be optimal during this time.

ACTIONS/INTERVENTIONS	RATIONALE
Review particular disease process, prognosis, and potential complications in clear concise terms, periodically repeating and updating information as necessary.	Providing information at the level of the client's/SO's understanding will reduce anxiety and misconceptions about what client is experiencing. Note: Research suggests nocturnal home hemodialysis (versus conventional HD) is associated with improved left ventricular function, decreased BP and pulse pressure, and reduced antihypertensive medication use.
Encourage and provide opportunity for questions.	Enhances learning process, promotes informed decision making, and reduces anxiety associated with the unknown.
Acknowledge that certain feelings/patterns of response are normal during course of therapy.	Client/SO may initially be hopeful and positive about the future, but as treatment continues and progress is less dramatic, they can become discouraged/depressed, and conflicts of dependence/independence may develop.
Stress necessity of reading all product labels (food/beverage and OTC drugs) and not taking medications/herbal supplements without prior approval of healthcare provider.	It is difficult to maintain electrolyte balance when exogenous intake is not factored into dietary restriction; e.g., hypercalcemia can result from routine supplement use in combination with increased dietary intake of calcium-fortified foods and medicines.
Stress importance of establishing and adhering to medication schedule reflecting the specific form of renal disease, timing of dialysis, and properties of the individual medications.	This is necessary to ensure that therapeutic levels of the drugs are reached and that toxic levels are avoided. *Note:* It is important that client remember to review/revise schedule as the regimen changes and to share with new providers (e.g., staff physician/RN if hospitalized).
Discuss significance of maintaining nutritious eating habits; preventing wide fluctuation of fluid/electrolyte balance; avoidance of crowds/people with infectious processes.	Depressed immune system, presence of anemia, invasive procedures, and malnutrition potentiate risk of infection.
Instruct client about epoetin (Epogen) or darbepoetin (Aransep) when indicated. Have client/SO demonstrate ability to administer and state adverse side effects and healthcare practices associated with this therapy.	Epogen is used for the management of the anemia associated with CRF/ESRD. The drug is given to increase and maintain RBC production, which can allow client to feel better and stronger. Darbepoetin is a non-natural recombinant protein than can stimulate RBC production, but the half-life is about three times longer than erythropoietin, resulting in less frequent dosing. Contraindications may include adverse side effects such as polycythemia/increased clotting, failure to administer correctly or have appropriate follow-up.
Identify healthcare/community resources; e.g., dialysis support group, social services, mental health clinic.	Knowledge and use of these resources assist client/SO to manage care more effectively. Interaction with others in similar situation provides opportunity for discussion of options and making informed choices; e.g., stopping dialysis, renal transplantation.

TEACHING: Procedure/Treatment (NIC)

ACTIONS/INTERVENTIONS	RATIONALE
Discuss procedures and purpose of dialysis in terms understandable to client. Repeat explanations as required.	A clear understanding of the purpose, process, and what is expected of client/SO facilitates their cooperation with regimen and may enhance outcomes.
Instruct client/SO in home dialysis as indicated:	Home dialysis is associated with better outcomes in general/better survival rates as dialysis is usually performed 5–7 days/week and is more intensive. This decreases fluctuations in fluid, solute, and electrolyte balance, more closely mimicking renal function. However, specific criteria for client/SO participation and training, home resources, and professional oversight must be met in order to consider this option.
Operation and maintenance of equipment (including vascular shunt), sources of supplies;	Information diminishes anxiety of the unknown and provides opportunity for client to be knowledgeable about own care.

ACTIONS/INTERVENTIONS	RATIONALE
Aseptic/clean technique;	Prevents contamination and reduces risk of infection.
Self-monitoring of effectiveness of procedure;	Provides information necessary to evaluate effects of therapy/need for change.
Management of potential complications;	Reduces concerns regarding personal well-being; supports efforts at self-care.
Contact persons;	Readily available support person can answer questions, troubleshoot problems, and facilitate timely medical intervention when indicated reducing risk/severity of complications. *Note:* Home dialysis clients usually are monitored by conventional dialysis center/interdisciplinary team.
Sources for supplies when away from home.	Home dialysis clients are often capable of travel (even overseas) with proper preplanning and support.

(Refer to Renal Dialysis: Peritoneal, following, or Hemodialysis, to complete the plan of care.)

POTENTIAL CONSIDERATIONS following acute hospitalization (dependent on client's age, physical condition/presence of complications, personal resources, and life responsibilities)

Fatigue—decreased metabolic energy production, states of discomfort, overwhelming psychologic or emotional demands, altered body chemistry.

excess Fluid Volume—fluid retention/excessive intake, inadequate therapeutic regimen.

risk for Infection—invasive procedures, decreased hemoglobin, chronic disease, malnutrition.

risk for ineffective Therapeutic Regimen Management—complexity of therapeutic regimen, economic difficulties, excessive demands made on individual/family.

risk for Caregiver Role Strain—severity of illness of care receiver, discharge of family member with significant home care needs, caregiver is spouse, presence of situational stressors.

RENAL DIALYSIS: PERITONEAL

Peritoneal dialysis (PD) can be used in ARF and in ESRD. The peritoneum serves as the semipermeable membrane permitting transfer of nitrogenous wastes/toxins and fluid from the blood into a dialysate solution. Fluid removal is controlled by adjusting the dextrose concentration in the dialysate (e.g., 1.5%, 2.5%, 4.25%) to create an osmotic gradient for water. Higher dextrose concentrations and more frequent exchanges increase the rate of fluid removal. Peritoneal dialysis is sometimes preferred over hemodialysis because it uses a simpler technique and provides more gradual physiological changes.

The manual single-bag method is usually done as an inpatient procedure with short dwell times of only 30–40 minutes and is repeated until desired effects are achieved. For long-term PD, a typical schedule calls for four exchanges a day, each with a dwell time of 4–6 hr.

The most commonly used type of long-term peritoneal dialysis is continuous ambulatory peritoneal dialysis (CAPD), which permits the client to manage the procedure at home with bag and gravity flow, using a prolonged dwell time at night and a total of three to five cycles daily and one long overnight dwell time, 7 days a week. No machinery is required. With CAPD, some clients experience problems with the long overnight dwell time because as dextrose in the solution crosses into body, it becomes glucose and starts to draw fluid from the peritoneal cavity back into the body, reducing the efficiency of the exchange. In this case, minicyclers may be helpful.

The different types of cycler-assisted PD are sometimes called automated peritoneal dialysis (APD). The APD machine controls the time of exchanges, drains the used solution, and fills the peritoneal cavity with new solution.

Continuous cycler-assisted peritoneal dialysis (CCPD) mechanically cycles shorter dwell times during the night (three to six cycles) with one 8-hour dwell time during daylight hours, increasing the client's independence. Nocturnal intermittent PD (NIPD) is like CCPD, only the number of overnight exchanges is greater (six to eight), and no exchange is performed during the day. An automated machine is required to warm and infuse, and then drain dialysate at preset intervals.

NURSING DIAGNOSIS: risk for excess Fluid Volume

Risk factors may include

Inadequate osmotic gradient of dialysate
Fluid retention (malpositioned or kinked/clotted catheter, bowel distention; peritonitis, scarring of peritoneum)
Excessive PO/IV intake

Possibly evidenced by

[Not applicable; presence of signs and symptoms establishes an *actual* diagnosis.]

DESIRED OUTCOMES/EVALUATION CRITERIA—CLIENT WILL:

Fluid Balance (NOC)

Demonstrate dialysate outflow exceeding/approximating infusion.
Experience no rapid weight gain, edema, or pulmonary congestion.

ACTIONS/INTERVENTIONS	RATIONALE
Peritoneal Dialysis Therapy (NIC)	
Independent	
Maintain a record of inflow/outflow volumes and cumulative fluid balance.	In most cases, the amount drained should equal or exceed the amount instilled. A positive balance indicates need of further evaluation.
Record serial weights, compare with I&O balance. Weigh client when abdomen is empty of dialysate (consistent reference point).	Serial body weights are an accurate indicator of fluid volume status. A positive fluid balance with an increase in weight indicates fluid retention.
Assess patency of catheter, noting difficulty in draining. Note presence of fibrin strings/plugs.	Slowing of flow rate/presence of fibrin suggests partial catheter occlusion requiring further evaluation/intervention.
Check tubing for kinks; note placement of bottles/bags. Anchor catheter so that adequate inflow/outflow is achieved.	Improper functioning of equipment may result in retained fluid in abdomen and insufficient clearance of toxins.
Turn from side to side, elevate the head of the bed, and apply gentle pressure to the abdomen.	May enhance outflow of fluid when catheter is malpositioned/obstructed by the omentum.
Note abdominal distention associated with decreased bowel sounds, changes in stool consistency, reports of constipation.	Bowel distention/constipation may impede outflow of effluent. (Refer to CP: Renal Dialysis; ND: risk for Constipation.)
Monitor BP and pulse, noting hypertension, bounding pulses, neck vein distention, peripheral edema; measure CVP if available.	Elevations indicate hypervolemia. Assess heart and breath sounds, noting S_3 and/or crackles, rhonchi. Fluid overload may potentiate HF/pulmonary edema.
Evaluate development of tachypnea, dyspnea, increased respiratory effort. Drain dialysate, and notify physician.	Abdominal distention/diaphragmatic compression may cause respiratory distress.
Assess for headache, muscle cramps, mental confusion, disorientation.	Symptoms suggest hyponatremia or water intoxication.
Collaborative	
Alter dialysate regimen as indicated.	Changes may be needed in the glucose or sodium concentration to facilitate efficient dialysis.

ACTIONS/INTERVENTIONS	RATIONALE
Monitor serum sodium.	Hypernatremia may be present, although serum levels may reflect dilutional effect of fluid volume overload.
Add heparin to initial dialysis runs; assist with irrigation of catheter with heparinized saline.	May be useful in preventing fibrin clot formation, which can obstruct peritoneal catheter.
Maintain fluid restriction as indicated.	Fluid restrictions may have to be continued to decrease fluid volume overload.

NURSING DIAGNOSIS: risk for deficient Fluid Volume

Risk factors may include

Use of hypertonic dialysate with excessive removal of fluid from circulating volume

Possibly evidenced by

[Not applicable; presence of signs and symptoms establishes an *actual* diagnosis.]

DESIRED OUTCOMES/EVALUATION CRITERIA—CLIENT WILL:

SYSTEMIC TOXIN CLEARANCE: Dialysis (NOC)

Achieve desired alteration in fluid volume and weight with BP and electrolyte levels within acceptable range.
Experience no symptoms of dehydration.

ACTIONS/INTERVENTIONS — RATIONALE

Peritoneal Dialysis Therapy (NIC)

Independent

ACTIONS/INTERVENTIONS	RATIONALE
Maintain record of inflow/outflow volumes and individual/cumulative fluid balance.	Provides information about the status of client's loss or gain at the end of each exchange.
Adhere to schedule for draining dialysate from abdomen.	Prolonged dwell times, especially when 4.5% glucose solution is used, may cause excessive fluid loss.
Weigh when abdomen is empty, following initial 6–10 runs, then as indicated.	Detects rate of fluid removal by comparison with baseline body weight.
Monitor BP (lying and sitting) and pulse. Note level of jugular pulsation.	Decreased BP, postural hypotension, and tachycardia are early signs of hypovolemia.
Note reports of dizziness, nausea, increasing thirst.	May indicate hypovolemia/hyperosmolar syndrome.
Inspect mucous membranes, evaluate skin turgor, peripheral pulses, capillary refill.	Dry mucous membranes, poor skin turgor and diminished pulses/capillary refill are indicators of dehydration and need for increased intake/changes in strength of dialysate.

Collaborative

ACTIONS/INTERVENTIONS	RATIONALE
Monitor laboratory studies as indicated; e.g.:	
Serum sodium and glucose levels;	Hypertonic solutions may cause hypernatremia by removing more water than sodium. In addition, dextrose may be absorbed from the dialysate, thereby elevating serum glucose.
Serum potassium levels.	Hypokalemia may occur and can cause cardiac dysrhythmias.

NURSING DIAGNOSIS: risk for Trauma

Risk factors may include

Catheter inserted into peritoneal cavity
Site near the bowel/bladder with potential for perforation during insertion or manipulation of the catheter

Possibly evidenced by

[Not applicable; presence of signs and symptoms establishes an *actual* diagnosis.]

DESIRED OUTCOMES/EVALUATION CRITERIA—CLIENT WILL:

Risk Control (NOC)

Experience no injury to bowel or bladder.

ACTIONS/INTERVENTIONS	RATIONALE
Peritoneal Dialysis Therapy (NIC)	
Independent	
Have client empty bladder before peritoneal catheter insertion if indwelling catheter not present.	An empty bladder is more distant from insertion site and reduces likelihood of being punctured during catheter insertion.
Anchor catheter/tubing with tape. Stress importance of client avoiding pulling/pushing on catheter. Restrain hands if indicated.	Reduces risk of trauma by manipulation of the catheter.
Note presence of fecal material in dialysate effluent or strong urge to defecate, accompanied by severe, watery diarrhea.	Suggests bowel perforation with mixing of dialysate and bowel contents.
Note reports of intense urge to void or large urine output following initiation of dialysis run. Test urine for sugar as indicated.	Suggests bladder perforation with dialysate leaking into bladder. Presence of glucose-containing dialysate in the bladder will elevate glucose level of urine.
Stop dialysis if there is evidence of bowel/bladder perforation, leaving peritoneal catheter in place.	Prompt action will prevent further injury. Immediate surgical repair may be required. Leaving catheter in place facilitates diagnosing/locating the perforation.

NURSING DIAGNOSIS: acute Pain

May be related to

Insertion of catheter through abdominal wall/catheter irritation, improper catheter placement
Irritation/infection within the peritoneal cavity
Infusion of cold or acidic dialysate, abdominal distention, rapid infusion of dialysate

Possibly evidenced by

Reports of pain
Self-focusing
Guarding/distraction behaviors, restlessness

DESIRED OUTCOMES/EVALUATION CRITERIA—CLIENT WILL:

Pain Level (NOC)

Verbalize decrease of pain/discomfort.
Demonstrate relaxed posture/facial expression; be able to sleep/rest appropriately.

ACTIONS/INTERVENTIONS	RATIONALE
Pain Management (NIC)	
Independent	
Investigate client's reports of pain; note intensity (0–10), location, and precipitating factors.	Assists in identification of source of pain and appropriate interventions.
Explain that initial discomfort usually subsides after the first few exchanges.	Information may reduce anxiety and promote relaxation during procedure.
Monitor for pain that begins during inflow and continues during equilibration phase. Slow infusion rate as indicated.	Pain occurs at these times if acidic dialysate causes chemical irritation of peritoneal membrane.
Note reports of discomfort that is most pronounced near the end of inflow and instill no more than 2000 mL of solution at a single time.	Likely the result of abdominal distention from dialysate. Amount of infusion may have to be decreased initially.
Prevent air from entering peritoneal cavity during infusion. Note report of pain in area of shoulder blade.	Inadvertent introduction of air into the abdomen irritates the diaphragm and results in referred pain to shoulder blade. This type of discomfort may also be reported during initiation of therapy/during infusions and usually is related to stretching/irritation of the diaphragm with abdominal distention. Smaller exchange volumes may be required until client adjusts.
Elevate head of bed at intervals. Turn client from side to side. Provide back care and tissue massage.	Position changes and gentle massage may relieve abdominal and general muscle discomfort.
Warm dialysate to body temperature before infusing.	Warming the solution increases the rate of urea removal by dilating peritoneal vessels. Cold dialysate causes vasoconstriction, which can cause discomfort and/or excessively lower the core body temperature, precipitating cardiac arrest.
Monitor for severe/continuous abdominal pain and temperature elevation (especially after dialysis has been discontinued).	May indicate developing peritonitis. (Refer to ND: risk for Infection, [peritonitis], following.)
Encourage use of relaxation techniques; e.g., deep-breathing exercises, guided imagery, visualization. Provide diversional activities.	Redirects attention, promotes sense of control.
Collaborative	
Administer analgesics.	Relieves pain and discomfort.
Add sodium hydroxide to dialysate, if indicated.	Occasionally used to alter pH if client is not tolerating acidic dialysate.

NURSING DIAGNOSIS: risk for Infection [peritonitis]

Risk factors may include

Contamination of the catheter during insertion, periodic changing of tubings/bags
Skin contaminants at catheter insertion site
Sterile peritonitis (response to the composition of dialysate)

Possibly evidenced by

[Not applicable; presence of signs and symptoms establishes an *actual* diagnosis.]

DESIRED OUTCOMES/EVALUATION CRITERIA—CLIENT WILL:

Risk Control (NOC)

Identify interventions to prevent/reduce risk of infection.
Experience no signs/symptoms of infection.

ACTIONS/INTERVENTIONS	RATIONALE
Infection Protection (NIC)	
Independent	
Observe meticulous aseptic techniques and wear masks during catheter insertion, dressing changes, and whenever the system is opened. Change tubings per protocol.	Prevents the introduction of organisms and airborne contamination that may cause infection (the most common complication of PD).
Change dressings as indicated, being careful not to dislodge the catheter. Note character, color, odor, or drainage from around insertion site.	Moist environment promotes bacterial growth. Purulent drainage at insertion site suggests presence of local infection, often involving skin organisms, which can be difficult to treat and sometimes require catheter removal and temporary HD. *Note:* Polyurethane adhesive film (e.g., blister film) dressings have been found to decrease amount of pressure on catheter and exit site as well as incidence of site infections.
Observe color and clarity of effluent.	Cloudy effluent is suggestive of peritoneal infection.
Apply povidone-iodine (Betadine) barrier in distal, clamped portion of catheter when intermittent dialysis therapy used.	Reduces risk of bacterial entry through catheter between dialysis treatments when catheter is disconnected from closed system.
Investigate reports of nausea/vomiting, increased/severe abdominal pain; rebound tenderness, fever, and leukocytosis.	Signs/symptoms suggesting peritonitis, requiring prompt intervention.
Collaborative	
Monitor WBC count of effluent.	Presence of WBCs initially may reflect normal response to a foreign substance; however, continued/new elevation suggests developing infection.
Obtain specimens of blood, effluent, and/or drainage from insertion site as indicated for culture/sensitivity.	Identifies types of organism(s) present, choice of interventions.
Monitor renal clearance/BUN, Cr.	Choice and dosage of antibiotics are influenced by level of renal function.
Administer antibiotics systemically or in dialysate as indicated.	Treats infection, prevents sepsis.

NURSING DIAGNOSIS: risk for ineffective Breathing Pattern

Risk factors may include

Abdominal pressure/restricted diaphragmatic excursion, rapid infusion of dialysate, pain
Inflammatory process (e.g., atelectasis/pneumonia)

Possibly evidenced by

[Not applicable; presence of signs and symptoms establishes an *actual* diagnosis.]

DESIRED OUTCOMES/EVALUATION CRITERIA—CLIENT WILL:

RESPIRATORY STATUS: Ventilation (NOC)

Display an effective respiratory pattern with clear breath sounds, ABGs within client's normal range.
Experience no signs of dyspnea/cyanosis.

ACTIONS/INTERVENTIONS	RATIONALE
Respiratory Monitoring (NIC)	
Independent	
Monitor respiratory rate/effort. Reduce infusion rate if dyspnea is present.	Tachypnea, dyspnea, shortness of breath, and shallow breathing during dialysis suggest diaphragmatic pressure from distended peritoneal cavity or may indicate developing complications.
Auscultate lungs, noting decreased, absent, or adventitious breath sounds; e.g., crackles/wheezes/rhonchi.	Decreased areas of ventilation suggest presence of atelectasis, whereas adventitious sounds may suggest fluid overload, retained secretions, or infection.
Note character, amount, and color of secretions.	Client is susceptible to pulmonary infections as a result of depressed cough reflex and respiratory effort, increased viscosity of secretions, as well as altered immune response and chronic/debilitating disease.
Elevate head of bed or have client sit up in chair. Promote deep-breathing exercises and coughing.	Facilitates chest expansion/ventilation and mobilization of secretions.
Collaborative	
Review ABGs/pulse oximetry and serial chest x-rays.	Changes in Pa_{O_2} and Pa_{CO_2} and appearance of infiltrates/congestion on chest x-ray suggest developing pulmonary problems.
Administer supplemental O_2 as indicated.	Maximizes oxygen for vascular uptake, preventing/lessening hypoxia.
Administer analgesics as indicated.	Alleviates pain, promotes comfortable breathing, maximal cough effort.

HEMODIALYSIS

In *hemodialysis* (HD), blood is shunted through an artificial kidney (dialyzer) for removal of toxins/excess fluid and then returned to the venous circulation. Hemodialysis is an efficient method for removing urea and other toxic products and correcting fluid and electrolyte imbalances but requires permanent arteriovenous access. Variations of HD include continuous renal replacement therapy (CRRT), a treatment for clients with acute renal failure where fluid and toxins are removed at a continuous and slower rate than intermittent HD. There are four commonly used types of CRRT, and blood is usually accessed via a central venous catheter.

This plan of care addresses the typical HD procedure, usually performed three times per week for 3–5 hr/procedure, requiring an arteriovenous (AV) access (e.g., primary AV fistula or synthetic graft), and may be carried out in the hospital, community dialysis center, or at home.

NURSING DIAGNOSIS: risk for Injury, [loss of vascular access]

Risk factors may include

Clotting; hemorrhage related to accidental disconnection; infection

Possibly evidenced by

[Not applicable; presence of signs and symptoms establishes an *actual* diagnosis.]

DESIRED OUTCOMES/EVALUATION CRITERIA—CLIENT WILL:

Hemodialysis Access (NOC)

Maintain patent vascular access.
Be free of infection.

ACTIONS/INTERVENTIONS	RATIONALE
Hemodialysis Therapy (NIC)	
Independent	
Clotting	
Monitor internal AV shunt patency at frequent intervals:	
Palpate for thrill;	Thrill is caused by turbulence of high-pressure arterial blood flow entering low-pressure venous system and should be palpable above venous exit site. If the thrill stops, or even feels different, this could indicate clotting. With early intervention, many clots can be dissolved or removed.
Auscultate for a bruit;	Bruit is the sound caused by the turbulence of arterial blood entering venous system and should be audible by stethoscope, although may be very faint. If the bruit gets higher in pitch, it could mean narrowing of the blood vessels; if it stops, clot may have formed.
Note color of blood and/or obvious separation of cells and serum;	Change of color from uniform medium red to dark purplish red suggests sluggish blood flow/early clotting. Separation in tubing is indicative of clotting. Very dark reddish-black blood next to clear yellow fluid indicates full clot formation.
Palpate skin around shunt for warmth.	Diminished blood flow results in "coolness" of shunt.
Notify physician and/or initiate declotting procedure if there is evidence of loss of shunt patency.	Rapid intervention may save access; however, declotting must be done by experienced personnel.
Evaluate reports of pain, numbness/tingling; note extremity swelling distal to access.	May indicate inadequate blood supply.
Avoid trauma to shunt; e.g., handle tubing gently, maintain cannula alignment. Limit activity of extremity. Avoid taking BP or drawing blood samples in shunt extremity. Instruct client not to sleep on side with shunt or carry packages, books, purse on affected extremity.	Decreases risk of clotting/disconnection.
Hemorrhage	
Attach two cannula clamps to shunt dressing. Have tourniquet available. If cannulas separate, clamp the arterial cannula first, then the venous. If tubing comes out of vessel, clamp cannula that is still in place and apply direct pressure to bleeding site. Place tourniquet above site or inflate BP cuff to pressure just above client's systolic BP.	Prevents massive blood loss while awaiting medical assistance if cannula separates or shunt is dislodged.

ACTIONS/INTERVENTIONS	RATIONALE
Infection	
Assess skin around vascular access, noting redness, swelling, local warmth, exudate, tenderness.	Signs of local infection, which can progress to sepsis if untreated.
Avoid contamination of access site. Use aseptic technique and masks when giving shunt care, applying/changing dressings, and when starting/completing dialysis process.	Prevents introduction of organisms that can cause infection.
Monitor temperature. Note presence of fever, chills, hypotension.	Signs of infection/sepsis requiring prompt medical intervention.
Collaborative	
Culture the site/obtain blood samples as indicated.	Determines presence of pathogens.
Monitor protime (PT), activated partial thromboplastin time (aPTT) as appropriate.	Provides information about coagulation status, identifies treatment needs, and evaluates effectiveness.
Administer medications as indicated; e.g.:	
Heparin (low-dose);	Infused on arterial side of filter to prevent clotting in the filter without systemic side effects.
Antibiotics (systemic and/or topical).	Prompt treatment of infection may save access, prevent sepsis.
Discuss use of acetylsalicylic acid (ASA), warfarin sodium (Coumadin) as appropriate.	Ongoing low-dose anticoagulation may be useful in maintaining patency of shunt.

NURSING DIAGNOSIS: risk for deficient Fluid Volume

Risk factors may include

Ultrafiltration
Fluid restrictions, actual blood loss (systemic heparinization or disconnection of the shunt)

Possibly evidenced by

[Not applicable; presence of signs and symptoms establishes an *actual* diagnosis.]

DESIRED OUTCOMES/EVALUATION CRITERIA—CLIENT WILL:

Hydration (NOC)

Maintain fluid balance as evidenced by stable/appropriate weight and vital signs, good skin turgor, moist mucous membranes, absence of bleeding.

ACTIONS/INTERVENTIONS	RATIONALE
Fluid Monitoring (NIC)	
Independent	
Measure all sources of I&O. Have client keep diary.	Aids in evaluating fluid status, especially when compared with weight. *Note:* Urine output is an inaccurate evaluation of renal function in dialysis clients. Some individuals have water output with little renal clearance of toxins, whereas others have oliguria or anuria.
Weigh daily, and before/after dialysis run.	Weight loss over precisely measured time is a measure of ultrafiltration and fluid removal. "Dry" weight (after dialysis session) determines how much extra fluid has been removed, and serves as a guide for subsequent dialysis run-time and solution.

ACTIONS/INTERVENTIONS	RATIONALE
Monitor BP, pulse, and hemodynamic pressures if available during dialysis.	Hypotension, tachycardia, falling hemodynamic pressures suggest volume depletion.

Hemodialysis Therapy (NIC)

Note/ascertain whether diuretics and/or antihypertensives are to be withheld.	Dialysis potentiates hypotensive effects if these drugs have been administered.
Verify continuity of shunt/access catheter.	Disconnected shunt/open access permits exsanguination.
Apply external shunt dressing. Permit no puncture of shunt.	Minimizes stress on cannula insertion site to reduce inadvertent dislodgement and bleeding from site.
Place client in a supine/Trendelenburg's position as necessary.	Maximizes venous return if hypotension occurs.
Assess for oozing or frank bleeding at access site, mucous membranes, or incisions/wounds. Hematest/guaiac stools, gastric drainage.	Systemic heparinization during dialysis increases clotting times and places client at risk for bleeding, especially during the first 4 hr after procedure.

Fluid Monitoring (NIC)

Collaborative

Monitor laboratory studies as indicated:	
Hb/Hct;	May be reduced because of anemia, hemodilution, or actual blood loss.
Serum electrolytes and pH;	Imbalances may require changes in the dialysate solution or supplemental replacement to achieve balance.
Clotting times; e.g., PT/aPTT, and platelet count.	Use of heparin to prevent clotting in blood lines and hemofilter alters coagulation and potentiates active bleeding.
Administer IV solutions (e.g., normal saline [NS])/volume expanders (e.g., albumin) during dialysis as indicated;	Saline/dextrose solutions, electrolytes, and $NaHCO_3$ may be infused in the venous side of continuous arteriovenous (CAV) hemofilter when high ultrafiltration rates are used for removal of extracellular fluid and toxic solutes. Volume expanders may be required during/following hemodialysis if sudden/marked hypotension occurs.
Blood/PRCs if needed.	Destruction of RBCs (hemolysis) by mechanical dialysis, hemorrhagic losses, decreased RBC production may result in profound/progressive anemia requiring corrective action.
Reduce rate of ultrafiltration during dialysis as indicated.	Reduces the amount of water being removed and may correct hypotension/hypovolemia.
Administer protamine sulfate as appropriate.	May be needed to return clotting times to normal or if heparin rebound occurs (up to 16 hr after hemodialysis).

NURSING DIAGNOSIS: risk for excess Fluid Volume

Risk factors may include

Rapid/excessive fluid intake: IV, blood, plasma expanders, saline given to support BP during dialysis

Possibly evidenced by

[Not applicable; presence of signs and symptoms establishes an *actual* diagnosis.]

DESIRED OUTCOMES/EVALUATION CRITERIA—CLIENT WILL:

Fluid Balance (NOC)

Maintain "dry weight" within client's normal range; be free of edema; have clear breath sounds and serum sodium levels within normal limits.

ACTIONS/INTERVENTIONS	RATIONALE
Fluid Management (NIC)	
Independent	
Measure all sources of I&O. Weigh routinely.	Aids in evaluating fluid status, especially when compared with weight. Weight gain between treatments should not exceed 0.5 kg/day.
Monitor BP, pulse.	Hypertension and tachycardia between hemodialysis runs may result from fluid overload and/or HF.
Note presence of peripheral/sacral edema, respiratory rales, dyspnea, orthopnea, distended neck veins, ECG changes indicative of ventricular hypertrophy.	Fluid volume excess due to inefficient dialysis or repeated hypervolemia between dialysis treatments may cause/exacerbate HF, as indicated by signs/symptoms of respiratory and/or systemic venous congestion.
Note changes in mentation. (Refer to CP: Renal Dialysis; ND: risk for disturbed Thought Processes.)	Fluid overload/hypervolemia may potentiate cerebral edema (disequilibrium syndrome).
Collaborative	
Monitor serum sodium levels. Restrict sodium intake as indicated.	High sodium levels are associated with fluid overload, edema, hypertension, and cardiac complications.
Restrict PO/IV fluid intake as indicated, spacing allowed fluids throughout a 24-hour period.	The intermittent nature of hemodialysis results in fluid retention/overload between procedures and may require fluid restriction. Spacing fluids helps reduce thirst.

URINARY DIVERSIONS/UROSTOMY (POSTOPERATIVE CARE)

Incontinent urinary diversions: These ostomies require permanent stoma care and external collecting devices.

Ileal conduit: Ureters are anastomosed to a segment of ileum and resected with the blood supply intact (usually 15–20 cm long). The proximal section is closed, and the distal end brought to skin opening to form a stoma (a passageway, not a storage reservoir).

Colonic conduit: This is a similar procedure using a segment of colon.

Ureterostomy: The ureter(s) is brought directly through the abdominal wall to form its own stoma.

Continent urinary diversions: Continent urinary reservoirs (CURs) have become one of the major options for clients to improve their quality of life regarding stoma care and the ability to sleep and travel. Two main continent alternatives are the *catheterizable urinary reservoir* and the *orthotopic neobladder.*

Kock reservoir or Indiana (ileocecal) pouch: A section of intestine is used to form a pouch inside the patient's abdomen, creating a reservoir that the patient periodically drains by inserting a catheter through the nipple valve, or one-way valve integrated into a stoma, thus negating the need for an external collecting device.

Orthotopic continent urinary diversion: Commonly referred to as *neobladder*, most closely resembles the normal urinary anatomy. A section of intestine is used to form a pouch inside the abdomen, creating a reservoir that is then attached to the urethra. The client can then urinate spontaneously; however, intermittent catheterization may be required to manage incomplete emptying of the reservoir.

This plan of care primarily addresses the nursing care of the client with incontinent urinary diversion with a permanent stoma and urine-collecting device.

CARE SETTING

Inpatient acute surgical unit.

RELATED CONCERNS

Cancer, page 857
Peritonitis, page 355
Psychosocial aspects of care, page 770
Surgical intervention, page 788

Client Assessment Database

Data depend on underlying problem, duration, and severity; e.g., malignant bladder tumor, congenital malformations, trauma, chronic infections, or intractable incontinence due to injury/disease of other body systems (e.g., multiple sclerosis). (Refer to appropriate CP.)

TEACHING/LEARNING

Discharge plan considerations: May require assistance with management of ostomy and acquisition of supplies.

Refer to section at end of plan for postdischarge considerations.

DIAGNOSTIC STUDIES

Intravenous pyelogram (IVP): Visualizes size/location of kidneys and ureters and rules out presence of tumors elsewhere in urinary tract.
Urine cytology: Detects tumor cells (cancer markers) in urine (for determining presence and type of tumor).
Cystoscopy with biopsy: Determines tumor location/stage of malignancy. Ultraviolet cystoscopy outlines bladder lesion.
Pelvic MRI or CT scan: Defines size of tumor mass, degree of pelvic spread.
Endoscopy: Evaluates intestines for use as conduit.
Conduitogram: Assesses length and emptying ability of the conduit and presence of stricture, obstruction, reflux, angulation, calculi, or tumor (may complicate or contraindicate use as a urinary diversion).
Bone scan: Determines presence of metastatic disease.
Bilateral pedal lymphangiogram: Determines involvement of pelvic nodes, where bladder tumor easily seeds because of close proximity.

NURSING PRIORITIES

1. Prevent complications.
2. Assist client/SO in physical and psychosocial adjustment.
3. Support independence in self-care.
4. Provide information about procedure/prognosis, treatment needs, potential complications, and resources.

DISCHARGE GOALS

1. Complications prevented/minimized.
2. Adjusting to perceived/actual changes.
3. Self-care needs met by self/with assistance as necessary.
4. Procedure/prognosis, therapeutic regimen, potential complications understood and sources of support identified.
5. Plan in place to meet needs after discharge.

NURSING DIAGNOSIS: risk for impaired Skin Integrity

Risk factors may include

Absence of sphincter at stoma [actual] with continuous flow of urine
Character/flow of urine from stoma
Reaction to product/chemicals; improper fitting of appliance or removal of adhesive

Possibly evidenced by

[Not applicable; presence of signs and symptoms establishes an *actual* diagnosis.]

DESIRED OUTCOMES/EVALUATION CRITERIA—CLIENT WILL:

TISSUE INTEGRITY: Skin and Mucous Membranes (NOC)

Maintain skin integrity.

Ostomy Self-Care (NOC)

Identify individual risk factors.
Demonstrate behaviors/techniques to promote healing/prevent skin breakdown.

ACTIONS/INTERVENTIONS	RATIONALE
Ostomy Care (NIC)	
Independent	
Inspect stoma/peristomal skin. Note irritation, bruises (dark, bluish color), rashes, status of sutures.	Monitors healing process/effectiveness of appliance and identifies areas of concern, need for further evaluation/intervention. Stoma should be pink or reddish similar to mucous membranes. Color changes may be temporary, but persistent changes may require surgical intervention. Early identification of stomal necrosis/ischemia or fungal infection provides for timely interventions to prevent skin necrosis.
Clean with water and pat dry (or use hair dryer on cool setting).	Maintaining a clean/dry area helps prevent skin breakdown.
Handle stoma gently to prevent irritation.	Mucosa has good blood supply and bleeds easily with rubbing or trauma.
Measure stoma periodically; e.g., each appliance change for first 6 weeks, then monthly times six.	As postoperative edema resolves, size of appliance must be altered to ensure proper fit so that urine is collected as it flows from the stoma and contact with the skin is prevented.
Apply effective sealant barrier; e.g., Skin Prep or similar product as recommended by appliance manufacturer.	Protects skin from pouch adhesive, enhances adhesiveness of pouch, and facilitates removal of pouch when necessary. *Note:* Some barriers are designed to be used without skin sealant.
Ensure opening for adhesive backing of pouch is at least 1/16 inch larger than the base of the stoma (Wound, Ostomy and Continence Nursing Society [WOCN] standard) with adequate adhesive area left to apply pouch.	Prevents trauma to the stoma tissue and protects the peristomal skin. Adequate adhesive area is important to maintain a seal. *Note:* Too tight a fit may cause stomal edema or stenosis.
Use a transparent, odor-proof drainable pouch. Keep gauze square/wick over stoma while cleansing area, and have client cough or strain before applying skin barrier wafer.	A transparent appliance during first 4–6 weeks allows easy observation of stoma and stents (when used) without necessity of removing appliance and irritating skin. Covering stoma prevents urine from wetting the peristomal area during pouch changes. Coughing empties distal portion of conduit, followed by a brief pause in drainage to facilitate application of appliance.
Avoid use of karaya-type appliances.	Will not protect skin because urine melts karaya.
Apply waterproof tape around pouch edges if desired.	Reinforces anchoring.
Connect collecting pouch to continuous bedside drainage system when necessary.	May be needed during times when rate of urine formation is increased; e.g., while IV fluids are administered. Weight of the urine can cause pouch to pull loose/leak when pouch becomes more than half full.
Cleanse ostomy pouch on a routine basis, using vinegar solution or commercial solution designed for this purpose.	Frequent pouch changes are irritating to the skin and should be avoided. Emptying and rinsing the pouch with vinegar or commercial solution not only removes bacteria but also deodorizes the pouch.
Change appliance every 3–5 days or as needed for leakage. Remove appliance gently while supporting skin. Use adhesive removers as indicated and wash off completely.	Prevents tissue irritation/destruction associated with "pulling" skin barrier wafer off.
Investigate reports of burning/itching around stoma.	Suggests peristomal irritation or possibly *Candida* infection, both requiring intervention. *Note:* Continuous exposure of skin to urine can cause hyperplasia around stoma, affecting pouch fit and increasing risk of infection.
Evaluate adhesive product and appliance fit on ongoing basis.	Provides opportunity for problem-solving. Determines need for further intervention.
Monitor for distention of lower abdomen (with ileal conduit), assess bowel sounds.	Intestinal distention can cause tension on new suture lines with possibility of rupture.

ACTIONS/INTERVENTIONS	RATIONALE
Collaborative	
Consult with enterostomal nurse.	Helpful in problem-solving and choosing products appropriate for client needs, considering stoma characteristics, client's physical/mental status, and financial resources. In the presence of persistent or recurring problems, the ostomy nurse has a wider range of knowledge and resources. *Note:* WOCN standards mandate that client be capable of changing an ostomy appliance before discharge, or receive home care until such time as client or caregivers are competent.
Apply antifungal spray or powder as indicated.	Assists in healing if peristomal irritation is caused by fungal infection. *Note:* These products can have potent side effects and should be used sparingly. Creams/ointments are to be avoided because they interfere with adhesion of the appliance.

NURSING DIAGNOSIS: disturbed Body Image

May be related to

Biophysical: presence of stoma, loss of control of urine elimination
Psychosocial: altered body structure
Disease process and associated treatment regimen; e.g., cancer

Possibly evidenced by

Verbalization of change in body image, fear of rejection/reaction of others, and negative feelings about body
Actual change in structure and/or function (ostomy)
Not touching/looking at stoma, refusal to participate in care

DESIRED OUTCOMES/EVALUATION CRITERIA—CLIENT WILL:

Body Image (NOC)

Demonstrate beginning acceptance by viewing/touching stoma and participating in self-care.
Verbalize feelings about stoma/illness; begin to deal constructively with situation.
Verbalize acceptance of self in situation, incorporating change into self-concept without negating self-esteem.

ACTIONS/INTERVENTIONS	RATIONALE
Body Image Enhancement (NIC)	
Independent	
Review reason for surgery and future expectations.	Client may find it easier to accept/deal with an ostomy done for chronic/long-term disease (e.g., intractable incontinence, infections) than for traumatic injury.
Ascertain whether counseling was initiated when the possibility and/or necessity of urinary diversion was first discussed.	Provides information about client's/SO's level of knowledge about individual situation and process of acceptance.

ACTIONS/INTERVENTIONS	RATIONALE
Answer all questions concerning urostomy and its function.	Establishes rapport and conveys interest/concern of caregiver. Provides additional information for client to consider.
Encourage client/SO to verbalize feelings. Acknowledge normality of feelings of anger, depression, and grief over loss. Discuss daily "ups and downs" that can occur after discharge.	Provides opportunity to deal with issues/misconceptions. Helps client/SO to realize that feelings experienced are not unusual and that feeling guilty for them is not necessary/helpful. Client needs to recognize feelings before they can be dealt with effectively.
Note behaviors of withdrawal, increased dependency, manipulation, or noninvolvement in care.	Suggestive of problems in adjustment that may require further evaluation and more extensive therapy. May reflect grief response to loss of body part/function and worry over acceptance by others and fear of further disability, or loss of life from cancer.
Provide opportunities for client/SO to view and touch stoma, using the moment to point out positive signs of healing, normal appearance, and so forth.	Although integration of stoma into body image can take months or even years, looking at the stoma and hearing comments (made in a normal, matter-of-fact manner) can help client with this acceptance. Touching stoma reassures client/SO that it is not fragile and that slight movements of stoma actually reflect normal peristalsis.
Provide opportunity for client to deal with ostomy through participation in self-care.	Independence in self-care helps improve self-esteem. In the case of a continent diversion, client needs the energy, ability, and time to intubate the stoma four times a day.
Maintain positive approach during care activities, avoiding expressions of disdain or revulsion. Do not take client's angry expressions personally.	Assists client/SO to accept body changes and feel all right about self. Anger is most often directed at the situation and lack of control individual has over what has happened (powerlessness), not the individual caregiver.
Plan/schedule care activities with client.	Promotes sense of control and gives message that client can handle this situation, enhancing self-esteem.
Discuss contacting ostomy/urostomy visitor and make arrangements for visit if client desires.	Can provide a good support system. Helps reinforce teaching (shared experiences) and facilitates acceptance of change as client realizes "life does go on" and can be relatively normal.
Discuss sexual functioning, medications that promote erection, and penile implant, if applicable, and alternative ways for sexual pleasuring. (Refer to ND: risk for Sexual Dysfunction.)	Client may experience anticipatory anxiety, fear of failure in relation to sex after surgery, usually because of ignorance, lack of knowledge. Surgery that removes the bladder and prostate (removed with the bladder) may disrupt parasympathetic nerve fibers that control erection in men, although newer techniques are available that may be used in individual cases to preserve nerve function.

NURSING DIAGNOSIS: acute Pain

May be related to

Physical factors; e.g., disruption of skin/tissues (incisions/drains)
Biologic: activity of disease process (cancer, trauma)
Psychologic factors; e.g., fear, anxiety

Possibly evidenced by

Reports of pain
Guarding/distraction behaviors, restlessness
Self-focusing
Autonomic responses; e.g., changes in vital signs

DESIRED OUTCOMES/EVALUATION CRITERIA—CLIENT WILL:

Pain Level (NOC)

Verbalize relief/control of pain.
Appear relaxed, able to sleep/rest appropriately.

Pain Control (NOC)

Perform general comfort measures.

ACTIONS/INTERVENTIONS	RATIONALE
Pain Management (NIC)	
Independent	
Assess pain, noting location, characteristics, intensity (0–10 scale).	Helps evaluate degree of discomfort and effectiveness of analgesia or may reveal developing complications; e.g., because abdominal pain usually subsides gradually by the third or fourth postoperative day, continued or increasing pain may reflect delayed healing, peristomal skin irritation, infection, intestinal obstruction.
Auscultate bowel sounds, note passage of flatus.	Indicates reestablishment of bowel function. Lack of return of bowel sounds/function within 72 hr may indicate presence of complication; e.g., peritonitis, hypokalemia, mechanical obstruction.
Note urine flow and characteristics.	Decreased flow may reflect urinary retention (due to edema) with increased pressure in upper urinary tract or leakage into peritoneal cavity (failure of anastomosis). Cloudy urine may be normal (presence of mucus) or indicate infectious process.
Encourage client to verbalize concerns. Active-listen these concerns and provide support by acceptance, remaining with client and giving appropriate information.	Reduction of anxiety/fear can promote relaxation and comfort.
Provide comfort measures; e.g., back rub, repositioning (using body support measures as needed). Assure client that position change will not injure stoma.	Reduces muscle tension, promotes relaxation, and may enhance coping abilities.
Encourage use of relaxation techniques; e.g., guided imagery, visualization, diversional activities.	Helps client rest more effectively and refocuses attention, which may enhance coping ability, reducing pain and discomfort.
Assist with ROM exercises and encourage early ambulation.	Reduces muscle/joint stiffness. Ambulation returns organs to normal position and promotes return of peristalsis/passage of flatus and feelings of general well-being.
Investigate and report abdominal muscle rigidity, involuntary guarding, and rebound tenderness.	Suggestive of peritoneal inflammation, requiring prompt medical intervention.
Collaborative	
Administer medications as indicated; e.g., narcotics, analgesics, patient-controlled analgesia (PCA).	Relieves pain, enhances comfort, and promotes rest. PCA may be more beneficial than intermittent analgesia, especially following radical resection.
Provide sitz baths if indicated.	Relieves local discomfort, reduces edema, and promotes healing of perineal wound associated with radical procedure.

ACTIONS/INTERVENTIONS	RATIONALE
Apply/monitor effects of transcutaneous electrical nerve stimulator (TENS) unit.	Cutaneous stimulation may be used to block transmission of pain stimulus.
Maintain patency of NG tube.	Decompresses stomach/intestines, prevents abdominal distention when intestinal function is impaired.

NURSING DIAGNOSIS: risk for Infection

Risk factors may include

Inadequate primary defenses (e.g., break in skin/incision; reflux of urine into urinary tract)

Possibly evidenced by

[Not applicable; presence of signs and symptoms establishes an *actual* diagnosis.]

DESIRED OUTCOMES/EVALUATION CRITERIA—CLIENT WILL:

Immune Status (NOC)

Achieve timely wound healing, be free of purulent drainage or erythema, and be afebrile.

KNOWLEDGE: Infection Control (NOC)

Verbalize understanding of individual causative/risk factors.
Demonstrate techniques, lifestyle changes to reduce risk.

ACTIONS/INTERVENTIONS — RATIONALE

Infection Protection (NIC)

Independent

ACTIONS/INTERVENTIONS	RATIONALE
Empty ostomy pouch when it becomes one-third full, once IV fluids and continuous pouch drainage have been discontinued.	Reduces risk of urinary reflux and maintains integrity of appliance seal if pouch does not have an antireflux valve.
Document urine characteristics, and note whether changes are associated with reports of flank pain.	Cloudy, odorous urine indicates infection (possibly pyelonephritis); however, urine normally contains mucus after a conduit procedure because of normal secretions of the intestine.
Test urine pH with Nitrazine paper (use fresh specimen, not from pouch); notify physician if greater than 6.5.	Urine is normally acidic, which discourages bacterial growth/UTIs. *Note:* Presence of alkaline urine also creates favorable environment for stone formation in presence of hypercalciuria.
Report sudden cessation of urethral drainage.	Constant drainage usually subsides within 10 days; however, abrupt cessation may indicate plugging and lead to abscess formation.
Note red rash around stoma.	Rash is most commonly caused by yeast. Urine leakage or allergy to appliance or products may also cause red, irritated areas.
Inspect incision line around stoma. Observe and document wound drainage, signs of incisional inflammation, systemic indicators of sepsis.	Provides baseline/comparative reference. Complications may include interrupted anastomosis of intestine/bowel or ureteral conduit, with leakage of bowel contents into abdomen or urine into peritoneal cavity.

ACTIONS/INTERVENTIONS	RATIONALE
Change dressings as indicated when used.	Moist dressings act as a wick to the wound and provide media for bacterial growth.
Assess skin-fold areas in groin, perineum, under arms and breasts.	Use of antibiotics and trapping of moisture in skin-fold areas increases risk of *Candida* infections.
Monitor vital signs.	An elevated temperature suggests incisional infection or UTI and/or respiratory complications.
Auscultate breath sounds.	Client is at high risk for development of respiratory complications because of length of time under anesthesia. Often this client is older and may already have a compromised immune system. Also, painful abdominal incisions cause client to breathe more shallowly than normal and to limit coughing effort. Accumulation of secretions in respiratory tract predisposes to atelectasis and infections.

Collaborative

Use pouch with antireflux valve if available.	Prevents backflow of urine into stoma, reducing risk of infection.
Obtain specimens of exudates, urine, sputum, blood as indicated.	Identifies source of infection/most effective treatment. Infected urine may cause pyelonephritis. *Note:* Urine specimen must be obtained from the conduit because the pouch is considered contaminated.
Administer medications as indicated; e.g.:	
Cephalosporins; e.g., cefoxitin (Mefoxin), cefazolin (Ancef);	Given to treat identified infection or may be given prophylactically, especially with history of recurrent pyelonephritis.
Antifungal powder;	Used to treat yeast infections around stoma.
Ascorbic acid/vitamin C.	Given to acidify urine, reduce bacterial growth/risk of infection. *Note:* Large doses of vitamin C can impair GI absorption of vitamin B_{12}, potentiating pernicious anemia.
Assist with injection of IV methylene blue.	Dye appearing in wound drainage signifies urine leakage into peritoneal cavity and need for surgical repair.

NURSING DIAGNOSIS: impaired Urinary Elimination

May be related to

Surgical diversion, tissue trauma, postoperative edema

Possibly evidenced by

Loss of continence
Changes in amount, character of urine; urinary retention

DESIRED OUTCOMES/EVALUATION CRITERIA—CLIENT WILL:

Urinary Elimination (NOC)

Display continuous flow of urine, with output adequate for individual situation.

ACTIONS/INTERVENTIONS — RATIONALE

Urinary Elimination Management (NIC)

Independent

ACTIONS/INTERVENTIONS	RATIONALE
Note presence of stents/ureteral catheters. Label "right" and "left" and observe urine flow through each.	Stents/ureteral catheters are placed during surgery to facilitate healing of internal anastomosis by keeping it urine free. It is necessary to verify that both kidneys/ureters are functional.

ACTIONS/INTERVENTIONS	RATIONALE
Record urinary output, investigate sudden reduction/cessation of urine flow.	Sudden decrease in urine flow may indicate obstruction/dysfunction (e.g., blockage by edema or mucus) or dehydration. *Note:* Reduced urinary output (not related to hypovolemia) associated with abdominal distention, fever, and clear/watery discharge from incision suggests urinary fistula, also requiring prompt intervention.
Observe and record color of urine. Note hematuria and/or bleeding from stoma.	Urine may be slightly pink, which should clear up in 2–3 days. Rubbing/washing stoma may cause temporary oozing because of vascular nature of tissues. Continued bleeding, frank blood in the pouch, or oozing around the base of stoma requires medical evaluation/intervention.
Position tubing and drainage pouch so that it allows unimpeded flow of urine. Monitor/protect placement of stents.	Blocked drainage allows pressure to build within urinary tract, risking anastomosis leakage and damage to renal parenchyma. *Note:* Stents inserted to maintain patency of ureters during period of postoperative edema may be inadvertently dislodged, compromising urine flow.
Demonstrate self-catheterization techniques and reservoir irrigations as appropriate.	Clients with continent diversions do not require an external collection device. Periodic catheterization empties the internal reservoir and reduces risk of injury from overdistention. Daily irrigations remove accumulated mucus from the reservoir. *Note:* Clients with Kock pouches connected to the urethra are instructed to void every 2 hr during the day and every 3 hr during the night. This is done by bearing down and applying hand pressure on the lower abdomen to aid in emptying the reservoir.
Encourage increased fluids and maintain accurate intake.	Maintains hydration and good urine flow.
Monitor vital signs. Assess peripheral pulses, skin turgor, capillary refill, and oral mucosa. Weigh daily.	Indicators of fluid balance. Reflects level of hydration and effectiveness of fluid replacement therapy.

Collaborative

ACTIONS/INTERVENTIONS	RATIONALE
Administer IV fluids as indicated.	Assists in maintaining hydration/adequate circulating volume and urinary flow.
Monitor electrolytes, ABGs, calcium.	Impaired renal function in client with intestinal conduit increases risk of severe electrolyte and/or acid-base problems; e.g., hyperchloremic acidosis. Elevated calcium levels increase risk of crystal/stone formation, affecting both urinary flow and tissue integrity.
Prepare for diagnostic testing, procedures as indicated.	Retrograde ileogram may be done to evaluate patency of conduit; nephrostomy tube or stents may be inserted to maintain urine flow until edema/obstruction is resolved.

NURSING DIAGNOSIS: risk for Sexual Dysfunction

Risk factors may include

Altered body structure/function, radical resection/treatment procedures
Vulnerability/psychologic concern about response of SO
Disruption of sexual response pattern; e.g., erection difficulty

Possibly evidenced by

[Not applicable; presence of signs and symptoms establishes an *actual* diagnosis.]

DESIRED OUTCOMES/EVALUATION CRITERIA—CLIENT WILL:

Sexual Functioning (NOC)

Verbalize understanding of relationship of physical condition to sexual problems.
Identify satisfying/acceptable sexual practices and explore alternative methods.
Resume sexual relationship as appropriate.

ACTIONS/INTERVENTIONS	RATIONALE
Sexual Counseling (NIC)	
Independent	
Ascertain client's/SO's sexual relationship before the disease and/or surgery. Identify future expectations and desires.	Mutilation and loss of privacy/control of a bodily function can affect client's view of personal sexuality. When coupled with the fear of rejection by SO, the desired level of intimacy can be greatly impaired. Sexual needs are very basic, and client will be rehabilitated more successfully when a satisfying sexual relationship is continued/developed.
Review with client/SO anatomy and physiology of sexual functioning in relation to own situation.	Understanding normal physiology helps client/SO understand the mechanisms of nerve damage and need for exploring alternative methods of satisfaction.
Reinforce information given by the physician. Encourage questions. Provide additional information as needed.	Reiteration of previously given information assists client/SO to hear and process the knowledge again, moving toward acceptance of individual limitations/restrictions and prognosis (e.g., that it may take up to 2 yr to regain potency after a radical procedure or that a penile prosthesis may be necessary).
Discuss resumption of sexual activity approximately 6 weeks after discharge, beginning slowly and progressing (e.g., cuddling/caressing until both partners are comfortable with body image/function changes). Include alternative methods of stimulation as appropriate.	Knowing what to expect in progress of recovery helps client avoid performance anxiety/reduce risk of "failure." If the couple is willing to try new ideas, this can assist with adjustment and may help achieve sexual fulfillment.
Encourage dialogue between client/SO. Suggest wearing pouch cover, T-shirt, or shortie nightgown.	Disguising urostomy appliance may aid in reducing feelings of self-consciousness, embarrassment during sexual activity.
Stress awareness of factors that might be distracting (e.g., unpleasant odors and pouch leakage).	Promotes resolution of solvable problems.
Encourage use of sense of humor.	Laughter can help individuals deal more effectively with difficult situation and promote a positive sexual experience.
Problem-solve alternative positions for coitus.	Minimizing awkwardness of appliance and physical discomfort can enhance satisfaction.
Discuss/role-play possible interactions or approaches when dealing with new sexual partners.	Rehearsal helps deal with actual situations when they arise, preventing self-consciousness about "different" body image.
Provide birth control information as appropriate and stress that impotence does not mean client is necessarily sterile.	Confusion about impotency and sterility can lead to an unwanted pregnancy.
Collaborative	
Arrange meeting with an ostomy visitor if appropriate.	Sharing of how these problems have been resolved by others can be helpful and reduce sense of isolation.
Refer to counseling/sex therapy as indicated.	If problems persist longer than several months after surgery, a trained therapist may be required to facilitate communication between client and SO.

NURSING DIAGNOSIS: deficient Knowledge [Learning Need] regarding condition, prognosis, treatment, self-care, and discharge needs

May be related to

Lack of exposure/recall; information misinterpretation
Unfamiliarity with information resources

Possibly evidenced by

Questions; statement of misconception/misinformation
Inaccurate follow-through of instruction/performance of urostomy care
Inappropriate or exaggerated behaviors (e.g., hostile, agitated, apathetic, withdrawn)

DESIRED OUTCOMES/EVALUATION CRITERIA—CLIENT WILL:

KNOWLEDGE: Disease Process (NOC)

Verbalize understanding of condition/disease process, prognosis, and potential complications.

Ostomy Self-Care (NOC)

Verbalize understanding of therapeutic needs.
Correctly perform necessary procedures, explain reasons for the action.
Initiate necessary lifestyle changes.

ACTIONS/INTERVENTIONS | RATIONALE

TEACHING: Disease Process (NIC)

Independent

ACTIONS/INTERVENTIONS	RATIONALE
Evaluate client's emotional and physical capabilities.	These factors affect client's ability to master tasks and willingness to assume responsibility for ostomy care.
Review anatomy, physiology, and implications of surgical intervention. Discuss future expectations.	Provides knowledge base from which client can make informed choices and an opportunity to clarify misconceptions regarding individual situation.
Include written/picture resources.	Provides references after discharge to support client efforts for independence in self-care.
Instruct client/SO in stomal care as appropriate. Allot time for return demonstrations and provide positive feedback for efforts.	Promotes positive management and reduces risk of improper ostomy care.
Ensure that stoma and appliance are odorless, nonleaking.	When client feels confident about urostomy, energy/attention can be focused on other tasks.
Demonstrate padding to absorb urethral drainage; ask client to report changes in amount, odor, character.	Small amount of leakage may continue for several weeks after prostate surgery with bladder left in place (temporary diversion procedure).
Recommend routine clipping/trimming of hair around stoma to edges of pouch adhesive.	Hair can be pulled out when the pouch is changed, causing irritation of hair follicles and increasing risk of local infection.
Encourage clients with Kock pouch to lengthen voiding interval by 1 hr each week unless discomfort noted.	Increases capacity of reservoir to achieve a more normal voiding pattern. Presence of discomfort suggests reservoir is full, necessitating prompt emptying.
Instruct client in a progressive exercise program to include Kegel's exercises and stop/start of urinary stream.	Improves tone of pelvic muscles and the external sphincter to enhance continence when client voids through urethra.
Encourage optimal nutrition.	Promotes wound healing, increases utilization of energy to facilitate tissue repair. Anorexia may be present for several months postoperatively, requiring conscious effort to meet nutritional needs.

ACTIONS/INTERVENTIONS	RATIONALE
Discuss use of acid-ash diet (e.g., cranberries, prunes, plums, cereals, rice, peanuts, noodles, cheese, poultry, fish); avoidance of salt substitutes, sodium bicarbonate, and antacids; and cautious use of products containing calcium.	May be useful in acidifying urine to decrease risk of infection and crystal/stone formation. Products containing bicarbonate/calcium potentiate risk of crystal/stone formation affecting both urinary flow and tissue integrity. *Note:* Use of sulfa drugs requires alkaline urine for optimal absorption, necessitating acid-ash diet/vitamin C supplements be withheld.
Discuss importance of maintaining normal weight.	Changes in weight can affect size of stoma/appliance fit. *Note:* Weight loss of 10–20 lb is not uncommon because of intestinal involvement and anorexia.
Stress necessity of increased fluid intake of at least 2–3 L/day; of cranberry juice or ascorbic acid/vitamin C tablets; avoidance of citrus fruits as indicated.	Maintains urinary output and promotes acidic urine to reduce risk of infection and stone formation. *Note:* Oranges/citrus fruits make urine alkaline and are therefore contraindicated. Large doses of vitamin C can inhibit vitamin B_{12} absorption, requiring periodic monitoring of vitamin B_{12} levels.
Discuss resumption of presurgery level of activity and possibility of sleep disturbance, anorexia, loss of interest in usual activities.	Client should be able to manage same degree of activity as previously enjoyed and in some cases increase activity level except for contact sports. "Homecoming depression" may occur, lasting for up to 3 months after surgery, requiring patience/support and ongoing evaluation.
Encourage regular activity/exercise program.	Immobility/inactivity increases urinary stasis and calcium shift out of bones, potentiating risk of stone formation and resultant urinary obstruction, infection.
Identify signs/symptoms requiring medical evaluation; e.g., changes in character, amount and flow of urine, unusual drainage from wound, fatigue/muscle weakness, anorexia, abdominal distention, confusion.	Early detection and prompt intervention of developing problems such as UTI, stricture, intestinal fistula may prevent more serious complications. Urinary electrolytes (especially chloride) are reabsorbed in the intestinal conduit, which leads to compensatory bicarbonate loss, lowered serum pH (metabolic acidosis), and potassium deficit.
Stress importance of follow-up appointments.	Monitors healing and disease process, provides opportunity for discussion of appliance problems, generalized health, and adaptation to condition. *Note:* Extensive surgery requires prolonged recuperation for regaining strength and endurance.
Identify community resources; e.g., United Ostomy Association, local ostomy support group, enterostomal therapist, visiting nurse, pharmacy/medical supply house.	Continued support after discharge is essential to facilitate the recovery process and client's independence in care. Enterostomal nurse can be very helpful in solving appliance problems and identifying alternatives to meet individual client needs.

POTENTIAL CONSIDERATIONS following acute hospitalization (dependent on client's age, physical condition/presence of complications, personal resources, and life responsibilities)

In addition to postsurgical concerns:

impaired Urinary Elimination—anatomic diversion.

situational low Self-Esteem—loss of/altered control of body function.

BENIGN PROSTATIC HYPERPLASIA (BPH)

Benign prostatic hyperplasia is characterized by progressive enlargement of the prostate gland (commonly seen in men older than age 50 years), causing varying degrees of urethral obstruction and restriction of urinary flow.

CARE SETTINGS

Community level, with more acute care provided during outpatient procedures.

RELATED CONCERNS

Prostatectomy, page 604
Psychosocial aspects of care, page 770
Renal failure: acute, page 541

Client Assessment Database

CIRCULATION

May exhibit: Elevated BP (renal effects of advanced enlargement)

ELIMINATION

May report:
Decreased force/caliber of urinary stream, dribbling
Hesitancy in initiating voiding
Inability to empty bladder completely, urgency and frequency of urination
Nocturia, dysuria, hematuria
Sitting to void, straining to initiate voiding
Recurrent UTIs, history of calculi (urinary stasis)
Chronic constipation (protrusion of prostate into rectum)

May exhibit:
Firm mass in lower abdomen (distended bladder), bladder tenderness
Inguinal hernia, hemorrhoids (result of increased abdominal pressure required to empty bladder against resistance)

FOOD/FLUID

May report:
Anorexia, nausea, vomiting
Recent weight loss

PAIN/DISCOMFORT

May report:
Suprapubic, flank, or back pain; sharp, intense (in acute prostatitis)
Low back pain

SAFETY

May report: Fever

SEXUALITY

May report:
Concerns about effects of condition/therapy on sexual abilities
Fear of incontinence/dribbling during intimacy
Decrease in force of ejaculatory contractions

May exhibit: Enlarged, tender prostate

TEACHING/LEARNING

May report:
Family history of cancer, hypertension, kidney disease
Use of antihypertensive or antidepressant medications, OTC cold/allergy medications containing sympathomimetics, urinary antibiotics or antibacterial agents
Use of nutrients/herbal supplements for self-treatment of BPH and urinary flow; e.g., saw palmetto, pygeum, pumpkin seed oil, or soy products

Discharge plan considerations: May need assistance with management of therapy; e.g., catheter

Refer to section at end of plan for postdischarge considerations.

DIAGNOSTIC STUDIES

Digital rectal exam (DRE): Prostate size and contour can be assessed, nodules evaluated, areas of suspected malignancy detected; also helps determine pelvic floor tone, presence or absence of fluctuance (i.e., prostate abscess) and pain/sensitivity of gland can be assessed.

Transrectal prostatic ultrasound (TRUS): Measures size of prostate and amount of residual urine, locates lesions unrelated to BPH. For client with elevated PSA levels, a TRUS-guided biopsy may be indicated.

Urinalysis: Yellow, dark brown, dark or bright red (bloody) in color; appearance may be cloudy, pH 7 or greater (suggests infection); bacteria, WBCs, RBCs may be present microscopically.

Urine culture: May reveal *Staphylococcus aureus, Proteus, Klebsiella, Pseudomonas,* or *Escherichia coli.*

Urine residual: Performed immediately after voiding to determine the severity of bladder decompensation (may be done by catheterization or by transabdominal ultrasound).

Urine cytology: To rule out bladder cancer.

Uroflowmetry: Helps distinguish poor bladder contractibility (detrusor underactivity) from bladder outlet obstruction (BOO) caused by smooth muscle hypertrophy.

IVP with postvoiding film: Shows delayed emptying of bladder/urine retention, varying degrees of urinary tract obstruction, and presence of prostatic enlargement, bladder diverticula, and abnormal thickening of bladder muscle.

Voiding cystourethrography: May be used instead of IVP to visualize bladder and urethra because it uses local dyes.

Cystourethroscopy: To view degree of prostatic enlargement and bladder wall changes (bladder diverticula).

Cystometrogram (CMG): Measures bladder pressures, evaluates detrusor muscle function and tone. Can be performed under fluoroscopy (videourodynamics) for clients with complex causes of outlet obstruction.

Prostate-specific antigen (PSA): Glycoprotein contained in the cytoplasm of prostatic epithelial cells, detected in the blood of adult men. Level is greatly increased in prostatic cancer but can also be elevated in BPH. *Note:* Research suggests elevated PSA levels with a low percentage of free PSA are more likely associated with prostate cancer than with a benign prostatic condition.

BUN/Cr: Elevated if renal function is compromised.

WBC: May be more than 11,000/mm^3, indicating infection if client is not immunosuppressed.

NURSING PRIORITIES

1. Relieve acute urinary retention.
2. Promote comfort.
3. Prevent complications.
4. Help client deal with psychosocial concerns.
5. Provide information about disease process/prognosis and treatment needs.

DISCHARGE GOALS

1. Voiding pattern normalized.
2. Pain/discomfort relieved.
3. Complications prevented/minimized.
4. Dealing with situation realistically.
5. Disease process/prognosis and therapeutic regimen understood.
6. Plan in place to meet needs after discharge.

NURSING DIAGNOSIS: [acute/chronic] Urinary Retention

May be related to

Mechanical obstruction; enlarged prostate
Decompensation of detrusor musculature
Inability of bladder to contract adequately

Possibly evidenced by

Frequency, hesitancy, inability to empty bladder completely; incontinence/dribbling
Bladder distention, residual urine

DESIRED OUTCOMES/EVALUATION CRITERIA—CLIENT WILL:

Urinary Elimination (NOC)

Void in sufficient amounts with no palpable bladder distention.
Demonstrate postvoid residuals of less than 50 mL, with absence of dribbling/overflow.

ACTIONS/INTERVENTIONS	RATIONALE
Urinary Retention Care (NIC)	
Independent	
Encourage client to void every 2–4 hr and when urge is noted.	May minimize urinary retention/overdistention of the bladder.
Ask client about stress incontinence when moving, sneezing, coughing, laughing, lifting objects.	High urethral pressure inhibits bladder emptying or can inhibit voiding until abdominal pressure increases enough for urine to be involuntarily lost.
Observe urinary stream, noting size and force.	Useful in evaluating degree of obstruction and choice of intervention.
Have client document time and amount of each voiding. Note diminished urinary output. Measure specific gravity as indicated.	Urinary retention increases pressure within the ureters and kidneys, which may cause renal insufficiency. Any deficit in blood flow to the kidney impairs its ability to filter and concentrate substances.
Percuss/palpate suprapubic area.	A distended bladder can be felt in the suprapubic area.
Encourage oral fluids up to 3000 mL daily, within cardiac tolerance, if indicated.	Increased circulating fluid maintains renal perfusion and flushes kidneys, bladder, and ureters of "sediment and bacteria." *Note:* Initially, fluids may be restricted to prevent bladder distention until adequate urinary flow is reestablished.
Monitor vital signs closely. Observe for hypertension, peripheral/dependent edema, changes in mentation. Weigh daily. Maintain accurate I&O.	Loss of kidney function results in decreased fluid elimination and accumulation of toxic wastes; may progress to complete renal shutdown.
Provide/encourage meticulous catheter and perineal care.	Reduces risk of ascending infection.
Recommend sitz bath as indicated.	Promotes muscle relaxation, decreases edema, and may enhance voiding effort.
Collaborative	
Administer medications as indicated:	Medications have long been used as a first-line therapy for clients with mild to moderate symptoms, chosen primarily because of the perceived reduced risk of adverse events and the desire to avoid surgery.
5-α-reductase inhibitors: e.g., finasteride (Proscar), dutasteride (Avodart);	Reduces the size of the prostate and decreases symptoms if taken long-term; however, side effects such as decreased libido and ejaculatory dysfunction may influence client's choice for long-term use.
Alpha-adrenergic antagonists; e.g., phenoxybenzamine (Dibenzyline), alfuzosin (UroXatral), terazosin (Hytrin), doxazosin (Cardura), tamsulosin (Flomax);	These agents block effects of postganglionic synapses that affect smooth muscle and exocrine glands. This action can decrease adverse urinary tract symptoms and increase urinary flow. Studies indicate that these drugs may be as effective as Proscar for outflow obstruction and may have fewer side effects in regard to sexual function.
Antispasmodics; e.g., oxybutynin (Ditropan);	Relieves bladder spasms related to irritation by the catheter.
Rectal suppositories (B&O);	Suppositories are absorbed easily through mucosa into bladder tissue to produce muscle relaxation/relieve spasms.
Antibiotics and antibacterials.	Given to combat infection. May be used prophylactically.
Catheterize for residual urine and leave indwelling catheter as indicated.	Relieves/prevents urinary retention and rules out presence of ureteral stricture. Coudé catheter may be required because the curved tip eases passage of the tube through the prostatic urethra. *Note:* Bladder decompression should be done with caution to observe for signs of adverse reaction; e.g., hematuria (rupture of blood vessels in the mucosa of the overdistended bladder) and syncope (excessive autonomic stimulation).

ACTIONS/INTERVENTIONS	RATIONALE
Irrigate catheter as indicated.	Maintains patency/urinary flow.
Monitor laboratory studies; e.g.:	
BUN, Cr, electrolytes;	Prostatic enlargement (obstruction) eventually causes dilation of upper urinary tract (ureters and kidneys), potentially impairing kidney function and leading to uremia.
Urinalysis and culture.	Urinary stasis potentiates bacterial growth, increasing risk of UTI.
Prepare for/assist with urinary drainage; e.g., cystostomy.	May be indicated to drain bladder during acute episode with azotemia or when surgery is contraindicated because of client's health status.
Prepare for procedures; e.g.:	
Heat therapies; e.g., laser, transurethral microwave thermotherapy (TUMT); radiofrequency/transurethral needle ablation (TUNA); high-intensity ultrasound; water-induced thermotherapy;	Most minimally invasive therapies rely on heat to cause destruction of prostatic tissue. Heat is delivered in a limited and controlled fashion to the central portion of the prostate. Treatment is often completed in a one-time procedure carried out in the physician's office. Long-term outcomes are variable in terms of adequately treating urinary tract symptoms.
Surgical procedures: Transurethral incision of the prostate (TUIP);	A procedure of almost equivalent efficacy to transurethral resection of the prostate (TURP) used for prostates with estimated resected tissue weight of 30 g or less. It may be performed instead of balloon dilation with better outcomes. Procedure can be done in ambulatory or short-stay settings. *Note:* Open prostate resection procedures (TURP) are typically performed on clients with very large prostate glands.
Balloon urethroplasty/transurethral dilation of the prostatic urethra;	Inflation of a balloon-tipped catheter within the obstructed area stretches the urethra and displaces prostatic tissue, to improve urinary flow. *Note:* This treatment mode has not been shown to be highly effective, and has largely been abandoned.
Urethral stent.	Placement of urethral stent is simple and immediately effective for restoring/maintaining patency of the urethral lumen. However, long-term failure rate is high, so this should be used only as a temporary measure until a more definitive procedure can be performed.

NURSING DIAGNOSIS: acute Pain

May be related to

Mucosal irritation: bladder distention, renal colic; urinary infection; radiation therapy

Possibly evidenced by

Reports of pain (bladder/rectal spasm)
Narrowed focus; altered muscle tone, grimacing; distraction behaviors, restlessness
Autonomic responses

DESIRED OUTCOMES/EVALUATION CRITERIA—CLIENT WILL:

Pain Level (NOC)

Report pain relieved/controlled.
Appear relaxed.
Be able to sleep/rest appropriately.

ACTIONS/INTERVENTIONS	RATIONALE
Pain Management (NIC)	
Independent	
Assess pain, noting location, intensity (scale of 0–10), characteristics, duration.	Provides information to aid in determining choice/effectiveness of interventions.
Tape drainage tube to thigh and catheter to the abdomen (if traction not required).	Prevents pull on the bladder and erosion of the penile-scrotal junction.
Recommend bedrest as indicated.	Bedrest may be needed initially during acute retention phase; however, early ambulation can help restore normal voiding patterns and relieve colicky pain.
Provide comfort measures; e.g., back rub, helping client assume position of comfort. Suggest use of relaxation/deep-breathing exercises, diversional activities.	Promotes relaxation, refocuses attention, and may enhance coping abilities.
Encourage use of sitz baths, warm soaks to perineum.	Promotes muscle relaxation.
Collaborative	
Insert catheter and attach to straight drainage as indicated.	Draining bladder reduces bladder tension and irritability.
Administer medications as indicated:	
Narcotics; e.g., meperidine (Demerol);	Given to relieve severe pain, provide physical and mental relaxation.
Antibacterials; e.g., methenamine hippurate (Hiprex);	Reduces bacteria present in urinary tract and those introduced by drainage system.
Antispasmodics and bladder sedatives; e.g., flavoxate (Urispas), oxybutynin (Ditropan).	Relieves bladder irritability.

NURSING DIAGNOSIS: risk for deficient Fluid Volume

Risk factors may include

Postobstructive diuresis from rapid drainage of a chronically overdistended bladder
Endocrine, electrolyte imbalances (renal dysfunction)

Possibly evidenced by

[Not applicable; presence of signs and symptoms establishes an *actual* diagnosis.]

DESIRED OUTCOMES/EVALUATION CRITERIA—CLIENT WILL:

Hydration (NOC)

Maintain adequate hydration as evidenced by stable vital signs, palpable peripheral pulses, good capillary refill, and moist mucous membranes.

ACTIONS/INTERVENTIONS	RATIONALE
Fluid Management (NIC)	
Independent	
Monitor output carefully. Note outputs of 100–200 mL/hr.	Rapid/sustained diuresis could cause client's total fluid volume to become depleted and limits sodium reabsorption in renal tubules.

ACTIONS/INTERVENTIONS	RATIONALE
Encourage increased oral intake based on individual needs.	Client may have restricted oral intake in an attempt to control urinary symptoms, reducing homeostatic reserves and increasing risk of dehydration/hypovolemia.
Monitor BP, pulse. Evaluate capillary refill and oral mucous membranes.	Enables early detection of and intervention for systemic hypovolemia.
Promote bedrest with head elevated.	Decreases cardiac workload, facilitating circulatory homeostasis.
Collaborative	
Monitor electrolyte levels, especially sodium.	As fluid is pulled from extracellular spaces, sodium may follow the shift, causing hyponatremia.
Administer IV fluids (hypertonic saline) as needed.	Replaces fluid and sodium losses to prevent/correct hypovolemia following outpatient procedures.

NURSING DIAGNOSIS: Fear/Anxiety [specify level]

May be related to

Change in health status: possibility of surgical procedure/malignancy
Embarrassment/loss of dignity associated with genital exposure before, during, and after treatment; concern about sexual ability

Possibly evidenced by

Increased tension, apprehension, worries
Expressed concerns regarding perceived changes
Fear of unspecific consequences

DESIRED OUTCOMES/EVALUATION CRITERIA—CLIENT WILL:

Anxiety [or] Fear Self-Control (NOC)

Appear relaxed.
Verbalize accurate knowledge of the situation.
Demonstrate appropriate range of feelings and lessened fear.
Report anxiety is reduced to a manageable level.

ACTIONS/INTERVENTIONS	RATIONALE
Anxiety Reduction (NIC)	
Independent	
Be available to client. Establish trusting relationship with client/SO.	Demonstrates concern and willingness to help. Encourages discussion of sensitive subjects.
Provide information about specific procedures and tests and what to expect afterward; e.g., catheter, bloody urine, bladder irritation. Be aware of how much information client wants.	Helps client understand purpose of what is being done, and reduces concerns associated with the unknown, including fear of cancer. However, overload of information is not helpful and may increase anxiety.
Maintain matter-of-fact attitude in doing procedures/dealing with client. Protect client's privacy.	Communicates acceptance and eases client's embarrassment.
Encourage client/SO to verbalize concerns and feelings.	Defines the problem, providing opportunity to answer questions, clarify misconceptions, and problem-solve solutions.

ACTIONS/INTERVENTIONS	RATIONALE
Reinforce previous information client has been given.	Allows client to deal with reality and strengthens trust in caregivers and information presented.

NURSING DIAGNOSIS: deficient Knowledge [Learning Need] regarding condition, prognosis, treatment, self-care, and discharge needs

May be related to

Lack of exposure/recall, information misinterpretation
Unfamiliarity with information resources
Concern about sensitive area

Possibly evidenced by

Questions, request for information, verbalization of the problem
Inappropriate behaviors; e.g., apathetic, withdrawn
Inaccurate follow-through of instructions, development of preventable complications

DESIRED OUTCOMES/EVALUATION CRITERIA—CLIENT WILL:

KNOWLEDGE: Disease Process (NOC)

Verbalize understanding of disease process/prognosis and potential complications.
Identify relationship of signs/symptoms to the disease process.

KNOWLEDGE: Treatment Regimen (NOC)

Verbalize understanding of therapeutic needs.
Initiate necessary lifestyle/behavior changes.
Participate in treatment regimen.

ACTIONS/INTERVENTIONS — RATIONALE

TEACHING: Disease Process (NIC)

Independent

ACTIONS/INTERVENTIONS	RATIONALE
Review disease process, client expectations.	Provides knowledge base from which client can make informed therapy choices.
Encourage verbalization of fears/feelings and concerns.	Helping client work through feelings can be vital to rehabilitation.
Give information that the condition is not sexually transmitted.	May be an unspoken fear.
Review drug therapy/use of herbal products and diet; e.g., increased fruits, soy beans.	Some clients may prefer to treat with complementary therapy because of decreased occurrence/lessened severity of side effects; e.g., impotence. *Note*: Nutrients known to inhibit prostate enlargement are zinc, soy protein, essential fatty acids, flaxseed, and lycopene. Herbal supplements that client may use are saw palmetto, pygeum, stinging nettle, and pumpkin seed oil.
Recommend avoiding spicy foods, coffee, alcohol, long automobile rides, rapid intake of fluids (particularly alcohol).	May cause prostatic irritation with resulting congestion. Sudden increase in urinary flow can cause bladder distention and loss of bladder tone, resulting in episodes of acute urinary retention.

ACTIONS/INTERVENTIONS	RATIONALE
Address sexual concerns; e.g., during acute episodes of prostatitis, intercourse is avoided, but may be helpful in treatment of chronic condition.	Sexual activity can increase pain during acute episodes but may serve as massaging agent in presence of chronic disease. *Note:* Medications such as finasteride (Proscar) are known to interfere with libido and erections. Alternatives include terazosin (Hytrin), doxazosin mesylate (Cardura), and tamsulosin (Flomax), which do not affect testosterone levels.
Provide information about sexual anatomy and function as it relates to prostatic enlargement. Encourage questions and promote a dialogue about concerns.	Having information about anatomy involved helps client understand the implications of proposed treatments because they might affect sexual performance.
Review signs/symptoms requiring medical evaluation; e.g., cloudy, odorous urine; diminished urinary output; inability to void; presence of fever/chills.	Prompt interventions may prevent more serious complications.
Discuss necessity of notifying other healthcare providers of diagnosis.	Reduces risk of inappropriate therapy; e.g., use of decongestants, anticholinergics, and antidepressants, which can increase urinary retention and may precipitate an acute episode.
Reinforce importance of medical follow-up for at least 6 months to 1 year, including rectal examination, urinalysis.	Recurrence of hypertrophy and/or infection (caused by same or different organisms) is not uncommon and requires changes in therapeutic regimen to prevent serious complications.

POTENTIAL CONSIDERATIONS following acute hospitalization (dependent on client's age, physical condition/presence of complications, personal resources, and life responsibilities)

[acute/chronic] Urinary Retention—urethral obstruction, decompensation of detrusor musculature, loss of bladder tone.

risk for Infection—urinary stasis, invasive procedure (periodic catheterization).

PROSTATECTOMY

Prostatectomy is the removal of the prostate gland. It is a surgical or laser procedure carried out to treat benign prostatic hypertrophy (BPH). Open surgical prostatectomy (either suprapubic or retropubic) is performed when the prostate is overly enlarged (>75 g), the bladder has been damaged, or when there are complicating factors (e.g., cancer). Surgical removal of the prostate is a major procedure with the potential side effects of any major surgical procedure; e.g., anesthesia complications, infection, pneumonia, blood clots.

Prostatectomy types include:

Laser: Obstructing prostatic tissue is vaporized with delivery of directed bursts of energy lasting from 30 to 60 seconds, causing the prostate to shrink. There is less bleeding and quicker recovery time than with TURP. Although laser prostatectomy is being done in routine practice, published data relative to the efficacy of the procedure are currently insufficient for long-term outcomes.

Transurethral resection of the prostate (TURP): Obstructive prostatic tissue of the medial lobe surrounding the urethra is removed by means of a resectoscope introduced through the urethra. TURP is the long-term treatment of choice for BPH.

Suprapubic/open prostatectomy: Obstructing prostatic tissue is removed through a low midline incision made through the bladder. This approach is preferred if bladder stones are present.

Retropubic prostatectomy: Hypertrophied prostatic tissue mass (located high in the pelvic region) is removed through a low abdominal incision without opening the bladder.

Perineal prostatectomy: Large prostatic masses low in the pelvic area are removed through an incision between the scrotum and the rectum. This more radical procedure is done for larger tumors/presence of nerve invasion.

CARE SETTING

Inpatient acute surgical unit.

RELATED CONCERNS

Benign prostatic hyperplasia (BPH), page 596
Cancer, page 857
Psychosocial aspects of care, page 770
Surgical intervention, page 788

Client Assessment Database

Refer to CP: Benign Prostatic Hyperplasia (BPH), p. 596, for assessment information.

Discharge plan considerations: Dependent upon type of procedure, needs may be minimal or client may require assistance with self-care needs, transportation, medical supplies, home maintanence

Refer to section at end of plan for postdischarge considerations.

NURSING PRIORITIES

1. Maintain homeostasis/hemodynamic stability.
2. Promote comfort.
3. Prevent complications.
4. Provide information about surgical procedure/prognosis, treatment, and rehabilitation needs.

DISCHARGE GOALS

1. Urinary flow restored/enhanced.
2. Pain relieved/controlled.
3. Complications prevented/minimized.
4. Procedure/prognosis, therapeutic regimen, and rehabilitation needs understood.
5. Plan in place to meet needs after discharge.

NURSING DIAGNOSIS: impaired Urinary Elimination

May be related to

Mechanical obstruction: blood clots, edema, trauma, surgical procedure
Pressure and irritation of catheter/balloon
Loss of bladder tone due to preoperative overdistention or continued decompression

Possibly evidenced by

Frequency, urgency, hesitancy, dysuria, incontinence, retention
Bladder fullness; suprapubic discomfort

DESIRED OUTCOMES/EVALUATION CRITERIA—CLIENT WILL:

Urinary Elimination (NOC)

Void normal amounts without retention.
Demonstrate behaviors to regain bladder/urinary control.

ACTIONS/INTERVENTIONS	RATIONALE
Urinary Elimination Management (NIC)	
Independent	
Assess urine output and catheter/drainage system, especially during bladder irrigation.	Retention can occur because of edema of the surgical area, blood clots, and bladder spasms.
Assist client to assume normal position to void; e.g., stand and walk to bathroom at frequent intervals after catheter is removed.	Encourages passage of urine and promotes sense of normality.
Record time, amount of voiding, and size of stream after catheter is removed. Note reports of bladder fullness; inability to void, urgency.	The catheter is usually removed 2–5 days after surgery, but voiding may continue to be a problem for some time because of urethral edema and loss of bladder tone.

ACTIONS/INTERVENTIONS	RATIONALE
Encourage client to void when urge is noted but not more than every 2–4 hr per protocol.	Voiding with urge prevents urinary retention. Limiting voids to every 4 hr (if tolerated) increases bladder tone and aids in bladder retraining.
Encourage fluid intake to 3000 mL as tolerated. Limit fluids in the evening once catheter is removed.	Maintains adequate hydration and renal perfusion for urinary flow. "Scheduling" fluid intake reduces need to void/interrupt sleep during the night.
Instruct client in perineal exercises; e.g., tightening buttocks, stopping and starting urine stream.	Helps regain bladder/sphincter/urinary control, minimizing incontinence.
Advise client that "dribbling" is to be expected after catheter is removed and should resolve as recuperation progresses. Provide/instruct in use of continence pads when indicated.	Information helps client deal with the problem. Postoperative incontinence is usually temporary, but stress incontinence (e.g., leaking urine when coughing, laughing, lifting) can persist indefinitely.
Collaborative	
Maintain continuous bladder irrigation (CBI), as indicated, in early postoperative period.	Flushes bladder of blood clots and debris to maintain patency of the catheter/urinary flow.
Measure residual volumes via suprapubic catheter, if present, or with Doppler ultrasound.	Monitors effectiveness of bladder emptying. Residuals more than 50 mL suggest need for continuation of catheter until bladder tone improves.

NURSING DIAGNOSIS: risk for deficient Fluid Volume

Risk factors may include

Vascular nature of surgical area, difficulty controlling bleeding
Restricted intake preoperatively
Postobstructive diuresis

Possibly evidenced by

[Not applicable; presence of signs and symptoms establishes an *actual* diagnosis.]

DESIRED OUTCOMES/EVALUATION CRITERIA—CLIENT WILL:

Hydration (NOC)

Maintain adequate hydration as evidenced by stable vital signs, palpable peripheral pulses, good capillary refill, moist mucous membranes, and appropriate urinary output.
Display no active bleeding.

ACTIONS/INTERVENTIONS	RATIONALE
Fluid Management (NIC)	
Independent	
Monitor I&O.	Indicator of fluid balance and replacement needs. With bladder irrigations, monitoring is essential for estimating blood loss and accurately assessing urine output. *Note:* Following release of urinary tract obstruction, marked diuresis may occur during initial recovery period.

ACTIONS/INTERVENTIONS	RATIONALE
Monitor vital signs, noting increased pulse and respiration, decreased BP, diaphoresis, pallor, delayed capillary refill, and dry mucous membranes.	Dehydration/hypovolemia requires prompt intervention to prevent impending shock. *Note:* Hypertension, bradycardia, and nausea/vomiting suggest "TURP syndrome," requiring immediate medical intervention.
Investigate restlessness, confusion, changes in behavior.	May reflect decreased cerebral perfusion (hypovolemia) or indicate cerebral edema from excessive solution absorbed into the venous sinusoids during TUR procedure (TURP syndrome).
Encourage fluid intake to 3000 mL/day unless contraindicated.	Flushes kidneys/bladder of bacteria and debris but may result in water intoxication/fluid overload if not monitored closely.

Bleeding Reduction (NIC)

Anchor catheter, avoid excessive manipulation.	Movement/pulling of catheter may cause bleeding or clot formation and plugging of the catheter, with bladder distention.
Observe catheter drainage, noting excessive/continued bleeding.	Bleeding is not unusual during first 24 hours (for all but the perineal approach). Continued/heavy bleeding or recurrence of active bleeding requires medical evaluation/intervention.
Evaluate color, consistency of urine; e.g.:	
Bright red with bright red clots;	Usually indicates arterial bleeding and requires aggressive therapy.
Dark burgundy with dark clots, increased viscosity;	Suggests venous source (the most common type of bleeding), which usually subsides on its own.
Bleeding with absence of clots.	May indicate blood dyscrasias or systemic clotting problems.
Inspect dressings/wound drains. Weigh dressings if indicated. Note hematoma formation.	Bleeding may be evident or sequestered within tissues of the perineum.
Avoid taking rectal temperatures and use of rectal tubes/enemas.	May result in referred irritation to prostatic bed and increased pressure on prostatic capsule with risk of bleeding.

Collaborative

Monitor laboratory studies as indicated; e.g.: Hb/Hct, RBCs;	Useful in evaluating blood losses/replacement needs.
Coagulation studies, platelet count.	May indicate developing complications; e.g., depletion of clotting factors, DIC.
Administer IV therapy/blood products as indicated.	May need additional fluids, if oral intake inadequate, or blood products if losses are excessive.
Maintain traction on indwelling catheter; tape catheter to inner thigh.	Traction on the 30-mL balloon positioned in the prostatic urethral fossa creates pressure on the arterial supply of the prostatic capsule to help prevent/control bleeding.
Release traction within 4–5 hr. Document period of application and release of traction if used.	Prolonged traction may cause permanent trauma/problems with urinary control.
Administer stool softeners, laxatives as indicated.	Prevention of constipation/straining for stool reduces risk of rectal-perineal bleeding.

NURSING DIAGNOSIS: risk for Infection

Risk factors may include

Invasive procedures: instrumentation during surgery, catheter, frequent bladder irrigation
Traumatized tissue, surgical incision (e.g., perineal)

Possibly evidenced by

[Not applicable; presence of signs and symptoms establishes an *actual* diagnosis.]

DESIRED OUTCOMES/EVALUATION CRITERIA—CLIENT WILL:

WOUND HEALING: Primary Intention (NOC)

Experience no signs of infection.
Achieve timely healing.

ACTIONS/INTERVENTIONS	RATIONALE
Infection Protection (NIC)	
Independent	
Maintain sterile catheter system; provide regular catheter/meatal care with soap and water, applying antibiotic ointment around catheter site.	Prevents introduction of bacteria and resultant infection/sepsis.
Ambulate with drainage bag dependent.	Avoids backward reflux of urine, which may introduce bacteria into the bladder.
Monitor vital signs, noting low-grade fever, chills, rapid pulse and respiration, restlessness, irritability, disorientation.	Client who has had cystoscopy and/or TURP is at increased risk for surgical/septic shock related to manipulation/instrumentation.
Observe drainage from wounds, around suprapubic catheter.	Presence of drains, suprapubic incision increases risk of infection, as indicated by erythema, purulent drainage.
Change dressings frequently (suprapubic/retropubic and perineal incisions), cleaning and drying skin thoroughly each time.	Wet dressings cause skin irritation and provide media for bacterial growth, increasing risk of wound infection.
Use ostomy-type skin barriers.	Provides protection for surrounding skin, preventing excoriation and reducing risk of infection.
Collaborative	
Administer antibiotics as indicated.	May be given prophylactically because of increased risk of infection with prostatectomy.

NURSING DIAGNOSIS: acute Pain

May be related to

Irritation of the bladder mucosa; reflex muscle spasm associated with surgical procedure and/or pressure from bladder balloon (traction)

Possibly evidenced by

Reports of painful bladder spasms
Facial grimacing, guarding, restlessness
Autonomic responses

DESIRED OUTCOMES/EVALUATION CRITERIA—CLIENT WILL:

Pain Level (NOC)

Report pain is relieved/controlled.
Appear relaxed, sleep/rest appropriately.

Pain Control (NOC)

Demonstrate use of relaxation skills and diversional activities as indicated for individual situation.

ACTIONS/INTERVENTIONS	RATIONALE
Pain Management (NIC)	
Independent	
Assess pain, noting location, intensity (0–10 scale), characteristics.	Changes in pain reports may indicate developing complications requiring further evaluation/intervention. *Note*: Sharp, intermittent pain with urge to void/passage of urine around catheter suggests bladder spasms, which tend to be more severe with suprapubic or TUR approaches (usually decrease by the end of 48 hr).
Maintain patency of catheter and drainage system. Keep tubings free of kinks and clots.	Maintaining a properly functioning catheter and drainage system decreases risk of bladder distention/spasm.
Promote intake of up to 3000 mL/day as tolerated.	Decreases irritation by maintaining a constant flow of fluid over the bladder mucosa.
Give client accurate information about catheter, drainage, and bladder spasms.	Allays anxiety and promotes cooperation with necessary procedures.
Provide comfort measures; e.g., position changes/back rub, therapeutic touch, and diversional activities. Encourage use of relaxation techniques, including deep breathing exercises, visualization, and guided imagery.	Reduces muscle tension, refocuses attention, and may enhance coping abilities.
Collaborative	
Provide sitz baths or heat lamp if indicated.	Promotes tissue perfusion and resolution of edema, and enhances healing (perineal approach).
Administer antispasmodics; e.g.:	
Oxybutynin (Ditropan), flavoxate (Urispas), B & O suppositories;	Relaxes smooth muscle to provide relief of spasms and associated pain.
Propantheline bromide (Pro-Banthine).	Relieves bladder spasms by anticholinergic action. Usually discontinued 24–48 hr before anticipated removal of catheter to promote normal bladder contraction.

NURSING DIAGNOSIS: risk for Sexual Dysfunction

Risk factors may include

Situational crisis (incontinence, leakage of urine after catheter removal, involvement of genital area)
Threat to self-concept/change in health status

Possibly evidenced by

[Not applicable; presence of signs and symptoms establishes an *actual* diagnosis.]

DESIRED OUTCOMES/EVALUATION CRITERIA—CLIENT WILL:

Sexual Functioning (NOC)

Report understanding of sexual function and alterations that may occur with surgery in individual situation.
Discuss concerns about possible changes in body image, sexual functioning with partner/SO and caregiver.
Demonstrate problem-solving skills regarding solutions to problems that occur.

ACTIONS/INTERVENTIONS	RATIONALE
Sexual Counseling (NIC)	
Independent	
Provide openings for client/SO to talk about concerns of incontinence and sexual functioning.	May have anxieties about the effects of surgery and may be hesitant about asking necessary questions. Anxiety may have affected ability to access information given previously.
Discuss basic anatomy. Be honest in answers to client's questions.	The nerve plexus that controls erection runs posteriorly to the prostate through the capsule. In procedures that do not involve the prostatic capsule, impotence and sterility usually are not consequences. Surgical procedure may not provide a permanent cure, and hypertrophy may recur.
Give accurate information about expectation of return of sexual function.	Physiologic impotence occurs when the perineal nerves are cut during radical procedures; with other approaches, sexual activity can usually be resumed within weeks. *Note:* Penile prosthesis may be recommended to facilitate erection and correct impotence following radical perineal procedure. Another option that may restore the ability to have an erection is the use of medications such as sildenafil citrate (Viagra).
Discuss retrograde ejaculation if transurethral/suprapubic approach is used.	Seminal fluid goes into the bladder and is excreted with the urine. This does not interfere with sexual functioning but will decrease fertility and cause urine to be cloudy.
Instruct in perineal and interruption/continuation of urinary stream exercises.	Tightening pelvic floor muscles (Kegel's exercises) prior to standing, coughing and sneezing promotes regaining bladder, and perhaps, erectile function.
Collaborative	
Refer to sexual counselor as indicated.	Persistent/unresolved problems may require professional intervention.

NURSING DIAGNOSIS: deficient Knowledge [Learning Need] regarding condition, prognosis, treatment, self-care, and discharge needs

May be related to

Lack of exposure/recall, information misinterpretation
Unfamiliarity with information resources

Possibly evidenced by

Questions, request for information, statement of misconception
Verbalization of the problem
Inaccurate follow-through of instruction, development of preventable complications

DESIRED OUTCOMES/EVALUATION CRITERIA—CLIENT WILL:

KNOWLEDGE: Disease Process (NOC)

Verbalize understanding of surgical procedure and potential complications.

KNOWLEDGE: Treatment Regimen (NOC)

Verbalize understanding of therapeutic needs.
Correctly perform necessary procedures and explain reasons for actions.
Initiate necessary lifestyle changes.
Participate in therapeutic regimen.

ACTIONS/INTERVENTIONS	RATIONALE
TEACHING: Disease Process (NIC)	
Independent	
Review implications of procedure and future expectations.	Provides knowledge base from which client can make informed choices.
Stress necessity of good nutrition; encourage inclusion of fruits, increased fiber in diet.	Promotes healing and prevents constipation, reducing risk of postoperative bleeding.
Discuss initial activity restrictions; e.g., avoidance of heavy lifting, strenuous exercise, prolonged sitting/long car trips, climbing more than two flights of stairs at a time.	Increased abdominal pressure/straining places stress on the bladder and prostate, potentiating risk of bleeding.
Encourage continuation of perineal exercises.	Facilitates urinary control and alleviation of incontinence.
Instruct in urinary catheter care if present. Identify source for supplies/support.	Promotes independence and competent self-care. (Catheter may be in place for several weeks post discharge.)
Instruct client to avoid tub baths after discharge.	Decreases the possibility of introduction of bacteria/infection, undue tension on incision.
Review signs/symptoms requiring medical evaluation; e.g., erythema, purulent drainage from wound sites; changes in character/amount of urine, presence of urgency/frequency; heavy bleeding, fever, or chills.	Prompt intervention may prevent serious complications. *Note:* Urine may appear cloudy for several weeks until postoperative healing occurs and may appear cloudy after intercourse because of retrograde ejaculation.
Provide written information to client/SO regarding recovery expectations and home management , as indicated (e.g., pain, incision care, catheter-related problems and care)	Anxiety related to hospitalization, procedure performed and associated diagnosis, fatigue, postoperative pain often makes it difficult for client to absorb necessary self-care information.
Stress importance of follow-up care; e.g., evaluation by primary healthcare provider, urologist/oncologist, and laboratory studies.	Monitoring and follow-up can reduce incidence of unaddressed complications. *Note*: PSA levels are monitored to assess for residual tumor. Persistent incontinence and/or other postoperative issues will require additional evaluation/treatment.
Provide information on available community resources; e.g., home-health services, medical equipment supply company, information/support persons.	Can be helpful in assisting client/SO in coping with challenges they are faced with following prostatectomy, whatever the reason for procedure (e.g., BPH, cancer, incontinence).

POTENTIAL CONSIDERATIONS following acute hospitalization (dependent on client's age, physical condition/presence of complications, personal resources, and life responsibilities)

In addition to postsurgical concerns:

impaired Urinary Elimination—loss of bladder tone, possible discharge with catheter in place.

Sexual Dysfunction—leakage of urine, loss of erectile function following radical procedure.

CP 10-1: TURP, hospital, ELOS: 3 Days Urology or Surgical Unit

ND and Categories of Care	Day 1____ (Day of Surgery)	Day 2____ (POD # 1)	Day 3____ (POD # 2)
Impaired urinary elimination R/T mechanical obstruction, loss of bladder tone, therapeutic intervention	Display urine output individually appropriate, few clots and catheter free-flowing	Verbalize understanding of home care needs, S/S to report to healthcare provider	Void normal amounts w/o retention Demonstrate behaviors to regain bladder/urinary control Plan in place to meet post-discharge needs
Referrals		Home Care	
Additional assessments	Characteristics of urinary drainage Urinary output q8hr Presence of spontaneous voiding	→ → →	Voiding frequency, character of urine Amount per void
Client education	Foley catheter function, hygiene	Perineal exercises Home care needs, activity/dietary restrictions, sexual concerns S/S to report to healthcare provider	→ Provide written instructions, schedule for follow-up visits
Additional nursing actions	Foley catheter to straight drain, irrigate/CBI per protocol Bedrest if CBI Bed flat × 8 if epidural anesthesia	→ D/C Stand to void q2–4hr Ambulate as tolerated Encourage fluids to 3 L/day as indicated	 → Per self q4hr → Ad lib →
Pain R/T increased frequency/force of ureteral contractions, tissue trauma, edema	Report pain relieved/controlled	→	→ Verbalize understanding of pain management post discharge
Additional assessments	Pain characteristics/changes, presence of bladder spasms Response to interventions	→ →	→ →
Medications Allergies:	Analgesic of choice IM/PO q4hr Antispasmodic prn	→ PO analgesic → D/C Stool softener/laxative	→ → →
Client education	Reporting of pain/effects of intervention Relaxation techniques		
Additional nursing actions	Routine comfort measures Anchor catheter, avoid manipulation Maintain potency of catheter	→ Sitz bath as indicated	→ →
Risk for deficient fluid volume, R/T nausea and vomiting, postobstructive diuresis	Maintain adequate hydration with VS stable, palpable pulses, good capillary refill, adequate urinary output Free of active bleeding	→ →	→ →
Diagnostic studies		Hb/Hct, RBC	
Additional assessments	Characteristics of catheter drainage VS per postoperative protocol Peripheral pulses, capillary refill, status of skin q8hr I&O q8hr Mental status/restlessness q4hr Temperature q8hr	→ Characteristics of urine → q8hr → → → q8hr →	→ → → D/C → D/C → D/C →
Medications	IV therapy/blood products as indicated	→ D/C	
Client education	Fluid needs/restrictions		
Additional nursing actions	Maintain catheter traction as indicated, release q4hr per protocol Begin PO fluids as tolerated	→ D/C → Advanced diet/fluids as tolerated	 →

UROLITHIASIS (RENAL CALCULI)

Renal calculi, or kidney stones, are formed of mineral deposits, predominant calcium oxalate and calcium phosphate. However, uric acid, struvite, and cystine are also calculus formers. Although renal calculi can form anywhere in the urinary tract, they are most commonly found in the renal pelvis and calyces. Renal calculi can remain asymptomatic until passed into a ureter and/or urine flow is obstructed, at which time the potential for renal damage is acute.

CARE SETTING

Often handled at the community level, however, acute episodes occasionally require inpatient treatment on a medical or surgical unit.

RELATED CONCERNS

Fluid and electrolyte imbalances, page 919
Metabolic acidosis (primary base bicarbonate deficiency), page 492
Metabolic alkalosis (primary base bicarbonate excess), page 495
Psychosocial aspects of care, page 770
Renal failure: acute, page 541

Client Assessment Database

Dependent on size, location, and etiology of calculi.

ACTIVITY/REST

May report: Sedentary occupation or occupation in which client is exposed to high environmental temperatures
Activity restrictions/immobility due to a preexisting condition (e.g., debilitating disease, spinal cord injury)

CIRCULATION

May exhibit: Elevated BP/pulse (pain, anxiety, kidney failure)
Warm, flushed skin, pallor

ELIMINATION

May report: History of recent/chronic UTI, previous obstruction (calculi)
Decreased urinary output, bladder fullness
Burning, urgency with urination
Diarrhea

May exhibit: Oliguria, hematuria, pyuria
Alterations in voiding pattern

FOOD/FLUID

May report: Nausea/vomiting, abdominal tenderness
Diet high in purines, calcium oxalate, and/or phosphates
Insufficient fluid intake, does not drink fluids well

May exhibit: Abdominal distention, decreased/absent bowel sounds
Vomiting

PAIN/DISCOMFORT

May report: Acute episode of excruciating, colicky pain with location depending on stone location; e.g., in the flank in the region of the costovertebral angle; may radiate to back, abdomen, and down to the groin/genitalia. Constant dull pain suggests calculi located in the renal pelvis or calyces.
May be described as acute, severe, and not relieved by positioning or any other measures

May exhibit: Guarding, distraction behaviors, self-focusing
Tenderness in renal areas on palpation

SAFETY

May report: Use of alcohol
Fever; chills

TEACHING/LEARNING

May report: Family history of kidney stones, kidney disease, hypertension, gout, chronic UTI, hereditary disease (renal tubular acidosis, cystinuria, hyperoxaluria)

History of small-bowel disease, previous abdominal surgery, hyperparathyroidism

Use of antibiotics, antihypertensives, sodium bicarbonate, allopurinol, phosphates, thiazides, excessive intake of calcium or vitamin D

Use of herbal remedies for kidney stones (e.g., valerian, skullcap, wild yam, khella, marshmallow, slippery elm)

Discharge plan considerations: May require dietary modifications, exercise program, pain management plan

Refer to section at end of plan for postdischarge considerations.

DIAGNOSTIC STUDIES

Urinalysis: Color may be yellow, dark brown, bloody. Commonly shows RBCs, WBCs, crystals (cystine, uric acid, calcium oxalate), casts, minerals, bacteria, pus. pH may be less than 5.0 (promotes cystine and uric acid stones) or higher than 7.5 (promotes magnesium, struvite, phosphate, or calcium phosphate stones).

Urine (24-hr): Measures urine volume and levels of acidity, calcium, sodium, uric acid, oxalate, citrate and creatinine.

Urine culture: May reveal UTI (*Staphylococcus aureus, Proteus, Klebsiella, Pseudomonas*) as cause for stone development (struvite or infection stone).

Biochemical survey: Elevated levels of magnesium, calcium, uric acid, phosphates, protein, electrolytes.

Serum and urine BUN/Cr: Abnormal (high in serum/low in urine) secondary to high obstructive stone in kidney causing ischemia/necrosis.

Serum chloride and bicarbonate levels: Elevation of chloride and decreased levels of bicarbonate suggest developing renal tubular acidosis.

CBC:

Hb/Hct: Abnormal if client is severely dehydrated, polycythemia is present (encourages precipitation of solids), or client is anemic (hemorrhage, kidney dysfunction/failure).

RBCs: Usually normal.

WBCs: May be increased, indicating infection/septicemia.

Parathyroid hormone (PTH): May be increased if kidney failure present. (PTH stimulates reabsorption of calcium from bones, increasing circulating serum and urine calcium levels.)

Kidney-ureters-bladder (KUB) radiographs: Shows presence of calculi and/or anatomic changes in the area of the kidneys or along the course of the ureter. May show small stones that can pass unnoticed, but KUB usually ordered on client reporting blood in urine or flank pain.

Kidney ultrasound: Screening test may determine obstructive changes and location of stone without the risk of kidney failure that can be induced by contrast medium.

Intrarenal doppler ultrasound: Improves the detection of early obstruction by evaluating for elevated resistive index (RI) in kidney with nondilated collecting system.

Intravenous urogram (IVU; also known as intravenous pylelogram [IVP]): Provides rapid confirmation of urolithiasis as a cause of abdominal or flank pain. Shows abnormalities in anatomical structures (distended ureter) and outline of calculi.

Cystoureteroscopy: Direct visualization of bladder and ureter may reveal stone and/or obstructive effects.

CT scan: Identifies/delineates calculi and other masses and kidney, ureteral, and bladder distention. Contrast is not used because it masks the stones.

NURSING PRIORITIES

1. Alleviate pain.
2. Maintain adequate renal functioning.
3. Prevent complications.
4. Provide information about disease process/prognosis and treatment needs.

DISCHARGE GOALS

1. Pain relieved/controlled.
2. Fluid/electrolyte balance maintained.
3. Complications prevented/minimized.
4. Disease process/prognosis and therapeutic regimen understood.
5. Plan in place to meet needs after discharge.

NURSING DIAGNOSIS: acute Pain

May be related to

Increased frequency/force of ureteral contractions
Tissue trauma, edema formation; cellular ischemia

Possibly evidenced by

Reports of colicky pain
Guarding/distraction behaviors, restlessness, moaning, self-focusing, facial mask of pain, muscle tension
Autonomic responses

DESIRED OUTCOMES/EVALUATION CRITERIA—CLIENT WILL:

Pain Level (NOC)

Report pain is relieved with spasms controlled.
Appear relaxed, able to sleep/rest appropriately.

ACTIONS/INTERVENTIONS	RATIONALE
Pain Management (NIC)	
Independent	
Document location, duration, intensity (0–10 scale), and radiation. Note nonverbal signs; e.g., elevated BP and pulse, restlessness, moaning, thrashing about.	Helps evaluate site of obstruction and progress of calculi movement. Flank pain suggests that stones are in the kidney area, upper ureter. Flank pain radiates to back, abdomen, groin, genitalia because of proximity of nerve plexus and blood vessels supplying other areas. Sudden, severe pain may precipitate apprehension, restlessness, severe anxiety.
Explain cause of pain and importance of notifying caregivers of changes in pain occurrence/characteristics.	Provides opportunity for timely administration of analgesia (helpful in enhancing client's coping ability and may reduce anxiety) and alerts caregivers to possibility of passing of stone/developing complications. Sudden cessation of pain usually indicates stone passage.
Provide comfort measures; e.g., back rub, restful environment.	Promotes relaxation, reduces muscle tension, and enhances coping.
Apply warm compresses to back.	Relieves muscle tension and may reduce reflex spasms.
Assist with/encourage use of focused breathing, guided imagery, diversional activities.	Redirects attention and aids in muscle relaxation.
Encourage/assist with frequent ambulation as indicated and increased fluid intake of at least 3–4 L/day within cardiac tolerance.	Renal colic can be worse in the supine position. Vigorous hydration promotes passing of stone, prevents urinary stasis, and aids in prevention of further stone formation.
Note reports of increased/persistent abdominal pain.	Complete obstruction of ureter can cause perforation and extravasation of urine into perirenal space. This represents an acute surgical emergency.

Collaborative:

Administer medications as indicated:

Narcotics; e.g., morphine sulfate (Astromorph, Duramorph), oral narcotic combination analgesics; e.g., oxycodone and acetaminophen (Percocet); nonsteroidal anti-inflammatory drugs (NSAIDs); e.g., ketorolac (Toradol), oral NSAIDs; e.g., ibuprofen (Motrin, Advil);	Narcotic and NSAID combination is often given intravenously during acute episode to quickly decrease ureteral colic and promote muscle/mental relaxation. Oral analgesics and NSAIDs are helpful to facilitate stone passage after acute attack.

ACTIONS/INTERVENTIONS	RATIONALE
Antispasmodics; e.g., flavoxate (Urispas), oxybutynin (Ditropan); calcium channel blocker; e.g., nifedipine (Adalat);	Decreases reflex spasm and relaxes ureteral smooth muscle, which facilitates stone passage.
Corticosteroids; e.g., prednisone (Deltasone).	May be used short-term to reduce tissue edema to facilitate movement of stone.
Maintain patency of catheters when used.	Prevents urinary stasis/retention, reduces risk of increased renal pressure and infection.

NURSING DIAGNOSIS: impaired Urinary Elimination

May be related to

Stimulation of the bladder by calculi, renal or ureteral irritation
Mechanical obstruction, inflammation

Possibly evidenced by

Urgency and frequency, oliguria (retention)
Hematuria

DESIRED OUTCOMES/EVALUATION CRITERIA—CLIENT WILL:

Urinary Elimination (NOC)

Void in normal amounts and usual pattern.
Experience no signs of obstruction.

ACTIONS/INTERVENTIONS	RATIONALE
Urinary Elimination Enhancement (NIC)	
Independent	
Monitor I&O and characteristics of urine.	Provides information about kidney function and presence of complications; e.g., infection and hemorrhage. Bleeding may indicate increased obstruction or irritation of ureter. *Note:* Hemorrhage due to ureteral ulceration is rare.
Determine client's normal voiding pattern and note variations.	Calculi may cause nerve excitability, which causes sensations of urgent need to void. Usually frequency and urgency increase as calculus nears ureterovesical junction.
Encourage increased fluid intake.	Increased hydration flushes bacteria, blood, and debris and may facilitate stone passage.
Strain all urine. Document any stones expelled and send to laboratory for analysis.	Retrieval of calculi allows identification of type of stone and influences choice of therapy.
Investigate reports of bladder fullness; palpate for suprapubic distention. Note decreased urine output, presence of periorbital/dependent edema.	Urinary retention may develop, causing tissue distention (bladder/kidney), and potentiates risk of infection, renal failure.
Observe for changes in mental status, behavior, or level of consciousness.	Accumulation of uremic wastes and electrolyte imbalances can be toxic to the CNS.

ACTIONS/INTERVENTIONS	RATIONALE
Collaborative	
Maintain patency of indwelling catheters (ureteral, urethral, or nephrostomy) when used.	May be required to facilitate urine flow/prevent retention and corresponding complications. Catheters are positioned above the stone to promote urethral dilation/stone passage. Continuous or intermittent irrigation can be carried out to flush kidneys/ureters and adjust pH of urine to permit dissolution of stone fragments following lithotripsy.
Administer medications as indicated; e.g.:	
Acetazolamide (Diamox), allopurinol (Zyloprim);	Increases urine pH (alkalinity) to reduce formation of acid stones. Antigout agents such as allopurinol (Zyloprim) also lower uric acid production and potential of stone formation.
Hydrochlorothiazide (Esidrix, HydroDIURIL), chlorthalidone (Hygroton);	Diuretics may be used to prevent urinary stasis and decrease calcium stone formation if not caused by underlying disease process such as primary hyperthyroidism or vitamin D abnormalities.
Penicillamine (Cuprimine), tiopronin (Thiola);	Drugs may be prescribed when cystine stones cannot be controlled by increasing fluid intake.
Ammonium chloride; potassium or sodium phosphate;	Reduces phosphate stone formation.
Antibiotics;	Presence of UTI/alkaline urine potentiates stone formation.
Potassium citrate (Polycitra-K), sodium bicarbonate.	Alkalinizing agents to dissolve/prevent reformation of some calculi.
Monitor laboratory studies; e.g., electrolytes, BUN, Cr;	Elevated BUN, Cr, and certain electrolytes indicate presence/degree of kidney dysfunction.
Urine culture and sensitivities.	Determines presence of UTI, which may be causing/complicating symptoms; determines antibiotic therapy.
Prepare client for/assist with endoscopic procedures; e.g.:	
Basket procedure; percutaneous ultrasonic lithotripsy; stent placement;	Calculi in the distal and mid ureter may be removed by fiberoptic ureteroscope that shatters the stone with a shock wave and captures it in a basketing catheter.
Extracorporeal shock wave lithotripsy (ESWL);	ESWL is the most frequently used outpatient procedure for treatment of stones that are not responsive to medical therapy. Kidney stones are pulverized by shock waves delivered from outside the body while client reclines in water bath or on soft cushion. ESWL is not ideal for large stones.
Percutaneous or open incision stone removal.	Surgery may be necessary to remove stone that is (1) too large to pass through ureters, (2) is caught in a difficult place, (3) blocks flow of urine, (4) causes ongoing urinary tract infection, (5) causes constant bleeding, and/or (6) is potentially damaging to kidney tissue. One advantage to the open procedure is that stone fragments are removed at surgery rather than relying on natural passage from the kidneys or urinary tract. Client may have a small drainage tube left in kidney or ureters during the healing process.

NURSING DIAGNOSIS: risk for deficient Fluid Volume

Risk factors may include

Nausea/vomiting (generalized abdominal and pelvic nerve irritation from renal or ureteral colic)
Postobstructive diuresis

Possibly evidenced by

[Not applicable; presence of signs or symptoms establishes an *actual* diagnosis.]

DESIRED OUTCOMES/EVALUATION CRITERIA—CLIENT WILL:

Hydration (NOC)

Maintain adequate fluid balance as evidenced by vital signs and weight within client's normal range, palpable peripheral pulses, moist mucous membranes, good skin turgor.

ACTIONS/INTERVENTIONS	RATIONALE
Fluid/Electrolyte Management (NIC)	
Independent	
Monitor I&O.	Comparing actual and anticipated output may aid in evaluating presence/degree of renal stasis/impairment. *Note:* Impaired kidney functioning and decreased urinary output can result in higher circulating volumes with signs/symptoms of HF.
Document incidence and note characteristics and frequency of vomiting and diarrhea, as well as accompanying or precipitating events.	Nausea/vomiting and diarrhea are commonly associated with renal colic because celiac ganglion serves both kidneys and stomach. Documentation may help rule out other abdominal occurrences as a cause for pain or pinpoint calculi.
Increase fluid intake to 3–4 L/day within cardiac tolerance.	Maintains fluid balance for homeostasis and "washing" action that may flush the stone(s) out. Dehydration and electrolyte imbalance may occur secondary to excessive fluid loss (vomiting and diarrhea).
Monitor vital signs. Evaluate pulses, capillary refill, skin turgor, and mucous membranes.	Indicators of hydration/circulating volume and need for intervention. *Note:* Decreased GFR stimulates production of renin, which acts to raise BP in an effort to increase renal blood flow.
Weigh daily.	Rapid weight changes suggests water loss/retention.
Collaborative	
Monitor Hb/Hct, electrolytes.	Assesses hydration and effectiveness of/need for interventions.
Administer IV fluids.	Maintains circulating volume (if oral intake is insufficient), promoting renal function.
Provide appropriate diet, clear liquids, bland foods as tolerated.	Easily digested foods decrease GI activity/irritation and help maintain fluid and nutritional balance.
Administer medications as indicated: antiemetics; e.g., prochlorperazine (Compazine).	Reduces nausea/vomiting.

NURSING DIAGNOSIS: deficient Knowledge [Learning Need] regarding condition, prognosis, treatment, self-care, and discharge needs

May be related to

Lack of exposure/recall; information misinterpretation
Unfamiliarity with information resources

Possibly evidenced by

Questions, request for information, statement of misconception
Inaccurate follow-through of instructions, development of preventable complications

DESIRED OUTCOMES/EVALUATION CRITERIA—CLIENT WILL:

KNOWLEDGE: Illness Care (NOC)

Verbalize understanding of disease process and potential complications.
Correlate symptoms with causative factors.
Verbalize understanding of therapeutic needs.
Initiate necessary lifestyle changes and participate in treatment regimen.

ACTIONS/INTERVENTIONS	RATIONALE
TEACHING: Disease Process (NIC)	
Independent	
Review disease process and future expectations.	Provides knowledge base from which client can make informed choices.
Stress importance of increased fluid intake; e.g., 3–4 L/day or as much as 6–8 L/day. Encourage client to notice dry mouth and excessive diuresis/diaphoresis and to increase fluid intake whether or not feeling thirsty.	Flushes renal system, decreasing opportunity for urinary stasis and stone formation. Increased fluid losses/dehydration require additional intake beyond usual daily needs.
Review dietary regimen, as individually appropriate:	Diet depends on the type of stone. Understanding reason for modifications provides opportunity for client to make informed choices, increases cooperation with regimen, and may prevent recurrence.
Low-purine diet; e.g., limited lean meat, turkey, legumes, whole grains, alcohol;	Decreases oral intake of uric acid precursors.
Low-oxalate diet; e.g., limited chocolate, caffeine-containing beverages, beets, nuts, rhubarb, strawberries, spinach, and wheat bran.	Reduces calcium-oxalate stone formation.
Limit calcium intake (to about 800 mg/day) when appropriate. Use calcium citrate when supplements are required;	Although not advocating high-calcium diets, researchers are urging that calcium limitation be reexamined. Research suggests that restricting dietary calcium is not helpful in reducing calcium stone formation, and may actually increase oxalate formation. Use of citrate is helpful in binding oxalate and improving calcium absorption.
Shorr regimen: low-calcium/phosphorus diet with aluminum carbonate gel 30–40 mL, 30 min pc and hs;	Prevents phosphoric calculi by forming an insoluble precipitate in the GI tract, reducing the load to the kidney nephrons. Also effective against other forms of calcium calculi. *Note:* May cause constipation.
Encourage foods rich in magnesium, and vitamins B and K.	These nutrients reduce stone formation
Discuss medication and herbal supplement regimen; avoidance of OTC drugs, and reading all product/food ingredient labels.	Drugs will be given to acidify or alkalize urine, depending on underlying cause of stone formation. Ingestion of products containing individually contraindicated ingredients (e.g., calcium, phosphorus) potentiates recurrence of stones. *Note*: Some herbal supplements (e.g., valerian, skullcap, wild yam, khella, marshmallow) are known to have anitspasmodic properties, or are soothing to irritated urinary tissues.
Encourage client to reveal all medications/herbals to physician, pharmacist.	To reduce risk of dangerous interactions, side effects.
Emphasize need for smoking cessation, when indicated.	Cigarette smoking may contribute to kidney stones because it increases urine levels of cadmium, a heavy metal.
Encourage regular activity/exercise program.	Inactivity contributes to stone formation through calcium shifts and urinary stasis.

ACTIONS/INTERVENTIONS	RATIONALE
Active-listen concerns about therapeutic regimen/lifestyle changes.	Helps client work through feelings and gain a sense of control over what is happening.
Identify signs/symptoms requiring medical evaluation; e.g., recurrent pain, hematuria, oliguria.	With increased probability of recurrence of stones, prompt interventions may prevent serious complications.
Demonstrate proper care of incisions/catheters if present.	Promotes competent self-care and independence.

POTENTIAL CONSIDERATIONS following acute hospitalizations (dependent on client's age, physical condition/presence of complications, personal resources, and life responsibilities)

impaired Urinary Elimination—recurrence of calculi.

11

CHAPTER

Women's Reproductive

HYSTERECTOMY

Hysterectomy is the surgical removal of the uterus, most commonly performed for malignancies and certain nonmalignant conditions (e.g., endometriosis, or fibroid tumors, pelvic relaxation with uterine prolapse) that lead to disabling levels of pain, discomfort, uterine bleeding, and emotional stress. The procedure can be done to control life-threatening bleeding/hemorrhage (obstetric or traumatic complication) and in the event of intractable pelvic infection or irreparable rupture of the uterus. The most common postoperative complications (i.e., atelectasis, pneumonia, paralytic ileus, deep vein thrombosis) are similar to any major surgery; however, even the prospect of hysterectomy is said to engender more stress than other comparable surgeries (Parker, 2003).

Abdominal hysterectomy types

Subtotal (partial): Body of the uterus is removed; cervical stump remains.
Total: Removal of the uterus and cervix.
Total with bilateral salpingo-oophorectomy: Removal of uterus, cervix, fallopian tubes, and ovaries is the treatment of choice for invasive cancer (11% of hysterectomies), fibroid tumors that are rapidly growing or produce severe abnormal bleeding (about one-third of all hysterectomies), and endometriosis invading other pelvic organs.
Total pelvic exenteration (TPE): A very complex and aggressive surgical procedure to treat invasive cervical cancer involving a radical hysterectomy with dissection of pelvic lymph nodes and bilateral salpingo-oophorectomy, total cystectomy, and abdominoperineal resection of the rectum. A colostomy and/or urinary conduit are created, and vaginal reconstruction may or may not be performed. These clients require intensive care during the initial postoperative period. (Refer to additional plans of care regarding fecal or urinary diversions as appropriate.)

Vaginal hysterectomy types

Vaginal hysterectomy or *laparoscopically assisted vaginal hysterectomy (LAVH):* Performed in certain conditions, such as uterine prolapse, cystocele/rectocele, carcinoma in situ, and high-risk obesity. Although research suggests that laparoscopic hysterectomy is associated with a higher rate of major complications, the procedures offer the advantages of less pain, no visible (or much smaller) scars, a shorter hospital stay, and shorter recovery period.

CARE SETTING

Inpatient acute surgical unit or short-stay unit, depending on type of procedure.

RELATED CONCERNS

Cancer, page 857
Psychosocial aspects of care, page 770
Surgical intervention, page 788 (for general considerations and interventions)
Thrombophlebitis: deep vein thrombosis, page 108

Client Assessment Database

Data depend on the underlying disease process/need for surgical intervention (e.g., cancer, prolapse, dysfunctional uterine bleeding, severe endometriosis, or pelvic infections unresponsive to medical management) and associated complications (e.g., anemia).

TEACHING/LEARNING

Discharge plan considerations: May need temporary help with transportation, homemaker/maintenance tasks

Refer to section at end of plan for postdischarge considerations.

DIAGNOSTIC STUDIES

Pelvic examination: May reveal uterine/other pelvic organ irregularities, such as masses, tender nodules, visual changes of cervix, requiring further diagnostic evaluation.

Pap smear: Cellular dysplasia reflects possibility of/presence of cancer.

Pelvic ultrasound or computed tomography (CT) scan: Aids in identifying size/location of pelvic mass.

Endovaginal ultrasound (EVUS): Evaluates for endometrial thickening.

Sonohysterogram: A saline-enhanced sonogram useful in delineating polyps and submucosal fibroids.

Hysteroscopy: Viewed by some to be the "gold standard." Uses fiberoptic viewing scope and a distending medium (such as carbon dioxide) to directly view the endometrial cavity. Cannot be used when cervical stenosis or active uterine bleeding present.

Laparoscopy: Done to visualize tumors, bleeding, known or suspected endometriosis. Biopsy may be performed or laser treatment for endometriosis. Rarely, exploratory laparotomy may be done for staging cancer or to assess effects of chemotherapy.

Endometrial sampling: *Dilation and curettage (D&C) with biopsy (endometrial/cervical):* Permits histopathological study of cells to determine presence/location of cancer.

Schiller's test (staining of cervix with iodine): Useful in identifying abnormal cells.

Complete blood count (CBC): Decreased hemoglobin (Hb) may reflect chronic anemia, whereas decreased hematocrit (Hct) suggests active blood loss. Elevated white blood cell (WBC) count may indicate inflammation/infectious process.

Sexually transmitted disease (STD) screen: Human papillomavirus (HPV) is present in 80% of clients with cervical cancer.

NURSING PRIORITIES

1. Support adaptation to change.
2. Prevent complications.
3. Provide information about procedure/prognosis and treatment needs.

DISCHARGE GOALS

1. Dealing realistically with situation.
2. Complications prevented/minimized.
3. Procedure/prognosis and therapeutic regimen understood.
4. Plan in place to meet needs after discharge.

[In addition to the NDs, see nursing actions/interventions listed in CP: Surgical Intervention]

NURSING DIAGNOSIS: situational low Self-Esteem

May be related to

Concerns about changes in femininity, effect on sexual relationship, inability to have children

Religious conflicts

Possibly evidenced by

Expressions of specific concerns/vague comments about result of surgery; fear of rejection or reaction of significant other (SO)

Withdrawal, depression

DESIRED OUTCOMES/EVALUATION CRITERIA—CLIENT WILL:

Self-Esteem (NOC)

Verbalize concerns and indicate healthy ways of dealing with them.

Verbalize acceptance of self in situation and adaptation to change in body/self-image.

ACTIONS/INTERVENTIONS	RATIONALE
Self-Esteem Enhancement (NIC)	
Independent	
Provide time to listen to concerns and fears of client /SO. Discuss client's perceptions of self related to anticipated changes and her specific lifestyle.	Research supports the idea that hysterectomy is physiologically and psychologically stressful for a woman, even when she desires the procedure. Although preoperative instruction and interaction are often performed at the community level, the postoperative care providers can convey interest and concern; and make opportunities for support, teaching and correction of misconceptions; e.g., loss of femininity and sexuality, weight gain, and menopausal body changes.
Provide accurate information, reinforcing information previously given.	Provides opportunity for client to question and assimilate information.
Ascertain individual strengths and identify previous positive coping behaviors.	Helpful to build on strengths already available for client to use in coping with current situation.
Provide open environment for client to discuss concerns about sexuality.	Promotes sharing of beliefs/values about sensitive subject, and identifies misconceptions/myths that may interfere with adjustment to situation. (Refer to ND: risk for Sexual Dysfunction.)
Collaborative	
Refer to pastoral staff, psychiatric clinical nurse specialist, other professionals for counseling as necessary.	May need additional help to resolve feelings about loss.

NURSING DIAGNOSIS: impaired Urinary Elimination/[acute] Urinary Retention

May be related to

Mechanical trauma, surgical manipulation, presence of local tissue edema, hematoma
Sensory/motor impairment: nerve paralysis

Possibly evidenced by

Sensation of bladder fullness, urgency
Small, frequent voiding or absence of urinary output
Overflow incontinence
Bladder distention

DESIRED OUTCOMES/EVALUATION CRITERIA—CLIENT WILL:

Urinary Elimination (NOC)

Empty bladder regularly and completely.

ACTIONS/INTERVENTIONS	RATIONALE
Urinary Elimination Management (NIC)	
Independent	
Note voiding pattern and monitor urinary output, once surgical catheter is removed.	May indicate urinary retention if voiding frequently in small/insufficient amounts (<100 mL).

ACTIONS/INTERVENTIONS	RATIONALE
Palpate bladder. Investigate reports of discomfort, fullness, inability to void.	Perception of bladder fullness, distention of bladder above symphysis pubis indicates urinary retention.
Provide routine voiding measures; e.g., privacy, normal position, running water in sink, pouring warm water over perineum.	Promotes relaxation of perineal muscles and may facilitate voiding efforts.
Provide/encourage good perineal cleansing and catheter care (when present).	Promotes cleanliness, reducing risk of ascending urinary tract infection (UTI).
Assess urine characteristics, noting color, clarity, odor.	Urinary retention, vaginal drainage, and possible presence of intermittent/indwelling catheter increase risk of infection, especially if client has perineal sutures.

Collaborative

Catheterize when indicated/per protocol if client is unable to void or is uncomfortable.	Edema or interference with nerve supply may cause bladder atony/urinary retention requiring decompression of the bladder. *Note:* Indwelling urethral or suprapubic catheter may be inserted intraoperatively if complications are anticipated.
Maintain patency of indwelling catheter; keep drainage tubing free of kinks.	Promotes free drainage of urine, reducing risk of urinary stasis/retention and infection.
Check residual urine volume after voiding as indicated.	May not be emptying bladder completely; retention of urine increases possibility for infection and is uncomfortable/painful.

NURSING DIAGNOSIS: risk for Constipation/Diarrhea

Risk factors may include

Physical factors: abdominal surgery, with manipulation of bowel, weakening of abdominal musculature
Pain/discomfort in abdomen or perineal area
Changes in dietary intake

Possibly evidenced by

[Not applicable; presence of signs and symptoms establishes an *actual* diagnosis.]

DESIRED OUTCOMES/EVALUATION CRITERIA—CLIENT WILL:

Bowel Elimination (NOC)

Display active bowel sounds/peristaltic activity.
Maintain usual pattern of elimination.

Bowel Management (NIC)

Independent

ACTIONS/INTERVENTIONS	RATIONALE
Auscultate bowel sounds. Note abdominal distention, presence of nausea/vomiting.	Indicators of presence/resolution of ileus, affecting choice of interventions.
Assist client with sitting on edge of bed and walking.	Early ambulation helps stimulate intestinal function and return of peristalsis.

ACTIONS/INTERVENTIONS	RATIONALE
Encourage adequate fluid intake, including fruit juices, when oral intake is resumed.	Promotes softer stool; may aid in stimulating peristalsis.
Provide sitz baths.	Promotes muscle relaxation, minimizes discomfort.
Collaborative	
Restrict oral intake as indicated.	Prevents nausea/vomiting until peristalsis returns (1–2 days).
Maintain nasogastric (NG) tube if present.	May be inserted in surgery to decompress stomach.
Provide clear/full liquids and advance to solid foods as tolerated.	When peristalsis begins, food and fluid intake promote resumption of normal bowel elimination.
Administer medications; e.g., stool softeners, mineral oil, laxatives, as indicated.	Promotes formation/passage of softer stool.

NURSING DIAGNOSIS: risk for ineffective Tissue Perfusion, (specify)

Risk factors may include

Hypovolemia
Reduction/interruption of blood flow: pelvic congestion, postoperative tissue inflammation, venous stasis
Intraoperative trauma or pressure on pelvic/calf vessels: lithotomy position during vaginal hysterectomy

Possibly evidenced by

[Not applicable; presence of signs and symptoms establishes an *actual* diagnosis.]

DESIRED OUTCOMES/EVALUATION CRITERIA—CLIENT WILL:

TISSUE PERFUSION: (Specify) (NOC)

Demonstrate adequate perfusion, as evidenced by stable vital signs, palpable pulses, good capillary refill, usual mentation, individually adequate urinary output.
Be free of edema, signs of thrombus formation.

ACTIONS/INTERVENTIONS	RATIONALE
Circulatory Care (NIC)	
Independent	
Monitor vital signs, palpate peripheral pulses and note capillary refill, assess urinary output/characteristics, evaluate changes in mentation.	Indicators of adequacy of systemic perfusion, fluid/blood needs, and developing complications.
Inspect dressings and perineal pads, noting color, amount, and odor of drainage. Weigh pads and compare with dry weight if client is bleeding heavily.	Proximity of large blood vessels to operative site and/or potential for alteration of clotting mechanism (e.g., cancer) increases risk of postoperative hemorrhage.
Turn client and encourage frequent coughing and deep-breathing exercises.	Prevents stasis of secretions and respiratory complications.
Avoid high-Fowler's position and pressure under the knees or crossing of legs.	Creates vascular stasis by increasing pelvic congestion and pooling of blood in the extremities, potentiating risk of thrombus formation.

ACTIONS/INTERVENTIONS	RATIONALE
Assist with/instruct in foot and leg exercises and ambulate as soon as able.	Movement enhances circulation and prevents stasis complications.
Note erythema, swelling of extremity, or reports of sudden chest pain with dyspnea.	May be indicative of development of thrombophlebitis/pulmonary embolus.

Collaborative

ACTIONS/INTERVENTIONS	RATIONALE
Administer IV fluids, blood products as indicated.	Replacement of blood losses maintains circulating volume and tissue perfusion.
Apply antiembolism stockings/ pneumatic compression stocking/boots (sequential compression devices [SCDs]).	Aids in venous return; reduces stasis and risk of thrombosis.
Assist with/encourage use of incentive spirometer.	Promotes lung expansion/minimizes atelectasis.

NURSING DIAGNOSIS: risk for Sexual Dysfunction

Risk factors may include

Altered body structure/function; e.g., shortening of vaginal canal, changes in hormone levels, decreased libido

Possible change in sexual response pattern; e.g., absence of rhythmic uterine contractions during orgasm, vaginal discomfort/pain (dyspareunia)

Possibly evidenced by

[Not applicable; presence of signs and symptoms establishes an *actual* diagnosis.]

DESIRED OUTCOMES/EVALUATION CRITERIA—CLIENT WILL:

Sexual Functioning (NOC)

Verbalize understanding of changes in sexual anatomy/function.

Discuss concerns about body image, sex role, desirability as a sexual partner with SO.

Identify satisfying/acceptable sexual practices and some alternative ways of dealing with sexual expression.

ACTIONS/INTERVENTIONS — RATIONALE

Sexual Counseling (NIC)

Independent

ACTIONS/INTERVENTIONS	RATIONALE
Listen to comments of client/SO.	Sexual concerns are often disguised as humor and/or offhand remarks.
Assess client's/SO's information regarding sexual anatomy/function and effects of surgical procedure.	May have misinformation/misconceptions that can affect adjustment. Negative expectations are associated with poor overall outcome. Changes in hormone levels can affect libido and/or decrease suppleness of the vagina. Although a shortened vagina can eventually stretch, intercourse initially may be uncomfortable/painful.
Identify cultural/value factors and conflicts present.	May affect return to satisfying sexual relationship.
Assist client to be aware of/deal with stage of grieving.	Acknowledging normal process of grieving for actual/perceived changes may enhance coping and facilitate resolution.

ACTIONS/INTERVENTIONS	RATIONALE
Encourage client to share thoughts/concerns with partner.	Open communication can identify areas of agreement/problems and promote discussion and resolution.
Problem-solve solutions to potential problems; e.g., postponing sexual intercourse when fatigued, substituting alternative means of expression, using positions that avoid pressure on abdominal incision, using vaginal lubricant.	Helps client return to desired/satisfying sexual activity.
Discuss expected physical sensations/discomforts, changes in response as appropriate to the individual.	Vaginal pain may be significant following vaginal procedure, or sensory loss may occur because of surgical trauma. Research data show a trend toward more problems with lubrication, arousal, and altered genital sensation after total hysterectomy as compared to vaginal hysterectomy, Altered hormone levels and loss of sensation of rhythmic contractions of the uterus during orgasm can impair sexual satisfaction for some women. *Note:* Many women experience few negative effects because fear of pregnancy is gone, and relief from symptoms often improves sexual pleasure.
Collaborative	
Refer to counselor/sex therapist as needed.	May need additional assistance to promote a satisfactory outcome.

NURSING DIAGNOSIS: risk for dysfunctional Grieving

Risk factors may include

Preloss psychologic symptoms; predisposition for anxiety and feelings of inadequacy
Frequency of major life events

Possibly evidenced by

[Not applicable; presence of signs and symptoms establishes an *actual* diagnosis.]

DESIRED OUTCOMES/EVALUATION CRITERIA—CLIENT WILL:

Grief Resolution (NOC)

Verbalize reality of perceived loss.
Report sense of acceptance and hope for future.

ACTIONS/INTERVENTIONS	RATIONALE
Grief Work Facilitation (NIC)	
Independent	
Provide open environment in which client feels free to realistically discuss feelings and concerns without confrontation.	Therapeutic communication skills such as active-listening, silence, being available, and acceptance provide opportunity and encourage client to talk freely and deal with the perceived loss. Provides opportunity for reflection aiding resolution and acceptance.
Determine client's perception and meaning of current and past losses. Note cultural factors/expectations.	Affects client's response and needs to be acknowledged in planning care. Perceptions and way of expressing self may be result of cultural expectations.

ACTIONS/INTERVENTIONS	RATIONALE
Assess emotional stress client is experiencing.	Being aware of what this operation means to client helps avoid inadvertent casualness or oversolicitude by care providers.
Encourage client to vent feelings appropriately, identifying meaning of loss.	Depending on the reason for the surgery (e.g., cancer or long-term heavy bleeding), the client may be frightened or relieved. She may mourn the loss of ability to fulfill her reproductive role whether or not she has borne children. She may also worry about her wholeness as a woman or have heard stories about problems others have had with the procedure.
Assist SOs to cope with client's responses.	Family may not share client's perspective and be intolerant, not recognizing needs of client.
Identify and problem-solve solutions to existing physical responses; e.g., eating, sleeping, activity levels, and sexual desire.	May need additional assistance to deal with the physical aspects of the potential for grieving.
Note withdrawn behavior, negative self-talk, overconcern with actual/perceived changes.	May indicate difficulty in working through the grief process and need for additional interventions/support.
Include family/SO as appropriate when determining future needs.	Depending on client desires/legal requirements, choices regarding future plans can provide guidance and peace of mind.
Discuss healthy ways of dealing with difficult situation.	Provides opportunity to look toward the future and incorporate perceived loss into lifestyle.

Collaborative

Refer to other resources; e.g., counseling, spiritual/pastoral care, psychotherapy as indicated.	May need additional help to prevent development of dysfunctional grieving and help client move toward a positive future.

NURSING DIAGNOSIS: deficient Knowledge [Learning Need] regarding condition, prognosis, treatment, self-care, and discharge needs

May be related to

Lack of exposure/recall
Information misinterpretation
Unfamiliarity with information resources

Possibly evidenced by

Questions/request for information, statement of misconception
Inaccurate follow-through of instructions, development of preventable complications

DESIRED OUTCOMES/EVALUATION CRITERIA—CLIENT WILL:

KNOWLEDGE: Disease Process (NOC)

Verbalize understanding of condition and potential complications.
Identify relationship of signs/symptoms related to surgical procedure and actions to deal with them.

KNOWLEDGE: Treatment Regimen (NOC)

Verbalize understanding of therapeutic needs.

ACTIONS/INTERVENTIONS	RATIONALE
TEACHING: Disease Process (NIC)	
Independent	
Review effects of surgical procedure and future expectations; e.g., client needs to know she will no longer menstruate or bear children, whether surgical menopause will occur, and the possible need for hormonal replacement.	Provides knowledge base from which client can make informed choices.
Discuss complexity of problems anticipated during recovery; e.g., emotional lability and expectation of feelings of depression/sadness, excessive fatigue, sleep disturbances, urinary problems.	Physical, emotional, and social factors can have a cumulative effect, which may delay recovery, especially if hysterectomy was performed because of cancer. Providing an opportunity for problem-solving may facilitate the process. Client/SO may benefit from the knowledge that a period of emotional lability is normal and expected during recovery.
Discuss resumption of activity. Encourage light activities initially, with frequent rest periods and increasing activities/exercise as tolerated. Stress importance of individual response in recuperation.	Client can expect to feel tired when she goes home and needs to plan a gradual resumption of activities, with return to work an individual matter. Prevents excessive fatigue; conserves energy for healing/tissue regeneration. *Note:* Some studies suggest that recovery from hysterectomy (especially when oophorectomy is done) may take up to four times as long as recovery from other major surgeries (12 months versus 3 months).
Identify individual restrictions; e.g., avoiding heavy lifting and strenuous activities (such as vacuuming, straining at stool), prolonged sitting/driving. Avoid tub baths/douching until physician allows.	Strenuous activity intensifies fatigue and may delay healing. Activities that increase intra-abdominal pressure can strain surgical repairs, and prolonged sitting potentiates risk of thrombus formation. Showers are permitted, but tub baths/douching may cause vaginal or incisional infections and are a safety hazard.
Encourage client to report bowel dysfunction (e.g., constipation, loss of urge to defecate, severe straining, incomplete evacuation, digital evacuation) to healthcare providers, if it occurs.	Constipation is a frequent symptom after hysterectomy, and may be related to undiagnosed irritable bowel syndrome (often present preoperatively) and/or be associated with the particular procedure performed (e.g., vaginal hysterectomy with posterior repair).
Discuss dietary modifications, medicinal bulk agents, stimulation by suppository, as indicated.	Postsurgical bowel dysfunction may be short-term or long-term and may require simple home management measures, or referral for medical intervention.
Review recommendations of resumption of sexual intercourse. (Refer to ND: risk for Sexual Dysfunction.)	When sexual activity is cleared by the physician, it is best to resume activity easily and gently, expressing sexual feelings in other ways or using alternative coital positions.
Identify dietary needs; e.g., high-quality protein, complex carbohydrates, additional iron. Include information about foods to include and avoid in managing menopausal symptoms.	Facilitates healing/tissue regeneration and helps correct anemia when present. Note: Certain vegetables (e.g., broccoli, cabbage, cauliflower, brussels sprouts, turnips) may have protective action against excessive estrogen effects. Some foods/substances to avoid/limit include rich dairy products, sugar, fried foods, caffeine, alcohol, nicotine.
Review hormone replacement therapy (HRT) and route (e.g., oral, injection, patch) when used. Clarify distinction between long-term HRT use for preventative therapy and short-term use for symptom relief.	Total hysterectomy with bilateral salpingo-oophorectomy (surgically induced menopause) requires replacement hormones. Benefits of HRT (particularly estrogen) include protection against osteoporosis and the amelioration of certain postmenapausal discomforts (e.g., sleep disturbance, hot flashes, mood disorders, memory and concentration, libido, and urinary symptoms). However, it is generally recognized that HRT is not cardioprotective, and risks may outweigh benefits.
Encourage taking prescribed drug(s) routinely (e.g., with meals or at bedtime) Determine when patch should be changed, wearing time altered.	Establishes routine for taking drug and reduces potential for discontinuing drug because of nausea (often an early side effect).

ACTIONS/INTERVENTIONS	RATIONALE
Discuss potential side effects; e.g., weight gain, increased skin pigmentation or acne, breast tenderness, headaches, photosensitivity.	Development of some side effects is expected but may require problem-solving in order for the client to continue the hormones, (e.g., change in dosage, change of delivery method, use of analgesics, sunscreen, sunglasses).
Recommend cessation of smoking, especially when receiving estrogen therapy.	Some studies suggest an increased risk of thrombophlebitis, myocardial infarction (MI), cerebrovascular accident (CVA), and pulmonary emboli associated with smoking and concurrent estrogen therapy.
Inquire if client is taking/planning to take vitamins/herbal supplements for menopause; e.g., vitamin C with bioflavonoids, calcium/magnesium, selenium, evening primrose oil, black cohosh, angelica, wild yam.	Client may express desire to use "natural hormones" and feel confused over choices. These substances are numerous and available, and have been the object of media attention. They should be reviewed in terms of expected action, potential interaction, or adverse effects (depending on client's particular situation/reason for hysterectomy).
Review incisional care when appropriate.	Facilitates competent self-care, promoting independence.
Stress importance of follow-up care.	Provides opportunity to ask questions, clear up misunderstandings, and detect developing complications. Note: Client needs to discuss with the physician her particular requirements for follow-up pelvic exams with Pap smear, once surgical healing has occurred. The need and rationale for these exams depends upon the client's reason for hysterectomy (e.g., benign fibroids vs cervical neoplasm).
Identify signs/symptoms requiring medical evaluation; e.g., fever/chills, change in character of vaginal/wound drainage, bright red bleeding.	Early recognition and treatment of developing complications such as infection/hemorrhage may prevent life-threatening situations. *Note:* Hemorrhage may occur as late as 2 weeks postoperatively.

POTENTIAL CONSIDERATIONS following acute hospitalization (dependent on client's age, physical condition/presence of complications, personal resources, and life responsibilities)

In addition to surgical and cancer concerns (if appropriate):

Sexual Dysfunction—altered body structure/function, changes in hormone levels, decreased libido, possible change in sexual response pattern, vaginal discomfort/pain (dyspareunia).

situational low Self-Esteem—concerns about changes in femininity, effect on sexual relationship, inability to have children, religious conflicts.

MASTECTOMY

The choice of treatment for breast cancer depends on tumor type, size, and location, as well as clinical characteristics (staging). Therapy may include surgical intervention with/without radiation, chemotherapy, and hormone therapy. Types of surgery are generally grouped into three categories: radical mastectomy, total mastectomy, and more limited procedures (e.g., segmental, lumpectomy).

Total (simple) mastectomy removes all breast tissue, but all or most axillary lymph nodes and chest muscles are left intact.

Modified radical mastectomy removes the entire breast, some or most lymph nodes, and sometimes the pectoralis minor chest muscles. Major chest muscles are left intact.

Radical (Halsted's) mastectomy is a procedure that is rarely performed because it requires removal of the entire breast, skin, major and minor pectoral muscles, axillary lymph nodes, and sometimes internal mammary or supraclavicular lymph nodes.

Lumpectomy is a limited procedure done on an outpatient basis where only the tumor and some surrounding tissue are removed. For most women with stage I or II breast cancer, breast conservation therapy (lumpectomy followed by radiation therapy) is as effective as mastectomy.

Breast reconstruction is often done at the time of cancer surgery because it does not compromise adjuvant treatment/interfere with cure of the cancer, and it improves the client's adjustment and acceptance. Some oncologists, however, prefer to postpone reconstruction until postprocedure therapy is completed to reduce the risk of postoperative complications.

CARE SETTING

Inpatient acute surgical unit.

RELATED CONCERNS

Cancer, page 857 (for additional nursing interventions regarding cancer treatment)
Psychosocial aspects of care, page 770
Surgical intervention, page 788

Client Assessment Database

ACTIVITY/REST

May report: Work, activity involving frequent/repetitive arm movements
Sleep style (e.g., sleeping on stomach)

CIRCULATION

May exhibit: Unilateral engorgement in affected arm (invaded lymph system)

EGO INTEGRITY

May report: Constant stressors in work/home life
Stress/fear involving diagnosis, prognosis, and future expectations

FOOD/FLUID

May report: Loss of appetite, recent weight loss

PAIN/DISCOMFORT

May report: Pain in advanced/metastatic disease (localized pain rarely occurs in early malignancy)
Some experience discomfort or "funny feeling" in breast tissue
Heavy, painful breasts premenstrually usually indicate fibrocystic disease

SAFETY

May exhibit: Nodular axillary masses
Edema, erythema of involved skin

SEXUALITY

May report: Presence of a breast lump (usually painless), changes in breast symmetry or size
Changes in breast skin (pitting, dimpling), color or temperature (redness), unusual nipple discharge, itching, burning, or retracted nipple or changes in vein pattern
History of early menarche (younger than age 12), late menopause (after age 50), late first pregnancy (after age 30)
Concerns about sexuality/intimacy

May exhibit: Change in breast contour/mass, asymmetry
Dimpling, puckering of skin; changes in skin color/texture; swelling, redness or heat in breast
Retraction of nipple, discharge from nipple (serous, serosanguinous, sanguineous, watery discharge increase likelihood of cancer, especially when accompanied by lump)

TEACHING/LEARNING

May report: Family history of genetically transmitted breast cancer includes those with multiple relatives with breast cancer (maternal and paternal), family history of ovarian cancer along with breast cancer, family history of bilateral or early-onset breast cancer, or breast cancer in a male relative. *Note:* Most breast cancer clients have no relatives with the disease, with only 5%–10% attributable to hereditary factors.
Previous unilateral breast cancer, endometrial or ovarian cancer

Discharge plan considerations: May need assistance with treatments/rehabilitation, decisions, self-care activities, homemaker/maintenance tasks

Refer to section at end of plan for postdischarge considerations.

DIAGNOSTIC STUDIES

Mammography: Visualizes internal structure of the breast; is capable of detecting nonpalpable cancers or tumors that are in early stages of development.

Computer-aided detection and diagnosis (CAD): Helps radiologist detect suspicious abnormalities on mammograms and diagnose more early-stage cancers than mammography alone.

Ductogram (galactogram): Determine cause of a nipple discharge. A fine plastic tube is placed into the opening of the duct at the nipple. A small amount of dye is injected that outlines the shape of the duct on an x-ray, and will show if there is a mass inside the duct.

Ultrasound: May be helpful in distinguishing between solid masses and cysts and in women whose breast tissue is dense; complements findings of mammography.

CT scan and magnetic resonance imaging (MRI): Scanning techniques can detect breast disease, especially larger masses, or tumors in small, dense breasts that are difficult to examine by mammography. These techniques are not suitable for routine screening and are not a substitute for mammography.

Positron emission tomography (PET): Helps detect malignant tissue outside the breast (metastasis); may help determine status of lymph nodes to reduce the need for biopsy.

Scintimammography: A radioactive tracer is injected into vein to detect breast cancer cells. It is helpful in evaluating abnormal mammograms, but is still considered experimental.

Breast biopsy (fine-needle aspiration, core sampling needle biopsy, or excisional): Provides definitive diagnosis of mass and is useful for histologic classification, staging, and selection of appropriate therapies.

Sentinel node biopsy: May eliminate need for axillary dissection in small breast tumors, limiting damage to lymph ducts and nerves.

Hormone receptor assays: Reveal whether cells of excised tumor or biopsy specimens contain hormone receptors (estrogen and progesterone). In malignant cells, the estrogen-plus receptor complex stimulates cell growth and division. About two-thirds of all women with breast cancer are estrogen-receptor positive and tend to respond favorably to the addition of hormone therapy, which extends the disease-free period and increases survival time.

HERr2/neu testing: About one-third of breast cancers have too much of a growth-promoting protein called HER2/neu. Cancer cells with too many copies of this gene tend to grow and spread more aggressively than other breast cancers. HER2/neu–positive breast cancers can be treated with a drug called Herceptin (trastuzumab) that prevents the HER2/neu protein from stimulating breast cancer cell growth.

Ploidy: Characteristic (marker) that refers to the amount of DNA cancer cells contain and helps predict how aggressive a cancer is likely to be. If there is a normal amount of DNA, the cells are said to be diploid. If the amount is abnormal, the cells are aneuploid. Aneuploid breast cancers tend to be faster growing and more likely to recur.

Cell proliferation rate: Assay measures cell proliferation in response to, e.g., certain growth factors, cytokines, mitogens, and nutrients. It can also be used for the analysis of cytotoxic compounds like anticancer drugs.

Chest x-ray, liver function studies, CBC, CT scan of abdomen (liver) and bone scan: Help determine presence and location of metastasis.

Breast cancer genes: Two tumor-suppressor genes, *BRCA-1* and *BRCA-2,* localized on chromosomes 17 and 13, respectively, are associated with a high risk of female beast cancer as well as ovarian cancer, male breast cancer (*BRCA2*), and other cancers. The tests may be performed on young women with more than one family member who has developed breast cancer at an early age.

NURSING PRIORITIES

1. Assist client/SO in dealing with stress of situation/prognosis.
2. Prevent complications.
3. Establish individualized rehabilitation program.
4. Provide information about disease process, procedure, prognosis, and treatment needs.

DISCHARGE GOALS

1. Dealing realistically with situation.
2. Complications prevented/minimized.
3. Exercise regimen initiated.
4. Disease process, surgical procedure, prognosis, and therapeutic regimen understood.
5. Plan in place to meet needs after discharge.

PREOPERATIVE

NURSING DIAGNOSIS: Fear/Anxiety [specify level]

May be related to

Threat of death; e.g., extent of disease
Threat to self-concept: change of body image; scarring, loss of body part, sexual attractiveness
Change in health status

Possibly evidenced by

Increased tension, apprehension, feelings of helplessness/inadequacy
Decreased self-assurance
Self-focus, restlessness, sympathetic stimulation
Expressed concerns regarding actual/anticipated changes in life

DESIRED OUTCOMES/EVALUATION CRITERIA—CLIENT WILL:

Fear [or] Anxiety Self-Control (NOC)

Acknowledge and discuss concerns.
Demonstrate appropriate range of feelings.
Report fear and anxiety are reduced to a manageable level.

ACTIONS/INTERVENTIONS	RATIONALE
Anxiety Reduction (NIC)	
Independent	
Ascertain what information client has about diagnosis, expected surgical intervention, and future therapies. Note presence of denial or extreme anxiety.	Provides knowledge base for the nurse to enable reinforcement of needed information, and helps identify client with high anxiety, low capacity for information processing, and need for special attention. *Note:* Denial may be useful as a coping method for a time, but extreme anxiety needs to be dealt with immediately.
Explain purpose and preparation for diagnostic tests.	Clear understanding of procedures and what is happening increases feelings of control and lessens anxiety.
Provide an atmosphere of concern, openness, and availability, as well as privacy for client/SO. Suggest that SO be present as much as possible/desired.	Time and privacy are needed to provide support, discuss feelings of anticipated loss and other concerns. Therapeutic communication skills, open questions, listening, and so forth facilitate this process.
Encourage questions and provide time for expression of fears. Tell client that stress related to breast cancer can persist for many months and to seek help/support.	Provides opportunity to identify and clarify misconceptions and offer emotional support.
Assess degree of support available to client. Give information about community resources, such as Reach to Recovery, YWCA Encore program. Encourage/provide for visit with a woman who has recovered from a similar surgery.	Can be a helpful resource when client is ready. A peer who has experienced the same process serves as a role model and can provide validity to the comments, hope for recovery/normal future.
Discuss role of rehabilitation after surgery.	Rehabilitation is an essential component of therapy intended to meet physical, social, emotional, and vocational needs so that client can achieve the best possible level of physical and emotional functioning.

POSTOPERATIVE

NURSING DIAGNOSIS: impaired Skin/Tissue Integrity

May be related to

Surgical removal of skin/tissue; altered circulation, presence of edema, drainage; changes in skin elasticity, sensation; tissue destruction (radiation)

Possibly evidenced by

Disruption of skin surface, destruction of skin layers/subcutaneous tissues

DESIRED OUTCOMES/EVALUATION CRITERIA—CLIENT WILL:

WOUND HEALING: Primary Intention (NOC)

Achieve timely wound healing, free of purulent drainage or erythema.
Demonstrate behaviors/techniques to promote healing/prevent complications.

ACTIONS/INTERVENTIONS	RATIONALE
Incision Site Care (NIC)	
Independent	
Assess dressings/wound for characteristics of drainage. Monitor amount of edema, redness, and pain in the incision.	Use of dressings depends on the extent of surgery and the type of wound closure. (Pressure dressings are usually applied initially and are reinforced, not changed.) Drainage occurs because of the trauma of the procedure and manipulation of the numerous blood vessels and lymphatics in the area.
Perform routine assessment of involved arm. Elevate hand/arm with shoulder positioned at appropriate angles (no more than 65 degrees of flexion, 45–65 degrees of abduction, 45–60 degrees of internal rotation) and forearm resting on wedge or pillow as indicated.	Preventing or minimizing edema reduces the discomfort and complications associated with it. Elevation of affected arm facilitates drainage and resolution of edema. *Note:* Lymphedema is present in 10%–30% of clients who have underarm lymph nodes removed. This may develop immediately after surgery or years later.
Monitor temperature.	Early recognition of developing infection enables rapid institution of treatment.
Place in semi-Fowler's position on back or unaffected side; avoid letting the affected arm dangle.	Assists with drainage of fluid through use of gravity.
Avoid measuring blood pressure (BP), injecting medications, or inserting IVs in affected arm.	Increases potential of constriction, infection, and lymphedema on affected side.
Inspect donor/graft site (if done) for color, blister formation; note drainage from donor site.	Color will be affected by availability of circulatory supply. Blister formation provides a site for bacterial growth/infection.
Assess wound drains, periodically noting amount and characteristics of drainage.	Drainage of accumulated fluids (e.g., lymph, blood) enhances healing and reduces the susceptibility to infection. Suction devices (e.g., Hemovac, Jackson-Pratt) are often inserted during surgery to maintain negative pressure in wound. Tubes are usually removed around the third day or when drainage ceases.
Encourage wearing of loose-fitting/nonconstrictive clothing. Tell client not to wear wristwatch or other jewelry on affected arm.	Reduces pressure on compromised tissues, which may improve circulation/healing and minimize lymphedema.
Collaborative	
Administer antibiotics as indicated.	May be given prophylactically or to treat specific infection and enhance healing.

NURSING DIAGNOSIS: acute Pain

May be related to

Surgical procedure; tissue trauma, interruption of nerves, dissection of muscles

Possibly evidenced by

Reports of stiffness, numbness in chest area, shoulder/arm pain, alteration of muscle tone
Self-focusing, distraction/guarding behaviors

DESIRED OUTCOMES/EVALUATION CRITERIA—CLIENT WILL:

Pain Level (NOC)

Express reduction in pain/discomfort.
Appear relaxed, able to sleep/rest appropriately.

ACTIONS/INTERVENTIONS	RATIONALE
Pain Management (NIC)	
Independent	
Assess reports of pain and stiffness, noting location, duration, and intensity (0–10 scale). Note reports of numbness and swelling. Be aware of verbal and nonverbal cues.	Aids in identifying degree of discomfort and need for/effectiveness of analgesia. The amount of tissue, muscle, and lymphatic system removed can affect the amount of pain experienced. Destruction of nerves in axillary region causes numbness in upper arm and scapular region, which may be more intolerable than surgical pain. *Note:* Pain in chest wall can occur from muscle tension, be affected by extremes in heat and cold, and continue for several months.
Discuss normality of phantom breast sensations.	Provides reassurance that sensations are not imaginary and that relief can be obtained.
Assist client to find position of comfort.	Elevation of arm, size of dressings, and presence of drains affect client's ability to relax and rest/sleep effectively.
Provide basic comfort measures (e.g., repositioning on back or unaffected side back rub) and diversional activities. Encourage early ambulation and use of relaxation techniques, guided imagery, therapeutic touch.	Promotes relaxation, helps refocus attention, and may enhance coping abilities.
Splint/support chest during coughing and deep-breathing exercises.	Facilitates participation in activity without undue discomfort.
Give appropriate pain medication on a regular schedule before pain is severe and before activities are scheduled.	Maintains comfort level and permits client to exercise arm and to ambulate without pain hindering efforts.
Collaborative	
Administer narcotics/analgesics as indicated.	Provides relief of discomfort/pain and facilitates rest, participation in postoperative therapy.

NURSING DIAGNOSIS: situational low Self-Esteem

May be related to

Biophysical: disfiguring surgical procedure
Psychosocial: concern about sexual attractiveness

Possibly evidenced by

Actual change in structure/body contour
Verbalization of fear of rejection or of reaction by others, change in social involvement
Negative feelings about body, preoccupation with change or loss, not looking at body, nonparticipation in therapy

DESIRED OUTCOMES/EVALUATION CRITERIA—CLIENT WILL:

Self-Esteem (NOC)

Demonstrate movement toward acceptance of self in situation.
Recognize and incorporate change into self-concept without negating self-esteem.
Set realistic goals and actively participate in therapy program.

ACTIONS/INTERVENTIONS	RATIONALE
Self-Esteem Enhancement (NIC)	
Independent	
Encourage questions about current situation and future expectations. Provide emotional support when surgical dressings are removed.	Loss of the breast causes many reactions, including feeling disfigured, fear of viewing scar, and fear of partner's reaction to change in body.
Identify role concerns as woman, wife, mother, career woman, and so forth.	May reveal how client's self-view has been altered.
Encourage client to express feelings; e.g., anger, hostility, and grief.	Loss of body part, disfigurement, and perceived loss of sexual desirability engender grieving process that needs to be dealt with so that client can make plans for the future. *Note:* Grief may resurface when subsequent procedures are done (e.g., fitting for prosthesis, reconstructive procedure) if postponed.
Discuss signs/symptoms of depression with client/SO.	Common reaction to this type of procedure that needs to be recognized and acknowledged to seek timely intervention as indicated.
Provide positive reinforcement for gains/improvement and participation in self-care/treatment program.	Encourages continuation of healthy behaviors.
Review possibilities for reconstructive surgery and/or prosthetic augmentation.	If feasible, reconstruction provides less disfiguring/"near-normal" cosmetic result. Variations in skin flap may be done for facilitation of reconstructive procedure, which is often performed at the same time as the mastectomy. The associated emotional boost may help client get through the more complex surgical recovery process and adjunctive therapies. *Note:* On occasion, reconstruction may not be done for 3–6 months. A prolonged delay may result in increased tension in relationships and impair client's incorporation of changes into self-concept.
Ascertain feelings/concerns of partner regarding sexual aspects, and provide information and support.	Negative responses directed at client may actually reflect partner's concern about hurting client, fear of cancer/death, difficulty in dealing with personality/behavior changes in client, or inability to look at operative area.

ACTIONS/INTERVENTIONS	RATIONALE
Discuss and refer to support groups, as appropriate.	Provides a place to exchange concerns and feelings with others who have had a similar experience, and identifies ways SO can facilitate client's recovery.

Collaborative

ACTIONS/INTERVENTIONS	RATIONALE
Provide temporary soft prosthesis, if indicated.	Prosthesis of nylon and Dacron fluff may be worn in bra until incision heals if reconstructive surgery is not performed at the time of mastectomy. This may promote social acceptance and allow client to feel more comfortable about body image at the time of discharge.

NURSING DIAGNOSIS: impaired physical Mobility

May be related to

Neuromuscular impairment; pain/discomfort; edema formation

Possibly evidenced by

Reluctance to attempt movement
Limited range-of-motion (ROM), decreased muscle mass/strength

DESIRED OUTCOMES/EVALUATION CRITERIA—CLIENT WILL:

Motivation (NOC)

Display willingness to participate in therapy.
Demonstrate techniques that enable resumption of activities.

Body Mechanics Performance (NOC)

Increase strength of affected body parts.

ACTIONS/INTERVENTIONS — RATIONALE

EXERCISE THERAPY: Muscle Control (NIC)

Independent

ACTIONS/INTERVENTIONS	RATIONALE
Elevate affected arm as indicated.	Promotes venous return, lessening possibility of lymphedema.
Begin passive ROM (e.g., flexion/extension of elbow, pronation/supination of wrist, clenching/extending fingers) as soon as possible.	Early postoperative exercises are usually started in the first 24 hr to prevent joint stiffness that can further limit movement/mobility.
Have client move fingers, noting sensations and color of hand on affected side.	Lack of movement may reflect problems with the intercostal brachial nerve, and discoloration can indicate impaired circulation.
Encourage client to use affected arm for personal hygiene; e.g., feeding, combing hair, washing face.	Increases circulation, helps minimize edema, and maintains strength and function of the arm and hand. These activities use the arm without abduction, which can stress the suture line in the early postoperative period.
Help with self-care activities as necessary.	Conserves client's energy, prevents undue fatigue.
Assist with ambulation and encourage correct posture.	Client will feel unbalanced and may need assistance until accustomed to change. Keeping back straight prevents shoulder from moving forward, avoiding permanent limitation in movement and posture.

ACTIONS/INTERVENTIONS	RATIONALE
Advance exercise as indicated; e.g., active extension of arm and rotation of shoulder while lying in bed, pendulum swings, rope turning, elevating arms to touch fingertips behind head.	Prevents joint stiffness, increases circulation, and maintains muscle tone of the shoulders and arm.
Recommend proper breathing technique of slow, deep breaths during exercise.	Contraction of abdominal muscles helps push fluid out of the cisterna chyli (a lymphatic reservoir) and through the thoracic duct, creating a vacuum effect enhancing drainage.
Progress to hand climbing (walking fingers up wall), clasping hands behind head, and full abduction exercises as soon as client can manage.	Because this group of exercises can cause excessive tension on the incision, they are usually delayed until healing process is well established.
Evaluate presence/degree of exercise-related pain and changes in joint mobility. Measure upper arm and forearm if edema develops.	Monitors progression/resolution of complications. May need to postpone increasing exercises and wait until further healing occurs.
Discuss types of exercises to be done at home to regain strength and enhance circulation in the affected arm.	Exercise program needs to be continued to regain optimal function of the affected side.
Coordinate exercise program into self-care and homemaker activities (e.g., dressing self, washing, dusting, mopping) and leisure activities, such as swimming.	Client is usually more willing to participate or finds it easier to maintain an exercise program that fits into lifestyle and accomplishes tasks as well.
Assist client to identify signs/symptoms of shoulder tension; e.g., inability to maintain posture, burning sensation in postscapular region. Instruct client to avoid sitting or holding arm in dependent position for extended periods.	Altered weight and support put tension on surrounding structures.

Collaborative

Administer medications as indicated, e.g.:	
Analgesics;	Pain needs to be controlled before exercise or client may not participate optimally and incentive to exercise may be lost.
Diuretics.	May be useful in treating and preventing fluid accumulation/lymphedema.
Maintain integrity of elastic bandages or custom-fitted pressure-gradient elastic sleeve.	Promotes venous return and decreases risk/effects of edema formation.
Refer to physical/occupational therapist, lymphedema clinic or specialist.	Provides individual exercise program. Assesses limitations/restrictions regarding employment requirements.

NURSING DIAGNOSIS: deficient Knowledge [Learning Need] regarding condition, prognosis, treatment, self-care, and discharge needs

May be related to

Lack of exposure/recall
Information misinterpretation

Possibly evidenced by

Questions/request for information, statement of misconception
Inaccurate follow-through of instructions, development of preventable complications

DESIRED OUTCOMES/EVALUATION CRITERIA—CLIENT WILL:

KNOWLEDGE: Illness Care (NOC)

Verbalize understanding of disease process and potential complications.
Perform necessary procedures correctly and explain reasons for actions.
Initiate necessary lifestyle changes and participate in treatment regimen.

ACTIONS/INTERVENTIONS	RATIONALE
TEACHING: Disease Process (NIC)	
Independent	
Review disease process, surgical procedure, and future expectations.	Provides knowledge base from which client can make informed choices, including participation in radiation/chemotherapy programs.
Review/have client demonstrate care of drains/wound sites.	Shorter hospital stays may result in discharge with drains in place, requiring more complex care by client/caregivers. Drains may be removed 7–10 days after surgery.
Recommend continuation of exercises, increasing program as healing progresses, for at least a year.	Enhances development of collateral lymphatic channels, reduces the tightening of scar tissue, and maintains muscle strength and function. *Note:* Moderation is important because strenuous activity/exercise increases heart rate and body temperature, which can potentially increase edema.
Discuss necessity for well-balanced, nutritious meals and adequate fluid intake.	Provides optimal nutrition and maintains circulating volume to enhance tissue regeneration/healing process.
Suggest alternating schedule of frequent rest and activity periods, especially in situations when sitting/standing is prolonged.	Prevents/limits fatigue, promotes healing, and enhances feelings of general well-being. Positions in which arm is dangling/extended intensify stress on structure lines, creating muscle tension/stiffness, and may interfere with healing.
Instruct client to protect hands and arms by wearing long sleeves and gloves when gardening, use thimble when sewing, use potholders when handling hot items, use plastic gloves when doing dishes, avoid lifting or moving heavy objects, and do not carry purse or wear jewelry/wristwatch on affected side.	Compromised lymphatic system causes tissues to be more susceptible to infection and/or injury, which may lead to lymphedema.
Demonstrate holding affected arm appropriately; e.g., not dangling the arm, swinging arms with elbows bent when walking, placing arm above heart level when sitting/lying down.	Helps prevent/minimize lymphedema and "frozen shoulder."
Warn against having blood withdrawn or receiving IV fluids/medications or BP measurements on the affected side.	May restrict the circulation and increase risk of infection when the lymphatic system is compromised.
Recommend wearing of a medical identification device.	Prevents unnecessary trauma (e.g., BP measurements, injections) to affected arm in emergency situations.
Demonstrate use of intermittent sequential pumping or low-stretch compression custom-made garments, as appropriate.	Occasionally used in managing lymphedema by promoting circulation and venous return.
Suggest gentle massage of healed incision with emollients.	Stimulates circulation, promotes elasticity of skin, and reduces discomfort associated with phantom breast sensations.
Recommend use of sexual positions that avoid pressure on chest wall. Encourage alternative forms of sexual expression (cuddling, touching) during initial healing process/while operative area is still tender.	Promotes feelings of femininity and sense of ability to resume sexual contact.
Encourage regular self-examination of remaining breast. Determine recommended schedule for mammography.	Identifies changes in breast tissue indicative of recurrent/new tumor development.
Stress importance of regular medical follow-up.	Other treatment may be required as adjunctive therapy, such as radiation. Recurrence of malignant breast tumors also can be identified and managed by oncologist.
Identify signs/symptoms requiring medical evaluation; e.g., breast or arm red, warm, and swollen; edema, purulent wound drainage; fever/chills.	Lymphangitis can occur as a result of infection, causing lymphedema.
Address additional concerns as indicated; e.g., ongoing therapies and expected and/or adverse side effects.	Medications such as tamoxifen (Nolvadex) used as follow-up to surgery/radiation require ongoing involvement in care.

POTENTIAL CONSIDERATIONS following acute hospitalization (dependent on client's age, physical condition/presence of complications, personal resources, and life responsibilities)

In addition to surgical and cancer concerns:

impaired Skin/Tissue Integrity—surgical removal of skin/tissue, altered circulation, presence of edema, drainage; changes in skin elasticity, sensation, tissue destruction (radiation).

situational low Self-Esteem—biophysical, disfiguring surgical procedure, concern about sexual attractiveness.

Self-Care Deficit (specify)—decreased strength/endurance, pain, muscular impairment.

CP 11–1 Sample CP: Mastectomy (Modified Radical), Hospital. ELOS: 2 days

ND and Categories Of Care	Day of Surgery____	Postop Day 1____	Postop Day 2____ (Discharge)
Impaired skin tissue integrity R/T therapeutic interventions	Display wound drainage w/in established limits (__mL) Maintain usual color, sensation, motion in fingers/hand	Participate in self-care activities/beginning exercise program Identify ways to maximize healing/minimize risk of injury to arm	Display early signs of healing w/minimal erythema, absence of purulent drainage, edema resolving Report plan in place to meet postdischarge needs
Referrals	Physical Therapist Occupational Therapist Home Care		
Additional assessments	Dressing/drainage q4hr	→ q8hr Wound characteristics	→
	Presence/degree of edema q8hr	→ qday & Measure upper arm/forearm if edema present	→
	Donor/graft site if used q4hr	→ q8hr	→D/C
	VS q1hr×4 → q4hr	→ q8hr	→q12hr
	I&O & JP drainage q8hr	→	→ Discharge w drain in place/ remove when less than 30ml/24 hrs
	Neurovascular check	→	
	__UE q1hr×4 → q4hr×2	→ q8hr	
Medications	Diuretic if edema present	→	→D/C
Client teaching	Protection of affected arm: shaving, use of deodorant/creams, activity limitations, avoidance of heat/cold, proper posture/positioning of arm, sexual positions to prevent pressure on chest wall, wearing loose-fitting clothing Graduated exercise program incorporating ADLs/homemaking activities	Wound care Gentle massage of healed incision General healthcare needs to promote healing, dietary intake, fluids, rest/pacing self Breast self-examination	Management of JP drain if not removed S/S to report to healthcare provider Use of medical alert device Provide written instructions, schedule for follow-up visits/additional treatment modalities
Additional nursing actions	Position per protocol; HOB elevated 30° or more	→	→
	BRP/chair w/assist	→ Ambulate/up ad lib	→
	Elevate affected arm	→	→
	Turn C, DB, incentive spirometry q2hr	→ DB/IS q2 hr WA	→
	Maintain elastic bandages/ custom-fitted pressure-gradient sleeve if used	→	→
	Reinforce dressing PRN	→ Assist w/ dressing chg	→ D/C dressing
	Encourage progressive exercises & ambulate as tolerated	→	→
	Advance diet as tolerated	→	→
Pain R/T tissue trauma, muscle dissection	Report pain reduced to manageable level	→	Verbalize understanding of therapeutic regimen
	Participate in activities to manage pain	→	→
Additional assessments	Pain characteristics/chges	→	→
	Response to interventions	→	→

ND and Categories Of Care	Day of Surgery____	Postop Day 1____	Postop Day 2____ (Discharge)
Medications: Allergies:	Analgesic of choice IV /PO	→ PO analgesic	→
Client education	Orient to unit/room Reporting of pain/effects of interventions Initial exercises of fingers/wrist of affected arm; ROM exercises of unaffected limbs Relaxation techniques Splinting of chest w/cough, DB, exercise	S/S of shoulder tension; possibility of phantom breast pain Progression of exercises as tolerated Home exercise program	Medication: dose, time/frequency, purpose, side effects
Additional nursing actions	Routine comfort measures Passive ROM/exercises per protocol Assist w/self-care	→ → Advance exercises as tolerated →	→ → →
Self-esteem, situational low R/T perceived disfigurement, psychosocial concerns	Verbalize feelings, verbal/nonverbal communication congruent	→ Participate in care/planning for future View incision	→ Verbalize acceptance of self → Plan in place to meet post discharge needs
Referrals	Social services Reach to Recovery		
Additional assessments	Response to surgical procedure by client and SO Availability/effectiveness of support systems	Future expectations, role concerns, usual coping strategies, past coping successes Understanding of diagnosis	
Client education	Postoperative routines Extent/outcome of surgical procedure Future treatment needs Use of/sources for temporary prosthesis Possibilities for reconstructive surgery/prosthetic augmentation	Community resources for client and SO	S/S to report to health-care provider (depression) Written information regarding diagnosis/treatment options
Additional nursing actions	Discuss normalcy of feelings Encourage participation in self-care at level of ability Provide positive reinforcement for participation in therapeutic regimen	Role-play ways of handling responses of others Provide support/answer questions when dressing removed	Identify options for managing home/work responsibilities; importance of taking time for self

12
CHAPTER

Orthopedic

FRACTURES

A *fracture* is a discontinuity or break in a bone. There are more than 150 fracture classifications. Five major types are as follows:

1. *Incomplete:* Fracture involves only a portion of the cross-section of the bone. One side breaks; the other usually just bends (greenstick).
2. *Complete:* Fracture line involves entire cross-section of the bone, and bone fragments are usually displaced.
3. *Closed:* The fracture does not extend through the skin.
4. *Open:* Bone fragments extend through the muscle and skin, which are potentially infected.
5. *Pathologic:* Fracture occurs in diseased bone (such as cancer, osteoporosis) with no or only minimal trauma.

Fracture treatment centers around three basic principles: reduction, immobilization or stabilization, and preservation of function. Reduction and immobilization can be achieved surgically (open reduction) or through nonsurgical (closed reduction) methods. Closed reduction methods include a wide range of interventions (e.g., simple braces or aluminum splints, plaster or fiberglass casts, metal braces, and/or traction devices). Stable fractures are usually treated with casting. Unstable fractures that are unlikely to reduce may require surgical fixation.

CARE SETTING

Most fractures are managed at the community level. Although a number of the interventions listed here are appropriate for this population, this plan of care addresses more complicated injuries encountered on an inpatient acute medical-surgical unit.

RELATED CONCERNS

Craniocerebral trauma (acute rehabilitative phase), page 218
Pneumonia, page 128
Psychosocia, aspects of care, page 770
Renal failure: acute, page 541
Spinal cord injury (acute rehabilitative phase), page 271
Surgical intervention, page 788
Thrombophlebitis: deep vein thrombosis, page 108

Client Assessment Database

Symptoms of fracture depend on the site, severity, type, and amount of damage to other structures.

ACTIVITY/REST

May report: Weakness, fatigue
Gait and/or mobility problems

May exhibit: Restricted/loss of function of affected part (may be immediate, because of the fracture, or develop secondarily from tissue swelling, pain)
Weakness (e.g., affected extremity or generalized)

CIRCULATION

May exhibit: Hypertension (occasionally seen as a response to acute pain/anxiety) or hypotension (severe blood loss)
Tachycardia (stress response, hypovolemia)
Pulse diminished/absent distal to injury in extremity
Delayed capillary refill, pallor of affected part
Tissue swelling, bruising, or hematoma mass at site of injury

ELIMINATION

May exhibit: Hematuria, sediment in urine, changes in output, acute renal failure (ARF) (with major skeletal muscle damage)

NEUROSENSORY

May report: Loss of/impaired motion or sensation
Muscle spasms, worsening over time
Numbness/tingling (paresthesias)

May exhibit: Local musculoskeletal deformities; e.g., abnormal angulation, posture changes, shortening of limbs, rotation, crepitation (grating sound with movement or touch), muscle spasms, visible weakness/loss of function
Giving way/collapse or locking of joints, dislocations
Agitation (may be related to pain/anxiety or other trauma)
Range-of-motion (ROM) deficits

PAIN/DISCOMFORT

May report: Sudden severe pain at the time of injury (may be localized to the area of tissue/skeletal damage and then become more diffuse; can diminish on immobilization); absence of pain suggests nerve damage
Muscle aching pain, spasms/cramping (after immobilization)

May exhibit: Guarding/distraction behaviors, restlessness
Self-focus

SAFETY

May report: Circumstances of incident that do not support type of injury incurred (suggestive of abuse)

May exhibit: Skin lacerations, tissue avulsion, bleeding, color changes
Localized swelling (may increase gradually or suddenly)
Use of alcohol or other drugs
Presence of fall-risk factors; e.g., age, osteoporosis, dementia, arthritis, other chronic conditions; preexisting (unrecognized) fracture

TEACHING/LEARNING

May report: Use of multiple medications (prescribed/over-the-counter [OTC]) with interactive effects

Discharge plan considerations: May require temporary assistance with transportation, self-care activities, and homemaker/maintenance tasks
May require additional therapy/rehabilitation post discharge, or possible placement in assisted-living/extended-care facility for a period of time

Refer to section at end of plan for postdischarge considerations.

DIAGNOSTIC STUDIES

Radiographic examinations: Determine location and extent of fractures/trauma; may reveal preexisting and yet undiagnosed fracture(s).
Bone scans, tomograms, computed tomography (CT)/magnetic resonance imaging (MRI) scans: Visualize fractures, bleeding, and soft-tissue damage; differentiate between stress/trauma fractures and bone neoplasms; and may be preferred diagnostic tool because of superior ability to image some types of injuries.
Arteriograms: May be done when occult vascular damage is suspected.
Complete blood count (CBC): Hematocrit (Hct) may be increased (hemoconcentration) or decreased (signifying hemorrhage at the fracture site or at distant organs in multiple trauma). Increased white blood cell (WBC) count is a normal stress response after trauma.
Urine creatinine (Cr) clearance: Muscle trauma increases load of Cr for renal clearance.
Coagulation profile: Alterations may occur because of blood loss, multiple transfusions, or liver injury.

NURSING PRIORITIES

1. Prevent further bone/tissue injury.
2. Alleviate pain.
3. Prevent complications.
4. Provide information about condition/prognosis and treatment needs.

DISCHARGE GOALS

1. Fracture stabilized.
2. Pain controlled.
3. Complications prevented/minimized.
4. Condition, prognosis, and therapeutic regimen understood.
5. Plan in place to meet needs after discharge.

NURSING DIAGNOSIS: risk for [additional] Trauma

Risk factors may include

Loss of skeletal integrity (fractures)/movement of bone fragments

Possibly evidenced by

[Not applicable; presence of signs and symptoms establishes an *actual* diagnosis.]

DESIRED OUTCOMES/EVALUATION CRITERIA—CLIENT WILL:

Bone Healing (NOC)

Maintain stabilization and alignment of fracture(s).
Display callus formation/beginning union at fracture site as appropriate.

Risk Control (NOC)

Demonstrate body mechanics that promote stability at fracture site.

ACTIONS/INTERVENTIONS	RATIONALE
Positioning (NIC)	
Independent	
Maintain bed rest/limb rest as indicated. Provide support of joints above and below fracture site, especially when moving/turning.	Provides stability, reducing possibility of disturbing alignment/muscle spasms, which enhances healing.
Cast Care: Wet (NIC)	
Support fracture site with pillows/folded blankets. Maintain neutral position of affected part with sandbags, splints, trochanter roll, footboard.	Prevents unnecessary movement and disruption of alignment. Proper placement of pillows also can prevent pressure deformities in the drying cast.
Use the palms of hands, not the fingertips, when touching the wet cast.	Fingertips can dent the cast before it is dry.
Obtain sufficient personnel for turning. Avoid using abduction bar for turning client with spica cast.	Hip/body or multiple casts can be extremely heavy and cumbersome. Failure to properly support limbs in casts may cause damage to cast or injury to client and staff.
Traction/Immobilization Care (NIC)	
Evaluate splinted extremity for edema resolution	Coaptation splint (e.g., Jones-Sugar tong) may be used to provide immobilization of fracture while excessive tissue swelling is present. As edema subsides, readjustment of splint or application of plaster/fiberglass cast may be required for continued alignment of fracture.

ACTIONS/INTERVENTIONS	RATIONALE
Maintain position/integrity of traction (e.g., Buck, Dunlop, Pearson, Russell).	Traction permits pull on the long axis of the fractured bone and overcomes muscle tension/shortening to facilitate alignment and union. Skeletal traction (pins, wires, tongs) permits use of greater weight for traction pull than can be applied to skin tissues.
Ascertain that all clamps are functional. Lubricate pulleys and check ropes for fraying. Secure and wrap knots with adhesive tape.	Ensures that traction setup is functioning properly to avoid interruption of fracture approximation.
Keep ropes unobstructed with weights hanging free, avoid lifting/releasing weights.	Optimal amount of traction weight is maintained. *Note:* Ensuring free movement of weights during repositioning of client avoids sudden excess pull on fracture with associated pain and muscle spasm.
Assist with placement of lifts under bed wheels if indicated.	Helps maintain proper client position and function of traction by providing counterbalance.
Position client so that appropriate pull is maintained on the long axis of the bone.	Promotes bone alignment and reduces risk of complications (e.g., delayed healing/nonunion).
Review restrictions imposed by therapy; e.g., not bending at waist/sitting up with Buck traction or not turning below the waist with Russell traction.	Maintains integrity of pull of traction.
Assess integrity of external fixation device.	Hoffman traction provides stabilization and rigid support for fractured bone without use of ropes, pulleys, or weights, thus allowing for greater client mobility/comfort and facilitating wound care. Loose or excessively tightened clamps/nuts can alter the compression of the frame, causing misalignment.

Collaborative

Review follow-up/serial x-rays.	Provides visual evidence of proper alignment or beginning callus formation/healing process to determine level of activity and need for changes in/additional therapy.
Initiate/maintain bone rehabilitation (e.g., early ambulation, weight bearing activities, soft tissue massage, and electrical stimulation if used.	Promotes bone growth and healing.

NURSING DIAGNOSIS: acute Pain

May be related to

Muscle spasms
Movement of bone fragments, edema, and injury to the soft tissue
Traction/immobility device
Stress, anxiety

Possibly evidenced by

Reports of pain
Distraction, self-focusing/narrowed focus, facial mask of pain
Guarding, protective behavior; alteration in muscle tone; autonomic responses

DESIRED OUTCOMES/EVALUATION CRITERIA—CLIENT WILL:

Pain Level (NOC)

Verbalize relief of pain.
Display relaxed manner, able to participate in activities, sleep/rest appropriately.

Pain Control (NOC)

Demonstrate use of relaxation skills and diversional activities as indicated for individual situation.

ACTIONS/INTERVENTIONS	RATIONALE
Pain Management (NIC)	
Independent	
Maintain immobilization of affected part by means of bedrest, cast, splint, traction. (Refer to ND: risk for [additional] Trauma.)	Relieves pain and prevents bone displacement/extension of tissue injury.
Elevate and support injured extremity.	Promotes venous return, decreases edema, and may reduce pain.
Avoid use of plastic sheets/pillows under limbs in cast.	Can increase discomfort by enhancing heat production in the drying cast.
Elevate bed covers, keep linens off toes.	Maintains body warmth without discomfort due to pressure of bedclothes on affected parts.
Evaluate/document reports of pain/discomfort, noting location and characteristics, including intensity (0–10 scale), relieving and aggravating factors. Note nonverbal pain cues (changes in vital signs and emotions/behavior). Listen to reports of family member/SO regarding client's pain.	Influences choice of/monitors effectiveness of interventions. Many factors, including level of anxiety, may affect perception of/reaction to pain. *Note:* Absence of pain expression does not necessarily mean lack of pain.
Encourage client to discuss problems related to injury.	Helps alleviate anxiety. Client may feel need to relive the accident experience.
Explain procedures before beginning them.	Allows client to prepare mentally for activity and to participate in controlling level of discomfort.
Medicate before care activities. Let client know it is important to request medication before pain becomes severe.	Promotes muscle relaxation and enhances participation.
Perform and supervise active/passive ROM exercises.	Maintains strength/mobility of unaffected muscles and facilitates resolution of inflammation in injured tissues.
Provide alternative comfort measures; e.g., massage, back rub, position changes.	Improves general circulation; reduces areas of local pressure and muscle fatigue.
Provide emotional support and encourage use of stress management techniques; e.g., progressive relaxation, deep-breathing exercises, visualization/guided imagery; provide therapeutic touch.	Refocuses attention, promotes sense of control, and may enhance coping abilities in the management of the stress of traumatic injury and pain, which is likely to persist for an extended period.
Identify diversional activities appropriate for client age, physical abilities, and personal preferences.	Prevents boredom, reduces muscle tension, and can increase muscle strength; may enhance coping abilities.
Investigate any reports of unusual/sudden pain or deep, progressive, and poorly localized pain unrelieved by analgesics.	May signal developing complications; e.g., infection, tissue ischemia, compartmental syndrome. (Refer to ND: risk for Peripheral Neurovascular Dysfunction, following.)
Collaborative	
Apply cold/ice pack first 24–72 hr and as necessary.	Reduces edema/hematoma formation, decreases pain sensation. *Note:* Length of application depends on degree of client comfort and as long as the skin is carefully protected.
Administer medications as indicated: narcotic and non-narcotic analgesics (e.g., morphine, meperidine [Demerol], hydrocodone [Vicodin]), injectable and oral nonsteroidal anti-inflammatory drugs (NSAIDs) (e.g., ketorolac [Toradol], ibuprofen [Motrin]), and/or muscle relaxants (e.g., cyclobenzaprine [Flexeril], carisoprodol [Soma]).	Given to reduce pain and/or muscle spasms. Studies of Toradol have proved it to be effective in alleviating bone pain, with longer action and fewer side effects than narcotic agents.

ACTIONS/INTERVENTIONS	RATIONALE
Maintain/monitor continuous IV/patient-controlled analgesia (PCA) using peripheral, epidural, or intrathecal routes of administration. Maintain safe and effective infusions/equipment.	Optimal pain management is essential to permit early mobilization and physical therapy, and to maintain adequate blood level of analgesia, preventing fluctuations in pain relief with associated muscle tension/spasms.

NURSING DIAGNOSIS: risk for Peripheral Neurovascular Dysfunction

Risk factors may include

Reduction/interruption of blood flow
Direct vascular injury, tissue trauma, excessive edema, thrombus formation
Hypovolemia

Possibly evidenced by

[Not applicable; presence of signs and symptoms establishes an *actual* diagnosis.]

DESIRED OUTCOMES/EVALUATION CRITERIA—CLIENT WILL:

TISSUE PERFUSION: Peripheral (NOC)

Maintain tissue perfusion as evidenced by palpable pulses, skin warm/dry, normal sensation, usual sensorium, stable vital signs, and adequate urinary output for individual situation.

ACTIONS/INTERVENTIONS — RATIONALE

Circulatory Precautions (NIC)

Independent

ACTIONS/INTERVENTIONS	RATIONALE
Remove jewelry from affected limb.	May restrict circulation when edema occurs.
Evaluate presence/quality of peripheral pulse distal to injury via palpation/Doppler. Compare with uninjured limb.	Decreased/absent pulse may reflect vascular injury and necessitates immediate medical evaluation of circulatory status. Be aware that occasionally a pulse may be palpated even though circulation is blocked by a soft clot through which pulsations may be felt. In addition, perfusion through larger arteries may continue after increased compartment pressure has collapsed the arteriole/venule circulation in the muscle.
Assess capillary return, skin color, and warmth distal to the fracture.	Return of color should be rapid (3–5 sec). White, cool skin indicates arterial impairment. Cyanosis suggests venous impairment. *Note:* Peripheral pulses, capillary refill, skin color, and sensation may be normal even in presence of compartmental syndrome because superficial circulation is usually not compromised.

CIRCULATORY CARE: Arterial [or] Venous Insufficiency (NIC)

ACTIONS/INTERVENTIONS	RATIONALE
Maintain elevation of injured extremity(ies) unless contraindicated by confirmed presence of compartment syndrome.	Promotes venous drainage/decreases edema. *Note:* In presence of increased compartment pressure, elevation of the extremity actually impedes arterial flow, decreasing perfusion.
Assess entire length of injured extremity for swelling/edema formation. Measure injured extremity and compare with uninjured extremity. Note appearance/spread of hematoma.	Increasing circumference of injured extremity may suggest general tissue swelling/edema but may reflect hemorrhage. *Note:* A 1-inch increase in an adult thigh can equal approximately 1 unit of sequestered blood.

ACTIONS/INTERVENTIONS	RATIONALE
Note reports of pain extreme for type of injury or increasing pain on passive movement of extremity, development of paresthesia, muscle tension/tenderness with erythema, and change in pulse quality distal to injury. Do not elevate extremity. Report symptoms to physician at once.	Continued bleeding/edema formation within a muscle enclosed by tight fascia can result in impaired blood flow and ischemic myositis or compartmental syndrome, necessitating emergency interventions to relieve pressure/restore circulation. *Note:* This condition constitutes a medical emergency and requires immediate intervention.
Investigate sudden signs of limb ischemia; e.g., decreased skin temperature, pallor, and increased pain.	Fracture dislocations of joints (especially the knee) may cause damage to adjacent arteries, with resulting loss of distal blood flow.
Encourage client to routinely exercise digits/joints distal to injury. Ambulate as soon as possible.	Enhances circulation and reduces pooling of blood, especially in the lower extremities.
Investigate tenderness, swelling, pain on dorsiflexion of foot (positive Homans' sign).	There is an increased potential for thrombophlebitis and pulmonary emboli in clients immobile for several days. *Note:* The absence of a positive Homans' sign is not a reliable indicator in many people, especially the elderly because they often have reduced pain sensation.
Monitor vital signs. Note signs of general pallor/cyanosis, cool skin, changes in mentation.	Inadequate circulating volume compromises systemic tissue perfusion.
Test stools/gastric aspirant for occult blood. Note continued bleeding at trauma/injection site(s) and oozing from mucous membranes.	Increased incidence of gastric bleeding accompanies fractures/trauma and may be related to stress or occasionally reflects a clotting disorder requiring further evaluation.

Pressure Management (NIC)

ACTIONS/INTERVENTIONS	RATIONALE
Perform neurovascular assessments, noting changes in motor/sensory function. Ask client to localize pain/discomfort.	Impaired feeling, numbness, tingling, increased/diffuse pain occur when circulation to nerves is inadequate or nerves are damaged.
Test sensation of peroneal nerve by pinch/pinprick in the dorsal web between the first and second toe, and assess ability to dorsiflex toes if indicated.	Length and position of peroneal nerve increase risk of its injury in the presence of leg fracture, edema/compartmental syndrome, or malposition of traction apparatus.
Assess tissues around cast edges for rough places/pressure points. Investigate reports of "burning sensation" under cast.	These factors may be the cause of or be indicative of tissue pressure/ischemia, leading to breakdown/necrosis.
Monitor position/location of supporting ring of splints or sling.	Traction apparatus can cause pressure on vessels/nerves, particularly in the axilla and groin, resulting in ischemia and possible permanent nerve damage.

CIRCULATORY CARE: Arterial [or] Venous Insufficiency (NIC)

Collaborative

ACTIONS/INTERVENTIONS	RATIONALE
Apply ice bags around fracture site for short periods of time on an intermittent basis for 24–72 hours.	Reduces edema/hematoma formation, which could impair circulation. *Note:* Length of application of cold therapy is usually 20–30 minutes at a time.
Monitor hemoglobin (Hb)/hematocrit (Hct), coagulation studies; e.g., prothrombin time (PT) levels.	Assists in calculation of blood loss and needs/effectiveness of replacement therapy. Coagulation deficits may occur secondary to major trauma, presence of fat emboli, or anticoagulant therapy.
Administer IV fluids/blood products as needed.	Maintains circulating volume, enhancing tissue perfusion.
Administer medications as indicated: Low-molecular-weight heparin or heparinoids; e.g., enoxaparin (Lovenox), dalteparin (Fragmin), ardeparin (Normiflo) if indicated.	Anticoagulants may be given prophylactically to reduce threat of deep venous thrombus.
Apply antiembolic hose/sequential pressure hose/compression boots as indicated.	Decreases venous pooling and may enhance venous return, thereby reducing risk of thrombus formation.

ACTIONS/INTERVENTIONS	RATIONALE
Pressure Management (NIC)	
Split/bivalve cast as needed. Be sure to cut through wadding down to the skin.	May be done on an emergency basis to relieve restriction and improve impaired circulation resulting from compression and edema formation in injured extremity. The wadding under the cast may also be restrictive.
Refer for/monitor intracompartmental pressures as appropriate.	Diagnosis of compartment syndrome requires advanced training and is typically performed by a specialist. It can be measured by means of handheld slit catheter. Values that are 10–30 mm Hg less than diastolic blood pressure indicate a probable compartment problem, requiring prompt medical attention.
Review electromyography (EMG)/nerve conduction velocity (NCV) studies.	May be performed to evaluate nerve injury/dysfunction and effect on muscle function (not typically done in the acute care setting).
Prepare for surgical intervention (e.g., fibulectomy/ fasciotomy) as indicated.	Failure to relieve pressure/correct compartmental syndrome within 4–6 hr of onset can result in severe contractures/loss of function and disfigurement of extremity distal to injury or even necessitate amputation.

NURSING DIAGNOSIS: risk for impaired Gas Exchange

Risk factors may include

Altered blood flow; blood/fat emboli
Alveolar/capillary membrane changes: interstitial, pulmonary edema, congestion

Possibly evidenced by

[Not applicable; presence of signs and symptoms establishes an *actual* diagnosis.]

DESIRED OUTCOMES/EVALUATION CRITERIA—CLIENT WILL:

RESPIRATORY STATUS: Gas Exchange (NOC)

Maintain adequate respiratory function, as evidenced by absence of dyspnea/cyanosis; respiratory rate and arterial blood gases (ABGs) within client's normal range.

ACTIONS/INTERVENTIONS	RATIONALE
Respiratory Monitoring (NIC)	
Independent	
Monitor respiratory rate and effort. Note stridor, use of accessory muscles, retractions, development of central cyanosis.	Tachypnea, dyspnea, and changes in mentation are early signs of respiratory insufficiency and may be the only indicator of developing pulmonary emboli in the early stage. Remaining signs/symptoms reflect advanced respiratory distress/impending failure.
Auscultate breath sounds, noting development of unequal, hyperresonant sounds; also note presence of crackles/rhonchi/wheezes and inspiratory crowing or croupy sounds.	Changes in/presence of adventitious breath sounds reflects developing respiratory complications; e.g., atelectasis, pneumonia, emboli, acute respiratory distress syndrome (ARDS). Inspiratory crowing reflects upper airway edema and is suggestive of fat emboli.

ACTIONS/INTERVENTIONS	RATIONALE
Handle injured tissues/bones gently, especially during first several days.	This may prevent the development of fat emboli (usually seen in first 12–72 hr), which are closely associated with fractures, especially of the long bones and pelvis.
Instruct and assist with deep-breathing and coughing exercises. Reposition frequently.	Promotes alveolar ventilation and perfusion. Repositioning promotes drainage of secretions and decreases congestion in dependent lung areas.
Note increasing restlessness, confusion, lethargy, stupor.	Impaired gas exchange/presence of pulmonary emboli can cause deterioration in client's level of consciousness as hypoxemia/acidosis develops.
Observe sputum for signs of blood.	Hemoptysis may occur with pulmonary emboli.
Inspect skin for petechiae above nipple line; in axilla, spreading to abdomen/trunk; buccal mucosa, hard palate; conjunctival sacs and retina.	This is the most characteristic sign of fat emboli, which may appear within 2–3 days after injury.

Collaborative

ACTIONS/INTERVENTIONS	RATIONALE
Instruct in/encourage regular use incentive spirometry.	Maximizes ventilation and minimizes atelectasis.
Administer supplemental oxygen if indicated.	Increases available O_2 for optimal tissue oxygenation.
Monitor respiratory indicators, e.g.: pulse oximetry/ serial ABGs;	Identifies situations in which oxygen desaturation is occurring, and reveals complications (e.g., impaired gas exchange/developing respiratory failure).
Laboratory studies; e.g., Hb, calcium, erythrocyte sedimentation rate (ESR), serum lipase, fat screen, platelets, as appropriate.	Anemia, hypocalcemia, elevated ESR and lipase levels, fat globules in blood/urine/sputum, and decreased platelet count (thrombocytopenia) are often associated with fat emboli.
Administer medications as indicated:	
Low-molecular-weight heparin or heparinoids; e.g., enoxaparin (Lovenox), dalteparin (Fragmin), ardeparin (Normiflo);	Used for prevention of thromboembolic phenomena, including deep vein thrombosis and pulmonary emboli.
Corticosteroids.	Steroids have been used with some success to prevent/treat fat embolus.

NURSING DIAGNOSIS: impaired physical Mobility

May be related to

Neuromuscular skeletal impairment, pain/discomfort, restrictive therapies (limb immobilization)
Psychologic immobility

Possibly evidenced by

Inability to move purposefully within the physical environment, imposed restrictions
Reluctance to attempt movement, limited ROM
Decreased muscle strength/control

DESIRED OUTCOMES/EVALUATION CRITERIA—CLIENT WILL:

Mobility (NOC)

Regain/maintain mobility at the highest possible level.
Maintain position of function.
Increase strength/function of affected and compensatory body parts.
Demonstrate techniques that enable resumption of activities, especially ADLs.

ACTIONS/INTERVENTIONS	RATIONALE
Bed Rest Care (NIC)	
Independent	
Assess degree of immobility produced by injury/treatment and note client's perception of immobility.	Client may be restricted by self-view/self-perception out of proportion with actual physical limitations, requiring information/interventions to promote progress toward wellness.
Encourage participation in diversional/recreational activities. Maintain stimulating environment; e.g., radio, TV, newspapers, personal possessions/pictures, clock, calendar, visits from family/friends.	Provides opportunity for release of energy, refocuses attention, enhances client's sense of self-control/self-worth, and aids in reducing social isolation.
Instruct client in/assist with active/passive ROM exercises of affected and unaffected extremities.	Increases blood flow to muscles and bone to improve muscle tone, maintain joint mobility; prevent contractures/atrophy and calcium resorption from disuse.
Encourage use of isometric exercises starting with the unaffected limb.	Isometrics contract muscles without bending joints or moving limbs and help maintain muscle strength and mass. *Note:* These exercises are contraindicated while acute bleeding/edema is present.
Provide footboard, wrist splints, trochanter/hand rolls as appropriate.	Useful in maintaining functional position of extremities, hands/feet, and preventing complications (e.g., contractures/footdrop).
Place in supine position periodically if possible when traction is used to stabilize lower limb fractures.	Reduces risk of flexion contracture of hip.
Instruct in/encourage use of trapeze and "post position" for lower limb fractures.	Facilitates movement during hygiene/skin care and linen changes; reduces discomfort of remaining flat in bed. "Post position" involves placing the uninjured foot flat on the bed with the knee bent while grasping the trapeze and lifting the body off the bed.
Assist with/encourage self-care activities (e.g., bathing, shaving).	Improves muscle strength and circulation, enhances client control in situation, and promotes self-directed wellness.
Provide/assist with mobility by means of wheelchair, walker, crutches, canes as soon as possible. Instruct in safe use of mobility aids.	Early mobility reduces complications of bedrest (e.g., phlebitis) and promotes healing and normalization of organ function. Learning the correct way to use aids is important to maintain optimal mobility and client safety.
Monitor blood pressure (BP) with resumption of activity. Note reports of dizziness.	Postural hypotension is a common problem following prolonged bedrest and may require specific interventions (e.g., tilt table with gradual elevation to upright position).
Reposition periodically and encourage coughing/deep-breathing exercises.	Prevents/reduces incidence of skin and respiratory complications (e.g., decubitus ulcer, atelectasis, pneumonia).
Auscultate bowel sounds. Monitor elimination habits and provide for regular bowel routine. Place on bedside commode, if feasible, or use fracture pan. Provide privacy.	Bedrest, use of analgesics, and changes in dietary habits can slow peristalsis and produce constipation. Nursing measures that facilitate elimination may prevent/limit complications. Fracture pan limits flexion of hips and lessens pressure on lumbar region/lower extremity cast.
Perform a thorough assessment of client's prior bowel habits.	Provides baseline for comparison with postsurgical concerns. Constipation in orthopedic clients is a major issue and needs immediate and ongoing attention.
Encourage increased fluid intake to 2000–3000 mL/day (within cardiac tolerance), including acid/ash juices.	Keeps the body well hydrated, decreasing risk of urinary infection, stone formation, and helps to prevent constipation.
Provide diet high in proteins, carbohydrates, vitamins, and minerals, limiting protein content until after first bowel movement.	In the presence of musculoskeletal injuries, early good feeding is needed as nutrients required for healing are rapidly depleted. This can have a profound effect on muscle mass, tone, and strength. *Note:* Protein foods increase contents in small bowel, resulting in gas formation and constipation. Therefore, gastrointestinal (GI) function should be fully restored before protein foods are increased.

ACTIONS/INTERVENTIONS	RATIONALE
Increase the amount of roughage/fiber in the diet. Limit gas-forming foods.	Adding bulk to stool helps prevent constipation. Gas-forming foods may cause abdominal distention, especially in presence of decreased intestinal motility.

Collaborative

Consult with physical/occupational therapist and/or rehabilitation specialist.	Useful in creating aggressive individualized activity/exercise program. Client may require long-term assistance with movement, strengthening, and weight-bearing activities, as well as use of adjuncts; e.g., walkers, crutches, canes; elevated toilet seats; pickup sticks/reachers; special eating utensils, help for women with actions such as hooking a brassiere.
Refer to dietitian/nutrition team as indicated.	Client with fractures, especially when associated with trauma, may have special nutritional considerations; e.g., may need enteral/parenteral feedings to maximize healing of tissues/bones.
Initiate bowel program (stool softeners, enemas, laxatives) as indicated.	Important to promote regular bowel evacuation and prevent constipation.
Refer to psychiatric clinical nurse specialist/therapist as indicated.	Client/SO may require more intensive treatment to deal with reality of current condition/prognosis, prolonged immobility, perceived loss of control.

NURSING DIAGNOSIS: actual/risk for impaired Skin/Tissue Integrity

May be related to

Puncture injury; compound fracture; surgical repair; insertion of traction pins, wires, screws
Altered sensation, circulation; accumulation of excretions/secretions
Physical immobilization

Possibly evidenced by (actual)

Reports of itching, pain, numbness, pressure in affected/surrounding area
Disruption of skin surface; invasion of body structures; destruction of skin layers/tissues

DESIRED OUTCOMES/EVALUATION CRITERIA—CLIENT WILL:

TISSUE INTEGRITY: Skin & Mucous Membranes (NOC)

Verbalize relief of discomfort.
Demonstrate behaviors/techniques to prevent skin breakdown/facilitate healing as indicated.
Achieve timely wound/lesion healing if present.

ACTIONS/INTERVENTIONS	RATIONALE
Skin Surveillance (NIC)	
Independent	
Examine the skin for open wounds, foreign bodies, rashes, bleeding, discoloration, duskiness, blanching.	Provides information regarding skin circulation and problems that may be caused by application and/or restriction of cast/splint or traction apparatus, or edema formation that may require further medical intervention.

ACTIONS/INTERVENTIONS	RATIONALE
Provide specialty beds and Geomatts as indicated.	Used for clients with high risk of skin breakdown, or in whom long-term immobility is expected.
Massage skin and bony prominences. Keep the bed linens dry and free of wrinkles. Place water pads/other padding under elbows/heels as indicated.	Reduces pressure on susceptible areas and risk of abrasions/skin breakdown.
Reposition frequently. Encourage use of trapeze if possible.	Lessens constant pressure on same areas and minimizes risk of skin breakdown. Use of trapeze may reduce risk of abrasions to elbows/heels.
Assess position of splint ring of traction device.	Improper positioning may cause skin injury/breakdown.

CAST CARE: Wet (NIC)

Plaster cast application and skin care:	
Cleanse skin with soap and water. Rub gently with alcohol and/or dust with small amount of a zinc or stearate powder;	Provides a dry, clean area for cast application. *Note:* Excess powder may cake when it comes in contact with water/perspiration.
Cut a length of stockinette to cover the area and extend several inches beyond the cast;	Useful for padding bony prominences, finishing cast edges, and protecting the skin.
Use palm of hand to apply, hold, or move cast and support on pillows after application; avoid using fingertips to hold cast;	Prevents indentations/flattening over bony prominences and weight-bearing areas (e.g., back of heels), which would cause abrasions/tissue trauma. An improperly shaped or dried cast is irritating to the underlying skin and may lead to circulatory impairment. Fingertips may dent the cast when it is wet.
Trim excess plaster from edges of cast as soon as casting is completed;	Uneven plaster is irritating to the skin and may result in abrasions.
Promote cast drying by removing bed linen, exposing to circulating air;	Prevents skin breakdown caused by prolonged moisture trapped under cast.
Observe for potential pressure areas, especially at the edges of and under the splint/cast;	Pressure can cause ulcerations, necrosis, and/or nerve palsies. These problems may be painless when nerve damage is present.
Pad (petal) the edges of the cast with waterproof tape;	Provides an effective barrier to cast flaking and moisture. Helps prevent breakdown of cast material at edges and reduces skin irritation/excoriation.
Cleanse excess plaster from skin while still wet, if possible;	Dry plaster may flake into completed cast and cause skin damage.
Protect cast and skin in perineal area. Provide frequent perineal care;	Prevents tissue breakdown and infection by fecal contamination.
Instruct client/SO to avoid inserting objects inside casts;	"Scratching an itch" may cause tissue injury.
Massage the skin around the cast edges with alcohol;	Has a drying effect, which toughens the skin. Creams and lotions are not recommended because excessive oils can seal cast perimeter, not allowing the cast to "breathe." Powders are not recommended because of potential for excessive accumulation inside the cast.
Turn frequently to include the uninvolved side, back, and prone positions (as tolerated) with client's feet over the end of the mattress.	Minimizes pressure on feet and around cast edges.

Traction/Immobilization Care (NIC)

Skin traction application and skin care:	
Cleanse the skin with warm, soapy water;	Reduces level of contaminants on skin.
Apply tincture of benzoin;	"Toughens" the skin for application of skin traction.
Apply commercial skin traction tapes (or make some with strips of moleskin/adhesive tape) lengthwise on opposite sides of the affected limb;	Traction tapes encircling a limb may compromise circulation.

ACTIONS/INTERVENTIONS	RATIONALE
Extend the tapes beyond the length of the limb;	Traction is inserted in line with the free ends of the tape.
Mark the line where the tapes extend beyond the extremity;	Allows for quick assessment of slippage.
Place protective padding under the limb and over bony prominences;	Minimizes pressure on these areas.
Wrap the limb circumference, including tapes and padding, with elastic bandages, being careful to wrap snugly but not too tightly;	Provides for appropriate traction pull without compromising circulation.
Palpate taped tissues daily and document any tenderness or pain;	If area under tapes is tender, suspect skin irritation, and prepare to remove the bandage system.
Remove skin traction every 24 hr per protocol, inspect and give skin care.	Maintains skin integrity.
Skeletal traction/fixation application and skin care:	
Bend wire ends or cover ends of wires/pins with rubber or cork protectors or needle caps;	Prevents injury to other body parts.
Pad slings/frame with sheepskin, foam.	Prevents excessive pressure on skin and promotes moisture evaporation that reduces risk of excoriation.

Pressure Management (NIC)

Collaborative

Provide foam mattress, sheepskins, flotation pads, or air mattress as indicated.	Because of immobilization of body parts, bony prominences other than those affected by the casting may suffer from decreased circulation.
Monovalve, bivalve, or cut a window in the cast, per protocol.	Allows the release of pressure and provides access for wound/skin care.

NURSING DIAGNOSIS: risk for Infection

Risk factors may include

Inadequate primary defenses: broken skin, traumatized tissues, environmental exposure

Invasive procedures, skeletal traction

Possibly evidenced by

[Not applicable; presence of signs and symptoms establishes an *actual* diagnosis.]

DESIRED OUTCOMES/EVALUATION CRITERIA—CLIENT WILL:

Infection Status (NOC)

Achieve timely wound healing, be free of purulent drainage or erythema, and be afebrile.

ACTIONS/INTERVENTIONS — RATIONALE

Infection Prevention (NIC)

Independent

Inspect the skin for preexisting irritation or breaks in continuity.	Pins or wires should not be inserted through skin infections, rashes, or abrasions (may lead to bone infection).

ACTIONS/INTERVENTIONS	RATIONALE
Assess pin sites/skin areas, noting reports of increased pain/burning sensation or presence of edema, erythema, foul odor, or drainage.	May indicate onset of local infection/tissue necrosis, which can lead to osteomyelitis.
Provide sterile pin/wound care according to protocol, and exercise meticulous hand washing.	May prevent cross-contamination and possibility of infection.
Instruct client not to touch the insertion sites.	Minimizes opportunity for contamination.
Line perineal cast edges with plastic wrap.	Damp, soiled casts can promote growth of bacteria.
Observe wounds for formation of bullae, crepitation, bronze discoloration of skin, frothy/fruity-smelling drainage.	Signs suggestive of gas gangrene infection.
Assess muscle tone, reflexes, and ability to speak.	Muscle rigidity, tonic spasms of jaw muscles, and dysphagia reflect development of tetanus.
Monitor vital signs. Note presence of chills, fever, malaise, changes in mentation.	Hypotension, confusion may be seen with gas gangrene; tachycardia and chills/fever reflect developing sepsis.
Investigate abrupt onset of pain/limitation of movement with localized edema/erythema in injured extremity.	May indicate development of osteomyelitis.
Institute prescribed isolation procedures.	Presence of purulent drainage requires wound/linen precautions to prevent cross-contamination.

Collaborative

Monitor laboratory/diagnostic studies, e.g.:	
Complete blood count (CBC);	Anemia may be noted with osteomyelitis; leukocytosis is usually present with infective processes.
ESR;	Elevated in osteomyelitis.
Cultures and sensitivity of wound/serum/bone;	Identifies infective organism and effective antimicrobial agent(s).
Radioisotope scans.	Hot spots signify increased areas of vascularity, indicative of osteomyelitis.
Administer medications as indicated, e.g.:	
IV/topical antibiotics;	Wide-spectrum antibiotics may be used prophylactically or may be geared toward a specific microorganism.
Tetanus toxoid.	Given prophylactically because the possibility of tetanus exists with any open wound. *Note:* Risk increases when injury/wound(s) occur in "field conditions" (outdoor/rural areas, work environment).
Provide wound/bone irrigations and apply warm/moist soaks as indicated.	Local debridement/cleansing of wounds reduces microorganisms and incidence of systemic infection. Continuous antimicrobial drip into bone may be necessary to treat osteomyelitis, especially if blood supply to bone is compromised.
Assist with procedures; e.g., incision/drainage, placement of drains, hyperbaric oxygen therapy.	Numerous procedures may be carried out in treatment of local infections, osteomyelitis, gas gangrene.
Prepare for surgery as indicated.	Sequestrectomy (removal of necrotic bone) is necessary to facilitate healing and prevent extension of infectious process.

NURSING DIAGNOSIS: deficient Knowledge [Learning Need] regarding condition, prognosis, treatment, self-care, and discharge needs

May be related to

Lack of exposure/recall
Information misinterpretation/unfamiliarity with information resources

Possibly evidenced by

Questions/request for information, statement of misconception
Inaccurate follow-through of instructions, development of preventable complications

DESIRED OUTCOMES/EVALUATION CRITERIA—CLIENT WILL:

KNOWLEDGE: Treatment Regimen (NOC)

Verbalize understanding of condition, prognosis, and potential complications.
Correctly perform necessary procedures and explain reasons for actions.

ACTIONS/INTERVENTIONS	RATIONALE
TEACHING: Disease Process (NIC)	
Independent	
Review pathology, prognosis, and future expectations.	Provides knowledge base from which client can make informed choices. *Note:* Internal fixation devices can ultimately compromise the bone's strength, and intramedullary nails/rods or plates may be removed at a future date.
Discuss dietary needs.	A low-fat diet with adequate quality protein and rich in calcium promotes healing and general well-being.
Discuss individual drug regimen as appropriate.	Proper use of pain medication and antiplatelet agents can reduce risk of complications. Long-term use of alendronate (Fosamax) may reduce risk of stress fractures. *Note:* Fosamax should be taken on an empty stomach with plain water because absorption of drug may be altered by food and some medications (e.g., antacids, calcium supplements).
Reinforce methods of mobility and ambulation as instructed by physical therapist when indicated.	Most fractures require casts, splints, or braces during the healing process. Further damage and delay in healing could occur secondary to improper use of ambulatory devices.
Suggest use of a backpack.	Provides place to carry necessary articles and leaves hands free to manipulate crutches; may prevent undue muscle fatigue when one arm is casted.
List activities client can perform independently and those that require assistance.	Organizes activities around need and who is available to provide help.
Identify available community services; e.g., rehabilitation team, home nursing/homemaker services.	Provides assistance to facilitate self-care and support independence. Promotes optimal self-care and recovery.
Encourage client to continue active exercises for the joints above and below the fracture.	Prevents joint stiffness, contractures, and muscle wasting, promoting earlier return to independence in activities of daily living (ADLs).
Discuss importance of clinical and therapy follow-up appointments.	Fracture healing may take as long as a year for completion, and client cooperation with the medical regimen facilitates proper union of bone. Physical therapy (PT)/occupational therapy (OT) may be indicated for exercises to maintain/strengthen muscles and improve function. Additional modalities such as low-intensity ultrasound may be used to stimulate healing of lower-forearm or lower-leg fractures.
Review proper pin/wound care.	Reduces risk of bone/tissue trauma and infection, which can progress to osteomyelitis.
Recommend cleaning external fixator device regularly.	Keeping device free of dust/contaminants reduces risk of infection.

ACTIONS/INTERVENTIONS	RATIONALE
Identify signs/symptoms requiring medical evaluation; e.g., severe pain, fever/chills, foul odors; changes in sensation, swelling, burning, numbness, tingling, skin discoloration, paralysis, white/cool toes or fingertips; warm spots, soft areas, cracks in cast.	Prompt intervention may reduce severity of complications such as infection/impaired circulation. *Note:* Some darkening of the skin (vascular congestion) may occur normally when walking on the casted extremity or using casted arm; however, this should resolve with rest and elevation.
Discuss care of "green" or wet cast.	Promotes proper curing to prevent cast deformities and associated misalignment/skin irritation. *Note:* Placing a "cooling" cast directly on rubber or plastic pillows traps heat and increases drying time.
Suggest the use of a blow-dryer to dry small areas of dampened cast.	Cautious use can hasten drying.
Demonstrate use of plastic bags to cover plaster cast during wet weather or while bathing. Clean soiled cast with a slightly dampened cloth and some scouring powder.	Protects from moisture, which softens the plaster and weakens the cast. *Note:* Fiberglass casts are being used more frequently. They also need to be thoroughly dried if they get wet to avoid developing mold, etc.
Emphasize importance of not adjusting clamps/nuts of external fixator device.	Tampering may alter compression and misalign fracture.
Recommend use of adaptive clothing.	Facilitates dressing/grooming activities.
Suggest ways to cover toes if appropriate; e.g., stockinette or soft socks.	Helps maintain warmth/protect from injury.
Discuss postcast removal instructions:	
Instruct client to continue exercises as permitted;	Reduces stiffness and improves strength and function of affected extremity.
Inform client that the skin under the cast is commonly mottled and covered with scales or crusts of dead skin;	It will be several weeks before normal appearance returns.
Wash the skin gently with soap, povidone-iodine (Betadine), or pHisoDerm, and water. Lubricate with a protective emollient;	New skin is extremely tender because it has been protected beneath a cast.
Inform client that muscles may appear flabby and atrophied (less muscle mass). Recommend supporting the joint above and below the affected part and the use of mobility aids; e.g., elastic bandages, splints, braces, crutches, walkers, or canes;	Muscle strength will be reduced and new or different aches and pains may occur for awhile secondary to loss of support.
Elevate the extremity as needed.	Swelling and edema tend to occur after cast removal.

POTENTIAL CONSIDERATIONS following acute hospitalization (dependent on client's age, physical condition/presence of complications, personal resources, and life responsibilities)

In addition to surgical considerations:

risk for Trauma—loss of skeletal integrity, weakness, balancing difficulties, reduced muscle coordination, lack of safety precautions, history of previous trauma.

impaired physical Mobility—neuromuscular skeletal impairment, pain/discomfort, restrictive therapies (limb immobilization); psychological immobility.

Self-Care Deficit—musculoskeletal impairment, decreased strength/endurance, pain.

risk for Infection—inadequate primary defenses: broken skin, traumatized tissues, environmental exposure, invasive procedures, skeletal traction.

AMPUTATION

In general, *amputation* of limbs is the result of peripheral vascular disease (most common cause in the United States), trauma (including battlefield wounds), malignant bone tumors, infections (e.g., osteomyelitis, gangrene), and congenital disorders. There are two types of amputations: (1) open or provisional, which requires subsequent revisions, and (2) closed (flap), where all the surgical revision is performed and the wound closed in one procedure. The type and level of amputation are determined entirely by the underlying condition (e.g., trauma vs peripheral vascular disease).

Upper-extremity amputations are generally due to trauma from industrial accidents. Reattachment surgery may be possible for fingers, hands, and arms. Lower-extremity amputations are performed much more frequently than upper-extremity amputations. Five levels are currently used in lower-extremity amputation: foot and ankle, below knee (BKA), knee disarticulation and above (thigh), knee-hip disarticulation, and hemipelvectomy and translumbar amputation.

General principles for amputation surgery involve appropriate management of skin, bone, nerves, and blood vessels. An optimal residual extremity is covered with well-vascularized muscle and skin. The use and early implementation of prosthetic devices are improving the long-term outcome for many clients with amputation. There are two basic types of prosthetic designs: (1) *exoskeletal* (outer plastic laminated skin with wood or urethane foam interiors) where the strength is provided by the outer layer; and (2) *endoskeletal* (aluminum, titanium, and other tubular materials form the inner structure [strength] and the external shape is removable, usually a sort of foam or skin-simulating material). New prosthetic devices are wonders of microengineering. For example: C-leg, a prosthesis that uses computer sensors and hydraulics, enables the client to move around nearly effortlessly.

For the purpose of this plan of care, amputation refers to the surgical/traumatic removal of a limb.

CARE SETTING

Inpatient acute surgical unit and subacute or rehabilitation unit.

RELATED CONCERNS

Cancer, page 857
Diabetes mellitus/diabetic ketoacidosis, page 412
Psychosocial aspects of care, page 770
Surgical intervention, page 788

Client Assessment Database

Data depend on underlying reason for surgical procedure; e.g., severe trauma, peripheral vascular/arterial occlusive disease, diabetic neuropathy, osteomyelitis, cancer.

ACTIVITY/REST

May report: Actual/anticipated limitations imposed by condition/amputation

CIRCULATION

May exhibit: Presence of edema; absent/diminished pulses in affected limb/digits

EGO INTEGRITY

May report: Concern about negative effects/anticipated changes in lifestyle, financial situation, reactions of others
Feelings of helplessness, powerlessness

May exhibit: Anxiety, apprehension, irritability, anger, fearfulness, withdrawal, grief, false cheerfulness

NEUROSENSORY

May report: Loss of sensation in affected area
Phantom pain

SAFETY

May exhibit: Necrotic/gangrenous area
Nonhealing wound, local infection

SEXUALITY

May report: Concerns about intimate relationships

SOCIAL INTERACTION

May report: Problems related to illness/condition
Concern about role function, reaction of others

TEACHING/LEARNING

Discharge plan considerations: May require assistance with wound care/supplies, adaptation to prosthesis/ambulatory devices, transportation, homemaker/maintenance tasks, possibly self-care activities and vocational retraining

Refer to section at end of plan for postdischarge considerations.

DIAGNOSTIC STUDIES

Studies depend on the underlying condition necessitating amputation and are used to determine the appropriate level for amputation.

X-rays: Identify skeletal abnormalities.

CT scan: Identifies soft-tissue and bone destruction, neoplastic lesions, osteomyelitis, hematoma formation.

Angiography and blood flow studies: Evaluate circulation/tissue perfusion problems and help predict potential for tissue healing after amputation.

Doppler ultrasound, laser Doppler flowmetry: Performed to assess and measure blood flow.

Transcutaneous oxygen pressure: Maps out areas of greater and lesser perfusion in the involved extremity.

Thermography: Measures temperature differences in an ischemic limb at two sites: at the skin and center of the bone. The lower the difference between the two readings, the greater the chance for healing.

Plethysmography: Segmental systolic BP measurements evaluate arterial blood flow.

ESR: Elevation indicates inflammatory response.

Wound cultures: Identify presence of infection and causative organism.

WBC count/differential: Elevation and "shift to left" suggest infectious process.

Biopsy: Confirms diagnosis of benign/malignant mass.

NURSING PRIORITIES

1. Support psychologic and physiological adjustment.
2. Alleviate pain.
3. Prevent complications.
4. Promote mobility/functional abilities.
5. Provide information about surgical procedure/prognosis and treatment needs.

DISCHARGE GOALS

1. Dealing with current situation realistically.
2. Pain relieved/controlled.
3. Complications prevented/minimized.
4. Mobility/function regained or compensated for.
5. Surgical procedure, prognosis, and therapeutic regimen understood.
6. Plan in place to meet needs after discharge.

NURSING DIAGNOSIS: situational low Self-Esteem

May be related to

Loss of body part/change in functional abilities

Possibly evidenced by

Anticipated changes in lifestyle, fear of rejection/reaction by others
Negative feelings about body, focus on past strength, function, or appearance
Feelings of helplessness, powerlessness
Preoccupation with missing body part, not looking at or touching stump
Perceived change in usual patterns of responsibility/physical capacity to resume role

DESIRED OUTCOMES/EVALUATION CRITERIA—CLIENT WILL:

Grief Resolution (NOC)

Begin to show adaptation and verbalize acceptance of self in situation (amputee).
Recognize and incorporate changes into self-concept in accurate manner without negating self-esteem.
Develop realistic plans for adapting to new role/role modifications.

ACTIONS/INTERVENTIONS	RATIONALE
Grief Work Facilitation (NIC)	
Independent	
Assess/consider client's preparation for and view of amputation.	Research shows that amputation poses serious threats to client's psychologic and psychosocial adjustment. Client who views amputation as life-saving or reconstructive may be able to accept the new self more quickly. Client with sudden traumatic amputation or who considers amputation to be the result of failure in other treatments is at greater risk for disturbances in self-concept.
Encourage expression of fears, negative feelings, and grief over loss of body part.	Venting emotions helps client begin to deal with the fact and reality of life without a limb.
Reinforce preoperative information including type/location of amputation, type of prosthetic fitting if appropriate (i.e., immediate, delayed), expected postoperative course, including pain control and rehabilitation.	Provides opportunity for client to question and assimilate information and begin to deal with changes in body image and function, which can facilitate postoperative recovery.
Assess degree of support available to client.	Sufficient support by SO and friends can facilitate rehabilitation process.
Discuss client's perceptions of self, related to change, and how client sees self in usual lifestyle/role functioning.	Aids in defining concerns in relation to previous lifestyle and facilitates problem solving. For example, client likely fears loss of independence, may lose ability to work, express sexuality, and may experience role/relationship changes.
Ascertain individual strengths and identify previous positive coping behaviors.	Helpful to build on strengths that are already available for client to use in coping with current situation.
Self-Esteem Enhancement (NIC)	
Encourage participation in ADLs. Provide opportunities to view/care for stump, using the moment to point out positive signs of healing.	Promotes independence and enhances feelings of self-worth. Although integration of stump into body image can take months or even years, looking at the stump and hearing positive comments (made in a normal, matter-of-fact manner) can help client with this acceptance.
Encourage/provide for visit by another amputee, especially one who is successfully rehabilitating.	A peer who has been through a similar experience serves as a role model and can provide validity to comments and hope for recovery and a normal future.
Provide open environment for client to discuss concerns about sexuality.	Promotes sharing of beliefs/values about sensitive subject, and identifies misconceptions/myths that may interfere with adjustment to situation.
Note withdrawn behavior, negative self-talk, use of denial, or overconcern with actual/perceived changes.	Identifies stage of grief/need for interventions.
Collaborative	
Discuss availability of various resources; e.g., psychiatric/sexual counseling, occupational therapist.	May need assistance for these concerns to facilitate optimal adaptation and rehabilitation.

NURSING DIAGNOSIS: acute Pain

May be related to

Physical injury/tissue and nerve trauma
Psychologic impact of loss of body part

Possibly evidenced by

Reports of pain
Narrowed self-focus
Autonomic responses, guarding/protective behavior

DESIRED OUTCOMES/EVALUATION CRITERIA—CLIENT WILL:

Pain Level (NOC)

Report pain is relieved/controlled.
Appear relaxed and able to rest/sleep appropriately.
Verbalize understanding of phantom pain and methods to provide relief.

ACTIONS/INTERVENTIONS	RATIONALE
Pain Management (NIC)	
Independent	
Document location and intensity of pain (0–10 scale). Investigate changes in pain characteristics; e.g., numbness, tingling.	Aids in evaluating need for and effectiveness of interventions. Changes may indicate developing complications; e.g., necrosis/infection.
Elevate affected part by raising foot of bed slightly or use of pillow/sling for upper-limb amputation.	Lessens edema formation by enhancing venous return; reduces muscle fatigue and skin/tissue pressure. *Note:* After initial 24 hr and in absence of edema, stump may be extended and kept flat.
Provide/promote general comfort measures (e.g., frequent turning, back rub) and diversional activities. Encourage use of stress management techniques (e.g., deep-breathing exercises, visualization, and guided imagery) and therapeutic touch.	Refocuses attention, promotes relaxation, may enhance coping abilities and may decrease occurrence of phantom-limb pain.
Investigate reports of progressive/poorly localized pain unrelieved by analgesics.	May indicate developing compartment syndrome, especially following traumatic injury. (Refer to CP: Fractures; ND: risk for Peripheral Neurovascular Dysfunction.)
Acknowledge reality of residual limb pain and phantom pain, and that various modalities will be tried for pain relief.	Residual limb pain is believed to come from injuries to nerves at the amputation site. At the ends of these injured nerve fibers, neuromas (bundles of nerve fibers) send out pain impulses in a random fashion, or when trapped (excessive compression) by other tissues such as muscle, or development of infectious process. In contrast, phantom pain is thought to originate in the part of the brain that controlled the limb before it was amputated. So the client experiences pain and sensation as if the limb were still in place. Phantom pain is often described as crushing, grinding or burning pain. It can occur immediately or may not start for several weeks. *Note:* Phantom pain is not well relieved by traditional pain medications.
Collaborative	
Administer medications, as indicated, (e.g., opioid analgesics: morphine [Astramorph, MS, MS Contin], meperidine [Demerol], combination agents: oxycodone with acetaminophen [Percocet]); anitinflammatory agents (e.g. acetaminophen [Tylenol], ibuprofen [Motrin]); antidepressants (e.g., amitriptyline [Elavil], nortriptyline [Pamelor]); antiseizure drugs (e.g., carbamazepine [Tegretol], gabapentin [Neurontin]); sedatives/antianxiety agents (e.g., diazepam [Valium], alprazolam [Xanax]); local/regional anesthetics e.g., novacaine (Marcaine).	Many medications and routes of administration may be used. In acute post amputation pain, opioid analgesics are the mainstay of pain management to reduce pain/muscle spasms. As surgical pain subsides, other medications will be added to manage more long-term conditions; e.g., antidepressants and antiseizure medications appear to be useful in the neuritic pain associated with phantom pain and sensations.
Instruct in/monitor use of patient-controlled analgesia (PCA).	PCA provides for continuous/timely drug administration, preventing fluctuations in pain level and muscle tension/spasms associated with surgical procedures.

ACTIONS/INTERVENTIONS	RATIONALE
Refer to interdisciplinary providers as appropriate; e.g., pain management specialist, physical therapist, prosthetist, orthopedic and neurosurgeon.	A multidisciplinary approach is required, and many therapy modalities may be needed both in the acute and the long term management of pain.
Discuss/monitor use of transcutaneous electrical nerve stimulation (TENS) of the stump.	For some individuals a TENS unit may be useful in treating retractable phantom limb pain, especially in combination with medications for neuropathic pain. *Note*: Stimulation of the intact (opposite) limb is often more effective, and an increase in phantom pain has been reported on occasion when TENS unit applied to stump.

NURSING DIAGNOSIS: risk for ineffective peripheral Tissue Perfusion

Risk factors may include

Reduced arterial/venous blood flow; tissue edema, hematoma formation
Hypovolemia

Possibly evidenced by

[Not applicable; presence of signs and symptoms establishes an *actual* diagnosis.]

DESIRED OUTCOMES/EVALUATION CRITERIA—CLIENT WILL:

TISSUE PERFUSION: Peripheral (NOC)

Maintain adequate tissue perfusion as evidenced by palpable peripheral pulses, warm/dry skin, and timely wound healing.

ACTIONS/INTERVENTIONS — RATIONALE

CIRCULATORY CARE: Arterial [or] Venous Insufficiency (NIC)

Independent

ACTIONS/INTERVENTIONS	RATIONALE
Monitor vital signs. Palpate peripheral pulses, noting strength and equality.	General indicators of circulatory status and adequacy of perfusion.
Perform periodic neurovascular assessments; e.g., sensation, movement, pulse, skin color, and temperature.	Amputation wound healing is a concern because most are performed for compromised circulation (e.g., PVD, damaged soft tissue due to trauma). Postoperative tissue edema, hematoma formation, or restrictive dressings may impair circulation to stump, resulting in tissue necrosis.
Note type of dressing used; e.g., soft, soft with pressure wrap, semirigid, rigid.	Postoperative dressing varies, each with advantages and disadvantages. For example, a soft dressing does not control edema. Adding a pressure wrap distributes pressure, but requires measures to avoid possible limb strangulation. Semirigid dressings (e.g., plaster splint, Unna bandage) or rigid dressings allow for decreased edema and immediate postoperative prosthesis with early ambulation, but limit access to wound and possible excessive pressure may lead to compromised healing.
Inspect dressings/drainage device, noting amount and characteristics of drainage.	Continued blood loss may indicate need for additional fluid replacement and evaluation for coagulation defect or surgical intervention to ligate bleeder.
Apply direct pressure to bleeding site if hemorrhage occurs. Contact physician immediately.	Direct pressure to bleeding site may be followed by application of a bulk dressing secured with an elastic wrap once bleeding is controlled.

ACTIONS/INTERVENTIONS	RATIONALE
Investigate reports of persistent/unusual pain in operative site.	Hematoma can form in muscle pocket under the flap, compromising circulation and intensifying pain.
Evaluate nonoperated lower limb for inflammation, positive Homans' sign.	Increased incidence of thrombus formation in clients with preexisting peripheral vascular disease/diabetic changes.
Encourage/assist with early ambulation.	Enhances circulation, helps prevent stasis and associated complications. Promotes sense of general well-being.

Collaborative

ACTIONS/INTERVENTIONS	RATIONALE
Administer IV fluids/blood products as indicated.	Maintains circulating volume to maximize tissue perfusion.
Apply antiembolic/sequential compression hose to nonoperated leg as indicated.	Enhances venous return, reducing venous pooling and risk of thrombophlebitis.
Administer low-dose anticoagulant as indicated.	May be useful in preventing thrombus formation without increasing risk of postoperative bleeding/hematoma formation.
Monitor laboratory studies, e.g.:	
Hb/Hct;	Indicators of hypovolemia/dehydration that can impair tissue perfusion.
PT/activated partial thromboplastin time (aPTT).	Evaluates need for/effectiveness of anticoagulant therapy and identifies developing complication; e.g., posttraumatic disseminated intravascular coagulation (DIC).

NURSING DIAGNOSIS: risk for Infection

Risk factors may include

Inadequate primary defenses (broken skin, traumatized tissue)
Invasive procedures; environmental exposure
Chronic disease, altered nutritional status

Possibly evidenced by

[Not applicable; presence of signs and symptoms establishes an *actual* diagnosis.]

DESIRED OUTCOMES/EVALUATION CRITERIA—CLIENT WILL:

WOUND HEALING: Primary Intention (NOC)

Achieve timely wound healing, be free of purulent drainage or erythema, and be afebrile.

ACTIONS/INTERVENTIONS — RATIONALE

Wound Care (NIC)

Independent

ACTIONS/INTERVENTIONS	RATIONALE
Maintain aseptic technique when changing dressings/caring for wound.	Minimizes opportunity for introduction of bacteria.
Inspect dressings and wound; note characteristics of drainage.	Early detection of developing infection provides opportunity for timely intervention and prevention of more serious complications (e.g., osteomyelitis).
Maintain patency and routinely empty drainage device.	Hemovac, Jackson-Pratt drains facilitate removal of drainage, promoting wound healing and reducing risk of infection.

ACTIONS/INTERVENTIONS	RATIONALE
Cover dressing with plastic when using the bedpan or if incontinent.	Prevents contamination in lower-limb amputation.
Expose stump to air, wash with mild soap and water after dressings are discontinued.	Maintains cleanliness, minimizes skin contaminants, and promotes healing of tender/fragile skin.
Monitor vital signs.	Temperature elevation/tachycardia may reflect developing sepsis.

Collaborative

Obtain wound/drainage cultures and sensitivities as appropriate.	Identifies presence of infection/specific organisms and appropriate therapy.
Administer antibiotics as indicated.	Wide-spectrum antibiotics may be used prophylactically, or antibiotic therapy may be geared toward specific organisms.

NURSING DIAGNOSIS: impaired physical Mobility

May be related to

Loss of a limb (particularly a lower extremity); pain/discomfort; perceptual impairment (altered sense of balance)

Possibly evidenced by

Reluctance to attempt movement
Impaired coordination; decreased muscle strength, control, and mass

DESIRED OUTCOMES/EVALUATION CRITERIA—CLIENT WILL:

Risk Control (NOC)

Verbalize understanding of individual situation, treatment regimen, and safety measures.
Maintain position of function as evidenced by absence of contractures.

Mobility (NOC)

Demonstrate techniques/behaviors that enable resumption of activities.
Display willingness to participate in activities.

ACTIONS/INTERVENTIONS	RATIONALE
Amputation Care (NIC)	
Independent	
Provide stump care on a routine basis; e.g., inspect area, cleanse and dry thoroughly, and rewrap stump with elastic bandage or air splint, or apply a stump shrinker (heavy stockinette sock), for "delayed" prosthesis.	Provides opportunity to evaluate healing and note complications (unless covered by immediate prosthesis). Wrapping stump controls edema and helps form stump into conical shape to facilitate fitting of prosthesis. *Note:* Air splint may be preferred, because it permits visual inspection of the wound.

ACTIONS/INTERVENTIONS	RATIONALE
Measure circumference periodically.	Measurement is done to estimate shrinkage to ensure proper fit of sock and prosthesis.
Rewrap stump immediately with an elastic bandage, elevate if "immediate/early" cast is accidentally dislodged. Prepare for reapplication of cast.	Edema will occur rapidly, and rehabilitation can be delayed.
Assist with specified ROM exercises for both the affected and unaffected limbs beginning early in postoperative stage.	Prevents contracture deformities, which can develop rapidly and could delay prosthesis usage.
Encourage active/isometric exercises for upper torso and unaffected limbs.	Increases muscle strength to facilitate transfers/ambulation and promote mobility and more normal lifestyle.
Provide trochanter rolls as indicated.	Prevents external rotation of lower-limb stump.
Instruct client to lie in prone position as tolerated at least twice a day with pillow under abdomen and lower-extremity stump.	Strengthens extensor muscles and prevents flexion contracture of the hip, which can begin to develop within 24 hr of sustained malpositioning.
Caution against keeping pillow under lower-extremity stump or allowing BKA limb to hang dependently over side of bed or chair.	Use of pillows can cause permanent flexion contracture of hip; a dependent position of stump impairs venous return and may increase edema formation.
Demonstrate/assist with transfer techniques and use of mobility aids; e.g., trapeze, crutches, or walker.	Facilitates self-care and client's independence. Proper transfer techniques prevent shearing abrasions/dermal injury related to "scooting."
Assist with ambulation.	Reduces potential for injury. Ambulation after lower-limb amputation depends on timing of prosthesis placement. For example: (1) Immediate postoperative fitting: A rigid plaster of Paris dressing is applied to the stump and a pylon and artificial foot are attached. Weight bearing begins within 24–48 hr. (2) Early postoperative fitting: Weight bearing does not occur until 10–30 days postoperatively. (3) Delayed fitting: More common in areas that do not have facilities available for immediate/early application of prosthesis or when the condition of the stump and/or client precludes these choices. With the advent of new medical techniques on the scene of the trauma, new surgical techniques, new occupational therapy techniques, and new component and prosthetic technology, it all begins when the stitches come out. Clients are fitted with prosthetics two weeks after their final amputation.
Help client continue preoperative muscle exercises as able/when allowed out of bed; e.g., client should (while holding on to chair for balance) perform abdomen-tightening exercises and knee bends; hop on foot; stand on toes.	Contributes to gaining improved sense of balance and strengthens compensatory body parts.
Instruct client in stump-conditioning exercises; e.g., pushing the stump against a pillow initially, then progressing to harder surface.	Hardens the stump by toughening the skin and altering feedback of resected nerves to facilitate use of prosthesis.

Collaborative

ACTIONS/INTERVENTIONS	RATIONALE
Refer to rehabilitation team; e.g., physical and occupational therapy, prosthetic specialists.	Provides for creation of exercise/activity program to meet individual needs and strengths, and identifies mobility functional aids to promote independence. Early use of a temporary prosthesis promotes activity and enhances general well-being/positive outlook. *Note:* Vocational counseling/retraining also may be indicated.
Provide foam/flotation mattress.	Reduces pressure on skin/tissues that can impair circulation, potentiating risk of tissue ischemia/breakdown.

NURSING DIAGNOSIS: deficient Knowledge [Learning Need] regarding condition, prognosis, treatment, self-care, and discharge needs

May be related to

Lack of exposure/recall
Information misinterpretation

Possibly evidenced by

Questions/request for information, verbalization of the problem
Inaccurate follow-through of instructions, development of preventable complications

DESIRED OUTCOMES/EVALUATION CRITERIA—CLIENT WILL:

KNOWLEDGE: Disease Process (NOC)

Verbalize understanding of condition/disease process and potential complications.

KNOWLEDGE: Treatment Regimen (NOC)

Verbalize understanding of therapeutic needs.
Correctly perform necessary procedures and explain reasons for the actions.
Initiate necessary lifestyle changes and participate in treatment regimen.

ACTIONS/INTERVENTIONS	RATIONALE
Amputation Care (NIC)	
Independent	
Review disease process/surgical procedure and future expectations.	Provides knowledge base from which client can make informed choices.
Instruct in dressing/wound care, inspection of stump using mirror to visualize all areas, skin massage, and appropriate wrapping of the stump.	Promotes competent self-care, facilitates healing and fitting of prosthesis and reduces potential for complications.
Discuss general stump care, e.g.:	
Wash daily with mild soap and water; rinse and pat dry. Do this daily, or more often if client sweats a lot, or in treating a rash or infection;	Hygiene of residual limb/stump is critical since most of the time it is enclosed in the socket or liner of prosthesis, rendering it more prone to skin breakdown and infection.
Massaging the stump after dressings are discontinued and suture line is healed;	Massage softens scar and prevents adherence to the bone, decreases tenderness, and stimulates circulation.
Avoiding use of alcohol-based lotions, or use of powders;	Although a small amount of lotion may be indicated if skin is dry, emollients/creams soften skin and may cause maceration when prosthesis is worn. Powder may cake, potentiating skin irritation.
Wearing only properly fitted, clean, wrinkle-free limb sock;	Stump may continue to shrink for up to 2 years, and an improperly fitting sock or one that is mended or dirty can cause skin irritation/breakdown.
Using clean cotton T-shirt under harness for upper-limb prosthesis;	Absorbs perspiration; prevents skin irritation from harness.
Review common problems and appropriate actions.	Problems can occur even when client is taking precautions; e.g., development of red/sore area that does not resolve when prosthesis is off, or blister caused by pressure between socket liner and skin. These problems need early medical follow-up if home interventions are not effective.

ACTIONS/INTERVENTIONS	RATIONALE
Stress importance of well-balanced diet and adequate fluid intake.	Provides needed nutrients for tissue regeneration/healing, aids in maintaining circulating volume and normal organ function, and aids in maintenance of proper weight (weight changes affect fit of prosthesis).
Recommend cessation of smoking. Offer referral resources for cessation programs.	Smoking potentiates peripheral vasoconstriction, impairing circulation and tissue oxygenation.
Review/demonstrate care of prosthetic device. Stress importance of routine maintenance/periodic refitting.	Ensures proper fit and alignment, reduces risk of complications, and prolongs life of prosthesis.
Encourage continuation of postoperative exercise program.	Enhances circulation/healing and function of affected part, facilitating adaptation to prosthetic device.
Identify techniques to manage phantom sensation and phantom pain. (Refer to ND: acute Pain.)	Persistent and/or recurring pain requires long-term management, with multiple strategies and modalities, including desensitization therapy, intermittent compression, medications, TENS, nerve blocks. *Note*: Electrical stimulation offers a short-term rerouting or stimulation of different nerve pathways, thus reducing the activity of the usual pain patterns.
Encourage taking care of whole self, body, mind, and spirit. Emphasize socialization, stress management, relaxation training, counseling.	Various techniques may be implemented, (e.g., relaxation breathing, exercises, visualization, biofeedback) to reduce muscle tension and enhance client's control of situation and coping abilities.
Identify signs/symptoms requiring medical evaluation; e.g., edema, erythema, increased/odorous drainage from incision, changes in sensation, movement, skin color, persistent phantom pain.	Prompt intervention may prevent serious complications and/or loss of function. *Note:* Chronic phantom-limb pain may indicate neuroma, requiring surgical resection.
Identify community and rehabilitation support; e.g., certified prosthetist-orthotist, amputee groups, home-care service, homemaker services, as needed.	Facilitates transfer to home, supports independence, and enhances coping.

POTENTIAL CONSIDERATIONS following acute hospitalization (dependent on client's age, physical condition/presence of complications, personal resources, and life responsibilities)

In addition to considerations in Surgical Intervention plan of care:

risk for Trauma—balancing difficulties/altered gait, muscle weakness, reduced muscle coordination, lack of safety precautions, hazards associated with use of assistive devices.

disturbed Body Image/situational low Self-Esteem—loss of body part, change in functional abilities.

Self-Care Deficit/impaired Home Maintenance (dependent on location of amputation)—musculoskeletal impairment, decreased strength/endurance, pain, depression.

TOTAL JOINT REPLACEMENT

Joint replacement is indicated for irreversibly damaged joints with loss of function and unremitting pain (e.g., degenerative and rheumatoid arthritis [RA]), selected fractures (e.g., hip/femoral neck), joint instability, and congenital hip disorders. Although joint replacement surgery can be performed on any joint except the spine, hip and knee replacements are the most common procedures. The prosthesis may be metallic or polyethylene (or a combination) implanted with methylmethacrylate cement, or it may be a porous, coated implant that encourages bony ingrowth.

CARE SETTING

Inpatient acute surgical unit and subacute or rehabilitation unit.

RELATED CONCERNS

Fractures, page 642
Psychosocial aspects of care, page 770
Rheumatoid arthritis, page 750

Sepsis/septicemia, page 701
Surgical intervention, page 788
Thrombophlebitis: deep vein thrombosis, page 108

Client Assessment Database

ACTIVITY/REST

May report: History of occupation/participation in sports activities that wear on particular joint
Difficulty walking, stiffness in joints (worse in the morning or after period of inactivity)
Fatigue, generalized and muscle weakness
Inability to participate in occupational/recreational activities at desired level
Interruption of sleep, delayed falling asleep/awakened by pain, does not feel well rested

May exhibit: Decreased ROM and muscle strength/tone

HYGIENE

May report: Difficulty performing ADLs
Use of special equipment/mobility devices
Need for assistance with some/all activities

NEUROSENSORY

May exhibit: Soft tissue swelling, nodules
Muscle spasm, stiffness, deformity
Impaired ROM of affected joints

PAIN/DISCOMFORT

May report: Pain (dull, aching, persistent) in affected joint(s), worsened by movement

SAFETY

May report: Traumatic injury/fractures affecting the joint
Congenital deformities
History of inflammatory, debilitating arthritis (RA or osteoarthritis); aseptic necrosis of the joint head

May exhibit: Distorted joints
Joint/tissue swelling, decreased ROM, changes in gait

TEACHING/LEARNING

May report: Current medication use; e.g., anti-inflammatory, analgesics/narcotics, steroids, hormone replacement therapy (HRT), bone resorption inhibitor (e.g., Fosamax), calcium supplements

Discharge plan considerations: May need assistance with transportation, self-care activities, homemaker/maintenance tasks, possible placement in rehab/extended-care facility for continued rehabilitation/assistance

Refer to section at end of plan for postdischarge considerations.

DIAGNOSTIC STUDIES

Radiographs: May reveal destruction of articular cartilage, bony demineralization, fractures, soft-tissue swelling; narrowing of joint space, joint subluxations or deformity.
Bone scan, CT/MRI: Determine extent of degeneration and rule out malignancy.

NURSING PRIORITIES

1. Prevent complications.
2. Promote optimal mobility.
3. Alleviate pain.
4. Provide information about diagnosis, prognosis, and treatment needs.

DISCHARGE GOALS

1. Complications prevented/minimized.
2. Mobility increased.
3. Pain relieved/controlled.
4. Diagnosis, prognosis, and therapeutic regimen understood.
5. Plan in place to meet needs after discharge.

NURSING DIAGNOSIS: risk for Infection

Risk factors may include

Inadequate primary defenses (broken skin, exposure of joint)
Inadequate secondary defenses/immunosuppression (long-term corticosteroid use, cancer)
Invasive procedures; surgical manipulation; implantation of foreign body
Decreased mobility

Possibly evidenced by

[Not applicable; presence of signs and symptoms establishes an *actual* diagnosis.]

DESIRED OUTCOMES/EVALUATION CRITERIA—CLIENT WILL:

Infection Status (NOC)

Achieve timely wound healing, be free of purulent drainage or erythema, and be afebrile.

ACTIONS/INTERVENTIONS	RATIONALE
Infection Protection (NIC)	
Independent	
Promote good handwashing by staff and client.	Reduces risk of cross-contamination.
Use strict aseptic or clean techniques as indicated to reinforce/change dressings and when handling drains. Instruct client not to touch/scratch incision.	Prevents contamination and risk of wound infection, which could require removal of prosthesis.
Maintain patency of drainage devices (e.g., Hemovac/Jackson-Pratt) when present. Note characteristics of wound drainage.	Reduces risk of infection by preventing accumulation of blood and secretions in the joint space (medium for bacterial growth). Purulent, nonserous, odorous drainage is indicative of infection, and continuous drainage from incision may reflect developing skin tract, which can potentiate infectious process.
Assess skin/incision color, temperature, and integrity; note presence of erythema/inflammation, loss of wound approximation.	Provides information about status of healing process and alerts staff to early signs of infection.
Investigate reports of increased incisional pain, changes in characteristics of pain.	Deep, dull, aching pain in operative area may indicate developing infection in joint. *Note*: Infection can be devastating, because joint cannot be saved once infection sets in and prosthetic loss will occur.
Monitor temperature. Note presence of chills.	Although temperature elevations are common in early postoperative phase, elevations occurring 5 or more days postoperatively and/or presence of chills usually requires intervention to prevent more serious complications; e.g., sepsis, osteomyelitis, tissue necrosis, and prosthetic failure.
Encourage fluid intake, high-protein diet with roughage.	Maintains fluid and nutritional balance to support tissue perfusion and provide nutrients necessary for cellular regeneration and tissue healing.
Collaborative	
Maintain reverse/protective isolation, if appropriate.	May be done initially to reduce contact with sources of possible infection, especially in elderly, immunosuppressed, or diabetic client.

ACTIONS/INTERVENTIONS	RATIONALE
Administer antibiotics as indicated.	Used prophylactically in the operating room and first 24 hours to prevent infection. Late infections may require IV antibiotic treatments for several weeks, in effort to save the prosthetic joint.

NURSING DIAGNOSIS: impaired physical Mobility

May be related to

Pain and discomfort, musculoskeletal impairment
Surgery/restrictive therapies

Possibly evidenced by

Reluctance to attempt movement, difficulty purposefully moving within the physical environment
Reports of pain/discomfort on movement
Limited ROM, decreased muscle strength/control

DESIRED OUTCOMES/EVALUATION CRITERIA—CLIENT WILL:

Mobility (NOC)

Maintain position of function, as evidenced by absence of contracture.
Display increased strength and function of affected joint and limb.
Participate in ADLs/rehabilitation program.

ACTIONS/INTERVENTIONS	RATIONALE
Positioning (NIC)	
Independent	
Maintain affected joint in prescribed position and body in alignment when in bed.	Provides for stabilization of prosthesis and reduces risk of injury during recovery from effects of anesthesia.
Medicate around the clock (or significantly before procedures/activities) so that client is able to participate.	Adequate analgesia is a priority to decrease pain, reduce muscle tension/spasm, and facilitate participation in therapy.
Turn on unoperated side using adequate number of personnel and maintaining operated extremity in prescribed alignment. Support position with pillows/wedges.	Prevents dislocation of hip prosthesis and prolonged skin/tissue pressure, reducing risk of tissue ischemia/breakdown.
Demonstrate/assist with transfer techniques and use of mobility aids; e.g., trapeze, walker, crutches, canes	Facilitates self-care and client's independence. Proper transfer techniques prevent shearing abrasions of skin and falls.
Determine upper body strength and need for equipment to assist with activities of daily living, as appropriate. Involve in exercise program.	Replacement of lower extremity joint requires increased use of upper extremities for transfer, for ADLs and desired activities, as well as use of ambulation devices.
Inspect skin, observe for reddened areas. Keep linens dry and wrinkle-free. Massage skin/bony prominences routinely. Protect operative heel, elevating whole length of leg with pillow and placing heel on water glove if burning sensation reported.	Prevents skin irritation/breakdown.

ACTIONS/INTERVENTIONS	RATIONALE
EXERCISE THERAPY: Joint Mobility (NIC)	
Perform/assist with ROM to unaffected joints.	Client with degenerative joint disease can quickly lose joint function during periods of restricted activity.
Promote participation in rehabilitative exercise program, e.g.:	
Total hip: Quadriceps and gluteal muscle setting, isometrics, leg lifts, dorsiflexion/ plantar flexion (ankle pumps) of the foot;	Strengthens muscle groups, increasing muscle tone and mass; stimulates circulation; prevents decubitus ulcers.
Total knee: Quadriceps setting, gluteal contraction, flexion/extension exercises, isometrics.	Active use of the joint may be painful but will not injure the joint. Continuous passive motion (CPM) exercise may be initiated on the knee joint postoperatively, although its use is dependent on the particular surgeon and individual's needs.
Observe appropriate limitations based on specific joint; e.g., avoid marked flexion/rotation of hip and flexion or hyperextension of leg; adhere to weight-bearing restrictions; wear knee immobilizer as indicated.	Joint stress is to be avoided at all times during stabilization period to prevent dislocation of new prosthesis.
Investigate sudden increase in pain and shortening of limb, as well as changes in skin color, temperature, and sensation.	May be indicative of slippage of prosthesis or other complication, requiring medical evaluation/intervention.
Encourage participation in ADLs.	Enhances self-esteem; promotes sense of control and independence.
Provide positive reinforcement for efforts.	Promotes a positive attitude and encourages involvement in therapy.

Collaborative

ACTIONS/INTERVENTIONS	RATIONALE
Consult with physical/occupational therapists and rehabilitation specialist.	Useful in creating individualized activity/exercise program. Client may require ongoing assistance with movement, strengthening, and weight-bearing activities, as well as use of adjuncts; e.g., walkers, crutches, canes, elevated toilet seat, pickup sticks, and so on.
Provide foam/flotation mattress.	Reduces skin/tissue pressure; limits feelings of fatigue and general discomfort.

NURSING DIAGNOSIS: risk for Peripheral Neurovascular Dysfunction

Risk factors may include

Orthopedic surgery, mechanical compression (e.g., dressing, brace, cast), vascular obstruction, immobilization

Possibly evidenced by

[Not applicable; presence of signs and symptoms establishes an *actual* diagnosis.]

DESIRED OUTCOMES/EVALUATION CRITERIA—CLIENT WILL:

TISSUE PERFUSION: Peripheral (NOC)

Maintain function as evidenced by sensation, movement within normal limits (WNL) for individual situation.
Demonstrate adequate tissue perfusion as evidenced by palpable pulses, brisk capillary refill, skin warm/dry, and normal color.

CIRCULATORY CARE: Arterial [or] Venous Insufficiency (NIC)

Independent

ACTIONS/INTERVENTIONS	RATIONALE
Palpate pulses. Evaluate capillary refill and skin color and temperature. Compare with nonoperated limb.	Diminished/absent pulses, delayed capillary refill time, pallor, blanching, cyanosis, and coldness of skin reflect diminished circulation/perfusion. Comparison with unoperated limb provides clues as to whether neurovascular problem is localized or generalized.
Assess motion and sensation of operated extremity.	Increasing pain, numbness/tingling, inability to perform expected movements (e.g., flex foot) suggests nerve injury, compromised circulation, or dislocation of prosthesis, requiring immediate intervention.
Test sensation of peroneal nerve by pinch/pinprick in the dorsal web between first and second toe, and assess ability to dorsiflex toes after hip/knee replacement.	Position and length of peroneal nerve increase risk of direct injury or compression by tissue edema/hematoma.
Monitor vital signs.	Tachycardia and falling BP may reflect response to hypovolemia/blood loss or suggest anaphylaxis related to absorption of methylmethacrylate into systemic circulation. *Note:* This occurs less often because of the advent of prosthetics with a porous layer that fosters ingrowth of bone instead of total reliance on adhesives to internally fix the device.
Monitor amount and characteristics of drainage on dressings/from suction device. Note swelling in operative area.	May indicate excessive bleeding/hematoma formation, which can potentiate neurovascular compromise. *Note:* Drainage following hip replacement may reach 1000 mL in early postoperative period, potentially affecting circulating volume.
Ensure that stabilizing devices (e.g., abduction pillow, splint device) are in correct position and are not exerting undue pressure on skin and underlying tissue. Avoid use of pillow or bed knee gatch under knees.	Reduces risk of pressure on underlying nerves or compromised circulation to extremities.
Evaluate for calf tenderness, positive Homans' sign, and inflammation.	Although clinical signs are often not reliable in this population, surveillance should be carried out. Early identification of thrombus development and intervention may prevent embolus formation.
Observe for signs of continued bleeding, oozing from puncture sites/mucous membranes, or ecchymosis following minimal trauma.	Depression of clotting mechanisms/sensitivity to anticoagulants may result in bleeding episodes that can affect red blood cell (RBC) level and circulating volume.

Collaborative

ACTIONS/INTERVENTIONS	RATIONALE
Administer IV fluids, blood/plasma expanders as needed.	Restores circulating volume to maintain perfusion. *Note:* Drainage collected from operative site during first 6–10 hr following procedure may be reinfused per protocol, reducing need for transfusion from unknown donor.
Monitor laboratory studies, e.g.:	
Hct;	Usually done 24–48 hr postoperatively for evaluation of blood loss, which can be quite large because of high vascularity of surgical site in hip replacement.
Coagulation studies.	Evaluates presence/degree of alteration in clotting mechanisms and effects of anticoagulant/antiplatelet agents when used.
Administer medications as indicated, e.g.: low-molecular-weight heparins, enoxaparin (Lovenox), dalteparin (Fragmin), tinzaparin (Innohep).	Anticoagulants/antiplatelet agents may be used routinely (prophylactically) to reduce risk of thrombophlebitis and pulmonary emboli. *Note*: Incidence of DVT without prophylaxis is around 50%–80% in client with knee replacement and 47%–64% in client with hip replacement. Studies have shown significant decrease in these numbers with prophylaxis.

ACTIONS/INTERVENTIONS	RATIONALE
Maintain intermittent compression stocking/compression boots when used.	Promotes venous return and prevents venous stasis, reducing risk of thrombus formation.
Apply cold/heat as indicated.	Ice packs are used initially to limit edema/hematoma formation. Heat may then be used to enhance circulation, facilitating resolution of tissue edema.
Prepare for surgical procedure as indicated.	Evacuation of hematoma, or revision of prosthesis may be required to correct compromised circulation.

NURSING DIAGNOSIS: acute Pain

May be related to

Injuring agents: biologic, physical/psychologic (e.g., muscle spasms, surgical procedure, preexisting chronic joint diseases, elderly age, anxiety)

Possibly evidenced by

Reports of pain; distraction/guarding behaviors
Narrowed focus/self-focusing
Alteration in muscle tone; autonomic responses

DESIRED OUTCOMES/EVALUATION CRITERIA—CLIENT WILL:

Pain Level (NOC)

Report pain relieved/controlled.
Appear relaxed, able to rest/sleep appropriately.

Pain Control (NOC)

Demonstrate use of relaxation skills and diversional activities as indicated by individual situation.

ACTIONS/INTERVENTIONS	RATIONALE
Pain Management (NIC)	
Independent	
Perform comprehensive assessment of pain, noting intensity (scale of 0–10), duration, and location. Determine if pain is at operative (or different) site, associated with range of motion, or weight bearing, associated with vascular compromise or fever.	Provides information on which to base and monitor effectiveness of interventions.
Maintain proper position of operated extremity.	Reduces muscle spasm and undue tension on new prosthesis and surrounding tissues.
Provide comfort measures (e.g., frequent repositioning, back rub) and diversional activities. Encourage stress management techniques (e.g., progressive relaxation, guided imagery, visualization, meditation). Provide therapeutic touch as appropriate.	Reduces muscle tension, refocuses attention, promotes sense of control, and may enhance coping abilities in the management of discomfort/pain, which can persist for an extended period.
Medicate on a regular schedule and before activities/procedures.	Reduces muscle tension; improves comfort, and facilitates participation.
Investigate reports of sudden, severe joint pain with muscle spasms and changes in joint mobility; sudden, severe chest pain with dyspnea and restlessness.	Early recognition of developing problems, such as dislocation of prosthesis or pulmonary emboli (blood/fat), provides opportunity for prompt intervention and prevention of more serious complications.

ACTIONS/INTERVENTIONS	RATIONALE
Collaborative	
Administer narcotics, analgesics, and muscle relaxants as indicated/around the clock. Instruct in/monitor use of PCA/epidural administration.	Relieves surgical pain and reduces muscle tension/spasm, which contributes to overall discomfort. Narcotic infusion (including epidural) may be given during first 24–48 hr, with oral analgesics added to pain management program as client progresses. *Note:* Use of ketorolac (Toradol) or other NSAIDs is contraindicated when client is receiving enoxaparin (Lovenox) therapy.
Apply ice packs as indicated.	Promotes vasoconstriction to reduce bleeding/tissue edema in surgical area and lessens perception of discomfort.
Initiate/maintain extremity mobilization: e.g., ambulation, physical therapy, exerciser/CPM device.	Increases circulation to affected muscles. Minimizes joint stiffness; relieves muscle spasms related to disuse.

NURSING DIAGNOSIS: risk for Constipation

Risk factors may include

Insufficient physical activity; decreased mobility, weakness
Insufficient fiber or fluid intake; dehydration, poor eating habits
Decreased gastrointestinal motility, effects of medications (anesthesia/opiate analgesics)
Environmental changes, inadequate toileting

Possibly evidenced by

[Not applicable; presence of signs and symptoms establishes an *actual* diagnosis.]

DESIRED OUTCOMES/EVALUATION CRITERIA—CLIENT WILL:

Bowel Elimination (NOC)

Maintain usual pattern of bowel functioning.
Demonstrate behaviors to prevent problem.

ACTIONS/INTERVENTIONS	RATIONALE
Bowel Management (NIC)	
Independent	
Identify individual risk factors. Determine current situation and possible impact on bowel function (e.g., surgery, use of medications affecting intestinal functioning [new and chronic use], age, weakness).	Constipation is one of the most frequent complaints following surgery and during rehabilitation. If left untreated, constipation can lead to nausea and vomiting, bowel obstruction, or even sepsis, especially in the elderly.
Auscultate abdomen for presence, location, and characteristics of bowel sounds.	Reflects activity of GI tract.
Determine usual elimination pattern (frequency), characteristics of stool (color, consistency, amount), and manner of constipation; e.g., use of laxatives.	Provides baseline for comparison, promotes recognition of changes, and helpful for establishing a preventative plan.
Evaluate usual dietary and fluid intake, compare with current intake.	Client's usual diet and fluid intake may be marginal at best in promoting healthy bowel functioning, especially when combined with current postsurgical status.

ACTIONS/INTERVENTIONS	RATIONALE
Promote increased fluid intake, including water and high-fiber fruit juices; offer warm stimulating fluids (e.g., coffee, tea, hot water).	Prevents dehydration, decreases reabsorption of water from the bowel promoting softer stool/facilitating passage of stool.
Encourage activity/exercise within client's limitation of activity. Assist with early mobility.	To stimulate/optimize GI function.
Provide privacy and routinely scheduled time for defecation based on usual pattern as appropriate (e.g., bedside commode/bathroom with elevated seat, after breakfast).	To facilitate return of normalcy in toileting routine.

Collaborative

Consult with dietitian/nutritionist as indicated.	Helpful in providing a diet with balanced fiber and bulk that client can continue after discharge to improve consistency of stool and facilitate its passage.
Implement bowel program: administer routine stool softeners (e.g., docusate [Colace]), stool stimulants (e.g., bisacodyl [Dulcolax]), sennosides (e.g., [Senokot, Ex-lax]), bulk-forming agents (e.g., polycarbophil [FiberCon]), psyllium (Metamucil), saline laxatives (e.g., magnesium citrate), and enemas as indicated.	Used to prevent or treat constipation.

NURSING DIAGNOSIS: deficient Knowledge [Learning Need] regarding condition, prognosis, treatment, self-care, and discharge needs

May be related to

Lack of exposure/recall
Information misinterpretation

Possibly evidenced by

Questions/request for information, statement of misconception
Inaccurate follow-through of instructions, development of preventable complications

DESIRED OUTCOMES/EVALUATION CRITERIA—CLIENT WILL:

KNOWLEDGE: Disease Process (NOC)

Verbalize understanding of surgical procedure and prognosis.
Correctly perform necessary procedures and explain reasons for the actions.

ACTIONS/INTERVENTIONS	RATIONALE
TEACHING: Disease Process (NIC)	
Independent	
Review disease process, surgical procedure, and future expectations.	Provides knowledge base from which client can make informed choices. The majority of total joint surgeries are elective and preoperative education is done in some form in the surgeon's office or in the admitting facility. Post-surgical review of process and expectations may be needed/desired.

ACTIONS/INTERVENTIONS	RATIONALE
Encourage alternating rest periods with activity.	Conserves energy for healing and prevents undue fatigue, which can increase risk of injury/fall.
Stress importance of continuing prescribed exercise/rehabilitation program within client's tolerance: crutch/cane walking, weight-bearing exercises, stationary bicycling, or swimming.	Increases muscle strength and joint mobility. Most clients will be involved in formal rehabilitation/outpatient, home care programs or be followed in extended-care facilities by physical therapists. Muscle aching indicates too much weight bearing or activity, signaling a need to cut back.
Review activity limitations, depending on joint replaced; e.g., for hip/knee—sitting for long periods or in low chair/toilet seat/recliner, jogging, jumping, excessive bending, lifting, twisting or crossing legs.	Prevents undue stress on implant. Long-term restrictions depend on individual situation/physician protocol.
Discuss need for safe environment in home (e.g., removing scatter rugs and unnecessary furniture) and use of assistive devices (e.g., hand rails in tub/toilet, raised toilet seat, cane for long walks).	Reduces risk of falls and excessive stress on joints.
Review/have client or caregiver demonstrate incisional/wound care.	Promotes independence in self-care, reducing risk of complications.
Identify signs/symptoms requiring medical evaluation; e.g., fever/chills, incisional inflammation, unusual wound drainage, pain in calf or upper thigh, or development of sore throat/dental infections.	Bacterial infections require prompt treatment to prevent progression to osteomyelitis in the operative area and prosthesis failure, which could occur at any time, even years later.
Review drug regimen; e.g., anticoagulants or antibiotics for invasive procedures (e.g., tooth extraction).	Prophylactic therapy may be necessary for a prolonged period after discharge to limit risk of thromboemboli/infection. Procedures known to cause bacteremia can lead to osteomyelitis and prosthesis failure.
Identify bleeding precautions, (e.g., use of soft toothbrush, electric razor, avoidance of trauma/forceful blowing of nose), and necessity of routine laboratory follow-up.	Reduces risk of therapy-induced bleeding/hemorrhage.
Encourage intake of balanced diet, including roughage and adequate fluids.	Enhances healing and feeling of general well-being. Promotes bowel and bladder function during period of altered activity.

POTENTIAL CONSIDERATIONS following acute hospitalization (dependent on client's age, physical condition/presence of complications, personal resources, and life responsibilities)

In addition to considerations in Surgical Intervention plan of care:

risk for Trauma—balancing difficulties/altered gait, weakness, lack of safety precautions, hazards associated with use of assistive devices.

risk for Constipation—insufficient physical activity/decreased mobility, weakness, insufficient fiber/fluid intake, poor eating habits.

Self-Care Deficit/ impaired Home Maintenance—musculoskeletal impairment, decreased strength/endurance, pain in operative site or other joints.

Sample CP: Total Hip Replacement, Hospital. ELOS: 4 Days Orthopedic or Surgical Unit

ND and Categories of Care	Day of Surgery ____	Day 1 ____	Day 2 ____	Day 3 ____	Day 4 ____ Discharge
Risk for infection R/T broken skin, exposure of joint, long-term steroid use, decreased mobility	Goals:				Display early signs of wound
	Participate in activities to reduce risk of postoperative infection	→	→	→	→ healing, free of erythema
		Free of purulent drainage	→	→	→ or drainage
		Be afrebile	→	→	→
				Verbalize understanding of healthcare needs to enhance healing, promote wellness	Plan in place to meet postdischarge needs, self-care
Diagnostics	Hb/Hct	→	Electrolytes if indicated		
	Pulse oximetry	→ D/C if stable			
Additional assessments	VS/Temp per postoperative protocol	→ q4hr	→ q8hr	→ bid unless elevated	→
	Breath sounds q8hr	→	→	→ bid	→
	Amount/characteristic of Hemovac drainage q8hr	→	→ D/C		
			Characteristics of wound/drainage qd and prn	→	→
Medications	IV antibiotics	→ D/C			
Allergies:	IV fluids/blood products	→	→ NS lock or D/C	→ D/C lock	
	Tylenol—Temp ≥ 101°F	→	→	→ D/C	
Client education	Disease process/surgical procedure		Dietary needs	Wound care	Provide written instructions for home care
	Handwashing technique, avoid touching of dressing/wound		S/S to report of health-care provider	Balancing rest/activity	
	Respiratory exercises, incentive spirometry				
Additional nursing actions	Aseptic/clean technique	→	→	→	→
	Protective isolation as indicated	→	→ D/C		
	Reinforce dressing	→	→ Change dressing qd and prn	→ D/C if incision dry	
				Clean incision bid	→
	Encourage PO fluids as tolerated	→	→	→	→
	T, C, B, DB, q2hr	→	Per self	→	→
	Incentive spirometry q2hr	→ q2hr WA	→ q4hr WA	→	→
	Supplemental O_2 as indicated	→ D/C if stable			
			High-calorie/protein diet WR	→	→

(Continued on following page)

Sample CP: Total Hip Replacement, Hospital. ELOS: 4 Days Orthopedic or Surgical Unit

ND and Categories of Care	Day of Surgery ____	Day 1 ____	Day 2 ____	Day 3 ____	Day 4 ____ Discharge
Impaired physical mobility R/T musculoskeletal impairment/discomfort, therapeutic restrictions				Independent in transfers	Independent in ambulation
	Maintain proper alignment and position of function	→	→	→	→
	Participate in rehabilitation/exercise program	→	→	→	
				Display increased strength/function of operated limb	→ Free of DT/thromboembolic complications Establish regular bladder/bowel elimination
Referrals		PT-assistive devices if not done preop	PT-exercises/ambulation	OT/rehabilitation specialist Social Services if placement indicated	Home care
Diagnostic studies		PT (coumadin use)	→	→	→ CBC w/platelets (if Lovenox used)
Additional assessments	Neurovascular status/alignment of operated leg per postoperative protocol	→ q4hr	→ q8hr	→ bid	→
	Skin (especially heels) q8hr or per protocol	→	→	→qd	→
	Voiding/urinary output q8hr	→	→	→ D/C	
	Bowel sounds q8hr	→	→ bid	→ qd	→ D/C
		Stool characteristics	→	→	→
Medications Allergies:	Coumadin (if Lovenox not ordered)	→ Daily order or	→	→	→
		Lovenox q12hr	→	→	→
	Stool softener/bowel program	→	→	→	→
Client education	Hip precautions Use of trapeze Initial exercises—ankle pumps, quad/gluteal sets	Transfer techniques	Use of mobility aids S/S to report to healthcare provider Self-administer Lovenox	Ambulation/weight-bearing exercises Activity level/restrictions post discharge Sexual concerns	Provide written instructions Home exercise program Coumadin dose, time, purpose, side effects, precautions, monitoring (if used)

Additional nursing actions	Bedrest/HOB elevated 30°	→ Chair/commode elevate operated leg	→ Chair ×3 ambulate with assistance	→ Ambulate ×3 with assistance as needed	→
	Pillow between knees	→	→	→ prn	→
	Turn per protocol q2hr	→	→	→	→
	ROM to nonoperated side q2hr	→	→ Per self	→	→
	Initial exercises q1hr WA	→	→	→	→
			Knee exercise ×5 q1hr WA	→ Leg strengthening	→
	SCDs to calves	→ While in bed	→	→ D/C if PT 1.3 or above	
	Total care	→ Assist w/care	→ Self-care	→	→ Shower as indicated
	Fracture pan	→ Elevated toilet seat	→	→	→
	Straight catheter if no void q8hr ×2	→ Insert Foley on #3 if no void	→ D/C Foley-male	→ D/C Foley-female	
	Foam/special mattress	→	→	→	→ Send home
Pain R/T therapeutic interventions, preexisting chronic joint disease	Verbalize pain within manageable level	→	→	→	→
		Participate in action to decrease pain	→	→	→
					Verbalize understanding of medications/modalities for pain management
					Demonstrate proper use of adjunct comfort measures
Additional assessments	Pain characteristics/changes	→	→	→	→
	Response to interventions	→	→	→	→
Medications Allergies: ______	PCA—narcotic of choice	→ D/C, begin PO if tolented	→ Acetaminophen prn for breakthrough pain	→	→
	Antiemetic prn	→ D/C			
	Muscle relaxant	→			
Client education	Orient to unit/room	Relaxation techniques, guided imagery, breathing exercises		Medications: dose, time, route, purpose, side effects	Written instructions for home care needs, equipment resources
	Proper use of PCA				
	Reporting of pain/effects of interventions				
Additional nursing actions	Maintain position/alignment of leg per protocol	→	→	→	→
	Ice pack to operated site	→ prn	→ D/C		
	Routine comfort measures prn	→	→	→	→

13

CHAPTER

Integumentary

BURNS: THERMAL/CHEMICAL/ELECTRICAL (ACUTE AND CONVALESCENT PHASES)

Each year, more than 1 million burn injuries occur in the United States; approximately 70,000 people require hospital care. Thermal burns, which are the most common type, occur because of fires, motor vehicle crashes, home fires, hot liquid spills, electrical malfunctions, and war. Survival rates have risen because of newer treatments and skin barrier development; however, moderate and severe burns account for many dollars spent on physical and psychologic rehabilitation.

Types of Burns

Thermal burns: Injuring agent can be flame, hot liquid, or contact with hot object. Flame burns are associated with smoke/inhalation injury.

Chemical burns: Occur from type/content of injuring agent, as well as concentration and temperature of agent.

Electrical burns: Occur from type/voltage of current that generates heat in proportion to resistance offered and travels the pathway of least resistance (i.e., nerves offer the least resistance and bones the greatest resistance). Underlying injury is more severe than visible injury.

Burn Wound Classification (Depth and Extent)

Superficial partial-thickness (first-degree) burns: Involve only the epidermis. Wounds appear bright pink to red with minimal edema and fine blisters if there are any blisters at all. The skin is often warm/dry.

Moderate partial-thickness (second-degree) burns: Involve the epidermis and dermis. Wounds appear red to pink with moderate edema and blisters that may be intact or draining.

Deep partial-thickness (second-degree) burns: Involve the deep dermis. Wounds appear pale pink to pale ivory with moderate edema and blisters. These wounds are dryer than moderate partial-thickness burns.

Full-thickness (third-degree) burns: Involve all layers of skin, subcutaneous fat, and may involve the muscle, nerves, and blood supply. Wound appearance varies from white to cherry red to brown or black, with blistering uncommon. These wounds have a dry, leathery texture. There is no pain in the center of these burns, but the edges of the burn wound may have heightened sensation.

Full-thickness/subdermal (fourth-degree) burns: Involve all skin layers plus muscle, organ tissue, and bone. Charring occurs.

CARE SETTING

The following adult clients are admitted for acute care and during the rehabilitation phase may be cared for in a subacute or rehabilitation unit: those with partial-thickness burns more than 10% total body surface area (TBSA) or whose age is considered high risk (older than 50 years and younger than 10 years); full-thickness burns more than 2% of TBSA; and clients with second- and third-degree burns of face, both hands, perineum, or both feet; or inhalation and all electrical burns, including lightning injury.

RELATED CONCERNS

Disaster considerations, page 890
Fluid and electrolyte imbalances, page 919
Metabolic acidosis (primary base bicarbonate deficiency), page 492
Psychosocial aspects of care, page 770
Respiratory acidosis (primary carbonic acid excess), page 194
Sepsis/septicemia, page 701
Surgical intervention, page 788

Total nutritional support: parenteral/enteral feeding, page 478
Upper gastrointestinal/esophageal bleeding, page 309

Client Assessment Database

Data depend on type, severity, and body surface area involved.

ACTIVITY/REST

May exhibit: Decreased strength, endurance
Limited range of motion (ROM) of involved areas
Impaired muscle mass, altered tone

CIRCULATION

May exhibit (with burn injury of more than 20% TBSA): Hypotension (shock)
Peripheral pulses diminished distal to extremity injury; generalized peripheral vasoconstriction with loss of pulses, mottling of skin, and coolness (electrical shock)
Tachycardia (shock/anxiety/pain)
Dysrhythmias (electrical shock)
Tissue edema formation (all burns)

EGO INTEGRITY

May report: Feeling scared, self-conscious, conspicuous, angry, embarrassed, different
Concerns about family, job, finances, disfigurement

May exhibit: Anxiety, crying, dependency, denial, withdrawal, hostility, aggressive behavior

ELIMINATION

May exhibit: Urinary output decreased/absent during emergent phase; color may be pink (hemochromogens from damaged red blood cells [RBCs]) or reddish black if myoglobin present, indicating deep-muscle damage
Diuresis (after capillary leak sealed and fluids mobilized back into circulation)
Bowel sounds decreased/absent, especially in cutaneous burns of more than 20%, because stress reduces gastric motility/peristalsis

FOOD/FLUID

May exhibit: Generalized tissue edema (swelling is rapid and may be extreme in early hours after injury)
Anorexia, nausea/vomiting

NEUROSENSORY

May report: Mixed areas of numbness, tingling, burning pain
Changes in vision, decreased visual acuity (electrical shock)

May exhibit: Changes in orientation, affect, behavior
Decreased deep tendon reflexes (DTRs), reflexes and sensation in injured extremities
Seizure activity (electrical shock)
Corneal lacerations, retinal damage (electrical shock)
Rupture of tympanic membrane (electrical shock)
Paralysis (electrical injury to nerve pathways)

PAIN/DISCOMFORT

May report: Pain varies; e.g., first-degree burns are extremely sensitive to touch, pressure, air movement, and temperature changes; second-degree moderate-thickness burns are very painful, whereas pain response in second-degree deep-thickness burns depends on intactness of nerve endings; third-degree burns are painless except along the edges of the burn wound

RESPIRATION

May report: Confinement in a closed space, prolonged exposure (possibility of inhalation injury)

May exhibit: Hoarseness, wheezy cough, carbonaceous particles on face/in sputum, drooling/inability to swallow oral secretions, and cyanosis (indicative of inhalation injury)
Thoracic excursion may be limited in presence of circumferential chest burns
Upper airway stridor/wheezes (obstruction due to laryngospasm, laryngeal edema)
Breath sounds: Crackles (pulmonary edema), stridor (laryngeal edema), profuse airway secretions/wheezing (rhonchi)

SAFETY

May exhibit: **Skin:**

General: Exact depth of tissue destruction may not be evident for 3–5 days because of the process of microvascular thrombosis in some wounds; unburned skin areas may be cool/clammy, pale, with slow capillary refill in the presence of decreased cardiac output as a result of fluid loss/shock state

Flame injury: There may be areas of mixed depth of injury because of varied intensity of heat produced by burning clothing; singed nasal hairs; dry, red mucosa of nose and mouth; blisters on posterior pharynx, circumoral and/or circumnasal edema

Chemical injury: Wound appearance varies according to causative agent; skin may be yellowish brown with soft leather-like texture; blisters, ulcers, necrosis, or thick eschar. (Injuries are generally deeper than they appear cutaneously, and tissue destruction can continue for up to 72 hours after injury.)

Electrical injury: The external cutaneous injury is usually much less than the underlying necrosis; appearance of wounds varies and may include entry/exit (explosive) wounds of current, arc burns from current moving in close proximity to body, and thermal burns due to ignition of clothing

Other: Presence of fractures/dislocations (concurrent falls, motor vehicle accident; tetanic muscle contractions due to electrical shock)

TEACHING/LEARNING

Discharge plan considerations: May require assistance with treatments, wound care/supplies, self-care activities, homemaker/maintenance tasks, transportation, finances, vocational counseling

Changes in physical layout of home or living facility other than home during prolonged rehabilitation

Refer to section at end of plan for postdischarge considerations.

DIAGNOSTIC STUDIES

Complete blood count (CBC): Initial increased hematocrit (Hct) suggests hemoconcentration due to fluid shift/loss. Later decreased Hct and RBCs may occur because of heat damage to vascular endothelium. Leukocytosis (decreased white blood cells [WBCs]) can occur because of loss of cells at wound site and inflammatory response to injury.

Arterial blood gases (ABGs): Baseline especially important with suspicion of inhalation injury. Reduced Pao_2/increased $Paco_2$ may be seen with carbon monoxide retention. Acidosis may occur because of reduced renal function and loss of compensatory respiratory mechanisms.

Carboxyhemoglobin (COHb): Elevation of more than 10% indicates carbon monoxide poisoning/inhalation injury.

Serum electrolytes: Potassium level may be initially elevated because of injured tissues/RBC destruction and decreased renal function; hypokalemia can occur when diuresis starts; magnesium level may be decreased. Sodium level may initially be decreased with body water losses; hypernatremia can occur later as renal conservation occurs.

Alkaline phosphatase: Elevated because of interstitial fluid shifts/impairment of sodium pump.

Serum glucose: Elevation reflects stress response.

Serum albumin: Albumin/globulin ratio may be reversed as a result of loss of protein in edema fluid.

Blood urea nitrogen (BUN)/creatinine (Cr): Elevation reflects decreased renal perfusion/function; however, Cr level can elevate because of tissue injury.

Urine: Presence of albumin, hemoglobin (Hb), and myoglobin indicates deep-tissue damage and protein loss (especially seen with serious electrical burns). Reddish black color of urine is due to presence of myoglobin.

Random urine sodium: More than 20 mEq/L indicates excessive fluid resuscitation; less than 10 mEq/L suggests inadequate fluid resuscitation.

Wound cultures: May be obtained for baseline data and repeated periodically.

Chest x-ray: May appear normal in early postburn period even with inhalation injury; however, a true inhalation injury presents as infiltrates, often progressing to whiteout on x-ray (acute respiratory distress syndrome [ARDS]).

Upper airway endoscopy/fiberoptic bronchoscopy: Useful in diagnosing extent of inhalation injury, when can be done immediately in the high-risk client; findings can include edema, hemorrhage, and/or ulceration of upper respiratory tract.

Flow volume loop: Provides noninvasive assessment of effects/extent of inhalation injury.

Xenon ventilation-perfusion lung scan: May be done to determine extent of inhalation injury.

Electrocardiogram (ECG): Signs of myocardial ischemia/dysrhythmias may occur with electrical burns.

Laser Doppler: Probes can be placed on a partial-thickness burn to monitor microvascular blood flow in dermis. The accuracy of burn depth diagnosis can range from 90% to 97%, but use of this technololgy is limited because scanners that can examine large burn areas are expensive and not readily available.

Photographs of burns: Provide documentation of burn wound and comparative baseline to evaluate healing.

Cardiac enzymes: Will provide an overview of the extent of muscle damage in the case of electrical injury.

NURSING PRIORITIES

1. Maintain patent airway/respiratory function.
2. Restore hemodynamic stability/circulating volume.
3. Alleviate pain.
4. Prevent complications.
5. Provide emotional support for client/significant other (SO).
6. Provide information about condition, prognosis, and treatment.

DISCHARGE GOALS

1. Homeostasis achieved.
2. Pain controlled/reduced.
3. Complications prevented/minimized.
4. Dealing with current situation realistically.
5. Condition/prognosis and therapeutic regimen understood.
6. Plan in place to meet needs after discharge.

NURSING DIAGNOSIS: risk for ineffective Airway Clearance

Risk factors may include

Tracheobronchial obstruction: mucosal edema and loss of ciliary action (smoke inhalation); circumferential full-thickness burns of the neck, thorax, and chest, with compression of the airway or limited chest excursion

Trauma: direct upper-airway injury by flame, steam, hot air, and chemicals/gases

Fluid shifts, pulmonary edema, decreased lung compliance

Possibly evidenced by

[Not applicable; presence of signs and symptoms establishes an *actual* diagnosis.]

DESIRED OUTCOMES/EVALUATION CRITERIA—CLIENT WILL:

RESPIRATORY STATUS: Airway Patency (NOC)

Demonstrate clear breath sounds, respiratory rate within normal range, be free of dyspnea/cyanosis.

ACTIONS/INTERVENTIONS	RATIONALE
Respiratory Monitoring (NIC)	
Independent	
Obtain history of injury. Note presence of preexisting respiratory conditions, history of smoking.	Causative burning agent, duration of exposure, and occurrence in closed or open space predict probability of inhalation injury. Type of material burned (such as wood, plastic, wool) suggests type of toxic gas exposure. Preexisting conditions increase the risk of respiratory complications.
Assess gag/swallow reflexes; note upper airway burns, drooling, inability to swallow, hoarseness, wheezy cough.	Suggestive of inhalation injury, which may develop over several days.
Monitor respiratory rate, rhythm, depth; note presence of pallor/cyanosis and carbonaceous or pink-tinged sputum.	Tachypnea, use of accessory muscles, presence of cyanosis, and changes in sputum suggest developing respiratory distress/pulmonary edema and need for medical intervention.
Auscultate lungs, noting stridor, wheezing/crackles, diminished breath sounds, brassy cough.	Airway obstruction/respiratory distress can occur very quickly or may be delayed; e.g., up to 3 days after burn.
Note presence of pallor or cherry-red color of unburned skin.	Suggests presence of hypoxemia or carbon monoxide.

ACTIONS/INTERVENTIONS	RATIONALE
Investigate changes in behavior/mentation; e.g., restlessness, agitation, confusion.	Although often related to pain, changes in consciousness may reflect developing, worsening hypoxia or effects of inhaled toxins (especially carbon monoxide).
Monitor 24-hr fluid balance, noting variations/changes.	Fluid shifts or excess fluid replacement increases risk of pulmonary edema. *Note:* Inhalation injury increases fluid demands as much as 35% or more because of edema and fluid shifts.

Airway Management (NIC)

Elevate head of bed. Avoid use of pillow under head, as indicated.	Promotes optimal lung expansion/respiratory function. When head/neck burns are present, a pillow can inhibit respiration, cause necrosis of burned ear cartilage, and promote neck contractures.
Encourage coughing/deep-breathing exercises and frequent position changes.	Promotes lung expansion, mobilization, and drainage of secretions.
Suction (if necessary) with extreme care, maintaining sterile technique.	Helps maintain clear airway, but should be done cautiously because of mucosal edema and inflammation. Sterile technique reduces risk of infection.
Promote voice rest, but assess ability to speak and/or swallow oral secretions periodically.	Increasing hoarseness/decreased ability to swallow suggests increasing tracheal edema and may indicate need for prompt intubation.

Collaborative

Administer humidified oxygen via appropriate mode; e.g., face mask.	Oxygen corrects hypoxemia/acidosis. Humidity decreases drying of respiratory tract and reduces viscosity of sputum.
Monitor continuous pulse oximetry and serial ABGs.	Baseline is essential for further assessment of respiratory status and as a guide to treatment. Pao_2 less than 50, $Paco_2$ greater than 50, and decreasing pH reflect smoke inhalation and developing pneumonia, ARDS.
Monitor COHb levels, if indicated.	Client with inhalation injury may be monitored for elevated carbon monoxide levels. If pH is below 7.4 along with elevated COHb, hyperbaric oxygenation may be considered.
Review serial chest x-rays.	Changes reflecting atelectasis/pulmonary edema may not occur for 2–3 days after burn.
Provide/assist with chest physiotherapy and incentive spirometry.	Chest physiotherapy drains dependent areas of the lung, and incentive spirometry may be done to improve lung expansion, thereby promoting respiratory function and reducing atelectasis. *Note*: Bronchoscopy may be done to remove endotrachael debris.
Prepare for/assist with intubation or tracheostomy, mechanical ventilation as indicated.	Intubation/mechanical support is required when airway edema or circumferential burn injury interferes with respiratory function/oxygenation. If client develops signs of respiratory failure or ARDS, mechanical ventilation and intensive respiratory care is required. (Refer to CP: Ventilatory Assistance [Mechanical].)

NURSING DIAGNOSIS: risk for deficient Fluid Volume

Risk factors may include

Loss of fluid through abnormal routes; e.g., burn wounds
Increased need: hypermetabolic state, insufficient intake
Hemorrhagic losses

Possibly evidenced by

[Not applicable; presence of signs and symptoms establishes an *actual* diagnosis.]

DESIRED OUTCOMES/EVALUATION CRITERIA—CLIENT WILL:

Hydration (NOC)

Demonstrate improved fluid balance as evidenced by individually adequate urinary output with normal specific gravity, stable vital signs, moist mucous membranes.

ACTIONS/INTERVENTIONS	RATIONALE
Shock Prevention (NIC)	
Independent	
Monitor vital signs, central venous pressure (CVP). Note capillary refill and strength of peripheral pulses.	Serves as a guide to fluid replacement needs and assesses cardiovascular response. *Note:* Invasive monitoring is indicated for clients with major burns, smoke inhalation, or preexisting cardiac disease, although there is an associated increased risk of infection, necessitating careful monitoring and care of insertion site.
Monitor urinary output and specific gravity. Observe urine color and Hematest as indicated.	Generally, fluid replacement should be titrated to ensure average urinary output of 30–50 mL/hr (in the adult). Urine can appear red to black (with massive muscle destruction) because of presence of blood and release of myoglobin. If gross myoglobinuria is present, minimum urinary output should be 75–100 mL/hr to reduce risk of tubular damage and renal failure.
Estimate wound drainage and insensible losses.	Increased capillary permeability, protein shifts, inflammatory process, and evaporative losses greatly affect circulating volume and urinary output, especially during initial 24–72 hours after burn injury.
Maintain cumulative record of amount and types of fluid intake.	Massive/rapid replacement with different types of fluids and fluctuations in rate of administration require close tabulation to prevent constituent imbalances or fluid overload.
Weigh daily.	Fluid replacement formulas partly depend on admission weight and subsequent changes. A 15%–20% weight gain can be anticipated in the first 72 hr during fluid replacement, with return to preburn weight approximately 10 days after burn.
Measure circumference of burned extremities as indicated.	May be helpful in estimating extent of edema/fluid shifts affecting circulating volume and urinary output.
Investigate changes in mentation.	Deterioration in the level of consciousness may indicate inadequate circulating volume/reduced cerebral perfusion.
Observe for gastric distention, hematemesis, tarry stools. Hematest nasogastric (NG) drainage and stools periodically.	Stress (Curling's) ulcer occurs in up to half of all severely burned clients and can occur as early as the first week. Clients with burns more than 20% TBSA are at risk for mucosal bleeding in the gastrointestinal (GI) tract during the acute phase because of decreased splanchnic blood flow and reflex paralytic ileus.
Collaborative	
Insert/maintain indwelling urinary catheter.	Allows for close observation of renal function and prevents urinary retention. Retention of urine with its by-products of tissue-cell destruction can lead to renal dysfunction and infection.

ACTIONS/INTERVENTIONS	RATIONALE
Insert/maintain large-bore IV catheter(s).	Accommodates rapid infusion of fluids.
Administer calculated IV replacement of fluids, electrolytes, plasma, albumin.	Fluid resuscitation replaces lost fluids/electrolytes and helps prevent complications; e.g., shock, acute tubular necrosis (ATN). Replacement formulas vary (e.g., Brooke, Evans, Parkland) but are based on extent of injury, amount of urinary output, and weight. *Note:* Once initial fluid resuscitation has been accomplished, a steady rate of fluid administration is preferred to boluses, which may increase interstitial fluid shifts and cardiopulmonary congestion.
Monitor laboratory studies (e.g., Hb/Hct, electrolytes, random urine sodium).	Identifies blood loss/RBC destruction and fluid and electrolyte replacement needs. Urine sodium less than 10 mEq/L suggests inadequate fluid resuscitation. *Note:* During first 24 hr after burn, hemoconcentration is common because of fluid shifts into the interstitial space.
Administer medications as indicated:	
Diuretics; e.g., mannitol (Osmitrol);	May be indicated to enhance urinary output and clear tubules of debris/prevent necrosis if acute renal failure (ARF) is present.
Potassium;	Although hyperkalemia often occurs during first 24–48 hours (tissue destruction), subsequent replacement may be necessary because of large urinary losses.
Antacids; e.g., calcium carbonate (Titralac), magaldrate (Riopan); histamine inhibitors; e.g., cimetidine (Tagamet)/ranitidine (Zantac).	Antacids may reduce gastric acidity; histamine inhibitors decrease production of hydrochloric acid to reduce risk of gastric irritation/bleeding.
Add electrolytes to water used for wound débridement, as indicated.	Washing solution that approximates tissue fluids may minimize osmotic fluid shifts.

NURSING DIAGNOSIS: acute Pain

May be related to

Destruction of skin/tissues, edema formation
Manipulation of injured tissues; e.g., wound débridement

Possibly evidenced by

Reports of pain
Narrowed focus, facial mask of pain
Alteration in muscle tone; autonomic responses
Distraction/guarding behaviors, anxiety/fear, restlessness, crying

DESIRED OUTCOMES/EVALUATION CRITERIA—CLIENT WILL:

Pain Level (NOC)

Report pain reduced/controlled.
Display relaxed facial expressions/body posture.

Pain Control (NOC)

Participate in activities and sleep/rest appropriately.

ACTIONS/INTERVENTIONS	RATIONALE
Pain Management (NIC)	
Independent	
Cover wounds as soon as possible unless open-air exposure burn care method required.	Temperature changes and air movement can cause great pain to exposed nerve endings.
Elevate burned extremities periodically.	Elevation may be required initially to reduce edema formation; thereafter, changes in position and elevation reduce discomfort and risk of joint contractures.
Provide bed cradle as indicated.	Elevation of linens off wounds may help reduce pain.
Wrap digits/extremities in position of function (avoiding flexed position of affected joints) using splints and footboards as necessary.	Position of function reduces deformities/contractures and promotes comfort. Although flexed position of injured joints may feel more comfortable, it can lead to flexion contractures.
Change position frequently and assist with active and passive range-of-motion (ROM) exercises as indicated.	Movement and exercise reduce joint stiffness and muscle fatigue, but type of exercise depends on location and extent of injury.
Maintain comfortable environmental temperature; provide heat lamps, heat-retaining body coverings.	Temperature regulation may be lost with major burns. External heat sources may be necessary to prevent chilling.
Assess reports of pain, noting location/character and intensity (0–10 scale).	Pain is nearly always present to some degree because of varying severity of tissue involvement/destruction but is usually most severe during dressing changes and débridement. Changes in location, character, and intensity of pain may indicate developing complications (e.g., limb ischemia) or herald improvement/return of nerve function/sensation.
Provide medication and/or place in hydrotherapy (as appropriate) before performing dressing changes and débridement.	Reduces severe physical and emotional distress associated with painful procedures.
Encourage expression of feelings about pain.	Verbalization allows outlet for emotions and may enhance coping mechanisms.
Involve client in determining schedule for activities, treatments, drug administration.	Enhances client's sense of control and strengthens coping mechanisms.
Explain procedures/provide frequent information as appropriate, especially during wound débridement.	Empathic support can help alleviate pain/promote relaxation. Knowing what to expect provides opportunity for client to prepare self and enhances sense of control.
Provide basic comfort measures; e.g., massage of uninjured areas, frequent position changes.	Promotes relaxation, reduces muscle tension and general fatigue.
Encourage use of stress management techniques; e.g., progressive relaxation, deep breathing, guided imagery, and visualization.	Refocuses attention, promotes relaxation, and enhances sense of control, which may reduce pharmacological dependency.
Provide diversional activities appropriate for age/condition.	Helps lessen concentration on pain experience and refocus attention.
Promote uninterrupted sleep periods.	Sleep deprivation can increase perception of pain/reduce coping abilities.
Collaborative	
Administer analgesics (narcotic and nonnarcotic) as indicated; e.g., morphine; fentanyl (Sublimaze, Ultiva), hydrocodone (Vicodin, Hycodan), oxycodone (OxyContin, Percocet).	The burned client may require around-the-clock medication and dose titration. IV method is often used initially to maximize drug effect. Concerns of client addiction or doubts regarding degree of pain experienced are not valid during emergent/acute phase of care, but narcotics should be decreased as soon as feasible and alternative methods for pain relief initiated.
Provide/instruct in use of patient-controlled analgesia (PCA).	PCA provides for timely drug administration, preventing fluctuations in intensity of pain, often at lower total dosage than would be given by conventional methods.

NURSING DIAGNOSIS: risk for Infection

Risk factors may include

Inadequate primary defenses: destruction of skin barrier, traumatized tissues
Inadequate secondary defenses: decreased Hb, suppressed inflammatory response
Environmental exposure, invasive procedures

Possibly evidenced by

[Not applicable; presence of signs and symptoms establishes an *actual* diagnosis.]

DESIRED OUTCOMES/EVALUATION CRITERIA—CLIENT WILL:

WOUND HEALING: Secondary Intention (NOC)

Achieve timely wound healing free of purulent exudate and be afebrile.

ACTIONS/INTERVENTIONS	RATIONALE
Infection Protection (NIC)	
Independent	
Implement appropriate isolation techniques as indicated.	Dependent on type/extent of wounds and the choice of wound treatment (e.g., open vs closed); isolation may range from simple wound/skin to complete or reverse to reduce risk of cross-contamination and exposure to multiple bacterial flora.
Emphasize/model good hand washing technique for all individuals coming in contact with client.	Prevents cross-contamination, reduces risk of acquired infection.
Use gowns, gloves, masks, and strict aseptic technique during direct wound care and provide sterile or freshly laundered bed linens/gowns.	Prevents exposure to infectious organisms.
Monitor/limit visitors, if necessary. If isolation is used, explain procedure to visitors. Supervise visitor adherence to protocol as indicated.	Prevents cross-contamination from visitors. Concern for risk of infection should be balanced against client's need for family support and socialization.
Wound Care (NIC)	
Shave/clip all hair from around burned areas to include a 1-inch border (excluding eyebrows). Shave facial hair (men) and shampoo head daily.	Hair is a good medium for bacterial growth; however, eyebrows act as a protective barrier for the eyes. Regular shampooing decreases bacterial fallout into burned areas.
Examine unburned areas (such as groin, neck creases, mucous membranes) and vaginal discharge routinely.	Opportunistic infections (e.g., yeast) frequently occur because of depression of the immune system and/or proliferation of normal body flora during systemic antibiotic therapy.
Provide special care for eyes; e.g., use eye covers and tear formulas as appropriate.	Eyes may be swollen shut and/or become infected by drainage from surrounding burns. If lids are burned, eye covers may be needed to prevent corneal damage.
Prevent skin-to-skin surface contact (e.g., wrap each burned finger/toe separately; do not allow burned ear to touch scalp).	Prevents adherence to surface it may be touching and encourages proper healing. *Note:* Ear cartilage has limited circulation and is prone to pressure necrosis.
Examine wounds daily, note/document changes in appearance, odor, or quantity of drainage.	Identifies presence of healing (granulation tissue) and provides for early detection of burn-wound infection. Infection in a partial-thickness burn may cause conversion of burn to full-thickness injury. *Note:* A strong sweet, musty smell at a graft site is indicative of *Pseudomonas.*

ACTIONS/INTERVENTIONS	RATIONALE
Monitor vital signs for fever, increased respiratory rate/depth in association with changes in sensorium, presence of diarrhea, decreased platelet count, and hyperglycemia with glycosuria.	Indicators of sepsis (often occurs with full-thickness burn) requiring prompt evaluation and intervention. *Note:* Changes in sensorium, bowel habits, and respiratory rate usually precede fever and alteration of laboratory studies.

Collaborative

Remove dressings and cleanse burned areas in a hydrotherapy/whirlpool tub or in a shower stall with handheld showerhead. Maintain temperature of water at 100°F (37.8°C). Wash areas with a mild cleansing agent or surgical soap.	Water softens and aids in removal of dressings and eschar (slough layer of dead skin or tissue). Sources vary as to whether bath or shower is best. Bath has advantage of water providing support for exercising extremities but may promote cross-contamination of wounds. Showering enhances wound inspection and prevents contamination from floating debris.
Excise and cover burn wounds quickly.	Early excision is known to reduce scarring and risk of infection, thereby facilitating healing.
Debride necrotic/loose tissue (including ruptured blisters) with scissors and forceps. Do not disturb intact blisters if they are smaller than 1–2 cm, do not interfere with joint function, and do not appear infected.	Promotes healing. Prevents autocontamination. Small, intact blisters help protect skin and increase rate of re-epithelialization unless the burn injury is the result of chemicals (in which case fluid contained in blisters may continue to cause tissue destruction).
Photograph wound initially and at periodic intervals.	Provides baseline and documentation of healing process.

Infection Protection (NIC)

Administer topical antimicrobial agents as indicated; e.g.:	The following agents help control bacterial growth and prevent drying of wound, which can cause further tissue destruction.
Silver sulfadiazine (Silvadene);	Still the most common topical antibiotic used in burn care, Silvadene is a broad-spectrum antimicrobial that may allow the wound to heal without need for skin grafting, is relatively painless but has intermediate, somewhat delayed eschar penetration. May cause rash or depression of WBCs.
Mafenide acetate (Sulfamylon) solution or mafenide HCl cream;	Antibiotic of choice with confirmed invasive burn wound infection that does not respond to Silvadene. Useful against gram-negative/gram-positive organisms, and some fungal species. The solution is painless, however the cream causes burning/pain on application and for 30 minutes thereafter. Can cause rash, and is contraindicated in metabolic acidosis.
Acticoat;	Acticoat is a non-adherent antimicrobial dressing that stays on the wound for up to 7 days, delivering a low concentration of nanocrystalline silver.
Aqueous silver nitrate;	Effective against *Staphylococcus aureus, Escherichia coli,* and *Pseudomonas aeruginosa,* but has poor eschar penetration, is painful, and may cause electrolyte imbalance. Dressings must be constantly saturated. Product stains skin/surfaces black.
Poloxamer 188 containing bacitracin and polymixin B;	This gel is effective against gram-positive organisms, does not interfere with re-ephithelializaton, and is generally used for tar and asphalt-based residues, other imbedded materials, and for superficial and facial burns.
Hydrogels; e.g., Transorb, Burnfree.	Useful for partial- and full-thickness burns; in rehydrating dry wound beds, and promoting autolytic debridement. May be used when infection is present.

ACTIONS/INTERVENTIONS	RATIONALE
Administer other medications as appropriate; e.g.;	
Subeschar clysis/systemic antibiotics;	Systemic antibiotics are given to control general infections identified by culture/sensitivity. Subeschar clysis has been found effective against pathogens in granulated tissues at the line of demarcation between viable/nonviable tissue, reducing risk of sepsis.
Tetanus toxoid or clostridial antitoxin as appropriate.	Tissue destruction/altered defense mechanisms increase risk of developing tetanus or gas gangrene, especially in deep burns such as those caused by electricity.
Place IV/invasive lines in nonburned area.	Decreased risk of infection at insertion site with possibility of progression to septicemia.
Obtain routine cultures and sensitivities of wounds/drainage.	Allows early recognition and specific treatment of wound infection.
Assist with excisional biopsies when infection is suspected.	Bacteria can colonize the wound surface without invading the underlying tissue; therefore, biopsies may be obtained for diagnosing infection.

NURSING DIAGNOSIS: ineffective Tissue Perfusion/risk for Peripheral Neurovascular Dysfunction

Risk factors may include

Reduction/interruption of arterial/venous blood flow; e.g., circumferential burns of extremities with resultant edema
Hypovolemia

Possibly evidenced by

[Not applicable; presence of signs and symptoms establishes an *actual* diagnosis.]

DESIRED OUTCOMES/EVALUATION CRITERIA—CLIENT WILL:

TISSUE PERFUSION: Peripheral (NOC)

Maintain palpable peripheral pulses of equal quality/strength; good capillary refill and skin color normal in uninjured areas.

ACTIONS/INTERVENTIONS	RATIONALE
CIRCULATORY CARE: Venous [or] Arterial (NIC)	
Independent	
Assess color, sensation, movement, peripheral pulses (via Doppler), and capillary refill on extremities with circumferential burns. Compare with findings of unaffected limb.	Edema formation can readily compress blood vessels, thereby impeding circulation and increasing venous stasis/edema. Comparisons with unaffected limbs aid in differentiating localized versus systemic problems (e.g., hypovolemia/decreased cardiac output).
Elevate affected extremities, as appropriate. Remove jewelry/arm band. Avoid taping around a burned extremity/digit.	Promotes systemic circulation/venous return and may reduce edema or other deleterious effects of constriction of edematous tissues. *Note*: Prolonged elevation can impair arterial perfusion if blood pressure (BP) falls or tissue pressures rise excessively.

ACTIONS/INTERVENTIONS	RATIONALE
Obtain BP in unburned extremity when possible. Remove BP cuff after each reading, as indicated.	If BP readings must be obtained on an injured extremity, leaving the cuff in place may increase edema formation/ reduce perfusion, and convert partial-thickness burn to a more serious injury.
Investigate reports of deep/throbbing ache, numbness.	Indicators of decreased perfusion and/or increased pressure within enclosed space, such as may occur with a circumferential burn of an extremity (compartmental syndrome).
Encourage active ROM exercises of unaffected body parts.	Promotes local and systemic circulation.
Investigate irregular pulses.	Cardiac dysrhythmias can occur as a result of electrolyte shifts, electrical injury, or release of myocardial depressant factor, compromising cardiac output/tissue perfusion.

Collaborative

Maintain fluid replacement per protocol. (Refer to ND: risk for deficient Fluid Volume.)	Maximizes circulating volume and tissue perfusion.
Monitor electrolytes, especially sodium, potassium, and calcium. Administer replacement therapy as indicated.	Losses/shifts of these electrolytes affect cellular membrane potential/excitability, thereby altering myocardial conductivity, potentiating risk of dysrhythmias, and reducing cardiac output and tissue perfusion.
Avoid use of IM/SC injections.	Altered tissue perfusion and edema formation impair drug absorption. Injections into potential donor sites may render them unusable because of hematoma formation.
Measure intracompartmental pressures as indicated. (Refer to CP: Fractures; ND: risk for Peripheral Neurovascular Dysfunction.)	Ischemic myositis may develop because of decreased perfusion.
Assist with/prepare for escharotomy/fasciotomy, as indicated.	Enhances circulation by relieving constriction caused by rigid, nonviable tissue (eschar) or edema formation.

NURSING DIAGNOSIS: imbalanced Nutrition: less than body requirements

May be related to

Hypermetabolic state (can be as much as 50%–60% higher than normal proportional to the severity of injury)
Protein catabolism
Anorexia, restricted oral intake

Possibly evidenced by

Decrease in total body weight, loss of muscle mass/subcutaneous fat, and development of negative nitrogen balance

DESIRED OUTCOMES/EVALUATION CRITERIA—CLIENT WILL:

Nutritional Status (NOC)

Demonstrate nutritional intake adequate to meet metabolic needs as evidenced by stable weight/muscle-mass measurements, positive nitrogen balance, and tissue regeneration.

ACTIONS/INTERVENTIONS	RATIONALE
Nutrition Therapy (NIC)	
Independent	
Auscultate bowel sounds, noting hypoactive/absent sounds.	Ileus is often associated with postburn period but usually subsides within 36–48 hr, at which time oral or intragastic feedings can be initiated.
Maintain strict calorie count. Weigh daily. Reassess percentage of open body surface area/wounds weekly.	Appropriate guides to proper caloric intake include 25 kcal/kg body weight, plus 40 kcal per percentage of TBSA burn in the adult. As burn wound heals, energy needs are reevaluated to calculate prescribed dietary formulas, and appropriate adjustments are made.
Monitor muscle mass/subcutaneous fat as indicated.	Indirect calorimetry, if available, may be useful in more accurately estimating body reserves/losses and effectiveness of therapy.
Provide small, frequent meals and snacks.	Helps prevent gastric distention/discomfort and may enhance intake.
Encourage client to view diet as a treatment and to make food/beverage choices high in calories/protein.	Calories and proteins are needed to meet metabolic needs, and promote wound healing.
Ascertain food likes/dislikes. Encourage SO to bring food from home as appropriate.	Provides client/SO sense of control; enhances participation in care and may improve intake.
Encourage client to sit up for meals and visit with others.	Sitting helps prevent aspiration and aids in proper digestion of food. Socialization promotes relaxation and may enhance intake.
Provide oral hygiene before meals.	Clean mouth/clear palate enhances taste and helps promote a good appetite.
Perform fingerstick glucose, urine testing as indicated.	Monitors for development of hyperglycemia related to hormonal changes/demands or use of hyperalimentation to meet caloric needs.
Collaborative	
Refer to dietitian/nutritional support team.	Useful in establishing individual nutritional needs (based on weight and body surface area of injury) and identifying appropriate routes.
Provide diet high in calories/protein with trace elements and vitamin supplements.	Calories (25 kcal/kg/day), proteins (up to 2G/k/day), and vitamins are needed to meet increased metabolic needs, maintain weight, and encourage tissue regeneration. Zero fat or minimal fat is preferred during early acute phase to minimize the susceptibility to infection.
Insert/maintain small feeding tube for enteral feedings and supplements if needed.	Provides continuous/supplemental feedings when client is unable to consume total daily calorie requirements orally. *Note:* Research supports use of early intragstric feedings as soon after admission as possible, since delayed enteral feeding (>18 hours) results in a high rate of gastroparesis and need for intravenous nutrition. Continuous tube feeding during the night increases calorie intake without decreasing appetite and oral intake during the day.
Administer parenteral nutritional solutions containing vitamins and minerals as indicated.	Total parenteral nutrition (TPN) maintains nutritional intake/meets metabolic needs in presence of severe complications or sustained esophageal/gastric injuries that do not permit enteral feedings. (Refer to CP: Total nutritional support: Parenteral/enteral feeding.)
Monitor laboratory studies; e.g., serum albumin/prealbumin, glucose, electrolytes, magnesium, BUN/Cr, calcium, inorganic phosphorus, transaminase, triglycerides.	Indicators of nutritional needs and adequacy of diet/therapy.
Administer insulin as indicated.	Elevated serum glucose levels may develop because of stress response to injury, high caloric intake, pancreatic fatigue.

NURSING DIAGNOSIS: impaired physical Mobility

May be related to

Neuromuscular impairment, pain/discomfort, decreased strength and endurance
Restrictive therapies, limb immobilization; contractures

Possibly evidenced by

Reluctance to move/inability to purposefully move
Limited ROM, decreased muscle strength control and/or mass

DESIRED OUTCOMES/EVALUATION CRITERIA—CLIENT WILL:

Mobility (NOC)

Maintain position of function as evidenced by absence of contractures.
Maintain or increase strength and function of affected and/or compensatory body part.

SELF-CARE: Activities of Daily Living (ADL) (NOC)

Verbalize and demonstrate willingness to participate in activities.
Demonstrate techniques/behaviors that enable resumption of activities.

ACTIONS/INTERVENTIONS	RATIONALE
Bed Rest Care (NIC)	
Independent	
Maintain proper body alignment with supports or splints, especially for burns over joints.	Promotes functional positioning of extremities and prevents contractures, which are more likely over joints.
Note circulation, motion, and sensation of digits frequently.	Edema may compromise circulation to extremities, potentiating tissue necrosis/development of contractures.
Initiate the rehabilitative phase on admission.	It is easier to enlist participation when client is aware of the possibilities that exist for recovery.
Perform ROM exercises consistently, initially passive, then active.	Prevents progressively tightening scar tissue and contractures, enhances maintenance of muscle/joint functioning and reduces loss of calcium from the bone.
Medicate for pain before activity/exercises.	Reduces muscle/tissue stiffness and tension, enabling client to be more active and facilitating participation.
Schedule treatments and care activities to provide periods of uninterrupted rest.	Increases client's strength and tolerance for activity.
Encourage family/SO support and assistance with ROM exercises.	Enables family/SO to be active in client care and provides more constant/consistent therapy.
Self-Care Assistance (NIC)	
Incorporate ADLs with physical therapy, hydrotherapy, and nursing care.	Combining activities produces improved results by enhancing effects of each.
Encourage client participation in all activities as individually able.	Promotes independence, enhances self-esteem, and facilitates recovery process.
Instruct and assist with mobility aids; e.g., cane, walker, crutches, as appropriate.	Promotes safe ambulation.

ACTIONS/INTERVENTIONS	RATIONALE
Bed Rest Care (NIC)	
Collaborative	
Provide foam, water/air mattress or kinetic therapy bed, as indicated.	Prevents prolonged pressure on tissues, reducing potential for tissue ischemia/necrosis and decubitus ulcer formation.
Maintain pressure garment when used.	Hypertrophic scarring can develop around grafted areas or at the site of deep partial-thickness wounds. Pressure dressings minimize scar tissue by keeping it flat, soft, and pliable, enhancing movement.
Consult with rehabilitation, physical, and occupational therapists.	Normally members of the burn team, these specialists provide integrated activity/exercise program and specific assistive devices based on individual needs. Consultation facilitates intensive long-term management of potential deficits.

NURSING DIAGNOSIS: impaired Skin Integrity, [grafts]

May be related to

Disruption of skin surface with destruction of skin layers (partial-/full-thickness burn) requiring grafting

Possibly evidenced by

Absence of viable tissue

DESIRED OUTCOMES/EVALUATION CRITERIA—CLIENT WILL:

WOUND HEALING: Secondary Intention (NOC)

Demonstrate tissue regeneration.
Achieve timely healing of burned areas.

ACTIONS/INTERVENTIONS	RATIONALE
Wound Care (NIC)	
Independent	
Preoperative	
Assess/document size, color, depth of wound, noting necrotic tissue and condition of surrounding skin.	Provides baseline information about need for skin grafting and possible clues about circulation in area to support graft.
Provide appropriate burn care and infection control measures. (Refer to ND: risk for Infection.)	Prepares tissues for grafting and reduces risk of infection/graft failure.
Collaborative	
Administer topical wound débridement ointment, as indicated:	
Enzymatic products: collangenase ointment (Santyl), papain (Accuzyme), as indicated.	Early débridement of burn eschar is beneficial to wound healing and some treatment centers suggest use of these products to promote healing. However, despite theoretical advantage, enzymatic débridement results have been highly variable.

ACTIONS/INTERVENTIONS	RATIONALE
Independent	
Postoperative	
Elevate grafted area if possible/appropriate.	Reduces swelling/limits risk of graft separation.
Maintain desired position and immobility of area when indicated.	Movement of tissue under graft can dislodge it, interfering with optimal healing.
Maintain dressings over newly grafted area and/or donor site as indicated; e.g., mesh, petroleum, nonadhesive.	Areas may be covered by translucent, nonreactive surface material (between graft and outer dressing) to eliminate shearing of new epithelium/protect healing tissue. The donor site is usually covered for 4–24 hr, then bulky dressings are removed and fine mesh gauze is left in place.
Keep skin free from pressure.	Promotes circulation and prevents ischemia/necrosis and graft failure.
Evaluate color of grafted and donor site(s); note presence/absence of healing.	Evaluates effectiveness of circulation and identifies developing complications.
Collaborative	
Maintain wound covering as indicated; e.g.:	
Biosynthetic dressing (Biobrane);	Biobrane membrane contains collagenous porcine peptides that adhere to wound surface until removed or sloughed off by spontaneous skin reepithelialization. Useful for eschar-free partial-thickness burns awaiting autografts because it can remain in place for longer periods of time and is permeable to topical antimicrobial agents.
Human fibroblast-derived temporary skin substitute (TransCyte);	Bioengineered skin substitute used on middermal burns after débridement and shows faster healing with less pain in prospective trials.
Nonbiologic synthetic dressings; e.g., contact layer dressing (Mepitel), hydrocolloid dressing (DuoDerm);	These dressings adhere to the skin to cover small partial-thickness burns and interact with wound exudate to form a soft gel that facilitates débridement.
Opsite, Acu-Derm.	Thin, transparent, elastic, waterproof, occlusive dressing (permeable to moisture and air) that is used to cover clean partial-thickness wounds and clean donor sites.
Wash sites with mild soap, rinse, and lubricate with cream (e.g., Nivea) several times daily after dressings are removed and healing is accomplished.	Newly grafted skin and healed donor sites require special care to maintain flexibility.
Aspirate blebs under sheet grafts with sterile needle or roll with sterile swab.	Fluid-filled blebs prevent graft adherence to underlying tissue, increasing risk of graft failure.
Prepare for/assist with surgical grafting or biological dressings; e.g.:	
Homograft (allograft);	Skin grafts obtained from living persons or cadavers are used as a temporary covering for extensive burns until individual's own skin is ready for grafting (test graft), to cover excised wounds immediately after escharotomy, or to protect granulation tissue.
Heterograft (xenograft, porcine);	Skin grafts may be carried out with animal skin for the same purposes as homografts or to cover meshed autografts.
Cultured epithelial autograft (CEA);	Skin graft obtained from uninjured part of client's own skin and prepared in a laboratory; may be full-thickness or partial-thickness. *Note:* This process takes 20–30 days from harvest to application. The new CEA sheets are one to six cell layers thick and thus are very fragile.
Artificial skin (Integra, Dermagraft-TC).	Wound coverings for full-thickness and deep partial-thickness burns provide a permanent, immediate covering that reproduces the skin's normal functions and stimulates the regeneration of dermal tissue.

NURSING DIAGNOSIS: Fear/Anxiety

May be related to

Situational crises: hospitalization/isolation procedures, interpersonal transmission and contagion, memory of the trauma experience, threat of death and/or disfigurement

Possibly evidenced by

Expressed concern regarding changes in life, fear of unspecific consequences
Apprehension, increased tension
Feelings of helplessness, uncertainty, decreased self-assurance
Sympathetic stimulation, extraneous movements, restlessness, insomnia

DESIRED OUTCOMES/EVALUATION CRITERIA—CLIENT WILL:

Fear [or] Anxiety Self-Control (NOC)

Verbalize awareness of feelings and healthy ways to deal with them.
Report anxiety/fear reduced to manageable level.
Demonstrate problem-solving skills, effective use of resources.

ACTIONS/INTERVENTIONS	RATIONALE
Anxiety Reduction (NIC)	
Independent	
Provide frequent explanations and information about care procedures. Repeat information as needed/desired.	Knowing what to expect usually reduces fear and anxiety, clarifies misconceptions, and promotes cooperation. *Note:* Because of the shock of the initial trauma, many people do not recall information provided during that time.
Demonstrate willingness to listen and talk to client when free of painful procedures.	Helps client/SO know that support is available and that healthcare provider is interested in the person, not just care of the burn.
Involve client/SO in decision-making process whenever possible. Provide time for questioning and repetition of proposed treatments.	Promotes sense of control and cooperation, decreasing feelings of helplessness/hopelessness.
Assess mental status, including mood/affect, comprehension of events, and content of thoughts; e.g., illusions or manifestations of terror/panic.	Initially, client may use denial and repression to reduce and filter information that might be overwhelming. Some clients display calm manner and alert mental status, representing dissociation from reality, which is also a protective mechanism.
Investigate changes in mentation and presence of hypervigilance, hallucinations, sleep disturbances (e.g., nightmares), agitation/apathy, disorientation, and labile affect, all of which may vary from moment to moment.	Indicators of extreme anxiety/delirium state in which client is literally fighting for life. Although cause can be psychologically based, pathologic life-threatening causes (e.g., shock, sepsis, hypoxia) must be ruled out.
Provide constant and consistent orientation.	Helps client stay in touch with surroundings and reality.
Encourage client to talk about the burn circumstances when ready.	Client may need to tell the story of what happened over and over to make some sense out of a terrifying situation. Adjustment to the impact of the trauma, grief over losses and disfigurement can easily lead to clinical depression, psychosis, and posttraumatic stress disorder (PTSD).
Explain to client what happened. Provide opportunity for questions and give open/honest answers.	Compassionate statements reflecting the reality of the situation can help client/SO acknowledge that reality and begin to deal with what has happened.

ACTIONS/INTERVENTIONS	RATIONALE
Identify previous methods of coping/handling of stressful situations.	Past successful behavior can be used to assist in dealing with the present situation.
Create a restful environment; use guided imagery and relaxation exercises.	Clients experience severe anxiety associated with burn trauma and treatment. These interventions are soothing and helpful for positive outcomes.
Assist the family to express their feelings of grief and guilt.	The family may initially be most concerned about client's dying and/or feel guilty, believing that in some way they could have prevented the incident.
Be empathetic and nonjudgmental in dealing with client and family.	Family relationships are disrupted; financial, lifestyle/role changes make this a difficult time for those involved with client, and they may react in many different ways.
Encourage family/SO to visit and discuss family happenings. Remind client of past and future events.	Maintains contact with a familiar reality, creating a sense of attachment and continuity of life.

Collaborative

Involve entire burn team in care from admission to discharge, including social worker and psychiatric resources.	Provides a wider support system and promotes continuity of care and coordination of activities.
Administer mild sedation as indicated; e.g., lorazepam (Ativan), alprazolam (Xanax), midazolam (Versed).	Antianxiety medications may be necessary for a brief period until client is more physically stable and internal locus of control is regained.

NURSING DIAGNOSIS: disturbed Body Image/ineffective Role Performance

May be related to

Situational crisis: traumatic event, dependent client role; disfigurement, pain

Possibly evidenced by

Negative feelings about body/self, fear of rejection/reaction by others
Focus on past appearance, abilities; preoccupation with change/loss
Change in physical capacity to resume role, change in social involvement

DESIRED OUTCOMES/EVALUATION CRITERIA—CLIENT WILL:

Body Image (NOC)

Incorporate changes into self-concept without negating self-esteem.
Verbalize acceptance of self in situation.

Role Performance (NOC)

Talk with family/SO about situation, changes that have occurred.
Develop realistic goals/plans for the future.

ACTIONS/INTERVENTIONS	RATIONALE
Body Image [or] Role Enhancement (NIC)	
Independent	
Assess meaning of loss/change to client/SO, including future expectations and impact of cultural/religious beliefs.	Traumatic episode results in sudden, unanticipated changes, creating feelings of grief over actual/perceived losses. This necessitates support to work through to optimal resolution.

ACTIONS/INTERVENTIONS	RATIONALE
Acknowledge and accept expression of feelings of frustration, dependency, anger, grief, and hostility. Note withdrawn behavior and use of denial.	Acceptance of these feelings as a normal response to what has occurred facilitates resolution. It is not helpful or possible to push client before he/she is ready to deal with situation. Denial may be prolonged and be an adaptive mechanism because client is not ready to cope with personal problems.
Set limits on maladaptive behavior (e.g., manipulative/aggressive). Maintain nonjudgmental attitude while giving care, and help client identify positive behaviors that will aid in recovery.	Client and SO tend to deal with this crisis in the same way in which they have dealt with problems in the past. Staff may find it difficult and frustrating to handle behavior that is disrupting/not helpful to recuperation but should realize that the behavior is usually directed toward the situation and not the care provider.
Be realistic and positive during treatments, in health teaching, and in setting goals within limitations.	Enhances trust and rapport between client and nurse.
Encourage client/SO to view wounds and assist with care as appropriate.	Promotes acceptance of reality of injury and of change in body and image of self as different.
Provide hope within parameters of individual situation; do not give false reassurance.	Promotes positive attitude and provides opportunity to set goals and plan for future based on reality.
Assist client to identify extent of actual change in appearance/body function.	Helps begin process of looking to the future and how life will be different.
Give positive reinforcement of progress and encourage endeavors toward attainment of rehabilitation goals.	Words of encouragement can support development of positive coping behaviors.
Show slides or pictures of burn care/other client outcomes, being selective in what is shown as appropriate to the individual situation. Encourage discussion of feelings about what client has seen.	Allows client/SO to be realistic in expectations. Also assists in demonstration of importance of/necessity for certain devices and procedures.
Encourage family interaction with each other and with rehabilitation team.	Maintains/opens lines of communication and provides ongoing support for client and family.
Provide support group for SO. Give information about how SO can be helpful to client.	Promotes ventilation of feelings and allows for more helpful responses to client.
Role-play social situations of concern to client.	Prepares client/SO for reactions of others and anticipates ways to deal with them.

Collaborative

Refer to physical/occupational therapy, vocational counselor, and psychiatric counseling; e.g., psychiatric clinical nurse specialist, social services, and psychologist, as needed.	Helpful in identifying ways/devices to regain and maintain independence. Client may need further assistance to resolve persistent emotional problems (e.g., posttrauma response).

NURSING DIAGNOSIS: deficient Knowledge [Learning Need] regarding condition, prognosis, treatment, self-care, and discharge needs

May be related to

Lack of exposure/recall
Information misinterpretation, unfamiliarity with resources

Possibly evidenced by

Questions/request for information, statement of misconception
Inaccurate follow-through of instructions, development of preventable complications

DESIRED OUTCOMES/EVALUATION CRITERIA—CLIENT WILL:

KNOWLEDGE: Disease Process (NOC)

Verbalize understanding of condition, prognosis, and potential complications.

KNOWLEDGE: Treatment Regimen (NOC)

Verbalize understanding of therapeutic needs.
Correctly perform necessary procedures and explain reasons for actions.
Initiate necessary lifestyle changes and participate in treatment regimen.

ACTIONS/INTERVENTIONS	RATIONALE
TEACHING: Disease Process (NIC)	
Independent	
Review condition, prognosis, and future expectations.	Provides knowledge base from which client can make informed choices.
Discuss client's expectations of returning home, to work, and to normal activities.	Client frequently has a difficult and prolonged adjustment after discharge. Problems often occur (e.g., sleep disturbances, nightmares, reliving the accident, difficulty with resumption of social interactions, intimacy/sexual activity, emotional lability) that interfere with successful adjustment to resuming normal life.
Review and have client/SO demonstrate proper burn, skin graft, and wound care techniques. Identify appropriate sources for outpatient care and supplies.	Promotes competent self-care after discharge, enhancing independence.
Discuss skin care; e.g., scar massage, use of non–perfume-containing moisturizers (e.g., Vaseline Intensive Care, Eucerin), sunscreens, and anti-itching medications (e.g., diphenhydramine [Benadryl], hydroxyzine [Atarax]).	Itching, blistering, and sensitivity of healing wounds/graft sites can be expected for an extended time, and injury can occur because of the lack of natural lubrication and fragility of the new tissue. *Note*: Sun block may be required for life because of potential for hyperpigmentation.
Explain scarring process and necessity for/proper use of silicone gel sheeting, static splint or pressure garments when used.	Helps minimize/treat hypertrophic scarring and contracture formation. Consistent use of the pressure garment over a long period can reduce the need for reconstructive surgery to release contractures and remove scars. *Note:* Studies show that client compliance is not easily attained and that client may wear garment inappropriately, with resultant failure to demonstrate a difference in scarring with pressure garment therapy.
Encourage continuation of prescribed exercise program and scheduled rest periods.	Maintains mobility, reduces complications, and prevents fatigue, facilitating recovery process.
Identify specific limitations of activity as individually appropriate.	Imposed restrictions depend on severity/location of injury and stage of healing.
Emphasize importance of sustained intake of high-protein/high-calorie meals and snacks.	Optimal nutrition enhances tissue regeneration and general feeling of well-being. *Note:* Client often needs to increase caloric intake to meet calorie and protein needs for healing.
Review medications, including purpose, dosage, route, and expected/reportable side effects.	Reiteration allows opportunity for client to ask questions and be sure understanding is accurate.
Advise client/SO of potential for exhaustion, boredom, emotional lability, adjustment problems. Provide information about possibility of discussion/interaction with appropriate professional counselors.	Provides perspective to some of the problems client/SO may encounter, and aids awareness that assistance is available when necessary.

ACTIONS/INTERVENTIONS	RATIONALE
Identify signs/symptoms requiring medical evaluation; e.g., inflammation, increase or changes in wound drainage, fever/chills, changes in pain characteristics, or loss of mobility/function.	Early detection of developing complications (e.g., infection, delayed healing) may prevent progression to more serious/life-threatening situations.
Stress necessity/importance of follow-up care/rehabilitation.	Long-term support with continual reevaluation and changes in therapy is required to achieve optimal recovery.
Provide phone number for contact person.	Provides easy access to treatment team to reinforce teaching, clarify misconceptions, and reduce potential for complications.
Identify community resources; e.g., skin/wound care professionals, crisis centers, recovery groups, mental health, Red Cross, visiting nurse, Ambli-Cab, homemaker service.	Facilitates transition to home, provides assistance with meeting individual needs, and supports independence.

POTENTIAL CONSIDERATIONS following acute hospitalization (dependent on client's age, physical condition/presence of complications, personal resources, and life responsibilities)

ineffective Coping—situational crisis, vulnerability.

risk for Disuse Syndrome—severe pain, prescribed immobilization/restrictive therapies.

situational low Self-Esteem—change in health status/independent functioning, perceived loss of control in some aspect of life.

ineffective Therapeutic Regimen Management—complexity of medical regimen, added demands made on individual/family, social support deficits.

Post-Trauma Syndrome—catastrophic accident/injury to self and possibly others.

14

CHAPTER

Systemic Infections and Immunologic Disorders

SEPSIS/SEPTICEMIA

Sepsis is a syndrome characterized by clinical signs and symptoms of systemic inflammatory response to infection that may progress along a continuum culminating in septic shock and multiorgan failure. *Septicemia* implies the presence of an infection of the blood caused by rapidly multiplying microorganisms or their toxins, which can result in profound physiologic changes and systemic sepsis. The pathogens can be bacteria, fungi, viruses, or rickettsiae. The most common causes of septicemia are Gram-negative bacteria (and endotoxins), staphylococci, and *Candida.* If the defense system of the body is not effective in controlling the invading microorganisms, septic shock may result, characterized by altered hemodynamics, impaired cellular function, and multiple system failure.

Clients at highest risk for bacteremia and septic shock include the elderly, infants, and immunosuppressed individuals. Factors associated with increased risk of developing sepsis include trauma to the gastrointestinal (GI) tract, perforation of the small intestine, surgery, chronic debilitating conditions (e.g., diabetes), use of invasive procedures and devices in the intensive care unit (ICU) setting (e.g., ventilators, invasive lines), and treatment with immunosuppressant drugs.

Recognizing the client at risk for developing sepsis is difficult owing to limited early signs and symptoms and because sepsis can progress subtly until sudden, overwhelming septic shock is present, affecting multiple organ systems. However, researchers have been assessing biomarkers that may more quickly identify the client at risk (e.g., C-reactive protein where inflammation is closely associated with coagulation).

Keys to identifying an individual with severe sepsis include the presence of (1) known or suspected infection, (2) two or more systemic inflammatory response syndrome (SIRS) criteria, (3) septic state that fails to respond to fluid resuscitation with development of perfusion abnormalities, and (4) sepsis in combination with failure of at least one body organ.

SIRS criteria include a proinflammtory response marked by tachycardia, hyperpnea, hypotension, hypoperfusion, oliguria, leukocytosis or leukopenia, fever or hypothermia, and possibly metabolic acidosis. SIRS characteristically does not include a documented source of bacteremia. Once end-organ damage begins (e.g., renal failure due to acute tubular necrosis [ATN]), the entity is no longer SIRS, and sepsis is progressing toward septic shock.

CARE SETTING

Although severely ill individuals will likely receive care in ICU, this plan addresses care on an inpatient acute medical-surgical unit.

RELATED CONCERNS

Acquired immunodeficiency syndrome (AIDS), page 726
Chronic obstructive pulmonary disease (COPD) and asthma, page 117
Disaster considerations, page 890
Fluid and electrolyte imbalances, page 919
Metabolic acidosis (primary base bicarbonate deficiency), page 495
Peritonitis, page 355
Pneumonia, page 128
Psychosocial aspects of care, page 770
Pulmonary tuberculosis (TB), page 184
Renal failure: acute, page 541
Surgical intervention, page 788
Total nutritional support: parenteral/enteral feeding, page 478
Ventilatory assistance (mechanical), page 170

Client Assessment Database

Data depend on the type, location, and duration of the infective process and organ involvement.

ACTIVITY/REST

May report: Fatigue, malaise

May exhibit: Mental status changes; e.g., withdrawn, lethargic
Respiration/heart rate increased with activity

CIRCULATION

May exhibit: Blood pressure (BP) normal/slightly low-normal range (as long as cardiac output remains elevated), profound hypotension (late stage)
Peripheral pulses bounding, rapid (hyperdynamic phase); weak/thready/easily obliterated, extreme tachycardia unless blunted by β-blockers/other medications (shock)
Heart sounds—development of S_3 and dysrhythmias suggest myocardial dysfunction, effects of acidosis/electrolyte imbalance
Skin warm, dry, flushed (vasodilation) or pale, cold, clammy, mottled (vasoconstriction)

ELIMINATION

May report: Burning with urination (UTI)

May exhibit: Urinary output decreased, concentrated; progressing to oliguria, anuria
Urine cloudy, malodorous

FOOD/FLUID

May report: Loss of appetite, nausea/vomiting

May exhibit: Weight loss, decreased subcutaneous fat/muscle mass (malnutrition)
Diminished/absent bowel sounds
Extremity and generalized edema

NEUROSENSORY

May report: Headache, dizziness, fainting

May exhibit: Restlessness, apprehension, confusion, disorientation, delirium/coma

PAIN/DISCOMFORT

May report: Abdominal tenderness, localized pain/discomfort
Generalized urticaria/pruritus

RESPIRATION

May report: Shortness of breath

May exhibit: Tachypnea with decreased respiratory depth, dyspnea, rapid labored respirations
Basilar crackles, rhonchi, wheezes (presence of pneumonia, developing pulmonary complications/onset of cardiac decompensation)

SAFETY

May report: History of recent/current infection, viral illness, cancer therapies, use of corticosteroids/other immunosuppressant medications

May exhibit: Temperature usually elevated (101°F or higher) but may be normal in elderly or compromised client; occasionally subnormal (lower than 98.6°F)
Shaking chills
Poor/delayed wound healing, purulent drainage, localized erythema
Macular erythematous rash, petechiae, oozing/bleeding from invasive line sites, wounds, mucous membranes

SEXUALITY

May report: Perineal pruritus
Recent childbirth/abortion

May exhibit: Maceration of vulva, purulent vaginal drainage

TEACHING/LEARNING

May report: Chronic/debilitating health problems; e.g., liver, renal, cardiac disease; cancer, diabetes mellitus (DM), alcoholism

History of splenectomy
Recent surgery/invasive procedures, traumatic wounds
Antibiotic use (recent or long-term)

Discharge plan considerations: May require assistance with wound care/supplies, treatments, self-care and homemaker tasks

Refer to section at end of plan for postdischarge considerations.

DIAGNOSTIC STUDIES

Cultures (wound, sputum, urine, blood): May identify causative organism(s). Sensitivity determines most effective drug choices. Catheter/intravascular line tips may need to be removed and cultured if the portal of entry is unknown. *Note:* Tests have value in identifying client with transition of disease process along a continuum (e.g., client with SIRS plus a positive culture has a diagnosis of sepsis; however, client can develop septic shock without displaying an identified bacterium by culture).

Complete blood count (CBC): Hematocrit (Hct) level may be elevated in hypovolemic states because of hemoconcentration. Leukopenia (decreased white blood cells [WBCs]) occurs early, followed by a rebound leukocytosis (15,000–30,000) with increased bands (shift to the left), indicating rapid production of immature WBCs. Neutrophils (also called granulocytes, polys, or polymorphonuclear neutrophils [PMNs]) may be elevated or depressed. Counts below 500/mL indicate immune system exhaustion. Platelets may be elevated initially as an acute-phase reactant.

Serum electrolytes: Various imbalances may occur because of acidosis, fluid shifts, and altered renal function.

Serologic markers:

Protein C: Study data suggests that almost all clients with severe sepsis have an acquired deficiency in protein C.

Procalcitonin: Peptide precursor to calcitonin rises with severity of illness, and increases more rapidly than C-reactive protein in client with sepsis.

C-reactive protein: An indicator of inflammation released by the liver in response to proinflammatory cytokines and is thought to recruit monocytes in early infection.

Clotting studies:

Platelets: Decreased levels (thrombocytopenia) can occur because of platelet aggregation.

Prothrombin time (PT)/activated partial thromboplastin time (aPTT): May be prolonged, indicating coagulopathy associated with liver ischemia, circulating toxins, shock state.

Fibrin degradation products: Often elevated; a condition associated with tendency to bleed.

Serum lactate: Elevated in metabolic acidosis, liver dysfunction, and shock, reflecting tissue hypoperfusion.

Serum glucose: Hyperglycemia occurs, reflecting gluconeogenesis and glycogenolysis in the liver in response to cellular starvation/alteration in metabolism.

Blood urea nitrogen (BUN)/Creatinine (Cr): Increased levels are associated with dehydration, renal impairment/failure, and liver dysfunction/failure.

Arterial blood gases (ABGs): Respiratory alkalosis and hypoxemia may occur early. In later states, hypoxemia, respiratory acidosis, lactic and metabolic acidosis occur because of failure of compensatory mechanisms.

Sublingual capnometry: Noninvasive technique that measures sublingual carbon dioxide can rapidly assess potential hypoperfusion.

Urinalysis: Presence of WBCs/bacteria suggests infection. Protein and red blood cells (RBCs) are often present.

Imaging studies: A variety of modalities are useful to document a clinically suspected focus of infection:

Radiographs: Abdominal and lower chest films indicating free air in the abdomen may suggest infection due to perforated abdominal/pelvic organ.

Ultrasound: Modality of choice when biliary tract source is suspected.

CT scan: Modality of choice when intra-abdominal abscess or other GI tract disorder is suspected origin.

Electrocardiogram (ECG): May show ST-segment and T-wave changes and dysrhythmias resembling myocardial infarction.

NURSING PRIORITIES

1. Eliminate infection.
2. Support tissue perfusion/circulatory volume.
3. Prevent complications.
4. Provide information about disease process, prognosis, and treatment needs.

DISCHARGE GOALS

1. Infection eliminated/controlled.
2. Homeostasis maintained.
3. Complications prevented/minimized.
4. Disease process, prognosis, and therapeutic regimen understood.
5. Plan in place to meet needs after discharge.

NURSING DIAGNOSIS: risk for Infection [progression of sepsis to septic shock, development of opportunistic infections]

Risk factors may include

Compromised immune system
Failure to recognize/treat infection and/or exercise proper preventive measures
Invasive procedures, environmental exposure (nosocomial)

Possibly evidenced by

[Not applicable; presence of signs and symptoms establishes an *actual* diagnosis.]

DESIRED OUTCOMES/EVALUATION CRITERIA—CLIENT WILL:

Infection Severity (NOC)

Achieve timely healing, be free of purulent secretions/drainage or erythema, and be afebrile.

ACTIONS/INTERVENTIONS	RATIONALE
Infection Control (NIC)	
Independent	
Understand the nurse's role in identifying client at risk and preventive interventions; e.g., hand disinfection, early removal of invasive tubes and catheters, 30-degree head elevation for client on ventilator, early nutrition.	The role of nurses in preventing the spread of severe sepsis is crucial because they are in the position to identify clients at the first signs of developing sepsis. The sooner that treatment of sepsis begins, the less likely that it will spread to involve organs and start a life-threatening cascade of events.
Wash hands with antibacterial soap before/after each care activity, even when gloves are used.	Reduces risk of cross-contamination because gloves may have unnoticeable defects, get torn or damaged during use. Some pathogens may survive on hands for 3+ hr after exposure. *Note:* Methicillin-resistant *Staphylococcus aureus* (MRSA) is most commonly transmitted via direct contact with healthcare workers who fail to wash hands between client contacts.
Provide isolation/monitor visitors as indicated.	Body substance isolation (BSI) should be used for all infectious clients. Wound/linen isolation and hand washing may be all that is required for draining wounds. Clients with diseases transmitted through air may also need airborne and droplet precautions. Reverse isolation/restriction of visitors may be needed to protect the immunosuppressed client.
Encourage/provide frequent position changes, deep-breathing/coughing exercises.	Good pulmonary toilet may reduce respiratory compromise.
Encourage client to cover mouth and nose with tissue during coughs/sneezes. Place in private room if indicated. Wear mask when providing direct care as appropriate.	Prevents spread of infection via airborne droplets.
Limit use of invasive devices/procedures when possible. Remove lines/devices when infection is present and replace if necessary.	Reduces number of sites for entry of opportunistic organisms.
Inspect wounds/site of invasive devices daily, paying particular attention to parenteral nutrition lines. Document signs of local inflammation/infection, changes in character of wound drainage, sputum, or urine.	Catheter-related bloodstream infections (CR-BSIs) are increasing in today's health-care world where central venous catheters are used in both acute and chronic care settings. Clinical signs (e.g., local inflammation or phlebitis) may provide clue to portal of entry, type of primary infecting organism(s), as well as early identification of secondary infections. *Note:* High nutrient content of total parenteral nutrition (TPN) provides excellent medium for bacterial growth.

ACTIONS/INTERVENTIONS	RATIONALE
Investigate reports of pain out of proportion to visible signs.	Pressure-like pain over area of cellulitis may indicate development of necrotizing fasciitis due to group A β-hemolytic streptococci (GABS), necessitating prompt intervention.
Maintain sterile technique when changing dressings, suctioning, providing site care; e.g., invasive line, urinary catheter.	Prevents/limits introduction of bacteria, reducing risk of nosocomial infection.
Wear gloves/gowns when caring for open wounds/anticipating direct contact with secretions or excretions.	Prevents spread of infection/cross-contamination.
Dispose of soiled dressings/materials in double bag.	Reduces contamination/soilage of area, limits spread of airborne organisms.
Note temperature trends and observe for shaking chills and profuse diaphoresis.	Fever (101°F–105°F/38.5°C–40°C) is the result of endotoxin effect on the hypothalamus and pyrogen-released endorphins. Hypothermia (lower than 96°F/36°C) is a grave sign reflecting advancing shock state, decreased tissue perfusion, and/or failure of the body's ability to mount a febrile response. Chills often precede temperature spikes in presence of generalized infection.
Monitor for signs of deterioration of condition/failure to improve with therapy.	May reflect inappropriate/inadequate antibiotic therapy or overgrowth of resistant or opportunistic organisms.
Inspect oral cavity for white plaques (thrush). Investigate reports of vaginal/perineal itching or burning.	Depression of immune system and use of antibiotics increase risk of secondary infections, particularly yeast.

Collaborative

Obtain specimens of urine, blood, sputum, wound, invasive lines/tubes as indicated for Gram stain, culture, and sensitivity.	Identification of portal of entry and organism causing the septicemia is crucial to effective treatment based on susceptibility to specific medications.
Monitor laboratory studies; e.g., WBC count with neutrophil and band counts.	The normal ratio of neutrophils to total WBCs is at least 50%; however, when WBC count is markedly decreased, calculating the absolute neutrophil count is more pertinent to evaluating immune status. Likewise, an initial elevation of band cells reflects the body's attempt to mount a response to the infection, whereas a decline indicates decompensation.
Administer medications as indicated:	
Anti-infective agents: broad-spectrum antibiotics; e.g., methicillin, imipenem and cilastatin (Primaxin), meropenem (Merrem), ticarcillin (Ticar), ticarcillin and clavulanate (Timentin), piperacillin and tazobactam (Zosyn), nafcillin (Nafcil), clindamycin (Cleocin), vancomycin (Vancocin); aminoglycosides; e.g., tobramycin (Nebcin), gentamicin (Garamycin); cephalosporins; e.g., cefotaxime (Claforan), ceftriaxone (Rocephin), cefuroxime (Zinacef); fluoroquinolones e.g., ciprofloxin (Cipro);	Specific antibiotics are determined by culture and sensitivity results, but therapy is usually initiated before obtaining results, using broad-spectrum antibiotics and/or based on most likely infecting organisms. Concomitant use of antimicrobials is often beneficial, but dosage must be balanced against renal function/clearance.
Immune globulins as appropriate;	May boost/provide temporary immunity to general infection or specific illness; e.g., varicella zoster, rabies.
Recombininant human APC (rhAPC) or drotrecogin α (activated) (Xigris).	Used to restore balance to the systemic irregularities (e.g., inflammation, coagulapathies) that occur during sepsis, and may reduce mortality in adult clients with severe sepsis who have a high risk of death.
Assist with/prepare for procedures; e.g., removal of infected devices, incision and drainage of wound, irrigation, application of warm/moist soaks as indicated.	Facilitates removal of infection sources, as well as purulent material/necrotic tissue to promote healing.
Prepare for hyperbaric therapy as appropriate.	Exposure to increased ambient oxygen tension enhances oxygen delivery to cells to combat anaerobic infections.

NURSING DIAGNOSIS: Hyperthermia

May be related to

Increased metabolic rate, illness
Dehydration
Direct effect of circulating endotoxins on the hypothalamus, altering temperature regulation

Possibly evidenced by

Increase in body temperature higher than normal range
Flushed skin, warm to touch
Increased respiratory rate, tachycardia

DESIRED OUTCOMES/EVALUATION CRITERIA—CLIENT WILL:

Thermoregulation (NOC)

Demonstrate temperature within normal range, be free of chills.
Experience no associated complications.

ACTIONS/INTERVENTIONS	RATIONALE
Fever Treatment (NIC)	
Independent	
Monitor client temperature (degree and pattern), note shaking chills/profuse diaphoresis.	Temperature of 102°F–106°F (38.9°C–41.1°C) suggests acute infectious disease process. Fever pattern may aid in diagnosis; e.g., sustained or continuous fever curves lasting more than 24 hr suggest pneumococcal pneumonia, scarlet or typhoid fever; remittent fever (varying only a few degrees in either direction) reflects pulmonary infections; intermittent curves or fever that returns to normal once in 24-hr period suggests septic episode, septic endocarditis, or tuberculosis (TB). Chills often precede temperature spikes. *Note:* Use of antipyretics alters fever patterns and may be restricted until diagnosis is made or if fever remains higher than 102°F (38.9°C).
Monitor environmental temperature, limit/add bed linens as indicated.	Room temperature/number of blankets should be altered to maintain near-normal body temperature.
Provide tepid sponge baths, avoid use of alcohol.	May help reduce fever. *Note.* Use of ice water/alcohol may cause chills, actually elevating temperature. In addition, alcohol is very drying to skin.
Collaborative	
Administer antipyretics; e.g., acetylsalicylic acid (ASA) (aspirin), acetaminophen (Tylenol).	Used to reduce fever by its central action on the hypothalamus; fever should be controlled in clients who are neutropenic or asplenic. However, fever may be beneficial in limiting growth of organisms and enhancing autodestruction of infected cells.
Provide cooling blanket as indicated.	Used to reduce fever, usually higher than 104°F–105°F (39.5°C–40°C), when brain damage/seizures can occur.

NURSING DIAGNOSIS: risk for ineffective Tissue Perfusion

Risk factors may include

Relative/actual hypovolemia
Reduction of arterial/venous blood flow: selective vasoconstriction, vascular occlusion (intimal damage/microemboli)

Possibly evidenced by

[Not applicable; presence of signs and symptoms establishes an *actual* diagnosis.]

DESIRED OUTCOMES/EVALUATION CRITERIA—CLIENT WILL:

Circulation Status (NOC)

Display adequate perfusion as evidenced by stable vital signs, palpable peripheral pulses, skin warm and dry, usual level of mentation, individually appropriate urinary output, and active bowel sounds.

ACTIONS/INTERVENTIONS	RATIONALE
Shock Prevention (NIC)	
Independent	
Maintain bedrest, assist with care activities.	Decreases myocardial workload and O_2 consumption, maximizing effectiveness of tissue perfusion.
Monitor trends in blood pressure (BP), especially noting progressive hypotension and widening pulse pressure.	Hypotension develops as microorganisms invade the bloodstream, stimulating release or activation of chemical and hormonal substances, which initially results in peripheral vasodilation, decreased systemic vascular resistance (SVR), and relative hypovolemia. As shock progresses, cardiac output becomes severely depressed due to major alterations in contractility and preload/afterload, producing profound hypotension.
Monitor heart rate, rhythm. Note dysrhythmias.	Tachycardia occurs because of sympathetic nervous system stimulation secondary to stress response and to compensate for the relative hypovolemia and hypotension. Cardiac dysrhythmias can occur as a result of hypoxia, acid-base/electrolyte imbalance and/or low-flow perfusion state.
Note quality/strength of peripheral pulses.	Initially, the pulse is strong/bounding because of increased cardiac output (CO). Pulse may become weak/thready as a result of sustained hypotension, decreased cardiac output, and peripheral vasoconstriction if the shock state progresses.
Assess respiratory rate, depth, and quality. Note onset of severe dyspnea.	Increased respirations occur in response to direct effects of endotoxins on the respiratory center in the brain, as well as developing hypoxia, stress, and fever. Respirations can become shallow as respiratory insufficiency develops, creating risk of acute respiratory failure. (Refer to ND: risk for impaired Gas Exchange.)
Investigate changes in sensorium; e.g., mental cloudiness, agitation, restlessness, personality changes, delirium, stupor, coma.	Changes reflect alterations in cerebral perfusion, hypoxemia, and/or acidosis.

ACTIONS/INTERVENTIONS	RATIONALE
Assess skin for changes in color, temperature, moisture.	Compensatory mechanisms of vasodilation results in warm, dry, pink skin, which is characteristic of hyperperfusion in hyperdynamic phase of early septic shock. If shock state progresses, compensatory vasoconstriction occurs, shunting blood to vital organs, reducing peripheral blood flow, and creating cool, clammy, pale/dusky skin.
Record hourly urinary output and specific gravity.	Decreasing urinary output with increased specific gravity indicates diminished renal perfusion related to fluid shifts and selective vasoconstriction. There may be transient polyuria during hyperdynamic phase (while cardiac output is elevated), but this may progress to oliguria. *Note:* Acute renal failure may herald development of hemolytic uremic syndrome (HUS) resulting from *Escherichia coli* infection (other manifestations include hemolytic anemia and thrombocytopenia).
Auscultate bowel sounds.	Reduced blood flow to the mesentery (splanchnic vasoconstriction) decreases peristalsis and may lead to paralytic ileus or possibly trigger multiple organ dysfunction syndrome (MODS).
Monitor gastric pH as indicated. Hematest gastric secretions/stools for occult blood.	Stress of illness and use of steroids increase risk of gastric mucosal erosion/bleeding.
Evaluate lower extremities for local tissue swelling, erythema, positive Homans's sign.	Venous stasis, changes in the coagulation processes, and infection may result in the development of thrombosis.
Maintain sequential compression stockings/boots (SCDs) as indicated.	Preventative measures for bedfast client to reduce lower extremity stasis complications.
Monitor for signs of bleeding; e.g., oozing from puncture sites/suture lines, petechiae, ecchymoses, hematuria, epistaxis, hemoptysis, hematemesis.	Coagulopathy/disseminated intravascular coagulation (DIC) may occur related to accelerated clotting in the microcirculation (activation of chemical mediators, vascular insufficiency, and cell destruction), creating a life-threatening hemorrhagic situation/multiple emboli.
Note drug effects, and monitor for signs of toxicity.	Massive doses of antibiotics are often ordered. These have potentially toxic effects when hepatic/renal perfusion is compromised.

Collaborative

Administer parenteral fluids. (Refer to ND: risk for deficient Fluid Volume, following.)	To maintain tissue perfusion, large amounts of fluid may be required to support circulating volume.
Administer drugs as indicated:	
Corticosteroids;	Although steroid therapy remains controversial, low-dose steroids may be given for the potential advantages of decreased capillary permeability, increased renal perfusion, and inhibition of microemboli formation. *Note*: Adrenal insufficiency occurs in between 25%–40% of clients with septic shock and is indicated by the need for vasopressors. Appropriate dosing of steroids provides support to dysfunctional adrenal glands and enhances vasomotor tone.
Inotropic agents/vasopressors; e.g. dopamine (Intropin), dobutamine (Dobutrex);	May be needed to improve organ perfusion and to maintain blood pressure during and after fluid treatment. *Note*: Client needing this level of support is critically ill and will be treated in the intensive care unit.
Low-molecular-weight heparin; e.g. enoxaparin (Lovenox), dalteparin (Fragmin), tinzaparin (Innohep); unfractionated heparin;	Given to prevent or treat deep vein thrombosis.
Histamine 2–receptor blockers; e.g., cimetidine (Tagamet), famotidine (Pepcid AC), nizatidine (Asid), rantidine (Zantac).	May be given to prevent/treat stress ulcers (common in this population).

ACTIONS/INTERVENTIONS	RATIONALE
Monitor laboratory studies; e.g., ABGs, lactate levels.	Development of respiratory/metabolic acidosis reflects loss of compensatory mechanisms; e.g., decreased renal perfusion/hydrogen excretion, and accumulation of lactic acid due to circulatory shunting and stagnation.
Provide supplemental O_2.	Maximizes oxygen available for cellular uptake.
Administer packed red blood cells (RBCs).	May be given to improve venous oxyhemoglobin saturation.
Maintain body temperature, using adjunctive aids as necessary. (Refer to ND: Hyperthermia.)	Temperature elevations increase metabolic/oxygen demands beyond cellular resources, hastening tissue ischemia/cellular destruction.
Assist with measurement of partial pressure of CO_2 in the gastric mucosa ($PrCO_2$) as indicated.	Gastric tonometry may be useful in diagnosing hypoperfusion of the gut before ischemic injury occurs, thus reducing risk of developing MODS.
Prepare for/transfer to critical care setting as indicated.	Progressive deterioration requires more aggressive therapy (e.g., hemodynamic monitoring and vasoactive drugs).

NURSING DIAGNOSIS: risk for deficient Fluid Volume

Risk factors may include

Marked increase in vascular compartment/massive vasodilation
Capillary permeability/fluid leaks into the interstitial space (third spacing)

Possibly evidenced by

[Not applicable; presence of signs and symptoms establishes an *actual* diagnosis.]

DESIRED OUTCOMES/EVALUATION CRITERIA—CLIENT WILL:

Hydration (NOC)

Maintain adequate circulatory volume as evidenced by vital signs within client's normal range, palpable peripheral pulses of good quality, and individually appropriate urinary output.

ACTIONS/INTERVENTIONS	RATIONALE
Shock Prevention (NIC)	
Independent	
Measure/record urinary output and specific gravity. Note cumulative intake and output (I&O) imbalances (including insensible losses), and correlate with daily weight. Encourage oral fluids to tolerance.	Decreasing urinary output with a high specific gravity suggests relative hypovolemia associated with vasodilation. Continued positive fluid balance with corresponding weight gain may indicate third spacing and tissue edema, suggesting need to alter fluid therapy/replacement components. *Note:* Excessive diarrhea may lead to a negative fluid balance.
Monitor BP and heart rate (HR). Measure central venous pressure (CVP) if used.	Reduction in the circulating fluid volume reduces BP/CVP, initiating compensatory mechanisms of tachycardia to improve cardiac output and increase systemic BP.
Palpate peripheral pulses.	Weak, easily obliterated pulses suggest hypovolemia.
Assess for dry mucous membranes, poor skin turgor, and thirst.	Hypovolemia/third spacing of fluid gives rise to signs of dehydration.

ACTIONS/INTERVENTIONS	RATIONALE
Observe for dependent/peripheral edema in sacrum, scrotum, back, legs.	Fluid losses from the vascular compartment into the interstitial space create tissue edema.

Collaborative

Administer IV fluids; e.g., isotonic crystalloids (D_5W, normal saline [NS], lactated Ringer's [LR]) and colloids (albumin, fresh frozen plasma) as indicated.	Fluid therapy is most effective early in the course of severe sepsis because as the condition worsens, there is greater dysfunction at the cellular level. Large volumes of fluid may be required to overcome relative hypovolemia (peripheral vasodilation), replace losses from increased capillary permeability (e.g., sequestration of fluid in the peritoneal cavity) and increased insensible sources (e.g., fever/diaphoresis).
Monitor laboratory values; e.g.:	
Hct/RBC count;	Evaluates changes in hydration/blood viscosity.
BUN/Cr.	Moderate elevations of BUN reflect dehydration; high values of BUN/Cr may indicate renal dysfunction/failure.
Monitor cardiac output as indicated.	CO (and other functional parameters, such as cardiac index, preload/afterload, contractility, and cardiac work) can be measured noninvasively using thoracic electrical bioimpedance (TEB) technique. Useful in determining therapeutic needs/effectiveness.

NURSING DIAGNOSIS: risk for impaired Gas Exchange

Risk factors may include

Altered O_2 supply: effects of endotoxins on the respiratory center in the medulla (resulting in hyperventilation/respiratory alkalosis); hypoventilation
Altered blood flow (changes in vascular resistance), alveolar-capillary membrane changes (increased capillary permeability leading to pulmonary congestion)
Interference with O_2 delivery/utilization in the tissues (endotoxin-induced damage to the cells/capillaries)

Possibly evidenced by

[Not applicable; presence of signs and symptoms establishes an *actual* diagnosis.]

DESIRED OUTCOMES/EVALUATION CRITERIA—CLIENT WILL:

RESPIRATORY STATUS: Gas Exchange (NOC)

Display ABGs and respiratory rate within client's normal range, with breath sounds clear and chest x-ray clear/improving.
Experience no dyspnea/cyanosis.

ACTIONS/INTERVENTIONS	RATIONALE
Respiratory Monitoring (NIC)	
Independent	
Maintain client airway. Place client in position of comfort with head of bed elevated 30–45 degrees.	Enhances lung expansion, reduces respiratory effort.

ACTIONS/INTERVENTIONS	RATIONALE
Monitor respiratory rate and depth. Note use of accessory muscles/work of breathing.	Rapid/shallow respirations occur because of hypoxemia, stress, and circulating endotoxins. Hypoventilation and dyspnea reflect ineffective compensatory mechanisms and are an indication that ventilatory support is needed.
Auscultate breath sounds. Note crackles, wheezes, areas of decreased/absent ventilation.	Respiratory distress and the presence of adventitious sounds are indicators of pulmonary congestion/interstitial edema, atelectasis. *Note:* Respiratory complications, including pneumonia and acute respiratory distress syndrome (ARDS), are prime causes of death.
Note presence of circumoral cyanosis.	Reflects inadequate central oxygenation/hypoxemia.
Investigate alterations in sensorium: agitation, confusion, personality changes, delirium, stupor, coma.	Cerebral function is very sensitive to decreases in oxygenation (e.g., hypoxemia, reduced perfusion).
Note cough and purulent sputum production.	Pneumonia is a common nosocomial infection that can occur by aspiration of oropharyngeal organisms or spread from other sites.
Reposition frequently. Encourage coughing and deep-breathing exercises. Suction as indicated.	Good pulmonary toilet is necessary for reducing ventilation/perfusion imbalance and for mobilizing and facilitating removal of secretions to maximize gas exchange.

Collaborative

Monitor ABGs/pulse oximetry.	Hypoxemia is related to decreased ventilation and pulmonary changes (e.g., interstitial edema, atelectasis, and pulmonary shunting) and increased oxygen demands caused by fever or infection. Respiratory acidosis (pH below 7.35 and $Paco_2$ higher than 40 mm Hg) occurs because of hypoventilation and ventilation-perfusion imbalance. As septic condition worsens, metabolic acidosis (pH below 7.35 and HCO_3 less than 22–24 mEq/L) develops as a result of buildup of lactic acid from anaerobic metabolism.
Administer supplemental O_2 via appropriate route; e.g., nasal cannula, mask, high-flow rebreathing mask.	Necessary for correction of hypoxemia with failing respiratory effort/progressing acidosis. *Note:* Intubation/mechanical ventilation may be required if respiratory failure develops.
Review serial chest x-rays.	Changes reflect progression/resolution of pulmonary complications; e.g., infiltrates/edema. *Note:* Changes in chest x-ray are usually 1–2 hr behind the clinical picture.

NURSING DIAGNOSIS: deficient Knowledge [Learning Need] regarding illness, prognosis, treatment, self-care, and discharge needs

May be related to

Lack of exposure/recall, information misinterpretation
Cognitive limitation

Possibly evidenced by

Questions/request for information, statement of misconception
Inaccurate follow-through of instructions, development of preventable complications

DESIRED OUTCOMES/EVALUATION CRITERIA—CLIENT WILL:

KNOWLEDGE: Infection Control (NOC)

Verbalize understanding of disease process, prognosis, and potential complications.
Correctly perform necessary procedures and explain reasons for the actions.
Initiate necessary lifestyle changes.
Verbalize understanding of therapeutic needs.
Participate in treatment regimen.

ACTIONS/INTERVENTIONS	RATIONALE
TEACHING: Disease Process (NIC)	
Independent	
Review disease process and future expectations.	Provides knowledge base from which client can make informed choices.
Review individual risk factors and mode of transmission/portal of entry of infections.	Steroid therapy, kidney/liver dysfunction, neoplastic disease, rheumatic heart disease, valve dysfunction, and diabetes may predispose to septicemia. Awareness of means of infection transmission provides opportunity to plan for/institute protective measures.
Provide information about drug therapy, interactions, side effects, and importance of adherence to regimen.	Promotes understanding of and enhances cooperation in treatment/prophylaxis, and reduces risk of recurrence and complications.
Discuss need for good nutritional intake/balanced diet.	Necessary for optimal healing, immune system enhancement, and general well-being.
Encourage adequate rest periods with scheduled activities.	Prevents fatigue, conserves energy, and facilitates recovery.
Review necessity of personal hygiene and environmental cleanliness, proper cooking techniques/food storage.	Helps control environmental exposure by diminishing the number of pathogens present. *Note:* Undercooked meat increases risk of exposure to *E. coli.*
Discuss proper use or avoidance of tampons with menstruating women as indicated.	Superabsorbent tampons/infrequent changing potentiate risk of *Staphylococcus aureus* infection (toxic shock syndrome).
Identify signs/symptoms requiring medical evaluation; e.g., persistent temperature elevation(s), tachycardia, syncope, rashes of unknown origin, unexplained fatigue, anorexia, increased thirst, and changes in bladder function.	Early recognition of developing/recurring infection allows for timely intervention and reduces risk for progression to life-threatening situation.
Stress importance of prophylactic immunization/antibiotic therapy as needed.	Used for prevention of infection dependent on individual risk factors; e.g., age, presence of chronic disease, immunosuppression.

POTENTIAL CONSIDERATIONS following acute hospitalization (dependent on client's age, physical condition/presence of complications, personal resources, and life responsibilities)

risk for recurrence/opportunistic Infection—stasis of body fluids, decreased hemoglobin, leukopenia, suppressed inflammatory response, use of anti-infective agents, increased environmental exposure, malnutrition.

imbalanced Nutrition: less than body requirements—increased energy needs (hypermetabolic state), anorexia, continuing GI dysfunction, side effects of medication.

Self-Care Deficit/ impaired Home Maintenance—decreased strength/endurance, pain/discomfort, inadequate support systems, unfamiliarity with neighborhood resources.

THE HIV-POSITIVE CLIENT

The individual identified as being HIV seropositive is one who is asymptomatic and who does not meet the Centers for Disease Control and Prevention (CDC) definition for AIDS. Studies reveal that persons with HIV-positive status may remain asymptomatic for 10 or more years. During the period of asymptomatic infection, the individual has the HIV in the blood and is contagious to others. Clients may live longer without symptoms if receiving highly active antiretroviral therapy (HAART) to reduce the viral load. After approximately a decade, especially in the undertreated individual, the immune system begins to decline and he or she develops symptoms of immune deficiency, a phase termed "symptomatic HIV infection." The individual might then develop AIDS-defining diseases.

With the inception of multiple drug regimens (using combinations of nucleoside reverse transcriptase inhibitors [NRTIs], protease inhibitors [PIs], or nonnucleoside reverse transcriptase inhibitors [NNRTIs]), the CD8+ CTL (cytotoxic T lymphocyte) and the CD4 count can be maintained at higher levels longer and the viral load minimized.

Controlling replication of HIV and lowering the viral load are the current focus of early intervention. Although imminent death is not a realistic concern, the client needs to make major behavioral and lifestyle changes to prolong life expectancy, and may have significant problems that require information and assistance. The person who is well supported medically may lead a productive life for an extended period.

At present, the rate of new infections is rapidly increasing among people of color, women in general (with the most common mode of transmission being heterosexual activity), and resurgence among young homosexual men who did not experience the losses of their predecessors and have a misconception regarding the efficacy of medications and therefore are engaging in unsafe sexual practices.

As medical interventions have improved, goals of treatment have changed. Early on, the goal of therapy was living longer. Now, healthier, longer lives are anticipated and expected, and a paradigm shift has occurred from staying alive to experiencing a good quality of life. New dosing regimens are addressing the issues of pill load (number of pills in each dose), dosing frequency, dietary restrictions, and adverse events, resulting in greater individualization of the medication regimen.

CARE SETTING

Community setting, although development of opportunistic infections may require occasional inpatient acute medical care.

RELATED FACTORS

Acquired immunodeficiency syndrome (AIDS), page 726
Extended care, page 810
Fluid and electrolyte imbalances, page 919
Pneumonia, page 128
Psychosocial aspects of care, page 770
Sepsis/septicemia, page 701

Client Assessment Database

Although client may be asymptomatic, refer to CP: AIDS for potential signs/symptoms.

Refer to section at end of plan for ongoing considerations.

DIAGNOSTIC STUDIES

Enzyme-linked immunosorbent assay (ELISA): A positive test result may be indicative of exposure to HIV but is not diagnostic. (Seroconversion can occur between 4 weeks and 6 months after exposure.)

Western blot test (blood/urine): Confirms diagnosis of HIV-1 in individuals with positive ELISA screening. (*Note:* In all other types of testing methods for Orasure, Standard, and Oraquick, the false-positive rate is 1%.)

Viral load tests:

Radioimmunoprecipitation–polymerase chain reaction (RI-PCR): Detects viral RNA levels as low as 50 copies/mL of plasma.

Branched DNA (bDNA) 3.0 assay: Has a wider range—50–500,000 copies/mL. (The RI-PCR range is 50–75,000/mL.)

Therapy can be initiated, or changes made in treatment approaches, based on rise of viral load or maintenance of a low viral load. This is currently the leading indicator of effectiveness of therapy.

CD8+ CTL (cytopathic suppressor cells): Current quantitative assays allow for rapid evaluation of levels. CD8+ (CTL) have been strongly implicated in the control of HIV-1 replications. At late stage of infection, CD8+ (CTL) numbers are reduced.

CD4+ lymphocyte count (previously T4 helper cells): Reduced. Client with counts below 500 benefit from antiretroviral therapy; counts equal to or below 200 define progression to AIDS. Levels are measured immediately before and again 4–8 weeks after initiation of antiretroviral therapy. Thus, it is used to diagnose HIV infection and progression and to monitor effects of drug therapy. The role of CD4+ T cells is unclear. CD4+ cells are a target for HIV infection and destruction. Some researchers postulate CD4+ cells are eliminated early. They may not contribute to host defense substantially in the late stages of disease.

Purified protein derivative (PPD): Used to screen for TB exposure. A positive result reflects current or prior exposure to TB. The criterion for positive PPD when immunodeficiency is present is 5-mm induration.

Serologies: *Rapid plasma reagin (RPR)/Venereal Disease Research Laboratory (VDRL):* Determines current/past exposure to syphilis and need for more specific testing. *Toxoplasma* and hepatitis B and C serologies are done.

Pap smear: Higher incidence (40%) of abnormal cells occurs in HIV-infected women. The critical role of Pap smear screening relates to its ability to detect precursor lesions that can precede the diagnosis of invasive carcinoma by several years.

Pelvic/genital examination: Identifies presence of lesions from sexually transmitted diseases (STDs), cervical and vaginal abnormalities.

Chemistries: Glucose levels elevated as a result of insulin resistance, and lipids rise as HIV infection progresses. Albumin/prealbumin and transferrin levels progressively decrease secondary to malabsorption/malnutrition.

CBC: Hemoglobin, RBC counts are decreased and abnormalities in iron metabolism can result in anemia, which occurs in 17% of asymptomatic clients with HIV and up to 85% of clients with advanced disease.

Chest x-ray: Abnormalities suggest presence of TB in PPD-positive, anergic, and/or symptomatic individuals. Diagnosis is then verified by sputum cultures or other tests, such as gallium scan.

NURSING PRIORITIES

1. Promote acceptance of reality of diagnosis/condition.
2. Support incorporation of behavioral/lifestyle changes to enhance well-being.
3. Provide information about disease process/prognosis and treatment needs.
4. Assist in developing plan and strategies to meet long-term medical, behavioral, and financial needs.

GOALS OF CARE

1. Dealing with current situation realistically.
2. Participating in and appropriately managing therapeutic regimen.
3. Diagnosis, prognosis, and therapeutic regimen understood.
4. Plan in place to meet medical, behavioral change, and financial needs.

NURSING DIAGNOSIS: impaired Adjustment

May be related to

Life-threatening, stigmatized condition/disease, incomplete/ongoing grieving
Assault to self-esteem, altered locus of control
Denial, negative attitudes toward health behavior
Inadequate support systems
Complex medication regimen and side effects (e.g., fatigue and depression)

Possibly evidenced by

Verbalization of nonacceptance/denial of diagnosis
Extended period of shock, disbelief, or anger regarding change in health status
Failure to take action to prevent further health problems
Inability to effectively manage medication regimen
Failure to achieve optimal sense of control

DESIRED OUTCOMES/EVALUATION CRITERIA—CLIENT WILL:

ACCEPTANCE: Health Status (NOC)

Verbalize reality and acceptance of condition.
Demonstrate increased trust and participation in development of plan of action.
Initiate lifestyle changes that will permit adaptation to present life situations.

ACTIONS/INTERVENTIONS	RATIONALE
Crisis Intervention (NIC)	
Independent	
Evaluate client's ability to understand events and realistically appraise situation.	Provides base to develop plan of action.
Identify real barriers to adjustment.	Promotes opportunity to deal appropriately with real problems in client's own situation.
Encourage expression of feelings, denial, shock, and fears. Listen without judgment, accepting client's expressions. Focus on positive outcomes.	It is important to convey belief in client's fears/feelings. By focusing on positive outcomes, client is encouraged to take charge of those areas in which changes can be made; e.g., managing medical regimen and behavior.
Challenge morbid thoughts and reframe into positive statements; e.g., "You know why the virus is going to kill me. I deserve to die for what I've done." Response: "The virus may or may not kill you. It's not smart enough to decide when you may die. The virus is 'just there.' It does not have a mind to know what you have or have not done."	Interrupts morbid thoughts and challenges client's self-deprecating ideas. As with any potentially terminal disease, this population is likely to experience depression and is at increased risk for suicide, necessitating ongoing evaluation.

ACTIONS/INTERVENTIONS	RATIONALE
Determine available resources and programs.	Helps identify what client needs and what might be immediately accessible. Addictive behaviors, ability of injection drug user to obtain clean "works," sexual myths, and perceptions of the need for condom use need to be addressed.
Assess social system, as well as presence of support, perception of losses, and stressors.	Partners, friends, and families will have individual responses depending on the individual's lifestyle, knowledge of HIV transmission, and belief systems. *Note*: Belief systems can include myths, e.g., HIV or religion, which can impact how the individual approaches the disease and the outcome.
Encourage client to participate in support groups.	Long-term support is critical to dealing with and effectively coping with the reality of being HIV positive and with frequent healthcare evaluations, medical treatments, and ongoing lifestyle changes.
Educate client about drug interactions, HIV, and emotions.	Fatigue and depression can be side effects of some medications and of the infection itself. Knowledge that these effects are usually of short duration can support informed choices/cooperation and promote hope.
Encourage continued or renewed use of familiar effective coping strategies.	Client is supported and given encouragement for past effective behaviors. Positive reinforcement enhances self-esteem.
Explore use and practice of new and different coping strategies.	Using new strategies is uncomfortable in the beginning, but practice fosters self-confidence.
Help client use humor to combat stigmatization of the disease.	Humor defuses the sense of secretiveness people may place on diagnosis of/dealing with HIV.
Reinforce structure in daily life. Include exercise as part of routine.	Routines help the person focus. Exercise improves sense of wellness and enhances immune response.
Discuss meaning of high-risk behavior (e.g., unprotected sexual activity or injection drug use with shared needles, failure to take medications), and address barriers to change.	Fear of disclosure, need to change usual behaviors, and the difficulty of doing so may prevent the individual from making the changes necessary to prevent transmission of disease and to manage lifestyle.
Assist client to set limits on sexually risky behaviors and explore ways client can achieve change.	Needs for love, comfort, and companionship that are met through sexual expression must be met safely through means that carry a reduced risk of HIV transmission.
Assist client to channel anger to healthy activities.	The increased energy of anger can be used to accomplish other tasks and enhance feelings of self-esteem.
Inform client about new medical advances/treatments.	Promotes hope and helps client make informed decisions.
Discuss issues of voluntary disclosure, personal responsibility, needs of others, and federal, state, and local reporting requirements.	Understanding responsibilities and consequences of disclosure is necessary for client to make informed decisions.

Collaborative

Refer to nurse practitioner/clinical nurse specialist, psychologist, social worker knowledgeable about HIV.	May need additional help adjusting to difficult situation.

NURSING DIAGNOSIS: Fatigue

May be related to

Decreased metabolic energy production, increased energy requirements (hypermetabolic state)
Overwhelming psychologic/emotional demands
Altered body chemistry: side effects of medications, insulin resistance

Possibly evidenced by

Verbalization of unremitting/overwhelming lack of energy
Inability to maintain usual routines, decreased performance, impaired ability to concentrate

DESIRED OUTCOMES/EVALUATION CRITERIA—CLIENT WILL:

Endurance (NOC)

Report improved sense of energy.
Participate in desired activities at level of ability.

Energy Conservation (NOC)

Identify individual areas of control and engage in energy conservation techniques.

ACTIONS/INTERVENTIONS	RATIONALE
Energy Management (NIC)	
Independent	
Assess sleep patterns and other factors that may be aggravating fatigue.	Multiple factors can cause/aggravate fatigue, including sleep deprivation, emotional distress, side effects of drugs, and developing central nervous system (CNS) disease.
Encourage timely evaluation of fatigue if new medications have been added to regimen.	Fatigue is present in variable degrees as part of HIV infection process, but is often aggravated by nutritional deficiencies and side effects of certain medications. For example, when protease inhibitors are added or changed, fatigue may worsen.
Discuss reality of client's feelings of exhaustion and identify limitations imposed by fatigue state. Note daily energy patterns—peaks and valleys.	Helpful in planning activities within tolerance levels. Clients often expect too much of themselves, believing that they should be able to do more.
Assist client to set realistic activity goals, determining individual priorities and responsibilities.	Client may need to alter priorities, delegate some responsibilities to manage fatigue and optimize performance.
Discuss energy conservation techniques; e.g., sitting instead of standing for activities as appropriate.	Enables client to become aware of ways in which energy expenditure can be maximized to complete necessary tasks.
Review importance of meeting individual nutritional needs.	Adequate nutrition is needed for optimizing energy production. (Refer to ND: imbalanced Nutrition: risk for less than body requirements, following.)
Encourage adequate rest periods during day, routine schedule for bedtime/arising, and scheduling activities during time of best energy.	Helps client recoup energy to manage desired activities.
Instruct in stress management techniques; e.g., breathing exercises, visualization, music and light therapy.	Reduction of stress factors in client's life can minimize energy output.
Identify available resources and support systems.	May require outside assistance with homemaking/maintenance activities, child care.

NURSING DIAGNOSIS: imbalanced Nutrition: risk for less than body requirements

Risk factors may include

Reported inadequate food intake less than recommended daily allowance
Lack of interest in food, anorexia, depression
Lack of information, misinformation, misconceptions

Limited resources (including finances)
Reported altered sensation of taste and smell, nausea and other side effects of medications
Sore, inflamed buccal cavity (e.g., thrush, cytomegalovirus [CMV] lesions)

Possibly evidenced by

[Not applicable; presence of signs and symptoms establishes an *actual* diagnosis.]

DESIRED OUTCOMES/EVALUATION CRITERIA—CLIENT WILL:

Nutritional Status (NOC)

Maintain adequate muscle mass.
Maintain stable weight.
Demonstrate laboratory values within normal limits.
Report improved energy level.

ACTIONS/INTERVENTIONS	RATIONALE
Nutritional Counseling (NIC)	
Independent	
Determine usual weight before client was diagnosed with HIV.	Early wasting is not readily determined by normal weight-to-height charts; therefore, determining current weight in relation to prediagnosis weight is more useful. Recent unexplained/involuntary weight loss may be a factor in seeking initial medical evaluation.
Weigh regularly and establish current anthropometric measurements. Measure resting energy expenditure (REE) using indirect calorimetry.	Helps assess/monitor wasting and determine nutritional needs (40% of HIV-positive clients show substantial weight loss). Indirect calorimetry is more accurate for calculating REE than Harris-Benedict equation, which underestimates the energy needs of these clients.
Determine client's current dietary pattern/intake and knowledge of nutrition. Use an in-depth dietary assessment tool.	Identification of these factors helps plan for individual needs. Clients with HIV infection have documented vitamin (e.g., vitamin B_{12}, folate) and trace mineral (e.g., zinc, magnesium, selenium) deficits. Alcohol and drug abuse can interfere with adequate intake.
Assess presence/degree of nausea and vomiting.	The causes of nausea and vomiting are numerous and are associated with medications, functional changes in GI system, and endocrine dysfunction. Protracted nausea and vomiting can debilitate a client, leading to loss of lean body mass, electrolyte imbalances, and further deterioration of immune function.
Ascertain current financial status, recent and/or anticipated changes in economic status. Explore related costs of a variety of foods.	Helps in planning for meeting nutritional needs, such as purchasing low-cost foods that are nutritionally packed, or client may need referral to financial aid to help with food stamps or obtaining meals.
Discuss/document nutritional side effects of medications.	Commonly used medications cause anorexia, altered taste, nausea and/or vomiting; some interfere with bone marrow production of RBCs, causing anemia. GI symptoms are common with over-the-counter (OTC) drugs like nonsteroidal anti-inflammatory drugs (NSAIDs), which also may contribute to anorexia.

ACTIONS/INTERVENTIONS	RATIONALE
Help client plan ways to maintain/ improve intake. Identify lactose-free supplements as appropriate. Provide information about nutritionally dense high-calorie, high-protein, high-vitamin, and high-mineral foods.	Having this information helps client understand importance of well-balanced diet. Some clients may try macrobiotic and other diets, believing the diarrhea is caused by lactose intolerance. Eliminating dairy products can have detrimental effects when these nutrient components are not replaced from other sources.
Stress importance of maintaining balanced/adequate nutritional intake and fluids rich with electrolytes; e.g., Gatorade or Pedialyte.	Client may be depressed and discouraged with changed health and social status and find it difficult to eat for many reasons. Knowing how important nutritionally balanced intake is to supporting the immune system and remaining healthy can motivate client to eat.
Assist client to formulate dietary plan, taking into consideration increased metabolic demands/energy needs and hyperlipidemia.	Provides guidance and feedback while promoting sense of control, enhancing self-esteem, and possibly improving intake. HIV infection is continuously stimulating the immune system, increasing metabolic rate and nutritional needs. *Note:* Use of protease inhibitors is known to elevate levels of glucose and lipids (especially triglycerides and cholesterol).
Recommend eating frequent small meals, avoiding cooking odors if bothersome, keeping room well ventilated, and removing noxious stimuli. Suggest use of spices, marinating red meat before cooking, and/or substituting other protein sources for red meat.	Reduces possible adverse stimuli or enhances palatability of food and may improve nutritional intake, which is needed to help client restore/maintain nutritional defenses.
Recommend environment conducive to eating. Emphasize importance of sharing mealtime with others. Identify someone who can join client for meals.	A quiet, relaxed/calm, unrushed setting and socialization can enhance appetite/food intake, especially when depression, neglect of self-care, and diminished appetite are present.
Explore complementary therapies/nonpharmacologic interventions, such as acupressure, progressive relaxation, and guided imagery to manage anorexia.	The goal of these interventions is to manage distressing symptoms that interfere with optimal nutritional intake.
Discuss use of *Lactobacillus acidophilus* replacement; e.g., LactAid dairy products and/or tablets/capsules.	HIV infection changes the structure of the gut wall, resulting in a decreased lactose level. Intolerance causes abdominal cramping, malabsorption, a bloated feeling, and diarrhea. Also, antibiotics taken for prevention of opportunistic infections cause changes in normal bowel flora, contributing to diarrhea.

Collaborative

ACTIONS/INTERVENTIONS	RATIONALE
Consult with dietitian, nutritional support team.	Provides assistance in planning nutritionally sound diet and identifying nutritional supplements to meet individual needs. Liquid supplements (e.g., Advera) have been specifically formulated for the GI manifestations common to the HIV-positive population.
Monitor laboratory values; e.g., hemoglobin (Hb), RBCs, albumin/prealbumin, total iron-binding capacity (TIBC), potassium, sodium.	These laboratory tests are important in monitoring the client's nutritional immune status and in identifying nutritional therapy needs. For example, decreased RBCs (anemia) may require additional interventions, such as use of epoetin (Epogen or Procrit) to stimulate RBC production.
Provide medications as indicated; e.g.,	
Dronabinol (Marinol), megestrol (Megace), cyproheptadine (Periactin);	Antiemetics/appetite stimulants can improve intake to prevent and correct dietary deficiencies. *Note:* Side effect of use of Megace may include impotence, necessitating change of drug as desired.
Antidiarrheal medications; e.g., diphenoxylate/atropine (Lomotil), octreotide (Sandostatin).	Diarrhea may be present because of altered GI flora and side effects of anti-infective agents. Treatment can correct malabsorption and enhance oral intake.
Consider use of acidophilus OTC products.	Can be useful in restoration of normal bowel flora.

NURSING DIAGNOSIS: deficient Knowledge [Learning Need] regarding disease, prognosis, treatment, self-care, and discharge needs

May be related to

Lack of exposure/recall
Information misinterpretation
Unfamiliarity with information resources
Cognitive limitation

Possibly evidenced by

Statement of misconception/request for information
Inaccurate follow-through of instructions, development of preventable complications
Inappropriate/exaggerated behaviors (e.g., hostile, agitated, hysterical, apathetic)

DESIRED OUTCOMES/EVALUATION CRITERIA—CLIENT WILL:

KNOWLEDGE: Disease Process (NOC)

Verbalize understanding of condition/disease process and potential complications.
Identify relationship of signs/symptoms to the disease process and correlate symptoms with causative factors.

KNOWLEDGE: Treatment Regimen (NOC)

Verbalize understanding of goals of treatment.
Initiate necessary lifestyle changes.
Participate in treatment regimen.

ACTIONS/INTERVENTIONS	RATIONALE
TEACHING: Learning Facilitation (NIC)	
Independent	
Assess emotional ability to assimilate information and understand instructions. Respect client's need to use denial coping techniques initially.	Initial shock and anxiety can block intake of information. Self-esteem, lifestyle, guilt, and denial of own responsibility in acquiring/transmitting disease become issues that must be dealt with. *Note:* Some initial denial may serve as a protective mechanism promoting more effective self-care.
Provide realistic, optimistic information during each contact with client.	Necessary to provide realistic hope because most clients have been exposed to some inaccurate information about AIDS or may have friends/lovers who have died of the disease.
Plan frequent short sessions for teaching. Include written information—a few pieces at each visit.	Client will likely feel overwhelmed and need time and repeated contacts to absorb information, the scope of and requirements for treating the infection. Written materials allow for later review and reinforcement of information presented.
Include SO/family in discussions and conferences as appropriate.	Provides opportunity to learn information first hand, ask questions, and provide support for client.
TEACHING: Disease Process (NIC)	
Determine current understanding and perception of diagnosis. Discuss difference between HIV positivity and AIDS.	Provides opportunity to clarify misconceptions/myths and make informed choices. People often believe that if they are positive for the virus, they have AIDS; having accurate information about the difference can alleviate fears and allow for development of an individualized plan of care.

ACTIONS/INTERVENTIONS	RATIONALE
Identify/problem-solve potential or actual barriers to accessing healthcare services.	Transportation, distance, child care, work schedule, homelessness/poverty, lack of insurance or finances are some of the issues that typically interfere with accessing needed primary care and prophylactic interventions.
Provide information about normal immune system/response and how HIV affects it, transmission of the virus, behaviors, and factors believed to increase probability of progression. Encourage questions.	Client needs to be aware of own personal risk and risk to others to make immediate and long-range decisions and establish a basis for goal setting. Also, establishes rapport and provides opportunity to identify concerns and assimilate information.
Review signs/symptoms that could be a consequence of HIV infection; e.g., mild fever, anorexia, weight loss, fatigue, night sweats, diarrhea, dry cough, rashes, headaches, and sleep disturbances.	Client may experience an acute illness 2–6 weeks after becoming infected; however, it is common for infection to be subclinical, with the individual simply feeling unwell.
Discuss management strategies for persistent signs/symptoms.	Client involvement in care increases cooperation and satisfaction with care.
Identify signs/symptoms that require medical evaluation; e.g., persistent fever, increasing cough or swollen lymph glands, profound fatigue unrelieved by rest, weight loss of 10 lb (or more) in less than 2 months, severe/persistent diarrhea, fever, blurred vision, skin discoloration or rash that persists or spreads, open sores anywhere, symptoms occurring with medication regimen.	Early recognition of progression of disease/development of opportunistic infections provides for timely intervention and may prevent more serious situations. *Note:* Most HIV-positive clients are now on medication regimens (usually at least three drugs) and must adhere to the dosages and schedules, which may be difficult and/or cause side effects that tempt client to alter or discontinue them without notifying the physician.
Stress necessity of regular follow-up care and evaluations including routine CD4 and HIV-RNA viral load counts, and any change in medication regimen (time, frequency, side effects).	Even though client may be asymptomatic, periodic evaluation may prevent development of complications, slow the progression of the disease, and assist with treatment decisions. *Note:* Clients who change medication dosage/frequency in response to side effects can create problems for medication adjustment later with increased viral load and drug resistance.
Discuss need for regular gynecologic examinations.	HIV-positive women experience a high prevalence of Pap smear, vaginal, and cervical abnormalities.
Discuss family planning issues, careful selection of oral contraceptives.	Various antiretroviral drugs have differing effects on ethinyl estradiol (EE) either enhancing or decreasing protective effectiveness.
Provide preconception counseling, giving information about risk of vertical transmission and ways to reduce the possibility of perinatal transmission.	The risk of viral rebound with adverse consequences to the fetus increases in women currently receiving treatment at the time of conception. Research shows that when antiretroviral treatment is initiated early in pregnancy, the neonatal transmission rate has dropped to less than 8% of live births. However, there is a lack of research regarding safety of antiretroviral therapy in pregnancy and its effect on the fetus. (Efavirenz is one exception; it is known to cause severe fetal malformation in monkeys.) The majority of drugs are category C (no clinical trial information) for therapy. For newly pregnant women, consider withholding medication until after the first trimester.
Refer to Antiretroviral Pregnancy Registry as appropriate.	Collection of information regarding women and pregnancy will increase data on teratogenic effects of medications/antiretrovirals.

TEACHING: Prescribed Medication (NIC)

Review drug therapies, including correct dosing/scheduling, side effects, monitoring tests/techniques, and adverse reactions as appropriate:	These drugs interfere with the HIV replication process, and early treatment may be considered when CD4 count is near 500, even if individual is asymptomatic. Side effects such as symptoms of peripheral neuropathy or pancreatitis necessitate prompt evaluation and possible discontinuation/change in therapy. *Note*: Medication management of HIV is now more individualized, targeting specific HIV isolates, identifying susceptibility, etc.

ACTIONS/INTERVENTIONS	RATIONALE
Antiretrovirals; e.g.: Enfuvirtide (ENF, T-20), emtricataline (FTC)-NRTI, azotzenavir (ATV) – PI, fosamprenevir (FPV) –908 – PI;	Currently, 12 antiretroviral agents have been approved by the Food and Drug Administration (FDA), all aimed at blocking replication of the HIV at some level. The drugs are generally given in groups of three because a multidrug regimen is more effective in reducing the viral load. (The goal is to maintain viral load at <500 copies/mL.)
Nucleoside reverse transcriptase inhibitors (NRTIs): zidovudine/ZDV (Retrovir, AZT), didanosine/ddI (Videx), zalcitabine/ddC, (Hivid), stavudine/d4T (Zerit), lamivudine/3TC (Epivir);	In the past, zidovudine was given alone and as a first-line treatment. Now the drug is usually given in a three-drug treatment regimen, along with another NRTI and a protease inhibitor. Zidovudine is, however, safe in preventing perinatal HIV infection, so it is an option for the pregnant client.
Protease inhibitors (PIs); e.g., indinavir/IDV (Crixivan), nelfinevir (Viracept), ritonavir/RTV (Norvir), saquinavir/SQV (Fortovase, Invirase), amprenavir/APV (Agenerase);	When combined with NRTIs, protease inhibitors control the HIV-RNA viral load by blocking viral replication at two different target sites in the replication process. Immune function is maintained with early intervention, or improved when initiated later.
Nonnucleoside reverse transcriptase inhibitors (NNRTIs); e.g., delavirdine/DLV (Rescriptor), nevirapine/NVP (Viramune), efavirenz/EFV (Sustiva);	These drugs inhibit viral replication by a different mechanism than NRTIs or PIs. They also are used in combination because using them alone seems to encourage drug resistance.
Anti-infectives; e.g., trimethoprim-sulfamethoxazole/TMP/SMX (Bactrim, Septra), azithromycin (Zithromax), clarithromycin (Biaxin), foscarnet (Foscavir), rifabutin (Mycobutin), isoniazid (INH), pyridoxine (Doxine).	Focus on prevention of commonly occurring opportunistic infections, such as *Pneumocystis carinii* pneumonia (PCP), cytomegalovirus (CMV), *Mycobacterium avium* complex (MAC), or TB may prolong general wellness. Primary prophylactic therapy aims to prevent or delay onset of symptoms of reactivated or newly acquired infection. The goal of secondary prophylaxis is to prevent or delay recurrent episodes of particular infection. Prophylaxis continues indefinitely as long as the drug is tolerated. *Note:* Many of these organisms (except those causing TB) are part of the normal body flora and are usually kept under control by the healthy immune system.
Provide information about clinical trials available as individually appropriate.	Scientific research requires HIV-positive test subjects. Participation may provide individual with a sense of contributing to body of knowledge/search for cure, in addition to no-cost monitoring and medications for those with limited financial resources.
Provide information about pharmaceutical company assistance programs.	Some medications are provided free or at reduced cost, based on income.

Risk Identification (NIC)

Assess potential for inappropriate/high-risk behavior; e.g., continued injection drug abuse, unsafe sexual practices. Stress need to avoid use of illicit injected drugs or, if unwilling to abstain, to avoid sharing needles and to clean works with bleach solution, rinsing carefully with water.	High denial/anger, drug addition may cause client to continue behaviors that are high risk for spread of the virus. Even moderate changes in lifestyle may reduce exposure to other infective agents that can cause additional stress to the immune system. *Note*: Client may intensify substance abuse as a means of denial.
Recommend exploring drug treatment resources; e.g., methadone clinics or substance abuse recovery groups or programs.	Programs could help reduce HIV transmission by reducing injection drug use when client substitutes (i.e., methadone) or recovers from drug use, or if safer injection and needle use techniques are learned. *Note*: Research suggests some women may decrease drug use/be amenable to rehabilitation in an attempt to improve relationships with children/family.

ACTIONS/INTERVENTIONS	RATIONALE
Stress necessity of, and methods for, practicing safer sex at all times.	Limits spread of virus and exposure to other STDs. A person's sexual expression and identity are threatened by the discovery of the diagnosis. Therefore, 40% or more of individuals with HIV may not reveal status to potential sexual partners, contributing to ongoing transmission. Women may not follow guidelines because partner refuses to use condoms.
Discuss active changes in sexual behaviors that client can make that may satisfy sexual needs.	Learning alternative forms of expression promotes a sense of responsibility and control. May reduce sexual tensions/promote normalcy in sexual relationships and reduce fear/guilt related to potential transmission of HIV. *Note:* Clients, particularly women, may fear partner will leave, resulting in loss of love and emotional/financial support.
Provide information about other necessary lifestyle changes and health maintenance factors:	Evidence suggests that specific dietary and lifestyle factors may slow the progression of HIV infection because they support a healthier immune system.
Avoid people with infections;	When the immune system is depressed, the person's ability to fight exposure to common communicable diseases is limited.
Exercise within ability, alternate rest periods with activity, and get adequate sleep;	Helps manage fatigue; maintains strength and sense of well-being. Exercise has also been shown to stimulate the immune system.
Eat regularly, even if appetite is reduced; try small, frequent meals and snacks of foods high in nutrition; discuss ways to control nausea/vomiting and improve appetite;	Physical and psychologic stressors increase metabolic needs; in addition, side effects of medication, presence of nausea/vomiting, and anorexia often limit oral intake. The result is nutritional deficits that can further impair the immune system.
Practice daily oral hygiene, use a soft toothbrush; examine mouth regularly for sores, white film, or changes in color; have regular dental checkups every 6 months;	Poor oral hygiene/dental care can affect oral intake adversely and increase the risk of opportunistic/systemic infections.
Examine skin for rashes, bruises, breaks in skin integrity.	May indicate developing complications/increased risk of infection.
Identify additional resources; e.g., support groups, peer counselors, and mental health professionals, case managers.	Client will experience a variety of emotional and psychologic responses to the diagnosis and its consequences and may need additional assistance and periodic reinforcement to promote optimal adjustment. *Note*: In early stages of HIV infection, focus may be on social services (e.g., help with housing, employment, legal issues, finances). Later, as disease progresses, the emphasis switches to medical and related community services.

NURSING DIAGNOSIS: risk for Social Isolation

Risk factors may include

Altered state of wellness, changes in physical appearance
Perceptions of unacceptable social or sexual behavior/values
Inadequate resources/fear of losing personal resources

Possibly evidenced by

[Not applicable; presence of signs and symptoms establishes an *actual* diagnosis.]

DESIRED OUTCOMES/EVALUATION CRITERIA— CLIENT WILL:

Social Support (NOC)

Identify stable system/individual(s).
Use resources for assistance as appropriate.
Express increased sense of self-esteem.

ACTIONS/INTERVENTIONS	RATIONALE
Support System Enhancement (NIC)	
Independent	
Determine client's response to condition, feelings about self, concerns/fears about response of others, sense of ability to control situation, sense of hope.	How the individual accepts and deals with the situation will help decide the plan of care and interventions.
Assess coping mechanisms/previous methods of dealing with life problems.	May reveal successful techniques that can be used in current situation.
Discuss concerns regarding employment/leisure involvement. Note potential problems involving finances, insurance, housing.	Clients with this potentially terminal illness that carries a stigma face major problems with possible loss of employment, medical insurance, housing, and care sources if they become unable to independently care for themselves.
Identify availability/stability of support systems including significant other (SO), immediate/extended family, community.	Crucial information to help client plan future care.
Encourage honesty in relationships as appropriate.	As a rule, acquaintances do not need to be informed of client's health status. However, information should be shared with close relationships (e.g., SO, family, sexual partners). Honesty can help identify stable support persons.
Encourage contact with SO, family, and friends.	Many clients fear telling SO, family, and friends for fear of rejection, and some clients withdraw as a result of tumultuous feelings. Contact promotes sense of support, concern, involvement, and understanding. Supporting loved ones as they learn of the diagnosis is beneficial and can provide optimism for the long-term.
Assist client to problem-solve solutions to short-term/imposed isolations (e.g., communicable disease measures, severely compromised immune system).	Anticipatory planning can defuse sense of isolation and loneliness that can accompany these situations.
Help client differentiate between isolation and loneliness/aloneness, which may be by choice.	Provides an opportunity for client to realize the control he or she has to make decisions about the choice to take care of self in regard to these issues.
Be alert to verbal/nonverbal cues; e.g., withdrawal, statements of despair, sense of aloneness. Determine presence/level of risk of suicidal thoughts.	Indicators of despair and suicidal ideation may be present. When these cues are acknowledged, client is usually willing to divulge thoughts and sense of isolation/hopelessness.
Collaborative	
Identify community resources, self-help groups, rehabilitation/drug cessation programs as indicated.	Provides opportunities for resolving problems that may contribute to sense of loneliness and isolation, transmission risks, and sense of guilt.
Refer to psychiatric clinical nurse specialist/psychiatrist as needed.	May require more in-depth support to deal with feelings, manage difficult situations.

NURSING DIAGNOSIS: ineffective [individual]/families Therapeutic Regimen Management

May be related to

Complexity of healthcare system/access to care, economic difficulties
Complexity of therapeutic regimen (e.g., confusing/difficult dosing schedule, duration of regimen)
Mistrust of regimen and/or healthcare personnel (client/provider interactions)
Health beliefs/cultural influences
Perceived seriousness/susceptibility/benefits of therapy
Decisional conflicts, powerlessness
Family conflict/crises

Possibly evidenced by

Expressed desire to manage situation more appropriately
Verbalized difficulty with regulation/integration of one or more prescribed regimens for treatment of illness and its effects
Failure to take actions to reduce risk factors for progression of illness and sequelae
Evidence of acceleration of illness symptoms/development of complications

DESIRED OUTCOMES/EVALUATION CRITERIA—CLIENT/FAMILY WILL:

TREATMENT BEHAVIOR: Illness or Injury (NOC)

Identify individual factors affecting management of regimen.
Accept personal responsibility for own actions and participate in problem-solving activities.
Develop contract for care with mutually agreeable goals for treatment and mechanisms for changing/terminating elements of plan.

ACTIONS/INTERVENTIONS	RATIONALE
Client Contracting (NIC)	
Independent	
Make time to listen to client concerns.	Promotes feelings of value and may identify additional factors that affect outcome of therapy. Timing of teaching needs to consider the stage of acceptance.
Note client's stage of acceptance of the diagnosis:	
Precontemplation stage;	Client has just learned of the diagnosis, and may not be able to participate in any discussions.
Contemplation stage;	Client can participate in/may initiate discussions of therapy. Encourages individual's responsibility to be involved with planning. Promotes increased sense of control and self esteem.
Action/maintenance stage.	Client is actively involved in understanding and managing own care.
Determine client's/SO's perception or understanding of regimen.	Identifies areas of confusion/conflict or lack of accurate information that may impede cooperation with regimen.
Assess perceived/actual barriers to accessing healthcare services and reasons for deviations from prescribed plan.	Provides opportunity to clarify actual problems and develop alternative plan acceptable to healthcare provider.
Instruct client carefully in all aspects of medication regimen, times, interaction with food, side effects;	Thorough understanding may enhance cooperation with regimen, help in identifying potential for compromise.
Provide written schedule;	Helpful for future reference.
Suggest placing doses of medications in various locations;	When client's routine is stable, and he or she engages in activities away from home, it is helpful to keep a supply of medications in more than one location (e.g., work, home of family/friends).
Recommend various methods to alert client to medication time, such as portable pill container, alarms;	Will assist busy or forgetful client to take medications at appropriate intervals.
Reduce dose frequency and number of pills when possible;	Increases ability to manage treatment regimen with little interference.
Stress importance of keeping healthcare provider informed of concerns and ability to continue prescribed medication regimen;	Drug levels quickly fall below therapeutic levels if one dose is missed. *Note:* Evidence suggests women tend to reduce or stop therapy secondary to side effects more frequently than men.

ACTIONS/INTERVENTIONS	RATIONALE
Notify healthcare provider immediately if unable to continue all antiretroviral medications (i.e., nausea/vomiting).	Reduces potential for drug resistance or increased viral load. Alternate medications may be available. Poor adherence or factors leading to discontinuation of an antiretroviral medication can impede future attempts to reduce viral load. Suboptimal drug exposure increases the potential for drug resistance.
Negotiate a therapy plan client can commit to. Include routines of awakening, meals, work schedule, and medication side effects.	The more individualized the plan is, the greater probability of adherence.
Assist client to develop realistic health goals and incorporate wellness activities and practices, i.e., exercise, smoking cessation, nutrition, vitamin supplements, into daily routine.	Multiple responsibilities and demands on the client's time, especially women, make it appear difficult to include any additional activities of self-care.
Review stress management skills.	Clients must balance self-care needs and needs of other family members, which may be conflicting.
Provide anticipatory guidance, possible occurrences and choices, if any, to prevent or delay complications.	Reduces crisis events. Provides time for client to prepare for known, usual or expected changes. Permits earlier initiation of therapies and decreases disruption of schedule.
Identify adaptive interventions valid for progressive long-term care needs.	Builds on coping strategies already effective for this individual.
Monitor adherence to prescribed medical regimen. Alter plan of care as needed.	Regimen is likely to be complicated and time consuming. Thoughtful changes in plan may help enhance cooperation.
Evaluate short term side effects and their interference with adherence to the medical regimen.	In the past, symptoms were considered part of having the disease and were accepted. Perception is that the side effect symptoms are the "main" effect. Improved options for better client care include the role of new HIV-1 protease inhibitors

Support System Enhancement (NIC)

Identify potential or actual support person(s). Include in teaching and problem-solving activities as appropriate.	Helpful in planning for future and current needs of person and family.
Help client develop strategies that can gain supportive persons.	The more support persons available, the lower the risk of support burnout.

Collaborative

Identify appropriate women's groups/services, social worker; financial resources, respite care, and other community programs.	Often female clients are single parents/caretakers for family. Groups can provide support and tangible help in dealing with issues of childcare, parenting, what to do when client is too ill to parent.
Refer to counselor/therapist, spiritual advisor as appropriate.	Opportunity to discuss concerns/fears may aid in problem-solving solutions and living with required changes.

POTENTIAL ONGOING CONSIDERATIONS (dependent on client's age, physical condition/presence of complications, person resources, and life responsibilities)

Fatigue—decreased metabolic energy production, increased energy requirements (hypermetabolic state).

imbalanced Nutrition: less than body requirements—increased metabolic demands/energy requirements, side effects of medication, anorexia, fatigue.

Decisional Conflict—unclear personal values/beliefs, perceived threat to value system, multiple or divergent sources of information, support system deficit, interference with decision making.

risk for Infection—depression of immune system, chronic disease, malnutrition, use of antimicrobial agents (superimposed infections; e.g., yeast).

ineffective [individual]/family Therapeutic Regimen Management—complexity of healthcare system/therapeutic regimen, perceived seriousness/susceptibility/benefits of therapy, family conflicts/crises.

ACQUIRED IMMUNODEFICIENCY SYNDROME (AIDS)

Acquired immunodeficiency syndrome (AIDS) is the final result of infection with a retrovirus, the human immunodeficiency virus (HIV). HIV infection is a progressive disease leading to AIDS, as defined by the Centers for Disease Control and Prevention (CDC) (January, 1994): "persons with CD4 cell count of under 200 (with or without symptoms of opportunistic infection) who are HIV-positive are diagnosed as having AIDS." The current focus of antiretroviral therapy (HAART) is to control viral replication and thus the viral load. The immune response is massive throughout the course of HIV disease. Research studies in 1995 showed that HIV initially replicates rapidly on a daily basis, and evidence suggests the cellular immune response is essential in limiting replication and rate of disease progression.

Health-related quality of life (HRQOL) is an important issue in the management of symptoms of severe HIV infection (e.g., anemia, pain, fatigue, weakness, sleep disorders, or gastrointestinal symptoms) and/or side effects of medications. Multiple medications and inconvenient dosing regimens can reduce a person's sense of control, independence, and general quality of life. During the winter of 1995–1996 landmark advancement occurred with the introduction of HIV protease inhibitors and combination antiretroviral therapy that resulted in significant reduction in mortality and HIV-related complications. In 2003, new medications were approved that are projected to increase adherence because of less frequent dosing, fewer pills each dose, and fewer side effects. These interventions that maximize quality of life are emerging as essential to improvement in treatment adherence.

In the United States, HAART has reduced the death rates sharply, but the rate of new infections remains above 40,000/year, with 2%–4% of those being multidrug-resistant HIV. Infected persons have been found to fall into certain high-risk categories: injection drug users, homosexual or bisexual men, hemophiliacs, sexual partners of aforementioned individuals, sexual partners of a person known to be HIV positive, prostitutes and their sexual partners, persons with any/several sexually transmitted diseases, individuals who have multiple sexual partners or who engage in unprotected intercourse, children born to infected mothers, and healthcare workers and other persons with occupational exposures.

CARE SETTING

The interventions listed here are appropriate for community care as well as inpatient or hospice setting. Most of the signs and symptoms and psychosocial issues happen long before inpatient care, which today is usually very short.

RELATED FACTORS

End of life/hospice care, page 880
Extended care, page 810
Fluid and electrolyte imbalances, page 919
The HIV-positive client, page 712
Psychosocial aspects of care, page 770
Sepsis/septicemia, page 701
Total nutritional support: parenteral/enteral feeding, page 478
Upper gastrointestinal/esophageal bleeding, page 309
Ventilatory assistance (mechanical), page 170

Client Assessment Database

Data depend on the organs/body tissues involved, the current viral load, and the specific opportunistic infection (OI) or cancer.

ACTIVITY/REST

May report: Reduced tolerance for usual activities, progressing to profound fatigue and malaise; weakness
Altered sleep patterns

May exhibit: Muscle weakness, wasting of muscle mass
Physiologic response to activity; e.g., changes in BP, HR, respirations

CIRCULATION

May report: Slow healing (if anemic); bleeding longer with injury

May exhibit: Tachycardia, postural BP changes
Decreased peripheral pulse volume
Pallor or cyanosis; delayed capillary refill

EGO INTEGRITY

May report: Stress factors related to lifestyle changes (specifically healthcare planning and regimen of multiple medications), losses; e.g., family support, relationships, independence, financial, spiritual concerns, and change in self-concept (loss of control/powerless)

Concern about appearance: Alopecia, disfiguring lesions, weight loss, altered distribution of body fat (associated with protease-inhibiting drug therapy), thinning of extremities, wrinkling of skin
Denial of diagnosis, feelings of hopelessness, helplessness, worthlessness, guilt, depression

May exhibit: Denial, anxiety, depression, fear, withdrawal
Angry behaviors, dejected body posture, crying, poor eye contact
Failure to keep appointments or multiple appointments for similar symptoms

ELIMINATION

May report: Difficult and painful elimination, rectal pain and itching
Intermittent, persistent, frequent diarrhea with or without abdominal cramping
Flank pain, burning on urination

May exhibit: Loose-formed to watery stools with or without mucus or blood; frequent, copious diarrhea
Abdominal tenderness
Rectal, perianal lesions or abscesses
Changes in urinary output, color, character
Urinary, bowel incontinence

FOOD/FLUID

May report: Anorexia, changes in taste of foods/food intolerance, nausea/vomiting
Rapid/progressive weight loss
Difficulty chewing and swallowing (sore mouth, tongue); dysphagia, retrosternal pain with swallowing
Food intolerance; e.g., diarrhea after dairy products, nausea, early satiation, bloating

May exhibit: Hyperactive bowel sounds
Abdominal distention (hepatosplenomegaly)
Weight loss, thin frame, decreased subcutaneous fat/muscle mass
Poor skin turgor
Lesions of the oral cavity, white patches, discoloration; poor dental/gum health, loss of teeth
Edema (generalized, dependent)

HYGIENE

May report: Inability to complete activities of daily living (ADLs) independently

May exhibit: Disheveled/unkempt appearance
Deficits in many or all personal care, self-care activities

NEUROSENSORY

May report: Fainting spells/dizziness; headache; stiff neck
Changes in mental status, loss of mental acuity/ability to solve problems, forgetfulness, poor concentration
Impaired sensation or sense of position and vibration
Muscle weakness, tremors, changes in visual acuity
Numbness, tingling in extremities (feet seem to display earliest changes)
Changes in visual acuity, light flashes/floaters, photophobia

May exhibit: Mental status changes ranging from confusion to dementia, delirium with sudden onset
Forgetfulness, poor concentration, decreased alertness, apathy, psychomotor retardation/slowed responses
Paranoid ideation, free-floating anxiety, unrealistic expectations
Abnormal reflexes, decreased muscle strength, ataxic gait
Fine/gross motor tremors, focal motor deficits, hemiparesis, seizures
Retinal hemorrhages and exudates (CMV retinitis); blindness

PAIN/DISCOMFORT

May report: Generalized/localized pain, aching and burning in feet
Headache
Pleuritic chest pain

May exhibit: Swelling of joints, painful nodules, tenderness
Decreased range of motion (ROM), gait changes/limp
Muscle guarding

RESPIRATION

May report: Frequent, persistent upper respiratory infections (URIs)
Progressive shortness of breath
Cough (ranging from mild to severe), nonproductive/productive of sputum (earliest sign of PCP may be a spasmodic cough on deep breathing)
Congestion or tightness in chest
History of exposure to/prior episode of active TB

May exhibit: Tachypnea, respiratory distress
Changes in breath sounds/adventitious breath sounds
Sputum yellow (in sputum-producing pneumonia)

SAFETY

May report: Exposure to infectious diseases; e.g., TB, STDs
History of other immune deficiency diseases; e.g., rheumatoid arthritis, cancer
History of frequent or multiple blood/blood product transfusions (e.g., hemophilia, major vascular surgery, traumatic incident)
History of falls, burns, episodes of fainting, slow-healing wounds
Easy bruising, prolonged bleeding, and hemorrhage (thrombocytopenia)
Suicidal/homicidal ideation with or without a plan

May exhibit: Recurrent fevers, low-grade, intermittent temperature elevations/spikes, night sweats
Changes in skin integrity; e.g., cuts, ulcerations, rashes (eczema, exanthemas, psoriasis); discolorations; changes in size/color of moles; unexplained, easy bruising; multiple injection scars (may be infected)
Rectal, perianal lesions or abscesses
Nodules, enlarged lymph nodes in two or more areas of the body (e.g., neck, axillae, groin)
Decline in general strength, muscle tone, changes in gait

SEXUALITY

May report: History of high-risk behavior; e.g., having sex with a partner who is HIV positive, multiple sexual partners, unprotected sexual activity, and anal sex
Loss of libido, too sick for sex, afraid to engage in any sexual activities
Inconsistent use of condoms
Use of birth control pills (enhanced susceptibility to virus in women who are exposed because of increased vaginal dryness/friability)

May exhibit: Pregnancy or risk for pregnancy (sexually active), pregnancy resulting in HIV-positive infant
Genitalia: Skin manifestations (e.g., herpes, warts), discharge

SOCIAL INTERACTION

May report: Problems related to diagnosis and treatment; e.g., loss of family/SO, friends, support; fear of telling others; fear of rejection/loss of income
Isolation, loneliness, close friends or sexual partners who have died of or are sick with AIDS
Questioning of ability to remain independent, unable to plan for needs

May exhibit: Changes in family/SO interaction pattern
Disorganized activities, difficulty with goal setting

TEACHING/LEARNING

May report: Failure to comply with treatment, continued high-risk behavior (e.g., unchanged sexual behavior or injection drug use)
Injection drug use/abuse, current smoking, alcohol abuse
Evidence of failure to improve from last hospitalization

Discharge plan considerations: Usually requires assistance with finances, medications and treatments, skin/wound care, equipment/supplies, transportation, food shopping and preparation, self-care, technical nursing procedures, homemaker/maintenance tasks, child care, changes in living arrangements

Refer to section at end of plan for postdischarge considerations.

DIAGNOSTIC STUDIES

CBC: Anemia and idiopathic thrombocytopenia (anemia occurs in up to 85% of clients with AIDS and may be profound). Leukopenia may be present; differential shift to the left suggests infectious process (PCP), although shift to the right may be noted.

PPD: Determines exposure and/or active TB disease. Of AIDS clients, 100% of those exposed to active *Mycobacterium tuberculosis* will develop the disease. Note: PPD may be negative because of anergy.

Serum antibody test: HIV screen by enzyme-linked immunosorbent assay (ELISA). (The current HIV test used in the United States is a combination HIV-1/HIV-2 test kit.)

Western blot test: Confirms diagnosis of HIV in blood and urine. (Clients are notified of status only after confirmation by Western blot.)

Viral load test:

RI-PCR: The most widely used test currently can detect viral RNA levels as low as 50 copies/mL of plasma with an upper limit of 75,000 copies/mL.

bDNA 3.0 assay: Has a wider range of 50–500,000 copies/mL. Therapy can be initiated, or changes made in treatment approaches, based on rise of viral load or maintenance of a low viral load. This is currently the leading indicator of effectiveness of therapy.

T-lymphocyte cells: Total count reduced.

CD4+ lymphocyte count: Immune system indicator that mediates several immune system processes and signals B cells to produce antibodies to foreign germs. Numbers less than 200 indicate severe immune deficiency response and diagnosis of AIDS.

T8+ CTL (cytopathic suppressor cells): Reversed ratio (2:1 or higher) of suppressor cells to helper cells (T8+ to T4+) indicates immune suppression.

PCR test: Detects HIV-DNA; most helpful in testing newborns of HIV-infected mothers. Infants carry maternal HIV antibodies and therefore test positive by ELISA and Western blot even though infant is not necessarily infected.

STD screening tests: Hepatitis B (HBV) envelope and core antibodies, hepatitis C (HVC), syphilis, and other common STDs (e.g., *Chlamydia*, gonococcus) may be positive.

Cultures: Histologic, cytologic studies of urine, blood, stool, spinal fluid, lesions, sputum, and secretions may be done to identify the opportunistic infection. Some of the most commonly identified are the following:

Protozoal and helminthic infections: PCP, cryptosporidiosis, toxoplasmosis.

Fungal infections: Candida albicans (candidiasis), *Cryptococcus neoformans* (cryptococcosis), *Histoplasma capsulatum* (histoplasmosis).

Bacterial infections: Mycobacterium avium-intracellulare (occurs with CD4 counts less than 50), miliary mycobacterial TB, *Shigella* (shigellosis), *Salmonella* (salmonellosis).

Viral infections: CMV (occurs with CD4 counts less than 50), herpes simplex, herpes zoster.

Neurologic studies; e.g., electroencephalogram (EEG), magnetic resonance imaging (MRI), computed tomography (CT) scans of the brain, electromyography (EMG)/nerve conduction studies: Indicated for changes in mentation, fever of undetermined origin, and/or changes in sensory/motor function to determine effects of HIV infection/opportunistic infections.

Chest radiographs: May initially be normal or may reveal progressive interstitial infiltrates secondary to advancing PCP (most common opportunistic disease) or other pulmonary complications/disease processes such as TB.

Pulmonary function tests: Useful in early detection of interstitial pneumonias.

Gallium scan: Diffuse pulmonary uptake occurs in PCP and other forms of pneumonia.

Biopsies: May be done for differential diagnosis of Kaposi's sarcoma (KS) or other neoplastic lesions.

Bronchoscopy/tracheobronchial washings: May be done with biopsy when PCP or lung malignancies are suspected (diagnostic confirming test for PCP).

Barium swallow, endoscopy, colonoscopy: May be done to identify opportunistic infection (e.g., *Candida,* CMV) or to stage KS in the GI system.

NURSING PRIORITIES

1. Prevent/minimize development of new infections.
2. Maintain homeostasis.
3. Promote comfort.
4. Support psychosocial adjustment.
5. Provide information about disease process/prognosis and treatment needs.

DISCHARGE GOALS/GOALS OF CARE

1. Infection prevented/resolved.
2. Complications prevented/minimized.
3. Pain/discomfort alleviated or controlled.
4. Client dealing with current situation realistically.
5. Diagnosis, prognosis, and therapeutic regimen understood.
6. Plan in place to meet ongoing needs.

NURSING DIAGNOSIS: risk for Infection [progression to sepsis/onset of new opportunistic infection]

Risk factors may include

Inadequate primary defenses: broken skin, traumatized tissue, stasis of body fluids
Depression of the immune system, chronic disease, malnutrition, use of antimicrobial agents
Environmental exposure, invasive techniques

Possibly evidenced by

[Not applicable; presence of signs and symptoms establishes an *actual* diagnosis.]

DESIRED OUTCOMES/EVALUATION CRITERIA—CLIENT WILL:

Infection Severity (NOC)

Achieve timely healing of wounds/lesions.
Be afebrile and free of purulent drainage/secretions and other signs of infectious conditions.

Risk Control (NOC)

Identify/participate in behaviors to reduce risk of infection.

ACTIONS/INTERVENTIONS	RATIONALE
Infection Control (NIC)	
Independent	
Assess client knowledge and ability to maintain opportunistic infection prophylactic regimen.	Multiple medication regimen is difficult to maintain over a long period of time. Clients may adjust medication regimen based on side effects experienced, contributing to inadequate prophylaxis, active disease, and resistance.
Wash hands before and after all care contacts. Instruct client/SO to wash hands as indicated.	Reduces risk of cross-contamination.
Provide a clean, well-ventilated environment. Screen visitors/staff for signs of infection and maintain isolation precautions as indicated.	Reduces number of pathogens presented to the immune system and reduces possibility of client contracting a nosocomial infection.
Discuss extent and rationale for isolation precautions and maintenance of personal hygiene.	Promotes cooperation with regimen and may lessen feelings of isolation.
Monitor vital signs, including temperature.	Provides information for baseline data; frequent temperature elevations/onset of new fever indicates that the body is responding to a new infectious process or that medications are not effectively controlling noncurable infections.
Assess respiratory rate/depth; note dry spasmodic cough on deep inspiration, changes in characteristics of sputum, and presence of wheezes/rhonchi. Initiate respiratory isolation when etiology of productive cough is unknown.	Respiratory congestion/distress may indicate developing PCP (the most common opportunistic disease in clients with CD4 count below 200); however, TB is on the rise and other fungal, viral, and bacterial infections may occur that compromise the respiratory system. *Note:* CMV and PCP can reside together in the lungs and, if treatment is not effective for PCP, the addition of CMV therapy may be effective.

ACTIONS/INTERVENTIONS	RATIONALE
Investigate reports of headache, stiff neck, and altered vision. Note changes in mentation and behavior. Monitor for nuchal rigidity/seizure activity.	Neurologic abnormalities are common and may be related to HIV or secondary infections. Symptoms may vary from subtle changes in mood/sensorium (personality changes or depression) to hallucinations, memory loss, severe dementias, seizures, and loss of vision. CNS infections (encephalitis is the most common) may be caused by protozoal and helminthic organisms or fungus.
Examine skin/oral mucous membranes for white patches or lesions. (Refer to ND: actual and/or risk for impaired Skin Integrity; impaired Oral Mucous Membrane.)	Oral candidiasis, KS, herpes, CMV, and cryptococcosis are common opportunistic diseases affecting the cutaneous membranes.
Clean client's nails frequently. File, rather than cut, and avoid trimming cuticles.	Reduces risk of transmission of pathogens through breaks in skin. *Note:* Fungal infections along the nail plate are common.
Monitor reports of heartburn, dysphagia, retrosternal pain on swallowing, increased abdominal cramping, profuse diarrhea.	Esophagitis may occur secondary to oral candidiasis, CMV, or herpes. Cryptosporidiosis is a parasitic infection responsible for watery diarrhea (often more than 15 L/day).
Inspect wounds/site of invasive devices, noting signs of local inflammation/infection.	Early identification/treatment of secondary infection may prevent sepsis.
Wear gloves and gowns during direct contact with secretions/excretions or any time there is a break in skin of caregiver's hands. Wear mask and protective eyewear to protect nose, mouth, and eyes from secretions during procedures (e.g., suctioning) or when splattering of blood may occur.	Use of masks, gowns, and gloves is required by Occupational Safety and Health Administration (OSHA, 1992) for direct contact with body fluids; e.g., sputum, blood/blood products, semen, vaginal secretions.
Dispose of needles/sharps in rigid, puncture-resistant containers.	Prevents accidental inoculation of caregivers. Use of needle cutters and recapping is not to be practiced. *Note:* Accidental needle sticks should be reported immediately, with follow-up evaluations done per protocol.
Label blood bags, body fluid containers, soiled dressings/linens, and package appropriately for disposal per isolation protocol.	Prevents cross-contamination and alerts appropriate personnel/departments to exercise specific hazardous materials procedures.
Clean up spills of body fluids/blood with bleach solution (1:10); add bleach to laundry.	Kills HIV and controls other microorganisms on surfaces.

Collaborative

ACTIONS/INTERVENTIONS	RATIONALE
Monitor laboratory studies; e.g.:	
CBC/differential;	Shifts in the differential and changes in WBC count indicate infectious process. Low WBC count or other changes in blood count may be related to treatments/medications.
Culture/sensitivity studies of lesions, blood, urine, and sputum.	May be done to diagnose complications and/or monitor effectiveness of medications.
Administer medications as indicated:	
Antiretrovirals; e.g.: Enfuvirtide (ENF, T-20), emtricataline (FTC)-NRTI, azotzenavir (ATV) – PI, fosamprenevir (FPV) – 908 – PI;	Currently, 12 antiretroviral agents have been approved by the Food and Drug Administration (FDA) (with approximately 20 more being tested) all aimed at blocking replication of the HIV virus at some level. The drugs are generally given in groups of three because a multidrug regimen is more effective in reducing the viral load. (The goal is to maintain viral load at <500 copies/mL.) Individual considerations are necessary when initiating, changing, interrupting or stopping treatment, or using salvage therapies (i.e., dropping T-cell counts necessitate changes to the failing regimen). *Note:* Studies reveal an increasing frequency of drug-resistant strains of HIV being transmitted to others.

ACTIONS/INTERVENTIONS	RATIONALE
Nucleoside reverse transcriptase inhibitors (NRTIs): zidovudine/ZDV (AZT, Retrovir), didanosine/ddI (Videx), zalcitabine/ddC (Hivid), stavudine/d4T (Zerit), lamivudine/3TC (Epivir), abacavir (Ziagen), entricitabine (FTC);	In the past, zidovudine was given alone and as a first-line treatment. The drug is now usually given in a three-drug treatment regimen. (Zidovudine has been found to be safe in preventing perinatal HIV infection so it is an option for the pregnant client.) *Note:* A new drug, Trizivir, combines Epivir, Retrovir, and Ziagen into one tablet that is taken twice daily.
Protease inhibitors; e.g., indinavir (Crixivan), nelfinavir (Viracept), ritonavir (Norvir), saquinavir (Fortovase, Invirase), atazanavir (ATV), fosamprenavir (FPV);	When combined with NRTIs, protease inhibitors effectively control the HIV-RNA viral load by blocking viral replication at two different target sites in the replication process. Immune function is maintained with early intervention, or improved when initiated later.
Nonnucleoside reverse transcriptase inhibitors (NNRTIs); e.g.: delavirdine (Rescriptor), nevirapine (Viramune), efavirenz (Sustiva);	Inhibit viral replication by a different mechanism than NRTIs. Using them alone seems to encourage drug resistance, so they are used in combination.
Anti-infectives/prophylaxis; e.g., trimethoprim-sulfamethoxazole/TMP/SMX (Bactrim, Septra), nystatin (Mycostatin), ketoconazole (Nizoral), pentamidine (Pentam, NebuPent), azithromycin (Zithromax), clarithromycin (Biaxin), rifabutin (Mycobutin), ganciclovir (Cytovene), foscarnet (Foscavir).	Managing opportunistic infections now includes prophylaxis to combat illnesses associated with them. For example, TMP/SMX is given to prevent PCP (pneumonia); Biaxin and Zithromax are recommended for prevention of MAC. Cytovene is used to prevent blindness/life-threatening dissemination of CMV. Foscavir can also be used to prevent CMV progression, but should be used with caution because it may cause renal toxicity.
Refer to/encourage cooperation with local epidemiology agency/public health.	Legal requirement. Accurate information facilitates tracking disease spread and groups affected.

NURSING DIAGNOSIS: risk for deficient Fluid Volume

Risk factors may include

Excessive losses: copious diarrhea, profuse sweating, vomiting
Hypermetabolic state, fever
Restricted intake: nausea, anorexia; lethargy

Possibly evidenced by

[Not applicable; presence of signs and symptoms establishes an *actual* diagnosis.]

DESIRED OUTCOMES/EVALUATION CRITERIA—CLIENT WILL:

Hydration (NOC)

Maintain hydration as evidenced by moist mucous membranes, good skin turgor, stable vital signs, individually adequate urinary output.

ACTIONS/INTERVENTIONS	RATIONALE
Fluid Management (NIC)	
Independent	
Monitor vital signs (including CVP if available). Note hypotension, including postural changes.	Indicators of circulating fluid volume.
Note temperature elevation and duration of febrile episode. Administer tepid sponge baths as indicated. Keep clothing and linens dry. Maintain comfortable environmental temperature.	Fever is one of the most frequent symptoms experienced by clients with HIV infections (97%). Increased metabolic demands and associated excessive diaphoresis result in increased insensible fluid losses and dehydration.

ACTIONS/INTERVENTIONS	RATIONALE
Assess skin turgor, mucous membranes, and thirst.	Indirect indicators of fluid status.
Measure urinary output and specific gravity. Measure/estimate amount of diarrheal loss. Note insensible losses.	Increased specific gravity/decreasing urinary output reflects altered renal perfusion/circulating volume. *Note:* Monitoring fluid balance is difficult in the presence of excessive GI/insensible losses.
Weigh as indicated.	Although weight loss may reflect muscle wasting, sudden fluctuations reflect state of hydration. Fluid losses associated with diarrhea can quickly create a crisis and become life-threatening.
Monitor oral intake and encourage fluids of at least 2500 mL/day.	Maintains fluid balance, reduces thirst, and keeps mucous membranes moist.
Make fluids easily accessible to client. Encourage use of fluids that are tolerable to client and that replace needed electrolytes; e.g., Gatorade, broth.	Enhances intake. Certain fluids may be too painful to consume (e.g., acidic juices) because of mouth lesions.
Eliminate foods potentiating diarrhea; e.g., spicy/high-fat foods, nuts, cabbage, milk products. Provide lactose-free supplements/products (e.g., Resource, Advera). Adjust rate/concentration of tube feedings if indicated.	May help reduce diarrhea. Use of lactose-free products helps control diarrhea in the lactose-intolerant client.
Encourage use of live culture yogurt or an OTC product *Lactobacillus acidophilus* (Lactaid).	Antibiotic therapies disrupt normal bowel flora balance, leading to diarrhea. *Note*: Must be taken 2 hr before or after antibiotic to prevent inactivation of live culture.

Collaborative

ACTIONS/INTERVENTIONS	RATIONALE
Administer fluids/electrolytes via feeding tube/IV as appropriate.	May be necessary to support/augment circulating volume, especially if oral intake is inadequate, nausea/vomiting persists.
Monitor laboratory studies as indicated; e.g.:	
Serum/urine electrolytes;	Alerts to possible electrolyte disturbances and determines replacement needs.
BUN/Cr;	Evaluates renal perfusion/function.
Stool specimen collection.	Bowel flora changes can occur with multiple or single antibiotic therapy.
Administer medications as indicated:	
Antiemetics; e.g., prochlorperazine maleate (Compazine), trimethobenzamide (Tigan), metoclopramide (Reglan);	Reduces incidence of vomiting to reduce further loss of fluids/electrolytes.
Antidiarrheals; e.g., diphenoxylate (Lomotil), loperamide (Imodium), paregoric; or antispasmodics; e.g., mepenzolate bromide (Cantil);	Decreases the amount and fluidity of stool; may reduce intestinal spasm and peristalsis. *Note*: Antibiotics may also be used to treat diarrhea if caused by infection.
Antipyretics; e.g., acetaminophen (Tylenol).	Helps reduce fever and hypermetabolic response, decreasing insensible losses. *Note:* Studies caution that Tylenol toxicity can occur more frequently in the client with AIDS, so it needs to be used with caution.
Maintain hypothermia blanket if used.	May be necessary when other measures fail to reduce excessive fever/insensible fluid losses.

NURSING DIAGNOSIS: ineffective Breathing Pattern/risk for impaired Gas Exchange

Risk factors may include

Muscular impairment (wasting of respiratory musculature), decreased energy/fatigue, decreased lung expansion

Retained secretions (tracheobronchial obstruction), infectious/inflammatory process; pain
Ventilation perfusion imbalance (PCP/other pneumonias, anemia)

Possibly evidenced by

[Not applicable; presence of signs and symptoms establishes an *actual* diagnosis.]

DESIRED OUTCOMES/EVALUATION CRITERIA—CLIENT WILL:

RESPIRATORY STATUS: Ventilation (NOC)

Maintain effective respiratory pattern.
Experience no dyspnea/cyanosis, with breath sounds and chest x-ray clear/improving and ABGs within client's normal range.

ACTIONS/INTERVENTIONS	RATIONALE
Respiratory Monitoring (NIC)	
Independent	
Auscultate breath sounds, noting areas of decreased/absent ventilation and presence of adventitious sounds; e.g., crackles, wheezes, rhonchi.	Suggests developing pulmonary complications/infection; e.g., atelectasis/pneumonia. *Note:* PCP is often advanced before changes in breath sounds occur.
Note rate/depth of respiration, use of accessory muscles, increased work of breathing, and presence of dyspnea, anxiety, cyanosis.	Tachypnea, cyanosis, restlessness, and increased work of breathing reflect respiratory distress and need for increased surveillance/medical intervention.
Assess changes in level of consciousness.	Hypoxemia can result in changes ranging from anxiety and confusion to unresponsiveness.
Investigate reports of chest pain.	Pleuritic chest pain may reflect nonspecific pneumonitis or pleural effusions associated with malignancies.
Ventilation Assistance (NIC)	
Elevate head of bed. Have client turn, cough, deep breathe as indicated.	Promotes optimal pulmonary function and reduces incidence of aspiration or infection due to atelectasis.
Suction airways as indicated, using sterile technique and observing safety precautions; e.g., mask, protective eyewear.	Assists in clearing the ventilatory passages, thereby facilitating gas exchange and preventing respiratory complications.
Allow adequate rest periods between care activities. Maintain a quiet environment.	Reduces oxygen consumption.
Collaborative	
Monitor/graph serial ABGs or pulse oximetry.	Indicators of respiratory status, treatment needs/effectiveness.
Review serial chest x-rays.	Presence of diffuse infiltrates may suggest pneumonia, whereas areas of congestion/consolidation may reflect other pulmonary complications; e.g., atelectasis or KS lesions.
Assist with/instruct in use of incentive spirometer. Provide chest physiotherapy; e.g., percussion, vibration, and postural drainage.	Encourages proper breathing technique and improves lung expansion. Loosens secretions, dislodges mucous plugs to promote airway clearance. *Note:* In the event of multiple skin lesions, chest physiotherapy may be discontinued.
Provide humidified supplemental O_2 via appropriate means; e.g., cannula, mask, intubation/mechanical ventilation.	Maintains effective ventilation/oxygenation to prevent/correct respiratory crisis.

ACTIONS/INTERVENTIONS	RATIONALE
Administer medications as indicated:	Choice of therapy depends on individual situation/infecting organism(s).
Antimicrobials; e.g.: trimethoprim-sulfamethoxazole (Bactrim, Septra), pentamidine isethionate (Pentam);	Although Bactrim (TMP/SMX) is the drug of choice for PCP, Pentam can be used in combination or alone when treatment with Bactrim is unsuccessful or contraindicated. *Note:* Bactrim may also be used prophylactically.
Foscarnet (Foscavir), ganciclovir (Cytovene);	Effective for treatment of pulmonary CMV infections. *Note:* CMV often coexists with PCP.
Clarithromycin (Biaxin), azithromycin (Zithromax), rifabutin (Mycobutin);	First-line therapy for treatment of MAC, a common bacterial infection that frequently disseminates to other organ systems.
Bronchodilators, expectorants, cough suppressants.	May be needed to improve/maintain airway patency or help clear secretions.
Prepare/assist with procedures as indicated; e.g., bronchoscopy.	May be required to clear mucous plugs, obtain specimens for diagnosis (biopsies/lavage).

NURSING DIAGNOSIS: risk for Injury, (hemorrhage)

Risk factors may include

Abnormal blood profile: decreased vitamin K absorption, alteration in hepatic function, presence of autoimmune antiplatelet antibodies, malignancies (KS), and/or circulating endotoxins (sepsis)

Possibly evidenced by

[Not applicable; presence of signs and symptoms establishes an *actual* diagnosis.]

DESIRED OUTCOMES/EVALUATION CRITERIA—CLIENT WILL:

Risk Control (NOC)

Display homeostasis as evidenced by absence of bleeding.

ACTIONS/INTERVENTIONS	RATIONALE
Bleeding Precautions (NIC)	
Independent	
Avoid injections, rectal temperatures/rectal tubes; administer rectal suppositories with caution.	Protects client from procedure-related causes of bleeding; i.e., insertion of thermometers, rectal tubes can damage or tear rectal mucosa. *Note:* Some medications may need to be given via suppository in spite of risk.
Maintain a safe environment; e.g., keep all necessary objects and call bell within client's reach and keep bed in low position.	Reduces accidental injury, which could result in bleeding.
Maintain bedrest/chair rest when platelets are below 10,000 or as individually appropriate. Assess medication regimen.	Reduces possibility of injury, although activity needs to be maintained. May need to discontinue or reduce dosage of a drug. *Note:* Client can have a surprisingly low platelet count without bleeding.
Hematest body fluids; e.g., urine, stool, vomitus, for occult blood.	Prompt detection of bleeding/initiation of therapy may prevent critical hemorrhage.
Observe for/report epistaxis, hemoptysis, hematuria, nonmenstrual vaginal bleeding, or oozing from lesions/body orifices/IV insertion sites.	Spontaneous bleeding may indicate development of DIC or immune thrombocytopenia, necessitating further evaluation and prompt intervention.

ACTIONS/INTERVENTIONS	RATIONALE
Monitor for changes in vital signs and skin color; e.g., BP, pulse, respirations, skin pallor/discoloration.	Presence of bleeding/hemorrhage may lead to circulatory failure/shock.
Evaluate change in level of consciousness.	May reflect cerebral bleeding.

Collaborative

Review laboratory studies; e.g., PT, aPTT, clotting time, platelets, Hb/Hct.	Detects alterations in clotting capability; identifies therapy needs. *Note:* Many individuals (up to 80%) display platelet count below 50,000 and may be asymptomatic, necessitating regular monitoring.
Administer blood products as indicated.	Transfusions may be required in the event of persistent/massive spontaneous bleeding.
Avoid use of aspirin products/NSAIDs, especially in presence of gastric lesions.	These medications reduce platelet aggregation, impairing/prolonging the coagulation process, and may cause further gastric irritation, increasing risk of bleeding. *Note*: Aspirin is contraindicated even short term because of its nonreversible effect on platelets.

NURSING DIAGNOSIS: imbalanced Nutrition: less than body requirements

May be related to

Inability or altered ability to ingest, digest, and/or metabolize nutrients: nausea/vomiting, hyperactive gag reflex, intestinal disturbances, GI tract infections, fatigue
Increased metabolic rate/nutritional needs (fever/infection)

Possibly evidenced by

Weight loss, decreased subcutaneous fat/muscle mass (wasting)
Lack of interest in food, aversion to eating, altered taste sensation
Abdominal cramping, hyperactive bowel sounds, diarrhea
Sore, inflamed buccal cavity
Abnormal laboratory results: vitamin/mineral and protein deficiencies, electrolyte imbalances

DESIRED OUTCOMES/EVALUATION CRITERIA—CLIENT WILL:

Nutritional Status (NOC)

Maintain weight or display weight gain toward desired goal.
Demonstrate positive nitrogen balance, be free of signs of malnutrition, and display improved energy level.

ACTIONS/INTERVENTIONS	RATIONALE
Nutritional Monitoring (NIC)	
Independent	
Assess ability to chew, taste, and swallow.	Lesions of the mouth, throat, and esophagus (often caused by candidiasis, herpes simplex, hairy leukoplakia, KS and other cancers) and metallic or other taste changes caused by medications may cause dysphagia, limiting client's ability to ingest food and reducing desire to eat.

ACTIONS/INTERVENTIONS	RATIONALE
Auscultate bowel sounds.	Hypermotility of intestinal tract is common and is associated with vomiting and diarrhea, which may affect choice of diet/route. *Note:* Lactose intolerance and malabsorption (e.g., with CMV, MAC, cryptosporidiosis) contribute to diarrhea and may necessitate change in diet/supplemental formula (e.g., Advera, Resource).
Weigh as indicated. Evaluate weight in terms of premorbid weight. Compare serial weights and anthropometric measurements.	Indicator of nutritional needs/adequacy of intake. *Note:* Because of immune suppression, some blood tests normally used for testing nutritional status are not useful.
Note drug side effects.	Prophylactic and therapeutic medications can have side effects affecting nutrition; e.g., ZDV (altered taste, nausea/vomiting), Bactrim (anorexia, glucose intolerance, glossitis), Pentam (altered taste and smell, nausea/vomiting, glucose intolerance), protease inhibitors (elevated lipids and blood sugar secondary to insulin resistance).

Nutritional Therapy (NIC)

ACTIONS/INTERVENTIONS	RATIONALE
Plan diet with client/SO, suggesting foods from home if appropriate. Provide small, frequent meals/snacks of nutritionally dense foods and nonacidic foods and beverages, with choice of foods palatable to client. Encourage high-calorie/nutritious foods, some of which may be considered appetite stimulants. Note time of day when appetite is best, and try to serve larger meal at that time.	Including client in planning gives a sense of control of environment and may enhance intake. Fulfilling cravings for noninstitutional food may also improve intake. *Note:* In this population, foods with a higher fat content may be recommended as tolerated to enhance taste and oral intake.
Limit food(s) that induce nausea/vomiting or are poorly tolerated by client with mouth sores/dysphagia. Avoid serving very hot liquids/foods. Serve foods that are easy to swallow; e.g., eggs, ice cream, cooked vegetables.	Pain in the mouth or fear of irritating oral lesions may cause client to be reluctant to eat. These measures may be helpful in increasing food intake.
Schedule medications between meals (if tolerated) and limit fluid intake with meals, unless fluid has nutritional value.	Gastric fullness diminishes appetite and food intake.
Encourage as much physical activity as possible.	May improve appetite and general feelings of well-being.
Provide frequent mouth care, observing secretion precautions. Avoid alcohol-containing mouthwashes.	Reduces discomfort associated with nausea/vomiting, oral lesions, mucosal dryness, and halitosis. Clean mouth may enhance appetite.
Provide rest period before meals. Avoid stressful procedures close to mealtime.	Minimizes fatigue; increases energy available for work of eating.
Remove existing noxious environmental stimuli or conditions that aggravate gag reflex.	Reduces stimulus of the vomiting center in the medulla.
Encourage client to sit up for meals.	Facilitates swallowing and reduces risk of aspiration.
Record ongoing caloric intake.	Identifies need for supplements or alternative feeding methods.

Collaborative

ACTIONS/INTERVENTIONS	RATIONALE
Review laboratory studies; e.g., BUN, glucose, liver function studies, electrolytes, protein, and albumin/prealbumin.	Indicates nutritional status and organ function, and identifies replacement needs. *Note:* Nutritional tests can be altered because of disease processes and response to some medications/therapies. (Multiple medications are metabolized by the liver and have potential for synergistic damage.)
Maintain NPO status when appropriate.	May be needed to reduce nausea/vomiting.
Insert/maintain nasogastric (NG) tube as indicated.	May be required to reduce vomiting or to administer tube feedings. *Note:* Esophageal irritation from existing infection (*Candida,* herpes, or KS) may provide site for secondary infections/trauma; therefore, NG tube should be used with caution.

ACTIONS/INTERVENTIONS	RATIONALE
Consult with dietitian/nutritional support team.	Provides for diet based on individual needs/appropriate route.
Administer enteral/parenteral feedings as indicated.	Enteral feedings are preferred because they cost less and carry less risk of exacerbating endocrine dysfunction than TPN. However, TPN may be required when oral/enteral feedings are not tolerated. TPN is reserved for those whose gut cannot absorb even an elemental formula (such as Vivonex) or those with severe refractory diarrhea.
Administer medications as indicated:	
Antiemetics; e.g., prochlorperazine (Compazine), promethazine (Phenergan), trimethobenzamide (Tigan);	Reduces incidence of nausea/vomiting, possibly enhancing oral intake.
Sucralfate (Carafate) suspension; mixture of Maalox, diphenhydramine (Benadryl), and lidocaine (Xylocaine);	Given with meals (swish and hold in mouth) to relieve mouth pain, enhance intake. Mixture may be swallowed in presence of pharyngeal/esophageal lesions.
Vitamin supplements;	Corrects vitamin deficiencies resulting from decreased food intake and/or disorders of digestion and absorption in the GI system. *Note:* Avoid megadoses; suggested supplemental level is two times the recommended daily allowance (RDA).
Appetite stimulants; e.g., dronabinol (Marinol), megestrol (Megace), oxandrolone (Oxandrin);	Marinol (an antiemetic) and Megace (an antineoplastic) act as appetite stimulants in the presence of AIDS. Oxandrin is currently being studied in clinical trials to boost appetite and improve muscle mass and strength.
TNF-α inhibitors; e.g., thalidomide;	Reduces elevated levels of tumor necrosis factor (TNF) present in chronic illness contributing to wasting/cachexia. Studies reveal a mean weight gain of 10% over 28 weeks of therapy.
Antidiarrheals; e.g., diphenoxylate (Lomotil), loperamide (Imodium), octreotide (Sandostatin);	Inhibit GI motility subsequently decreasing diarrhea. Imodium or Sandostatin is effective treatment for secretory diarrhea (secretion of water and electrolytes by intestinal epithelium).
Antibiotic therapy; e.g., ketoconazole (Nizoral), fluconazole (Diflucan).	May be given to treat/prevent infections involving the GI tract.

NURSING DIAGNOSIS: acute/chronic Pain

May be related to

Tissue inflammation/destruction: infections, internal/external cutaneous lesions, rectal excoriation, malignancies, necrosis
Peripheral neuropathies, myalgias, and arthralgias
Abdominal cramping

Possibly evidenced by

Reports of pain
Self-focusing, narrowed focus, guarding behaviors
Alteration in muscle tone, muscle cramping, ataxia, muscle weakness, paresthesias, paralysis
Autonomic responses, restlessness

DESIRED OUTCOMES/EVALUATION CRITERIA—CLIENT WILL:

Pain Level (NOC)

Report pain relieved/controlled.
Demonstrate relaxed posture/facial expression.
Be able to sleep/rest appropriately.

ACTIONS/INTERVENTIONS	RATIONALE
Pain Management (NIC)	
Independent	
Assess pain reports, noting location, intensity (0–10 scale), frequency, and time of onset. Note nonverbal cues; e.g., restlessness, tachycardia, grimacing.	Indicates need for/effectiveness of interventions and may signal development/resolution of complications. *Note:* Chronic pain does not produce autonomic changes; however, acute and chronic pain can coexist.
Instruct/encourage client to report pain as it develops rather then waiting until level is severe.	Efficacy of comfort measures and medications is improved with timely intervention.
Encourage verbalization of feelings.	Can reduce anxiety and fear and thereby reduce perception of intensity of pain.
Provide diversional activities; e.g., reading, visiting, music/television.	Refocuses attention; may enhance coping abilities.
Perform palliative measures; e.g., repositioning, massage, ROM of affected joints.	Promotes relaxation/decreases muscle tension.
Instruct client in/encourage use of visualization, guided imagery, progressive relaxation, deep-breathing techniques, meditation, and mindfulness.	Promotes relaxation and feeling of well-being. May decrease the need for narcotic analgesics (CNS depressants) when a neuro/motor degenerative process is already involved. May not be successful in presence of dementia, even when dementia is minor. *Note:* Mindfulness is the skill of staying in the here and now.
Provide oral care. (Refer to ND: impaired Oral Mucous Membrane.)	Oral ulcerations/lesions may cause severe discomfort.
Apply warm/moist packs to pentamidine injection/IV sites for 20 min after administration.	These injections are known to cause pain and sterile abscesses.
Collaborative	
Administer analgesics/antipyretics, narcotic analgesics. Use patient-controlled analgesia (PCA) or provide around-the-clock analgesia with rescue doses prn.	Provides relief of pain/discomfort; reduces fever. PCA or around-the-clock medication keeps the blood level of analgesia stable, preventing cyclic undermedication or overmedication. *Note:* Drugs such as Ativan may be used to potentiate effects of analgesics.

NURSING DIAGNOSIS: actual and/or risk for impaired Skin Integrity

Risk factors may include

Decreased level of activity/immobility, altered sensation, skeletal prominence, changes in skin turgor
Malnutrition, altered metabolic state

May be related to (actual)

Immunologic deficit: AIDS-related dermatitis; viral, bacterial, and fungal infections (e.g., herpes, *Pseudomonas, Candida*); opportunistic disease processes (e.g., KS)
Excretions/secretions

Possibly evidenced by

Skin lesions, ulcerations, decubitus ulcer formation

DESIRED OUTCOMES/EVALUATION CRITERIA—CLIENT WILL:

Risk Control (NOC)

Be free of/display improvement in wound/lesion healing.

TISSUE INTEGRITY: Skin & Mucous Membranes (NOC)

Demonstrate behaviors/techniques to prevent skin breakdown/promote healing.

ACTIONS/INTERVENTIONS	RATIONALE
Skin Surveillance (NIC)	
Independent	
Assess skin daily. Note color, turgor, circulation, and sensation. Describe/measure lesions and observe changes.	Establishes comparative baseline providing opportunity for timely intervention.
Maintain/instruct in good skin hygiene; e.g., wash thoroughly, pat dry carefully, and gently massage with lotion or appropriate cream.	Maintaining clean, dry skin provides a barrier to infection. Patting skin dry instead of rubbing reduces risk of dermal trauma to dry/fragile skin. Massaging increases circulation to the skin and promotes comfort. *Note:* Isolation precautions are required when extensive or open cutaneous lesions are present.
Reposition frequently. Use turn sheet as needed. Encourage periodic weight shifts. Protect bony prominences with pillows, heel/elbow pads, sheepskin.	Reduces stress on pressure points, improves blood flow to tissues, and promotes healing.
Maintain clean, dry, wrinkle-free linen, preferably soft cotton fabric.	Skin friction caused by movement over wet/wrinkled or rough sheets leads to irritation of fragile skin and increases risk of infection.
Encourage ambulation/out of bed as tolerated.	Decreases pressure on skin from prolonged bedrest.
Cleanse perianal area by removing stool with water and mineral oil or commercial product. Avoid use of toilet paper if vesicles are present. Apply protective creams; e.g., zinc oxide, A & D ointment.	Prevents maceration caused by diarrhea and keeps perianal lesions dry. *Note:* Use of toilet paper may abrade lesions.
File nails regularly.	Long/rough nails increase risk of dermal damage.
Cover open pressure ulcers with sterile dressings or protective barrier; e.g., Tegaderm, DuoDerm, as indicated.	May reduce bacterial contamination, promote healing.
Collaborative	
Provide foam/flotation/alternate pressure mattress or bed.	Reduces pressure on skin, tissue, and lesions, decreasing tissue ischemia.
Obtain cultures of open skin lesions.	Identifies pathogens and appropriate treatment choices.
Apply/administer topical/systemic drugs as indicated.	Used in treatment of skin lesions. Use of agents such as Prederm spray can stimulate circulation, enhancing healing process. *Note:* When multidose ointments are used, care must be taken to avoid cross-contamination.
Provide wound care as indicated; e.g.,	
Cover ulcerated KS lesions with wet-to-wet dressings or antibiotic ointment and nonstick dressing (e.g., Telfa);	Protects ulcerated areas from contamination and promotes healing.
Use Tegasorb Thin or other absorbing product as indicated.	If the wound/ulcer is moist with exudate/discharge, these products keep the wound slightly moist with no maceration of periwound tissue.
Refer to physical therapy for regular exercise/activity program.	Promotes improved muscle tone and skin health.

NURSING DIAGNOSIS: impaired Oral Mucous Membrane

May be related to

Immunologic deficit and presence of lesion-causing pathogens; e.g., *Candida,* herpes, KS
Dehydration, malnutrition
Ineffective oral hygiene
Side effects of drugs, chemotherapy

Possibly evidenced by

Open ulcerated lesions, vesicles
Oral pain/discomfort
Stomatitis; leukoplakia, gingivitis, carious teeth

DESIRED OUTCOMES/EVALUATION CRITERIA—CLIENT WILL:

Oral Hygiene (NOC)

Display intact mucous membranes, which are pink, moist, and free of inflammation/ulcerations.

Risk Control (NOC)

Demonstrate techniques to restore/maintain integrity of oral mucosa.

ACTIONS/INTERVENTIONS	RATIONALE
Oral Health Restoration (NIC)	
Independent	
Assess mucous membranes/document all oral lesions. Note reports of pain, swelling, difficulty with chewing/swallowing.	Edema, open lesions, and crusting on oral mucous membranes and throat may cause pain and difficulty with chewing/swallowing.
Provide oral care daily and after food intake, using soft toothbrush, nonabrasive toothpaste, nonalcohol mouthwash, floss, and lip moisturizer.	Alleviates discomfort, prevents acid formation associated with retained food particles, and promotes feeling of well-being.
Rinse oral mucosal lesions with saline/dilute hydrogen peroxide or baking soda solutions.	Reduces spread of lesions and encrustations from candidiasis, and promotes comfort.
Suggest use of sugarless gum/candy or commercial salivary substitute.	Stimulates flow of saliva to neutralize acids and protect mucous membranes. Sorbitol in some artificially sweetened products can increase risk for loose stools.
Plan diet to avoid salty, spicy, abrasive, and acidic foods or beverages. Check for temperature tolerance of foods. Offer cool/cold smooth foods.	Abrasive foods may open healing lesions. Open lesions are painful and aggravated by salt, spice, acidic foods/beverages. Extreme cold or heat can cause pain to sensitive mucous membranes.
Encourage oral intake of at least 2500 mL/day.	Maintains hydration; prevents drying of oral cavity.
Encourage client to refrain from smoking.	Smoke is drying and irritating to mucous membranes.
Collaborative	
Obtain culture specimens of lesions.	Reveals causative agents and identifies appropriate therapies.
Administer medications, as indicated; e.g., nystatin (Mycostatin), ketoconazole (Nizoral);	Specific drug choice depends on particular infecting organism(s); e.g., *Candida.*
TNF-α inhibitor; e.g., thalidomide.	Effective in treatment of oral lesions due to recurrent stomatitis.
Apply mixture of Maalox, diphenhydramine (Benadryl), and lidocaine (Xylocaine) to oral lesions.	Reduces local pain of *Candida* and other oral lesions.
Refer for dental consultation, if appropriate.	May require additional therapy to prevent dental losses.

NURSING DIAGNOSIS: Fatigue

May be related to

Decreased metabolic energy production, increased energy requirements (hypermetabolic state)
Overwhelming psychological/emotional demands
Altered body chemistry: side effects of medication, chemotherapy, insulin resistance

Possibly evidenced by

Unremitting/overwhelming lack of energy, inability to maintain usual routines, decreased performance, impaired ability to concentrate, lethargy/listlessness
Disinterest in surroundings

DESIRED OUTCOMES/EVALUATION CRITERIA—CLIENT WILL:

Endurance (NOC)

Report improved sense of energy.
Perform ADLs, with assistance as necessary.
Participate in desired activities at level of ability.

ACTIONS/INTERVENTIONS	RATIONALE
Energy Management (NIC)	
Independent	
Assess sleep patterns and note changes in thought processes/behaviors.	Multiple factors can aggravate fatigue, including sleep deprivation, emotional distress, side effects of drugs/chemotherapies, and developing CNS disease.
Recommend scheduling activities for periods when client has most energy. Plan care to allow for rest periods. Involve client/SO in schedule planning.	Planning allows client to be active during times when energy level is higher, which may restore a feeling of well-being and a sense of control. Frequent rest periods are needed to restore/conserve energy.
Establish realistic activity goals with client.	Provides for a sense of control and feelings of accomplishment. Prevents discouragement from fatigue of overactivity.
Encourage client to do whatever possible; e.g., self-care, sit in chair, short walks. Increase activity level as indicated.	Prevents severe deconditioning, and may conserve strength, increase stamina, and enable client to become more active.
Identify energy conservation techniques; e.g., sitting, breaking ADLs into manageable segments. Keep travelways clear of furniture. Provide/assist with ambulation/self-care needs as appropriate.	Weakness may make ADLs almost impossible for client to complete. Protects client from injury during activities.
Monitor physiological response to activity; e.g., changes in BP, respiratory rate, or heart rate.	Tolerance varies greatly, depending on the stage of the disease process, nutrition state, fluid balance, and number/type of opportunistic diseases.
Encourage nutritional intake. (Refer to ND: imbalanced Nutrition: less than body requirements.)	Adequate intake/utilization of nutrients is necessary to meet increased energy needs for activity. *Note:* Continuous stimulation of the immune system by HIV infection contributes to a hypermetabolic state.
Collaborative	
Refer to physical/occupational therapy.	Programmed daily exercises and activities help client maintain/increase strength and muscle tone, enhance sense of well-being.

ACTIONS/INTERVENTIONS	RATIONALE
Refer to community resources; e.g., grocery delivery/Meals on Wheels, house cleaning/home maintenance services, home care agency.	Provides assistance in areas of individual need as ability to care for self becomes more difficult.
Provide supplemental O_2 as indicated.	Presence of anemia/hypoxemia reduces oxygen available for cellular uptake and contributes to fatigue.

NURSING DIAGNOSIS: disturbed Thought Processes

May be related to

Hypoxemia, CNS infection by HIV, brain malignancies, and/or disseminated systemic opportunistic infection, cerebrovascular accident (CVA)/hemorrhage; vasculitis

Alteration of drug metabolism/excretion, accumulation of toxic elements, renal failure, severe electrolyte imbalance, hepatic insufficiency

Possibly evidenced by

Altered attention span; distractibility

Memory deficit

Disorientation; cognitive dissonance; delusional thinking

Sleep disturbances

Impaired ability to make decisions/problem-solve; inability to follow complex commands/mental tasks, loss of impulse control

DESIRED OUTCOMES/EVALUATION CRITERIA—CLIENT WILL:

Cognition (NOC)

Maintain usual reality orientation and optimal cognitive functioning.

ACTIONS/INTERVENTIONS	RATIONALE
Cognitive Stimulation (NIC)	
Independent	
Assess mental and neurological status using appropriate tools.	Establishes functional level at time of admission and provides baseline for future comparison.
Consider effects of emotional distress; e.g., anxiety, grief, anger.	May contribute to reduced alertness, confusion, withdrawal, and hypoactivity, requiring further evaluation and intervention.
Monitor medication regimen and usage.	Actions and interactions of various medications, prolonged drug half-life/altered excretion rates result in cumulative effects, potentiating risk of toxic reactions. Some drugs may have adverse side effects; e.g., haloperidol (Haldol) can seriously impair motor function in clients with AIDS dementia complex.
Investigate changes in personality, response to stimuli, orientation/level of consciousness; or development of headache, nuchal rigidity, vomiting, fever, seizure activity.	Changes may occur for numerous reasons, including development/exacerbation of opportunistic diseases/CNS infection. *Note:* Early detection and treatment of CNS infection may limit permanent impairment of cognition.
Maintain a pleasant environment with appropriate auditory, visual, and cognitive stimuli.	Providing normal environmental stimuli can help in maintaining some sense of reality orientation.

ACTIONS/INTERVENTIONS	RATIONALE
Provide cues for reorientation; e.g., radio, television, calendars, clocks, room with an outside view. Use client's name; identify yourself. Maintain consistent personnel and structured schedules as appropriate.	Frequent reorientation to place and time may be necessary, especially during fever/acute CNS involvement. Sense of continuity may reduce associated anxiety.
Discuss use of datebooks, lists, other devices to keep track of activities.	These techniques help client manage problems for forgetfulness.
Encourage family/SO to socalize and provide reorientation with current news, family events.	Familiar contacts are often helpful in maintaining reality orientation, especially if client is hallucinating.
Encourage client to do as much as possible; e.g., dress and groom, see friends.	Can help maintain mental abilities for longer period.
Provide support for SO. Encourage discussion of concerns and fears.	Bizarre behavior/deterioration of abilities may be very frightening for SO and makes management of care/dealing with situation difficult. SO may feel a loss of control as stress, anxiety, burnout, and anticipatory grieving impair coping abilities.
Provide information about care on an ongoing basis. Answer questions simply and honestly. Repeat explanations as needed.	Can reduce anxiety and fear of unknown; can enhance client's understanding and involvement/cooperation in treatment when possible.

Cognitive Restructuring (NIC)

Reduce provocative/noxious stimuli. Maintain bedrest in quiet, darkened room if indicated.	If client is prone to agitation, violent behavior, or seizures, reducing external stimuli may be helpful.
Decrease noise, especially at night.	Promotes sleep, reducing cognitive symptoms and effects of sleep deprivation.
Set limits on maladaptive/abusive behavior; avoid open-ended choices.	Provides sense of security/stability in an otherwise confusing situation.
Maintain safe environment; e.g., excess furniture out of the way, call bell within client's reach, bed in low position/rails up; restriction of smoking (unless monitored by caregiver/SO), seizure precautions, soft restraints if indicated.	Decreases the possibility of client injury.
Discuss causes/future expectations and treatment if dementia is diagnosed. Use concrete terms.	Obtaining information that ZDV has been shown to improve cognition can provide hope and control for losses.

Collaborative

Assist with diagnostic studies; e.g., MRI, CT scan, spinal tap, and monitor laboratory studies as indicated; e.g., BUN/Cr, electrolytes, ABGs.	Choice of tests/studies depends on clinical manifestations and index of suspicion, because changes in mental status may reflect a wide variety of causative factors; e.g., CMV meningitis/encephalitis, drug toxicity, electrolyte imbalances, and altered organ function.
Administer medications as indicated:	
Amphotericin B (Fungizone);	Antifungal useful in treatment of cryptococcosis meningitis.
ZDV (Retrovir) and other antiretrovirals alone or in combination;	Shown to improve neurological and mental functioning for undetermined period of time.
Antipsychotics; e.g., haloperidol (Haldol), and/or antianxiety agents; e.g., lorazepam (Ativan).	Cautious use may help with problems of sleeplessness, emotional lability, hallucinations, suspiciousness, and agitation.
Provide controlled environment/behavioral management.	Team approach may be required to protect client when mental impairment (e.g., delusions) threatens client safety.
Refer to counseling as indicated.	May help client gain control in presence of thought disturbances or psychotic symptoms.

NURSING DIAGNOSIS: Anxiety [specify level]/Fear

May be related to

Threat to self-concept, threat of death, change in health/socioeconomic status, role functioning
Interpersonal transmission and contagion
Separation from support system
Fear of transmission of the disease to family/loved ones

Possibly evidenced by

Increased tension, apprehension, feelings of helplessness/hopelessness
Expressed concern regarding changes in life
Fear of unspecific consequences
Somatic complaints, insomnia, sympathetic stimulation, restlessness

DESIRED OUTCOMES/EVALUATION CRITERIA—CLIENT WILL:

Anxiety [or] Fear Self-Control (NOC)

Verbalize awareness of feelings and healthy ways to deal with them.
Display appropriate range of feelings and lessened fear/anxiety.
Demonstrate problem-solving skills.
Use resources effectively.

ACTIONS/INTERVENTIONS	RATIONALE
Anxiety Reduction (NIC)	
Independent	
Assure client of confidentiality within limits of situation.	Provides reassurance and opportunity for client to problem-solve solutions to anticipated situations.
Maintain frequent contact with client. Talk with and touch client. Limit use of isolation clothing and masks.	Provides assurance that client is not alone or rejected; conveys respect for and acceptance of the person, fostering trust.
Provide accurate, consistent information regarding prognosis. Avoid arguing about client's perceptions of the situation.	Can reduce anxiety and enable client to make decisions/choices based on realities.
Be alert to signs of denial/depression (e.g., withdrawal; angry, inappropriate remarks). Determine presence of suicidal ideation and assess potential on a scale of 1–10.	Client may use defense mechanism of denial and continue to hope that diagnosis is inaccurate. Feelings of guilt and spiritual distress may cause client to become withdrawn and believe that suicide is a viable alternative. Although client may be too "sick" to have enough energy to implement thoughts, ideation must be taken seriously and appropriate intervention initiated.
Provide open environment in which client feels safe to discuss feelings or to refrain from talking.	Helps client feel accepted in present condition without feeling judged, and promotes sense of dignity and control.
Permit expressions of anger, fear, despair without confrontation. Give information that feelings are normal and are to be appropriately expressed.	Acceptance of feelings allows client to begin to deal with situation.
Recognize and support the stage client/family is at in the grieving process. (Refer to CP: Cancer, ND: anticipatory Grieving.)	Choice of interventions is dictated by stage of grief, coping behaviors; e.g., anger/withdrawal, denial.
Explain procedures, providing opportunity for questions and honest answers. Arrange for someone to stay with client during anxiety-producing procedures and consultations.	Accurate information allows client to deal more effectively with the reality of the situation, thereby reducing anxiety and fear of the unknown.

ACTIONS/INTERVENTIONS	RATIONALE
Identify and encourage client interaction with support systems. Encourage verbalization/interaction with family/SO.	Reduces feelings of isolation. If family support systems are not available, outside sources may be needed immediately; e.g., local AIDS task force.
Provide reliable and consistent information and support for SO.	Allows for better interpersonal interaction and reduction of anxiety and fear.
Include SO as indicated when major decisions are to be made.	Ensures a support system for client, and allows SO the chance to participate in client's life. *Note:* If client, family, and SO are in conflict, separate care consultations and visiting times may be needed.
Discuss Advance Directives, end-of-life desires/needs. Review specific wishes and explain various options clearly.	May assist client/SO to plan realistically for terminal stages and death. *Note*: Many individuals do not understand medical terminology/options e.g., PEG tube for short- or long-term feeding.

Collaborative

Refer to psychiatric counseling (e.g., psychiatric clinical nurse specialist, psychiatrist, social worker).	May require further assistance in dealing with diagnosis/prognosis, especially when suicidal thoughts are present.
Provide contact with other resources as indicated; e.g.:	
Spiritual advisor;	Provides opportunity for addressing spiritual concerns.
Hospice staff.	May help relieve anxiety regarding end-of-life care and support for client/SO.

NURSING DIAGNOSIS: Social Isolation

May be related to

Altered state of wellness, changes in physical appearance, alterations in mental status
Perceptions of unacceptable social or sexual behavior/values
Inadequate personal resources/support systems
Physical isolation

Possibly evidenced by

Expressed feeling of aloneness imposed by others, feelings of rejection
Absence of supportive SO: partners, family, acquaintances/friends

DESIRED OUTCOMES/EVALUATION CRITERIA—CLIENT WILL:

Social Support (NOC)

Identify supportive individual(s).
Use resources for assistance.

Social Involvement (NOC)

Participate in activities/programs at level of ability/desire.

ACTIONS/INTERVENTIONS	RATIONALE
Support System Enhancement (NIC)	
Independent	
Ascertain client's perception of situation.	Isolation may be partly self-imposed because client fears rejection/reaction of others.
Spend time talking with client during and between care activities. Be supportive, allowing for verbalization. Treat with dignity and regard for client's feelings.	Client may experience physical isolation as a result of current medical status and some degree of social isolation secondary to diagnosis of AIDS.
Limit/avoid use of mask, gown, and gloves when possible; e.g., when talking to client.	Reduces client's sense of physical isolation and provides positive social contact, which may enhance self-esteem and decrease negative behaviors.
Identify support systems available to client, including presence of/relationship with immediate and extended family.	When client has assistance from SO, feelings of loneliness and rejection are diminished. *Note:* Client may not receive usual/needed support for coping with life-threatening illness and associated grief because of fear and lack of understanding (AIDS hysteria).
Explain isolation precautions/procedures to client and SO.	Gloves, gowns, mask are not routinely required with a diagnosis of AIDS except when contact with secretions/excretions is expected. Misuse of these barriers enhances feelings of emotional and physical isolation. When precautions are necessary, explanations help client understand reasons for procedure and provide feeling of inclusion in what is happening.
Encourage open visitation (as able), telephone contacts, and social activities within tolerated level.	Participation with others can foster a feeling of belonging.
Encourage active role of contact with SO.	Helps reestablish a feeling of participation in a social relationship. May lessen likelihood of suicide attempts.
Develop a plan of action with client: Look at available resources; support healthy behaviors. Help client problem-solve solution to short-term/imposed isolation.	Having a plan promotes a sense of control over own life and gives client something to look forward to/actions to accomplish.
Be alert to verbal/nonverbal cues; e.g., withdrawal, statements of despair, sense of aloneness. Ask client if thoughts of suicide are being entertained.	Indicators of despair and suicidal ideation are often present. When these cues are acknowledged by the caregiver, client is usually willing to talk about thoughts of suicide and sense of isolation and hopelessness.
Collaborative	
Refer to resources; e.g., social services counselors, and AIDS organizations/projects (local and national).	Establishes support systems; may reduce feelings of isolation.
Provide for placement in sheltered community when necessary.	May need more specific care when unable to be maintained at home or when SO cannot manage care.

NURSING DIAGNOSIS: Powerlessness

May be related to

Confirmed diagnosis of a potentially terminal disease, incomplete grieving process
Social ramifications of AIDS, alteration in body image/desired lifestyle, advancing CNS involvement

Possibly evidenced by

Feelings of loss of control over own life
Depression over physical deterioration that occurs despite client compliance with regimen

Anger, apathy, withdrawal, passivity
Dependence on others for care/decision making, resulting in resentment, anger, guilt

DESIRED OUTCOMES/EVALUATION CRITERIA—CLIENT WILL:

HEALTH BELIEFS: Perceived Control (NOC)

Acknowledge feelings and healthy ways to deal with them.
Verbalize some sense of control over present situation.
Make choices related to care and be involved in self-care.

ACTIONS/INTERVENTIONS	RATIONALE
Self-Responsibility Facilitation (NIC)	
Independent	
Identify factors that contribute to client's feelings of powerlessness; e.g., diagnosis of a terminal illness, lack of support systems, lack of knowledge about present situation.	Clients with AIDS are usually aware of the current literature and prognosis unless newly diagnosed. Powerlessness is most prevalent in a client newly diagnosed with HIV and when dying with AIDS. Fear of AIDS (by the general population and the client's family/SO) is the most profound cause of client's isolation. For some homosexual clients, this may be the first time that the family has been made aware that client lives an alternative lifestyle.
Assess degree of feelings of helplessness; e.g., verbal/nonverbal expressions indicating lack of control ("It won't make any difference"), flat affect, and lack of communication.	Determines the status of the individual client and allows for appropriate intervention when client is immobilized by depressed feelings.
Encourage active role in planning activities, establishing realistic/attainable daily goals. Encourage client control and responsibility as much as possible. Identify things that client can and cannot control.	May enhance feelings of control and self-worth and sense of personal responsibility.
Encourage Advance Directives/Living Will and durable medical power of attorney documents, with specific and precise instructions regarding acceptable and unacceptable procedures to prolong life.	Many factors associated with the treatments used in this debilitating and often fatal disease process place client at the mercy of medical personnel and other unknown people who may be making decisions for and about client without regard for client's wishes, increasing loss of independence.
Discuss desires/assist with planning for funeral as appropriate.	The individual can gain a sense of completion and value to his or her life when he or she decides to be involved in planning this final ceremony. This provides an opportunity to include things that are of importance to the person.

NURSING DIAGNOSIS: deficient Knowledge [Learning Need] regarding disease, prognosis, current therapies, and self-care needs

May be related to

Lack of exposure/recall, information misinterpretation
Cognitive limitation
Unfamiliarity with information resources

Possibly evidenced by

Questions/request for information, statement of misconception
Inaccurate follow-through of instructions, development of preventable complications

DESIRED OUTCOMES/EVALUATION CRITERIA—CLIENT WILL:

KNOWLEDGE: Disease Process (NOC)

Verbalize understanding of condition/disease process and potential complications.
Identify relationship of signs/symptoms to the disease process and correlate symptoms with causative factors.

KNOWLEDGE: Treatment Regimen (NOC)

Verbalize understanding of therapeutic needs.
Correctly perform necessary procedures and explain reasons for actions.
Initiate necessary lifestyle changes and participate in treatment regimen.

ACTIONS/INTERVENTIONS	RATIONALE
TEACHING: Disease Process (NIC)	
Independent	
Review disease process and future expectations.	Provides knowledge base from which client can make informed choices.
Determine level of independence/dependence and physical condition. Note extent of care and support available from family/SO and need for supplemental caregivers.	Helps plan amount of care and symptom management required and need for additional resources.
Review modes of transmission of disease, especially if newly diagnosed.	Corrects myths and misconceptions; promotes safety for client/others. Accurate epidemiological data are important in targeting prevention interventions.
Instruct client and caregivers concerning infection control; e.g.: using good handwashing techniques for everyone (client, family, caregivers); using gloves when handling bedpans, dressings/soiled linens; wearing mask if client has productive cough; placing soiled/wet linens in plastic bag and separating from family laundry, washing with detergent and hot water; cleaning surfaces with bleach/water solution of 1:10 ratio, disinfecting toilet bowl/bedpan with full-strength bleach; preparing client's food in clean area; washing dishes/utensils in hot soapy water (can be washed with the family dishes).	Reduces risk of transmission of diseases; promotes wellness in presence of reduced ability of immune system to control level of flora.
Stress necessity of daily skin care, including inspecting skin folds, pressure points, and perineum, and of providing adequate cleansing and protective measures; e.g., ointments, padding.	Healthy skin provides barrier to infection. Measures to prevent skin disruption and associated complications are critical.
Ascertain that client/SO can perform necessary oral and dental care. Review procedures as indicated. Encourage regular dental care.	The oral mucosa can quickly exhibit severe, progressive complications. Studies indicate that 65% of AIDS clients have some oral symptoms. Therefore, prevention and early intervention are critical.
Review dietary needs (high-protein and high-calorie) and ways to improve intake when anorexia, diarrhea, weakness, depression interfere with intake.	Promotes adequate nutrition necessary for healing and support of immune system, enhances feeling of well-being.
Discuss medication regimen, interactions, and side effects.	Enhances cooperation with/increases probability of success with therapeutic regimen. (Refer to CP: The HIV-Positive Client, ND: ineffective [individual]/family Therapeutic Regimen Management.)
Provide information about symptom management that complements medical regimen; e.g., with intermittent diarrhea, take diphenoxylate (Lomotil) before going to social event.	Provides client with increased sense of control, reduces risk of embarrassment, and promotes comfort.

ACTIONS/INTERVENTIONS	RATIONALE
Stress importance of adequate rest.	Helps manage fatigue; enhances coping abilities and energy level.
Encourage activity/exercise at level that client can tolerate.	Stimulates release of endorphins in the brain, enhancing sense of well-being.
Stress necessity of continued healthcare and follow-up.	Provides opportunity for altering regimen to meet individual/changing needs.
Recommend cessation of smoking.	Smoking increases risk of respiratory infections and can further impair immune system.
Identify signs/symptoms requiring medical evaluation; e.g., persistent fever/night sweats, swollen glands, continued weight loss, diarrhea, skin blotches/lesions, headache, chest pain/dyspnea.	Early recognition of developing complications and timely interventions may prevent progression to life-threatening situation.
Identify community resources; e.g., hospice/residential care centers, visiting nurse, home care services, Meals on Wheels, peer group support.	Facilitates transfer from acute care setting for recovery/independence or end-of-life care.

POTENTIAL CONSIDERATIONS in addition to the nursing diagnoses listed in the plan of care.

anticipatory Grieving—loss of physiologic/psychologic well-being, social/lifestyle changes, loss of SO/family, probability of premature death.

ineffective Protection—abnormal blood profile (anemia, thrombocytopenia, coagulation), inadequate nutrition, drug therapies (e.g., antineoplastic, immune), chronic disease.

Caregiver Role Strain—illness severity of care receiver, significant home care needs, caregiver health impairment, marginal family adaptation or dysfunction, presence of situational stressors, lack of respite for caregiver, caregiver's competing role commitments.

RHEUMATOID ARTHRITIS

Rheumatoid arthritis (RA) is a chronic, systemic inflammatory disease involving connective tissue and characterized by destruction and proliferation of the synovial membrane, resulting in joint destruction, ankylosis, and deformity. Although the cause is unknown, researchers speculate that a virus may initially trigger the body's immune response, which then becomes chronically activated and turns on itself (autoimmune response). Immunologic mechanisms appear to play an important role in the initiation and perpetuation of the disease, in which spontaneous remissions and unpredictable exacerbations occur. RA is a disorder of the immune system and, as such, is a whole-body disease that can extend beyond the joints, affecting other organ systems, such as the skin and eyes.

RA affects people differently. For some people it lasts only a few months or a year or two and then resolves without causing any noticeable damage. Some people have mild or moderate forms of the disease, with periods of exacerbation (called flares) and remission. Others have a severe form of the disease that is active most of the time, lasts for years or a lifetime and leads to serious joint damage and disability.

CARE SETTINGS

Community level unless surgical procedure is required.

RELATED CONCERNS

Psychosocial aspects of care, page 770
Total joint replacement, page 667

Client Assessment Database

Data depend on severity and involvement of other organs (e.g., eyes, heart, lungs, kidneys), stage (i.e., acute exacerbation or remission), and coexistence of other forms of arthritis/autoimmune diseases.

ACTIVITY/REST

May report: Joint pain and tenderness worsened by movement and stress placed on joint; morning stiffness (duration often 1 hr or more), usually occurs symmetrically

Functional limitations affecting ADLs, desired lifestyle, leisure time, and occupation
Fatigue; sleep disturbances

May exhibit: Malaise
Impaired ROM of joints, particularly hand (fingers and wrist), hips, knees, ankles, elbows, and shoulders
Muscle atrophy, joint and muscle contractures/deformities
Decreased muscle strength, altered gait/posture

CARDIOVASCULAR

May report: Intermittent pallor, cyanosis, then redness of fingers/toes before color returns to normal (Raynaud's phenomenon)

EGO INTEGRITY

May report: Acute/chronic stress factors (e.g., financial, employment, disability, relationship factors)
Hopelessness and powerlessness (incapacitating situation)
Threat to self-concept, body image, personal identity (e.g., dependence on others)

FOOD/FLUID

May report: Inability to obtain/consume adequate food/fluids (temporomandibular joint [TMJ] involvement)
Anorexia, nausea

May exhibit: Weight loss
Dryness of oral mucous membranes, decreased oral secretions, dental caries (Sjögren's syndrome)

HYGIENE

May report: Varying difficulty performing self-care activities; dependence on others

NEUROSENSORY

May report: Numbness/tingling of hands and feet, loss of sensation in fingers

May exhibit: Symmetrical joint swelling

PAIN/DISCOMFORT

May report: Acute episodes of pain (may/may not be accompanied by soft-tissue swelling in joints), symmetrical pattern involving joints on both sides of the body
Chronic aching pain and stiffness with mornings most difficult

May exhibit: Red, swollen, hot joints (during acute exacerbations)

SAFETY

May report: Difficulty managing homemaker/maintenance tasks
Persistent low-grade fever
Dryness of eyes and mucous membranes

May exhibit: Pale, shiny, taut skin; subcutaneous rounded, nontender nodules; lesions, leg ulcers
Skin/periarticular local warmth, erythema
Decreased muscle strength, altered gait, reduced ROM

SEXUALITY

May report: Difficulty engaging in sexual activity as desired/abstinence

SOCIAL INTERACTION

May report: Impaired interactions with family/others, change in roles, isolation

TEACHING/LEARNING

May report: Familial history of RA (in juvenile onset)
Usual onset between ages 25 and 50, ratio of women to men 3:1
Use of health foods, vitamins, untested arthritis "cures"
History of pericarditis, valvular lesions, pulmonary fibrosis, pleuritis

Discharge plan considerations: May require assistance with transportation, self-care activities, and homemaker/maintenance tasks; changes in physical layout of home

Refer to section at end of plan for postdischarge considerations.

DIAGNOSTIC STUDIES

Inflammatory markers:

Cyclic citrullinated peptide (also called anti-CCP) antibody test: Useful in detecting early RA. If both CCP and RF are positive, it is likely the client has a more severe form of the disease.

Rheumatoid factor (RF): Positive in more than 80% of cases, but may become positive later in disease process than CCP (Rose-Waaler test).

Erythrocyte sedimentation rate (ESR): Usually greatly increased (80–100 mm/hr). May return to normal as symptoms improve.

Antinuclear antibody (ANA) titer: Screening test for rheumatic disorders, elevated in 25%–30% of RA clients. Follow-up tests are needed for the specific rheumatic disorders; e.g., anti-RNP is used for differential diagnosis of systemic rheumatic disease.

C-reactive protein (CRP): Test of protein produced only when inflammation is present; may be elevated with RA, but is not specific to RA.

Latex fixation: Positive in 75% of typical cases.

Agglutination reactions: Positive in more than 50% of typical cases.

Serum complement: C_3 and C_4 increased in acute onset (inflammatory response). Immune disorder/exhaustion results in depressed total complement levels.

CBC: Usually reveals moderate anemia (in approximately 80% of clients). WBC is elevated when inflammatory processes are present.

Immunoglobulin (Ig) (IgM and IgG): Elevation strongly suggests autoimmune process as cause for RA.

Radiographs of involved joints: Reveals soft-tissue swelling, erosion of joints and osteoporosis of adjacent bone (early changes) progressing to bone cyst formation, narrowing of joint space, and subluxation. Concurrent osteoarthritic changes may be noted.

CT/MRI scans (joints and cervical spine): Identifies inflamed synovium. MRI may be necessary to demonstrate cord compression.

Direct arthroscopy: Visualization of area reveals bone irregularities/degeneration of joint.

Synovial/fluid aspirate: May reveal volume greater than normal; opaque, cloudy, yellow appearance (inflammatory response, bleeding, degenerative waste products); elevated levels of WBCs and leukocytes; decreased viscosity and complement (C_3 and C_4).

Synovial membrane biopsy: Reveals inflammatory changes and development of pannus (inflamed synovial granulation tissue).

NURSING PRIORITIES

1. Alleviate pain.
2. Increase mobility.
3. Promote positive self-concept.
4. Support independence.
5. Provide information about disease process/prognosis and treatment needs.

DISCHARGE GOALS

1. Pain relieved/controlled.
2. Client is dealing realistically with current situation.
3. Client is managing ADLs by self/with assistance as appropriate.
4. Disease process/prognosis and therapeutic regimen understood.
5. Plan in place to meet needs after discharge.

NURSING DIAGNOSIS: acute/chronic Pain

May be related to

Injuring agents: distention of tissues by accumulation of fluid/inflammatory process, destruction of joint

Possibly evidenced by

Reports of pain/discomfort, fatigue
Self-narrowed focus
Distraction behaviors/autonomic responses
Guarding/protective behavior

DESIRED OUTCOMES/EVALUATION CRITERIA—CLIENT WILL:

Pain Level (NOC)

Report pain is relieved/controlled.
Appear relaxed, able to sleep/rest and participate in activities appropriately.

Pain Control (NOC)

Follow prescribed pharmacologic regimen.
Incorporate relaxation skills and diversional activities into pain control program.

ACTIONS/INTERVENTIONS	RATIONALE
Pain Management (NIC)	
Independent	
Investigate reports of pain, noting location and intensity (using 0–10/similar scale). Note precipitating factors and nonverbal pain cues.	Self-report should be the primary source of pain assessment in determining pain management needs and effectiveness of program.
Recommend/provide firm mattress or bedboard, small pillow. Elevate linens with bed cradle as needed.	Soft/sagging mattress, large pillows prevent maintenance of proper body alignment, placing stress on affected joints. Elevation of bed linens reduces pressure on inflamed/painful joints.
Suggest client assume position of comfort while in bed or sitting in chair. Promote bed rest when indicated, but resume movement as soon as possible.	In severe disease/acute exacerbation, total bedrest may be necessary (until objective and subjective improvements are noted) to limit pain/injury to joint. *Note*: Immobility is known to worsen arthritis pain and stiffness.
Place/monitor use of pillows, sandbags, trochanter rolls, splints.	Rests painful joints and maintains neutral position. *Note:* Use of splints can decrease pain and may reduce damage to joint; however, prolonged inactivity can result in loss of joint mobility/function.
Encourage frequent changes of position. Assist client to move in bed, supporting affected joints above and below, avoiding jerky movements.	Prevents general fatigue and joint stiffness. Stabilizes joint, decreasing joint movement and associated pain.
Recommend that client take warm bath or shower on arising and/or at bedtime. Apply warm, moist compresses to affected joints several times a day. Monitor water temperature of compresses, baths, and so on.	Heat promotes muscle relaxation and mobility, decreases pain, and relieves morning stiffness. Sensitivity to heat may be diminished and dermal injury may occur.
Provide gentle massage.	Promotes relaxation/reduces muscle tension.
Encourage use of stress management techniques; e.g., progressive relaxation, biofeedback, visualization, guided imagery, self-hypnosis, and controlled breathing. Provide therapeutic touch.	Promotes relaxation, provides sense of control, and may enhance coping abilities.
Involve in diversional activities appropriate for individual situation.	Refocuses attention, provides stimulation, and enhances self-esteem and feelings of general well-being.
Medicate before planned activities/exercises as indicated.	Promotes relaxation, reduces muscle tension/spasms, facilitating participation in therapy.
Monitor for development of skin rash in clients using COX-2 inhibitors, especially those allergic to sulfur.	Severe/life threatening skin reactions (e.g., toxic epidermal necrolysis, Stevens-Johnson syndrome, and erythema multiforme) may develop within the first two weeks of treatment or later on, indicating need for prompt discontinuation of medication.

ACTIONS/INTERVENTIONS	RATIONALE
Collaborative	
Administer medications as indicated; e.g.:	Because irreversible joint damage occurs within the first 2 years, early diagnosis and intervention is necessary. Medications are the mainstay of treatment. DMARDs may be started immediately, but due to their slow onset of action, NSAIDs and glucocorticoids may be prescribed until the antirheumatic drugs take effect.
Disease-modifying antirheumatic drugs (DMARD); e.g., methotrexate (Rheumatrex), cyclosprine (Neoral), hydroxychloroquine (Plaquenil), sulfasalazine (Azulfidine); gold compounds; e.g., auranofin (Ridaura), azathioprine (Imuran), leflunomide (Arava);	These slow-onset drugs (3–12 weeks) vary in action and may be used in combinations to reduce pain and swelling, lessening arthritic symptoms over time.
Biologicals; e.g., etanercept (Enbrel), infliximab (Remicade), adalimumab (Humira); interleukin-1 receptor agonist; e.g., anakinra (Kinaret);	These injectable drugs are the first genetically engineered medications for arthritis. These anti-TNF compounds block inflammation and rapidly decrease pain and joint swelling. Enbrel is self-injected weekly and may be used in combination with methotrexate. Humira can be self-injected every other week. Remicade is administered IV at 2- to 6-week intervals initially, then 1- to 3-month intervals. *Note:* Injection site reactions are the most common side effect noted with Humira and Kinaret, but drug discontinuation is uncommon.
Salicylates; e.g., aspirin (ASA, buffered and plain) (Acuprin, Ecotrin, ZORprin);	One of the mainstays of treatment until the 1990s, ASA is still used to exert an anti-inflammatory and mild analgesic effect, decreasing stiffness and increasing mobility. ASA must be taken regularly to sustain a therapeutic blood level. Research indicates that ASA has the lowest toxicity index of commonly prescribed NSAIDs.
Nonsteroidal anti-inflammatory drugs (NSAIDs); e.g., ibuprofen (Advil, Motrin), naproxen (Aleve, Naprosyn), sulindac (Clinoril), prioxicam (Feldene), fenoprofen (Nalfon), diclofenac (Voltaren), ketoprofen (Orudis), ketorolac (Toradol), nabumetone (Relafen);	These drugs control mild to moderate pain and inflammation by inhibition of prostaglandin synthesis and allow for improvement in mobility and function.
Glucocorticosteroids; e.g., prednisone (Deltasone), methylprednisolone (Depo-Medrol), dexamethasone (Decadron);	Low-dose oral glucocorticosteroids should be considered for short-term use, especially in the first 2 years, as drugs modify the immune response and suppress inflammation and progression of joint erosion.
COX-2 inhibitors; e.g., celecoxib (Celebrex), rofecoxib (Vioxx), valdecoxib (Bextra);	A new class of medication, COX-2 inhibitors interfere with prostaglandin production, similarly to NSAIDs, but are less likely to harm the stomach lining or kidneys. May be used in combination with other medications. *Note:* Recent controversy about these drugs resulted in Vioxx being withdrawn from the market, then restored by the FDA. These drugs should be used with caution in clients with significant hypertension, renal disease, heart disease, or at high risk for cardiac involvement.
Tetracyclines; e.g., minocycline (Minocin);	Characteristics of anti-inflammatory and immune modifier effects coupled with ability to block metalloproteinases (associated with joint destruction) have resulted in modest benefits in research studies.
D-Penicillamine (Cuprimine);	May control systemic effects of RA synovitis and scleroderma if other therapies have not been successful. High rate of side effects (e.g., thrombocytopenia, leukopenia, aplastic anemia) necessitates close monitoring. *Note:* Drug should be given between meals because drug absorption is impaired by food, as well as antacids and iron products.
Antacids; e.g., misoprostol (Cytotec), omeprazole (Prilosec);	Given with NSAID agents to minimize gastric irritation/discomfort, reducing risk of GI bleed.

ACTIONS/INTERVENTIONS	RATIONALE
Narcotic analgesics; e.g., morphine, oxycodone, hydrocodone combinations.	Although narcotics are generally contraindicated because of chronic nature of condition, short-term use of these products may be required to control severe pain during periods of acute exacerbation. *Note:* Codeine and propoxyphene (Darvon) products should be avoided because of their side effects and limited analgesic effectiveness.
Assist with physical therapies; e.g., paraffin glove, whirlpool baths.	Provides sustained heat to reduce pain and improve ROM of affected joints.
Apply ice or cold packs when indicated.	Cold may relieve pain and swelling during acute episodes.
Instruct in use/monitor effect of transcutaneous electrical nerve stimulator (TENS) unit if used.	Constant low-level electrical stimulus blocks transmission of pain sensations.
Assist with other modalities as indicated; e.g., blood filtration.	Prosorba Column is a device similar to a kidney dialysis machine that removes substances from blood plasma that contribute to joint swelling and pain. The plasma is then returned to the client's blood stream. The offending antibodies are gone, decreasing the immune response.
Prepare for surgical interventions; e.g., synovectomy, total joint replacement, joint fusion; tunnel release procedures, tendon repair.	Corrective surgical procedures may be indicated to reduce pain and/or improve joint function and mobility.

NURSING DIAGNOSIS: impaired physical Mobility/impaired Walking

May be related to

Skeletal deformity
Pain, discomfort
Intolerance to activity, decreased muscle strength

Possibly evidenced by

Reluctance to attempt movement/inability to purposefully move within the physical environment
Limited ROM, impaired coordination, decreased muscle strength/control and mass (late stages)

DESIRED OUTCOMES/EVALUATION CRITERIA—CLIENT WILL:

Mobility (NOC)

Maintain position of function with absence/limitation of contractures.
Maintain or increase strength and function of affected and/or compensatory body part.
Demonstrate techniques/behaviors that enable resumption/continuation of activities.

ACTIONS/INTERVENTIONS	RATIONALE
EXERCISE THERAPY: Joint Mobility (NIC)	
Independent	
Evaluate/continuously monitor degree of joint inflammation/pain.	Level of activity/exercise depends on progression/resolution of inflammatory process.

ACTIONS/INTERVENTIONS	RATIONALE
Maintain bedrest/chair rest when indicated. Schedule activities providing frequent rest periods and uninterrupted nighttime sleep.	Person with RA needs a good balance between rest and exercise, with more rest when disease is active and more exercise when it is not. Systemic rest is mandatory during acute exacerbations and important throughout all phases of disease to reduce fatigue, improve strength.
Assist with active/passive ROM and resistive exercises and isometrics when able.	Maintains/improves joint function, muscle strength, and general stamina. *Note:* Inadequate exercise leads to joint stiffening, whereas excessive activity can damage joints.
Encourage client to maintain upright and erect posture when sitting, standing, walking.	Maximizes joint function, maintains mobility.
Discuss/provide safety needs; e.g., raised chairs/toilet seat, use of handrails in tub/shower and toilet, proper use of mobility aids/wheelchair safety.	Helps prevent accidental injuries/falls.

Positioning (NIC)

Reposition frequently using adequate personnel. Demonstrate/assist with transfer techniques and use of mobility aids; e.g., walker, cane, trapeze.	Relieves pressure on tissues and promotes circulation. Facilitates self-care and client's independence. Proper transfer techniques prevent shearing abrasions of skin.
Position with pillows, sandbags, trochanter roll. Provide joint support with splints.	Promotes joint stability (reducing risk of injury) and maintains proper joint position and body alignment, minimizing contractures.
Suggest using small/thin pillow under neck.	Prevents flexion of neck.

Collaborative

Provide foam/alternating pressure mattress.	Decreases pressure on fragile tissues to reduce risks of immobility/development of decubitus ulcers.

EXERCISE THERAPY: Joint Mobility (NIC)

Consult with physical/occupational therapists and vocational specialist.	Useful in formulating exercise/activity program based on individual needs in identifying and reducing impairments in range of motion, flexibility, strength and endurance, and to instruct in joint protection strategies and mobility devices/adjuncts.

SELF-CARE ASSISTANCE: IADL (NIC)

Determine appropriateness of/ability to use scooter or special enhancements to automobile (e.g., hand controls, wide mirrors).	Facilitates movement within the environment, decreases fatigue, promotes independence.

NURSING DIAGNOSIS: disturbed Body Image/ineffective Role Performance

May be related to

Changes in ability to perform usual tasks
Increased energy expenditure, impaired mobility

Possibly evidenced by

Change in structure/function of affected parts
Negative self-talk, focus on past strength/function, appearance
Change in lifestyle/physical ability to resume roles, loss of employment, dependence on SO for assistance
Change in social involvement; sense of isolation
Feelings of helplessness, hopelessness

DESIRED OUTCOMES/EVALUATION CRITERIA—CLIENT WILL:

PSYCHOSOCIAL ADJUSTMENT: Life Change (NOC)

Verbalize increased confidence in ability to deal with illness, changes in lifestyle, and possible limitations.
Formulate realistic goals/plans for future.

ACTIONS/INTERVENTIONS	RATIONALE
Body Image [or] Role Enhancement (NIC)	
Independent	
Encourage verbalization about concerns of disease process, future expectations.	Provides opportunity to identify fears/misconceptions and deal with them directly.
Discuss meaning of loss/change to client/SO. Ascertain how client views self in usual lifestyle functioning, including sexual aspects.	Identifying how illness affects perception of self and interactions with others will determine need for further intervention/counseling.
Discuss client's perception of how SO perceives limitations.	Verbal/nonverbal cues from SO may have a major impact on how client views self.
Acknowledge and accept feelings of grief, hostility, dependency.	Constant pain is wearing, and feelings of anger and hostility are common. Acceptance provides feedback that feelings are normal.
Note withdrawn behavior, use of denial, or overconcern with body/changes.	May suggest emotional exhaustion or maladaptive coping methods, requiring more in-depth intervention/psychologic support.
Set limits on maladaptive behavior. Assist client to identify positive behaviors that will aid in coping.	Helps client maintain self-control, which enhances self-esteem.
Involve client in planning care and scheduling activities.	Enhances feelings of competency/self-worth, encourages independence and participation in therapy.
Assist with grooming needs as necessary.	Maintaining appearance enhances self-image.
Give positive reinforcement for accomplishments.	Allows client to feel good about self. Reinforces positive behavior. Enhances confidence.
Collaborative	
Refer to psychiatric counseling; e.g., psychiatric clinical nurse specialist, psychiatrist/psychologist, social worker.	Client/SO may require ongoing support to deal with long-term/debilitating process.
Administer medications as indicated; e.g., antianxiety and mood-elevating drugs.	May be needed in presence of severe depression until client develops more effective coping skills.

NURSING DIAGNOSIS: Self-Care Deficit (specify)

May be related to

Musculoskeletal impairment, decreased strength/endurance, pain on movement
Depression

Possibly evidenced by

Inability to manage ADLs (feeding, bathing, dressing, and/or toileting)

DESIRED OUTCOMES/EVALUATION CRITERIA—CLIENT WILL:

SELF-CARE: Activities of Daily Living (ADL) (NOC)

Perform self-care activities at a level consistent with individual capabilities.

SELF-CARE: Instrumental Activities of Daily Living (IADL) (NOC)

Demonstrate techniques/lifestyle changes to meet self-care needs.
Identify personal/community resources that can provide needed assistance.

ACTIONS/INTERVENTIONS	RATIONALE
Self-Care Assistance (NIC)	
Independent	
Determine usual level of functioning (Functional Level Classification 0–4) before onset/exacerbation of illness and potential changes now anticipated.	May be able to continue usual activities with necessary adaptations to current limitations.
Maintain mobility, pain control, and exercise program.	Support physical/emotional independence.
Assess barriers to participation in self-care. Identify/plan for environmental modifications.	Prepares for increased independence, which enhances self-esteem.
Allow client sufficient time to complete tasks to fullest extent of ability. Capitalize on individual strengths.	May need more time to complete tasks by self but provides an opportunity for greater sense of self-confidence and self-worth.
Collaborative	
Consult with rehabilitation specialists; e.g., occupational therapist.	Helpful in determining assistive devices to meet individual needs; e.g., button hooks, long-handled shoehorn, reacher, hand-held shower head.
Arrange home-health evaluation before discharge, with follow-up afterward.	Identifies problems that may be encountered because of current level of disability. Provides for more successful team efforts with others who are involved in care; e.g., occupational therapy team.
Arrange for consult with other agencies; e.g., Meals on Wheels, home care service, nutritionist.	May need additional kinds of assistance to continue in home setting.

NURSING DIAGNOSIS: risk for impaired Home Maintenance

Risk factors may include

Long-term degenerative disease process
Inadequate support systems

Possibly evidenced by

[Not applicable; presence of signs and symptoms establishes an *actual* diagnosis.]

DESIRED OUTCOMES/EVALUATION CRITERIA—CLIENT WILL:

SELF-CARE: Instrumental Activities of Daily Living (IADL) (NOC)

Maintain safe, growth-promoting environment.
Demonstrate appropriate, effective use of resources.

ACTIONS/INTERVENTIONS	RATIONALE
Home Maintenance Assistance (NIC)	
Independent	
Determine level of physical functioning using Functional Level Classification 0–4.	Identifies degree of assistance/support required. For example, the level 0 client is completely able to perform usual activities of daily living (self-care, vocational, and avocational), whereas the level 4 client is limited in all these areas and does not participate in activity.
Evaluate environment to assess ability to care for self.	Determines feasibility of remaining in/changing home layout to meet individual needs.
Determine financial resources to meet needs of individual situation. Identify support systems available to client; e.g., extended family, friends/neighbors.	Availability of personal resources and community supports will affect ability to problem-solve and choice of solutions.
Develop plan for maintaining a clean, healthful environment; e.g., sharing of household repair/tasks between family members or by contract services.	Ensures that needs will be met on an ongoing basis.
Identify sources for necessary equipment; e.g., lifts, elevated toilet seat, wheelchair/scooter.	Provides opportunity to acquire equipment before discharge.
Collaborative	
Coordinate home evaluation by occupational therapist/rehabilitation team.	Useful for identifying adaptive equipment, ways to modify tasks to maintain independence.
Identify/meet with community resources; e.g., visiting nurse, homemaker service, social services, senior citizens' groups.	Can facilitate transfer to/support continuation in home setting.

NURSING DIAGNOSIS: deficient Knowledge [Learning Need] regarding disease, prognosis, treatment, self-care, and discharge needs

May be related to

Lack of exposure/recall
Information misinterpretation

Possibly evidenced by

Questions/request for information, statement of misconception
Inaccurate follow-through of instructions, development of preventable complications

DESIRED OUTCOMES/EVALUATION CRITERIA—CLIENT WILL:

KNOWLEDGE: Disease Process (NOC)

Verbalize understanding of condition/prognosis, and potential complications.

KNOWLEDGE: Treatment Regimen (NOC)

Verbalize understanding of therapeutic needs.
Develop a plan for self-care, including lifestyle modifications consistent with mobility and/or activity restrictions.

ACTIONS/INTERVENTIONS	RATIONALE
TEACHING: Disease Process (NIC)	
Independent	
Review disease process, prognosis, and future expectations.	Provides knowledge base from which client can make informed choices.
Discuss client's role in management of disease process through nutrition, medication, and balanced program of exercise and rest.	Goal of disease control is to suppress inflammation in joints/other tissues to maintain joint function and prevent deformities.
Assist in planning a realistic and integrated schedule of activity, rest, personal care, drug administration, physical therapy, and stress management.	Provides structure and defuses anxiety when managing a complex chronic disease process.
Identify individually appropriate exercise program components; e.g., swimming, stationary bike, nonimpact aerobics.	Can increase client's energy level and mental alertness, minimize functional limitations. Program needs to be customized based on joints involved/client's general condition to maximize effect and reduce risk of injury.
Stress importance of continued pharmacotherapeutic management.	Benefits of drug therapy depend on correct dosage; e.g., aspirin must be taken regularly to sustain therapeutic blood levels of 18–25 mg/dL.
Recommend use of enteric-coated/buffered aspirin or nonacetylated salicylates; e.g., choline salicylate (Arthropan) or choline magnesium trisalicylate (Trilisate).	Coated/buffered preparations ingested with food minimize gastric irritation, reducing risk of bleeding/hemorrhage. *Note:* Nonacetylated products have a longer half-life, requiring less frequent administration in addition to producing less gastric irritation.
Suggest taking medications, such as NSAIDs, with meals, milk products, or antacids and at bedtime.	Limits gastric irritation. Reduction of pain at hs enhances sleep, and increased blood level decreases early-morning stiffness.
Identify adverse drug effects; e.g., tinnitus, gastric intolerance, GI bleeding, purpuric rash.	Prolonged, maximal doses of aspirin may result in overdose. Tinnitus usually indicates high therapeutic blood levels. If tinnitus occurs, the dosage is usually decreased by 1 tablet every 2–3 days until it stops.
Stress importance of reading product labels and refraining from OTC drug usage without prior medical approval.	Many products (e.g., cold remedies, antidiarrheals) contain hidden salicylates that increase risk of drug overdose/harmful side effects.
Review importance of balanced diet with foods high in vitamins, protein, and iron.	Promotes general well-being and tissue repair/regeneration.
Encourage obese client to lose weight, and supply with weight reduction information as appropriate.	Weight loss reduces stress on joints, especially hips, knees, ankles, feet.
Provide information about/resources for assistive devices; e.g., wheeled dolly/wagon for moving items, pickup sticks, lightweight dishes and pans, raised toilet seat, safety handlebars.	Reduces force exerted on joints and enables individual to participate more comfortably in needed/desired activities.
Discuss energy-saving techniques; e.g. sitting instead of standing to prepare meals, shower, shave/apply make-up.	Prevents fatigue; facilitates self-care and independence.
Encourage maintenance of correct body position and posture both at rest and during activity; e.g., keeping joints extended, not flexed, wearing splints for prescribed periods, avoiding remaining in a single position for extended periods, positioning hands near center of body during use, and sliding rather than lifting objects when possible.	Good body mechanics must become a part of client's lifestyle to lessen joint stress and pain.
Review safety issues related to mobility devices, especially electric scooters. Suggest use of a pennant when traveling on open streets.	Ability to travel over uneven surfaces or gravel/soft ground is dependent upon specific scooter model. In addition, speed and safe maneuvering is equally important for the driver and other individuals in the vicinity. A pennant can be seen by other motorists.
Review necessity of frequent inspection of skin and meticulous skin care under splints, casts, supporting devices. Demonstrate proper padding.	Reduces risk of skin irritation/breakdown.

ACTIONS/INTERVENTIONS	RATIONALE
Discuss necessity of medical follow-up/laboratory studies; e.g., ESR, salicylate levels, PT.	Drug therapy requires frequent assessment/refinement to ensure optimal effect and to prevent overdose/dangerous side effects; e.g., aspirin prolongs PT, increasing risk of bleeding.
Provide for sexual and childbirth counseling as necessary.	Information about different positions and techniques and/or other options for sexual fulfillment may enhance personal relationships and feelings of self-worth/self-esteem. *Note:* A large number of clients with RA are in childbearing years and need counseling, support, and medical interventions.
Identify community resources; e.g., chapters of National Institute of Arthritis and Muscular and Skin Diseases (NIAMS), Arthritis Foundation.	Assistance/support from others promotes maximal recovery.

POTENTIAL CONSIDERATIONS following acute hospitalization (dependent on client's age, physical condition/presence of complications, personal resources, and life responsibilities)

Fatigue—increased energy requirements to perform ADLs, states of discomfort.

chronic Pain—accumulation of fluid/inflammation, destruction of joint.

impaired physical Mobility—skeletal deformity, pain/discomfort, decreased muscle strength, intolerance to activity.

Self-Care Deficit/ impaired Home Maintenance—musculoskeletal impairment, decreased strength/endurance, pain on movement, inadequate support systems, insufficient finances, unfamiliarity with neighborhood resources.

TRANSPLANTATION CONSIDERATIONS (POSTOPERATIVE AND LIFELONG)

The contemporary practice of medicine includes transplantation of tissues, partial organs, and whole organs. With current technology and knowledge of immune responses at the molecular level, transplantation is becoming commonplace. The most frequently transplanted organs are the kidney, liver, and heart. In addition, successful bone, heart valve, cartilage, vein, and cornea transplantations are performed on a daily basis. Heart transplantation has successfully moved from the experimental to the conventional domain of therapy, and many other transplants are moving into that domain as well, including bone marrow, stem cell, and pancreatic islet cell transplantation.

The major problem to be overcome is the immunologic response of the client to donor tissues. The ability of the immune system to distinguish self from nonself is crucial to its proper functioning; therefore, in the process of transplantation, the donor/nonself can be rejected. The three forms of rejection are (1) hyperactive or hyperacute (within minutes to hours) is rare, (2) acute (usually within 3–6 months), and (3) chronic (occurring months or years after transplant).

General postoperative care is similar to that for any other major abdominal or cardiothoracic surgery; however, special considerations necessitate meticulous measures to prevent infection and identify early signs of rejection.

CARE SETTING

Post-ICU plan of care addresses early recovery and long-term postdischarge community/clinic follow-up phases.

RELATED CONCERNS

Refer to (1) specific surgical plans of care for general considerations (e.g., cardiac surgery) and (2) organ-specific plans (e.g., heart failure, renal failure, cirrhosis, hepatitis) relative to issues of target organ problems following transplantation.

Peritonitis, page 355
Psychosocial aspects of care, page 770
Sepsis/septicemia, page 701
Surgical intervention, page 788
Thrombophlebitis: deep vein thrombosis, page 108

Client Assessment Database

Refer to specific plans of care for data reflecting specific organ failure necessitating transplantation.

EGO INTEGRITY

May report: Feelings of anxiety, fearfulness

Multiple stressors: Impact of condition on personal relationships, ability to perform expected/needed roles, loss of control, required lifestyle changes, financial concerns, cost of procedure/future treatment needs, uncertainty of outcomes/personal mortality, spiritual conflicts, waiting period for suitable donation

Concerns about changes in appearance (e.g., bloating, jaundice, major scars), esthetic side effects of immunosuppressant medications

Spiritual questioning (e.g., "Why me?" "Why should I benefit from someone else's death?")

May exhibit: Anxiety, delirium, depression; cognitive and emotional behavioral changes

SEXUALITY

May report: Loss of libido

Concerns regarding sexual activity

SOCIAL INTERACTIONS

May report: Reactions of family members

Conflicts regarding family member(s) ability/willingness to participate; e.g., financial, organ/bone marrow donation, postprocedure support

Concern about benefiting from other person's death

Concern for family member who must take on new responsibilities as roles shift

TEACHING/LEARNING

May report: Previous illnesses, hospitalizations, surgeries

Lack of improvement/deterioration in condition

Beliefs about transplantation; previous noncompliance with medical treatment

History of/current dependencies (e.g., alcohol/drug use) resulting in organ failure

Discharge plan considerations: May need assistance with ADLs; shopping, transportation, ambulation; managing medication regimen

Refer to section at end of plan for postdischarge considerations.

DIAGNOSTIC STUDIES (DEPENDENT ON SPECIFIC ORGAN INVOLVEMENT)

General preoperative screening studies include:

Donor matching: Studies include blood type, human leukocyte antigen (HLA) antibody screen.

CT/MRI scan: Reveals status of body systems and organs, including size, shape, and general function of major blood vessels; organ size for best match with donor organ; and potential sources of postoperative complications. Rules out presence of cancer, which would contraindicate transplantation.

Total-body bone scan: Evaluates status of skeletal system to determine presence/absence of bone cancer.

Specific blood and tissue typing: As may be required for donor-recipient matching.

Dental evaluation: To rule out oral infection or abscessed teeth. Dental work may be required prior to transplantation procedures.

Ear, nose, and throat evaluation: To rule out sinus infection.

Renal function studies (e.g., IV pyelogram, creatinine clearance): Determines functional status of kidneys.

Pulmonary function studies: Determines lung function and/or limitations that may complicate recovery.

CBC: Identifies anemia, which can reduce oxygen-carrying capacity, and other blood factors that may affect recovery.

Biochemical studies: Various tests done as indicated in addition to electrolytes, immune status.

Screening tests: To detect presence/type of hepatitis; HIV, viral titer (e.g., CMV, herpes).

ECG: Screens cardiac status; e.g., electrical conduction/dysrhythmias, signs of infarcts/hypertrophy.

NURSING PRIORITIES

1. Prevent infection.
2. Maximize organ function.
3. Promote independent functioning.
4. Support family involvement and coping.

DISCHARGE GOALS

1. Free of signs of infection.
2. Signs of rejection absent/minimized.
3. New organ function adequate.
4. Usual activities resumed.

5. Client/family education plan established.
6. Plan in place to meet individual needs following discharge.

NURSING DIAGNOSIS: risk for Infection

Risk factors may include

Medically induced immunosuppression, suppressed inflammatory response
Antibiotic therapy
Invasive procedures, broken skin/traumatized tissue
Effects of chronic/debilitating disease

Possibly evidenced by

[Not applicable; presence of signs and symptoms establishes an *actual* diagnosis.]

DESIRED OUTCOMES/EVALUATION CRITERIA—CLIENT WILL:

Infection Severity (NOC)

Be free of signs of infection.
Achieve timely wound healing.

CLIENT/CAREGIVER WILL:

Risk Control (NOC)

Demonstrate techniques, lifestyle changes to promote safe environment.

ACTIONS/INTERVENTIONS	RATIONALE
Infection Protection (NIC)	
Independent	
Screen visitors/staff for signs of infection; make sure nurse caring for client with new transplant is not caring for another client with infection. Maintain protective isolation as indicated.	Reduces possibility of client's contracting a nosocomial infection. *Note:* Total isolation is usually restricted to clients with lung transplants or individuals with neutropenia.
Demonstrate and emphasize importance of proper hand-washing techniques by client and caregivers.	First-line defense against infection/cross-contamination.
Inspect all incisions/puncture sites. Evaluate healing progress.	Promotes early identification of onset of infection and prompt intervention.
Provide meticulous care of invasive lines, incisions, wounds. Remove invasive devices as soon as possible.	Minimizes potential for bacteria to reduce exposure/risk of infection.
Encourage deep breathing, coughing.	Mobilizes respiratory secretions and reduces risk of respiratory problems.
Provide/assist with frequent oral hygiene.	Meticulous attention to oral mucosa is necessary because immunosuppression/antibiotic therapies increase risk of opportunistic oral/mucosal infections.
Obtain sterile specimens of wound drainage as appropriate.	Identifying organism allows for appropriate treatment.
Collaborative	
Monitor laboratory tests; e.g., WBC count, blood glucose.	An upward trend from baseline could signal infection; however, a low WBC count may result from immunosuppressant therapy or from a viral infection. *Note*: Use of some medications (e.g., corticosteroids) increases risk of insulin resistance, and tight glucose control is required in postoperative period to reduce risk of deep wound infections.

ACTIONS/INTERVENTIONS	RATIONALE
Administer antimicrobials as indicated; e.g., levofloxacin (Levaquin), cefazolin (Ancef), cefepime (Maxipime), vancomycin (Lyphocin), ciprofloxacin (Cipro).	Antibiotics may be used to treat infections, but all must be monitored for side effects and drug interactions with cyclosporine and other immunosuppressants required to prevent organ rejection.

NURSING DIAGNOSIS: Anxiety [specify level]/Fear

May be related to

Unconscious conflict about essential values/beliefs
Situational crises, interpersonal transmission/contagion
Threat to self-concept [perceived or actual], organ rejection, threat of death
Side effects of steroids and/or cyclosporine

Possibly evidenced by

Increased tension, apprehension, uncertainty
Expressed concerns
Somatic complaints
Sympathetic stimulation

DESIRED OUTCOMES/EVALUATION CRITERIA—CLIENT WILL:

Anxiety [or] Fear Self-Control (NOC)

Appear relaxed and report anxiety is reduced to a manageable level.
Verbalize awareness of feelings.
Identify healthy ways to deal with anxiety.
Use resources/support systems effectively.

ACTIONS/INTERVENTIONS	RATIONALE
Anxiety Reduction (NIC)	
Independent	
Discuss client's post-transplant expectations and fears, including physical appearance, lifestyle changes, and concern about recurrence of disease/condition that precipitated the need for the transplant.	Depending on past experience and exposure to others with transplants, client may have unrealistic ideas and real concerns about what may happen (e.g., rejection of received organ, effects of required medications, limitations associated with immunosuppression). Even with effective preoperative teaching, client will continue to have new concerns or suppressed thoughts and beliefs, which can surface during recovery; e.g., recurrence of disease (such as hepatitis C) in the transplanted organ or chronic rejection.
Encourage client to discuss feelings and concerns about situation and to express fears.	Helps identify issues and can lead to problem solving. Client may experience anxiety about many things (e.g., physical limitations, cognitive changes, role changes in family). These anxieties change frequently; some are persistent, and new ones arise. Serious anxiety, delirium, and depression are the most commonly reported postoperative psychiatric problems.
Discuss beliefs/concerns that are commonly held regarding source of organ.	Cultural/spiritual beliefs may lead client to question whether organ from someone of another race or particular group may change own sense of self-identity/sexuality. *Note:* Some clients may use denial to deal with concerns about the organ donor. A lack of interest or curiosity about the donor may indicate donor denial.

ACTIONS/INTERVENTIONS	RATIONALE
Answer client's questions about donor honestly, but refrain from providing unrequested information.	Excess information may add to survivor guilt, distracting client from focusing on business of recovery.
Identify/encourage use of previously successful coping behaviors.	Prolonged nature of stressors can erode coping abilities, discussion regarding previous successes may promote repetition of more effective behaviors.
Help client focus on one "problem" at a time.	Dealing with one issue at a time seems to make it more manageable. Provides sense of success and opportunity to build on each success.
Discuss possibility and normalcy of mood swings.	Feelings of euphoria and depression are not uncommon, especially in the early postoperative period and can be managed to a large extent by presence, quiet environment and rest. Medication may be required to promote client safety and comfort.
Encourage open communication between SO/family and client within safe environment.	Free expression of feelings/beliefs can lead to clarification and problem-solving of different views. When concerns or beliefs are hidden from one another, additional stress/adverse effects may result.
Provide opportunity for client and SO/family to meet with other(s) who have experienced a similar and successful transplant.	Sharing experiences and hearing about successes and universal problems can lessen client's/SO's anxieties, promote hope, and provide a role model.
Identify possible actions to limit physical effects or manifestations of long-term steroid/cyclosporine use.	Learning about clothing styles, makeup techniques, use of bleach or mild depilatory to reduce facial hair can enhance client's appearance and reduce anxiety about social rejection.

Collaborative

ACTIONS/INTERVENTIONS	RATIONALE
Refer to spiritual advisor as indicated.	Facing one's mortality may provoke feelings of anxiety and questions about one's spiritual beliefs and practices.
Refer to social worker, other professionals as indicated.	Provides assistance with readjustment to life following major life event.

NURSING DIAGNOSIS: risk for ineffective Coping/compromised/disabled family Coping

Risk factors may include

Situational crises, family disorganization and role changes
Prolonged disease exhausting supportive capacity of SO/family

Possibly evidenced by

[Not applicable; presence of signs and symptoms establishes an *actual* diagnosis.]

DESIRED OUTCOMES/EVALUATION CRITERIA—CLIENT/FAMILY WILL:

Coping [or] Family Coping (NOC)

Assess current situation accurately.
Verbalize awareness of own coping abilities.
Meet psychologic needs as evidenced by appropriate expression of feelings, identifying options and resources.

ACTIONS/INTERVENTIONS	RATIONALE
Coping Enhancement [or] Family Integrity Promotion (NIC)	
Independent	
Encourage and support client/family in evaluating lifestyle. Discuss implications for the future.	Helps client/family evaluate and choose activities that are important and begin to adjust to new lifestyle of wellness. *Note:* Transplant clients sometimes cannot evaluate the seriousness of their condition or do not comprehend the risks or benefits involved in transplantation. Acceptance into a transplant program is often a major stressful event as it signals a "last treatment option." Additionally, there may be denial about the impact of long-term post-transplantation treatment requirements (i.e., use of immunosuppressant drugs, biopsies, blood tests, and clinic visits).
Assess client's/family's current functional status and note how transplant is affecting ability to cope.	Provides a starting point to identify needs and plan care. The client's SO/family have been dealing with client's chronic disease, experiencing the uncertainty of organ waiting period, and protracted postoperative recovery course. They are the family members who also face a complicated medical regimen after the client's discharge, factors which place demands on their life routines, time, energy, finances, and relationships.
Determine additional outside stressors (e.g., family, social, work environment, or nursing/healthcare management).	Illness and treatment demands may affect all areas of life, and problems need to be addressed and resolved to enable client and SO to manage current situation optimally.
Provide ongoing information about expected progression of recuperation and potential course of recovery.	Knowing what to expect helps individuals cope more effectively, encourages planning for future needs/lifestyle changes. *Note:* These clients normally require a longer postoperative recovery period because of effects of medication regimen, opportunistic infections, or episodes of organ rejection.
Discuss normalcy of/monitor progression through states of acceptance of transplanted organ: Foreign body stage—organ feels strange, separate from own body; Partial internalization stage—protective of organ, restricts movement/activity, excessive concern regarding organ function/fragility; Complete internalization—acceptance of organ into self-concept, discusses organ only in response to direct questioning.	Sense that organ is "outside" body can be very frightening, while fixation on organ can be irritating to others. Understanding normalcy of feelings is reassuring. *Note:* Movement through stages is variable and regression is common, especially during early post-transplant period.
Have individual/SO list previous methods of dealing with life problems and outcomes of actions.	Promotes problem solving in current situation, allows individual to build on past successes.
Active-listen and identify individual's perceptions of what is happening, how transplant has affected view of self-family member.	Helps those involved to recognize own feelings and concerns regarding use of an organ from someone who died.
Encourage discussion between client/family regarding future expectations.	Period of dependence during illness, concerns over possible organ rejection/life-threatening complications may lead to conflicts regarding client's return to an independent role.
Collaborative	
Involve in individual/family support groups.	Provides role models, source of practical advice, and emotional support to aid in problem-solving.
Refer to spiritual resource and/or psychiatric clinical nurse specialist/psychiatrist, social worker as indicated.	May be helpful in resolving lingering/difficult concerns. *Note:* During waiting period for transplant, relationships with family members may have been strained as a result of the varied stressors involved and because clients tend to feel closer to members of the healthcare team and other individuals sharing the same experiences.

NURSING DIAGNOSIS: deficient Knowledge [Learning Need] regarding prognosis, therapeutic regimen, self-care, and discharge needs

May be related to

Lack of exposure/recall
Information misinterpretation
Unfamiliarity with information resources
Cognitive limitation

Possibly evidenced by

Request for information; statement of misconception
Development of preventable complication

DESIRED OUTCOMES/EVALUATION CRITERIA—CLIENT WILL:

KNOWLEDGE: Health Behaviors [or] Health Resources (NOC)

Describe measures to reduce individual risk factors to recovery/general well-being.
Initiate necessary lifestyle changes and participate in treatment regimen.
Identify community resources.
Develop plan to meet follow-up care needs.
Assume responsibility for own learning and begin to look for information and ask questions.

For routine postoperative instructions, refer to CP: Surgical Intervention.

ACTIONS/INTERVENTIONS	RATIONALE
TEACHING: Disease Process (NIC)	
Independent	
Include SO/family in teaching.	Successful recovery and long-term wellness require a coordinated effort by client and those regularly involved with client.
Provide information via multiple media, including written format, depending on level of comprehension. Include presentations by various members of the transplant team as appropriate.	Enhances learning experience and provides references for postdischarge review/verification of recall. Use of team members; e.g., dietitian, physical/occupational therapists, provides for personalization of teaching plan to meet individual needs.
Review general signs/symptoms of rejection and infection (e.g., general malaise/fatigue, dyspnea, sudden weight gain, fever/chills, sore throat, delayed healing of wound, nausea/vomiting, syncope). Review indicators specific to transplanted organ (e.g., liver rejection: pain in liver or back, lighter-colored stools, jaundice, dark-colored urine).	Prompt recognition and timely intervention may limit severity of complication. Acute rejection usually develops within days of transplant or may be delayed for a number of months. If detected early, rejection process can be minimized or reversed with changes in drug regimen. *Note:* Chronic rejection developing after months/years is generally irreversible (seldom seen following liver transplantation).
Emphasize necessity/verify client ability to adhere to medical regimen and appropriate follow-up, including periodic laboratory tests (e.g., drug levels, lipid panels, organ function studies), routine examinations (e.g., dental, gynecologic), and specialty examinations (e.g., ophthalmologic, gastroenterologic). Anticipate problems and participate in problem-solving with client/SO.	Because the incidence of medication noncompliance is a major cause (at least 50%) of post-transplant complications and mortality, the client/SO needs to understand that adherence to regimen is imperative (e.g., dosing, timing, length of time after transplant, addition of this medication regimen to others client requires, physical/cognitive demands of routine). Routine follow-up/care by healthcare providers is necessary to maximize general well-being and to monitor effects of long-term medication regimen on other organ systems (e.g., nephrotoxic effects). Specialty examinations aid in monitoring new organ function and effect on other systems. Additionally, steroids (when used) may cause changes in visual acuity or development of cataracts/glaucoma.

ACTIONS/INTERVENTIONS	RATIONALE
Recommend that results of laboratory tests/diagnostic studies done locally be faxed to transplant center.	Long-term care is very complex and requires coordination and cooperation between all healthcare providers.
Discuss need to seek medical attention earlier than was probably done in the past.	Generally a "wait and see" attitude can be detrimental because a delay in treatment could result in organ damage/rejection.
Discuss managing immunosuppressant therapy, including "do's and don'ts" of specific medications, anticipated and adverse effects, interaction with other drugs, appropriate use of OTC products; adjustment of prescribed medication dosage during periods of stress, or with gradual decrease in immunosuppression over months/years, as appropriate.	Multiple medications, often a triple therapy such as cyclosporine or tacrolimus (Prograf), sirolimus (Rapamune) are typically required on an ongoing/lifelong basis to prevent organ rejection. Additional drugs may be needed to manage side and adverse effects of immunosuppressant therapy (e.g., infection, weight gain, nausea, diarrhea, osteoporosis, peptic ulcers, hypertension).
Encourage client/SO to maintain a working relationship with transplant team. Include family members, caregivers in education sessions and discharge planning as appropriate.	Promotes understanding and cooperation among those providing medical and psychologic support in care of client.
Recommend wearing an identification tag (e.g., bracelet, necklace).	In emergencies, provides immediate information to care providers relative to surgical/transplant history and medication regimen.
Identify community resources, including transplant club/support groups.	Provides opportunity for client and SO(s) to share experiences with others who are going through the same process. Providing anticipatory guidance may enhance problem solving.
Discuss self-monitoring routine and record keeping; e.g., chart temperature per protocol (before breakfast/dinner and when not feeling well), weigh daily before breakfast (in like clothing, same scale), blood pressure/pulse, changes in medication dosage, changes in health status/functional ability.	Helps care providers identify individual needs/development of complications.
Recommend frequent oral/dental care and periodic visual inspection of oral mucosa and gums.	Immunosuppression increases susceptibility to common opportunistic infections affecting the mouth (e.g., *Candida*, herpes simplex). Ongoing drug regimen, such as cyclosporine, can cause hypertrophy of gums, or Rapamune can cause ulcerations of the oral mucosa.
Review dietary needs. Determine optimal weight; discuss expected changes associated with medication regimen.	Requirements of normal healing, as well as effects of current stress, medications, and preoperative debilitation, can exacerbate nutritional deficiencies/imbalances and cause excessive weight loss; however, undesired weight gain can also occur because food tastes better, dietary restrictions are eliminated, and prednisone stimulates appetite.
Identify risk factors/additional safety concerns relative to infections; e.g., avoid changing cat litter box or use of live virus vaccines, use gloves when gardening, and take proper care of wounds/tissue trauma.	Awareness of possible risks (including unusual sources) enables client/family to plan for avoidance. Cat litter can transmit infectious agents such as *Listeria.* Steroid-induced skin fragility increases risk of injury from minor trauma as a result of thinning of the skin/immunosuppression.
Discuss necessity of handling skin carefully, avoiding strong sunlight and using sunblock with SPF of 15 or higher.	Steroid therapy results in skin fragility, sun sensitivity, and risk of developing skin cancers.
Review common postoperative care needs; e.g., routine wound care, need for adequate rest, avoidance of heavy lifting/physical labor or exercise (including contact sports), and activities that stretch or put pressure on incision; when/how to resume driving and sexual activity; dietary and fluid needs/restrictions.	Reduces likelihood of complications, aids client/SO in determining appropriateness of activities, and enhances client's sense of control and personal responsibility for altering activity level. *Note:* General advice for early phase: "If it hurts, don't do it."
Provide information about potential sexual dysfunction and encourage open communication for future discussion/support as needed.	Decreased libido, erectile dysfunction, and impaired orgasmic ability often occur because of medication regimen, low hormone levels, impaired blood flow, fear of harm to transplanted organ, or emotional disturbances. Initially client may be too focused on survival to address sexual issues/concerns.

ACTIONS/INTERVENTIONS	RATIONALE
Encourage continuation of preillness daily routines and activities as appropriate.	Enhances general well-being. Promotes focus on returning to "normal life," reducing sense that everything is different now.
Discuss participation in planned endurance and strength training exercise programs and inform about Transplant Olympics as appropriate/desired.	Restores strength, promotes sense of well-being and self-esteem, reduces risk of osteoporosis and inappropriate weight gain, and decreases hypertension.
Identify employment concerns/risks specific to particular transplanted organ, job responsibilities, and workplace environment.	Provides opportunity to problem-solve, plan for modifications, or seek alternative options.
Discuss travel needs; e.g., notify team contact person in advance regarding plans, hand carry medications when traveling by airplane, locate transplant center nearest to travel destination before leaving home.	Frees client to be involved in travel if desired. May need special instructions/precautions, depending on travel destination.
Stress importance of notifying future care providers of medication regimen.	Status of immune system functioning may require prophylactic therapy for procedures (such as antibiotics with dental care).

POTENTIAL CONSIDERATONS following acute hospitalization (depending on client's age, physical condition/presence of complications, personal resources, and life responsibilities)

ineffective Therapeutic Regimen Management—postdischarge concern, complexity of therapeutic regimen, side effects of medications, economic difficulties, prolonged nature of treatment.

risk for Infection—immunosuppression, antibiotic therapy.

ineffective Protection—drug therapies (corticosteroid, immune).

deficient Knowledge [Learning Need}—participation in support groups, ongoing care in collaboration with transplant team, gradual decrease of immunosuppression over months and years.

15
CHAPTER

General

PSYCHOSOCIAL ASPECTS OF CARE

The emotional response of the client during illness is of extreme importance. The mind-body-spirit connection is well established; it is known, for example, that when a physiologic response occurs, there is a corresponding psychologic response. Also, there are physiologic conditions that have a psychologic component; for example, the emotional instability associated with steroid therapy or Cushing's syndrome or the irritability of hypoglycemia. Rapid growth in the field of psychoneuroimmunology regularly provides new information about these issues.

With expanding technology in healthcare, ethical issues are being hotly debated. Although the stress of illness is well recognized, the effect on the individual is unpredictable. It is not necessarily the event that creates problems, but rather the client's perception of and response to the event, which may result in unmet psychologic needs that drain energy resources needed for healing. The caregivers', clients', and significant others' (SOs) values, sensitivity to different cultures, and language barriers (including difficulties that people have in talking about their bodies) affect the care a client expects and receives.

CARE SETTING

Any setting in which nursing contact occurs/care is provided.

RELATED CONCERNS

This is an aspect of all care and plans of care.

Assessment Factors to Be Considered

INDIVIDUAL

Age and gender
Religious affiliation: Church attendance, importance of religion in client's life, belief in life after death
Level of knowledge/education, how the individual accesses and incorporates information; e.g., auditory, visual, kinesthetic
Client's dominant language/literacy, knowledge and use of other languages, style of speech
Patterns of communication with SOs, with healthcare givers
Perception of body and its functions: In health, illness, this illness/situation
How does client define and perceive illness?
How is client experiencing illness versus what illness actually is?
Emotional response to current treatment/hospitalization
Past experience with illness, hospitalization, and healthcare systems
Emotional reactions in feeling (sensory) terms; e.g., states, "I feel scared."
Behavior when anxious, afraid, impatient, withdrawn, or angry

SIGNIFICANT OTHERS

Marital status, SOs, nuclear/extended family, recurring or patterned relationships
Family development cycle: Just married, children (young, adolescent, leaving/returning home), retired
What are the interaction processes within the family?
Client's role in family tasks and functions
How are SOs affected by the illness and prognosis?
Lifestyle differences that need to be considered: Dietary, spiritual, sexual preference, other community (e.g., religious order, commune, retirement center)

SOCIOECONOMIC

Employment; finances
Environmental factors: residence, work, and recreation; out of usual environment (on vacation, visiting)

Social class, value system
Social acceptability of disease/condition (e.g., sexually transmitted diseases [STDs], HIV, obesity, substance abuse)

CULTURAL

Ethnic background, heritage and residence/local
Beliefs regarding caring and curing
Health-seeking behaviors, illness referral system
Values related to health and treatment
Cultural factors related to illness in general and to pain response

DISEASE (ILLNESS)

Kind/cause of illness; how has it been treated/how should it be treated? Anticipated response to treatment; client's/SO's expectations
Is this an acute or chronic condition, is it inherited, what is the threat to self/others?
If terminal illness, what do the client and SO know and anticipate?
Is the condition "appropriate" to the afflicted individual; e.g., multiple sclerosis, diabetes mellitus (DM), cancer (*Note*: Some theories suggest certain personalities are more prone to certain illnesses.)
Illness related to personality factors, such as type A (may be myth or valid relative to management of stressors); high-risk behaviors

NURSE RELATED

Basic knowledge of human responses and how the current situation is related to response of the individual
Basic knowledge of biologic, psychologic, social, cultural, and religious issues
Knowledge and use of therapeutic communication skills
Knowledge of own value and belief system, including prejudices, biases
Willingness to look at own behavior in relation to interaction with others and make changes as necessary
Respect of client's privacy, confidentiality, human needs

NURSING PRIORITIES

1. Encourage effective coping skills of client/SO.
2. Reduce anxiety/fear.
3. Facilitate integration of self-concept and body-image changes.
4. Support grieving process.
5. Promote safe environment/client well-being.

DISCHARGE GOALS

1. Client/family dealing realistically with current situation.
2. Reports anxiety/fear manageable.
3. Progressing through stages of grieving.
4. Safe environment maintained.
5. Plan in place to meet needs after discharge.

NURSING DIAGNOSIS: ineffective Coping/decisional Conflict (specify)

May be related to

Gender differences in coping strategies
Situational crises/personal vulnerability, multiple life changes/maturational crises, age/developmental stage, uncertainty
Inadequate level of confidence in ability to cope, perception of control, high degree of threat, inadequate resources available
No vacations/inadequate relaxation
Impairment of nervous system, memory loss, impaired adaptive behaviors and problem-solving skills
Severe pain/overwhelming threat to self
Unclear personal values/beliefs; perceived threat to value system, lack of experience/interference with decision-making; lack of relevant information
Support system deficit, multiple or divergent sources of information

Possibly evidenced by

Verbalization of inability to cope/ask for help, inappropriate use of defense mechanisms, inability to meet role expectations, basic needs, problem-solve
Muscular tension, frequent headaches/neckaches
Report of chronic worry, fatigue, insomnia, anxiety/depression; poor concentration
Poor self-esteem
Alteration in social participation, change in usual communication patterns, verbal manipulation
High illness/accident rate, overeating, excessive smoking/drinking
Destructive behavior toward self or others, risk taking
Uncertainty about choices, vacillation between alternative actions, delayed decision making
Self-focusing, feeling of distress/questioning personal values and beliefs while attempting a decision

DESIRED OUTCOMES/EVALUATION CRITERIA—CLIENT WILL:

Coping (NOC)

Identify ineffective coping behaviors and consequences.
Verbalize awareness of own coping/problem-solving abilities.
Meet psychologic needs as evidenced by appropriate expression of feelings, identification of options, and use of resources.

Decision-Making (NOC)

Make decisions and express satisfaction with choices.

ACTIONS/INTERVENTIONS	RATIONALE
Coping Enhancement (NIC)	
Independent	
Review pathophysiology affecting the client and extent of feelings of hopelessness/helplessness/loss of control over life, level of anxiety, perception of situation.	Indicators of degree of disequilibrium and need for intervention to prevent or resolve the crisis. Studies suggest that up to 85% of all physically ill people are depressed to some degree. Impairment of normal functioning for more than 2 weeks, especially in presence of chronic condition, may reflect depression, requiring further evaluation.
Establish therapeutic nurse-client relationship.	Client may feel freer in the context of this relationship to verbalize feelings of helplessness/powerlessness and to discuss changes that may be necessary in the client's life.
Note expressions of indecision, dependence on others, and inability to manage own activities of daily living (ADLs).	May indicate need to lean on others for a time. Early recognition and intervention can help client regain equilibrium.
Assess presence of positive coping skills/inner strengths; e.g., use of relaxation techniques, willingness to express feelings, use of support systems.	When the individual has coping skills that have been successful in the past, they may be used in the current situation to relieve tension and preserve the individual's sense of control. However, limitations of condition may impact choices available to client; e.g., playing musical instrument to relieve stress may not be possible for individual with tremors or hemiparesis, but listening to tapes/CDs may provide some degree of comfort.
Encourage client to talk about what is happening at this time and what has occurred to precipitate feelings of helplessness and anxiety.	Provides clues to assist client to develop coping and regain equilibrium.

ACTIONS/INTERVENTIONS	RATIONALE
Evaluate ability to understand events. Correct misperceptions, provide factual information.	Assists in identification and correction of perception of reality and enables problem-solving to begin.
Provide quiet, nonstimulating environment. Determine what client needs, and provide if possible. Give simple, factual information about what client can expect and repeat as necessary.	Decreases anxiety and provides control for the client during crisis situation.
Allow client to be dependent in the beginning, with gradual resumption of independence in ADLs, self-care, and other activities. Make opportunities for client to make simple decisions about care/other activities when possible, accepting choice not to do so.	Promotes feelings of security (client will know nurse will provide safety). As control is regained, client has the opportunity to develop adaptive coping/problem-solving skills.
Accept verbal expressions of anger, setting limits on maladaptive behavior.	Verbalizing angry feelings is an important process for resolution of grief and loss. However, preventing destructive actions (such as striking out at others) preserves client's self-esteem.
Discuss feelings of self-blame/projection of blame on others.	Although these mechanisms may be protective at the moment of crisis, they eventually are counterproductive and intensify feelings of helplessness and hopelessness.
Note expressions of inability to find meaning in life/reason for living, feelings of futility or alienation from God.	Crisis situation may evoke questioning of spiritual beliefs, affecting ability to cope with current situation and plan for the future.
Promote safe and hopeful environment, as needed. Identify positive aspects of this experience and assist client to view it as a learning opportunity.	May be helpful while client regains inner control. The ability to learn from the current situation can provide skills for moving forward.
Provide support for client to problem-solve solutions for current situation. Provide information and reinforce reality as client begins to ask questions; look at what is happening.	Helping client/SO to brainstorm possible solutions (giving consideration to the pros and cons of each) promotes feelings of self-control/esteem.
Provide for gradual implementation and continuation of necessary behavior/lifestyle changes. Reinforce positive adaptation/new coping behaviors.	Reduces anxiety of sudden change and allows for developing new and creative solutions.

Collaborative

Refer to other resources as necessary (e.g., clergy, psychiatric clinical nurse specialist/psychiatrist, family/marital therapist, addiction support groups).	Additional assistance may be needed to help client resolve problems/make decisions.

NURSING DIAGNOSIS: risk for compromised family Coping

May be related to

Inadequate or incorrect information or understanding by a primary person, unrealistic expectations
Temporary family disorganization and role changes, feel that caregiving interferes with other important roles in their lives
Prolonged disease/disability progression that exhausts the supportive capacity of family members

Possibly evidenced by

[Not applicable; presence of signs and symptoms establishes an *actual* diagnosis.]

DESIRED OUTCOMES/EVALUATION CRITERIA—FAMILY WILL:

Family Coping (NOC)

Identify resources within themselves to deal with situation.
Visit regularly and participate positively in care of client, within limits of abilities.
Express more realistic understanding and expectations of the client.
Provide opportunity for client to deal with situation in own way.

ACTIONS/INTERVENTIONS	RATIONALE
Family Involvement Promotion (NIC)	
Independent	
Establish rapport and acknowledge difficulty of the situation for the family.	May assist family to accept what is happening and be willing to share problems with caregivers.
Determine current knowledge/perception of the situation.	Lack of information or unrealistic perceptions can interfere with family members'/client's response to illness situation.
Assess level of anxiety present in family/SO.	Anxiety level needs to be dealt with before problem-solving can begin. Individuals may be so preoccupied with own reactions to situation that they are unable to respond to another's needs.
Evaluate preillness/current behaviors that are interfering with the care/recovery of the client.	Information about family problems (e.g., divorce/separation, financial limitations, substance use) will be helpful in determining options and developing an appropriate plan of care.
Discuss underlying reasons for client behaviors with family.	When family members know why client is behaving in different ways, it helps them understand and accept/deal with situation.
Assist family/client to understand "who owns the problem" and who is responsible for resolution. Avoid placing blame or guilt.	When these boundaries are defined, each individual can begin to take care of own self and stop taking care of others in inappropriate ways.
Reframe negative expressions into positives whenever possible.	Promotes more hopeful attitude and helps family/client look toward the future.
Involve SO in information giving, problem-solving, and care of client as feasible. Identify other ways of demonstrating support while maintaining client's independence.	Information can reduce feelings of helplessness. Involvement in care enhances feelings of control and self-worth.
Collaborative	
Refer to appropriate resources for assistance as indicated (e.g., counseling, psychotherapy, financial, spiritual).	May need additional assistance in resolving family issues.

NURSING DIAGNOSIS: readiness for enhanced family Coping

May be related to

Basic needs sufficiently gratified and adaptive tasks effectively addressed to enable goals of self-actualization to surface
Willingness to deal with one's own needs and to begin to problem-solve with the client

Possibly evidenced by

Family member attempting to describe growth impact of crisis on his/her own values, priorities, goals, or relationships
Family member moving in direction of health-promoting and enriching lifestyle and generally choosing experiences that optimize wellness

DESIRED OUTCOMES/EVALUATION CRITERIA—FAMILY WILL:

Family Functioning (NOC)

Express willingness to look at own role in family's growth.
Undertake tasks leading to change.
Verbalize feelings of self-confidence and satisfaction with progress being made.

ACTIONS/INTERVENTIONS	RATIONALE
Family Support (NIC)	
Independent	
Provide opportunities for family to talk with client and/or caregiver(s).	Reduces anxiety and allows expression of what has been learned and how they are managing, as well as opportunity to make plans for the future and share support.
Listen to family's expressions of hope, planning, effect on relationships/life, change of values.	Provides clues to avenues to explore for assistance with growth.
Provide opportunities for and instruction in how SOs can care for client. Discuss ways in which they can support client in meeting own needs.	Enhances feelings of control and involvement in situation in which SOs cannot do many things. Also provides opportunity to learn how to be most helpful when client is discharged from care.
Provide a role model with which family may identify.	Having a positive example can help with adoption of new behaviors to promote growth.
Discuss importance of open communication. Role play effective communication skills of active-listening, "I-messages," and problem solving.	Helps individuals to express needs and wants in ways that will develop family cohesiveness. Promotes solutions in which everyone wins.
Encourage family to learn new and effective ways of dealing with feelings.	Effective recognition and expression of feelings clarify situation for involved individuals.
Encourage seeking support appropriately. Give information about available persons and agencies.	Permission to seek help as needed allows them to choose to take advantage of available assistance/resources.
Collaborative	
Refer to specific support group(s) as indicated.	Provides opportunities for sharing experiences, provides mutual support and practical problem solving, and can aid in decreasing alienation and helplessness.

NURSING DIAGNOSIS: Anxiety [specify level]/Fear

May be related to

Unconscious conflict about essential goals and values of life, unmet needs
Situational/maturational crises, interpersonal transmission and contagion, stress
Threat of death (perceived or actual)

Threat to or change in health status (exposure to toxins, progressive/debilitating disease, terminal illness), interaction patterns, role function/status, environment (safety), economic status
Familial association/heredity
Separation from support system; knowledge deficit
Sensory impairment; environmental stimuli; substance abuse

Possibly evidenced by

Behavioral: Expressed concerns due to change in life events, diminished productivity, insomnia
Poor eye contact, glancing about, scanning and vigilance
Restlessness, extraneous movement, fidgeting
Affective: Irritability, jittery, overexcited, rattled, regretful, anguish
Painful and persistent increased helplessness, feeling of inadequacy, uncertainty
Scared, distressed, apprehensive, worried, increased wariness
Physiologic: Reports of increased tension, feelings of helplessness, inadequacy; apprehension, uncertainty, being scared, overexcited
Facial tension, sympathetic/parasympathetic stimulation (quivering voice, trembling, insomnia), extraneous movements (e.g., foot shuffling, hand/arm movements)
Cognitive: Blocking of thought, impaired attention, confusion, forgetfulness, rumination, difficulty concentrating
Dread of an identifiable problem recognized by the client, fear of unspecific consequences, tendency to blame others
Focus on self, fight/flight behavior

DESIRED OUTCOMES/EVALUATION CRITERIA—CLIENT WILL:

Anxiety [or] Fear Self-Control (NOC)

Acknowledge and discuss fears/concerns.
Appear relaxed and report anxiety is reduced to a manageable level.
Verbalize awareness of feelings of anxiety and healthy ways to deal with them.
Demonstrate problem-solving and use resources effectively.

ACTIONS/INTERVENTIONS	RATIONALE
Anxiety Reduction (NIC)	
Independent	
Note palpitations, elevated pulse/respiratory rate.	Changes in vital signs may suggest the degree of anxiety the client is experiencing or reflect the impact of physiologic factors; e.g., endocrine imbalances.
Acknowledge fear/anxieties. Validate observations with client; e.g., "You seem to be afraid?"	Feelings are real, and it is helpful to bring them out in the open so they can be discussed and dealt with.
Assess degree/reality of threat to client and level of anxiety (e.g., mild, moderate, severe) by observing behavior such as clenched hands, wide eyes, startle response, furrowed brow, clinging to family/staff, or physical/verbal lashing out.	Individual responses can vary according to cultural beliefs/traditions and culturally learned patterns. Distorted perceptions of the situation may magnify feelings.
Note narrowed focus of attention (e.g., client concentrates on one thing at a time).	Narrowed focus usually reflects extreme fear/panic.
Observe speech content, vocabulary, and communication patterns; e.g., rapid/slow, pressured speech, words commonly used, repetition, use of humor/laughter, swearing.	Provides clues about such factors as the level of anxiety, ability to comprehend what is currently happening, cognition difficulties, and possible language differences.

ACTIONS/INTERVENTIONS	RATIONALE
Assess severity of pain when present. Delay gathering of information if pain is severe.	Severe pain and anxiety leave little energy for critical thinking and other activities.
Determine client's/SO's perception(s) of the situation.	Regardless of the reality of the situation, perception affects how each individual deals with the illness/stress.
Acknowledge reality of the situation as the client sees it, without challenging the belief.	Client may need to deny reality until ready to deal with it. It is not helpful to force the client to face facts.
Evaluate coping/defense mechanisms being used to deal with the perceived or real threat.	May be dealing well with the situation at the moment; e.g., denial and regression may be helpful coping mechanisms for a time. However, use of such mechanisms diverts energy the client needs for healing, and problems need to be dealt with at some point in time.
Review coping mechanisms used in the past; e.g., problem-solving skills, recognizing/asking for help.	Provides opportunity to build on resources the client/SO may have used successfully.
Assist client to use the energy of anxiety for coping with the situation when possible.	Moderate anxiety heightens awareness and can help motivate the client to focus on dealing with problems.
Maintain frequent contact with the client/SO. Be available for listening and talking as needed.	Establishes rapport, promotes expression of feelings, and helps client and SO look at realities of the illness/treatment without confronting issues they are not ready to deal with.
Acknowledge feelings as expressed (e.g., use of active-listening, reflection). If actions are unacceptable, take necessary steps to control/deal with behavior. (Refer to ND: risk for Violence.)	Often acknowledging feelings enables client to deal more appropriately with situation. May need chemical/physical control for brief periods.
Identify ways in which client can get help when needed, including telephone numbers of contact persons.	Provides assurance that staff/resources are available for assistance/support.
Stay with or arrange to have someone stay with client as indicated.	Continuous support may help client regain internal locus of control and reduce anxiety/fear to a manageable level.
Provide accurate information as appropriate and when requested by the client/SO. Answer questions freely and honestly and in language that is understandable by all. Repeat information as necessary; correct misconceptions.	Complex and/or anxiety-provoking information can be given in manageable amounts over an extended period. As opportunities arise and facts are given, individuals will accept what they are ready for. *Note:* Words/phrases may have different meanings for each individual; therefore, clarification is necessary to ensure understanding.
Avoid empty reassurances, with statements of "everything will be all right." Instead, provide specific information; e.g., "Your heart rate is regular, your pain is being easily controlled, and that is what we want," or "Your CD4 count has been stable for the last three visits."	It is not possible for the nurse to know how the specific situation will be resolved, and false reassurances may be interpreted as lack of understanding or honesty, further isolating the client. Sharing observations used in assessing condition/prognosis provides opportunity for client/SO to feel reassured.
Note expressions of concern/anger about treatment or staff.	Anxiety about self and outcome may be masked by comments or angry outbursts directed at therapy/caregivers.
Ask client/SO to identify what he or she can/cannot do about what is happening.	Assists in identifying areas in which control can be exercised and those in which control is not possible.
Provide as much order and predictability as possible in scheduling care/activities, visitors.	Helps client anticipate and prepare for difficult treatments/movements, as well as look forward to pleasant occurrences.
Instruct in ways to use positive self-talk; e.g., "I can manage this pain for now," or "My cancer is shrinking."	Internal dialogue is often negative. When this is shared out loud, the client becomes aware and can be directed in the use of positive self-talk, which can help reduce anxiety.
Encourage client to develop regular exercise/activity program.	Has been shown to raise endorphin levels to enhance sense of well-being and help reduce level of anxiety.
Encourage/instruct in guided imagery/ relaxation methods (e.g., imaging a pleasant place, use of music/tapes, deep breathing, meditation, and mindfulness).	Promotes release of endorphins and aids in developing internal locus of control, reducing anxiety. May enhance coping skills, allowing body to go about its work of healing. *Note:* Mindfulness is a method of being in the here and now, concentrating on what is happening in the moment.

ACTIONS/INTERVENTIONS	RATIONALE
Provide touch, terapeutic touch, massage, and other adjunctive therapies as indicated.	Aids in meeting basic human need, decreasing sense of isolation, and assisting client to feel less anxious. *Note:* Therapeutic touch requires the nurse to have specific knowledge and experience to use the hands to correct energy field disturbances by redirecting human energies to help or heal.

Collaborative

Administer medications as needed: e.g., Antianxiety agents: diazepam (Valium), clorazepate (Tranxene), chlordiazepoxide (Librium); benzodiazepines: alprazolam (Xanax); oxazepam (Serax), lorazepam (Ativan), temazepam (Restoril); SSRIs: fluoxetine (Prozac), sertraline (Zoloft), fluvoxamine (Luvox), citalopram HAABr (Celexa), paroxetine HCL (Paxil); Other: buspirone (BuSpar), doxepin (Adapin, Sinequan).	Antianxiety agents and/or antidepressants may be useful for brief periods to assist the client/SO to reduce anxiety to manageable levels, providing opportunity for initiation of client's own coping skills. *Note:* Use of selective serotonin reuptake inhibitors (SSRIs) such as Prozac, Zoloft have been associated with sexual function complaints. Alternatives may need to be considered. Also, ethnic variations affecting psychotropic drugs require close monitoring to determine therapeutic dosage. For example, East Asians and blacks may be more sensitive/react faster, have higher plasma drug levels, and have increased risk of side effects, necessitating lower dosage than whites in general.

NURSING DIAGNOSIS: situational low Self-Esteem

May be related to

Biophysical, psychosocial, cognitive, perceptual, cultural, and/or spiritual crisis; e.g., changes in health status/body image, role performance, personal identity, loss of control of some aspect of life
Maturational transitions; developmental changes (specify)
Behavior inconsistent with values
Perceived/anticipated failure at life event(s), lack of recognition/rewards

Possibly evidenced by

Rationalizes away/rejects positive feedback, negative self-appraisal in response to life events
Verbalization of negative feelings about the self (helplessness, uselessness); focus on past abilities, strengths, function, or appearance; preoccupation with change/loss
Evaluates self as unable to handle situations/events, hesitant to try new things/situations, difficulty making decisions
Fear of rejection/reaction by others, projection of blame/responsibility for problems

DESIRED OUTCOMES/EVALUATION CRITERIA—CLIENT WILL:

Self-Esteem (NOC)

Verbalize realistic view and acceptance of self in situation.
Identify existing strengths and view self as capable person.
Recognize and incorporate change into self-concept in accurate manner without negating self-worth.
Demonstrate adaptation to changes/events that have occurred as evidenced by setting of realistic goals and active participation in work/play/personal relationships.

ACTIONS/INTERVENTIONS	RATIONALE
Self-Esteem Enhancement (NIC)	
Independent	
Ask how the client would like to be addressed.	Shows courtesy/respect and acknowledges person.
Identify SO from whom the client derives comfort and who should be notified in case of emergency.	Allows provisions to be made for specific person(s) to visit or remain close, and provides needed support for client. *Note:* May or may not be legal next of kin.
Identify basic sense of self-esteem, image client has of existential, physical, psychologic self. Identify locus of control.	May provide insight into whether this is a single episode or recurrent/chronic situation and can help determine needs and treatment plan. Determining whether the individual's locus of control is internal or external facilitates choosing most effective interventions.
Determine client's perception of threat to self.	Client's perception is more important than what is really happening and needs to be dealt with before reality can be addressed.
Active-listen client concerns and fears.	Conveys sense of caring and can be helpful in identifying the client's needs, problems, and coping strategies and how effective they are. Provides opportunity to develop and begin a problem-solving process.
Encourage verbalization of feelings, accepting what is said.	Helps client/SO begin to adapt to change and reduces anxiety about altered function/lifestyle.
Discuss stages of grief and the importance of grief work. (Refer to ND: Grieving [specify].)	Grieving is a necessary step for integration of change/loss into self-concept.
Provide nonthreatening environment, listen and accept client as presented.	Promotes feelings of safety, encouraging verbalization.
Observe nonverbal communication; e.g., body posture and movements, eye contact, gestures, use of touch.	Nonverbal language is a large portion of communication and therefore is extremely important. How the person uses touch provides information about how it is accepted and how comfortable the individual is with being touched.
Reflect back to the client what has been said; e.g., "It upset you when he told you that."	Clarification and verification of what has been heard promotes understanding and allows client to validate information, otherwise assumptions may be inaccurate.
Observe and describe behavior in objective terms.	All behavior has meaning, some of which is obvious and some of which needs to be identified. This is a process of educated guesswork and requires validation by the client.
Identify age and developmental level.	Age is an indicator of the stage of life client is experiencing; e.g., adolescence, middle age. However, developmental level may be more important than chronologic age in anticipating and identifying some of the client's needs. Some degree of regression occurs during illness, depending on many factors such as the normal coping skills of the individual, the severity of the illness, and family/cultural expectations.
Discuss client's view of body image and how illness/condition might affect it.	The client's perception of a change in body image may occur suddenly or over time (e.g., actual loss of a body part through injury/surgery, or a perceived loss, such as a heart attack) or be a continuous subtle process (e.g., chronic illness, eating disorders, or aging). Awareness can alert the nurse to the need for appropriate interventions tailored to the individual need.
Encourage discussion of physical changes in a simple, direct, and factual manner. Give realistic feedback and discuss future options; e.g., rehabilitation services.	Provides opportunity to begin incorporating actual changes in an accepting and hopeful atmosphere.
Acknowledge efforts at problem-solving, resolution of current situation, and future planning.	Provides encouragement and reinforces continuation of desired behaviors.
Recognize client's pace for adaptation to demands of current situation.	Failure to acknowledge client's need to take time and/or pressuring client to "get on with it" conveys a lack of acceptance of the person as an individual and may result in feelings of lowered self-esteem.

ACTIONS/INTERVENTIONS	RATIONALE
Introduce tasks at client's level of functioning, progressing to more complex activities as tolerated.	Provides opportunity for client to experience successes, reaffirming capabilities and enhancing self-worth.
Ascertain how the client sees own role within the family system; e.g., breadwinner, homemaker, husband/wife.	Illness may create a temporary or permanent problem in role expectations. Sexual role and how the client views self in relation to the current illness also play important parts in recovery.
Assist client/SO with clarifying expected roles and those that may need to be relinquished or altered.	Provides opportunity to identify misconceptions and begin to look at options; promotes reality orientation.
Determine client awareness of own responsibility for dealing with situation, personal growth.	Conveys confidence in client's ability to cope. When client acknowledges own part in planning and carrying out treatment plan, he or she has more investment in following through on decisions that have been made.
Assess impact of condition/surgery on sexuality.	Sexuality encompasses the whole person in the total environment. Many times problems of illness are superimposed on already existing problems of sexuality and can affect client's sense of self-worth. Some problems are more obvious than others, such as illness involving the reproductive parts of the body. Others are less obvious, such as sexual values, role in family; e.g., mother, wage earner, single parent.
Be alert to comments and innuendos, which may mean the client has a concern in the area of sexuality.	People are often reluctant and/or embarrassed to ask direct questions about sexual/sexuality concerns.
Be aware of caregiver's feelings about dealing with the subject of sexuality.	Nurses/caregivers are often as reluctant and embarrassed in dealing with sexuality issues as most clients. (Refer to CP: Extended Care, ND: ineffective Sexuality Pattern/Sexual Dysfunction.)

Collaborative

Provide information and referral to hospital and community resources.	Enables client/SO to be in contact with interested groups with access to assistive and supportive devices, services, and counseling.
Support participation in group/community activities; e.g., assertiveness classes, volunteer work, support groups.	Promotes skills of coping and sense of self-worth. Provides role models and facilitates problem-solving.
Refer to psychiatric support/therapy group, social services, as indicated.	May be needed to assist client/SO to achieve optimal recovery.
Refer to appropriate resources for sex therapy as need indicates.	May be someone with comfort level and knowledge who is available, or may be necessary to refer to professional resources for additional guidance and support.

NURSING DIAGNOSIS: Grieving [specify]

May be related to

Potential/actual or perceived object loss (may include people, possessions, job, status, home, ideals, parts and processes of the body), chronic and/or fatal illness

Thwarted grieving response to a loss, lack of resolution of previous grieving response/absence of anticipatory grieving

Preloss neuroticism, psychologic symptoms, frequency of major life events, predisposition for anxiety and feelings of inadequacy

Past psychiatric or mental health treatment

Possibly evidenced by

Verbal expression of distress/unresolved issues, difficulty in expressing loss, denial of loss

Altered eating habits, sleep/dream patterns, activity levels, libido
Crying, labile affect, feelings of sorrow, guilt, anger
Alterations in concentration and/or pursuit of tasks, developmental regression; difficulty taking on new or different roles
Persistent anxiety, depression, prolonged difficulty coping, feelings of inadequacy, dependency, self criticism

DESIRED OUTCOMES/EVALUATION CRITERIA—CLIENT WILL:

Grief Resolution (NOC)

Identify and express feelings freely/effectively.
Verbalize a sense of progress toward resolution of the grief and hope for the future.
Function at an acceptable level, participate in work and ADLs as appropriate.

ACTIONS/INTERVENTIONS	RATIONALE
Grief Work Facilitation (NIC)	
Independent	
Provide open environment in which client feels free to realistically discuss feelings and concerns.	Therapeutic communication skills such as active-listening, silence, being available, and acceptance provide opportunity and encourage the client to talk freely and deal with the perceived/actual loss.
Determine client perception and meaning of loss (current and past). Note cultural religious factors/expectations.	Affects client's responses and needs to be acknowledged in planning care.
Identify stage of grieving and effect on functioning:	Awareness allows for appropriate choice of interventions because individuals handle grief in many different ways.
Denial: Be aware of avoidance behaviors; anger, withdrawal, and so forth. Allow client to talk about what he or she chooses, and do not try to force client to "face the facts";	Denying the reality of diagnosis and/or prognosis is an important phase in which the client protects self from the pain and reality of the threat of loss. Each person does this in an individual manner based on previous experiences with loss and cultural/religious factors.
Anger: Note behaviors of withdrawal, lack of cooperation, and direct expression of anger. Be alert to body language and check meaning with client, noting congruency with verbalizations. Encourage/allow verbalization of anger, acknowledge feelings, set limits regarding destructive behavior;	Denial gives way to feelings of anger, rage, guilt, and resentment. Client may find it difficult to express anger directly and may feel guilty about normal feelings of anger. Although staff may have difficulty dealing with angry behaviors, acceptance allows client to work through the anger and move on to more effective coping behaviors.
Bargaining: Be aware of statements such as ". . . if I do this, my problem will be fixed." Allow verbalization without confrontation about realities;	Bargaining with care providers or God often occurs and may be helpful in beginning resolution and acceptance. Client may be working through feelings of guilt about things done or undone.
Depression: Give client permission to be where he or she is. Provide hope within parameters of individual situation without giving false reassurance. Provide comfort and availability, as well as caring for physical needs;	When client can no longer deny the reality of the loss, feelings of helplessness and hopelessness replace feelings of anger. The client needs information that this is a normal progression of feelings.
Acceptance: Respect client's needs and wishes for quiet, privacy, and/or talking.	Having worked through the denial, anger, and depression, client often prefers to be alone and may not want to talk much at this point. Client may still cling to hope, which can be sustaining through whatever is currently happening.
Active-listen client's concerns and be available for help as necessary.	The process of grieving does not proceed in an orderly fashion, but fluctuates with various aspects of all stages present at one time or another. If process is dysfunctional or prolonged, more aggressive interventions may be required to facilitate the process.

ACTIONS/INTERVENTIONS	RATIONALE
Determine quality of interactions with others, including family members.	Although periods of withdrawal/loneliness usually accompany grieving, persistent isolation may indicate deepening depression, necessitating further evaluation/intervention. *Note:* Family/SO may not be dysfunctional but may be intolerant of client's behaviors.
Identify and problem-solve solutions to existing physical responses; e.g., eating, sleeping, activity levels, and sexual desire.	May need additional assistance to deal with the physical aspects of grieving.
Assess needs of SO and assist as indicated.	Identification of problems indicating dysfunctional grieving allows for individual interventions.
Include family/SO as appropriate when determining future needs.	Depending on client desires/legal requirements, choices regarding future plans (e.g., living situation, continuation of care, end-of-life decisions, funeral arrangements) can provide guidance and peace of mind.
Discuss healthy ways of dealing with difficult situation.	Provides opportunity to look toward the future and plan for family's/SO's needs (e.g., for life after loss).

Collaborative

Refer to other resources; e.g., support groups, counseling, spiritual/pastoral care, psychotherapy as indicated.	May need additional help to resolve grief, make plans, and look toward the future.

NURSING DIAGNOSIS: risk for impaired Religiosity

Risk factors may include

Physical: Sickness/illness, pain
Psychologic factors: Ineffective support/coping with condition, personal disaster/crisis, lack of security, anxiety, fear of death, use of religion to manipulate
Sociocultural: Barriers to practicing religion (cultural and environmental)
Lack of social integration, lack of social/cultural interaction
Spiritual: Spiritual crises, suffering
Developmental and situational: Life transitons, aging; end-stage life crises

Possibly evidenced by

[Not applicable; presence of signs and symptoms establishes an *actual* diagnosis.]

DESIRED OUTCOMES/EVALUATION CRITERIA — CLIENT WILL:

Spiritual Health (NOC)

Express ability to once again participate in beliefs and rituals of desired religion.
Discuss beliefs/values about spiritual/religious issues.
Attend religious/worship services of choice as desired.
Verbalize concerns about end-of-life issues and fear of death.

ACTIONS/INTERVENTIONS	RATIONALE
Spiritual Suppot (NIC)	
Independent	
Listen to client's/SO's reports and expressions of anger/concern, alienation from God. Note sense of guilt or retribution.	May be suffering from severe/terminal illness or accident straining resources and affecting client's ability to cope. Perception of guilt may cause spiritual crisis/suffering resulting in rejection of religious activities/symbols.

ACTIONS/INTERVENTIONS	RATIONALE
Discuss differences between grief and guilt and help client to identify and deal with each. Point out consequences of actions based on guilt.	As client recognizes consequences of actions, they can be discussed, and desire to change may enhance new coping skills, avoid acting out of false guilt, and enable client to resume desired religious activities.
Use therapeutic communication skills of reflection and active-listening.	Communicates acceptance and enables client to find own solutions to concerns.
Encourage expression of feelings about illness/condition, death.	Allows client to identify how feelings are impacting situation and deal with them appropriately.
Determine sense of futility, feelings of hopelessness, lack of motivation to help self.	Indicators that client may see no, or only limited, options/alternatives or personal choices available and lack energy to deal with situation.
Assess extent of depression client may be experiencing.	Some studies suggest that a focus on religion may protect against depression.
Note recent changes in behavior; e.g., withdrawal from others/religious activities, dependence on alcohol or medications.	Helpful in determining severity/duration of situation and possible need for additional referrals, such as substance withdrawal. Lack of connectedness with self/others impairs ability to trust others or feel worthy of trust from others/God.
Suggest use of journaling/reminiscence.	Promotes life review. Can assist in clarifying values/ideas, recognizing and resolving feelings/situation and identifying reasons for resuming desired religious activities.
Encourage client to identify SO(s) and others (e.g., spiritual advisor, parish nurse) who can provide needed support.	Ongoing support is required to enhance sense of connectedness and strengthen religious ties as desired.

Religious Ritual Enhancement (NIC)

Identify client's religious affiliation, associated rituals, and beliefs.	Helps determine individual's needs and possible resources if desired.
Make time for nonjudgmental discussion of philosophical issues related to religious belief patterns and customs.	Open communication can assist client to check reality of perceptions and identify personal options and willingness to resume desired activities.
Discuss desire to continue/reconnect with previous belief patterns and customs.	Enables client to identify barriers to participating in desired activities and take appropriate actions to resume them.
Involve client in refining heathcare goals and therapeutic regimen as appropriate.	Identifies role illness is playing in current concerns about ability to/appropriateness of participating in desired religious activities.
Provide privacy for meditation/prayer, performance of rituals as appropriate.	Allows client to engage in spitirual activites in own way without fear of interruption/judgment of others.
Explore alternatives/modifications of ritual based on setting and individual needs/limitations.	Assists client to develop new ways of expressing religious beliefs/satisfying these needs.

Collaborative

Refer to spiritual resources as indicated e.g., spiritual advisor who has qualifications/experience in dealing with specific problems individual is concerned about, facility's chaplain or visiting clergy, parish nurse.	Provides answers to spiritual questions, assists in the journey of self-discovery, can help client learn to accept/forgive self, and engage in desired rituals.

NURSING DIAGNOSIS: risk for ineffective Therapeutic Regimen Management

Risk factors may include

Complexity of therapeutic regimen, knowledge deficits, inadequate number and types of cues to action

Decisional conflicts: client/family value system, health beliefs, spiritual values, cultural influences, ethical concerns, perceived seriousness
Perceived barriers, economic difficulties, side effects of therapy, mistrust of regimen and/or healthcare personnel, complexity of healthcare system
Family patterns of healthcare, family conflict, powerlessness

Possibly evidenced by

[Not applicable; presence of signs and symptoms establishes an *actual* diagnosis.]

DESIRED OUTCOMES/EVALUATION CRITERIA—CLIENT WILL:

TREATMENT BEHAVIOR: Illness or Injury (NOC)

Participate in the development of goals and treatment plan.
Verbalize accurate knowledge of disease and understanding of treatment regimen.
Demonstrate behaviors/changes in lifestyle necessary to incorporate/maintain therapeutic regimen in daily life.
Identify/use available resources.

ACTIONS/INTERVENTIONS	RATIONALE
Values Clarification (NIC)	
Independent	
Review client's/SO's knowledge and understanding of the need for treatment/medication, as well as consequences of actions and choices. Note ability to comprehend information, including literacy, level of education, primary language.	Provides opportunities to clarify viewpoints/misconceptions. Verifies that client/SO has accurate/factual information with which to make informed choices.
Be aware of developmental and chronological age.	Impacts ability to understand own needs/incorporate into treatment regimen.
Determine cultural, spiritual, and health beliefs and ethical concerns.	Provides insight into thoughts/factors related to individual situation. Beliefs will affect client's perception of situation and participation in treatment regimen. Treatment may be incongruent with client's social/cultural lifestyle and perceived role/responsibilities.
Self-Modification Assistance (NIC)	
Review treatment plan with client/SO.	Provides opportunities to exchange accurate information and to clarify viewpoints/misconceptions.
Contract with client for participation in care.	Client who agrees to own responsibility is more apt to adhere to treatment plan.
Establish graduated goals or modified regimen as necessary; work out alternate solutions.	Promotes client involvement/ independence; provides opportunity for compromise and may enhance cooperation with regimen. When client participates in setting goals, there is a sense of investment that encourages cooperation and willingness to follow through with the program.
Assess availability/use of support systems. Identify additional resources as appropriate.	Access to/proper use of helpful resources can assist client in meeting treatment goals and provide purpose for living. Presence of caring, empathic family/SO(s) can help client in process of recovery.
Determine potential problems that may/do interfere with treatment, including lack of financial/personal resources, lack of availability of providers. Assess level of anxiety, locus of control, sense of powerlessness.	Many factors may be involved in behavior that is disruptive to the treatment regimen (e.g., fear of hospitalization/treatment, denial of situation consequences, suspicion about healthcare system, physical factors, such as pain, hypoxemia, chemical imbalance).

ACTIONS/INTERVENTIONS	RATIONALE
Note length of illness/prognosis.	Clients tend to become passive and dependent in long-term, debilitating illness.
Listen to/active-listen client's reports and comments.	Conveys message of concern, belief in individual's capabilities to resolve situation in positive manner.
Develop a system for self-monitoring. Share data pertinent to client's condition; e.g., laboratory results, blood pressure (BP) readings.	Provides a sense of control; enables client to follow own progress and make informed choices.
Have same personnel care for client as much as possible.	Enables relationship to develop in which the client can begin to trust/participate in care.
Accept client's choice/point of view even if it appears to be self-destructive; e.g., decision to continue smoking.	Client has the right to make own decisions, and acceptance may give a sense of control, which can help client look more clearly at consequences. Confrontation is not beneficial and may actually be detrimental to future cooperation and goal achievement.
Be aware of own/caregiver's response to client's treatment choices (e.g., refusal of blood or chemotherapy, living will/advance directives).	Negative feelings regarding these choices may create power struggles and be expressed in judgmental behaviors that block or interfere with client's wishes, comfort, and/or care. *Note:* If resolution cannot be found, providers have the right to terminate their services with appropriate notice.

NURSING DIAGNOSIS: risk for self-directed/other-directed Violence

Risk factors may include

Neurologic impairment (e.g., positive EEG, ACT, MRI, neurologic findings, head trauma, seizure disorders)
Cognitive impairment (e.g., decreased intellectual functioning, learning disabilities, attention deficit disorder)
Hormonal imbalance, toxic reactions to medication, pathologic intoxication, substance abuse/withdrawal, physical health (chronic/terminal illness)
Attempt to deal with the threat to self-concept that illness can represent, suicidal ideation/behavior, depression, impulsivity, suicidal plan (clear and specific lethality, method, and availability of destructive means)
History of violence against others, violent antisocial behavior, childhood abuse, witnessing family violence

[Possible indicators]

Emotional status (hopelessness, despair, increased anxiety, panic, anger, hostility)
Suspicion of others, paranoid ideation, delusions, hallucinations
Body language: rigid posture, clenched fists, facial expressions
Increased motor activity, excitement, irritability, agitation
Overt and aggressive acts, self-destructive behavior
Verbal clues (e.g. talking about death, "better off without me," asking questions about lethal dosages of drugs)
Behavioral clues (e.g., writing forlorn notes, giving away personal items)

DESIRED OUTCOMES/EVALUATION CRITERIA—CLIENT WILL:

Impulse Self-Control (NOC)

Acknowledge realities of the situation.
Verbalize understanding of reason(s) for behavior/precipitating factors.
Express increased self-concept.
Demonstrate self-control, as evidenced by relaxed posture, nonviolent behavior.

ACTIONS/INTERVENTIONS	RATIONALE
Mood Management (NIC)	
Independent	
Observe for early signs of distress and investigate possible causes.	Irritability, pacing, shouting/cursing, lack of cooperation, and demanding behavior may all be signs of increasing anxiety or indicate change in health status of confused client that requires further evaluation.
Maintain straightforward communication and assist client to learn assertive rather than manipulative, nonassertive/aggressive behavior.	Avoids reinforcing manipulative behavior and enhances positive interactions with others, accomplishing the goal of getting needs met in acceptable ways.
Help client identify more adequate solutions/behaviors (e.g., motor activities/exercise). Redirect/provide directions for actions client can take.	Promotes release of energies in acceptable ways. Redirecting confused client can minimize escalation of agitation. (Refer to CP: Dementia of the Alzheimer's Type/Vascular Dementia.)
Give as much autonomy as is possible in the situation.	Enhances feelings of power and control in a situation in which many things are not within individual's control.
Monitor for suicidal/homicidal intent; e.g., morbid or anxious feelings while with the client, thoughts expressed by/warning from the client, "It doesn't matter, I'd be better off dead"; mood swings, putting affairs in order, previous suicide attempt.	Indicators of need for further assessment, evaluation, and intervention/psychiatric care.
Assess suicidal intent (1–10 scale) by asking directly if client is thinking of killing self, has plan, means, and so on.	Provides guidelines for necessity/urgency of interventions. Direct questioning is most helpful when done in a caring, concerned manner.
Acknowledge reality of suicide/homicide as an option. Discuss consequences of actions if client were to follow through on intent. Ask how it will help client resolve problems.	Client is often focused on suicide (or homicide) as the "only" option and this response provides an opening to look at and discuss other options. *Note:* Be aware of own responsibility under Tarasoff's rule to warn possible victim(s) when client is expressing homicidal ideation.
Accept client's anger without reacting on an emotional basis.	Responding with anger is not helpful in resolving the situation and may result in escalating client's behavior. Anger is usually not directed at the nurse, but at the situation, feelings of powerlessness, etc.
Remain calm and state limits on behavior in a firm manner. Be truthful and nonjudgmental.	Understanding that helplessness and fear underlie this behavior aides in choosing appropriate response.
Assume that the client has control and is responsible for own behavior.	Often enables the individual to exercise control. *Note:* When violent behavior is the result of drugs, client may not be able to respond appropriately.
Identify conditions that may interfere with ability to control own behavior.	Acute or chronic brain syndrome, drug-induced or postsurgical confusion may precipitate violent behavior that is difficult to control.
ENVIRONMENTAL MANAGEMENT: Violence Prevention (NIC)	
Provide protection within the environment; e.g., constant observation, removal of objects that might be used to harm self/others.	May need more structure to maintain control until own internal locus of control is regained.
Tell client to "stop."	May be sufficient to help client control own actions if exhibiting hostile actions. *Note:* Client is often afraid of own actions and wants staff to set limits.
Use an organized team approach when necessary to subdue client with force. Tell client clearly and concisely what is happening.	Knowing and practicing these actions before they are needed helps prevent untoward problems. Keeping client informed can help client to regain internal control.
Hold client; place in restraints or seclusion if necessary. Do so in a calm, positive, nonstimulating/nonpunitive manner.	As a last resort, physical restraint may be necessary while the client regains control. *Note:* These measures are meant to protect client, not punish the behavior.
Apply and adjust restraint devices properly.	It is important to maintain body alignment and client safety and comfort.

ACTIONS/INTERVENTIONS	RATIONALE
Document precise reason for restraints, actions taken, doctor's order. Check restraints frequently per facility protocol, each time documenting the condition and how long the restraints are used.	Restraints are to be used for very specific reasons, which need to be clearly documented to avoid overuse or misuse, and to ensure client safety.
Collaborative	
Refer to psychiatric resource(s), e.g., psychiatric clinical nurse specialist, psychiatrist, psychologist, social worker, and classes such as anger management.	More in-depth assistance may be needed to deal with client and defuse situation. Learning new ways to deal with feelings can provide opportunity for individual to manage life in a more optimal way.
Administer medications; e.g., antianxiety/antipsychotic agents, sedatives, narcotics.	May be indicated to quiet/control behavior. *Note:* May need to be withheld if they are suspected to be the cause of/contribute to the behavior.

NURSING DIAGNOSIS: risk for Post-Trauma Syndrome

Risk factors may include

Events outside the range of usual human experience: serious accidents or motor vehicle crashes/tragic occurrence involving multiple deaths, natural or manmade disasters (e.g., floods, earthquakes, tornadoes, airplane crashes), wars, epidemics
Physical/psychosocial abuse, being held prisoner of war or criminal victimization (torture), rape
Witnessing mutilation, violent death, or other horrors

Possibly evidenced by

[Not applicable; presence of signs and symptoms establishes an *actual* diagnosis.]

DESIRED OUTCOMES/EVALUATION CRITERIA—CLIENT WILL:

Coping (NOC)

Verbalize reduced stress.
Demonstrate ability to deal with emotional reactions in an individually appropriate manner.
Express own feelings/reactions; avoid projection.
Demonstrate appropriate changes in lifestyle/getting support from SO/friends as needed.
Participate in plans for follow-up care/counseling.

ACTIONS/INTERVENTIONS	RATIONALE
Crisis Intervention (NIC)	
Independent	
Determine when traumatic event(s) occurred: present or past.	Manifestations of acute and chronic posttrauma responses may require different interventions. *Note:* Event may encompass many forms of trauma, including the diagnosis of life-threatening illness.
Assess physical trauma, if present, and individual reaction to occurrence; e.g., physical symptoms such as numbness, headache, tightness in chest, and psychologic responses of anger, shock, acute anxiety, confusion, denial.	Provides information with which to develop plan of care, make informed choices.

ACTIONS/INTERVENTIONS	RATIONALE
Evaluate behavior (e.g., calm or agitated, excited/hysterical, inappropriate laughter, crying), expressions of disbelief and/or self-blame.	Indicators of extent of individual response to traumatic incident and degree of disorganization.
Note ethnic background/cultural and religious perceptions and beliefs about the event.	May influence client's response to what has happened; e.g., may believe it is retribution from God.
Assess signs/stage of grieving.	Client may be suffering from sense of loss of self and/or others.
Tell client that painful emotional reactions are normal. Phrase this information in neutral terms: "You may or may not experience . . . ."	Understanding that experiencing these uncomfortable feelings is not unusual after traumatic event may reduce client's anxiety/fear of "going crazy" and enhance coping.
Discuss things client can do to feel better; e.g., physical exercise alternated with relaxation, keeping busy with normal activities, talking to others, acknowledging that it is all right to feel upset, writing about the experience in a journal; being kind to self.	Enhances sense of control and helps client achieve resolution of uncomfortable feelings. Often when the client begins these activities within the first 24 hr of the event, further therapy may not be required.
Assist with learning stress management techniques.	Promotes sense of control and ability to handle existing problems.
Identify supportive persons for client.	Having positive support systems/role models can help client reach optimal recovery.
None signs of severe/prolonged depression; frequency of flashbacks/nightmares; presence of chronic pain, somatic complaints.	If client did not deal with trauma when it occurred, behavioral manifestations may reveal extent of problem in the present.
Help client identify factors that may have created a vulnerable situation/increased likelihood for event.	Even though individual may not be responsible for what has happened, he or she may have placed self at risk/engaged in activities potentiating negative outcome. Changes in behaviors/lifestyle may decrease potential for recurrence.

Collaborative

Refer to support groups, counselors/therapists for further therapy; e.g., psychotherapy (in conjunction with medications), implosive therapy, flooding, hypnosis, eye movement desensitization, and reprocessing (EMDR), rolfing, memory work, or cognitive restructuring, as indicated.	Client may need more in-depth assistance from sensitive, trained individuals who are skilled in dealing with these problems to prevent progression to/treat development of post-trauma syndrome.

POTENTIAL CONSIDERATIONS

Refer to primary diagnosis for postdischarge concerns.

SURGICAL INTERVENTION

Surgery may be required to diagnose or cure a specific disease process, correct a structural deformity, restore a functional process, or reduce the level of dysfunction/pain. Although surgery is generally elective or preplanned, potentially life-threatening conditions can arise, requiring emergency intervention. Absence or limitation of preoperative preparation and teaching increases the need for postoperative support in addition to managing underlying medical conditions.

CARE SETTING

May be inpatient on a surgical unit or outpatient/short-stay in an ambulatory surgical setting.

RELATED CONCERNS

Alcohol: acute withdrawal, page 831
Cancer, page 857
Diabetes mellitus/diabetic ketoacidosis, page 412
Fluid and electrolyte imbalance, page 919
Pneumothorax/hemothorax, page 150
Metabolic acidosis (primary base bicarbonate deficiency), page 492
Metabolic alkalosis (primary base bicarbonate excess), page 495
Peritonitis, page 355

Pneumonia, page 128
Psychosocial aspects of care, page 770
Respiratory acidosis, page 194
Respiratory alkalosis (primary), page 198
Sepsis/septicemia, page 701
Thrombophlebitis: deep vein thrombosis, page 108
Total nutritional support: parenteral/enteral feeding, page 478

Also refer to plan of care for specific surgical procedure performed.

Client Assessment Database

Data depend on the duration/severity of underlying problem and involvement of other body systems. Refer to specific plans of care for data and diagnostic studies relevant to the procedure and additional nursing diagnoses.

CIRCULATION

May report: History of cardiac problems, heart failure (HF), pulmonary edema, peripheral vascular disease, or vascular stasis (increases risk of thrombus formation)

May exhibit: Changes in heart rate (sympathetic stimulation)

EGO INTEGRITY

May report: Feelings of anxiety, fear, anger, apathy
Multiple stress factors; e.g., financial, relationship, lifestyle

May exhibit: Restlessness, increased tension/irritability
Sympathetic stimulation; e.g., changes in HR, respiratory rate

ELIMINATION

May report: History of kidney/bladder conditions, use of diuretics/laxatives
Change in bowel habits

May exhibit: Abdominal tenderness, distention
Absence of bowel elimination
Decreased or absence of urinary elimination

FOOD/FLUID

May report: Pancreatic insufficiency/diabetes mellitus (DM) (predisposing to hypoglycemia/ketoacidosis)
Use of diuretics

May exhibit: Malnutrition (including obesity)
Dry mucous membranes (limited intake/nothing-by-mouth [NPO] preoperatively)

RESPIRATION

May report: Infections, chronic conditions/cough, smoking

May exhibit: Changes in respiratory rate (respiratory pathology or sympathetic stimulation)

SAFETY

May report: Differences in personal identifiers, procedure type and/or site when compared to verification tools; i.e., consent, history and physical examination (H&P), surgery schedule
Allergies or sensitivities to medications, iodine, food, tape, latex, and solution(s)
Immune deficiencies (increases risk of systemic infections and delayed healing)
Presence of cancer/recent cancer therapy
Family history of malignant hyperthermia/reaction to anesthesia, autoimmune diseases
History of hepatic disease (affects drug detoxification and may alter coagulation)
History of blood transfusion(s)/transfusion reaction

May exhibit: Presence of existing infectious process, fever

TEACHING/LEARNING

May report: Use of medications such as anticoagulants, steroids, nonsteroidal anti-inflammatories, antibiotics, antihypertensives, cardiotonic glycosides, antidysrhythmics, bronchodilators, diuretics, decongestants, analgesics, anti-inflammatories, anticonvulsants, or antipsychotics/antianxiety agents, as well as over-the-counter (OTC) medications, herbal supplements (e.g., garlic, ginseng, *Gingko biloba,* ginger, feverfew—risk of excessive postoperative bleeding), or alcohol or other drugs of abuse (risk of liver damage affecting coagulation and choice of anesthesia, as well as potential for postoperative withdrawal)

Discharge plan considerations: May require temporary assistance with transportation, dressing(s)/supplies, self-care, and homemaker/maintenance tasks
Possible placement in rehabilitation/extended care facility

Refer to section at end of plan for postdischarge considerations.

DIAGNOSTIC STUDIES

General preoperative requirements may include: Complete blood count (CBC), prothrombin time (PT)/activated partial thromboplastin time (aPTT), chest x-ray. Other studies depend on type of operative procedure, underlying medical conditions, current medications, age, and weight. These tests may include blood urea nitrogen (BUN), creatinine (Cr), glucose, arterial blood gases (ABGs), electrolytes, liver function, thyroid, nutritional studies, electrocardiogram (ECG). Deviations from normal should be corrected if possible for safe administration of anesthetic agents.

CBC: An elevated white blood cell (WBC) count is indicative of inflammatory process (may be diagnostic; e.g., appendicitis); decreased WBC count suggests viral processes (requiring evaluation because immune system may be dysfunctional). Low hemoglobin (Hb) suggests anemia/blood loss (impairs tissue oxygenation and reduces the Hb available to bind with inhalation anesthetics); may suggest need for crossmatch/blood transfusion. An elevated hematocrit (Hct) may indicate dehydration; decreased Hct suggests fluid overload.

Electrolytes: Imbalances impair organ function; e.g., decreased potassium affects cardiac muscle contractility, leading to decreased cardiac output.

ABGs: Evaluates current respiratory status, which may be especially important in smokers, clients with chronic lung diseases.

Coagulation times: May be prolonged, interfering with intraoperative/postoperative hemostasis; hypercoagulation increases risk of thrombosis formation, especially in conjunction with dehydration and decreased mobility associated with surgery.

Urinalysis: Presence of WBCs or bacteria indicates infection. Elevated specific gravity may reflect dehydration.

Pregnancy test: Positive results affect timing of procedure and choice of pharmacologic agents.

Chest x-ray: Should be free of infiltrates, pneumonia; used for identification of masses and chronic obstructive pulmonary disease (COPD).

ECG: Abnormal findings require attention before administering anesthetics.

NURSING PRIORITIES

1. Assure correct client, procedure, and site.
2. Reduce anxiety and emotional trauma.
3. Provide for physical safety.
4. Prevent complications.
5. Alleviate pain.
6. Facilitate recovery process.
7. Provide information about disease process/surgical procedure, prognosis, and treatment needs.

DISCHARGE GOALS

1. Client dealing realistically with current situation.
2. Injury prevented.
3. Complications prevented/minimized.
4. Pain relieved/controlled.
5. Wound healing/organ function progressing toward normal.
6. Disease process/surgical procedure, prognosis, and therapeutic regimen understood.
7. Plan in place to meet needs after discharge.

PERIOPERATIVE

NURSING DIAGNOSIS: deficient Knowledge [Learning Need] regarding condition, prognosis, treatment, self-care, and discharge needs

May be related to

Lack of exposure/recall, information misinterpretation
Unfamiliarity with information resources

Possibly evidenced by

Statement of the problem/concerns, misconceptions
Request for information
Inappropriate, exaggerated behaviors (e.g., agitated, apathetic, hostile)
Inaccurate follow-through of instructions/development of preventable complications

DESIRED OUTCOMES/EVALUATION CRITERIA—CLIENT WILL:

KNOWLEDGE: Treatment Procedure(s) (NOC)

Verbalize understanding of disease process/perioperative process and postoperative expectations.
Correctly perform necessary procedures and explain reasons for the actions.
Initiate necessary lifestyle changes and participate in treatment regimen.

ACTIONS/INTERVENTIONS	RATIONALE
TEACHING: Preoperative (NIC)	
Independent	
Assess client's level of understanding.	Facilitates planning of preoperative teaching program, identifies content needs.
Review specific pathology and anticipated surgical procedure. Verify correct client, procedure, and marked site and that appropriate consent has been signed.	Provides knowledge base from which client can make informed therapy choices and consent appropriate for correct procedure and site. Presents opportunity to clarify misconceptions.
Use institution's Universal Protocol for Preventing Wrong Site, Wrong Procedure and Wrong Person Surgery, and resource teaching materials, audiovisuals as available.	Institution's Universal Protocol for and completion of specific checklists will minimize risk of error. Specifically designed materials can facilitate the client's learning.
Implement individualized preoperative teaching program:	
Preoperative/postoperative procedures and expectations, urinary and bowel changes, dietary considerations, activity levels/transfers, respiratory/cardiovascular exercises; anticipated IV lines and tubes (e.g., nasogastric [NG] tubes, drains, and catheters);	Enhances client's understanding/control and can relieve stress related to the unknown/unexpected.
Preoperative instructions; e.g., bowel prep, NPO time, shower/skin preparation, which routine medications to take/hold; e.g., prophylactic antibiotics, or anticoagulants, anesthesia premedication;	Helps reduce the possibility of postoperative complications and promotes a rapid return to normal body function. *Note:* In some instances, liquids and medications are allowed up to 2 hr before scheduled procedure.
Intraoperative client safety; e.g., positional needs due to arthritis, previous injury, or current mobility; not crossing legs during procedures performed under local/light anesthesia;	Reduced risk of complications/untoward outcomes, such as muscular, nerve, or joint soreness (e.g., injury to the peroneal and tibial nerves with postoperative pain in the calves and feet).
Expected/transient reactions (e.g., low backache, localized numbness and reddening or skin indentations);	Minor effects of immobilization/positioning should resolve in 24 hr. If they persist, medical evaluation is required.
Inform client/SO about timely arrival on surgical day, itinerary, physician/SO communications.	Logistical information about preoperative preparation time, operating room (OR) schedule and locations (e.g., recovery room, postoperative room assignment), as well as where and when the surgeon will communicate with SO relieves stress and miscommunications, preventing confusion and doubt over client's well-being.

ACTIONS/INTERVENTIONS	RATIONALE
Discuss/develop individual postoperative pain management plan. Identify misconceptions client may have and provide appropriate information. Including use of 0–10 pain assessment scale.	Increases likelihood of successful pain management. Some clients may expect to be pain-free or fear becoming addicted to narcotic agents.
Provide opportunity to practice coughing, deep-breathing, and muscular exercises.	Enhances learning and continuation of activity postoperatively.

NURSING DIAGNOSIS: Fear/Anxiety [specify level]

May be related to

Situational crisis (including wrong client, procedure or site error), unfamiliarity with environment
Change in health status, threat of death
Separation from usual support systems

Possibly evidenced by

Increased tension, apprehension, decreased self-assurance, behavior regression
Expressed concern regarding changes, fear of consequences
Facial tension, restlessness, focus on self
Sympathetic stimulation

DESIRED OUTCOMES/EVALUATION CRITERIA—CLIENT WILL:

Anxiety [or] Fear Self-Control (NOC)

Acknowledge feelings and identify healthy ways to deal with them.
Appear relaxed, able to rest/sleep appropriately.
Report decreased fear and anxiety reduced to a manageable level.
Demonstrate ability to carry out procedure requirements.

ACTIONS/INTERVENTIONS	RATIONALE
Preoperative Coordination (NIC)	
Independent	
Provide preoperative education, including intentional repetitive verification of client identifiers, procedure, marked site steps and surgical "time out" process. Visit with operating room (OR) personnel before surgery when possible. Discuss/demonstrate routine procedures and processes that may frighten/concern client; e.g., masks, lights, IVs, BP cuff, electrodes, bovie pad, feel of oxygen cannula/mask on nose or face, autoclave and suction noises, child crying.	Can provide reassurance that client safety precautions are constantly ongoing, alleviate client's anxiety, as well as provide information for formulating intraoperative care. Acknowledges that foreign environment may be frightening, alleviates associated fears. Decreased anxiety level reduces elevation of glucocorticosteroid levels, which can interfere with healing.
Inform client/SO of nurse's intraoperative advocate role.	Develops trust/rapport, decreasing fear of loss of control in a foreign environment. Provides patient/SO with contact person.
Assure client anticipating local/spinal anesthesia that drowsiness/sleep occurs, that more sedation may be requested and will be given if needed, and that surgical drapes will block view of the operative field.	Reduces concerns that client may "see" the procedure.

ACTIONS/INTERVENTIONS	RATIONALE
Surgical Preparation (NIC)	
Identify fear levels that may necessitate postponement of surgical procedure.	Overwhelming or persistent fears result in excessive stress reaction, increasing glucocorticosteroid levels, potentiating risk of adverse reaction to procedure and anesthetic agents and imparing healing.
Validate source of fear. Provide accurate factual information. Active-listen concerns.	Identification of specific fear helps client deal realistically with it; e.g., misidentification/wrong operation, dismemberment, disfigurement, loss of dignity/control, or being awake/aware with local anesthesia. Client may have misinterpreted preoperative information or have misinformation regarding surgery/disease process. Fears regarding previous experiences of self/family/acquaintances may be unresolved.
Note expressions of distress/feelings of helplessness, preoccupation with anticipated change/loss, choked feelings.	Client may already be grieving for the loss represented by the anticipated surgical procedure/diagnosis/prognosis of illness.
Introduce client to staff at time of transfer to operating suite.	Establishes rapport and psychologic comfort with operative team.
Verbalize and document client identifiers to surgery schedule, client identification band, chart, marked site, and signed operative consent for surgical procedure according to facility's protocol and checklist.	Provides for positive identification, reducing fear that wrong procedure may be done as well as minimizing risk for wrong procedure and site.
Prevent unnecessary body exposure during transfer and in OR suite.	Preserves client's modesty, reduces fear of loss of dignity and inability to exercise control, and reinforces nurse advocacy role.
Give simple, concise directions/explanations to sedated client. Review environmental concerns as needed.	Impairment of thought processes makes it difficult for client to understand lengthy instructions.
Control external stimuli.	Extraneous noises and commotion may accelerate anxiety.

Collaborative

ACTIONS/INTERVENTIONS	RATIONALE
Refer to surgeon, anesthesiologist, clinical manager, pastoral spiritual care, psychiatric clinical nurse specialist, psychiatric counseling if indicated.	Further evaluation/counseling may be desired or required for client to deal with fear, especially concerning life-threatening conditions, serious and/or high-risk procedures.
Discuss postponement/cancellation of surgery with physician, anesthesiologist, client, and family as appropriate.	May be necessary if overwhelming fears are not reduced/resolved.
Refer wrong client, procedure, site or implant discrepancies to surgeon, anesthesiologist, and appropriate persons.	Discrepancies must be corrected and verified by surgeon, client/SO prior to OR entry.
Administer medications as indicated; e.g.:	
Sedatives, hypnotics;	Used to promote sleep the evening before surgery; may enhance coping abilities.
IV antianxiety agents;	May be provided in the outpatient admitting/preoperative holding area to reduce nervousness and provide comfort. *Note:* Respiratory depression/bradycardia may occur, necessitating prompt intervention.
Administer antacids, H_2 blocker, preoperatively as indicated.	Neutralizes gastric acidity and may reduce risk of aspiration/severity of pneumonia should aspiration occur, especially in obese/pregnant clients in whom there is an 85% risk of mortality with aspiration. *Note*: Ranitidine (Zantac) has been found to reduce postoperative infections in acute colorectal surgery.

NURSING DIAGNOSIS: risk for perioperative positioning Injury

Risk factors may include

Disorientation, sensory/perceptual disturbances due to anesthesia
Immobilization, musculoskeletal impairments
Obesity/emaciation, edema

Possibly evidenced by

[Not applicable; presence of signs and symptoms establishes an *actual* diagnosis]

DESIRED OUTCOMES/EVALUATION CRITERIA—CLIENT WILL:

Physical Injury Severity (NOC)

Be free of injury related to perioperative disorientation.
Be free of untoward skin/tissue injury or changes lasting beyond 24–48 hr following procedure.
Report resolution of localized numbness, tingling, or changes in sensation related to positioning within 24–48 hr as appropriate.

ACTIONS/INTERVENTIONS	RATIONALE
Positioning Intraoperative (NIC)	
Independent	
Note anticipated length of procedure and customary position. Provide for potential complications.	Supine position may cause low back pain and skin pressure at heels/elbows/sacrum; lateral chest position can cause shoulder and neck pain, plus eye and ear injury on the client's downside.
Review client's history, noting age, weight/height, nutritional status, physical limitation/preexisting conditions that may affect choice of position and skin/tissue integrity during surgery.	Many conditions (e.g., lack of subcutaneous padding in elderly person, arthritis, thoracic outlet/cubital tunnel syndrome, diabetes, obesity, presence of abdominal stoma, peripheral vascular disease, level of hydration, temperature of extremities) can make individual prone to injury.
Stabilize both client cart and OR table when transferring client to and from OR table, using an adequate number of personnel for transfer and support of extremities.	Unstabilized cart/table can separate, causing client to fall. Both side rails must be in the down position for caregiver(s) to assist client transfer and prevent loss of balance.
Anticipate movement of extraneous lines and tubes during the transfer and secure or guide them into position.	Prevents undue tension and dislocation of IV lines, NG tubes, catheters, and chest tubes; maintains gravity drainage when appropriate.
Secure client on OR table with safety belt and arm protection as appropriate, explaining necessity for safety precaustions.	OR tables and arm boards are narrow, placing client at risk for injury, especially during fasciculation. Client may become resistive or combative when sedated or emerging from anesthesia, furthering potential for injury.
Protect body from contact with metal parts of the operating table.	Reduces risk of electrical injury.
Prepare equipment and padding for required position, according to operative procedure and client's specific needs. Pay special attention to pressure points of bony prominences (e.g., arms, ankles) and neurovascular pressure points and soft tissue (e.g., breasts, knees).	Depending on individual client's size, weight, and preexisting conditions, extra padding materials may be required to protect bony prominences, prevent circulatory compromise/nerve pressure, or allow for optimum chest expansion for ventilation.

ACTIONS/INTERVENTIONS	RATIONALE
Position extremities so they may be periodically checked for safety, circulation, nerve pressure, and alignment. Monitor peripheral pulses, skin color/temperature.	Prevents accidental trauma; e.g., hands, fingers, and toes could inadvertently be scraped, pinched, or amputated by moving table attachments; positional pressure of brachial plexus, peroneal, and ulnar nerves can cause serious neurovascular problems with extremities; prolonged plantar flexion may result in footdrop.
Place legs in stirrups simultaneously (when lithotomy position used), adjusting stirrup height to client's legs, maintaining symmetrical position. Pad popliteal space and heels/feet as indicated.	Prevents muscle strain, reduces risk of hip dislocation in elderly clients. Padding helps prevent peroneal and tibial nerve damage. *Note:* Prolonged positioning in stirrups may lead to compartment syndrome in calf muscles.
Provide foot board/elevate drapes off toes, decrease blanket weight on extremities. Avoid/monitor equipment and instrumentation placement on trunk/extremities during procedure.	Pressure may cause neural, circulatory, and skin integrity disruption.
Reposition slowly at transfer from table and to bed.	Myocardial depressant effect of various agents increases risk of hypotension and/or bradycardia. Controlling movement enhances volume accommodation.
Determine specific postoperative positioning guidelines; e.g., elevation of head of bed following spinal anesthesia, or nose and throat surgery, turn to unoperated side following pneumonectomy.	Reduces risk of postoperative complications; e.g., headache associated with migration of spinal anesthesia, or loss of maximal respiratory effort.

Collaborative

Recommend position changes to anesthesiologist and/or surgeon as appropriate.	Close attention to proper positioning can prevent muscle strain, nerve damage, circulatory compromise, and undue pressure on skin/bony prominences. Although the anesthesiologist is responsible for positioning, the nurse may be able to see/have more time to note client needs, and provide assistance.

NURSING DIAGNOSIS: risk for Injury

Risk factors may include

Wrong client, procedure, site, implants, equipment or materials
Interactive conditions between individual and environment
External environment; e.g., physical design, structure of environment, exposure to equipment, instrumentation, positioning, use of pharmaceutical agents
Internal environment; e.g., tissue hypoxia, abnormal blood profile/altered clotting factors, broken skin

Possibly evidenced by

[Not applicable; presence of signs and symptoms establishes an *actual* diagnosis]

DESIRED OUTCOMES/EVALUATION CRITERIA—CAREGIVER WILL:

Risk Control (NOC)

Implement surgical Universal "Time Out" Protocol
Identify individual risk factors.
Modify environment as indicated to enhance safety and use resources appropriately.

ACTIONS/INTERVENTIONS	RATIONALE
Surgical Precautions (NIC)	
Independent	
Remove dentures, partial plates or bridges, preoperatively per protocol. Inform anesthesiologist of problems with natural teeth; e.g., loose teeth.	Foreign bodies may be aspirated during endotracheal intubation/extubation.
Remove prosthetics, other devices preoperatively or after induction, depending on sensory/perceptual alterations and mobility impairment.	Contact lenses may cause corneal abrasions while under anesthesia; eyeglasses and hearing aids are obstructive and may break; however, clients may feel more in control of environment if hearing and visual aids are left on as long as possible. Artificial limbs may be damaged and skin integrity impaired if left on.
Remove jewelry preoperatively. Tape over, or isolate from skin according to institution protocol. Remove piercing hardware.	Metals conduct electrical current and provide an electrocautery hazard. Piercings may be "snagged," resulting in soft-tissue injury. In addition, loss or damage to client's personal property can easily occur in the foreign environment. *Note:* In some cases (e.g., arthritic knuckles), it may not be possible to remove rings without cutting them off. In this situation, applying tape over the ring may prevent client from "catching" ring and prevent loss of stone or damage to finger.
Verify client identity and scheduled operative procedure by comparing client chart, arm band, and surgical schedule. Verbally ascertain correct name, procedure, operative site, and physician.	Ensures correct client, procedure, and appropriate extremity/side.
Document allergies, including risk for adverse reaction to latex, tape, and prep solutions.	Reduces risk for allergic responses that may impair skin integrity or lead to life-threatening systemic reactions.
Give simple and concise directions to the sedated client.	Impairment of thought process makes it difficult for client to understand lengthy directions.
Prevent pooling of prep solutions under and around client.	Antiseptic solutions may chemically burn skin, as well as conduct electricity.
Assist with induction as needed; e.g., stand by to apply cricoid pressure during intubation or stabilize position during lumbar puncture for spinal block.	Facilitates safe administration of anesthesia.
Verify electrical safety of equipment used in surgical procedure; e.g., intact cords, grounds, medical engineering verification labels.	Malfunction of equipment can occur during the operative procedure, causing not only delays and unnecessary anesthesia but also injury or death; e.g., short circuits, faulty grounds, laser malfunctions, or laser misalignment. Periodic electrical safety checks are imperative for all OR equipment.
Place dispersive electrode (electrocautery pad) over largest available muscle mass closest to surgical site, ensuring its contact.	Provides for shortest distance and maximum conductivity to ground to prevent electrical burns.
Confirm and document correct sponge, instrument, needle, and blade counts.	Foreign bodies remaining in body cavities at closure may result in inflammation, infection, perforation, and abscess formation, and disastrous complications that can lead to death.
Laser Precautions (NIC)	
Verify credentials of laser operators for specific wavelength laser required for particular procedure.	Because of the potential hazards of laser, physician and equipment operators must be certified in the use and safety requirements of specific wavelength laser and procedure; i.e., open, endoscopic, abdominal, laryngeal, intrauterine.
Confirm presence of fire extinguishers and wet fire smothering materials when lasers are used intraoperatively.	Laser beam may inadvertently contact and ignite combustibles outside of surgical site; e.g., drapes, sponges.
Apply client and personnel eye protection before laser activation.	Eye protection for specific laser wavelength must be used to prevent injury.

ACTIONS/INTERVENTIONS	RATIONALE
Protect surrounding skin and anatomy appropriately; i.e., wet towels, sponges, dams, cottonoids.	Prevents inadvertent skin integrity disruption, hair ignition, and adjacent anatomy injury in area of laser beam use.

Specimen Management (NIC)

ACTIONS/INTERVENTIONS	RATIONALE
Handle, label, and document specimens appropriately, ensuring proper medium and transport for tests required.	The OR nurse advocate must properly identify specimens to client, site, and test to ensure validity and maximum client outcome. Loss or mislabeling of specimens renders the surgical procedure fruitless and grossly compromises further treatment and client outcome. Frozen sections, preserved or fresh examination, and cultures all have different medium and transfer requirements.

Fluid Management (NIC)

ACTIONS/INTERVENTIONS	RATIONALE
Observe intake and output (I&O) during procedure. Anticipate need for volume replacement/rapid infusion via infusion pumps and set up appropriately. Ascertain that pumps are functioning accurately.	Potential for fluid volume deficit or excess exists, affecting safety of anesthesia, tissue perfusion, organ function, and client well-being.

Collaborative

ACTIONS/INTERVENTIONS	RATIONALE
Administer IV fluids, blood/blood components, and medications, e.g., aprotinin (Trasylol), desmopressin (DDAVP), as indicated.	Maintains homeostasis and adequate level of sedation/muscle relaxation to produce optimal surgical outcome. *Note*: Trasylol or DDAVP may be given before or during procedure to reduce blood loss/promote clotting.
Collect autologous blood intraoperatively as appropriate.	Blood lost intraoperatively may be collected, filtered, and reinfused either intraoperatively or postoperatively. A continuous, closed circuit must be maintained for the procedure to be acceptable for use by Jehovah's Witnesses. *Note:* Alternatively, red blood cell (RBC) production may be increased by the administration of epoetin (Epogen, Procrit) for up to 3 weeks preoperatively, reducing the need for blood transfusion whether autologous or donated.

Surgical Precautions (NIC)

ACTIONS/INTERVENTIONS	RATIONALE
Validate surgical field medications and dosages with surgeon and anesthesiologist. Including local anesthetics with/without epinephrine in regional blocks.	Prevents administration of contraindicated medications or inappropriate dosages. *Note*: Excessive doses of local anesthetic agents may potentiate cardiovascular compromise.

NURSING DIAGNOSIS: risk for Infection

Risk factors may include

Broken skin, traumatized tissues, stasis of body fluids
Presence of pathogens/contaminants, environmental exposure, invasive procedures

Possibly evidenced by

[Not applicable; presence of signs and symptoms establishes an *actual* diagnosis]

DESIRED OUTCOMES/EVALUATION CRITERIA—CAREGIVER WILL:

KNOWLEDGE: Infection Control (NOC)

Identify individual risk factors and interventions to reduce potential for infection.
Maintain safe aseptic environment.

ACTIONS/INTERVENTIONS	RATIONALE
INFECTION CONTROL: Intraoperative (NIC)	
Independent	
Adhere to facility infection control, sterilization, and aseptic policies/procedures.	Established mechanisms designed to prevent infection.
Verify sterility of all items used in procedure as event related.	Prepackaged items may appear to be sterile; however, each item must be scrutinized for manufacturer's sterility statement or central sterile processing indicators, package integrity, environmental effect on package, and delivery techniques. *Note*: Package sterilization and expiration dates, lot/serial numbers must be documented on implant items for further follow-up if necessary.
Review laboratory studies for systemic infections and scrutinize operative area for possibility of localized infections.	Increased WBC count may indicate ongoing infection, which the operative procedure will alleviate (e.g., appendicitis, abscess, inflammation from trauma). Presence of local or systemic infection may contraindicate or adversely affect the surgical procedure and/or anesthesia e.g., upper respiratory infection (URI) , urinary tract infection (UTI), skin lesions, or unknown infections.
Verify that preoperative skin, vaginal, and bowel cleansing procedures have been done as needed depending on specific surgical procedure.	Cleansing reduces bacterial counts on the skin, vaginal mucosa, and alimentary tract.
Prepare operative site according to specific procedures.	Minimizes bacterial counts at operative site.
Examine skin for breaks or irritation, signs of infection.	Disruptions of skin integrity at or near the operative site are sources of contamination to the incision. Careful shaving/clipping as close as possible to incision time will prevent skin abrasions which potentiate skin infection.
Maintain dependent gravity drainage of indwelling catheters, tubes, and/or positive pressure of parenteral or irrigation lines.	Prevents stasis and reflux of body fluids.
Identify breaks in aseptic technique and resolve immediately on occurrence.	Contamination by environmental/personnel contact renders the sterile field unsterile, thereby increasing the risk of infection.
Utilize Universal Precautions, containing contaminated fluids/materials to specific site in operating room suite, and dispose of according to facility protocol.	Containment of blood and body fluids, tissue, and materials in contact with an infected wound/client will prevent spread of infection to environment and other clients or personnel.
Apply sterile dressing.	Prevents environmental contamination of fresh wound.
Monitor blood glucose levels of diabetic clients as indicated.	Depending on length of procedure and type of IV fluids infused, intervention may be required to maintain preferred glucose levels.
Collaborative	
Provide and document copious wound irrigation; e.g., saline, water, antibiotic, or antiseptic.	May be used intraoperatively to reduce bacterial counts at surgical site and cleanse the wound of debris; e.g., bone, ischemic tissue, bowel contaminants, toxins.
Obtain specimens for cultures/Gram stain.	Immediate identification of infective organism type by Gram stain allows prompt treatment, while more specific identification by cultures can be obtained in hours/days.
Administer antibiotics as indicated.	May be given prophylactically for suspected infection or contamination.

NURSING DIAGNOSIS: risk for imbalanced Body Temperature

Risk factors may include

Exposure to cool environment
Use of medications, anesthetic agents
Extremes of age, weight; dehydration

Possibly evidenced by

[Not applicable; presence of signs and symptoms establishes an *actual* diagnosis]

DESIRED OUTCOMES/EVALUATION CRITERIA— CLIENT WILL:

Thermoregulation (NOC)

Maintain body temperature within normal range.

ACTIONS/INTERVENTIONS	RATIONALE
TEMPERATURE REGULATION: Intraoperative (NIC)	
Independent	
Note preoperative temperature related to age and disease process.	Used as baseline for monitoring intraoperative temperature. Preoperative temperature elevations may be indicative of disease process; e.g., appendicitis, abscess, or systemic disease requiring perioperative treatment. *Note:* Effects of aging on hypothalamus may decrease fever response to infection.
Assess environmental temperature and modify as needed; e.g., provide warming blankets, increase room temperature.	Manipulating ambient air around client will prevent heat loss.
Cover skin areas outside of operative field.	Heat losses will occur as skin and mucosa are exposed to cool environmental temperatures; e.g., legs, arms, head, mucosa.
Provide cooling measures for client with preoperative or intraoperative temperature elevations.	Cool irrigations, exposure of skin surfaces to air, cooling blanket may be required to decrease temperature.
Increase ambient room temperature (e.g., to 78°F or 80°F) at conclusion of procedure.	Minimizes client heat loss when drapes are removed and client is prepared for transfer.
Apply warming blankets at emergence from anesthesia.	Inhalation anesthetics depress the hypothalamus, resulting in poor body temperature regulation.
Collaborative	
Monitor temperature throughout intraoperative phase.	Continuous warm/cool humidified inhalation anesthetics are used to maintain humidity and temperature balance within the tracheobronchial tree. Temperature fluctuations may indicate adverse response to anesthesia. *Note:* Use of atropine or scopolamine may further increase temperature.
Malignant Hyperthermia Precautions (NIC)	
Respond promptly to symptoms of malignant hyperthermia (MH); i.e., rapid temperature elevation/persistent high fever:	Prompt recognition and immediate action to control temperature is necessary to prevent serious complications/death.
Provide iced saline to all body surfaces and orifices;	Iced solution lavage of body surfaces and cavities will reduce body temperature.

ACTIONS/INTERVENTIONS	RATIONALE
Obtain dantrolene (Dantrium) for IV administration per protocol.	Immediate action to control temperature is necessary to prevent intense catabolic process associated with malignant hyperthermia.

POSTOPERATIVE

NURSING DIAGNOSIS: Ineffective Breathing Pattern

May be related to

Neuromuscular, perceptual/cognitive impairment
Decreased lung expansion, energy
Tracheobronchial obstruction

Possibly evidenced by

Changes in respiratory rate and depth
Reduced vital capacity, apnea, cyanosis, noisy respirations

DESIRED OUTCOMES/EVALUATION CRITERIA—CLIENT WILL:

Respiratory Status: Ventilation (NOC)

Establish a normal/effective respiratory pattern free of cyanosis or other signs of hypoxia.

ACTIONS/INTERVENTIONS — RATIONALE

Postanesthesia Care (NIC)

Independent

ACTIONS/INTERVENTIONS	RATIONALE
Maintain client airway by head tilt, jaw hyperextension, oral pharyngeal airway.	Prevents airway obstruction.
Auscultate breath sounds. Listen for gurgling, wheezing, crowing, and/or silence after extubation.	Lack of breath sounds is indicative of obstruction by mucus or tongue and may be corrected by positioning and/or suctioning. Diminished breath sounds suggest atelectasis. Wheezing indicates bronchospasm, whereas crowing or silence reflects partial to total laryngospasm.
Observe respiratory rate and depth, chest expansion, use of accessory muscles, retraction or flaring of nostrils, skin color; note airflow.	Ascertains effectiveness of respirations immediately so corrective measures can be initiated.
Monitor vital signs continuously.	Increased respirations, tachycardia, and/or bradycardia suggests hypoxia.
Position client appropriately, depending on respiratory effort and type of surgery.	Head elevation and left lateral Sims' position prevents aspiration of secretions/vomitus; enhances ventilation to lower lobes and relieves pressure on diaphragm
Observe for return of muscle function, especially respiratory.	After administration of intraoperative muscle relaxants, return of muscle function occurs first to the diaphragm, intercostals, and larynx; followed by large muscle groups, neck, shoulders, and abdominal muscles; then by midsize muscles, tongue, pharynx, extensors, and flexors; and finally by eyes, mouth, face, and fingers.

ACTIONS/INTERVENTIONS	RATIONALE
Initiate "stir-up" (turn, cough, deep breathe) regimen as soon as client is reactive and continue in the postoperative period.	Active deep ventilation inflates alveoli, breaks up secretions, increases O_2 transfer, and removes anesthetic gases; coughing enhances removal of secretions from the pulmonary system. *Note:* Respiratory muscles weaken and atrophy with age, possibly hampering elderly client's ability to cough or deep breathe effectively.
Observe for excessive somnolence.	Narcotic-induced respiratory depression or presence of muscle relaxants in the body may be cyclical in recurrence, creating sine-wave pattern of depression and reemergence from anesthesia. In addition, thiopental sodium (Pentothal) is absorbed in the fatty tissues, and, as circulation improves, it may be redistributed throughout the bloodstream.
Elevate head of bed as appropriate to surgical procedure. Get out of bed as soon as possible.	Promotes maximal expansion of lungs, decreasing risk of pulmonary complications.
Suction as necessary.	Airway obstruction can occur as a result of blood or mucus in throat or trachea.

Collaborative

Administer supplemental O_2 as indicated.	Maximizes oxygen for uptake to bind with Hb in place of anesthetic gases to enhance removal of inhalation agents.
Administer IV medications; e.g., naloxone (Narcan), doxapram (Dopram), or neostigmine (Prostigmin).	Narcan reverses narcotic-induced central nervous system (CNS) depression; Dopram stimulates respiratory muscles. The effects of both drugs are cyclic in nature and respiratory depression may return. Prostigmin reverses nonpolarizing muscle blockers.
Provide/maintain ventilator assistance.	Depending on cause of respiratory depression or type of surgery (e.g., pulmonary, extensive abdominal, cardiac), endotracheal tube (ET) may be left in place and mechanical ventilation maintained for a time.
Assist with use of respiratory aids; e.g., incentive spirometer.	Maximal respiratory efforts reduce potential for atelectasis and infection.

NURSING DIAGNOSIS: disturbed Sensory-Perception, (specify)/disturbed Thought Processes

May be related to

Chemical alteration: use of pharmaceutical agents, hypoxia
Therapeutically restricted environments, excessive sensory stimuli
Physiologic stress

Possibly evidenced by

Disorientation to person, place, time; change in usual response to stimuli; impaired ability to concentrate, reason, make decisions
Motor incoordination

DESIRED OUTCOMES/EVALUATION CRITERIA—CLIENT WILL:

Cognition (NOC)

Regain usual level of consciousness/mentation.
Recognize limitations and seek assistance as necessary.

ACTIONS/INTERVENTIONS	RATIONALE
Postanesthesia Care (NIC)	
Independent	
Reorient client continuously when emerging from anesthesia; confirm that surgery is completed.	As client regains consciousness, support and assurance of current physical status will help alleviate anxiety.
Speak in normal, clear voice without shouting, being aware of what you are saying. Minimize discussion of negatives (e.g., client/personnel problems) within client's hearing. Explain procedures and environmental events even if client does not seem aware.	The nurse cannot tell when client is aware, but it is thought that the sense of hearing returns before client appears fully awake, so it is important not to say things that may be misinterpreted. Providing factual information helps client preserve dignity and prepare for next recuperative activity.
Evaluate sensation/movement of extremities and trunk as appropriate.	Return of function following local or spinal nerve blocks depends on type/amount of agent used and duration of procedure.
Use bed rail padding, medical protective devices as necessary.	Provides for client safety/protection from environment during emergence state. Prevents injury to head and extremities if client becomes combative while disoriented.
Secure parenteral lines, ET tube, catheters, if present, and check for patency.	Disoriented client may pull on lines and drainage systems, disconnecting or kinking them.
Maintain quiet, calm environment.	External stimuli, such as noise, lights, touch, may cause psychic aberrations when dissociative anesthetics (e.g., ketamine) have been administered.
Investigate changes in sensorium.	Continued confusion, specific to pediatric and geriatric age groups, may reflect drug interactions, hypoxia, anxiety, pain, electrolyte imbalances, or fear.
Observe for hallucinations, delusions, depression, or an excited state.	May develop following trauma and indicate delirium, or may reflect "sundowner's syndrome" in elderly client. In client who has used alcohol/drugs to excess, may suggest impending delirium tremens.
Reassess sensory, motor and cognitive function thoroughly before discharge.	Phase II recovery/ambulatory surgical client must be able to care for self with the help of SO (if available) to prevent personal injury after discharge.
Collaborative	
Evaluate need for extended stay in postoperative recovery area or need for additional nursing care before discharge as appropriate.	Disorientation may persist, and SO may not be able to protect the client at home.
Contact/refer to case manager for alternate care options.	May not be ready/able to care for self, especially if no SO/family available to provide necessary assistance.

NURSING DIAGNOSIS: risk for deficient Fluid Volume

Risk factors may include

Restriction of oral intake (disease process/medical procedure/presence of nausea)
Loss of fluid through abnormal routes; e.g., indwelling tubes, drains; normal routes; e.g., vomiting
Loss of vascular integrity, changes in clotting ability
Extremes of age and weight

Possibly evidenced by

[Not applicable; presence of signs and symptoms establishes an *actual* diagnosis]

DESIRED OUTCOMES/EVALUATION CRITERIA—CLIENT WILL:

Hydration (NOC)

Demonstrate adequate fluid balance, as evidenced by stable vital signs, palpable pulses of good quality, normal skin turgor, moist mucous membranes, and individually appropriate urinary output.

ACTIONS/INTERVENTIONS	RATIONALE
Fluid Management (NIC)	
Independent	
Measure and record I&O (including tubes and drains). Calculate urine specific gravity as appropriate. Review intraoperative record for potential causes of imbalance.	Accurate documentation helps identify fluid losses/replacement needs and influences choice of interventions. *Note:* Ability to concentrate urine declines with age, increasing renal losses despite general fluid deficit.
Assess urinary output specifically for type of operative procedure done.	May be decreased or absent after procedures on the genitourinary system and/or adjacent structures (e.g., ureteroplasty, ureterolithotomy, abdominal or vaginal hysterectomy), indicating malfunction or obstruction of the urinary system.
Provide voiding assistance measures as needed; e.g., privacy, sitting position, running water in sink, pouring warm water over perineum.	Promotes relaxation of perineal muscles and may facilitate voiding efforts.
Monitor vital signs, noting changes in blood pressure, heart rate and rhythm, and respirations. Calculate pulse pressure.	Hypotension, tachycardia, increased respirations may indicate fluid deficit; e.g., dehydration/hypovolemia. Although a drop in blood pressure is generally a late sign of fluid deficit (hemorrhagic loss), widening of the pulse pressure may occur early, followed by narrowing as bleeding continues and systolic BP begins to fall.
Note presence of nausea/vomiting.	Women, obese clients, and those prone to motion sickness have a higher risk of postoperative nausea/vomiting. In addition, the longer the duration of anesthesia, the greater the risk for nausea. *Note:* Nausea occurring during first 12–24 hr postoperatively is frequently related to anesthesia (including regional anesthesia). Nausea persisting more than 3 days postoperatively may be related to the choice of narcotic for pain control or other drug therapy.
Inspect dressings, drainage devices at regular intervals. Assess wound for swelling.	Excessive bleeding can lead to hypovolemia/circulatory collapse. Local swelling may indicate hematoma formation/hemorrhage. *Note:* Bleeding into a cavity (e.g., retroperitoneal) may be hidden and diagnosed only via vital sign depression, client reports of pressure sensation in affected area.
Monitor skin temperature, palpate peripheral pulses.	Cool/clammy skin, weak pulses indicate decreased peripheral circulation and need for additional fluid replacement.
Collaborative	
Administer parenteral fluids, blood products (including autologous collection), and/or plasma expanders as indicated. Increase IV rate if needed.	Replaces documented fluid loss. Timely replacement of circulating volume decreases potential for complications of deficit; e.g., electrolyte imbalance, dehydration, cardiovascular collapse. *Note:* Increased volume may be required initially to support circulating volume/prevent hypotension because of decreased vasomotor tone following halothane (Fluothane) administration.

ACTIONS/INTERVENTIONS	RATIONALE
Insert/maintain urinary catheter with or without urimeter as necessary.	Provides mechanism for accurate monitoring of urinary output.
Resume oral intake gradually, or begin enteral feeding as indicated.	Following surgical procedures not involving the gastrointestional (GI) tract, the small bowel may be capable of absorbing nutrients regardless of absence of bowel sounds reflecting GI motility. If no evidence of abdominal distention, mechanical obstruction, or GI bleeding, early enteral feeding can hasten resolution of postoperative ileus and reduce risk of infection. As ileus resolves, oral fluids can be started.
Administer medications as appropriate e.g.:	
Antiemetics;	Relieves nausea/vomiting, which may impair intake and add to fluid losses. *Note:* Naloxone (Narcan) may relieve nausea related to use of anesthesthetic agents; e.g., morphine (Duramorph), fentanyl citrate (Sublimaze).
Epoetin alfa, vitamins B_{12}/C, folic acid.	Medications used to stimulate production of RBCs is begun preoperatively and may be administered postoperatively as well.
Monitor laboratory studies; e.g., Hb/Hct, electrolytes. Compare preoperative and postoperative blood studies.	Indicators of hydration/circulating volume. Preoperative anemia and/or low Hct combined with unreplaced fluid losses intraoperatively will further potentiate deficit.

NURSING DIAGNOSIS: acute Pain

May be related to

Disruption of skin, tissue, and muscle integrity; musculoskeletal/bone trauma
Presence of tubes and drains

Possibly evidenced by

Reports of pain
Alteration in muscle tone, facial mask of pain
Distraction/guarding/protective behaviors
Self-focusing, narrowed focus
Autonomic responses

DESIRED OUTCOMES/EVALUATION CRITERIA—CLIENT WILL:

Pain Level (NOC)

Report pain relieved/controlled.
Appear relaxed, able to rest/sleep and participate in activities appropriately.

ACTIONS/INTERVENTIONS	RATIONALE
Pain Management (NIC)	
Independent	
Note client's age, weight, coexisting medical/psychologic conditions, idiosyncratic sensitivity to analgesics, and intraoperative course (e.g., size/location of incision, drain placement, anesthetic agents used).	Approach to postoperative pain management is based on multiple variable factors. *Note*: Administration of the anticonvulsant lamotrigine (Lamictal) before spinal anesthesia reduces analgesic use and lowers pain-scale ratings in the postoperative client.

ACTIONS/INTERVENTIONS	RATIONALE
Review intraoperative/recovery room record for type of anesthesia and medications previously administered.	Presence of narcotics and droperidol in system potentiates narcotic analgesia, whereas inhalation anesthetics have no analgesic effects. In addition, intraoperative local/regional blocks have varying duration; e.g., 1–2 hr for regionals or up to 2–6 hr for locals.
Evaluate pain regularly (e.g., every 2 hr × 12) noting characteristics, location, and intensity (0–10 scale). Emphasize client's responsibility for reporting pain/relief of pain completely.	Provides information about need for/effectiveness of interventions. *Note:* It may not always be possible to eliminate pain; however, analgesics should reduce pain to a tolerable level. A frontal and/or occipital headache may develop 24–72 hr following spinal anesthesia, necessitating recumbent position, increased fluid intake, and notification of the anesthesiologist for alternative pain relief plan.
Note presence of anxiety/fear, and relate with nature of and preparation for procedure.	Concern about the unknown (e.g., outcome of a biopsy) and/or inadequate preparation (e.g., emergency appendectomy) can heighten client's perception of pain.
Assess vital signs, noting tachycardia, hypertension, and increased respiration, even if client denies pain.	Changes in these vital signs often indicate acute pain and discomfort. *Note:* Some clients may have a slightly lowered BP, which returns to normal range after pain relief is achieved.
Assess causes of possible discomfort other than operative procedure.	Discomfort can be caused/aggravated by presence of nonpatent indwelling catheters, NG tube, parenteral lines (bladder pain, gastric fluid and gas accumulation, and infiltration of IV fluids/medications).
Provide information about transitory nature of discomfort, as appropriate.	Understanding the cause of the discomfort (e.g., sore muscles from administration of succinylcholine may persist up to 48 hr postoperatively; sinus headache associated with nitrous oxide and sore throat due to intubation are transitory) provides emotional reassurance. *Note:* Paresthesia of body parts suggests nerve injury. Symptoms may last hours or months and require additional evaluation.
Reposition as indicated; e.g., semi-Fowler's; lateral Sims'.	May relieve pain and enhance circulation. Semi-Fowler's position relieves abdominal muscle tension and arthritic back muscle tension, whereas lateral Sims' will relieve dorsal pressures.
Provide additional comfort measures; e.g., backrub, heat/cold applications.	Improves circulation, reduces muscle tension and anxiety associated with pain. Enhances sense of well-being.
Encourage use of relaxation techniques; e.g., deep-breathing exercises, guided imagery, visualization, music.	Relieves muscle and emotional tension; enhances sense of control and may improve coping abilities.
Provide regular oral care, occasional ice chips/sips of fluids as tolerated.	Reduces discomfort associated with dry mucous membranes due to anesthetic agents, oral restrictions.
Document effectiveness and side/adverse effects of analgesia.	Respirations may decrease on administration of narcotic, and synergistic effects with anesthetic agents may occur. *Note:* Migration of epidural analgesia toward head (cephalad diffusion) may cause respiratory depression or excessive sedation.

Collaborative

Administer medications as indicated:

Analgesics IV (after reviewing anesthesia record for contraindications and/or presence of agents that may potentiate analgesia);	Analgesics given IV reach the pain centers immediately, providing more effective relief with small doses of medication. IM administration takes longer, and its effectiveness depends on absorption rates and circulation. *Note:* Narcotic dosage should be reduced by one-fourth to one-third after use of fentanyl (Innovar) or droperidol (Inapsine) to prevent profound tranquilization during first 10 hr postoperatively.
Provide around-the-clock analgesia with intermittent rescue doses;	Research supports need to administer analgesics around the clock initially to prevent rather than merely treat pain.

ACTIONS/INTERVENTIONS	RATIONALE
Patient-controlled analgesia (PCA) or epidural analgesia (PCEA);	Use of PCA necessitates detailed client instruction. PCA must be monitored closely, but is considered very effective in managing acute postoperative pain with smaller amounts of narcotic and increased client satisfaction.
Local anesthetics; e.g., epidural block/infusion;	Analgesics may be injected into the operative site, or nerves to the site may be kept blocked in the immediate postoperative phase to prevent severe pain. *Note:* Continuous epidural infusions may be used for 1–5 days following procedures that are known to cause severe pain (e.g., certain types of thoracic or abdominal surgery).
Nonsteroidal anti-inflammatory drugs (NSAIDs); e.g., aspirin, ketorolate (Toradol), diflunisal (Dolobid), naproxen (Anaprox).	Useful for mild to moderate pain or as adjuncts to opioid therapy when pain is moderate to severe. Allows for a lower dosage of narcotics, reducing potential for side effects. Use alternating schedule with NSAIDs administered between opioid doses so peak effect occurs at a different time. *Note*: May be contraindicated because of effects on coagulation.
Monitor use/effectiveness of transcutaneous electrical nerve stimulation (TENS).	TENS may be useful in reducing pain and amount of medication required postoperatively.

NURSING DIAGNOSIS: impaired Skin/Tissue Integrity

May be related to

Mechanical interruption of skin/tissues
Altered circulation, effects of medication, accumulation of drainage, altered metabolic state

Possibly evidenced by

Disruption of skin surface/layers and tissues

DESIRED OUTCOMES/EVALUATION CRITERIA—CLIENT WILL:

WOUND HEALING: Primary Intention (NOC)

Achieve timely wound healing.

KNOWLEDGE: Treatment Regimen (NOC)

Demonstrate behaviors/techniques to promote healing and to prevent complications.

ACTIONS/INTERVENTIONS	RATIONALE
Incision Site Care (NIC)	
Independent	
Reinforce initial dressing/change as indicated. Use strict aseptic techniques.	Protects wound from mechanical injury and contamination. Prevents accumulation of fluids that may cause excoriation. *Note:* Studies suggest clean techniques may be sufficient, but additional research is required before protocols are revised.

ACTIONS/INTERVENTIONS	RATIONALE
Gently remove tape (in direction of hair growth) and dressings when changing.	Reduces risk of skin trauma and disruption of wound.
Apply skin sealants/barriers before tape if needed. Use paper/silk (hypoallergenic) tape or Montgomery straps/elastic netting for dressings requiring frequent changing.	Reduces potential for skin trauma/abrasions and provides additional protection for delicate skin/tissues.
Check tension of dressings. Apply tape at center of incision to outer margin of dressing. Avoid wrapping tape around extremity.	Prevent tape skin abrasions. Wrapping tape can impair/occlude circulation to wound and to distal portion of extremity.
Inspect incision regularly, noting characteristics and integrity. Note clients at risk for delayed healing; e.g., presence of chronic obstructive pulmonary disease (COPD), anemia, obesity/malnutrition, DM, hematoma formation, vomiting, ETOH (ethyl alcohol) withdrawal; use of steroid therapy; advanced age.	Early recognition of delayed healing/developing complications may prevent a more serious situation. Incisions may heal more slowly in clients with comorbidity, or the elderly in whom reduced cardiac output decreases capillary blood flow.
Assess amounts and characteristics of drainage.	Decreasing drainage suggests evolution of healing process, whereas continued drainage or presence of bloody/odoriferous exudate suggests complications (e.g., fistula formation, hemorrhage, infection).
Maintain patency of drainage tubes; apply collection bag over drains/incisions in presence of copious or caustic drainage.	Facilitates approximation of wound edges; reduces risk of infection and chemical injury to skin/tissues.
Elevate operative area as appropriate.	Promotes venous return and limits edema formation. *Note:* Elevation in presence of venous insufficiency may be detrimental.
Splint abdominal and chest incisions/area with pillow or pad during coughing/movement.	Equalizes pressure on the wound, minimizing risk of dehiscence/rupture— especially important during stage I healing (first 3–4 days) and for incisions closed with adhesives.
Caution client not to touch incision.	Prevents contamination of area.
Cleanse skin surface (if needed) with diluted hydrogen peroxide solution, or running water and mild soap after incision is sealed.	Reduces skin contaminants; aids in removal of drainage/exudate.
Monitor blood glucose levels of diabetic clients as indicated.	These clients are at higher risk for nosocomial infections and delayed healing, and the risk increases if glucose level exceeds 220 mg/dL on the first postoperative day.

Collaborative

Apply ice if appropriate.	Reduces edema formation that may cause undue pressure on incision during initial postoperative period.
Use abdominal binder if indicated.	Provides additional support for high-risk incisions (e.g., obese client).

Wound Care (NIC)

Irrigate wound; assist with debridement as needed.	Removes infectious exudate/necrotic tissue to promote healing.
Monitor/maintain dressings; e.g., hydrogel, vacuum dressing.	May be used to hasten healing in large, draining wound/fistula, to increase client comfort, and to reduce frequency of dressing changes. Also allows drainage to be measured more accurately and analyzed for pH and electrolyte content as appropriate.

NURSING DIAGNOSIS: risk for ineffective Tissue Perfusion

Risk factors may include

Interruption of flow: arterial, venous
Hypovolemia

Possibly evidenced by

[Not applicable; presence of signs and symptoms establishes an *actual* diagnosis]

DESIRED OUTCOMES/EVALUATION CRITERIA—CLIENT WILL:

Circulation Status (NOC)

Demonstrate adequate perfusion evidenced by stable vital signs, peripheral pulses present and strong, skin warm/dry, usual mentation and individually appropriate urinary output.

ACTIONS/INTERVENTIONS	RATIONALE
Hypovolemia Management (NIC)	
Independent	
Change position slowly initially.	Vasoconstrictor mechanisms are depressed and quick movement may lead to orthostatic hypotension, especially in the early postoperative period.
Monitor vital signs; palpate peripheral pulses; note skin temperature/color and capillary refill. Evaluate urinary output/time of voiding. Document dysrhythmias.	Indicators of adequacy of circulating volume and tissue perfusion/organ function. Effects of medications/electrolyte imbalances may create dysrhythmias, impairing cardiac output and tissue perfusion.
Investigate changes in mentation/failure to achieve usual mental state.	May reflect a number of problems such as inadequate clearance of anesthetic agent, oversedation (pain medication), hypoventilation, hypovolemia, or intraoperative complications (e.g., emboli).
Embolus Precautions (NIC)	
Assist with ROM exercises, including active ankle/leg exercises.	Stimulates peripheral circulation; aids in preventing venous stasis to reduce risk of thrombus formation.
Encourage/assist with early ambulation.	Enhances circulation and return of normal organ function.
Avoid use of knee gatch/pillow under knees. Caution client against crossing legs or sitting with legs dependent for prolonged period.	Prevents stasis of venous circulation and reduces risk of thrombophlebitis.
Assess lower extremities for erythema, edema, calf tenderness (positive Homans' sign).	Circulation may be restricted by some positions used during surgery, whereas anesthetics and decreased activity alter vasomotor tone, potentiating vascular pooling and increasing risks of thrombus formation.
Collaborative	
Apply antiembolic hose/SCDs as indicated.	Promotes venous return and prevents venous stasis of legs to reduce risk of thrombosis.
Hypovolemia Management (NIC)	
Administer IV fluids/blood products as needed.	Maintains circulating volume, supports perfusion.

NURSING DIAGNOSIS: deficient Knowledge [Learning Need] regarding condition/situation, prognosis, treatment, self care, and discharge needs

May be related to

Lack of exposure/lack of recall, information misinterpretation
Unfamiliarity with information resources
Cognitive limitation

Possibly evidenced by

Questions/request for information; statement of misconception
Inaccurate follow-through of instructions/development of preventable complications

DESIRED OUTCOMES/EVALUATION CRITERIA—CLIENT WILL:

KNOWLEDGE: Disease Process (NOC)

Verbalize understanding of condition, effects of procedure and potential complications.

KNOWLEDGE: Treatment Regimen (NOC)

Verbalize understanding of therapeutic needs.
Correctly perform necessary procedures and explain reasons for actions.
Initiate necessary lifestyle changes and participate in treatment regimen.

ACTIONS/INTERVENTIONS	RATIONALE
TREATMENT: Disease Process (NIC)	
Independent	
Review specific surgery performed/procedure done and future expectations.	Provides knowledge base from which client can make informed choices.
Review and have client/SO demonstrate dressing/incision/tube care when indicated. Identify source for supplies.	Promotes competent self-care and enhances independence. *Note*: For incisions closed with a surgical zipper, patient should be instructed as to when is is appropriate to peel off the device.
Stress avoidance of environmental risk factors; e.g., exposure to crowds/persons with infections.	Reduces potential for acquired infections.
Discuss drug therapy, including use of prescribed and OTC analgesics, and resumption of herbal supplements.	Enhances cooperation with regimen, reduces risk of adverse reactions/untoward effects. *Note:* Herbal preparations such as garlic, ginseng, *Gingko biloba,* ginger, feverfew increase the risk of postoperative bleeding and are contraindicated for several days following surgery.
Identify specific activity limitations.	Prevents undue strain on operative site.
Recommend planned/progressive exercise.	Promotes return of normal function and enhances feelings of general well-being.
Schedule adequate rest periods.	Prevents fatigue and conserves energy for healing.
Review importance of nutritious diet and adequate fluid intake.	Provides elements necessary for tissue regeneration/healing and support of tissue perfusion and organ function.
Encourage cessation of smoking.	Smoking increases risk of pulmonary infections, causes vasoconstriction, and reduces oxygen-binding capacity of blood, affecting cellular perfusion and potentially impairing healing.

ACTIONS/INTERVENTIONS	RATIONALE
Identify signs/symptoms requiring medical evaluation; e.g., nausea/vomiting; difficulty voiding; fever; continued/odoriferous wound drainage; incisional swelling, erythema, or separation of edges; unresolved or changes in characteristics of pain.	Early recognition and treatment of developing complications (e.g., ileus, urinary retention, infection, delayed healing) may prevent progression to more serious or life-threatening situation.
Stress necessity of follow-up visits with providers, including therapists, laboratory.	Monitors progress of healing and evaluates effectiveness of regimen.
Include SO in teaching program/discharge planning. Provide written instructions/teaching materials. Instruct in use of and arrange for special equipment.	Provides additional resources for reference after discharge. Promotes effective self-care.
Identify available resources; e.g., homecare services, visiting nurse, Meals on Wheels, outpatient therapy, contact phone number for questions.	Enhances support for client during recovery period and provides additional evaluation of ongoing needs/new concerns.

POTENTIAL CONSIDERATIONS following surgical procedure (dependent on client's age, physical condition/presence of complications, personal resources, and life responsibilities)

Fatigue—increased energy requirements to perform activities of daily living, states of discomfort.

risk for Infection—broken skin, traumatized tissues, stasis of body fluids, presence of pathogens/contaminants, environmental exposure, invasive procedures.

Self-Care Deficit/ impaired Home Maintenance—decreased strength/endurance, pain/discomfort, unfamiliarity with neighborhood resources, inadequate support systems.

Refer also to appropriate plans of care regarding underlying condition/specific surgical procedure for additional considerations.

EXTENDED CARE

Clients in the acute care setting may be discharged to an extended-care facility. Clients requiring relatively short-term rehabilitation and those needing long-term care/permanent nursing care are included in this group. The level of care and needs of the client (e.g., physical, occupational, rehabilitation therapy; IV and respiratory support) are frequently the deciding factors in the choice of placement. Although elderly people are the primary population in extended-care facilities, increasing numbers of younger individuals are requiring care for debilitating conditions when they cannot be managed in the home setting.

RELATED CONCERNS

Acquired immunodeficiency syndrome (AIDS), page 726
Cancer, page 857
Cerebrovascular accident/stroke, page 236
Dementia of the Alzheimer's type/vascular dementia, page 945
End of life/hospice care, page 880
Multiple sclerosis, page 291
Psychosocial aspects of care, page 770
Spinal cord injury, page 271
Surgical intervention, page 788
Ventilatory assistance (mechanical), page 170

Client Assessment Database

Data depend on underlying physical/psychosocial conditions necessitating continuation of structured care.

TEACHING/LEARNING

Discharge plan considerations: May require assistance with treatments, self-care activities, health maintenance, nutritional support

Refer to section at end of plan for postdischarge considerations.

Diagnostic Studies: Dependent on age, general health, and medical condition.
CBC: Reveals problems such as infection, anemia, other abnormalities.
Chemistry profile: Evaluates general organ function/imbalances. Age-related changes include decreased serum albumin, up to 20% increase in alkaline phosphatase, decreased urine creatinine clearance.
Urinalysis: Provides information about kidney function; determines presence of urinary tract infection (UTI) or DM. *Note*: Bacteria are common in some populations, especially the elderly and bedridden, reflecting urinary stasis.
Pulse oximetry: Determines oxygenation, respiratory function.
Communicable disease screens: To rule out TB, HIV, venereal disease, hepatitis.
Drug screen: As indicated by usage to identify therapeutic or toxic levels.
Visual acuity testing: Identifies cataracts/other vision problems.
Tonometer test: Measures intraocular pressure.
Chest radiographs: Reveals size of heart, lung abnormalities/disease conditions, changes of the large blood vessels and bony structure of the chest.
ECG: Provides baseline data, detects abnormalities; e.g., ST segment and T wave changes, atrial and ventricular dysrhythmias, and various heart blocks are common in the elderly.

NURSING PRIORITIES

1. Promote physiologic and psychologic well-being.
2. Provide for security and safety.
3. Prevent complications of disease and/or aging process.
4. Promote effective coping skills and independence.
5. Encourage continuation of healthy habits, participation in plan of care to meet individual needs and wishes.

DISCHARGE GOALS

1. Client dealing realistically with current situation.
2. Homeostasis maintained.
3. Injury prevented.
4. Complications prevented/minimized.
5. Client meeting ADLs by self/with assistance as necessary.
6. Plan in place to meet needs after discharge as appropriate.

NURSING DIAGNOSIS: risk for Relocation Stress Syndrome

Risk factors may include

Decreased psychosocial or physical health status
Temporary/permanent move that may be voluntary/involuntary
Past, current, recent losses
Feelings of powerlessness
Lack of predeparture counseling
Unpredictability of experience

Possibly evidenced by

[Not applicable; presence of signs and symptoms establishes an *actual* diagnosis]

DESIRED OUTCOMES/EVALUATION CRITERIA—CLIENT WILL:

Anxiety Level (NOC)

Demonstrate appropriate range of feelings and appear relaxed.

Psychosocial Adjustment: Life Change (NOC)

Verbalize understanding of reasons for change as able.
Participate in routine and special/social events as capable.
Verbalize acceptance of situation.

ACTIONS/INTERVENTIONS	RATIONALE
Relocation Stress Reduction (NIC)	
Independent	
Provide client/SO with a copy of "A Patient's Bill of Rights" and review it with them. Discuss facility's rules; e.g., visitors, off-grounds visits, personal property.	Provides information that can foster confidence that individual rights do continue in this setting and the client is still "his or her own person" and has some control over what happens.
Ascertain if client has completed Advance Directives. Provide information as appropriate.	Assures client/family wishes will be known to provide direction to caregivers.
Determine client/SO attitude toward admission to facility and expectations for the future.	If this is expected to be a temporary placement, client/SO concerns will be different than if placement is permanent. When client is giving up own home and way of life, feelings of helplessness, loss, and grief are to be expected.
Help family/SO to be honest with client regarding admission. Be clear about actions/events.	Family may have difficulty dealing with decision/reality of permanent placement and may avoid discussing situation with client. Honesty decreases "surprises," assists in maintaining trust, and may enhance coping.
Identify support person(s) important to client and include in care activities, mealtime, and so on, as appropriate.	During adjustment period/times of stress, client may benefit from presence of trusted individual who can provide reassurance and reduce sense of isolation.
Assess level of anxiety and discuss reasons when possible.	Identifying specific problems enables individual to deal more realistically with them and care provider to intervene as necessary; e.g., client who is being neglected or abused or has unrelieved pain may be very anxious and afraid or unable to verbalize.
Develop nurse-client relationship.	Trusting relationships among client/SO/staff promotes optimal care and support.
Make time to listen to client about concerns, and encourage free expression of feelings; e.g., anger, hostility, fear, and loneliness.	Being available in this way allows client to feel accepted, begin to acknowledge and deal with feelings related to circumstances of admission.
Acknowledge reality of situation and feelings of client. Accept expressions of anger while limiting aggressive, acting-out behavior.	Permission to express feelings allows for beginning resolution. Acceptance promotes sense of self-worth. *Note*: Psychosocial and/or physiologic disturbances can occur as a result of transfer from one environment to another, especially if the move is unexpected/involuntary.
Identify strengths and successful coping behaviors and incorporate into problem-solving.	Building on past successes increases likelihood of positive outcome in present situation. Enhances sense of control and management of current deficits.
Orient to physical aspects of facility, schedules, and activities. Introduce to roommate(s) and staff. Give explanation of roles.	Getting acquainted is an important part of admission. Knowledge of where things are and whom client can expect assistance from can be helpful in reducing anxiety.
Determine client's usual schedule and incorporate into facility routine as much as possible.	Consistency provides reassurance and may lessen confusion and enhance cooperation.
Provide above information in written or audiovisual form as well.	Overload of information is difficult to remember. Client can refer to written or audiovisual materials as needed to refresh memory/learn new information.
Give careful thought to room placement. Provide help and encouragement in placing client's own belongings around room. Do not transfer from one room to another without client approval/documentable need.	Location, roommate compatibility, and place for personal belongings are important considerations for helping the client feel "at home." Changes are often met with resistance and can result in emotional upset and decline in physical condition. *Note*: Persons with severe behavioral problems/cognitive dysfunctions may require a private room.
Note behavior, presence of suspiciousness/paranoia, irritability, defensiveness. Compare to SO's description of customary responses.	Increased stress, physical discomfort, and fatigue may temporarily exacerbate mental deterioration (cognitive inaccessibility) and further impair communication (social inaccessibility). This represents a catastrophic episode that can escalate into a panic state and violence.

ACTIONS/INTERVENTIONS	RATIONALE
Be aware of escalating anxiety, presence of delirium. Look for possible causes.	Common causes of delirium include drug toxicity, electrolyte imbalances, withdrawal states (alcohol, other drugs), pain/trauma (especially hip fractures), and advanced disease resulting in organ failure.

Collaborative

ACTIONS/INTERVENTIONS	RATIONALE
Refer to social service or other appropriate agency for assistance. Have case manager, social worker discuss ramifications of Medicare/Medicaid if client is eligible for these resources.	Often client is not aware of the resources available, and providing current information about individual coverage/limitations and other possible sources of support will assist with adjustment to new situation.

NURSING DIAGNOSIS: anticipatory Grieving

May be related to

Perceived, actual, or potential loss of physiopsychosocial well-being, personal possessions, or SO; cultural beliefs about aging/debilitation

Possibly evidenced by

Denial of feelings, depression, sorrow, guilt
Alterations in the activity level, sleep patterns, eating habits, libido

DESIRED OUTCOMES/EVALUATION CRITERIA—CLIENT WILL:

Grief Resolution (NOC)

Identify and express feelings appropriately.
Progress through the grieving process.
Enjoy the present and plan for the future, one day at a time.

Grief Work Facilitation (NIC)

Independent

ACTIONS/INTERVENTIONS	RATIONALE
Assess emotional state. Note cultural beliefs, expectations.	Anxiety and depression are common reactions to changes/losses associated with long-term illness or debilitating condition. In addition, changes in neurotransmitter levels (e.g., increased monoamine oxidase [MAO] and serotonin levels with decreased norepinephrine) may potentiate depression in elderly clients. Personal expectations may affect response to change.
Make time to listen to the client. Encourage free expression of hopeless feelings and desire to die.	It is more helpful to allow these feelings to be expressed and dealt with than to deny or ignore them.
Assess suicidal potential.	May be related to physical disease, social isolation, and grief. *Note:* Studies indicate women are three times as likely to attempt suicide; however, men are three times as likely to succeed.
Involve SO in discussions and activities to the level of their willingness.	When SOs are involved, there is more potential for successful problem-solving. *Note:* SO may not be available or may not choose to be involved.

ACTIONS/INTERVENTIONS	RATIONALE
Provide liberal touching/hugs as individually accepted.	Conveys sense of concern/closeness to reduce feelings of isolation and enhance sense of self-worth. *Note*: Touch may be viewed as a threat by some clients and escalate feelings of anger.
Identify spiritual concerns. Discuss available resources and encourage participation in religious activities as appropriate.	Search for meaning is common to those facing changes in life. Participation in religious/spiritual activities can provide sense of direction and peace of mind.
Assist with/plan for specifics as necessary (e.g., Advance Directives to determine code status/Living Will wishes, making of will, funeral arrangements if appropriate).	Having these issues resolved can help client/SO deal with the grieving process and may provide peace of mind.

Collaborative

Refer to other resources as indicated; e.g., spiritual advisor/parish nurse, case manager/social worker.	May need further assistance to resolve some problems.

NURSING DIAGNOSIS: impaired Memory/disturbed Thought Processes

May be related to

Physiologic changes of aging, loss of cells/brain atrophy, decreased blood supply, altered sensory input
Pain, effects of medications
Psychologic conflicts: Disrupted life pattern

Possibly evidenced by

Slower reaction times, gradual memory loss, altered attention span; disorientation; inability to follow
Altered sleep patterns
Personality changes

DESIRED OUTCOMES/EVALUATION CRITERIA—CLIENT WILL:

Cognition (NOC)

Maintain/improve usual reality orientation.

Distorted Thought Self-Control (NOC)

Recognize changes in thinking and behavior.
Identify interventions to deal effectively with situation/deficits.

ACTIONS/INTERVENTIONS — RATIONALE

Cognitive Stimulation (NIC)

Independent

ACTIONS/INTERVENTIONS	RATIONALE
Allow adequate time for client to respond to questions/comments and to make decisions.	Reaction time may be slowed with aging (changes in metabolism/cerebral blood flow) or with brain injuries and some neuromuscular conditions.
Discuss happenings of the past. Place familiar objects in room. Encourage the display of photographs/photo albums, frequent visits from SO/friends.	Events of the past may be more readily recalled by the elderly client, because long-term memory usually remains intact. Reminiscence/life review and companionship are beneficial to clients.

ACTIONS/INTERVENTIONS	RATIONALE
Note client's problem of short-term memory loss, and provide with aids (e.g., calendars, clocks, room signs, pictures) to assist in continual reorientation.	Short-term memory loss presents a challenge for nursing care, especially if the client cannot remember such things as how to use the call bell or how to get to the bathroom. This problem is not in client's control but may be less frustrating if simple reminders are used. It may be helpful for older person (and family) to know that short-term memory loss is common and is not necessarily a sign of "senility."
Evaluate individual stress level and deal with it appropriately.	Stress level may be greatly increased because of recent losses; e.g., poor health, death of spouse/companion, loss of home. In addition, some conflicts that occur with age come from previously unresolved problems that may need to be dealt with now.
Assess physical status/psychiatric symptoms. Institute interventions appropriate to findings.	Not all mental changes are the result of aging, and it is important to rule out physical causes before accepting these as unchangeable. May be pain (often unreported/ underestimated), metabolic, toxic, drug-induced (e.g., antiparkinson agents, tricyclic antidepressants), or the result of infectious, cardiac, or respiratory disorders.
Reorient to person/place and time as appropriate.	Helps client maintain focus.
Have client repeat verbal/written instructions.	Verifies hearing/ability to read and comprehend.
Note cyclic changes in mentation/behavior; e.g., evening confusion, picking at bedclothes, pacing, shouting, wandering aimlessly.	"Sundowner syndrome" may occur in response to visual/hearing deficits enhanced by declining light, fatigue, inflexible institution schedules, peak/trough drug levels, dehydration, and electrolyte imbalances.
Involve in regular exercise, activity, and diversional programs.	Promotes release of endorphins, enhancing sense of well-being, and can improve thinking abilities. *Note*: Studies suggest withdrawn and inactive clients are at greater risk of evening confusion.
Schedule at least one rest period per day.	Prevents fatigue; enhances general well-being.
Provide brighter lighting in room/area by midafternoon (e.g., 3 pm) or earlier on cloudy/winter days.	Maximizes visual perception; may limit evening confusion.
Turn off lights at bedtime. Provide night lights where appropriate.	Reinforces "sleep time" while meeting safety needs.
Support client's involvement in own care. Provide opportunity for choices on a daily basis.	Choice is a necessary component in everyday life. Cognitively impaired clients may respond with aggressive behavior as they lose control in their lives.

Collaborative

Review results of laboratory/diagnostic tests; e.g., electrolytes, thyroid studies, full drug screen, computerized tomography (CT) scan.	Aids in establishing cause of changes in mentation and determining treatment options. *Note*: These tests can identify the causes of dementia in 90% of the cases.
Administer medications as indicated; e.g., tacrine (Cognex), donepazil (Aricept).	These drugs may fight dementia by blocking chemical breakdown of acetylcholine and improving cholinergic function. Aricept has been shown to improve intellectual ability and daily functioning in mild to moderate Alzheimer's disease (as assessed by Alzheimer's Disease Assessment Scale [ADAS-Cog]). (Refer to CP: Dementia of the Alzheimer's Type/Vascular Dementia.)

NURSING DIAGNOSIS: compromised family Coping

May be related to

Placement of family member in extended care facility
Temporary family disorganization and role changes
Situational/transitional crises SO may be facing
Client providing little support for SO
Prolonged disease or disability progression that exhausts the supportive capacity of SOs

Possibly evidenced by

SO describes significant preoccupation with personal reactions; e.g., fear, anticipatory grief, guilt, anxiety
SO attempts assistive/supportive behaviors with unsatisfactory results
SO withdraws from client
SO displays protective behavior disproportionate (too little or too much) to client's abilities/need for autonomy

DESIRED OUTCOMES/EVALUATION CRITERIA—FAMILY WILL:

Family Coping (NOC)

Identify/verbalize resources within themselves to deal with the situation.
Interact appropriately with the client and staff, providing support and assistance as indicated.
Verbalize knowledge and understanding of situation.

ACTIONS/INTERVENTIONS	RATIONALE
Family Support (NIC)	
Independent	
Introduce staff and provide SO with information about facility and care. Be available for questions. Provide tour of facility.	Helpful to establish beginning relationships. Offers opportunities for enhancing feelings of involvement.
Determine involvement and availability of family/SO.	Clarifies expectations and abilities, identifies needs.
Encourage SO participation in care at level of desire and capability and within limits of safety. Include in social events/celebrations.	Helps family to feel at ease and allows them to feel supportive and a part of the client's life.
Accept choices of SO regarding level of involvement in care.	Families may choose to ignore client or may project feelings of guilt regarding placing client in facility by criticizing staff. *Note*: Feelings of dissatisfaction with the staff may be transferred back to the client.
Evaluate SO's/caregiver's level of stress/coping abilities, especially before planning for discharge.	Caring for/about clients with chronic/debilitating conditions places a heavy strain on SO. Although support groups may be very helpful, learning stress management techniques may be more effective in strengthening individual coping as the focus is on the SO rather than the SO-client relationship.
Support the caregiver with attention, compassion, time, respect, honesty, advocacy, and understanding.	Nursing interventions need to prepare the caregivers for the challenges they face, and meet their needs for compassion and caring.
Identify availability and use of community support systems.	Helps determine areas of need and provides information regarding additional resources to enhance coping.
Be aware of staff's own feelings of anger and frustration about client's/SO's choices and goals that differ from those of staff, and deal with them appropriately.	Group care conferences or individual counseling may be helpful in problem-solving.
Collaborative	
Inform SO of services available to them (meal tickets, family cooking time, group care conference, visiting nurse, caseworker, social services).	Promotes feeling of involvement; eases transition in adjustment to client's admission to homecare or facility care.
Advise caregivers of resources available, such as Eldercare Locator, Seniornet, Today's Caregiver, Caregiver Network, Inc.	Helps nurses, clients, and caregivers feel supported and able to provide more skillful care.

NURSING DIAGNOSIS: risk for Poisoning, [drug toxicity]

Risk factors may include

Reduced metabolism; impaired circulation; precarious physiologic balance, presence of multiple diseases/organ involvement
Use of multiple prescribed/OTC drugs

Possibly evidenced by

[Not applicable; presence of signs and symptoms establishes an *actual* diagnosis.]

DESIRED OUTCOMES/EVALUATION CRITERIA—CLIENT WILL:

RISK CONTROL: Drug Use (NOC)

Maintain prescribed drug regimen free of untoward side effects.

ACTIONS/INTERVENTIONS	RATIONALE
Medication Management (NIC)	
Independent	
Determine allergies, medication and other drug use history.	Helps avoid repetition/creation of problems.
Review resources (e.g., drug manuals, pharmacist) for information about toxic symptoms and side effects. List drug actions and interactions and idiosyncrasies; e.g., medications that are given with or without foods, as well as those that should not be crushed.	Provides information about drugs being taken and identifies possible interactions. Toxicity can be increased in the debilitated and older client with symptoms not as apparent.
Discuss self-administration of/access to OTC products.	Limits interference with prescribed regimen/desired drug action and organ function. May prevent inadvertent overdosing/toxic reactions. *Note*: Appropriate use of OTC products kept at bedside or via free access at nurses' station fosters independence and enhances sense of control and self-esteem.
Identify swallowing problems or reluctance to take tablets or capsules.	May not be able to or want to take medication.
Give pills in a spoonful of soft foods; e.g., applesauce, ice cream; or use liquid form of medication if available.	Ensures proper dosage if client is unable to/does not like to swallow pills.
Open capsules or crush tablets only when appropriate.	Should not be done unless absolutely necessary because this may alter absorption of medications; e.g. enteric-coated tablets may be absorbed in stomach when crushed, instead of in the intestines.
Make sure medication has been swallowed.	Ensures effective therapeutic use of medication and prevents pill hoarding.
Observe for changes in condition/behavior.	Behavior may be only indication of drug toxicity, and early identification of problems provides for appropriate intervention. *Note*: Elderly individuals have increased sensitivity to anticholinergic effects of medications; therefore, use of anticholinergics, antiparkinson agents, benzodiazepines, CNS depressants, and tricyclic antidepressants may cause delirium/confusion.
Use discretion in the administration of sedatives.	A quiet place where the client can pace, or seclusion, may be more helpful. If client is destructive or excessively disruptive, pharmacological or mechanical control measures may be required. Convenience of the staff is never a reason for sedating client; however, client safety and rights of other clients need to be taken into consideration.

ACTIONS/INTERVENTIONS	RATIONALE
Collaborative	
Review drug regimen routinely with physician and pharmacist.	Provides opportunity to alter therapy (e.g., reduce dosage, discontinue medications) as client's needs and organ functions change.
Obtain serum drug levels as indicated.	Determines therapeutic/toxicity levels.

NURSING DIAGNOSIS: impaired verbal Communication

May be related to

Degenerative changes (e.g., reduced cerebral circulation, hearing loss); progressive neurologic disease (e.g., Parkinson's disease, Alzheimer's disease)
Laryngectomy/tracheostomy; stroke, traumatic brain injury

Possibly evidenced by

Impaired articulation; difficulty with phonation; inability to modulate speech, find words, name, or identify objects (aphasia, dysarthria)
Diminished hearing ability

DESIRED OUTCOMES/EVALUATION CRITERIA—CLIENT WILL:

Communication (NOC)

Establish method of communication by which needs can be expressed.
Demonstrate congruent verbal and nonverbal communication.

ACTIONS/INTERVENTIONS	RATIONALE
COMMUNICATION ENHANCEMENT: Speech Deficit (NIC)	
Independent	
Assess reason for lack of communication, including CNS and neuromuscular functioning, gag/swallow reflexes, hearing, teeth/mouth problems.	Identification of the problem is essential to appropriate intervention. Sometimes clients do not want to talk, may think they talk when they do not, may expect others to know what they want, may not be able to comprehend or be understood.
Determine whether client is bilingual and what language is primary.	With declining cerebral function/diminished thought processes, increased level of stress, client may mix languages/revert to original language.
Investigate how SO communicates with the client.	Provide opportunity to develop/continue effective communication patterns, which have already been established.
Assess client knowledge base and level of comprehension. Treat the client as an adult, avoiding pity and impatience.	Knowing how much to expect of the client can help to avoid frustration and unreasonable demands for performance. However, having an expectation that the client will understand may help raise level of performance.
Establish therapeutic nurse-client relationship through Active-Listening, being available for problem solving.	Aids in dealing with communication problems.
Make client aware of presence when entering the room by speaking, turning a light off and on/touching client or mattress as appropriate.	Getting attention is the first step in communication.
Make eye contact, place self at or below client's level, and speak face to face.	Conveys interest and promotes contact.

ACTIONS/INTERVENTIONS	RATIONALE
Speak slowly and distinctly, using simple sentences, yes-or-no questions. Avoid speaking loudly or shouting. Supplement with written communication when possible/needed. Allow sufficient time for reply; remain relaxed with client.	Assists in comprehension and overall communication. Client may respond poorly to high-pitched sounds; shouting also obscures consonants and amplifies vowels.
Use other creative measures to assist in communication; e.g., picture chart/alphabet board, sign language, lip reading when appropriate.	Many options are available, depending on individual situation. *Note*: Sign language also may be used effectively with other than hearing-impaired individuals.

COMMUNICATION ENHANCEMENT: Hearing Deficit (NIC)

Check ears for excess cerumen.	Hardened earwax may decrease hearing acuity and causes tinnitus.
Ascertain if client has/uses hearing aid.	Client may have, but not use, hearing aid (e.g., may not fit well, may need batteries).
Be aware that behavioral problems may be associated with hearing loss.	Anger, explosive temper outbursts, frustration, embarrassment, depression, withdrawal, and paranoia may be attempts to deal with communication problems.

Collaborative

Refer to speech therapists, ear/nose/throat physician, or for audiometry as needed.	Determines extent of hearing loss and whether a hearing aid is appropriate. May be helpful to a client and staff in improving communication. *Note*: Some sources believe 90% of the clients in extended care facilities have some degree of hearing loss (presbycusis) because this is a common age change. Hearing aids are most effective with conductive losses and may help with sensorineural losses.

NURSING DIAGNOSIS: disturbed Sleep Pattern

May be related to

Internal factors: illness, psychologic stress, inactivity
External factors: environmental changes, facility routines

Possibly evidenced by

Reports of difficulty in falling asleep/not feeling well-rested
Interrupted sleep, awakening earlier than desired
Change in behavior/performance, increasing irritability, listlessness

DESIRED OUTCOMES/EVALUATION CRITERIA—CLIENT WILL:

Sleep (NOC)

Report improvement in sleep/rest pattern.
Verbalize increased sense of well-being and feeling rested.

ACTIONS/INTERVENTIONS — RATIONALE

Sleep Enhancement (NIC)

Independent

ACTIONS/INTERVENTIONS	RATIONALE
Ascertain usual sleep habits and changes that are occurring.	Determines need for action and helps identify appropriate interventions.

ACTIONS/INTERVENTIONS	RATIONALE
Provide comfortable bedding and some of own possessions; e.g., pillow, afghan.	Increases comfort for sleep and physiologic/psychologic support.
Establish new sleep routine incorporating old pattern and new environment.	When new routine contains as many aspects of old habits as possible, stress and related anxiety may be reduced, enhancing sleep.
Match with roommate who has similar sleep patterns and nocturnal needs.	Decreases likelihood that "night owl" roommate may delay client's falling asleep or create interruptions that cause awakening.
Encourage some light physical activity during the day. Make sure client stops activity several hours before bedtime as individually appropriate.	Daytime activity can help client expend energy and be ready for nighttime sleep; however, continuation of activity close to bedtime may act as a stimulant, delaying sleep.
Promote bedtime comfort regimens; e.g., warm bath and massage, a glass of warm milk, wine/brandy at bedtime.	Promotes a relaxing, soothing effect. *Note*: Milk has soporific qualities, enhancing synthesis of serotonin, a neurotransmitter that helps client fall asleep faster and sleep longer.
Instruct in relaxation measures.	Helps induce sleep.
Reduce noise and light.	Provides atmosphere conducive to sleep.
Encourage position of comfort, assist in turning.	Repositioning alters areas of pressure and promotes rest.
Lower bed and position one side against wall when possible. Avoid use of side rails.	May have fear of falling because of change in size and height of bed. *Note*: Side rails place client at risk for falling when climbing over rails or possible entrapment.
Avoid/limit interruptions (e.g., awakening for medications or therapies).	Uninterrupted sleep is more restful, and client may be unable to return to sleep when wakened.

Collaborative

Administer sedatives, hypnotics with caution as indicated.	May be given to help client sleep/rest during transition period from home to new setting. *Note*: Avoid habitual use because these drugs decrease REM (rapid eye movement) sleep time.

NURSING DIAGNOSIS: altered Nutrition: less/more than body requirements

May be related to

Impaired dentition, dulling of senses of smell and taste
Cognitive limitations, depression
Inability to feed self effectively
Sedentary activity level

Possibly evidenced by

Reported/observed dysfunctional eating patterns
Weight under/over ideal for height and frame
Poor muscle tone, pale conjunctiva/mucous membranes
Signs/symptoms of vitamin/protein deficits, electrolyte imbalances

DESIRED OUTCOMES/EVALUATION CRITERIA—CLIENT WILL:

Nutritional Status (NOC)

Maintain normal weight or progress toward weight goal with normalization of laboratory values and be free of signs of malnutrition/obesity.
Demonstrate eating patterns/behaviors to maintain appropriate weight.

ACTIONS/INTERVENTIONS	RATIONALE
Nutrition Management (NIC)	
Independent	
Assess causes of weight loss/gain; e.g., dysphagia due to decreased saliva production, neurogenic/psychogenic disturbances, tumors, muscular dysfunction, altered senses of smell and taste, or dysfunctional eating patterns related to depression.	Aids in creating plan of care/choice of interventions. *Note*: In elderly clients saliva secretion may be decreased by as much as 66%, taste buds atrophy with reduced sensitivity to sweet and salt.
Check state of client's dental health periodically, including fit and condition of dentures, if present.	Oral infections/dental problems, shrinking gums, reaction of client's oral mucous membranes and saliva (associated with medications/treatments), loss of teeth or ill-fitting dentures can all decrease client's ability to chew.
Weigh on admission and on a regular basis.	Monitors nutritional state and effectiveness of interventions.
Monitor total caloric intake as indicated.	If dietary plan is ineffective in meeting individual goals, calorie count/food diary may help identify problem areas.
Observe condition of skin; note muscle wasting, brittle nails, dry, lifeless hair, and signs of poor healing.	Reflects lack of adequate nutrition.
Evaluate activity pattern.	Extremes of exercise (e.g., sedentary life, continuous pacing) affect caloric needs.
Incorporate favorite foods and maintain as near-normal food consistency as possible; e.g., soft or finely ground food with gravy or liquid added. Avoid baby food whenever possible.	Aids in maintaining intake, especially when mouth and dental problems exist. Baby food is often unpalatable and can decrease appetite and lower self-esteem.
Encourage the use of spices (other than sodium) to client's personal taste.	Reduction in number and acuity of taste buds results in food tasting bland and decreases enjoyment of food and desire to eat.
Provide small, frequent feedings as indicated.	Decreased gastric motility causes client to feel full and reduces intake.
Serve hot foods hot and cold foods cold.	Foods served at the proper temperature are more palatable, and enjoyment may increase appetite.
Promote a pleasant environment for eating, with company if possible.	Eating is in part a social event, and appetite can improve with increased socialization.
Have healthy snack foods (e.g., cheese, crackers, soup, fruit) available on a 24-hr basis.	Helps meet individual needs and enhances intake with caloric recommendations.
Plan for social events; provide for snacks even when working to reduce total calories.	Eating is part of socialization, and being able to respond to body's needs enhances sense of control and willingness to participate in dietary program.
Encourage exercise and activity program within individual ability.	Promotes sense of well-being and may improve appetite.
Collaborative	
Consult with dietitian.	Aids in establishing specific nutritional program to meet individual client needs.
Provide balanced diet with individually appropriate protein, complex carbohydrates, and calories. Include supplements between meals as indicated.	Adjustments may be needed to deal with the body's decreased ability to process protein, as well as decreased metabolic rate and levels of activity. *Note*: Reduced production of salivary ptyalin inhibits digestion of complex carbohydrates in elderly individuals affecting dietary plan. In addition, delayed insulin release by the pancreas and reduced peripheral sensitivity to insulin decrease glucose tolerance.
Administer vitamin/mineral supplements as appropriate.	With age, renal and other regulatory systems cannot compensate as well for errors in intake. Mineral requirements change as hormone levels, metabolism, and GI function change. In addition, absorption can be impaired by medication use and chronic illness.
Refer for dental care routinely and as needed.	Maintenance of oral/dental health and good dentition can enhance intake.

NURSING DIAGNOSIS: Self-Care Deficit: (specify)

May be related to

Depression, discouragement, loss of mobility, general debilitation, perceptual/cognitive impairment

Possibly evidenced by

Inability to manage ADLs, unkempt appearance

DESIRED OUTCOMES/EVALUATION CRITERIA—CLIENT WILL:

Self-Care: Activities of Daily Living (ADL) (NOC)

Perform self-care activities within level of own ability.
Demonstrate techniques/lifestyle changes to meet own needs.
Use resources effectively.

ACTIONS/INTERVENTIONS	RATIONALE
Self-Care Assistance (NIC)	
Independent	
Determine current capabilities (0–4 scale) and barriers to participation in self-care.	Comprehensive functional assessment includes independent performance of basic ADLs, social activities, sensory abilities, cognition, and ability to ambulate.
Involve client in formulation of plan of care at level of ability.	Enhances sense of control and aids in cooperation and maintenance of independence.
Encourage self-care. Work within present abilities; do not pressure client, but encourage client to reach beyond current capabilities. Provide adequate time for client to complete tasks. Have expectation of improvement and assist as needed.	Doing for oneself enhances feeling of self-worth. Failure can produce discouragement and depression.
Provide and promote privacy, including during bathing/showering.	Modesty may lead to reluctance to participate in care or perform activities in the presence of others.
Use specialized equipment as needed; e.g., tub transfer seat, grab bars, raised toilet seat.	Enhances ability to move/perform activities safely.
Give tub bath, using walk-in tub, or two-person or mechanical lift if necessary. Use shower chair and spray attachment as appropriate. Avoid chilling.	Provides safety for those who cannot get into the tub alone. Shower may be more feasible for some clients, though it may be less beneficial/desirable to the client. Elderly/debilitated clients are more prone to chilling.
Shampoo/style hair as needed. Provide/assist with manicure.	Aids in maintaining appearance. Shampooing may be required more/less frequently than bathing schedule.
Encourage use of barber/beauty salon if client is able.	Enhances self-image and self-esteem, preserving dignity of the client.
Acquire clothing with modified fasteners as indicated.	Use of Velcro instead of buttons/shoe laces can facilitate process of dressing/undressing.
Encourage/assist with routine mouth/teeth care daily. Promote/provide denture care on a regular basis (e.g. cleaning, disinfecting, storage, repair, use of dental adhesive). Use alternate oral hygiene measures as indicated (e.g. suction toothbrush, backward-bent toothbrush, chlorhexidine and fluoride mouthrinses, regular suctioning).	Reduces risk of gum disease/tooth loss, enhances oral health, promotes proper fitting and use of dentures.

ACTIONS/INTERVENTIONS	RATIONALE
Collaborative	
Consult with physical/occupational therapists and rehabilitation specialist.	Useful in establishing exercise/activity program and in identifying assistive devices to meet individual needs/safety concerns and in facilitating independence.

NURSING DIAGNOSIS: risk for impaired Skin Integrity

Risk factors may include

General debilitation, reduced mobility, changes in skin and muscle mass associated with aging, sensory/motor deficits
Altered circulation, edema, poor nutrition
Excretions/secretions (bladder and bowel incontinence)
Problems with self-care

Possibly evidenced by

[Not applicable; presence of signs and symptoms establishes an *actual* diagnosis.]

DESIRED OUTCOMES/EVALUATION CRITERIA—CLIENT WILL:

Risk Control (NOC)

Maintain intact skin.
Identify individual risk factors.
Demonstrate behaviors/techniques to prevent skin breakdown/facilitate healing.

ACTIONS/INTERVENTIONS	RATIONALE
Skin Surveillance (NIC)	
Independent	
Inspect skin, tissues, and mucous membranes routinely.	Provides opportunity for early intervention in potential high-risk population, who may have thin, less elastic, and more fragile skin and tissues.
Anticipate and use preventive measures in clients who are at risk for skin breakdown, such as anyone who is thin, obese, aging, or debilitated.	Decubitus ulcers are difficult to heal, and prevention is the best treatment.
Assess nutritional status and initiate corrective measures as indicated. Provide balanced diet; e.g., adequate protein, vitamins, and minerals.	A positive nitrogen balance and improved nutritional state can help prevent skin breakdown and promote ulcer healing. *Note*: May need additional calories and protein if draining ulcer present.
Maintain strict skin hygiene, using mild, nondetergent soap (if any), drying gently and thoroughly, and lubricating with lotion or emollient.	A daily bath is usually not necessary in elderly clients because there is atrophy of sebaceous and sweat glands, and bathing may create dry skin problems. However, as epidermis thins with age, cleansing and use of lubricants is needed to keep skin soft/pliable and protect susceptible skin from breakdown.
Change position frequently in bed and chair. Recommend 10 min of exercise each hour and/or perform passive ROM.	Improves circulation, muscle tone, and joint motion and promotes client participation.
Use a rotation schedule in turning client. Use draw/turn sheet. Pay close attention to client's comfort level.	Allows for longer periods free of pressure; prevents shearing or tearing motions that can damage fragile tissues. *Note*: Use of prone position depends on client tolerance and should be maintained for only a short time.

ACTIONS/INTERVENTIONS	RATIONALE
Massage bony prominences gently with lotion or cream.	Enhances circulation to tissues, increases vascular tone, and reduces tissue edema. *Note*: Contraindicated if area is pink/red because cellular damage may occur. Gentle massage around area may stimulate circulation to impaired tissues.
Keep sheets and bedclothes clean, dry, and free from wrinkles, crumbs, and other irritating material.	Avoids friction/abrasion injury of skin.
Use elbow/heel protectors, foam/water or gel pads, sheepskin for positioning in bed and when up in chair.	Reduces risk of tissue abrasions and decreases pressure that can impair cellular blood flow. Promotes circulation of air along skin surface to dissipate heat/moisture.
Provide for safety during ambulation, using appropriate adaptive devices; e.g., walker, cane.	Loss of muscle strength and flexibility and physical disease process/debilitation may result in impaired coordination.
Limit exposure to temperature extremes/use of heating pad or ice pack.	Decreased sensitivity to pain/heat/cold increases risk of tissue trauma.
Examine feet and nails routinely and provide foot and nail care as indicated:	Foot problems are common among clients who are elderly, diabetic, bedfast, and/or debilitated.
Keep nails cut short and smooth;	Jagged, rough nails can cause tissue damage/infection.
Use lotion, softening cream on feet;	Prevents drying/cracking of skin; promotes maintenance of healthy skin.
Check for fissures between toes, swab with hydrogen peroxide or dust with antiseptic powder, and place a wisp of cotton between the toes;	Prevents spread of infection and/or tissue injury.
Rub feet with witch hazel or a mentholated preparation and have client wear lightweight cotton stockings.	Even though rash may not be present, burning and itching may be a problem. *Note*: Witch hazel may be contraindicated if skin is dry.
Inspect skin surface/folds (especially when incontinence pad/pants are used) and bony prominences routinely. Increase preventive measures when reddened areas are noticed.	Skin breakdown can occur quickly with potential for infection and necrosis, possibly involving muscle and bone. There is increased risk of redness/irritation around legs due to elastic bands in adult incontinence pads/pants.
Continue regimen for redness and irritation when break in skin occurs.	Aggressive measures are important because decubitus ulcers can develop in a matter of a few hours.
Observe for decubitus ulcer development, and treat immediately according to protocol.	Timely intervention may prevent extensive damage.

Collaborative

Provide waterbed, alternating pressure/egg-crate or gel mattress, and pad for chair.	Provides protection and improved circulation by decreasing amount of pressure on tissues.
Monitor Hb/Hct and blood glucose levels.	Anemia, dehydration, and elevated glucose levels are factors in skin breakdown and can impair healing.
Refer to podiatrist as indicated.	May need professional care for such problems as ingrown toenails, corns, bony changes, skin/tissue ulceration.
Provide whirlpool treatments as appropriate.	Increases circulation and has a debriding action.
Assist with topical applications; e.g., hydrogel dressings, skin barrier dressings (Duoderm, Op-Site), collagenase therapy, absorbable gelatin sponges (Gelfoam), aerosol sprays.	Although there are differing opinions about the efficacy of these agents, individual or combination use may enhance healing.
Administer nutritional supplements and vitamins as indicated.	Aids in healing/cellular regeneration.
Prepare for/assist with skin grafting (Refer to CP: Burns, ND: impaired Skin Integrity.)	May be required to close large ulcers.

NURSING DIAGNOSIS: risk for altered Urinary Elimination

Risk factors may include

Changes in fluid/nutritional pattern
Neuromuscular changes
Perceptual/cognitive impairment

Possibly evidenced by

[Not applicable; presence of signs and symptoms establishes an *actual* diagnosis.]

DESIRED OUTCOMES/EVALUATION CRITERIA—CLIENT WILL:

Urinary Elimination (NOC)

Maintain/regain effective pattern of elimination.
Initiate necessary lifestyle changes.
Participate in treatment regimen to correct/control situation; e.g., bladder training program or use of indwelling catheter.

ACTIONS/INTERVENTIONS	RATIONALE
Urinary Elimination Management (NIC)	
Independent	
Monitor voiding pattern. Identify possible reasons for changes; e.g., disorientation, neuromuscular impairment, psychotropic medications.	This information is essential to plan for care and influences choice of individual interventions. Nocturia, frequency, and urgency are common because bladder capacity and/or tone are affected. Bladder pelvic muscles and sphincter tone may also be affected.
Palpate bladder. Observe for "overflow" voiding, determine frequency and timing of dribbling/voiding.	Bladder distention indicates urinary retention, which may cause incontinence and infection.
Promote fluid intake of 2000–3000 mL/day within cardiac tolerance; include fruit juices, especially cranberry juice. Schedule fluid intake times appropriately.	Maintains adequate hydration and promotes kidney function. Acid-ash juices act as an internal pH acidifier, retarding bacterial growth. *Note*: Client may decrease fluid intake in an attempt to control incontinence, and become dehydrated. Instead, fluids may be scheduled to decrease frequency of incontinence (e.g., limit fluids after 6 pm to reduce need to void during the night).
Institute bladder program (including scheduled voiding times, Kegel's exercise) involving client and staff in a positive manner.	Regular toileting times may help control incontinence. Program is more apt to be successful when positive attitudes and cooperation are present.
Assist client to sit upright on bedpan/commode if not able to use bedside commode.	Provides functional position for voiding.
Provide/encourage perineal care daily and as needed.	Reduces risk of contamination/ascending infection.
Use adult incontinence pads/pants during day if needed. Keep client clean and dry. Provide frequent skin care.	When training is unsuccessful, this is the preferred method of management. *Note*: Avoiding use of incontinence pads during night exposes skin to air, reducing risk of irritation.
Avoid verbal or nonverbal signs of rejection, disgust, or disapproval over failures.	Expressions of disapproval lower self-esteem and are not helpful to a successful program.
Provide regular catheter care and maintain patency if indwelling catheter is present.	Prevents infection and/or minimizes reflux.

NTERVENTIONS	RATIONALE
ive	
medications as indicated; e.g.:	
tynin chloride (Ditropan); tolterodine tartrate l);	Promotes bladder sphincter control.
in C, methenamine mandelate (Mandelamine).	Bladder pH acidifiers retard bacterial growth.
Maintain indwelling catheter/provide intermittent catheterization.	May be used if continence cannot be maintained to prevent skin breakdown and resultant problems.
Irrigate catheter with acetic acid, if indicated.	May be done to maintain acid pH and retard bacterial growth.

NURSING DIAGNOSIS: risk for Constipation/Diarrhea

Risk factors may include

Changes in/inadequate nutrition or fluid intake, poor muscle tone, change in level of activity
Medication side effects
Perceptual/cognitive impairment, depression
Lack of privacy

Possibly evidenced by

[Not applicable; presence of signs and symptoms establishes an *actual* diagnosis.]

DESIRED OUTCOMES/EVALUATION CRITERIA—CLIENT WILL:

Bowel Elimination (NOC)

Establish/maintain normal patterns of bowel functioning.
Demonstrate changes in lifestyle as necessitated by risk or contributing factors.
Participate in bowel program, as indicated.

ACTIONS/INTERVENTIONS	RATIONALE
Bowel Management (NIC)	
Independent	
Ascertain usual bowel pattern and aids used (e.g., previous long-term laxative use). Compare with current routine.	Determines extent of problem and indicates need for/type of interventions appropriate. Many clients may already be laxative-dependent, and it is important to re-establish as near-normal functioning as possible.
Assess reasons for problems, rule out medical causes; e.g., bowel obstruction, cancer, hemorrhoids, drugs, impaction.	Identification/treatment of underlying medical condition is necessary to achieve optimal bowel function.
Determine presence of food/drug sensitivities.	May contribute to diarrhea.
Institute individualized program of exercise, rest, diet, and bowel retraining.	Depends on the needs of the client. Loss of muscular tone reduces peristalsis or may impair control of rectal sphincter.
Provide diet high in bulk in the form of whole-grain cereals, breads, fresh fruits (especially prunes, plums).	Improves stool consistency, promotes evacuation.
Decrease or eliminate foods such as dairy products.	These foods are known to be constipating.
Encourage increased fluid intake.	Promotes normal stool consistency.
Use adult incontinence pads/pants, if needed. Keep client clean and dry. Provide frequent perineal care. Apply skin protective ointment to anal area.	Prevents skin breakdown.

ACTIONS/INTERVENTIONS	RATIONALE
Keep air freshener in room/at bedside or in bathroom.	Limits noxious odors and may help reduce client embarrassment/concern.
Give emotional support to client. Avoid "blaming" (talk/actions) if incontinence occurs.	Decreases feelings of frustration and embarrassment.

Collaborative

ACTIONS/INTERVENTIONS	RATIONALE
Administer medications as indicated:	
Bulk-providers/stool softeners; e.g., Metamucil;	Promotes regularity by increasing bulk and/or improving stool consistency.
Camphorated tincture of opium (Paregoric), diphenoxylate with atropine (Lomotil).	May be needed on a short-term basis when diarrhea persists.

NURSING DIAGNOSIS: impaired physical Mobility/risk for Falls

May be related to

Decreased strength and endurance, neuromuscular impairment
Pain/discomfort
Perceptual/cognitive impairment

Possibly evidenced by

Impaired coordination, limited ROM, decreased muscle mass, strength, control
Reluctance to attempt movement, inability to purposefully move

DESIRED OUTCOMES/EVALUATION CRITERIA—CLIENT WILL:

Mobility (NOC)

Maintain/increase strength and function of affected body parts.
Verbalize willingness to, and participate in, desired activities.
Demonstrate techniques/behaviors that enable continuation or resumption of activities.

Environmental Management (NIC)

Independent

ACTIONS/INTERVENTIONS	RATIONALE
Determine functional ability (0–4 scale) and reasons for impairment.	Identifies need for/degree of intervention required.
Note emotional/behavioral responses to altered ability.	Physical changes and loss of independence often create feelings of anxiety, anger, frustration, and depression that may be manifested as reluctance to engage in activity.
Plan activities/visits with adequate rest periods as necessary.	Can limit/prevent fatigue; conserve energy for continued participation.
Encourage participation in self-care, occupational/recreational activities.	Promotes independence and self-esteem; may enhance willingness to participate.
Provide chairs with firm, high seats and lifting chairs when indicated.	Facilitates rising from seated position.

ACTIONS/INTERVENTIONS	RATIONALE
Fall Prevention (NIC)	
Perform initial and ongoing fall-risk assessment, including fall history, gait and balance assessment, cognition, use of mobility adjuncts, environmental conditions.	Information can help determine client's potential for falling and identify which risk factors can be modified (e.g. medications, uncorrected sensory impairments, poorly fitting shoes).
Assist with transfers and ambulation if indicated; show client/SO ways to move safely.	Prevents accidental falls/injury, especially in the client with altered gait, generalized weakness, orthostatic hypotension, fatigue, and vision disturbances.
Obtain supportive shoes and well-fitting, nonskid slippers.	Assists client to walk with a firm step/maintain sense of balance and prevents slipping.
Remove clutter, wires/cords, scatter rugs, and extraneous furniture from pathways. Keep floors dry.	Reduces risk of falling/injuring self.
Encourage use of hand rails in hallway, stairwells, and bathrooms. Keep bed height in low position.	Promotes independence in mobility; reduces risk of falls.
Review safe use of mobility aids/adjunctive devices; e.g., walker, braces, prosthetics.	Facilitates activity, reduces risk of injury.
Provide for environmental changes to meet visual deficiencies:	Prevents accidents and reduces sense of sensory deprivation. If client is visually impaired, may need assistance and ongoing orientation to surroundings.
Keep areas well lighted. Accompany and keep close to client when in unfamiliar areas;	Provides for safety and psychologic comfort.
Avoid use of physical restraints;	Studies show that older adults who are restrained (particularly when visually or cognitively impaired) are more likely to experience a fall than those who are not restrained.
Speak to client when entering the room, and let client know when leaving;	Special actions help client who cannot see to know when someone is there.
Encourage client with glasses/contacts to wear them. Be sure glasses are kept clean. Determine reason if glasses are not being worn.	Optimal visual acuity facilitates participation in activities and reduces risk of falls/injury. Client may not be wearing glasses because they need adjustment or change in correction.
Collaborative	
Arrange for regular eye examinations.	Identifies development/progression of vision problem (e.g., myopia, hyperopia, presbyopia, astigmatism, cataract, glaucoma, tunnel vision, loss of peripheral fields, blindness) and specific options for care.
Consult with physical/occupational therapists, rehabilitation specialist.	Useful in creating individual exercise/activity program and identifying adjunctive aids. *Note*: Even in the elderly population, inclusion of moderate weight-lifting in the exercise program can improve and maintain the cardiovascular system, decrease obesity and blood pressure, improve bone density, balance, and muscle tone/strength.

NURSING DIAGNOSIS: deficient Diversional Activity

May be related to

Environmental lack of diversional activity, long-term care requirements
Physical limitations, psychologic condition; e.g., depression

Possibly evidenced by

Statements of boredom, depression, lack of energy
Disinterest, lethargy, withdrawn behavior, hostility

DESIRED OUTCOMES/EVALUATION CRITERIA—CLIENT WILL:

Leisure Participation (NOC)

Recognize own response and initiate appropriate coping actions.
Engage in satisfying activities within personal limitations.

ACTIONS/INTERVENTIONS	RATIONALE
Activity Therapy (NIC)	
Independent	
Determine avocation/hobbies client previously pursued. Incorporate activities, if appropriate, into present program.	Encourages involvement and helps to stimulate client mentally/physically to improve overall condition and sense of well-being.
Encourage participation in mix of activities/stimuli; e.g., music, news program, educational presentations, crafts, social interactions, as appropriate.	Offering different activities helps client to try out new ideas and develop new interests. Activities need to be personally meaningful for the client to derive the most enjoyment from them (e.g., talking or Braille books for the blind, closed-caption TV broadcasts for the deaf/hearing impaired).
Provide change of scenery when possible, alter personal environment, encourage trips to shop/participate in local/family events.	Stimulates energy and provides new outlook for client.
Collaborative	
Refer to occupational therapist, activity director.	Can introduce and design new programs to provide positive stimuli for the client.

NURSING DIAGNOSIS: risk for ineffective Sexuality Pattern

Risk factors may include

Biophychosocial alteration of sexuality
Interference in psychologic/physical well-being, self-image
Lack of privacy/SO

Possibly evidenced by

[Not applicable; presence of signs and symptoms establishes an *actual* diagnosis.]

DESIRED OUTCOMES/EVALUATION CRITERIA—CLIENT WILL:

Role Performance (NOC)

Verbalize knowledge and understanding of sexual limitations, difficulties, or changes that have occurred.
Demonstrate improved communication and relationship skills.
Identify appropriate options to meet needs.

ACTIONS/INTERVENTIONS	RATIONALE
Sexual Counseling (NIC)	
Independent	
Note client/SO cues regarding sexuality.	May be concerned that condition/environmental restrictions may interfere with sexual function or ability, but is afraid to ask directly.
Determine cultural and religious/value factors and conflicts that may be present.	Affects client's perception of existing problems and response of others (e.g., family, staff, other residents). Provides starting point for discussion and problem solving.
Assess developmental and lifestyle issues.	Factors such as menopause and aging, adolescence, and young adulthood need to be taken into consideration with regard to sexual concerns about illness and long-term care.
Provide atmosphere in which discussion of sexuality is encouraged/permitted.	When concerns are identified and discussed, problem solving can begin.
Provide privacy for client/SO.	Demonstrates acceptance of need for intimacy and provides opportunity to continue previous patterns of interaction as much as possible.
Collaborative	
Refer to sex counselor/therapist, family therapy when indicated.	May require additional assistance for resolution of problems.

NURSING DIAGNOSIS: ineffective Health Maintenance

May be related to

Lack of, or significant alteration in, communication skills
Complete or partial lack of gross and/or fine motor skills
Perceptual/cognitive impairment, lack of ability to make deliberate/thoughtful judgments
Lack of material resources

Possibly evidenced by

Demonstrated lack of knowledge regarding basic health practices
Reported/observed inability to take responsibility for meeting basic health needs, impairment of personal support system
Demonstrated lack of behaviors adaptive to internal or external environmental changes

DESIRED OUTCOMES/EVALUATION CRITERIA—CLIENT/CAREGIVER WILL:

PARTICIPATION: Health Care Decisions (NOC)

Verbalize understanding of factors contributing to current situation.
Adopt lifestyle changes supporting individual healthcare goals.
Assume responsibility for own healthcare needs when possible.

ACTIONS/INTERVENTIONS	RATIONALE
Health Education (NIC)	
Independent	
Assess level of adaptive behavior, knowledge, and skills about health maintenance, environment, and safety.	Identifies areas of concern/need and aids in choice of interventions.

ACTIONS/INTERVENTIONS	RATIONALE
Provide information about individual healthcare needs.	Provides knowledge base and encourages participation in decision-making.
Develop plan with client/SO for self-care incorporating existing disabilities adapting and organizing care.	Assists client/caregiver to maintain and manage desired level of independence when possible.
Maintain adequate hydration and balanced diet with sufficient protein intake.	Promotes general well-being and aids in disease prevention.
Schedule adequate rest with progressive activity program.	Prevents fatigue and enhances general well-being.
Promote good hand washing and personal hygiene. Use aseptic techniques as necessary.	Prevents contamination/cross-contamination, reducing risk of illness/infection.
Protect from exposure to infections, avoid extremes of temperature. Recommend the wearing of masks/other interventions as indicated.	With age, immune protective responses slow down and physiologic reactions to temperature extremes may be impaired. As organ function decreases (especially thymus gland) and natural antibodies decline, clients are at increased risk for infection. Staff and/or visitors with colds or other infections may expose client to these illnesses.
Encourage cessation of smoking.	Smokers are prone to bronchitis and ineffective clearing of secretions.
Encourage reporting of signs/symptoms as they occur.	Provides opportunity for early recognition of developing complications and timely intervention to prevent serious illness.

Health System Guidance (NIC)

Note client's previous use of professional services, and continue as appropriate. Include in choice of new healthcare providers as able.	Preserves continuity and promotes independence in meeting own healthcare needs.
Observe for/monitor changes in vital signs; e.g., temperature elevation.	Early identification of onset of illness allows for timely intervention and may prevent serious complications. *Note*: Elderly persons often display subnormal temperatures, so presence of a low-grade fever may be of serious concern.

Collaborative

Identify resources for/administer medications as indicated:	
Immunizations; e.g., *Haemophilus influenzae* (flu), pneumonia;	Reduces risk of acquiring contagious/potentially life-threatening diseases.
Antibiotics.	May be used prophylactically, depending on individual disease process/risk factors and to treat infections.
Schedule preventive/routine healthcare appointments based on individual needs; e.g., with cardiologist, podiatrist, ophthalmologist, dentist.	Promotes optimal recovery/maintenance of health.
Refer to support services as indicated; e.g., home health care agency, durable medical equipment company, Senior Resources, social services, national hospice organization, Alzheimer's Disease and Related Disorders Association, AARP, Center for Health Care Ethics, Choice in Dying, American Bar Association, Commission on Legal Problems of the Elderly, Internet Resources, Adult Protective Services.	Many community resources are available, and often untapped, to make life and care of the individual easier.

POTENTIAL CONSIDERATIONS following discharge from care facility.

Refer to plan of care for diagnosis that required admission.

ALCOHOL: ACUTE WITHDRAWAL

Alcohol, a CNS depressant drug, is used socially in our society for many reasons: to enhance the flavor of food, to encourage relaxation and conviviality, for celebrations, and as a sacred ritual in some religious ceremonies. Therapeutically, it is the major ingredient in many OTC/prescription medications. It can be harmless, enjoyable, and sometimes beneficial when used responsibly and in moderation. Like other mind-altering drugs, however, it has the potential for misuse and, in fact, is the most widely abused drug in the United States (research suggests 5%–10% of the adult population) and is potentially fatal with a blood alcohol level (BAL) of .40 or greater. Recently, heightened awareness of the dangers of binge drinking has occurred following the deaths of several young college students. Although programs aimed at informing people of the potential lethality of this behavior have been instituted, many people continue to ignore the possibility.

The spectrum of alcohol withdrawal symptoms ranges from minor symptoms (e.g., insomnia and tremulousness) to severe complications (e.g., withdrawal seizures and delirium tremens [DTs]).

CARE SETTING

May be inpatient on a behavioral unit or outpatient in community programs. Although clients are not generally admitted to the acute care setting with this diagnosis, withdrawal from alcohol may occur secondarily during hospitalization for other illnesses/conditions. A short hospital stay may be required during the acute phase because of severity of general condition, or a delayed discharge from acute care can be the result of alcohol withdrawal beginning within 6–48 hr of admission.

RELATED CONCERNS

Cirrhosis of the liver, page 453
Heart failure, page 47
Psychosocial aspects of care, page 770
Substance dependence/abuse rehabilitation, page 843
Upper gastrointestinal/esophageal bleeding, page 309

Client Assessment Database

Data depend on the duration/extent of use of alcohol, concurrent use of other drugs, degree of organ involvement, and presence of other pathology.

ACTIVITY/REST

May report: Difficulty sleeping, not feeling well rested

CIRCULATION

May exhibit: Generalized tissue edema (due to protein deficiencies)
Peripheral pulses weak, irregular, or rapid
Hypertension common in early withdrawal stage but may become labile/progress to hypotension
Tachycardia common during acute withdrawal; numerous dysrhythmias may be identified

EGO INTEGRITY

May report: Feelings of guilt/shame; defensiveness about drinking
Denial, rationalization
Multiple stressors/losses (relationships, employment, finances)
Use of alcohol to deal with life stressors, boredom

ELIMINATION

May report: Diarrhea
May exhibit: Bowel sounds varied (may reflect gastric complications; e.g., hemorrhage)

FOOD/FLUID

May report: Nausea/vomiting; food intolerance
May exhibit: Gastric distention, ascites, liver enlargement (seen in cirrhosis)
Muscle wasting, dry/dull hair, swollen salivary glands, inflamed buccal cavity, capillary fragility (malnutrition)
Bowel sounds varied (reflecting malnutrition, electrolyte imbalances, general bowel dysfunction)

NEUROSENSORY

May report: "Internal shakes"
Headache, dizziness, blurred vision; "blackouts"
May exhibit: Psychopathology; e.g., paranoid schizophrenia, major depression (may indicate dual diagnosis)
Level of consciousness/orientation varies; e.g., confusion, stupor, hyperactivity, distorted thought processes, slurred/incoherent speech
Memory loss/confabulation

Affect/mood/behavior: May be fearful, anxious, easily startled, inappropriate, silly, euphoric, irritable, physically/verbally abusive, depressed, and/or paranoid
Hallucinations may be visual, tactile, olfactory, or auditory; e.g., client may be picking items out of air or responding verbally to unseen person/voices
Eye examination—nystagmus (associated with cranial nerve palsy); pupil constriction (may indicate CNS depression); arcus senilis—ringlike opacity of the cornea (although normal in aging populations, suggests alcohol-related changes in younger clients)
Fine motor tremors of face, tongue, and hands; seizures (commonly grand mal)
Gait unsteady (ataxia), may be due to thiamine deficiency or cerebellar degeneration (Wernicke's encephalopathy)

PAIN/DISCOMFORT

May report: Constant upper abdominal pain and tenderness radiating to the back (pancreatic inflammation)

RESPIRATION

May report: History of smoking, recurrent/chronic respiratory problems
May exhibit: Tachypnea (hyperactive state of alcohol withdrawal)
Cheyne-Stokes respirations or respiratory depression
Breath sounds diminished, adventitious sounds (suggests pulmonary complications; e.g., respiratory depression, pneumonia)

SAFETY

May report: History of recurrent trauma such as falls, fractures, lacerations, burns, blackouts, or motor vehicle crashes
May exhibit: Skin: Flushed face/palms of hands; scars, ecchymotic areas; cigarette burns on fingers, spider nevus (impaired portal circulation), fissures at corners of mouth (vitamin deficiency)
Fractures healed or new (signs of recent/recurrent trauma)
Temperature elevation (dehydration and sympathetic stimulation), flushing/diaphoresis (suggests presence of infection)
Suicidal ideation/suicide attempts (some research suggests alcoholic suicide attempts are 30% higher than national average for general population)

SOCIAL INTERACTION

May report: Frequent sick days off from work/school, fighting with others, arrests, e.g., disorderly conduct, motor vehicle violations/driving under the influence (DUI). (Legal involvement with increased DUIs/accidents are commonly used to differentiate abuse from addiction.)
Denial that alcohol intake has any significant effect on present condition
Dysfunctional family system of origin (generational involvement), problems in current relationships, often alienated from family when problem is chronic
Mood changes affecting interactions with others

TEACHING/LEARNING

May report: Family history of alcoholism
History of alcohol and/or other drug use/abuse, tobacco use
Ignorance and/or denial of addiction to alcohol, or inability to cut down or stop drinking despite repeated efforts, previous periods of abstinence/withdrawal
Large amount of alcohol consumed in last 24–48 hr ("bingeing")
Previous hospitalizations for alcoholism/alcohol-related diseases; e.g., cirrhosis, esophageal varices
Discharge plan considerations: May require assistance to maintain abstinence and begin to participate in rehabilitation program

Refer to section at end of plan for postdischarge considerations.

DIAGNOSTIC STUDIES

Blood alcohol/drug levels: Blood alcohol level (BAL) may/may not be severely elevated, depending on amount consumed, time between consumption and testing, and the degree of tolerance, which varies widely. In the absence of elevated alcohol tolerance, blood levels in excess of 100 mg/dL are associated with ataxia; at 200 mg/dL, the client is drowsy and confused; respiratory depression occurs with blood levels of 400 mg/dL and death is possible. In addition to alcohol, numerous controlled substances may be identified in a polydrug screen; e.g., amphetamine, cocaine, morphine, oxycodone (Percodan), methaqualone (Quaalude). *Note*: The mixture of methamphetamine and alcohol is of concern because methamphetamine is fast acting and clears from the system quickly, leaving the client to collapse from the alcohol.

CBC: Decreased Hb/Hct may reflect such problems as iron-deficiency anemia or acute/chronic GI bleeding. WBC count may be increased with infection or decreased if immunosuppressed.

Glucose/ketones: Hyperglycemia/hypoglycemia may be present, related to pancreatitis, malnutrition, or depletion of liver glycogen stores. Ketoacidosis may be present with/without metabolic acidosis.

Electrolytes: Hypokalemia and hypomagnesemia are common.

Liver function tests: Lactate dehydrogenase (LDH), aspartate aminotransferase (AST), alanine aminotransferase (ALT), and amylase may be elevated, reflecting liver or pancreatic damage.

Nutritional tests: Albumin is low and total protein may be decreased. Vitamin deficiencies are usually present, reflecting malnutrition/malabsorption.

Other screening studies (e.g., hepatitis, HIV, TB): Depend on general condition, individual risk factors, and care setting.

Urinalysis: Infection may be identified; ketones may be present, related to breakdown of fatty acids in malnutrition (pseudodiabetic condition).

Chest radiography: May reveal right lower lobe pneumonia (common manifestation may be related to malnutrition, depressed immune system, aspiration) or chronic lung disorders associated with tobacco use.

ECG: Dysrhythmias, cardiomyopathies, and/or ischemia may be present because of direct effect of alcohol on the cardiac muscle and/or conduction system, as well as effects of electrolyte imbalance.

Addiction Severity Index (ASI): An assessment tool that produces a "problem severity profile" of the client, including chemical, medical, psychologic, legal, family/social, and employment/support aspects, indicating areas of treatment needs.

Clinical Institute Withdrawal Assessment (CIWA): Provides a clinical quantification of the severity of the alcohol withdrawal syndrome and can be rapidly administered at the bedside. Scores of 9–15 points correspond with moderate withdrawal, and scores >15 correspond to severe withdrawal symptoms and increased risk of DTs and seizures.

NURSING PRIORITIES

1. Maintain physiologic stability during acute withdrawal phase.
2. Promote client safety.
3. Provide appropriate referral and follow-up.
4. Encourage/support SO involvement in "intervention" (confrontation) process.
5. Provide information about condition/prognosis and treatment needs.

DISCHARGE GOALS

1. Homeostasis achieved.
2. Complications prevented/resolved.
3. Sobriety being maintained on a day-to-day basis.
4. Ongoing participation in rehabilitation program/attending group therapy; e.g., Alcoholics Anonymous.
5. Condition, prognosis, and therapeutic regimen understood.
6. Plan in place to meet needs after discharge.

This plan of care is to be used in conjunction with CP: Substance Dependence/Abuse Rehabilitation.

NURSING DIAGNOSIS: risk for ineffective Breathing Pattern

Risk factors may include

Direct effect of alcohol toxicity on respiratory center and/or sedative drugs given to decrease alcohol withdrawal symptoms
Tracheobronchial obstruction
Presence of chronic respiratory problems, inflammatory process
Decreased energy/fatigue

Possibly evidenced by

[Not applicable; presence of signs and symptoms establishes an *actual* diagnosis]

DESIRED OUTCOMES/EVALUATION CRITERIA—CLIENT WILL:

Respiratory Status: Ventilation (NOC)

Maintain effective breathing pattern with respiratory rate within normal range, lungs clear, and free of cyanosis or other signs/symptoms of hypoxia.

ACTIONS/INTERVENTIONS	RATIONALE
Respiratory Monitoring (NIC)	
Independent	
Monitor respiratory rate/depth and pattern as indicated. Note periods of apnea, Cheyne-Stokes respirations.	Frequent assessment is important because toxicity levels may change rapidly. Hyperventilation is common during acute withdrawal phase. Kussmaul's respirations are sometimes present because of acidotic state associated with vomiting and malnutrition. However, marked respiratory depression can occur because of CNS depressant effects of alcohol if acute intoxication is present. This may be compounded by drugs used to control alcohol withdrawal symptoms (AWS).
Auscultate breath sounds. Note presence of adventitious sounds; e.g., rhonchi, wheezes.	Client is at risk for atelectasis related to hypoventilation and pneumonia. Right lower lobe pneumonia is common in alcohol-debilitated clients and is often due to chronic aspiration. Chronic lung diseases are also common; e.g., emphysema, bronchitis.
Airway Management (NIC)	
Elevate head of bed.	Decreases potential for aspiration; lowers diaphragm, enhancing lung inflation.
Encourage cough/deep-breathing exercises and frequent position changes.	Facilitates lung expansion and mobilization of secretions to reduce risk of atelectasis/pneumonia.
Have suction equipment, airway adjuncts available.	Sedative effects of alcohol/drugs potentiate risk of aspiration, relaxation of oropharyngeal muscles, and respiratory depression, requiring intervention to prevent respiratory arrest.
Collaborative	
Administer supplemental oxygen if necessary.	Hypoxia may occur with CNS/respiratory depression.
Review serial chest x-rays, ABGs/pulse oximetry as available/indicated.	Monitors presence of secondary complications such as atelectasis/pneumonia; evaluates effectiveness of respiratory effort, identifies therapy needs.

NURSING DIAGNOSIS: risk for decreased Cardiac Output

Risk factors may include

Direct effect of alcohol on the heart muscle
Altered systemic vascular resistance
Electrical alterations in rate, rhythm, conduction

Possibly evidenced by

[Not applicable; presence of signs and symptoms establishes an *actual* diagnosis]

DESIRED OUTCOMES/EVALUATION CRITERIA—CLIENT WILL:

Circulation Status (NOC)

Display vital signs within client's normal range, absence of/reduced frequency of dysrhythmias.
Demonstrate an increase in activity tolerance.

ACTIONS/INTERVENTIONS	RATIONALE
Hemodynamic Regulation (NIC)	
Independent	
Monitor vital signs frequently during acute withdrawal.	Hypertension frequently occurs in acute withdrawal phase. Extreme hyperexcitability, accompanied by catecholamine release and increased peripheral vascular resistance, raises BP and heart rate; however, BP may become labile/progress to hypotension. *Note:* Client may have underlying cardiovascular disease, which is compounded by alcohol withdrawal.
Monitor cardiac rate/rhythm. Document irregularities/dysrhythmias.	Long-term alcohol abuse may result in cardiomyopathy/HF. Tachycardia is common because of sympathetic response to increased circulating catecholamines. Irregularities/dysrhythmias may develop with electrolyte shifts/imbalance. All of these may have an adverse effect on cardiac function/output.
Monitor body temperature.	Elevation may occur because of sympathetic stimulation, dehydration, and/or infections, causing vasodilation and compromising venous return/cardiac output.
Monitor I&O. Note 24-hr fluid balance.	Preexisting dehydration, vomiting, fever, and diaphoresis may result in decreased circulating volume that can compromise cardiovascular function. *Note:* Hydration is difficult to assess in the alcoholic client because the usual indicators are not reliable, and overhydration is a risk in the presence of compromised cardiac function.
Be prepared for/assist in cardiopulmonary resuscitation.	Causes of death during acute withdrawal stages include cardiac dysrhythmias, respiratory depression/arrest, oversedation, excessive psychomotor activity, severe dehydration or overhydration, and massive infections. Mortality for unrecognized/untreated DTs may be as high as 25%.
Collaborative	
Monitor laboratory studies; e.g., serum electrolyte levels, RBCs, platelets.	Electrolyte imbalances; e.g., potassium/magnesium, potentiate risk of cardiac dysrhythmias and CNS excitability. Anemia may be present and platelets can be decreased in late stage alcoholism due to liver dysfunction.
Administer fluids and electrolytes, as indicated.	Severe alcohol withdrawal causes the client to be susceptible to excessive fluid losses (associated with fever, diaphoresis, and vomiting) and electrolyte imbalances, especially potassium, magnesium, and glucose.
Administer medications as indicated; e.g.:	
Clonidine (Catapres), atenolol (Tenormin);	Although the use of benzodiazepines is often sufficient to control hypertension during initial withdrawal from alcohol, some clients may require more specific therapy. *Note:* Atenolol and other β-adrenergic blockers may speed up the withdrawal process and eliminate tremors, as well as lower the heart rate, blood pressure, and body temperature.
Potassium.	Corrects deficits that can result in life-threatening dysrhythmias.

NURSING DIAGNOSIS: risk for Injury, [specify]

Risk factors may include

Cessation of alcohol intake with varied autonomic nervous system responses to the system's suddenly altered state
Involuntary clonic/tonic muscle activity (seizures)
Equilibrium/balancing difficulties, reduced muscle and hand/eye coordination

Possibly evidenced by

[Not applicable; presence of signs and symptoms establishes an *actual* diagnosis]

DESIRED OUTCOMES/EVALUATION CRITERIA—CLIENT WILL:

Risk Control (NOC)

Demonstrate absence of untoward effects of withdrawal.
Experience no physical injury.

ACTIONS/INTERVENTIONS	RATIONALE
SUBSTANCE USE TREATMENT: Alcohol Withdrawal (NIC)	
Independent	
Identify stage of AWS (alcohol withdrawal syndrome) using CIWA; i.e., stage I is associated with signs/symptoms of hyperactivity (e.g., tremors, sleeplessness, nausea/vomiting, diaphoresis, tachycardia, hypertension), stage II is manifested by increased hyperactivity plus hallucinations and/or seizure activity; stage III symptoms include DTs and extreme autonomic hyperactivity with profound confusion, anxiety, insomnia, fever.	Alcohol withdrawal usually begins 3–36 hr after the last drink. Prompt recognition and intervention may halt progression of symptoms and enhance recovery/improve prognosis. In addition, recurrence/progression of symptoms indicates need for changes in drug therapy/more intense treatment to prevent death. DTs may not present until 2–3 days after last alcohol intake, usually lasting 1–5 days, but may persist for up to 10 days.
Monitor/document seizure activity. Maintain patent airway. Provide environmental safety; e.g., padded side rails, bed in low position.	Grand mal seizures are most common and may be related to decreased magnesium levels, hypoglycemia, elevated blood alcohol, or history of head trauma/preexisting seizure disorder. *Note:* In absence of history of/other pathology causing seizures, they usually stop spontaneously, requiring only symptomatic treatment. (Antiepileptic drugs are not indicated for alcohol withdrawal seizures.)
Check deep-tendon reflexes. Assess gait if possible. Palpate upper arm to discern actual withdrawal versus medication-seeking behavior.	Reflexes may be depressed, absent, or hyperactive. Peripheral neuropathies are common, especially in malnourished client. Ataxia (gait disturbance) is associated with Wernicke's syndrome (thiamine deficiency) and cerebellar degeneration. Three ways to assess whether the client is having actual withdrawal tremors are (1) have the client stick out his or her tongue— it will be tremulous; (2) feel the client's upper arm—withdrawal tremors can be felt bone deep; (3) have the client visually track a pencil—there will be observable nystagmus. Vital signs may also be elevated. *Note*: The client does not have to be sober to be in withdrawal.
Assist with ambulation and self-care activities as needed.	Prevents falls with resultant injury.
Provide for environmental safety when indicated. (Refer to ND: disturbed Sensory Perception, [specify], following.)	May be required when equilibrium, hand/eye coordination problems exist.

ACTIONS/INTERVENTIONS	RATIONALE
Collaborative	
Administer medications as indicated; e.g.:	
Benzodiazepines (BZDs); e.g., chlordiazepoxide (Librium, Libritabs, Mitran), diazepam (Valium, Diazemuls, Diastat), lorazapam (Ativan), clonazepate (Tranxene);	BZDs are commonly used to control neuronal hyperactivity because of their minimal respiratory and cardiac depression and anticonvulsant properties. Studies have also shown that these drugs can prevent progression to more severe states of withdrawal. IV/PO administration is preferred route because IM absorption is unpredictable. Muscle-relaxant qualities are particularly helpful to client in controlling "the shakes," trembling, and ataxic quality of movements. Client may initially require large doses to achieve desired effect, and then drugs may be tapered and discontinued, usually within 96 hr. *Note:* These agents are used cautiously in clients with known hepatic disease because they are metabolized by the liver. In this situation, oxazepam (Serax) may be drug of choice because of shorter half-life.
Haloperidol (Haldol);	May be used in conjunction with BZDs for clients experiencing agitation and hallucinations, although used with caution as it can lower seizure threshold.
Thiamine;	Thiamine deficiency (common in alcohol abuse) may lead to neuritis, Wernecke's syndrome, and/or Korsakoff's psychosis.
Magnesium sulfate.	Reduces tremors and seizure activity by decreasing neuromuscular excitability.

NURSING DIAGNOSIS: disturbed Sensory Perception (specify)

May be related to

Chemical alteration: Exogenous (e.g., alcohol consumption/sudden cessation) and endogenous (e.g., electrolyte imbalance, elevated ammonia and BUN)
Sleep deprivation
Psychologic stress (anxiety/fear)

Possibly evidenced by

Disorientation to time, place, person, or situation
Changes in usual response to stimuli; exaggerated emotional responses, change in behavior
Bizarre thinking
Listlessness, irritability, apprehension, activity associated with visual/auditory hallucinations
Fear/anxiety

DESIRED OUTCOMES/EVALUATION CRITERIA—CLIENT WILL:

Cognition (NOC)

Regain/maintain usual level of consciousness.

Distorted Thought Self-Control (NOC)

Report absence of/reduced hallucinations.
Identify external factors that affect sensory-perceptual abilities.

ACTIONS/INTERVENTIONS	RATIONALE
SUBSTANCE USE TREATMENT: Alcohol Withdrawal (NIC)	
Independent	
Assess level of consciousness, ability to speak, response to stimuli/commands.	Speech may be garbled, confused, or slurred. Response to commands may reveal inability to concentrate, impaired judgment, or muscle coordination deficits.
Observe behavioral responses; e.g., hyperactivity, disorientation, confusion, sleeplessness, irritability.	Hyperactivity related to CNS disturbances may escalate rapidly. Sleeplessness is common due to loss of sedative effect gained from alcohol usually consumed before bedtime. Sleep deprivation may aggravate disorientation/confusion. Progression of symptoms may indicate impending hallucinations (stage II) or DTs (stage III).
Note onset of hallucinations, Document as auditory, visual, and/or tactile.	Auditory hallucinations are reported to be more frightening/threatening to client. Visual hallucinations occur more at night and often include insects, animals, or faces of friends/enemies. Clients are frequently observed "picking the air." Yelling may occur if client is calling for help from perceived threat (usually seen in stage III AWS).
Provide quiet environment. Speak in calm, quiet voice. Regulate lighting as indicated. Turn off radio/TV during sleep.	Reduces external stimuli during hyperactive stage. Client may become more delirious when surroundings cannot be seen, but some respond better to quiet, darkened room.
Provide care by same personnel whenever possible.	Promotes recognition of caregivers and a sense of consistency, which may reduce fear.
Encourage SO to stay with client whenever possible.	May have a calming effect, and may provide a reorienting influence.
Reorient frequently to person, place, time, and surrounding environment as indicated.	May reduce confusion; prevent/limit misinterpretation of external stimuli.
Avoid bedside discussion about client or topics unrelated to the client that do not include the client.	Client may hear and misinterpret conversation, which can aggravate hallucinations.
Provide environmental safety; e.g., place bed in low position, leave doors in full open or closed position, observe frequently, place call light/bell within reach, remove articles that can harm client.	Client may have distorted sense of reality or be fearful or suicidal, requiring protection from self.
Collaborative	
Provide seclusion, restraints as necessary.	Clients with excessive psychomotor activity, severe hallucinations, violent behavior, and/or suicidal gestures may respond better to seclusion. Restraints are usually ineffective and add to client's agitation, but occasionally may be required to prevent self-harm.
Monitor laboratory studies; e.g., electrolytes, magnesium levels, liver function studies, ammonia, BUN, glucose, ABGs.	Changes in organ function may precipitate or potentiate sensory-perceptual deficits. Electrolyte imbalance is common. Liver function is often impaired in the chronic alcoholic, and ammonia intoxication can occur if the liver is unable to convert ammonia to urea. Ketoacidosis is sometimes present without glycosuria; however, hyperglycemia or hypoglycemia may occur, suggesting pancreatitis or impaired gluconeogenesis in the liver. Hypoxemia and hypercarbia are common manifestations in chronic alcoholics who are also heavy smokers.
Administer medications as indicated; e.g.:	
Antianxiety agents as indicated. (Refer to ND: Anxiety [severe/panic]/Fear), following.);	Reduces hyperactivity, promoting relaxation/sleep. Drugs that have little effect on dreaming may be desired to allow dream recovery (REM rebound) to occur, which has previously been suppressed by alcohol use.
Thiamine, vitamins C and B complex, multivitamins, Stresstabs.	Vitamins may be depleted because of insufficient intake and malabsorption. Vitamin deficiency (especially thiamine) is associated with ataxia, loss of eye movement and pupillary response, palpitations, postural hypotension, and exertional dyspnea.

NURSING DIAGNOSIS: Anxiety [severe/panic]/Fear

May be related to

Cessation of alcohol intake/physiologic withdrawal
Situational crisis (hospitalization)
Threat to self-concept, perceived threat of death

Possibly evidenced by

Feelings of inadequacy, shame, self-disgust, and remorse
Increased helplessness/hopelessness with loss of control of own life
Increased tension, apprehension
Fear of unspecified consequences; identifies object of fear

DESIRED OUTCOMES/EVALUATION CRITERIA—CLIENT WILL:

Anxiety [or] Fear Self-Control (NOC)

Verbalize reduction of fear and anxiety to an acceptable and manageable level.
Express sense of regaining some control of situation/life.
Demonstrate problem-solving skills and use resources effectively.

ACTIONS/INTERVENTIONS	RATIONALE
Anxiety Reduction (NIC)	
Independent	
Identify cause of anxiety, involving client in the process. Explain that alcohol withdrawal increases anxiety and uneasiness. Reassess level of anxiety on an ongoing basis.	Person in acute phase of withdrawal may be unable to identify and/or accept what is happening. Anxiety may be physiologically or environmentally caused. Continued alcohol toxicity will be manifested by increased anxiety and agitation as effects of medication wear off.
Develop a trusting relationship through frequent contact, being honest and nonjudgmental. Project an accepting attitude about alcoholism.	Provides client with a sense of humanness, helping to decrease paranoia and distrust. Client will be able to detect biased or condescending attitude of caregivers.
Discuss use of harm (risk) reduction programs that include (1) skills to strengthen client's personal anti-drinking commitment, (2) peer discussion groups, (3) SO component to encourage reinforcement of messages client is receiving, (4) long-term focus with age-appropriate booster sessions, (5) strengthening community norms against alcohol/other drug use.	Have been found to be helpful in decreasing alcohol and drug use.
Inform client about what you plan to do and why. Include client in planning process and provide choices when possible.	Enhances sense of trust, and explanation may increase cooperation/reduce anxiety. Provides sense of control over self in circumstance where loss of control is a significant factor. *Note:* Feelings of self-worth are intensified when one is treated as a worthwhile person.
Reorient frequently. (Refer to ND: disturbed Sensory Perception.)	Client may experience periods of confusion, resulting in increased anxiety.
Collaborative	
Administer medications as indicated; e.g.:	
Benzodiazepines; e.g., chlordiazepoxide (Librium), diazepam (Valium);	Antianxiety agents are given during acute withdrawal to help client relax, be less hyperactive, and feel more in control.
Barbiturates; e.g., phenobarbital, or possibly secobarbital (Seconal), pentobarbital (Nembutal).	These drugs are sometimes used to treat or prevent alcohol withdrawal seizures, but need to be used with caution because they are respiratory depressants and REM sleep cycle inhibitors.

ACTIONS/INTERVENTIONS	RATIONALE
Arrange "intervention" (confrontation) in controlled setting.	Process wherein SO/family members, supported by staff, provide information about how client's drinking and behavior have affected each one of them, helps client acknowledge that drinking is a problem and has resulted in current situational crisis.
Provide consultation for referral to detoxification/crisis center for ongoing treatment program as soon as medically stable (e.g., oriented to reality).	Client is more likely to contract for treatment while still hurting and experiencing fear and anxiety from last drinking episode. Motivation decreases as well-being increases and person again feels able to control the problem. Direct contact with available treatment resources provides realistic picture of help. Decreases time for client to "think about it"/change mind or restructure and strengthen denial systems.

POTENTIAL CONSIDERATIONS following acute care (dependent on client's age, physical condition/presence of complications, personal resources, and life responsibilities)

Refer to: Substance Abuse/Rehabilitation plan of care, and plans of care for any specific underlying medical condition(s).

Sample CP: Alcohol Withdrawal Program. ELOS: 5 Days Behavioral Unit

ND and Categories of Care	Time Dimension	Goals/Actions	Time Dimension	Goals/Actions	Time Dimension	Goals/Actions
Risk for Injury (varied autonomic and sensory responses)	Day 1	Verbalize understanding of unit policies, procedures, and safety concerns relative to individual needs Cooperate with therapeutic regimen	Day 3 Day 4	Vital signs stable I&O balanced Display marked decrease in objective symptoms	Day 5	Be free of injury resulting from ETOH withdrawal Display no objective symptoms of withdrawal
Referrals	Day 1	RN-NP or MD If indicated: Internist Cardiologist Neurologist				
Diagnostic studies	Day 1	BA level Drug screen (urine and blood) If indicated: CXR Pulse oximetry ECG	Day 2	SMA 20 Serum Mg, amylase RPR UA ↑	Day 4	Repeat of selected studies as indicated
Additional assessments	Day 1 Day 1–4 Ongoing Stage I Stage II Stage III	VS, temp, respiratory status/breath sounds q4h I&O q8h Motor activity, body language, verbalizations, need for/type of restraint Withdrawal symptoms: Tremors, N/V, hypertension, tachycardia, diaphoresis, sleeplessness Increased hyperactivity, hallucinations, seizure activity Extreme autonomic hyperactivity, profound confusion, anxiety, fever	Day 2–3	VS q8h if stable	Day 4–5	VS qd

(Continued on the following page)

Sample CP: Alcohol Withdrawal Program. ELOS: 5 Days Behavioral Unit *(Continued)*

ND and Categories of Care	Time Dimension	Goals/Actions	Time Dimension	Goals/Actions	Time Dimension	Goals/Actions
Medications Allergies: ________	Day 1 Day 1–4 Day 2	Librium 200 mg PO Thiamine 100 mg IM Librium 160 mg PO	Day 3 Day 4	Librium 120 mg PO Librium 80 mg PO	Day 5	Librium 40 mg PO
Client education	Day 1	Orient to room/unit, schedule, procedures	Day 3–4	Need for ongoing therapy Goals/availability of AA program	Day 5	Schedule of follow-up visits if indicated
Additional nursing actions	Day 1	Bed rest 12 hr if in withdrawal Position change, HOB elevated; C, DB exercises if on bed rest	Day 3–5	Activity as tolerated		
	Day 1–2	Assist with ambulation, self-care as needed Encourage fluids if free of N/V				
	Ongoing	Provide environmental safety measures, seizure precautions as indicated Reorient as needed				
Ineffective Coping R/T personal vulnerability, situational crisis, inadequate coping methods	Day 1–5	Participate in development/evaluation of treatment plan	Day 3	Verbalize understanding of relationship of ETOH abuse to current situation	Day 5	Plan in place to meet needs postdischarge
	Day 2–5	Interact in group sessions	Day 4	Identify/make contact with potential resources, support groups		
Referrals	Day 1 Day 2–5	Psychiatrist Group sessions	Day 4	Community classes: Assertiveness training Stress management		
Additional assessments	Day 1	Understanding of current situation Drinking pattern, previous withdrawal, other drug use, attitudes toward substance use History of violence	Day 2–3	Previous coping strategies/consequences Perception of drug use on life, employment, legal issues		
	Day 1–2	Relationships with others: personal, work/school Readiness for group activities	Day 3–5	Congruency of actions based on insight		
Medications			Day 5	Naltrexone 50 mg/day if indicated		
Client education	Day 1	Physical effects of ETOH abuse	Day 3–5	Human behavior and interactions with others/transactional analysis (TA)	Day 5	Medication dose, frequency, side effects Written instructions for therapeutic program
	Day 1–2	Types/use of relaxation techniques				
	Day 2	Consequences of ETOH abuse	Day 4–5	Community resources for self/family Identify goals for change		

(Continued on the following page)

ND and Categories of Care	Time Dimension	Goals/Actions	Time Dimension	Goals/Actions	Time Dimension	Goals/Actions
Additional nursing actions	Day 1–5	Support client's taking responsibility for own recovery Provide consistent approach/ expectations for behavior Set limits/confront inappropriate behaviors	Day 2–5	Discuss alternative solutions Provide positive feedback for efforts Support during confrontation by peer group Encourage verbalization of feelings, personal reflection		
Altered nutrition: less than body requirements R/T poor intake, effects of ETOH on digestive system, and hyper-metabolic response to withdrawal	Day 2–5	Select foods appropriately to meet individual dietary needs	Day 4	Verbalize understandings of effects of ETOH abuse and reduced dietary intake on nutritional status	Day 5	Display stable weight or initial weight gain as appropriate, and laboratory results WNL
Referrals	Day 1 and prn	Dietitian				
Diagnostic studies	Day 1	CBC, liver function studies Serum albumin, transferrin	Day 2–5	Fingerstick glucose prn		
Additional assessments	Day 1	Weight, skin turgor, condition of mucous membranes, muscle tone			Day 5	Weight
	Day 1–2	Bowel sounds, characteristics of stools				
	Day 1–5	Appetite, dietary intake				
Medications	Day 1–5	Antacid ac and hs Imodium 2 mg prn	Day 2–5	Multivitamin 1tab/qd		
Client education	Day 1–2	Individual nutritional needs	Day 4	Principles of nutrition, foods for maintenance of wellness		
Additional nursing actions	Day 1	Liquid/bland diet as tolerated	Day 2–5	Advance diet as tolerated		
	Day 1–5	Encourage small, frequent, nutritious meals/snacks Encourage good oral hygiene pc and hs				

SUBSTANCE DEPENDENCE/ABUSE REHABILITATION

Many drugs and volatile substances are subject to abuse. This disorder is a continuum of phases incorporating a cluster of cognitive, behavioral, and physiologic symptoms that include loss of control over use of the substance and a continued use of the substance despite adverse consequences. A number of factors have been implicated in the predisposition to abuse a substance: biologic, biochemical, psychologic (including developmental), personality, sociocultural and conditioning, and cultural and ethnic influences. While no single theory adequately explains the etiology of this problem, many treatment approaches, such as Alcoholics Anonymous (AA) and harm reduction, are being successful.

CARE SETTING

Inpatient stay on behavioral unit or outpatient care in a day program or community agency.

RELATED CONCERNS

Alcohol: acute withdrawal, page 831
Psychosocial aspects of care, page 770

Client Assessment Database

Depends on substances involved, duration of use, and organs affected.
A comprehensive assessment should include questions regarding factors that protect and minimize the risk of substance use. These factors are grouped into five general domains:

1. Community (e.g., availability of substances)
2. Family (e.g., discipline, conflict, attitudes, communication)
3. Peer/individual (e.g., the individual's delinquency, perception of risk, friends' attitudes and use of substances)
4. Work/school (e.g., attendance, performance, grades)
5. General (e.g., participation in activities, religious beliefs)

TEACHING/LEARNING

Discharge plan considerations: May need assistance with long-range plan for recovery

Refer to section at end of plan for postdischarge considerations.

DIAGNOSTIC STUDIES

Serum, urine, and/or hair drug screens: Identifies drug(s) being used, including usual drugs of abuse (e.g., alcohol, heroin, marijuana, cocaine, inhalants). Newer designer drugs, e.g., ketamine and ecstasy, are often not screened for because of the expense.

Screening for use/relapse: Variety of tools may be used (e.g., alcohol use disorders screening test [AUDIT], alcohol abuse/dependence screener [CAGE], drug abuse/dependence screener [DAST])

Addiction Severity Index (ASI) assessment tool: Produces a "problem severity profile" of the client, including chemical, medical, psychologic, legal, family/social, and employment/support aspects, indicating areas of treatment needs.

Other screening studies (e.g., hepatitis, HIV, TB): Depends on general condition, individual risk factors, and care setting.

NURSING PRIORITIES

1. Provide support for decision to stop substance use/harm reduction.
2. Strengthen individual coping skills.
3. Facilitate learning of new ways to reduce anxiety.
4. Promote family involvement in rehabilitation program.
5. Facilitate family growth/development.
6. Provide information about condition, prognosis, and treatment needs.

DISCHARGE GOALS

1. Responsibility for own life and behavior assumed.
2. Plan to maintain substance-free life formulated.
3. Family relationships/enabling issues being addressed.
4. Treatment program successfully begun.
5. Condition, prognosis, and therapeutic regimen understood.
6. Plan in place to meet needs after discharge.

NURSING DIAGNOSIS: Denial

May be related to

Personal vulnerability, difficulty handling new situations
Previous ineffective/inadequate coping skills with substitution of drug(s)
Learned response patterns, cultural factors, personal/family value systems

Possibly evidenced by

Delay in seeking or refusal of healthcare attention to the detriment of health/life
Does not perceive personal relevance of symptoms or danger or admit impact of condition on life pattern; projection of blame/responsibility for problems
Use of manipulation to avoid responsibility for self

DESIRED OUTCOMES/EVALUATION CRITERIA—CLIENT WILL:

ACCEPTANCE: Health Status (NOC)

Verbalize awareness of relationship of substance abuse to current situation.
Engage in therapeutic program.
Verbalize acceptance of responsibility for own behavior.

ACTIONS/INTERVENTIONS	RATIONALE
Behavior Modification (NIC)	
Independent	
Ascertain by what name client would like to be addressed.	Shows courtesy and respect, giving client a sense of orientation and control.
Convey attitude of acceptance, separating individual from unacceptable behavior.	Promotes feelings of dignity and self-worth.
Ascertain reason for beginning abstinence, involvement in therapy.	Provides insight into client's willingness to commit to long-term behavioral change, and whether client even believes that he or she can change. (Denial is one of the strongest and most resistant symptoms of substance abuse.) The decision to quit is an important step to success in therapy.
Review definition of drug dependence and categories of symptoms (e.g., patterns of use, impairment caused by use, tolerance to substance).	This information helps client make decisions regarding acceptance of problem and treatment choices.
Answer questions honestly and provide factual information. Keep your word when agreements are made.	Creates trust, which is the basis of the therapeutic relationship.
Provide information about addictive use versus experimental, occasional use; biochemical/genetic disorder theory (genetic predisposition, use activated by environment; compulsive desire.)	Progression of use continuum is from experimental/recreational to addictive use. Comprehending this process is important in combating denial. Education may relieve client's guilt and blame and may help awareness of recurring addictive characteristics.
Discuss current life situation and impact of substance use.	First step in decreasing use of denial is for client to see the relationship between substance use and personal problems.
Confront and examine denial/rationalization in peer group. Use confrontation with caring.	Because denial is the major defense mechanism in addictive disease, confrontation by peers can help the client accept the reality of adverse consequences of behaviors and that drug use is a major problem. Caring attitude preserves self-concept and helps decrease defensive response.
Provide information regarding effects of addiction on mood/personality.	Individuals often mistake effects of addiction and use this to justify or excuse drug use.
Remain nonjudgmental. Be alert to changes in behavior; e.g., restlessness, increased tension.	Confrontation can lead to increased agitation, which may compromise safety of client/staff.
Provide positive feedback for expressing awareness of denial in self/others.	Necessary to enhance self-esteem and to reinforce insight into behavior.
Maintain firm expectation that client attend recovery support/therapy groups regularly.	Attendance is related to admitting need for help, to working with denial, and for maintenance of a long-term drug-free existence.
Encourage and support client's taking responsibility for own recovery (e.g., development of alternative behaviors to drug urge/use). Assist client to learn own responsibility for recovering.	Denial can be replaced with positive action when client accepts the reality of own responsibility.
Be aware of own enabling behaviors.	Caregiving lends itself to "taking care" of clients that can backfire in substance abuse treatment.

NURSING DIAGNOSIS: ineffective Coping

May be related to

Personal vulnerability
Negative role modeling, inadequate support systems
Previous ineffective/inadequate coping skills with substitution of drug(s)

Possibly evidenced by

Impaired adaptive behavior and problem-solving skills
Decreased ability to handle stress of illness/hospitalization
Financial affairs in disarray, employment/school difficulties (e.g., losing time on job/not maintaining steady employment; poor work/school performances, on-the-job injuries)
Verbalization of inability to cope/ask for help

DESIRED OUTCOMES/EVALUATION CRITERIA—CLIENT WILL:

Substance Addiction Consequences (NOC)

Identify consequences of using substance as a method of coping.

Coping (NOC)

Identify other ineffective coping behaviors.
Engage in effective coping skills/problem solving.
Initiate necessary lifestyle changes.

ACTIONS/INTERVENTIONS	RATIONALE
Substance Use Treatment (NIC)	
Independent	
Review program rules, philosophy expectations.	Having information provides opportunity for client to cooperate and function as a member of the group/milieu, enhancing sense of control and sense of success.
Determine understanding of current situation and previous/other methods of coping with life's problems.	Provides information about degree of denial, acceptance of personal responsibility/commitment to change; identifies coping skills that may be used in present situation.
Set limits and confront efforts to get caregiver to grant special privileges, making excuses for not following through on behaviors agreed on, and attempting to continue drug use. Avoid use of labels, such as lying.	Client has learned manipulative behavior throughout life and needs to learn a new way of getting needs met. Following through on consequences of failure to maintain limits can help the client to change ineffective behaviors. Use of labels promotes negative attitudes that can impede therapeutic relationships.
Be aware of staff attitudes, feelings, and enabling behaviors.	Lack of understanding, judgmental/enabling behaviors can result in inaccurate data collection and nontherapeutic approaches.
Encourage verbalization of feelings, fears, and anxiety.	May help client begin to come to terms with long-unresolved issues.
Explore alternative coping strategies.	Client may have little or no knowledge of adaptive responses to stress and needs to learn other options for managing time, feelings, and relationships without drugs.
Assist client to learn/encourage use of relaxation skills, guided imagery, visualizations.	Helps client relax, develop new ways to deal with stress, problem-solve.
Structure diversional activity that relates to recovery (e.g., social activity within support group), wherein issues of being chemically free are examined.	Discovery of alternative methods of coping with drug hunger can remind client that addiction is a lifelong process and opportunity for changing patterns is available.
Use peer support to examine ways of coping with drug hunger.	Self-help groups (e.g., AA, Narcotics Anonymous, Crystal Methamphetamine Anonymous) are valuable for learning and promoting abstinence in each member, using understanding and support as well as peer pressure. *Note*: Methamphetamine is increasing in use.

ACTIONS/INTERVENTIONS	RATIONALE
Identify possible/actual triggers for relapse. Encourage client to use the acronym HALT (Am I hungry, angry, lonely, or tired?).	Employment/financial stressors, isolation, unhealthy relationships/being around substance-using friends, hearing certain songs, premenstrual syndrome—the list of possibilities depends on the individual. Being aware of the triggers provides an opportunity to plan for ways to avoid/deal with them.
Encourage involvement in therapeutic writing. Have client begin journaling or writing autobiography.	Therapeutic writing/journaling can enhance participation in treatment; serves as a release for grief, anger, and stress; provides a useful tool for monitoring client's safety; and can be used to evaluate client's progress. Autobiographical activity provides an opportunity for client to remember and identify sequence of events in his or her life that relate to current situation.
Discuss client's plans for living without drugs.	Provides opportunity to develop/refine plans. Devising a comprehensive strategy for avoiding relapses helps client into maintenance phase of behavioral change.

Collaborative

ACTIONS/INTERVENTIONS	RATIONALE
Administer medications as indicated; e.g.:	
Disulfiram (Antabuse);	This drug can be helpful in maintaining abstinence from alcohol while other therapy is undertaken. By inhibiting alcohol oxidation, the drug leads to an accumulation of acetaldehyde with a highly unpleasant reaction if alcohol is consumed.
Metronidazole (Flagyl);	Increasingly used to maintain abstinence from alcohol instead of Antabuse. It has the same GI distress effects but fewer cardiac concerns and less cost.
Acamprosate (Campral EC);	Helps prevent relapses in alcoholism by lowering receptors for the excitatory neurotransmitter glutamate. This agent may become drug of choice because it does not make the user sick if alcohol is consumed; it has no sedative, antianxiety, muscle relaxant or antidepressant properties and produces no withdrawal symptoms.
Buprenorphine (Buprex, Subutex, Suboxone);	Used in the treatment of opioid addiction. At low doses it produces sufficient agonist effect to enable opioid-addicted individuals to discontinue the misuse of opioids without experiencing withdrawal symptoms. This drug carries a lower risk of abuse, dependence, and side effects compared to full opioid agonists.
Methadone (Dolophine), levo-α-acetymethadol (LAAM);	Methadone is thought to blunt the craving for/diminish the effects of opioids and is used to assist in withdrawal and long-term maintenance programs. It can allow the individual to maintain daily activities and ultimately withdraw from drug use. LAAM is a long-acting synthetic μ agonist thought to be a safe and effective alternative to methadone maintenance. Harm-reduction needs to be considered versus the possibility of exchanging one addiction for another.
Naltrexone (Trexan), nalmefine (Revex).	Used to suppress craving for opioids and may help prevent relapse in the client abusing alcohol. Current research suggests that naltrexone suppresses urge to continue drinking by interfering with alcohol-induced release of endorphins.
Encourage involvement with self-help associations; e.g., Alcoholics/Narcotics Anonymous.	Puts client in direct contact with support system necessary for managing sobriety/drug-free life.
Refer to community/social resources e.g., housing assistance, employment agencies, childcare, food stamps, alternative schooling.	Dealing with life problems in a proactive way enhances coping abilities, reduces sense of isolation and hopelessness, and decreases risk of relapse.

NURSING DIAGNOSIS: Powerlessness

May be related to

Substance addiction with/without periods of abstinence
Episodic compulsive indulgence; attempts at recovery
Lifestyle of helplessness

Possibly evidenced by

Ineffective recovery attempts, statements of inability to stop behavior/requests for help
Continuous/constant thinking about drug and/or obtaining drug
Alteration in personal, occupational, and social life

DESIRED OUTCOMES/EVALUATION CRITERIA—CLIENT WILL:

HEALTH BELIEFS: Perceived Control (NOC)

Admit inability to control drug habit, surrender to powerlessness over addiction.
Verbalize acceptance of need for treatment and awareness that willpower alone cannot control abstinence.
Engage in peer support.
Demonstrate active participation in program.
Regain and maintain healthy state with a drug-free lifestyle.

ACTIONS/INTERVENTIONS	RATIONALE
Self-Responsibility Facilitation (NIC)	
Independent	
Use crisis intervention techniques to initiate behavior changes:	May need to use emergency commitments or other legal holds for the client's safety. Client may be more amenable to acceptance of need for treatment at this time.
Assist client to recognize problem exists. Discuss in a caring, nonjudgmental manner how drug has interfered with life;	In the precontemplation phase, the client has not yet identified that drug use is problematic. While client is hurting, it is easier to admit substance use has created negative consequences.
Involve client in development of treatment plan, using problem-solving process in which client identifies goals for change and agrees to desired outcomes;	During the contemplation phase, the client realizes a problem exists and is thinking about a change of behavior. The client is committed to the outcomes when the decision-making process involves solutions that are promulgated by the individual.
Discuss alternative solutions;	Brainstorming helps creatively identify possibilities and provides sense of control. During the preparation phase, minor action may be taken as individual organizes resources for definitive change.
Assist in selecting most appropriate alternative;	As possibilities are discussed, the most useful solution becomes clear.
Support decision and implementation of selected alternative(s).	Helps the client persevere in process of change. During the action phase, the client engages in a sustained effort to maintain sobriety, and mechanisms are put in place to support abstinence.
Explore support in peer group. Encourage sharing about drug hunger, situations that increase the desire to indulge, ways that substance has influenced life.	Client may need assistance in expressing self, speaking about powerlessness, and admitting need for help in order to face up to problem and begin resolution.

ACTIONS/INTERVENTIONS	RATIONALE
Assist client to learn ways to enhance health and structure healthy diversion from drug use (e.g., maintaining a balanced diet, getting adequate rest, exercise [e.g., walking, slow/long distance running]; and acupuncture, biofeedback, deep meditative techniques).	Learning to empower self in constructive areas can strengthen ability to continue recovery. These activities help restore natural biochemical balance, aid detoxification, and manage stress, anxiety, use of free time. These diversions can increase self-confidence, thereby improving self-esteem. *Note:* Exercise promotes release of endorphins, creating a feeling of well-being.
Provide information regarding understanding of human behavior and interactions with others; e.g., transactional analysis.	Understanding these concepts can help the client to begin to deal with past problems/losses and prevent repeating ineffective coping behaviors and self-fulfilling prophecies.
Assist client in self-examination of spirituality, faith.	Although not mandatory for recovery, surrendering to and faith in a power greater than oneself has been found to be effective for many individuals in substance recovery; may decrease sense of powerlessness.
Instruct in and role-play assertive communication skills.	Effective in helping refrain from use, to stop contact with users and dealers, to build healthy relationships, regain control of own life.
Provide treatment information on an ongoing basis.	Helps client know what to expect, and creates opportunity for client to be a part of what is happening and make informed choices about participation/outcomes.

Collaborative

Refer to/assist with making contact with programs for ongoing treatment needs; e.g., partial hospitalization drug treatment programs, Narcotics/Alcoholics Anonymous, peer support group.	Continuing treatment is essential to positive outcome. Follow-through may be easier once initial contact has been made.

NURSING DIAGNOSIS: altered Nutrition: less than body requirements

May be related to

Insufficient dietary intake to meet metabolic needs for psychologic, physiologic, or economic reasons

Possibly evidenced by

Weight loss, weight below norm for height/body build, decreased subcutaneous fat/muscle mass
Reported altered taste sensation, lack of interest in food
Poor muscle tone
Sore, inflamed buccal cavity
Laboratory evidence of protein/vitamin deficiencies

DESIRED OUTCOMES/EVALUATION CRITERIA—CLIENT WILL:

Nutritional Status (NOC)

Demonstrate progressive weight gain toward goal with normalization of laboratory values and absence of signs of malnutrition.

KNOWLEDGE: Treatment Regimen (NOC)

Verbalize understanding of effects of substance abuse, reduced dietary intake on nutritional status.
Demonstrate behaviors, lifestyle changes to regain and maintain appropriate weight.

ACTIONS/INTERVENTIONS	RATIONALE
Nutrition Therapy (NIC)	
Independent	
Assess height/weight, age, body build, strength, activity/rest level. Note condition of oral cavity.	Provides information about individual on which to base caloric needs/dietary plan. Type of diet/foods may be affected by condition of mucous membranes and teeth.
Take anthropometric measurements; e.g., triceps skinfold, when available.	Calculates subcutaneous fat and muscle mass to aid in determining dietary needs.
Note total daily calorie intake. Recommend client maintain a diary of intake, as well as times and patterns of eating.	Information will help identify nutritional needs/deficiencies.
Evaluate energy expenditure (e.g., pacing or sedentary), and establish an individualized exercise program.	Activity level affects nutritional needs. Exercise enhances muscle tone, may stimulate appetite.
Provide opportunity to choose foods/snacks to meet dietary plan.	Enhances participation/sense of control, may promote resolution of nutritional deficiencies, and helps evaluate client's understanding of dietary teaching.
Recommend monitoring weight weekly.	Provides information regarding effectiveness of dietary plan.
Collaborative	
Consult with dietitian.	Useful in establishing individual dietary needs/plan and provides additional resource for learning.
Review laboratory studies as indicated, (e.g., glucose, serum albumin/prealbumin, electrolytes).	Identifies anemias, electrolyte imbalances, and other abnormalities that may be present, requiring specific therapy.
Refer for dental consultation as necessary.	Teeth are essential to good nutritional intake and dental hygiene/care is often a neglected area in this population.

NURSING DIAGNOSIS: chronic low Self-Esteem

May be related to

Social stigma attached to substance abuse, expectation that one controls behavior
Negative role models, abuse/neglect, dysfunctional family system
Life choices perpetuating failure, situational crisis with loss of control over life events
Biochemical body change (e.g., withdrawal from alcohol/other drugs)

Possibly evidenced by

Self-negating verbalization, expressions of shame/guilt
Evaluation of self as unable to deal with events, confusion about self, purpose or direction in life
Rationalizing away/rejecting positive feedback about self

DESIRED OUTCOMES/EVALUATION CRITERIA—CLIENT WILL:

Self-Esteem (NOC)

Identify feelings and underlying dynamics for negative perception of self.
Verbalize acceptance of self as is and an increased sense of self-worth.
Set goals and participate in realistic planning for lifestyle changes necessary to live without drugs.

ACTIONS/INTERVENTIONS	RATIONALE
Self-Esteem Enhancement (NIC)	
Independent	
Provide opportunity for and encourage verbalization/discussion of individual situation.	Client often has difficulty expressing self, even more difficulty accepting the degree of importance substance has assumed in life and its relationship to present situation.
Assess mental status. Note presence of other psychiatric disorders (dual diagnosis).	Many clients use substances in an attempt to obtain relief from depression or anxiety, which may predate use and/or be the result of substance use. Approximately 60% of substance-dependent clients have underlying psychologic problems, and treatment for both is imperative to achieve/maintain abstinence.
Spend time with client. Discuss client's behavior/use of substance in a nonjudgmental way.	The nurse's presence conveys acceptance of the individual as a worthwhile person.
Provide grief counseling as indicated.	Discussion provides opportunity for insight into the problems abuse has created for the client. Life losses secondary to alcohol/drug abuse problems need to be addressed to enable client to move on with rehabilitation.
Provide reinforcement for positive actions and encourage client to accept this input.	Failure and lack of self-esteem have been problems for this client, who needs to learn to accept self as an individual with positive attributes.
Observe family interactions/SO dynamics and level of support.	Substance abuse is a family disease, and how the members act and react to the client's behavior affects the course of the disease and how client sees self. Many unconsciously become "enablers," helping the individual to cover up the consequences of the abuse. (Refer to ND: dysfunctional Family Processes: alcoholism, following.)
Encourage expression of feelings of guilt, shame, and anger.	The client often has lost respect for self and believes that the situation is hopeless. Expression of these feelings helps client begin to accept responsibility for self and take steps to make changes.
Help client acknowledge that substance use is the problem and that problems can be dealt with without the use of drugs. Confront the use of defenses; e.g., denial, projection, rationalization.	When drugs can no longer be blamed for the problems that exist, client can begin to deal with the problems and live without substance use. Confrontation helps client accept the reality of the problems as they exist.
Ask client to list and review past accomplishments and positive happenings.	There are things in everyone's life that have been successful. Often when self-esteem is low, it is difficult to remember these successes or to view them as successes.
Use techniques of role rehearsal.	Assists client to practice developing skills to cope with new role as a person who no longer uses or needs drugs to handle life's problems.
Collaborative	
Involve client in group therapy.	Group sharing helps encourage verbalization because other members of group are in various stages of abstinence from drugs and can address the client's concerns/denial. The client can gain new skills, hope, and a sense of family/community from group participation.
Formulate plan to treat other mental illness problems.	Clients who seek relief for other mental health problems through drugs will continue to do so once discharged. Both the substance use and the mental health problems need to be treated together to maximize abstinence potential. Treatment may be difficult because of difficulty of taking initiative, thinking realistically, and problem-solving. Behavioral methods seem to be most helpful.

ACTIONS/INTERVENTIONS	RATIONALE
Administer antipsychotic medications, quetiapine (Serequel), olanzapine (Zyprexa/Zydis), as necessary.	Prolonged/profound psychosis following lysergic acid diethylamide (LSD) or phencyclidine (PCP) use can be treated with these drugs because it is probably the result of an underlying functional psychosis that has now emerged. Methamphetamine psychosis often does not reverse. *Note:* Avoid the use of phenothiazines because they may decrease seizure threshold and cause hypotension in the presence of LSD/PCP use.
Monitor for diabetes, weight gain, and dyslipidemia.	Atypical antipsychotics (e.g., Zyprexa) are associated with these effects and should be monitored closely for changes in glucose control. Measurement of fasting blood glucose at the beginning of therapy and periodical monitoring during therapy are recommended.

NURSING DIAGNOSIS: dysfunctional Family Processes: alcoholism [substance abuse]

May be related to

Abuse of substance(s), resistance to treatment
Family history of substance abuse
Addictive personality
Inadequate coping skills, lack of problem-solving skills

Possibly evidenced by

Anxiety, anger/suppressed rage, shame, and embarrassment
Emotional isolation/loneliness, vulnerability, repressed emotions
Disturbed family dynamics, closed communication systems, ineffective spousal communication and marital problems
Altered role function/disruption of family roles
Manipulation, dependency, criticizing, rationalization/denial of problems
Enabling to maintain drinking (substance abuse), refusal to get help/inability to accept and receive help appropriately

DESIRED OUTCOMES/EVALUATION CRITERIA—FAMILY WILL:

Family Coping (NOC)

Verbalize understanding of dynamics of enabling behaviors.
Participate in individual family programs.
Identify ineffective coping behaviors and consequences.
Initiate and plan for necessary lifestyle changes.
Take action to change self-destructive behaviors/alter behaviors that contribute to partner's/SO's addiction.

ACTIONS/INTERVENTIONS	RATIONALE
Substance Use Treatment (NIC)	
Independent	
Review family history, explore roles of family members, circumstances involving drug use, strengths, areas for growth.	Determines areas for focus, potential for change.

ACTIONS/INTERVENTIONS	RATIONALE
Explore how the SO has coped with the client's habit (e.g., denial, repression, rationalization, hurt, loneliness, projection).	The person who enables also suffers from the same feelings as the client and uses ineffective methods for dealing with the situation, necessitating help in learning new/effective coping skills.
Determine understanding of current situation and previous methods of coping with life's problems.	Provides information on which to base present plan of care.
Assess current level of functioning of family members.	Affects individual's ability to cope with situation.
Determine extent of enabling behaviors being evidenced by family members, explore with each individual and client.	Enabling is doing for the client what he or she needs to do for self (rescuing). People want to be helpful and do not want to feel powerless to help their loved one stop substance use and change the behavior that is so destructive. However, the substance abuser often relies on others to cover up own inability to cope with daily responsibilities.
Provide information about enabling behavior, addictive disease characteristics for both user and nonuser.	Awareness and knowledge of behaviors (e.g., avoiding and shielding, taking over responsibilities, rationalizing, and subserving) provide opportunity for individuals to begin the process of change.
Identify and discuss sabotage behaviors of family members.	Even though family member(s) may verbalize a desire for the individual to become substance free, the reality of interactive dynamics is that they may unconsciously not want the individual to recover because this would affect the family member's/members' own role in the relationship. Additionally, they may receive sympathy/attention from others (secondary gain).
Encourage participation in therapeutic writing; e.g., journaling (narrative), guided or focused.	Serves as a release for feelings (e.g., anger, grief, stress), helps move individuals forward in treatment process.
Provide factual information to client and family about the effects of addictive behaviors on the family and what to expect after discharge.	Many clients/SOs are not aware of the nature of addiction. If client is using legally obtained drugs, he or she may believe this does not constitute abuse.
Encourage family members to be aware of their own feelings, look at the situation with perspective and objectivity. They can ask themselves: "Am I being conned? Am I acting out of fear, shame, guilt, or anger? Do I have a need to control?"	When the enabling family members become aware of their own actions that perpetuate the addict's problems, they need to decide to change themselves. If they change, the client can then face the consequences of his or her own actions and may choose to get well.
Provide support for enabling partner(s). Encourage group work.	Families/SOs need support to produce change as much as the person who is addicted.
Assist the client's partner to become aware that client's abstinence and drug use are not the partner's responsibility.	Partners need to learn that user's habit may or may not change despite partner's involvement in treatment.
Help the recovering (former user) partner who is enabling to distinguish between destructive aspects of behavior and genuine motivation to aid the user.	Enabling behavior can be partner's attempts at personal survival.
Note how partner relates to the treatment team/staff.	Determines enabling style. A parallel exists between how partner relates to user and to staff, based on partner's feelings about self and situation.
Explore conflicting feelings the enabling partner may have about treatment; e.g., feelings similar to those of abuser (blend of anger, guilt, fear, exhaustion, embarrassment, loneliness, distrust, grief, and possibly relief).	Useful in establishing the need for therapy for the partner. This individual's own identity may have been lost, she or he may fear self-disclosure to staff, and may have difficulty giving up the dependent relationship.
Involve family in discharge referral plans.	Drug abuse is a family illness. Because the family has been so involved in dealing with the substance abuse behavior, family members need help adjusting to the new behavior of sobriety/abstinence. Incidence of recovery is almost doubled when the family is treated along with the client.
Be aware of staff's enabling behaviors and feelings about client and enabling partners.	Lack of understanding of enabling can result in nontherapeutic approaches to clients and their families.

ACTIONS/INTERVENTIONS	RATIONALE
Collaborative	
Involve in substance abuse treatment plan.	Can be voluntary, court ordered, or via Department of Human Services involvement.
Encourage involvement with self-help associations, Alcoholics/Narcotics Anonymous, Al-Anon, Alateen, and professional family therapy.	Puts client/family in direct contact with support systems necessary for continued sobriety and to assist with problem resolution.

NURSING DIAGNOSIS: Sexual Dysfunction

May be related to

Altered body function: Neurologic damage and debilitating effects of drug use (particularly alcohol and opiates)

Possibly evidenced by

Progressive interference with sexual functioning
In men: a significant degree of testicular atrophy is noted (testes are smaller and softer than normal), gynecomastia (breast enlargement), impotence/decreased sperm counts
In women: loss of body hair, thin soft skin, and spider angioma (elevated estrogen), amenorrhea/increase in miscarriages

DESIRED OUTCOMES/EVALUATION CRITERIA—CLIENT WILL:

Substance Addiction Consequences (NOC)

Verbally acknowledge effects of drug use on sexual functioning/reproduction.

Sexual Functioning (NOC)

Identify interventions to correct/overcome individual situation.

ACTIONS/INTERVENTIONS	RATIONALE
Sexual Counseling (NIC)	
Independent	
Ascertain client's beliefs and expectations. Have client describe problem in own words.	Determines level of knowledge, identifies misperceptions, level of concern regarding STDs, level of risk reduction, and specific learning needs.
Encourage and accept individual expressions of concern.	Most people find it difficult to talk about this sensitive subject and may not ask directly for information.
Provide education opportunity (e.g., pamphlets, consultation with appropriate persons) for client to learn effects of drug on sexual functioning.	Much of denial and hesitancy to seek treatment may be reduced as a result of sufficient and appropriate information.
Provide information about individual's condition.	Sexual functioning may have been affected by drug (alcohol) itself and/or psychologic factors (such as stress or depression). Information can assist client to understand own situation and identify actions to be taken.
Assess drinking/drug history of pregnant client. Provide information about effects of substance abuse on the reproductive system/fetus (e.g., increased risk of premature birth, brain damage, and fetal malformation).	Awareness of the negative effects of alcohol/other drugs on reproduction may motivate client to stop using drug(s). When client is pregnant, identification of potential problems aids in planning for future fetal needs/concerns.

ACTIONS/INTERVENTIONS	RATIONALE
Discuss prognosis for sexual dysfunction; e.g., impotence/low sexual desire.	In about 50% of cases, impotence is reversed with abstinence from drug(s); in 25%, the return to normal functioning is delayed; and approximately 25% remain impotent.

Collaborative

Refer for sexual counseling if indicated.	Couple may need additional assistance to resolve more severe problems/situations. Client may have difficulty adjusting if drug has improved sexual experience (e.g., heroin decreases dyspareunia in women/premature ejaculation in men). Furthermore, the client may have engaged enjoyably in bizarre, erotic sexual behavior under influence of the stimulant drug; client may have found no substitute for the drug, may have driven a partner away, and may have no motivation to adjust to sexual experience without drugs.
Review results of sonogram if pregnant.	Assesses fetal growth and development to identify possibility of fetal alcohol syndrome/other drug harmful effects and future needs. There are concerns about placental abruption with the use of methamphetamine and cocaine.

NURSING DIAGNOSIS: deficient Knowledge [Learning Need] regarding condition, prognosis, treatment, self care, and discharge needs

May be related to

Lack of information, information misinterpretation
Cognitive limitations/interference with learning (other mental illness problems/organic brain syndrome), lack of recall

Possibly evidenced by

Statements of concern, questions/misconceptions
Inaccurate follow-through of instructions/development of preventable complications
Continued use in spite of complications/adverse consequences

DESIRED OUTCOMES/EVALUATION CRITERIA—CLIENT WILL:

KNOWLEDGE: Substance Abuse Control (NOC)

Verbalize understanding of own condition/disease process, prognosis, and potential complications.
Verbalize understanding of therapeutic needs.
Identify/initiate necessary lifestyle changes to remain drug free.
Participate in treatment program including plan for follow-up/long-term care.

ACTIONS/INTERVENTIONS	RATIONALE
Learning Facilitation (NIC)	
Independent	
Be aware of and deal with anxiety of client and family members.	Anxiety can interfere with ability to hear and assimilate information.
Provide an active role for the client/SO in the learning process; e.g., discussions, group participation, role-playing.	Learning is enhanced when persons are actively involved.

ACTIONS/INTERVENTIONS	RATIONALE
Provide written and verbal information as indicated. Include list of articles, books, Internet sites, special TV programs related to client/family needs and encourage reading and discussing what they learn.	Helps client/SO make informed choices about future and can be a useful addition to other therapeutic approaches.
Assess client's knowledge of own situation; e.g., disease, complications, and needed changes in lifestyle.	Assists in planning for long-range changes necessary for maintaining sobriety/drug-free status. Client may have street knowledge of the drug but be ignorant of medical facts.
Pace learning activities to individual needs.	Facilitates learning because information is more readily assimilated when timing is considered.

TEACHING: Disease Process (NIC)

Review condition and prognosis/future expectations.	Provides knowledge base from which client can make informed choices.
Discuss relationship of drug use to current situation.	Often client has misperception (denial) of real reason for admission to the medical (psychiatric) setting.
Educate about effects of specific drug(s) used; e.g., PCP is deposited in body fat and may reactivate (flashbacks) even after long interval of abstinence; alcohol use may result in mental deterioration, liver involvement/damage; cocaine can damage postcapillary vessels and increase platelet aggregation, promoting thromboses and infarction of skin/internal organs, causing localized atrophie blanche or sclerodermatous lesions.	Information will help client understand possible long-term effects of drug use.
Discuss potential for reemergence of withdrawal symptoms in stimulant abuse as early as 3 months or as late as 9–12 months after discontinuing use.	Even though intoxication may have passed, client may manifest denial, drug hunger, and periods of "flare-up," wherein there is a delayed recurrence of withdrawal symptoms (e.g., anxiety; depression; irritability; sleep disturbance; compulsiveness with food, especially sugars).
Inform client of effects of disulfiram (Antabuse) in combination with alcohol intake and importance of avoiding use of alcohol-containing products; e.g., cough syrups, foods/candy, mouthwash, aftershave, cologne.	Interaction of alcohol and Antabuse results in nausea and hypotension, which may produce fatal shock. Individuals on Antabuse are sensitive to alcohol on a continuum, with some being able to drink while taking the drug and others having a reaction with only slight exposure. Reactions also appear to be dose-related.
Review specific aftercare needs; e.g., PCP user should drink cranberry juice and continue use of ascorbic acid; alcohol abuser with liver damage should refrain from drugs/anesthetics or use of household cleaning products that are detoxified in the liver.	Promotes individualized care related to specific situation. Cranberry juice and ascorbic acid enhance clearance of PCP from the system. Substances that have the potential for liver damage are more dangerous in the presence of an already damaged liver.
Discuss variety of helpful organizations and programs that are available for assistance/referral such as AA, Dual Recovery Anonymous, Narcotics Anonymous.	Long-term support is necessary to maintain optimal recovery. Psychosocial needs and other issues may need to be addressed.

POTENTIAL CONSIDERATIONS following acute care (dependent on client's age, physical condition/presence of complications, personal resources, and life responsibilities)

ineffective [individual]/family Therapeutic Regimen Management—decisional conflicts, excessive demands made on individual or family, family conflict, perceived seriousness/benefits.

ineffective Coping—vulnerability, situational crises, multiple life changes, inadequate relaxation, inadequate/loss of support systems.

readiness for enhanced family Coping—needs sufficiently gratified and adaptive tasks effectively addressed to enable goals of self-actualization to surface.

(Physical needs depend on substance effect on organ systems—refer to appropriate medical plans of care for additional considerations.)

CANCER

Cancer is a general term used to describe a disturbance of cellular growth and refers to a group of diseases and not a single disease entity. There are currently more than 150 different known types of cancer. Because cancer is a cellular disease, it can arise from any body tissue, with manifestations that result from failure to control the proliferation and maturation of cells.

There are four main classifications of cancer according to tissue type: (1) lymphomas (cancers originating in infection-fighting organs), (2) leukemias (cancers originating in blood-forming organs), (3) sarcomas (cancers originating in bones, muscle, or connective tissue), and (4) carcinomas (cancers originating in epithelial cells). Within these broad categories, a cancer is classified by histology, stage, and grade.

Through years of observation and documentation, it has been noted that the metastatic behavior of cancers varies according to the primary site of diagnosis. This behavior pattern is known as the "natural history." An example is the metastatic pattern for primary breast cancer: breast-bone-lung-liver-brain. Knowledge of the etiology and natural history of a cancer type is important in planning the client's care and in evaluating the client's progress, prognosis, and physical complaints.

CARE SETTING

Cancer centers may focus on staging and major treatment modalities for complex cancers. Treatment for managing adverse effects such as malnutrition and infection may take place in short-stay, ambulatory, or community settings. More cancer clients are receiving care at home because of personal choice and healthcare costs.

RELATED CONCERNS

End of life/hospice care, page 880
Fecal diversion: postoperative care of ileostomy and colostomy, page 338
Hysterectomy, page 621
Leukemias, page 523
Lung cancer (postoperative care), page 141
Lymphomas, page 532
Mastectomy, page 630
Prostatectomy, page 604
Psychosocial aspects of care, page 770
Radical neck surgery: laryngectomy (postoperative care), page 157
Sepsis/septicemia, page 701
Total nutritional support: parenteral/enteral feeding, page 478
Urinary diversion/urostomy (postoperative care), page 585

Client Assessment Database

Depends on organs/tissues involved and stage of disease.

Refer to appropriate plans of care for additional assessment information.

ACTIVITY/REST

May report: Weakness and/or fatigue
Changes in rest pattern and usual hours of sleep per night; presence of factors affecting sleep; e.g., pain, anxiety, night sweats
Limitations of participation in hobbies, exercise, usual activities

CIRCULATION

May report: Palpitations, chest pain on exertion
May exhibit: Changes in BP, fluctuations in heart rate

EGO INTEGRITY

May report: Stress factors (financial, job, role changes) and ways of handling stress (e.g., smoking, drinking, delay in seeking treatment, religious/spiritual belief)
Concern about changes in appearance; e.g., alopecia, disfiguring lesions, surgery, profound weight loss, edema and/or weight gain
Denial of diagnosis, feelings of powerlessness, hopelessness, helplessness, worthlessness, guilt, loss of control, depression
May exhibit: Denial, withdrawal, anger

ELIMINATION

May report: Changes in bowel pattern; e.g., blood in stools, pain with defecation, constipation
Changes in urinary elimination; e.g., pain or burning on urination, hematuria, frequent urination

May exhibit: Changes in bowel sounds, abdominal distention, diarrhea, dysuria, frequency, incontinence

FOOD/FLUID

May report: Poor dietary habits (e.g., low-fiber, high-fat, additives, preservatives)
Anorexia, nausea/vomiting; difficulty swallowing, mouth sores
Food intolerances

May exhibit: Changes in weight, severe weight loss, cachexia, wasting of muscle mass
Changes in skin moisture/turgor, edema
Ulcerations of oral mucosa

NEUROSENSORY

May report: Dizziness, syncope, lack of coordination, unstable balance
Numbness/tingling of extremities, sensation of coldness, difficulty performing fine motor skills (i.e., buttoning shirt)

PAIN/DISCOMFORT

May report: No pain, or varying degrees; e.g., mild discomfort to severe pain (associated with disease process)

RESPIRATION

May report: Smoking (tobacco, marijuana), living with someone who smokes
Asbestos or dust exposure (e.g., coal, sandstone)
History of chronic respiratory disease
Dyspnea with exertion

SAFETY

May report: Exposure to toxic chemicals, carcinogens (occupation/profession or environment)
Excessive/prolonged sun exposure

May exhibit: Skin rashes, ulcerations; dry, leather-like skin

SEXUALITY

May report: Sexual concerns; e.g., impact on relationship, change in level of satisfaction, impotence
Nulligravida greater than 30 years of age, multigravida, multiple sex partners, early sexual activity, genital herpes, exposure to HPV (human papillomavirus)

SOCIAL INTERACTION

May report: Inadequate/weak support system
Marital history (regarding in-home satisfaction, support, or help)
Concerns about role function/responsibility

TEACHING/LEARNING

May report: Family history of cancer; e.g., multiple family members/mother, grandmother, aunt or sister with breast cancer
Primary site, date discovered/diagnosed
Metastatic disease: Additional sites involved (if none, natural history of primary will provide important information for looking for metastasis)
Treatment history: Previous treatment for cancer—place and treatments given

Discharge plan considerations: May require assistance with finances, medications/treatments, wound care/supplies, transportation, food shopping and preparation, self-care, homemaker/maintenance tasks, provision for child care, changes in living facilities/hospice

Refer to section at end of plan for postdischarge considerations.

DIAGNOSTIC STUDIES

Test selection depends on history, clinical manifestations, and index of suspicion for a particular cancer.
Endoscopy: Used for direct visualization of body organs/cavities to detect abnormalities.

Scans (e.g., magnetic resonance imaging [MRI], CT, gallium, positron emission tomography [PET]) and ultrasound: May be done for diagnostic purposes, identification of metastasis, and evaluation of response to treatment.

Biopsy (fine-needle aspiration [FNA], needle core, incisional/excisional): Done to differentiate diagnosis and delineate treatment and may be taken from various sites; e.g., bone marrow, skin, or organ. Example: Bone marrow is done in myeloproliferative diseases for diagnosis; in solid tumors for staging.

Tumor markers (substances produced and secreted by tumor cells and found in serum, e.g., carcinoembryonic antigen [CEA], prostate-specific antigen [PSA], α-fetoprotein (AFP), human chorionic gonadotropin [hCG], CA15-3, CA19-9, CA125): Helpful in diagnosing cancer but more useful as prognostic indicator and/or therapeutic monitor. For example, CA125 levels are monitored in ovarian cancer. Often these levels are high prior to surgery. The levels should be lower after surgery and with a response to chemotherapy. If the cancer begins to grow, usually the CA125 level will begin to increase before any other signs or symptoms are evident.

Hormone receptors: Estrogen and progesterone receptors are assays done on breast tissue to provide information about whether or not hormonal manipulation would be therapeutic in breast cancer treatment/control. *Note:* Any hormone may be elevated because many cancers secrete inappropriate hormones (ectopic hormone secretion).

Her-2/neu ***amplification:*** *Her-2/neu* is a cellular proto-oncogene that stimulates cell growth. Amplification (a large number of these receptors found on the cell surface) results in more aggressive breast cancers and usually worse prognosis with earlier appearance of metastatic disease.

Gene mutations: *BRCA-1* and *BRCA-2* function as tumor suppressor genes. If these genes are mutated, there may be an increased lifetime risk of acquiring breast, ovarian, prostatic, and possibly other cancers.

Screening chemistry tests, e.g., electrolytes (sodium, potassium, calcium), renal tests (BUN/Cr), liver tests (bilirubin, AST, alkaline phosphatase, LDH), bone tests (calcium): Depend on individual condition, risk factors.

CBC with differential and platelets: May reveal anemia, changes in RBCs and WBCs; reduced or increased platelets.

Chest x-ray: Screens for primary or metastatic disease of lungs.

NURSING PRIORITIES

1. Support adaptation and independence.
2. Promote comfort.
3. Maintain optimal physiologic functioning.
4. Prevent complications.
5. Provide information about disease process/condition, prognosis, and treatment needs.

DISCHARGE GOALS

1. Client is dealing with current situation realistically.
2. Pain alleviated/controlled.
3. Homeostasis achieved.
4. Complications prevented/minimized.
5. Disease process/condition, prognosis, and therapeutic choices and regimen understood.
6. Plan in place to meet needs after discharge.

NURSING DIAGNOSIS: Fear/Anxiety (specify level)

May be related to

Situational crisis (cancer)
Threat to/change in health/socioeconomic status, role functioning, interaction patterns
Threat of death
Separation from family (hospitalization, treatments), interpersonal transmission/contagion of feelings

Possibly evidenced by

Increased tension, shakiness, apprehension, restlessness, insomnia
Expressed concerns regarding changes in life events
Feelings of helplessness, hopelessness, inadequacy
Sympathetic stimulation, somatic complaints

DESIRED OUTCOMES/EVALUATION CRITERIA—CLIENT WILL:

Fear [or] Anxiety Self-Control (NOC)

Display appropriate range of feelings and lessened fear.
Appear relaxed and report anxiety is reduced to a manageable level.
Demonstrate use of effective coping mechanisms and active participation in treatment regimen.

ACTIONS/INTERVENTIONS	RATIONALE
Anxiety Reduction (NIC)	
Independent	
Review client's/SO's previous experience with cancer. Determine what the doctor has told client and what conclusion client has reached.	Clarifies client's perceptions; assists in identification of fear(s) and misconceptions based on diagnosis and experience with cancer.
Encourage client to share thoughts and feelings.	Provides opportunity to examine realistic fears and misconceptions about diagnosis.
Provide open environment in which client feels safe to discuss feelings or to refrain from talking.	Helps client feel accepted in present condition without feeling judged and promotes sense of dignity and control.
Maintain frequent contact with client. Talk with and touch client as appropriate.	Provides assurance that the client is not alone or rejected; conveys respect for and acceptance of the person, fostering trust.
Be aware of effects of isolation on client when required by immunosuppression or radiation implant. Limit use of isolation clothing/masks as possible.	Sensory deprivation may result when sufficient stimulation is not available and may intensify feelings of anxiety/fear and alienation.
Assist client/SO in recognizing and clarifying fears to begin developing coping strategies for dealing with these fears.	Coping skills are often stressed after diagnosis and during different phases of treatment. Support and counseling are often necessary to enable individual to recognize and deal with fear and to realize that control/coping strategies are available.
Provide accurate, consistent information regarding diagnosis and prognosis. Avoid arguing about client's perceptions of situation.	Can reduce anxiety and enable client to make decisions/choices based on realities.
Permit expressions of anger, fear, despair without confrontation. Give information that feelings are normal and are to be appropriately expressed.	Acceptance of feelings allows client to begin to deal with situation.
Explain the recommended treatment, its purpose, and potential side effects. Help client prepare for treatments.	The goal of cancer treatment is to destroy malignant cells while minimizing damage to normal ones. Treatment may include surgery (curative, preventive, palliative), as well as chemotherapy, radiation (internal, external), or newer/organ-specific treatments such as whole-body hyperthermia or biotherapy. Bone marrow or peripheral progenitor cell (stem cell) transplant may be recommended for some types of cancer.
Explain procedures, providing opportunity for questions and honest answers. Stay with client during anxiety-producing procedures and consultations.	Accurate information allows client to deal more effectively with reality of situation, thereby reducing anxiety and fear of the unknown.
Provide primary and consistent caregivers whenever possible.	May help reduce anxiety by fostering therapeutic relationship and facilitating continuity of care.

ACTIONS/INTERVENTIONS	RATIONALE
Promote calm, quiet environment.	Facilitates rest, conserves energy, and may enhance coping abilities.
Identify stage/degree of grief client and SO are currently experiencing. (Refer to ND: anticipatory Grieving, following.)	Choice of interventions is dictated by stage of grief, coping behaviors; e.g., anger/withdrawal, denial.
Note ineffective coping; e.g., poor social interactions, helplessness, giving up everyday functions and usual sources of gratification.	Identifies individual problems and provides support for client/SO in using effective coping skills.
Be alert to signs of denial/depression; e.g., withdrawal, anger, inappropriate remarks. Determine presence of suicidal ideation and assess potential on a scale of 1–10.	Client may use defense mechanism of denial and express hope that diagnosis is inaccurate. Feelings of guilt, spiritual distress, physical symptoms, or lack of cure may cause the client to become withdrawn and believe that suicide is a viable alternative.
Encourage and foster client interaction with support systems.	Reduces feelings of isolation. If family support systems are not available, outside sources may be needed immediately; e.g., local cancer support groups.
Provide reliable and consistent information and support for SO.	Allows for better interpersonal interaction and reduction of anxiety and fear.
Include SO as indicated/client desires when major decisions are to be made.	Provides a support system for the client and allows the SO to be involved appropriately.

Collaborative

Administer antianxiety medications, e.g., lorazepam (Ativan), alprazolam (Xanax), as indicated.	May be useful for brief periods of time to help client handle feelings of anxiety related to diagnosis/situation and/or during periods of high stress.
Refer to additional resources for counseling/support as needed.	May be useful from time to time to assist client/SO in dealing with anxiety.

NURSING DIAGNOSIS: anticipatory Grieving

May be related to

Anticipated loss of physiologic well-being (e.g., loss of body part; change in body function), change in lifestyle
Perceived potential death of client

Possibly evidenced by

Changes in eating habits, alterations in sleep patterns, activity levels, libido, and communication patterns
Denial of potential loss, choked feelings, anger

DESIRED OUTCOMES/EVALUATION CRITERIA—CLIENT WILL:

Grief Resolution (NOC)

Identify and express feelings appropriately.
Continue normal life activities, looking toward/planning for the future, one day at a time.
Verbalize reality/acceptance of situation.

ACTIONS/INTERVENTIONS	RATIONALE
Grief Work Facilitation (NIC)	
Independent	
Expect initial shock and disbelief following diagnosis of cancer and/or traumatizing procedures (e.g., disfiguring surgery, colostomy, amputation).	Few clients are fully prepared for the reality of the changes that can occur.
Assess client/SO for stage of grief currently being experienced. Explain process as appropriate.	Knowledge about the grieving process reinforces the normality of feelings/reactions being experienced and can help client deal more effectively with them.
Provide open, nonjudgmental environment. Use therapeutic communication skills of active-listening, acknowledgment, and so on.	Promotes and encourages realistic dialogue about feelings and concerns.
Encourage verbalization of thoughts/concerns and accept expressions of sadness, anger, rejection. Acknowledge normality of these feelings.	Client may feel supported in expression of feelings by the understanding that deep and often conflicting emotions are normal and experienced by others in this difficult situation.
Be aware of mood swings, evidence of conflict, expressions of anger/hostility, and other acting-out behavior. Set limits on inappropriate behavior, redirect negative thinking.	May be client's way of expressing/dealing with feelings of despair/spiritual distress reflecting ineffective coping and need for additional interventions. Preventing destructive actions enables client to maintain control and sense of self-esteem.
Note signs of debilitating depression. Ask client direct questions about state of mind. Listen for statements of despair, guilt, hopelessness; e.g., "nothing to live for."	Studies show that many cancer clients are at high risk for suicide. They are especially vulnerable when recently diagnosed and/or discharged from hospital.
Reinforce teaching regarding disease process and treatments. Be honest; do not give false hope while providing emotional support.	Client/SO benefit from factual information. Honest answers promote trust and provide reassurance that correct information will be given.
Review past life experiences, role changes, and coping skills.	Opportunity to identify skills that may help individuals cope with grief of current situation more effectively.
Hope Instillation (NIC)	
Identify positive aspects of the situation.	Possibility of remission and slow progression of disease and/or new therapies can offer hope for the future.
Discuss ways client/SO can plan together for the future. Encourage setting of realistic goals.	Having a part in problem-solving/planning can provide a sense of control over anticipated events.
Assist client/SO to identify strengths in self/situation and support systems.	Recognizing these resources provides opportunity to work through feelings of grief.
Encourage participation in care and treatment decisions.	Allows client to retain some control over life.
Refer to appropriate counselor as needed (e.g., psychiatric clinical nurse specialist, social worker, hospice counselor, psychologist, clergy).	Can help alleviate distress or palliate feelings of grief to facilitate coping and foster growth.
Refer to visiting nurse, home health agency as needed, or hospice program, if appropriate.	Provides support in meeting physical and emotional needs of client/SO, and can supplement the care family and friends are able to give.

Refer to CP: End of Life/Hospice Care, ND: anticipatory Grieving/death Anxiety, for additional interventions.

NURSING DIAGNOSIS: situational low Self-Esteem

May be related to

Biophysical: disfiguring surgery, chemotherapy or radiotherapy side effects; e.g., loss of hair, nausea/vomiting, weight loss, anorexia, impotence, sterility, overwhelming fatigue, uncontrolled pain

Psychosocial: threat of death, feelings of lack of control and doubt regarding acceptance by others, fear and anxiety

Possibly evidenced by

Verbalization of change in lifestyle, fear of rejection/reaction of others, negative feelings about body, feelings of helplessness, hopelessness, powerlessness
Preoccupation with change or loss
Not taking responsibility for self-care, lack of follow-through
Change in self-perception/other's perception of role

DESIRED OUTCOMES/EVALUATION CRITERIA—CLIENT WILL:

Self-Esteem (NOC)

Verbalize understanding of body changes, acceptance of self in situation.
Begin to develop coping mechanisms to deal effectively with problems.
Demonstrate adaptation to changes/events that have occurred as evidenced by setting of realistic goals and active participation in work/play/personal relationships as appropriate.

ACTIONS/INTERVENTIONS	RATIONALE
Chemotherapy [or] Radiation Therapy Management (NIC)	
Independent	
Discuss with client/SO how the diagnosis and treatment are affecting the client's personal life/home and work activities.	Aids in defining concerns to begin problem-solving process.
Review anticipated side effects associated with a particular treatment, including possible effects on sexual activity and sense of attractiveness/desirability; e.g., alopecia, disfiguring surgery. Tell client that not all side effects occur and that others may be minimized/controlled.	Anticipatory guidance can help client/SO begin the process of adaptation to new state and to prepare for some side effects; e.g., buy a wig before radiation, schedule time off from work as indicated. (Refer to ND: risk for ineffective Sexuality Patterns.)
Encourage discussion of/problem-solve concerns about effects of cancer/treatments on role as homemaker, wage earner, parent, and so forth.	May help reduce problems that interfere with acceptance of treatment or aggravate progression of disease.
Acknowledge difficulties client may be experiencing. Give information that counseling is often necessary and important in the adaptation process.	Validates reality of client's feelings and gives permission to take whatever measures are necessary to cope with what is happening.
Evaluate support structures available to and used by client/SO.	Helps with planning for care while hospitalized and after discharge.
Provide emotional support for client/SO during diagnostic tests and treatment phase.	Although some clients adapt/adjust to cancer effects or side effects of therapy, many need additional support during this period.
Use touch during interactions, if acceptable to client, and maintain eye contact.	Affirmation of individuality and acceptance is important in reducing client's feelings of insecurity and self-doubt.
Collaborative	
Refer client/SO to supportive group programs (e.g., I Can Cope, Reach to Recovery, Encore).	Group support is usually very beneficial for both client and SO, providing contact with other clients with cancer at various levels of treatment and/or recovery, validating feelings, and assisting with problem-solving.

ACTIONS/INTERVENTIONS	RATIONALE
Refer for professional counseling as indicated.	May be necessary to regain and maintain a positive psychosocial structure if client/SO support systems are deteriorating.

NURSING DIAGNOSIS: acute/chronic Pain

May be related to

Disease process (compression/destruction of nerve tissue, infiltration of nerves or their vascular supply, obstruction of a nerve pathway, inflammation)
Side effects of various cancer therapy agents

Possibly evidenced by

Reports of pain
Self-focusing/narrowed focus
Alteration in muscle tone; facial mask of pain
Distraction/guarding behaviors
Autonomic responses, restlessness (acute pain)

DESIRED OUTCOMES/EVALUATION CRITERIA—CLIENT WILL:

Pain Level (NOC)

Report maximal pain relief/control with minimal interference with ADLs.

Pain Control (NOC)

Follow prescribed pharmacologic regimen.
Demonstrate use of relaxation skills and diversional activities as indicated for individual situation.

ACTIONS/INTERVENTIONS	RATIONALE
Pain Management (NIC)	
Independent	
Determine pain history, e.g., location of pain, frequency, duration, and intensity using numeric rating scale (0–10 scale), or verbal rating scale ("no pain" to "excruciating pain") and relief measures used. Believe client's report.	Information provides baseline data to evaluate need for/effectiveness of interventions. Pain of more than 6 mo duration constitutes chronic pain, which may affect therapeutic choices. Recurrent episodes of acute pain can occur within chronic pain, requiring increased level of intervention. *Note:* The pain experience is an individualized one composed of both physical and emotional responses.
Determine timing/precipitants of "breakthrough" pain when using around-the-clock agents, whether oral, IV, topical, transmucosal, epidural, or patch medications.	Pain may occur near the end of the dose interval, indicating need for higher dose or shorter dose interval. Pain may be precipitated by identifiable triggers, or occur spontaneously, requiring use of short half-life agents for rescue or supplemental doses.
Evaluate/be aware of painful effects of particular therapies; i.e., surgery, radiation, chemotherapy, biotherapy. Provide information to client/SO about what to expect.	A wide range of discomforts are common (e.g., incisional pain, burning skin, low back pain, mouth sores, headaches), depending on the procedure/agent being used. Pain is also associated with invasive procedures to diagnose/treat cancer.

ACTIONS/INTERVENTIONS	RATIONALE
Provide nonpharmacologic comfort measures (e.g., massage, repositioning, backrub) and diversional activities (e.g., music, television).	Promotes relaxation and helps refocus attention.
Encourage use of stress management skills/complementary therapies (e.g., relaxation techniques, visualization, guided imagery, biofeedback, laughter, music, aromatherapy, and therapeutic touch).	Enables client to participate actively in nondrug treatment of pain and enhances sense of control. Pain produces stress and, in conjunction with muscle tension and internal stressors, increases client's focus on self, which in turn increases the level of pain.
Provide cutaneous stimulation; e.g., heat/cold, massage.	May decrease inflammation, muscle spasms, reducing associated pain. *Note:* Heat may increase bleeding/edema following acute injury, whereas cold may further reduce perfusion to ischemic tissues.
Be aware of barriers to cancer pain management related to client, as well as the healthcare system.	Clients may be reluctant to report pain for reasons such as fear that disease is worse; worry about unmanageable side effects of pain medications; beliefs that pain has meaning, such as "God wills it," they should overcome it, or that pain is merited or deserved for some reason. Healthcare system problems include factors such as inadequate assessment of pain, concern about controlled substances/client addiction, inadequate reimbursement/cost of treatment modalities.
Evaluate pain relief/control at regular intervals. Adjust medication regimen as necessary.	Goal is maximum pain control with minimum interference with ADLs. *Note:* Opioid tolerance requires ongoing readjustment of dosage and use of combination therapy.
Inform client/SO of the expected therapeutic effects and discuss management of side effects.	This information helps establish realistic expectations, confidence in own ability to handle what happens.

Collaborative

ACTIONS/INTERVENTIONS	RATIONALE
Discuss use of additional alternative/complementary therapies; e.g., acupuncture/acupressure.	May provide reduction/relief of pain without drug-related side effects.
Develop individualized pain management plan with the client and physician. Provide written copy of plan to client, family/SO, and care providers.	An organized plan beginning with the simplest dosage schedules and least invasive modalities improves chance for pain control. Particularly with chronic pain, client/SO must be active participant in pain management and all care providers need to be consistent.
Administer analgesics as indicated; e.g.:	A wide range of analgesics and associated agents may be employed around-the-clock to manage pain. *Note:* Addiction to or dependency on drug is not a concern.
Opioids; e.g., codeine, morphine (MSContin), oxycodone (oxycontin), hydrocodone (Vicodin), hydromorphone (Dilaudid), methadone (Dolophine), fentanyl (Duragesic), oxymorphone (Numorphan);	Effective for localized and generalized moderate to severe pain, with long-acting/controlled-release forms available. Routes of administration include oral, transmucosal, transdermal, nasal, rectal, and infusions (subcutaneous, IV, epidural, intrathecal), which may be delivered via PCA. IM use is not recommended because absorption is not reliable, in addition to being painful and inconvenient. Note: Fentanyl citrate (Oralet) is a transmucosal agent that is stroked on the inner cheek and absorbed through the mucosa. It was developed to control breakthrough pain in clients using sustained release preparations of fentanyl (patch).
Acetaminophen (Tylenol) and nonsteroidal anti-inflammatory drugs (NSAIDs), including aspirin, ibuprofen (Motrin, Advil), peroxicam (Feldene), indomethacin (Indocin);	Adjuvant drugs are useful for mild to moderate pain and can be combined with opioid and other modalities.
Corticosteroids, e.g., dexamethasone (Decadron); prednisone;	May be effective in controlling pain associated with inflammatory process (e.g., metastatic bone pain, acute spinal cord compression, and neuropathic pain).

ACTIONS/INTERVENTIONS	RATIONALE
Anticonvulsants; e.g., phenytoin (Dilantin), valproic acid (Depakote), clonazepam (Klonopin), gabapentin (Neurontin);	Useful for peripheral pain syndromes associated with neuropathic pain, especially shooting pain.
Tricyclic antidepressants; e.g., amitriptyline (Elavil), imipramine (Tofranil), doxepin (Sinequan), trazodone (Desyrel);	Effective for neuropathic pain (e.g., tingling, burning pain) and pain resulting from surgery, chemotherapy, or nerve infiltration.
Antihistamines; e.g., hydroxyzine (Atarax, Vistaril);	Mild anxiolytic agent with sedative and analgesic properties. May produce additive analgesia with therapeutic doses of opioids and may be beneficial in limiting opioid-induced nausea/vomiting.
Radioisotopes; e.g., strontium-89 (Metastron), Samarium SM 153 lexidronam (Quadramet);	Effective in treating pain resulting from osteoblastic metastatic bone lesions. Drug onset is about 1 wk with duration of 2–4 months. May help reduce dosage of opioid analgesics. *Note:* Bone marrow/WBC and platelet counts may be suppressed for up to 8 wk after cessation of the drug.
Bisphosphonates; e.g., Pamidronate (Aredia), zoledronic acid (Zometa).	Specific inhibitors of osteoclastic activity that treat hypercalcemia and reduce bone pain and fractures (especially in multiple myeloma, breast, and prostate cancer).
Provide/instruct in use of PCA as appropriate.	Provides for timely drug administration, preventing fluctuations in intensity of pain, often at lower total dosage than would be given by conventional methods.
Instruct in use of electrical stimulation (e.g., TENS) unit.	TENS blocks nerve transmission of pain stimulus, providing reduction/relief of pain without drug-related side effects. Can be used in combination with other modalities.
Prepare for/assist with procedures; e.g., nerve blocks, cordotomy, commissural myelotomy, radiation therapy.	May be used in severe/intractable pain unresponsive to other measures. *Note:* Radiation is especially useful for bone metastasis and may provide fast onset of pain relief even with only one treatment.
Refer to structured support group, psychiatric clinical nurse specialist, psychologist, spiritual advisor for counseling as indicated.	May be necessary to reduce anxiety and enhance client's coping skills, decreasing level of pain. *Note:* Hypnosis can heighten awareness and help to focus concentration to decrease perception of pain.

NURSING DIAGNOSIS: imbalanced Nutrition: less than body requirements

May be related to

Hypermetabolic state associated with cancer
Consequences of chemotherapy, radiation, surgery; e.g., anorexia, gastric irritation, taste distortions, nausea
Emotional distress, fatigue, poorly controlled pain

Possibly evidenced by

Reported inadequate food intake, altered taste sensation, loss of interest in food, perceived/actual inability to ingest food, vomiting
Body weight 20% or more under ideal for height and frame, decreased subcutaneous fat/muscle mass
Sore, inflamed buccal cavity
Diarrhea and/or constipation, abdominal cramping

DESIRED OUTCOMES/EVALUATION CRITERIA—CLIENT WILL:

Nutritional Status (NOC)

Demonstrate stable weight/progressive weight gain toward goal with normalization of laboratory values and be free of signs of malnutrition.

KNOWLEDGE: Diet (NOC)

Verbalize understanding of individual interferences to adequate intake.
Participate in specific interventions to stimulate appetite/increase dietary intake.

ACTIONS/INTERVENTIONS	RATIONALE
Nutrition Therapy (NIC)	
Independent	
Monitor daily food intake, have client keep food diary as indicated.	Identifies nutritional strengths/deficiencies.
Measure height, weight, and tricep skinfold thickness (or other anthropometric measurements as appropriate). Ascertain amount of recent weight loss. Weigh daily or as indicated.	If these measurements fall below minimum standards, client's chief source of stored energy (fat tissue) is depleted.
Assess skin/mucous membranes for pallor, delayed wound healing, enlarged parotid glands.	Helps in identification of protein-calorie malnutrition, especially when weight and anthropometric measurements are less than normal.
Encourage client to eat high-calorie, nutrient-rich diet, with adequate fluid intake. Encourage use of supplements and frequent/smaller meals spaced throughout the day.	Metabolic tissue needs are increased as well as fluids (to eliminate waste products). Supplements can play an important role in maintaining adequate caloric and protein intake.
Create pleasant dining atmosphere; encourage client to share meals with family/friends.	Makes mealtime more enjoyable, which may enhance intake.
Encourage open communication regarding anorexia.	Often a source of emotional distress, especially for SO who wants to feed client frequently. When client refuses, SO may feel rejected/frustrated.
Chemotherapy Management (NIC)	
Adjust diet before and immediately after treatment; e.g., clear, cool liquids, light/bland foods, candied ginger, dry crackers, toast, carbonated drinks. Give liquids 1 hr before or 1 hr after meals.	The effectiveness of diet adjustment is very individualized in relief of post-therapy nausea. Clients must experiment to find best solution/combination. Avoiding fluids during meals minimizes becoming "full" too quickly.
Control environmental factors (e.g., strong/noxious odors or noise). Avoid overly sweet, fatty, or spicy foods.	Can trigger nausea/vomiting response.
Encourage use of relaxation techniques, visualization, guided imagery, moderate exercise before meals.	May prevent onset or reduce severity of nausea, decrease anorexia, and enable client to increase oral intake.
Identify the client who experiences anticipatory nausea/vomiting and take appropriate measures.	Psychogenic nausea/vomiting occurring before chemotherapy generally does not respond to antiemetic drugs. Change of treatment environment or client routine on treatment day may be effective.
Evaluate effectiveness of antiemetic agents.	Individuals respond differently to all medications. First-line antiemetics may not work, requiring alteration in or use of combination drug therapy.
Hematest stools, gastric secretions.	Certain therapies (e.g., antimetabolites) inhibit renewal of epithelial cells lining the GI tract, which may cause changes ranging from mild erythema to severe ulceration with bleeding.
Collaborative	
Review laboratory studies as indicated; e.g., total lymphocyte count, serum transferrin, and albumin/prealbumin.	Helps identify the degree of biochemical imbalance/malnutrition and influences choice of dietary interventions. *Note:* Anticancer treatments can also alter nutrition studies, so all results must be correlated with the client's clinical status.

ACTIONS/INTERVENTIONS	RATIONALE
Administer medications as indicated:	
5-HT3 receptor antagonists; e.g., ondansetron (Zofran), granisetron (Kytril), palonosetron (Aloxi); NK-1 receptor antagonist aprepitant (Emend); phenothiazines; e.g., prochlorperazine (Compazine), thiethylperazine (Torecan); antidopaminergics; e.g., metoclopramide (Reglan); antihistamines; e.g., diphenhydramine (Benadryl); cannabinoid dronabinol (Marinol);	Most antiemetics act to interfere with stimulation of true vomiting center, and chemoreceptor trigger zone agents also act peripherally to inhibit reverse peristalsis. These medications are often prescribed routinely before, during, and after chemotherapy to prevent nausea and vomiting.
Corticosteroids; e.g., dexamethasone (Decadron); cannabinoids; e.g., 9-tetrahydrocannabinol (dronabinol, [Marinol]); benzodiazepines; e.g., lorazepam (Ativan); butyrophenones; e.g., haloperidol (Haldol), droperidol (Inapsine);	Combination therapy (e.g., Torecan with Decadron and/or Ativan) is often more effective than single agents. *Note:* Recent studies report that the legal agent Marinol did not provide the same level of relief from nausea and vomiting as did medicinal marijuana. However, because of legal implications and availability of legal medications, medicinal use of marijuana continues to be widely restricted.
Vitamins, especially A, D, E, and B_6;	Prevents deficit related to decreased absorption of fat-soluble vitamins. Deficiency of B_6 can contribute to/exacerbate depression, irritability, neuropathy.
Antacids and/or proton pump inhibitors; e.g., esomeprazole (Nexium), lansoprazole (Prevacid), pantoprazole (Protonix).	Minimizes gastric irritation, decreases nausea, and reduces risk of mucosal ulceration.
Administer antiemetic on a regular schedule before/during and after administration of antineoplastic agent as appropriate.	Nausea/vomiting are frequently the most disabling and psychologically stressful side effects of chemotherapy.

Nutrition Therapy (NIC)

ACTIONS/INTERVENTIONS	RATIONALE
Refer to dietitian/nutritional support team.	Provides for specific dietary plan to meet individual needs and reduce problems associated with protein/calorie malnutrition and micronutrient deficiencies.
Insert/maintain NG or feeding tube for enteric feedings, or central line for total parenteral nutrition (TPN) if indicated.	In the presence of severe malnutrition (e.g., loss of 25%–30% body weight in 2 months) or if client has been NPO for 5 days and is unlikely to be able to eat for another week, tube feeding or TPN may be necessary to meet nutritional needs. *Note:* TPN is used with caution because it is associated with a more than fourfold increase in the risk of significant infection.

NURSING DIAGNOSIS: risk for deficient Fluid Volume

Risk factors may include

Excessive losses through normal routes (e.g., vomiting, diarrhea) and/or abnormal routes (e.g., indwelling tubes, wounds)
Hypermetabolic state
Impaired intake of fluids

Possibly evidenced by

[Not applicable; presence of signs and symptoms establishes an *actual* diagnosis]

DESIRED OUTCOMES/EVALUATION CRITERIA—CLIENT WILL:

Hydration (NOC)

Display adequate fluid balance as evidenced by stable vital signs, moist mucous membranes, good skin turgor, prompt capillary refill, and individually adequate urinary output.

ACTIONS/INTERVENTIONS	RATIONALE
Fluid/Electrolyte Management (NIC)	
Independent	
Monitor I&O and specific gravity; include all output sources; e.g., emesis, diarrhea, draining wounds. Calculate 24-hr balance.	Continued negative fluid balance, decreasing renal output, and concentration of urine suggest developing dehydration and need for increased fluid replacement.
Weigh as indicated.	Sensitive measurement of fluctuations in fluid balance.
Monitor vital signs. Evaluate peripheral pulses, capillary refill.	Reflects adequacy of circulating volume.
Assess skin turgor and moisture of mucous membranes. Note reports of thirst.	Indirect indicators of hydration status/degree of deficit.
Encourage increased fluid intake to 3000 mL/day as individually appropriate/tolerated.	Assists in maintenance of fluid requirements and reduces risk of harmful side effects; e.g., hemorrhagic cystitis in client receiving cyclophosphamide (Cytoxan).
Observe for bleeding tendencies; e.g., oozing from mucous membranes, puncture sites; presence of ecchymosis or petechiae.	Early identification of problems (which may occur as a result of cancer and/or therapies) allows for prompt intervention.
Minimize venipunctures (e.g., combine IV starts with blood draws). Encourage client to consider central venous catheter placement.	Reduces potential for hemorrhage and infection associated with repeated venous puncture.
Avoid trauma and apply pressure to puncture sites.	Reduces potential for bleeding/hematoma formation.
Collaborative	
Provide IV fluids as indicated.	Given for general hydration and to dilute antineoplastic drugs and reduce adverse side effects; e.g., nausea/vomiting or nephrotoxicity.
Administer antiemetic therapy. (Refer to ND: imbalanced Nutrition: less than body requirements.)	Alleviation of nausea/vomiting decreases gastric losses and allows for increased oral intake.
Monitor laboratory studies; e.g., CBC, electrolytes, serum albumin.	Provides information about level of hydration and corresponding deficits. *Note:* Malnutrition and effects of decreased albumin levels potentiates fluid shifts/edema formation.
Administer transfusions as indicated; e.g.:	
RBCs;	May be needed to restore blood count and prevent manifestations of anemia often present in cancer clients; e.g., tachycardia, tachypnea, dizziness, and weakness.
Platelets.	Thrombocytopenia (which may occur as a side effect of chemotherapy, radiation, or cancer process) increases the risk of bleeding from mucous membranes and other body sites. Spontaneous bleeding may occur with platelet count of 5000.
Avoid use of aspirin, gastric irritants, platelet inhibitors or herbs, such as gensing, green tea, garlic, ginger, ginkgo, or willow bark.	Negatively affect clotting mechanism and/or potentiate risk of bleeding.

NURSING DIAGNOSIS: Fatigue

May be related to

Decreased metabolic energy production, increased energy requirements (hypermetabolic state and effects of treatment)
Overwhelming psychologic/emotional demands
Altered body chemistry: side effects of pain and other medications, chemotherapy, radiation therapy, biotherapy

Possibly evidenced by

Unremitting/overwhelming lack of energy, inability to maintain usual routines, decreased performance, impaired ability to concentrate, lethargy/listlessness
Disinterest in surroundings

DESIRED OUTCOMES/EVALUATION CRITERIA—CLIENT WILL:

Endurance (NOC)

Report improved sense of energy.
Perform ADLs and participate in desired activities at level of ability.

ACTIONS/INTERVENTIONS	RATIONALE
Energy Management (NIC)	
Independent	
Have client rate fatigue, using a numeric scale, if possible, and the time of day when it is most severe.	Helps in developing a plan for managing fatigue.
Plan care to allow for rest periods. Schedule activities for periods when client has most energy. Involve client/SO in schedule planning.	Frequent rest periods and/or naps are needed to restore/conserve energy. Planning will allow client to be active during times when energy level is higher, which may restore a feeling of well-being and a sense of control.
Establish realistic activity goals with client.	Provides for a sense of control and feelings of accomplishment.
Assist with self-care needs when indicated; keep bed in low position, pathways clear of furniture; assist with ambulation.	Weakness may make ADLs difficult to complete or place the client at risk for injury during activities.
Encourage client to do whatever possible; e.g., self-bathing, sitting up in chair, walking. Increase activity level as individual is able.	Enhances strength/stamina and enables client to become more active without undue fatigue.
Encourage aerobic exercise, as client is able with goal of 30 minutes/day.	Aerobic exercise minimizes fatigue, increases strength/stamina, stimulates release of natural endorphins which promotes sense of well-being.
Monitor physiologic response to activity; e.g., changes in BP or heart/respiratory rate.	Tolerance varies greatly depending on the stage of the disease process, nutrition state, fluid balance, and reaction to therapeutic regimen.
Perform pain assessment and provide pain management.	Poorly managed cancer pain can contribute to fatigue.
Encourage nutritional intake. (Refer to ND: imbalanced Nutrition: less than body requirements.)	Adequate intake/use of nutrients is necessary to meet energy needs and build energy reserves for activity.
Encourage adequate fluid intake. (Refer to ND: risk for deficient Fluid Volume.)	Prevents dehydration (which increases fatigue).
Collaborative	
Provide supplemental oxygen as indicated.	Presence of anemia/hypoxemia reduces O_2 available for cellular uptake and contributes to fatigue.
Refer to physical/occupational therapy.	Programmed daily exercises and activities help client maintain/increase strength and muscle tone, enhance sense of well-being. Use of adaptive devices may help conserve energy.

NURSING DIAGNOSIS: risk for Infection

Risk factors may include

Inadequate secondary defenses and immunosuppression; e.g., bone marrow suppression (dose-limiting side effect of both chemotherapy and radiation)
Malnutrition, chronic disease process
Invasive procedures

Possibly evidenced by

[Not applicable; presence of signs and symptoms establishes an *actual* diagnosis]

DESIRED OUTCOMES/EVALUATION CRITERIA—CLIENT WILL:

Immune Status (NOC)

Remain afebrile and achieve timely healing as appropriate.

KNOWLEDGE: Infection Control (NOC)

Identify and participate in interventions to prevent/reduce risk of infection.

ACTIONS/INTERVENTIONS	RATIONALE
Infection Protection (NIC)	
Independent	
Promote good handwashing procedures by staff and visitors. Screen/limit visitors who may have infections. Place in reverse isolation as indicated.	Protects client from sources of infection, such as visitors and staff who may have an upper respiratory infection (URI).
Emphasize personal hygiene (encourage to bathe daily).	Limits potential sources of infection and/or secondary overgrowth.
Monitor temperature.	Temperature elevation may occur (if not masked by corticosteroids or anti-inflammatory drugs) because of various factors; e.g., chemotherapy side effects, disease process, or infection. Early identification of infectious process enables appropriate therapy to be started promptly.
Encourage fluids. (Refer to ND: risk for deficient Fluid Volume.)	Adequate fluid intake enhances immune system and aids natural defense mechanisms.
Assess all systems (e.g., skin, respiratory, genitourinary) for signs/symptoms of infection on a continual basis.	Early recognition and intervention may prevent progression to more serious situation/sepsis.
Reposition frequently, keep linens dry and wrinkle free.	Reduces pressure and irritation to tissues and may prevent skin breakdown (potential site for bacterial growth).
Promote adequate rest/exercise periods.	Limits fatigue, yet encourages sufficient movement to prevent stasis complications; e.g., pneumonia, decubitus ulcers, and thrombus formation.
Stress importance of good oral hygiene.	Development of stomatitis increases risk of infection/secondary overgrowth.
Avoid/limit invasive procedures. Adhere to aseptic techniques.	Reduces risk of contamination, limits portal of entry for infectious agents.
Collaborative	
Monitor CBC with differential WBC and granulocyte count and platelets as indicated.	Bone marrow activity may be inhibited by effects of chemotherapy, the disease state, or radiation therapy.

ACTIONS/INTERVENTIONS	RATIONALE
	Monitoring status of myelosuppression is important for preventing further complications (e.g., infection, anemia, or hemorrhage) and scheduling drug delivery. *Note:* The nadir (point of lowest drop in blood count) is usually seen 7–10 days after administration of chemotherapy.
Obtain cultures as indicated.	Identifies causative organism(s) and appropriate therapy.
Administer antibiotics as indicated.	May be used to treat identified infection or given prophylactically in immunocompromised client.

NURSING DIAGNOSIS: risk for impaired Oral Mucous Membranes

Risk factors may include

Side effect of some chemotherapeutic agents (e.g., antimetabolites) and radiation
Dehydration, malnutrition, NPO restrictions for more than 24 hr

Possibly evidenced by

[Not applicable; presence of signs and symptoms establishes an *actual* diagnosis]

DESIRED OUTCOMES/EVALUATION CRITERIA—CLIENT WILL:

Oral Hygiene (NOC)

Display intact mucous membranes, which are pink, moist, and free of inflammation/ulcerations.

Self-Care Oral Hygiene (NOC)

Verbalize understanding of causative factors.
Demonstrate techniques to maintain/restore integrity of oral mucosa.

ACTIONS/INTERVENTIONS	RATIONALE
Oral Health Maintenance (NIC)	
Independent	
Assess dental health and oral hygiene periodically.	Identifies prophylactic treatment needs before initiation of chemotherapy or radiation and provides baseline data of current oral hygiene for future comparison.
Encourage client to assess oral cavity daily, noting changes in mucous membrane integrity (e.g., dry, reddened). Note reports of burning in the mouth, changes in voice quality, ability to swallow, sense of taste, development of thick/viscous saliva, blood-tinged emesis.	Inflammation of the oral mucosa (stomatitis) generally occurs 7–14 days after treatment begins, but signs may be seen as early as day 3 or 4, especially if there are any preexisting oral problems. The range of response extends from mild erythema to severe ulceration, and may extend the length of the GI tract (mucositis), which can be very painful, can inhibit oral intake, and is potentially life threatening. Early identification enables prompt treatment.
Discuss with client areas needing improvement and demonstrate methods for good oral care.	Good care is critical during treatment to control stomatitis complications.
Initiate/recommend oral hygiene program to include:	
Avoidance of commercial mouthwashes, lemon/glycerine swabs;	Products containing alcohol or phenol may exacerbate mucous membrane dryness/irritation.
Use of mouthwash made from warm water with salt and baking soda. A dilute solution of hydrogen peroxide may be used for bleeding or infected tissue.	May be soothing to the membranes. Rinsing before meals may improve the client's sense of taste. Rinsing after meals and at bedtime dilutes oral acids and relieves xerostomia.

ACTIONS/INTERVENTIONS	RATIONALE
Brush with soft toothbrush or foam swab;	Prevents trauma to delicate/fragile tissues. *Note:* Toothbrush should be changed at least every 3 months.
Floss gently or use WaterPik cautiously;	Removes food particles that can promote bacterial growth. *Note:* Water under pressure has the potential to injure gums/force bacteria under gum line.
Keep lips moist with lip gloss or balm, K-Y Jelly, Chapstick;	Promotes comfort and prevents drying/cracking of tissues.
Encourage use of mints/hard candy or artificial saliva (Ora-Lube, Salivart) as indicated.	Stimulates secretions/provides moisture to maintain integrity of mucous membranes, especially in presence of dehydration/reduced saliva production.
Instruct regarding dietary changes: e.g., avoid hot or spicy foods, acidic juices; suggest use of straw; ingest soft or blenderized foods, popsicles, and ice cream as tolerated.	Severe stomatitis may interfere with nutritional and fluid intake leading to negative nitrogen balance or dehydration. Dietary modifications may make foods easier to swallow and may feel soothing.
Encourage fluid intake as individually tolerated.	Adequate hydration helps keep mucous membranes moist, preventing drying/cracking.
Discuss limitation of smoking and alcohol intake.	May cause further irritation and dryness of mucous membranes. *Note*: May need to compromise if these activities are important to client's emotional status.
Monitor for and explain to client signs of oral superinfection (e.g., thrush).	Early recognition provides opportunity for prompt treatment.

Collaborative

Refer to dentist before initiating chemotherapy or head/neck radiation.	Prophylactic examination and repair work before therapy reduce risk of infection.
Culture suspicious oral lesions.	Identifies organism(s) responsible for oral infections and suggests appropriate drug therapy.
Administer medications as indicated; e.g.:	
Analgesic rinses (e.g., mixture of Koatin, pectin, diphenhydramine [Benadryl], and topical lidocaine [Xylocaine]);	Aggressive analgesia program may be required to relieve intense pain. *Note:* Rinse should be used as a swish-and-spit rather than a gargle, which could anesthetize client's gag reflex.
Antifungal mouthwash preparation, e.g., nystatin (Mycostatin), and antibacterial Biotane;	May be needed to treat/prevent secondary oral infections, such as *Candida, Pseudomonas,* herpes simplex.
Antinausea agents;	When given before beginning mouth care regimen, may prevent nausea associated with oral stimulation.
Opioid analgesics: e.g., hydromophone (Dilaudid), morphine.	May be required for acute episodes of moderate to severe oral pain.

NURSING DIAGNOSIS: risk for impaired Skin/Tissue Integrity

Risk factors may include

Effects of radiation and chemotherapy
Immunologic deficit
Altered nutritional state, anemia

Possibly evidenced by

[Not applicable; presence of signs and symptoms establishes an *actual* diagnosis]

DESIRED OUTCOMES/EVALUATION CRITERIA—CLIENT WILL:

Risk Control (NOC)

Identify interventions appropriate for specific condition.
Participate in techniques to prevent complications/promote healing as appropriate.

ACTIONS/INTERVENTIONS	RATIONALE
Chemotherapy [or] Radiation Therapy Management (NIC)	
Independent	
Assess skin frequently for side effects of cancer therapy; note breakdown/delayed wound healing. Emphasize importance of reporting open areas to caregiver.	A reddening and/or tanning effect (radiation reaction) may develop within the field of radiation. Dry desquamation (dryness and pruritus), moist desquamation (blistering), ulceration, hair loss, loss of dermis and sweat glands may also be noted. In addition, skin reactions (e.g., allergic rashes, hyperpigmentation, pruritus, and alopecia) may occur with some chemotherapy agents.
Bathe with lukewarm water and mild soap.	Maintains cleanliness without irritating the skin.
Encourage client to avoid vigorous rubbing and scratching and to pat skin dry instead of rubbing.	Helps prevent skin friction/trauma to sensitive tissues.
Turn/reposition frequently.	Promotes circulation and prevents undue pressure on skin/tissues.
Review skin care protocol for client receiving radiation therapy:	Designed to minimize trauma to area of radiation therapy.
Avoid rubbing or use of soap, lotions, creams, ointments, powders or deodorants on area; avoid applying heat or attempting to wash off marks/tattoos placed on skin to identify area of irradiation;	Can potentiate or otherwise interfere with radiation delivery. May actually increase irritation/reaction.
Recommend wearing soft, loose cotton clothing; have female client avoid wearing bra if it creates pressure;	Skin is very sensitive during and after treatment, and all irritation should be avoided to prevent dermal injury.
Apply cornstarch, Aquaphor, Lubriderm, Eucerin (or other recommended water-soluble moisturizing gel) to area twice daily as needed;	Helps control dampness or pruritus. Maintenance care is required until skin/tissues have regenerated and are back to normal.
Encourage liberal use of sunscreen/block and breathable, protective clothing.	Protects skin from ultraviolet rays and reduces risk of recall reactions.
Review skin care protocol for client receiving chemotherapy; e.g.:	
Use appropriate peripheral or central venous catheter, dilute anticancer drug per protocol and ascertain that IV is infusing well;	Reduces risk of tissue irritation/extravasation of agent into tissues.
Instruct client to notify caregiver promptly of discomfort at IV insertion site;	Development of irritation indicates need for alteration of rate/dilution of chemotherapy and/or change of IV site to prevent more serious reaction.
Assess skin/IV site and vein for erythema, edema, tenderness; weltlike patches, itching/burning, swelling, soreness, blisters progressing to ulceration/tissue necrosis.	Presence of phlebitis, vein flare (localized reaction), or extravasation requires immediate discontinuation of antineoplastic agent and medical intervention.
Wash skin immediately with soap and water if antineoplastic agents are spilled on unprotected skin (client or caregiver).	Dilutes drug to reduce risk of skin irritation/chemical burn.
Advise clients receiving 5-fluorouracil (5-FU) and methotrexate to avoid sun exposure. Withhold methotrexate if sunburn present.	Sun can cause exacerbation of burn spotting (a side effect of 5-FU) or can cause a red "flash" area with methotrexate, which can exacerbate drug's effect.
Review expected dermatologic side effects seen with chemotherapy; e.g., rash, hyperpigmentation, and peeling of skin on palms.	Anticipatory guidance helps decrease concern if side effects do occur.
Inform client that if alopecia occurs, hair could grow back after completion of chemotherapy, but may/may not grow back after radiation therapy.	Anticipatory guidance may help adjustment to/preparation for baldness. Men are often as sensitive to hair loss as women. Radiation's effect on hair follicles may be permanent, depending on rad dosage.

ACTIONS/INTERVENTIONS	RATIONALE
Collaborative	
Administer appropriate antidote if extravasation of IV should occur; e.g.:	Reduces local tissue damage.
Dimethyl sulfoxide (DMSO);	Some studies suggest benefit with topical DMSO for mitomycin and doxorubicin (Adriamycin). *Note:* Injection of diphenhydramine (Benadryl) may relieve symptoms of vein flare.
Hyaluronidase (Wydase);	Injected subcutaneously for vincristine (Oncovin), vinblastine (Velban), etoposide (VP16), vindesine (Eldisine), vinorelbine (Navelbine), teniposide (Vm26), and paclitaxel (Taxol) infiltration.
Thiosulfate.	Injected subcutaneously for nitrogen mustard and large amounts (greater than 20 mL) of concentrated cisplatin.
Apply ice pack/warm compresses per protocol.	Controversial intervention depends on type of agent used. Ice restricts blood flow, keeping drug localized, whereas heat enhances dispersion of neoplastic drug/antidote, minimizing tissue damage.

NURSING DIAGNOSIS: risk for Constipation/Diarrhea

Risk factors may include

Irritation of the GI mucosa from either chemotherapy or radiation therapy, malabsorption of fat
Hormone-secreting tumor, carcinoma of colon
Poor fluid intake, low-bulk diet, lack of exercise, use of opiates/narcotics

Possibly evidenced by

[Not applicable; presence of signs and symptoms establishes an *actual* diagnosis]

DESIRED OUTCOMES/EVALUATION CRITERIA—CLIENT WILL:

Bowel Elimination (NOC)

Maintain usual bowel consistency/pattern.
Verbalize understanding of factors and appropriate interventions/solutions related to individual situation.

ACTIONS/INTERVENTIONS	RATIONALE
Bowel Management (NIC)	
Independent	
Ascertain usual elimination habits.	Data required as baseline for future evaluation of therapeutic needs/effectiveness.
Assess bowel sounds and monitor/record bowel movements (BMs) including frequency, consistency (particularly during first 3–5 days of vinca alkaloid therapy).	Defines problem, i.e., diarrhea, constipation. *Note:* Constipation is one of the earliest manifestations of neurotoxicity.
Monitor I&O and weight.	Dehydration, weight loss, and electrolyte imbalance are complications of diarrhea. Inadequate fluid intake may potentiate constipation.
Encourage adequate fluid intake (e.g., 2000 mL/24 hr), increased fiber in diet, regular exercise.	May reduce potential for constipation by improving stool consistency and stimulating peristalsis, can prevent dehydration associated with diarrhea.

ACTIONS/INTERVENTIONS	RATIONALE
Provide small, frequent meals of foods low in residue (if not contraindicated), maintaining needed protein and carbohydrates (e.g., eggs, cooked cereal, bland cooked vegetables).	Reduces gastric irritation. Use of low-fiber foods can decrease irritability and provide bowel rest when diarrhea present.
Adjust diet as appropriate: avoid foods high in fat (e.g., butter, fried foods, nuts), foods with high-fiber content, those known to cause diarrhea or gas (e.g., cabbage, baked beans, chili), food/fluids high in caffeine, or extremely hot or cold food/fluids.	GI stimulants that may increase gastric motility/frequency of stools.
Check for impaction if client has not had bowel movement (BM) in 3 days or if abdominal distention, cramping, headache are present.	Further interventions/alternative bowel care may be needed.

Collaborative

Monitor laboratory studies as indicated; e.g., electrolytes.	Electrolyte imbalances may be the result of/contribute to altered GI function.
Administer IV fluids;	Prevents dehydration, dilutes chemotherapy agents to diminish side effects.
Antidiarrheal agents;	May be indicated to control severe diarrhea.
Stool softeners, laxatives, enemas as indicated.	Prophylactic use may prevent further complications in some clients (e.g., those who will receive vinca alkaloid, have poor bowel pattern before treatment, or have decreased motility).

NURSING DIAGNOSIS: risk for ineffective Sexuality Pattern

Risk factors may include

Knowledge/skill deficit about alternative responses to health-related transitions, altered body function/structure, illness, and medical treatment
Overwhelming fatigue
Fear and anxiety
Lack of privacy/SO

Possibly evidenced by

[Not applicable; presence of signs and symptoms establishes an *actual* diagnosis]

DESIRED OUTCOMES/EVALUATION CRITERIA—CLIENT WILL:

Role Performance (NOC)

Verbalize understanding of effects of cancer and therapeutic regimen on sexuality and measures to correct/deal with problems.
Maintain sexual activity at a desired level as possible.

ACTIONS/INTERVENTIONS	RATIONALE
Sexual Counseling (NIC)	
Independent	
Discuss with client/SO the nature of sexuality and reactions when it is altered or threatened. Provide information about normality of these problems and that many people find it helpful to seek assistance with adaptation process.	Acknowledges legitimacy of the problem. Sexuality encompasses the way men and women view themselves as individuals and how they relate between and among themselves in every area of life.

ACTIONS/INTERVENTIONS	RATIONALE
Advise client of side effects of prescribed cancer treatment that are known to affect sexuality.	Anticipatory guidance can help client and SO begin the process of adaptation to new state.
Provide private time for hospitalized client. Knock on door and receive permission from client/SO before entering.	Sexual needs do not end because the client is hospitalized. Intimacy needs continue and an open and accepting attiude for the expression of those needs is essential.

Collaborative

Refer to sex therapist as indicated.	May require additional assistance in dealing with situation.

NURSING DIAGNOSIS: risk for interrupted Family Processes

Risk factors may include

Situational/transitional crises: long-term illness, change in roles/economic status
Developmental: anticipated loss of a family member

Possibly evidenced by

[Not applicable; presence of signs and symptoms establishes an *actual* diagnosis]

DESIRED OUTCOMES/EVALUATION CRITERIA—FAMILY WILL:

Family Coping (NOC)

Express feelings freely.
Demonstrate individual involvement in problem-solving process directed at appropriate solutions for the situation.
Encourage and allow member who is ill to handle situation in own way.

ACTIONS/INTERVENTIONS — RATIONALE

Family Process Maintenance (NIC)

Independent

ACTIONS/INTERVENTIONS	RATIONALE
Note components of family, presence of extended family, and others; e.g., friends/neighbors.	Helps client and caregiver know who is available to assist with care/provide respite and support.
Identify patterns of communication in family and patterns of interaction between family members.	Provides information about effectiveness of communication and identifies problems that may interfere with family's ability to assist client and adjust positively to diagnosis/treatment of cancer.
Assess role expectations of family members and encourage discussion about them.	Each person may see the situation in own individual manner, and clear identification and sharing of these expectations promote understanding.
Assess energy direction; e.g., are efforts at resolution/problem solving purposeful or scattered?	Provides clues about interventions that may be appropriate to assist client and family in directing energies in a more effective manner.
Note cultural/religious beliefs.	Affects client/SO reaction and adjustment to diagnosis, treatment, and outcome of cancer.
Listen for expressions of helplessness.	Helpless feelings may contribute to difficulty adjusting to diagnosis of cancer and cooperating with treatment regimen.
Deal with family members in a warm, caring, respectful way. Provide information (verbal/written), and reinforce as necessary.	Provides feelings of empathy and promotes individual's sense of worth and competence in ability to handle current situation.

ACTIONS/INTERVENTIONS	RATIONALE
Encourage appropriate expressions of anger without reacting negatively to them.	Feelings of anger are to be expected when individuals are dealing with the difficult/potentially fatal illness of cancer. Appropriate expression enables progress toward resolution of the stages of the grieving process.
Acknowledge difficulties of the situation; e.g., diagnosis and treatment of cancer, possibility of death.	Communicates acceptance of the reality the client/family are facing.
Identify and encourage use of previous successful coping behaviors.	Most people have developed effective coping skills that can be useful in dealing with current situation.
Stress importance of continuous open dialogue between family members.	Promotes understanding and assists family members to maintain clear communication and resolve problems effectively.

Collaborative

Refer to support groups, clergy, family therapy as indicated.	May need additional assistance to resolve problems of disorganization that may accompany diagnosis of potentially terminal illness (cancer).

NURSING DIAGNOSIS: deficient Knowledge [Learning Need] regarding illness, prognosis, treatment, self care, and discharge needs

May be related to

Lack of exposure/recall, information misinterpretation, myths
Unfamiliarity with information resources
Cognitive limitation

Possibly evidenced by

Questions/request for information, verbalization of problem
Statement of misconception
Inaccurate follow-through of instructions/development of preventable complications

DESIRED OUTCOMES/EVALUATION CRITERIA—CLIENT WILL:

KNOWLEDGE: Disease Process (NOC)

Verbalize accurate information about diagnosis, prognosis, and potential complications at own level of readiness.

KNOWLEDGE: Treatment Regimen (NOC)

Verbalize understanding of therapeutic needs.
Correctly perform necessary procedures and explain reasons for the actions.
Initiate necessary lifestyle changes and participate in treatment regimen.
Identify/use available resources appropriately.

ACTIONS/INTERVENTIONS | RATIONALE

TEACHING: Disease Process (NIC)

Independent

ACTIONS/INTERVENTIONS	RATIONALE
Review with client/SO understanding of specific diagnosis, treatment alternatives, and future expectations.	Validates current level of understanding, identifies learning needs, and provides knowledge base from which client can make informed decisions.

ACTIONS/INTERVENTIONS	RATIONALE
Determine client's perception of cancer and cancer treatment(s), ask about client's own/previous experience or experience with other people who have (or had) cancer.	Aids in identification of ideas, attitudes, fears, misconceptions, and gaps in knowledge about cancer.
Provide clear, accurate information in a factual but sensitive manner. Answer questions specifically, but do not bombard with unessential details.	Helps with adjustment to the diagnosis of cancer by providing needed information along with time to absorb it. *Note:* Rate and method of giving information may need to be altered to decrease client's anxiety and enhance ability to assimilate information.
Provide anticipatory guidance with client/SO regarding treatment protocol, length of therapy, expected results, possible side effects. Be honest with client.	Client has the "right to know" (be informed) and participate in decision tree. Accurate and concise information helps to dispel fears and anxiety, helps clarify the expected routine, and enables client to maintain some degree of control.
Ask client for verbal feedback, and correct misconceptions about individual's type of cancer and treatment.	Misconceptions about cancer may be more disturbing than facts and can interfere with treatments/delay healing.
Outline normally expected limitations (if any) on ADLs (e.g., difficulty cooking meals when nauseated/fatigued, limit sun exposure, alcohol intake; loss of work time because of effects of treatments).	Enables client/SO to begin to put limitations into perspective and plan/adapt as indicated.
Provide written materials about cancer, treatment, and available support systems.	Anxiety and preoccupation with thoughts about life and death often interfere with client's ability to assimilate adequate information. Written, take-home materials provide reinforcement and clarification about information as client needs it.
Review specific medication regimen and use of OTC drugs.	Enhances ability to manage self-care and avoid potential complications, drug reactions/interactions.
Address specific home care needs; e.g., ability to live alone, perform necessary treatments/procedures, and acquire supplies.	Provides information regarding changes that may be needed in current plan of care to meet therapeutic needs.
Do predischarge home evaluation as indicated.	Aids in transition to home setting by providing information about needed changes in physical layout, acquisition of needed supplies.
Refer to community resources as indicated: e.g., social services, home health agencies, Meals on Wheels, local American Cancer Society chapter, respite care, hospice center/services.	Promotes competent self-care and optimal independence. Maintains client in desired/home setting.
Review with client/SO the importance of maintaining optimal nutritional status.	Promotes well-being, facilitates recovery, and is critical in enabling the client to tolerate treatments.
Encourage diet variations and experimentation in meal planning and food preparation; e.g., cooking with sweet juices, wine; serving foods cold or at room temperature as appropriate (ice cream, egg salad).	Creativity may enhance flavor and intake, especially when protein foods taste bitter.
Recommend cookbooks that are designed for cancer clients.	Helps provide specific menu/recipe ideas.
Recommend increased fluid intake and fiber in diet, as well as routine exercise.	Improves consistency of stool and stimulates peristalsis.
Instruct client to assess oral mucous membranes routinely, noting erythema, ulceration.	Early recognition of problems promotes early intervention, minimizing complications that may impair oral intake and provide avenue for systemic infection.
Advise client concerning skin and hair care: e.g., avoid harsh shampoos, hair dyes, permanents, salt water, chlorinated water; avoid exposure to strong wind and extreme heat or cold; avoid sun exposure to target area for 1 yr after end of radiation treatments; and regularly apply sunblock (SPF 15 or greater).	Prevents additional hair damage and skin irritation, may prevent recall reactions.
Review signs/symptoms requiring medical evaluation (depending on individual situation); e.g., infection, delayed healing, drug reactions, increased pain; or	Early identification and treatment may limit severity of complications. *Note*: The use of central venous access devices for various therapies, (e.g., chemotherapy, TPN,

ACTIONS/INTERVENTIONS	RATIONALE
swelling of face/eyes/lips, hands/arms that may worsen when lying down, dyspnea/cough, headache, and visual disturbances suggestive of superior vena cava syndrome (SVCS).	or antibiotic administration) may cause local vein trauma leading to SVCS days, months, or even years after catheter insertion.
Stress importance of continuing medical follow-up.	Provides ongoing monitoring of progression/resolution of disease process and opportunity for timely diagnosis and treatment of complications and early detection of second malignancies. *Note:* Some complications can develop long after therapy is completed; e.g., pathologic fractures, radiation cystitis/nephritis, or pneumonitis. Periodic thyroid function tests are indicated for clients with radiation to the neck/upper chest because hypothyroidism may develop.
Encourage periodic review of advance directives. Promote inclusion of family/SO in decision-making process.	Client/family/SO need to re-evaluate choices as condition changes (for better/worse) and treatment options become available or are exhausted.

POTENTIAL CONSIDERATIONS following acute hospitalization (dependent on client's age, physical condition/presence of complications, personal resources, and life responsibilities)

In addition to Potential Considerations in specific plans of care (e.g., leukemia, mastectomy):

ineffective Coping—situational crises, vulnerability.

Self-Care Deficit/ impaired Home Maintenance—decreased strength/endurance, pain/discomfort, depression, insufficient finances, unfamiliarity with neighborhood resources, inadequate support systems.

risk for Caregiver Role Strain—illness severity of care receiver, significant home care needs, situational stressors, complexity/amount of caregiving tasks.

acute/chronic Pain—disease process (compression/destruction of nerve tissue, infiltration of nerves, or their vascular supply, obstruction of a nerve pathway, inflammation).

ineffective Therapeutic Regimen Management—complexity of therapeutic regimen, economic difficulties, decisional conflict, perceived barriers, powerlessness, social support deficits.

END OF LIFE/HOSPICE CARE

Nursing care involves the support of general well-being of our clients, the provision of episodic acute care and rehabilitation, and when a return to health is not possible, a peaceful death. Dying is a profound transition for the individual. As healthcare providers, we become skilled in nursing and medical science, but the care of the dying person encompasses much more. Certain aspects of this care are taking on more importance for clients, families, and healthcare providers. These include pain and other symptom management and psychologic, spiritual, and grief/bereavement support.

Recent studies have identified barriers to end of life care, including client or family member's avoidance of death, influence of managed care on end of life care, and lack of continuity of care across settings. In addition, if the dying client requires a lengthy period of care or complicated physical care, there is the likelihood of caregiver fatigue (psychologic and physical) that can compromise the care provided.

The best opportunity for quality end of life care occurs when clients facing death, and their families, have time to consider the meaning of their lives, make plans, and shape the course of their living while preparing for death.

CARE SETTING

Hospice is an idea (not dependent on a particular place or facility) of moving from curative to supportive care for the dying client. Although much of the care of the dying is still provided by nurses in hospitals (primarily in oncology and critical care areas), other care settings are becoming more common; e.g., the home, assisted living/extended care setting, or hospice inpatient unit.

RELATED CONCERNS

Cancer, page 857
Extended care, page 810
Psychosocial aspects of care, page 770
Care plan(s) reflecting underlying pathology of terminal condition

Client Assessment Database

Data depend on underlying terminal condition and involvement of other body systems.

EGO INTEGRITY

May report: Stress related to recent changes in ability to care for self and decision to accept hospice services
Feelings of helplessness/hopelessness, sorrow, anger; choked feelings
Fear of the dying process, loss of physical and/or mental abilities
Concern about impact of death on SO/family
Inner conflict about beliefs, meaning of life/death
Financial concerns, lack of preparation (e.g., will, power of attorney, funeral)

May exhibit: Deep sadness, crying, anxiety, apathy
Altered communication patterns, social isolation, withdrawal

SOCIAL INTERACTION

May report: Apprehension about caregiver's ability to provide care
Changes in family roles/usual patterns of responsibility

May exhibit: Difficulty adapting to changes imposed by condition/dying process

NURSING PRIORITIES

1. Control pain.
2. Prevent/manage complications.
3. Maintain quality of life as possible.
4. Plans in place to meet client's/family's last wishes (e.g., care setting, Advance Directives, will, funeral).

NURSING DIAGNOSIS: acute/chronic Pain

May be related to

Injuring agents (biologic, chemical, physical, psychologic)
Chronic physical disability

Possibly evidenced by

Verbal/coded report, preoccupation with pain
Changes in appetite/eating, weight; sleep patterns; altered ability to continue desired activities; fatigue
Guarded/protective behavior, distraction behavior (pacing/repetitive activities, reduced interaction with others)
Facial mask, expressive behavior (restlessness, moaning, crying, irritability), self-focusing, narrowed focus (altered time perception, impaired thought processes)
Alteration in muscle tone (varies from flaccid to rigid)
Autonomic responses (diaphoresis, changes in BP, respiration, pulse), sympathetic mediated responses (temperature, cold, changes of body position, hypersensitivity)

DESIRED OUTCOMES/EVALUATION CRITERIA—CLIENT WILL:

Pain Control (NOC)

Report pain is relieved/controlled.
Verbalize methods that provide relief.
Follow prescribed pharmacological regimen.
Demonstrate use of relaxation skills and diversional activities as indicated.

FAMILY/SO(S) WILL:

Cooperate in pain management program.

ACTIONS/INTERVENTIONS	RATIONALE
Pain Management (NIC)	
Independent	
Perform a comprehensive pain evaluation, including location, characteristics, onset/duration, frequency, quality, severity (e.g., 0–10 scale), and precipitating/aggravating factors. Note cultural issues impacting reporting and expression of pain. Determine client's acceptable level of pain.	Provides baseline information from which a realistic plan can be developed, keeping in mind that verbal/behavioral cues may have little direct relationship to the degree of pain perceived. *Note:* Often client does not feel the need to be completely pain free but is able to be more functional when pain is at lower level on the pain scale.
Determine possible pathophysiologic/psychologic causes of pain (e.g., inflammation, fractures, cancer process, surgery, grief, fear/anxiety, delirium).	Pain is associated with many factors that may be interactive and increase the degree of pain experienced.
Assess client's perception of pain (being aware of client's cognitive status) along with behavioral and psychologic responses. Determine client's attitude toward/use of pain medications and locus of control (internal/external).	Helps identify client's needs, ability to adequately express self, and pain control methods found to be helpful or not helpful in the past. *Note:* Individuals with external locus of control may take little or no responsibility for pain management.
Encourage client/family to express feelings/concerns about narcotic use.	Inaccurate information regarding drug use/fear of addiction or oversedation may impair pain control efforts.
Verify current and past analgesic/narcotic drug use (including alcohol).	May provide insight into what has/has not worked in the past or may impact therapy plan.
Assess degree of personal adjustment to diagnosis, such as anger, irritability, withdrawal, acceptance.	These factors are variable and often affect the perception of pain/ability to cope and need for pain management.
Discuss with SO(s) ways in which they can assist client and reduce precipitating factors.	Promotes involvement in care and belief that there are things they can do to help.
Identify specific signs/symptoms and changes in pain requiring notification of healthcare provider/medical intervention.	Unrelieved pain may be associated with progression of terminal disease process, or be associated with complications that require medical management.
Involve caregivers in identifying effective comfort measures for client; e.g., use of nonacidic fluids, oral swabs/lip salve, skin/perineal care, enema. Instruct in use of oxygen/suction equipment as appropriate.	Managing troubling symptoms such as nausea, dry mouth, dyspnea, constipation can reduce client's suffering and family anxiety, improving quality of life and allowing client/family to focus on other issues.
Demonstrate/encourage use of relaxation techniques; e.g., guided imagery, tapes/music, meditation.	May reduce need for/can supplement analgesic therapy, especially during periods when client desires to minimize sedative effects of medication.
Monitor for/discuss possibility of changes in mental status; e.g., agitation, confusion, restlessness.	Although causes of deterioration are numerous in terminal stages, early recognition and management of the psychologic component is an integral part of pain management.
Collaborative	
Establish pain management plan with client, family, and healthcare providers, including options for management of breakthrough pain.	Inadequate pain management remains one of the most significant deficiencies in the care of the dying client. A stepwise plan (analgesic ladder) developed in advance increases client's level of trust that comfort will be maintained, reducing anxiety.
Schedule/administer analgesics as indicated to maximal dosage. Notify physician if regimen is inadequate to meet pain control goal.	Helps maintain "acceptable" level of pain. Modifications of drug dosage/combinations may be required.
Instruct client, family/caregiver in use of sustained-release formulations, around-the-clock dosing, breakthrough pain management and technology (e.g., pump or PCA) for pain control.	By understanding and managing these factors, pain relief can be enhanced and quality of life improved.
Review medicinal options to treat constipation.	Various "cocktails" are available to stimulate bowel function, reduce associated discomfort.

Refer to CP: Cancer, ND: acute/chronic Pain for additional interventions.

NURSING DIAGNOSIS: Activity Intolerance/Fatigue

May be related to

Generalized weakness
Bedrest or immobility, progressive disease state/debilitating condition
Imbalance between oxygen supply and demand
Cognitive deficits/emotional status, secondary to underlying disease process/ depression
Pain, extreme stress

Possibly evidenced by

Report of lack of energy, inability to maintain usual routines
Verbalizes no desire and/or lack of interest in activity
Lethargic, drowsy; decreased performance
Disinterested in surroundings/introspection

DESIRED OUTCOMES/EVALUATION CRITERIA—CLIENT WILL:

Energy Conservation (NOC)

Identify negative factors affecting performance and eliminate/reduce their effects when possible.
Adapt lifestyle to energy level.
Verbalize understanding of potential loss of ability in relation to existing condition.

Endurance (NOC)

Maintain or achieve slight increase in activity tolerance evidenced by acceptable level of fatigue/weakness.
Remain free of preventable discomfort and/or complications.

ACTIONS/INTERVENTIONS	RATIONALE
Energy Management (NIC)	
Independent	
Assess sleep patterns and note changes in thought processes/behaviors.	Multiple factors can aggravate fatigue, including sleep deprivation, emotional distress, side effects of medication, and progression of disease process.
Recommend scheduling activities for periods when client has most energy. Adjust activities as necessary, reducing intensity level/discontinuing activities as indicated.	Prevents overexertion, allows for some activity within client ability.
Encourage client to do whatever possible; e.g., self-care, sit in chair, visit with family/friends.	Provides for sense of control and feeling of accomplishment.
Instruct client/family/caregiver in energy conservation techniques. Stress necessity of allowing for frequent rest periods following activities.	Enhances performance while conserving limited energy, preventing increase in level of fatigue.
Demonstrate proper performance of ADLs, ambulation/ position changes. Identify safety issues; e.g., use of assistive devices, temperature of bath water, keeping travelways clear of furniture.	Protects client/caregiver from injury during activities.

ACTIONS/INTERVENTIONS	RATIONALE
Encourage nutritional intake/use of supplements as appropriate.	Necessary to meet energy needs for activity.
Document cardiopulmonary response to activity (i.e., weakness, fatigue, dyspnea, arrhythmias, and diaphoresis).	Can provide guidelines for participation in activities.
Monitor breath sounds. Note feelings of panic/air hunger.	Hypoxemia increases sense of fatigue, impairs ability to function.

Collaborative

Provide supplemental oxygen as indicated and monitor response.	Increases oxygenation. Evaluates effectiveness of therapy.

NURSING DIAGNOSIS: anticipatory Grieving/death Anxiety

May be related to

Anticipated loss of physiologic well-being (e.g., change in body function)
Perceived death of client

Possibly evidenced by

Changes in eating habits, alterations in sleep patterns, activity levels, libido, and communication patterns
Denial of potential loss, choked feelings, anger
Fear of the process of dying; loss of physical and/or mental abilities
Negative death images or unpleasant thought about any event related to death or dying; anticipated pain related to dying
Powerlessness over issues related to dying, total loss of control over any aspect of one's own death, inability to problem-solve
Worrying about impact of one's own death on SOs, being the cause of other's grief and suffering, concerns of overworking the caregiver as terminal illness incapacitates

DESIRED OUTCOMES/EVALUATION CRITERIA—CLIENT WILL:

Grief Resolution (NOC)

Identify and express feelings appropriately.
Continue normal life activities, looking toward/planning for the future, one day at a time.
Verbalize understanding of the dying process and feelings of being supported in grief work.

Dignified Life Closure (NOC)

Experience personal empowerment in spiritual strength and resources to find meaning and purpose in grief and loss.

FAMILY WILL:

Grief Resolution (NOC)

Verbalize understanding of the stages of grief and loss; ventilate conflicts and feelings related to illness and death.

ACTIONS/INTERVENTIONS	RATIONALE
Grief Work Facilitation (NIC)	
Independent	
Facilitate development of a trusting relationship with client/family.	Trust is necessary before client/family can feel free to open personal lines of communication with the hospice team and address sensitive issues.
Assess client/SO for stage of grief currently being experienced. Explain process as appropriate.	Knowledge about the grieving process reinforces the normality of feelings/reactions being experienced and can help client deal more effectively with them.
Provide open, nonjudgmental environment. Use therapeutic communication skills of active-listening, acknowledgment, and so on.	Promotes and encourages realistic dialogue about feelings and concerns.
Encourage verbalization of thoughts/concerns and accept expressions of sadness, anger, rejection. Acknowledge normality of these feelings.	Client may feel supported in expression of feelings by the understanding that deep and often conflicting emotions are normal and experienced by others in this difficult situation.
Be aware of mood swings, hostility, and other acting-out behavior. Set limits on inappropriate behavior, redirect negative thinking.	Indicators of ineffective coping and need for additional interventions. Preventing destructive actions enables client to maintain control and sense of self-esteem.
Monitor for signs of debilitating depression; e.g., statements of hopelessness, desire to "end it now." Ask client direct questions about state of mind.	Client may be especially vulnerable when recently diagnosed with end-stage disease process and/or when discharged from hospital. Fear of loss of control/concerns about managing pain effectively may cause client to consider suicide.
Reinforce teaching regarding disease process and treatments and provide information as requested/appropriate about dying. Be honest; do not give false hope while providing emotional support.	Client/SO benefit from factual information. Individuals may ask direct questions about death, and honest answers promote trust and provide reassurance that correct information will be given.
Review past life experiences, role changes, sexuality concerns, and coping skills. Promote an environment conducive to talking about things that interest client.	Opportunity to identify skills that may help individuals cope with grief of current situation more effectively. *Note:* Issues of sexuality remain important at this stage; e.g., feelings of masculinity/femininity, giving up role within family (caretaker/provider), ability to maintain sexual activity (if desired).
Investigate evidence of conflict; expressions of anger; and statements of despair, guilt, hopelessness, inability to grieve.	Interpersonal conflicts/angry behavior may be client's/SO's way of expressing or dealing with feelings of despair/spiritual distress, necessitating further evaluation and support.
Determine way that client/SO understand and respond to death; e.g., cultural expectations, learned behaviors, experience with death (close family members/friends), beliefs about life after death, faith in a Higher Power (God).	These factors affect how each individual faces death and influences how they may respond and interact.
Assist client/SO to identify strengths in self/situation and support systems.	Recognizing these resources provides opportunity to work through feelings of grief.
Be aware of own feelings about death. Accept whatever methods client/SO have chosen to help each other through the process.	Caregiver's anxiety and unwillingness to accept reality of possibility of own death may block ability to be helpful to client/SO, necessitating enlisting the aid of others to provide needed support.
Dying Care (NIC)	
Provide open environment for discussion with client/SO (when appropriate) about desires/plans pertaining to death; e.g., making will, burial arrangements, tissue donation, death benefits, insurance, time for family gatherings, how to spend remaining time.	If client/SO are mutually aware of impending death, they may more easily deal with unfinished business or desired activities. Having a part in problem-solving/planning can provide a sense of control over anticipated events.
Encourage participation in care and treatment decisions.	Allows client to retain some control over life.

ACTIONS/INTERVENTIONS	RATIONALE
Visit frequently and provide physical contact as appropriate/desired, or provide frequent phone support as appropriate for setting. Arrange for care provider/support person to stay with client as needed.	Helps reduce feelings of isolation and abandonment.
Provide time for acceptance, final farewell, and arrangements for memorial/funeral service according to individual spiritual/cultural/ethnic needs.	Accommodation of personal/family wishes helps reduce anxiety and may promote sense of peace.

Collaborative

Determine spiritual needs/conflicts and refer to appropriate team members including clergy/spiritual advisor, parish nurse.	Providing for spiritual needs, forgiveness, prayer, devotional materials, or sacraments as requested can relieve spiritual pain and provide a sense of peace. (Refer to ND: risk for Spiritual Distress.)
Refer to appropriate counselor as needed (e.g., psychiatric clinical nurse specialist, social worker, psychologist, pastoral support).	Compassion and support can help alleviate distress or palliate feelings of grief to facilitate coping and foster growth.
Refer to visiting nurse, home health agency if hospice services not available.	Provides support in meeting physical and emotional needs of client/SO, and can supplement the care family and friends are able to give.
Identify need for/appropriate timing of anti-depressants/anxiety medications.	May alleviate distress, enhance coping, especially for clients not requiring analgesics.

NURSING DIAGNOSIS: compromised [or] disabled family Coping/Caregiver Role Strain

May be related to

Inadequate or incorrect information or understanding by a primary person, unrealistic expectations
Temporary preoccupation by significant person who is trying to manage emotional conflicts and personal suffering and is unable to perceive or to act effectively with regard to client's needs; does not have enough resources to provide the care needed
Temporary family disorganization and role changes, feel that caregiving interferes with other important roles in their lives
Client providing little support in turn for the primary person
Prolonged disease/disability progression that exhausts the supportive capacity of significant persons
Significant person with chronically unexpressed feelings of guilt, anxiety, hostility, despair
Highly ambivalent family relationships, feel stress or nervousness in their relationship with the care receiver

Possibly evidenced by

Client expressing/confirming a concern or complaint about SO's response to client's health problem, despair about family reactions/lack of involvement, history of poor relationship between caregiver and care receiver
Neglectful relationships with other family members
Inability to complete caregiving tasks, altered caregiver health status
SO describing preoccupation about personal reactions; displaying intolerance, abandonment, rejection; caregiver not developmentally ready for caregiver role
SO attempting assistive/supportive behaviors with less than satisfactory results, withdrawing or entering into limited or temporary personal communication with client,

displaying protective behavior disproportionate (too little or too much) to client's abilities or need for autonomy
Apprehension about future regarding care receiver's health and the caregiver's ability to provide care

DESIRED OUTCOMES/EVALUATION CRITERIA—FAMILY/CAREGIVER WILL:

CAREGIVER PERFORMANCE: Direct [or] Indirect Care (NOC)

Identify resources within themselves to deal with situation.
Participate positively in care of client, within limits of abilities.
Engage in problem-solving with direct care providers to meet client's individual needs.

Caregiver-Patient Relationship (NOC)

Express more realistic understanding and expectations of client.
Provide opportunity for client to deal with situation in own way.

ACTIONS/INTERVENTIONS	RATIONALE
Family Involvement Promotion (NIC)	
Independent	
Assess level of anxiety present in family/SO.	Anxiety level needs to be dealt with before problem-solving can begin. Individuals may be so preoccupied with own reactions to situation that they are unable to respond to another's needs.
Establish rapport and acknowledge difficulty of the situation for the family.	May assist SO to accept what is happening and be willing to share problems with healthcare providers.
Determine level of impairment of perceptual/cognitive/physical abilities. Evaluate pre-illness/current behaviors that may be interfering with the care of client.	Information about family problems (e.g., divorce/separation, alcoholism/other drug abuse, abusive situation) will be helpful in determining options and developing an appropriate plan of care.
Note client's emotional/behavioral responses resulting from increasing weakness and dependency (e.g., hallucinations, delusions, hostility, withdrawal, depression).	Approaching death is most stressful when client/family coping responses are strained, resulting in increased frustration, guilt, and anguish.
Discuss underlying reasons for client behaviors with family.	When family members know why client is behaving differently, it may help them understand and accept/deal with unusual behaviors.
Assist family/client to understand "who owns the problem" and who is responsible for resolution. Avoid placing blame or guilt.	When these boundaries are defined, each individual can begin to take care of own self and stop taking care of others in inappropriate ways.
Determine current knowledge/perception of the situation.	Provides information on which to begin planning care and make informed decisions. Lack of information or unrealistic perceptions can interfere with caregiver's/care receiver's response to illness situation.
Assess current actions of SO and how they are received by client.	SO may be trying to be helpful, but actions are not perceived as being helpful by client. SO may be withdrawn or too protective.
Facilitate family conference (include all family members as appropriate). Provide/reinforce information about terminal illness/death and future family needs.	Knowledge can help the family prepare for eventualities and deal with the actual death process. Increases understanding of necessary activities/steps to be taken to deal with funeral preparations, legal/financial concerns, and survivor issues.

ACTIONS/INTERVENTIONS	RATIONALE
Caregiver Support (NIC)	
Determine caregiver's level of commitment, responsibility, and involvement in care. Use assessment tool, such as Burden Interview, to further clarify caregiver's abilities, when appropriate.	Progressive/terminal care taxes caregiver and may alter ability to meet client's/own needs.
Ascertain caregiver's understanding and acceptance of client's wishes/advance directives.	If caregiver is not in total agreement with client's wishes, role strain may be intensified as specific decisions are made regarding care/termination of therapies.
Involve SO in information giving, problem-solving, and care of client as appropriate. Instruct in medication administration techniques, needed treatments, appropriate complementary and alternative therapies; e.g., massage, herbs, aromatherapy, relaxation techniques. Ascertain adeptness with required equipment.	Information can reduce feelings of helplessness and uselessness. Helping a client/family find comfort is often more important than adhering to strict routines. However, family caregivers need to feel confident with specific care activities and equipment. *Note*: Use of complementary and alternative medicine (CAM) is increasing for pain/symptom relief with lessened side effects.
Provide positive feedback for efforts.	Helps caregiver recognize/feel valued for contribution to care.
Stress importance of self-nurturing; e.g., personal needs, social contacts.	Taking time for self can help lessen risk of being overwhelmed by situation.
Identify/schedule alternative care resources, e.g., family, friends, sitter, respite services, as needed.	As client's condition worsens, primary caregiver will require additional help from other sources to maintain client at home as desired while still meeting own needs for rest and personal time.
Collaborative	
Refer to appropriate resources for assistance as indicated (e.g., counseling, psychotherapy, financial, spiritual, respite care).	May need additional assistance in resolving family issues/making peace and maintaining personal well-being.
Arrange for appropriate prescriptions for SO (e.g., sedative/hypnotic).	Mild medication may be beneficial in reducing anxiety/promoting sleep, which in turn can enhance coping ability.

NURSING DIAGNOSIS: risk for Spiritual Distress

Risk factors may include

Physical or psychologic stress, energy-consuming anxiety
Situational losses
Blocks to self-love, low self-esteem, inability to forgive

Possibly evidenced by

[Not applicable; presence of signs and symptoms establishes an *actual* diagnosis.]

DESIRED OUTCOMES/EVALUATION CRITERIA—CLIENT/SO WILL:

Dignified Life Closure (NOC)

Identify meaning and purpose in one's life that reinforces hope, peace, and contentment.
Verbalize acceptance of self as being worthy, not deserving of illness/death.
Identify and use resources appropriately.

ACTIONS/INTERVENTIONS	RATIONALE
Spiritual Support (NIC)	
Independent	
Listen to client/SOs reports/expressions of anger/concern.	May reveal many conflicting thoughts and beliefs; e.g., that illness/situation is a punishment for wrongdoing, or that death is desirable or feared. Dying client faces momentous losses of physical control and function, of independence, of relationships, of possibilities, and ultimately of life itself. To family members and friends, the loss of a loved one causes great stress and temporarily impairs concentration, decision making, and work performance.
Determine client's religious/spiritual orientation, current involvement, presence of conflicts in current circumstances.	Provides insight as to where client currently is and what hopes for the future may be. *Note*: Individuals reporting high spirituality were less hopeless, had less desire to hasten their deaths, and had less suicidal ideation.
Assess sense of self-concept, worth, ability to enter into/maintain loving relationships.	Necessary to provide firm foundation for growth and guiding client/family through life closure and completion tasks.
Explore meaning/interpretation and relationship of spirituality, life/death, and illness to client's spiritual centeredness.	Identifying the meaning of these issues may be helpful in forming or stating a belief system that enables client to move forward. Comfort can be gained when family and friends share client's beliefs and support search for spiritual knowledge.
Explore ways that spirituality/religious practices have affected client's life; e.g. music, prayer, service to others.	Allows client to explore spiritual needs and decide what fits own view, and provides support for dealing with current situation.
Determine support systems available to and used by client/SO.	May help identify strengths and weaknesses in relationship dynamics that the client/SOs may want to address; e.g. expressing love, forgiveness, support.
Encourage client to be introspective in search for peace and harmony.	Finding peace within will carry over to relationships with others and one's outlook on life and death.
Establish environment that promotes free expression of feelings and concerns.	May help identify the real need of the day. For example, the dying person may not hope for cure or postponement of death, but rather that on the next day he or she will feel better with fewer physical and emotional discomforts.
Have client/SO identify and prioritize current/immediate needs as regards faith, influence, and community.	Helps them focus on what needs to be done and identify manageable steps to take.
Make time for nonjudgmental discussion of cultural and philosophic issues/questions about spiritual impact of illness and/or impending death.	Spiritual or religious practices (customs) and rituals often play important roles, especially at a time of such significant transition in life.
Discuss difference between grief and guilt and help client to identify and deal with each, assuming responsibility for own actions.	Identifies persons at risk for complicated grief and bereavement and its associated depression and complications. May provide opportunities for resolution.
Use therapeutic communication skills of gentle stillness, reflection, conveying respect through tone of voice and body language, and active-listening.	Encourages client/SO to identify and express end of life concerns, hopes, fears, and expectations openly and honestly in a caring milieu.
Review coping skills used and their effectiveness in current situation.	Helps client/SO remember and call upon strengths that have been helpful in other situations. May free the client to be "more" creative, loving, and into the experience of well being.
Suggest use of story telling, journaling, or taping thoughts.	Helps client explore and find own solutions to concerns. Identifies strengths to incorporate into plan and techniques needing revision.
Determine how involved in physical care the family members want to be. Establish with client/SO wishes for the moment of death.	Clarification of specific wishes can be helpful in reducing stress and allow for needed differences in response.

ACTIONS/INTERVENTIONS	RATIONALE
Collaborative	
Encourage participation in desired religious activities, prayer, meditation, contact with minister/spiritual advisor/grief counselor.	May prove beneficial to both client and family members in reflecting on life and death issues. Can assist in clarifying values/ideas, recognizing and resolving feelings and promote comfort. Validating one's beliefs in an external way can support and strengthen the inner self.

Refer to CP: Psychologic Aspects of Care, ND: risk for impaired Religiosity for additional interventions.

DISASTER CONSIDERATIONS

Physical effects of a catastrophic event can vary depending on the type of disaster. For example, explosive devices, transportation accidents, hurricanes, or floods might result in burns and crush injuries; release of chemical agents or use of biologic weapons/reemerging infections (e.g., pandemic influenza) causing mass infections may result in various physical problems depending on the agent involved.

Disaster/extreme events can exacerbate any chronic condition, such as heart or lung problems, and/or precipitate emergent conditions such as premature births, seizures, and psychiatric conditions, panic disorders, and suicidal thoughts.

Following any disaster, those involved, victims, rescuers, and the surrounding community, suffer from a variety of responses. The bigger the disaster/catastrophe, the greater the number of people involved and the wider the effect. With the playing and replaying of the events, the effects can be magnified and people far removed from the scene may also suffer.

CARE SETTING

Wherever disaster occurs, to include triage areas, aid stations, clinics, hospital/emergency centers, shelters.

RELATED CONCERNS

Burns: thermal/chemical/electrical, page 680
Craniocerebral trauma, page 218
Fractures, page 642
Pneumonia, page 128
Sepsis/septicemia, page 701
Psychosocial aspects of care, page 770

Client Assessment Database

Data depend on specific injuries incurred/presence of chronic conditions (refer to specific plans of care for appropriate data reflecting e.g., burns, multiple trauma, cardiac and respiratory conditions, and so forth).

ACTIVITY/REST

May report: Sleep disturbances, recurrent intrusive dreams of the event, nightmares, difficulty in falling or staying asleep, hypersomnia (intrusive thoughts, flashbacks)
Fatigue, listlessness

CIRCULATION

May report: Palpitations or tachycardia
Sweating, hot flashes, or chills

May exhibit: Cold, clammy hands
Increased blood pressure (anxiety), decreased blood pressure (dehydration/hypovolemia)

EGO INTEGRITY

May report: Excessive worry about event, avoidance of circumstances/locations associated with incident
Sense of inner turmoil
Dry mouth, upset stomach, lump in throat
Threat to physical integrity or self-concept
Questioning of God's purpose/abandonment

May exhibit: Facial expression in keeping with level of anxiety (furrowed brow, strained face, eyelid twitch)

ELIMINATION

May report: Frequent urination, diarrhea

FOOD/FLUID

May report: Lack of interest in food, dysfunctional eating pattern
Nausea, vomiting

NEUROSENSORY

May report: Anticipation of misfortune to self or others, feeling stuck
Absence of other mental disorder

May exhibit: Motor tension, shakiness, jitteriness, trembling, easily startled
Apprehensive expectation, rumination
Excessive vigilance/hyperattentiveness; distractibility, difficulty concentrating, irritability, impatience, psychic numbing

PAIN/DISCOMFORT

May report: Muscle aches, headaches, chest pain (in addition to pain related to physical injuries/conditions)

RESPIRATORY

May report: Shortness of breath, smothering sensation

May exhibit: Increased respiratory rate

SEXUALITY

May report: Decreased libido

SOCIAL INTERACTIONS

May report: Concern for well-being of others
Questioning own actions/survival
Difficulty participating in social settings, reluctance to engage in usual activities/work

TEACHING/LEARNING

Discharge plan considerations: Dependent on individual situation, level of support, and available resources

DIAGNOSTIC STUDIES

Dependent on injuring agent/exposure and availability of resources for testing/procedures.

NURSING PRIORITIES

1. Prevent/treat life-threatening conditions.
2. Prevent further injury/spread of infection.
3. Support efforts to cope with situation.
4. Facilitate integration of event.
5. Assist community in preparing for future occurrences.

DISCHARGE GOALS

1. Free of preventable complications.
2. Anxiety/fear reduced to a manageable level.
3. Beginning to cope effectively with situation.
4. Plan in place to meet needs after discharge.
5. Community preparedness enhanced.

NURSING DIAGNOSIS: risk for/actual Injury (trauma, suffocation, poisoning)

Risk factors may include

Biologic (immunization level of community, presence of microorganism)
Contact with chemical pollutants, poisonous agents
Exposure to open flame/flammable material
Acceleration/deceleration forces
Contamination of food or water

Possibly evidenced by

[Not applicable; presence of signs and symptoms establishes an *actual* diagnosis.]

DESIRED OUTCOMES/EVALUATION CRITERIA—CLIENT/CAREGIVERS WILL:

Physical Injury Severity (NOC)

Minimize degree of/prevent further injury.

Personal Safety Behavior (NOC)

Verbalize understanding of condition/specific needs.
Identify interventions appropriate to situation.
Demonstrate behaviors necessary to protect self from further injury.
Accept responsibility for own care and follow up as individually able.

ACTIONS/INTERVENTIONS	RATIONALE
TRIAGE: Disaster (NIC)	
Independent	
Acquire information about nature of emergency, accident, or disaster.	Identifies basic resource needs and helps to prepare staff for appropriate level of response based on customary injuries/healthcare needs usually associated with specific event.
Prepare area and equipment, check and restock supplies.	Assists in providing safe medical and nursing care in anticipation of emergency need.
Assist in prioritizing (triaging) clients for treatment. Monitor for/treat life-threatening injuries.	Promotes efficient care of those who can be medically treated, and maximizes use of resources.
Determine primary needs/specific complaints of client. Check for medical alert tag.	Information necessary for triaging to appropriate services.
Obtain additional medical information including preexisting conditions, allergies, current medication. Perform more in-depth assessment as time allows/condition warrants.	Provides for assessment and treatment of conditions that might not be evident initially.
Determine client's developmental level, decision-making ability, level of cognition, and competence.	Affects treatment plan regarding issues of informed consent, self-care, client teaching, and discharge.
Evaluate individual's response to event, mood, coping abilities, personal vulnerability.	People react to traumatic situations in many ways and may exhibit a wide range of responses, from no visible response to wild emotions. This may result in carelessness/increased risk-taking without considerations of consequences, or inability to act on own behalf (including protecting self).
Ascertain knowledge of needs/injury prevention and motivation to prevent further injury.	Indicator of need for information, assistance with making positive changes, promoting safety, and sense of security.

ACTIONS/INTERVENTIONS	RATIONALE
Discuss importance of self-monitoring of conditions/emotions that can contribute to occurrence of injury (e.g., shock state, ignoring basic needs, fatigue, anger, irritability).	Recognizing these factors and dealing with them appropriately (including seeking support/assistance) can reduce individual risks.
Note socioeconomic status/availability and use of resources.	May determine ability to access help for identified problems.

Collaborative

ACTIONS/INTERVENTIONS	RATIONALE
Work with other agencies (e.g., law enforcement, fire department, Red Cross, ambulance/EMT), as indicated. Follow prearranged roles when participating in a community disaster plan.	During a disaster, many people are involved with care of victims. Most communities have disaster plans in which nurses will participate.
Identify/manage life-threatening situations (e.g., airway problems, bleeding, diminished consciousness).	Stabilization of medical condition necessary before proceeding with additional therapies.

TRIAGE: Emergency Care (NIC)

ACTIONS/INTERVENTIONS	RATIONALE
Obtain/assist with diagnostic studies as indicated.	Choice of studies is dependent on individual situation and availability of resources.
Provide therapeutic interventions as individually appropriate. (Refer to specific CPs; e.g., Burns, Fractures, Crainocerebral Trauma, Myocardial Infarction, COPD, Ventilatory Assistance [mechanical].)	Specific needs of client and the level of care available at a particular site determine response.
Provide written instructions/list of resources for later review.	Client/SO(s) are generally not able to assimilate information at time of crisis, and may want/need reinforcement or additional information.
Identify community resources including shelter, neighbors/friends, and government agencies available for assistance.	May need assistance/ongoing monitoring postdischarge to deal with self-care needs as well as safe housing and other life requirements. *Note:* Release of client without active support increases personal risk because of possibility of unrecognized or subacute injury/delayed psychologic response.
Refer to other resources as indicated (e.g., counseling/psychotherapy).	Immediate "debriefing"/counseling is beneficial for dealing with crisis to enhance ability to meet own needs.

NURSING DIAGNOSIS: risk for Infection

Risk factors may include

Environmental exposure, inadequate acquired immunity
Trauma/tissue destruction, invasive procedures
Chronic disease, malnutrition
Insufficient knowledge to avoid exposure to pathogens

Possibly evidenced by

[Not applicable; presence of signs and symptoms establishes an *actual* diagnosis.]

DESIRED OUTCOMES/EVALUATION CRITERIA—CLIENT WILL:

Risk Control (NOC)

Verbalize understanding of individual exposure/risk factor(s).
Identify interventions to prevent/reduce risk of infection.

Infection Severity (NOC)

Be free of/demonstrate resolution of infection.

ACTIONS/INTERVENTIONS	RATIONALE
Infection Control (NIC)	
Independent	
Note risk factors for occurrence of infection (e.g., environmental exposure, compromised host, traumatic injury/loss of skin integrity). Determine proximity to incident. Be aware of incubation period for various diseases.	Understanding nature/properties of infectious agents and individual's exposure determines choice of therapeutic intervention. *Note:* Those upwind of an aerosol release of a biologic agent may have little or no exposure to the agent. (Refer to Chart 15–1, at end of plan of care, for pertinent information.)
Observe for signs and symptoms of infective agent and sepsis (systemic infection); fever, chills, diaphoresis, altered level of consciousness, positive blood cultures. Investigate presence of rash.	Initial symptoms of some agents include fever, fatigue, joint aches, and headache similar to influenza and the infection may be misdiagnosed as an influenza-like infection (ILI) unless healthcare providers maintain an index of suspicion and obtain additional diagnostic studies.
Practice and demonstrate proper handwashing technique.	First-line defense to limit spread of infections.
Provide for infection precautions/isolation as indicated (e.g., standard precautions of gown/gloves/face shield or goggles, respiratory mask/filter, reverse or negative pressure room).	Reduces risk of cross-contamination to staff, visitors, and other clients.
Group/cohort individuals with same diagnosis/exposure as resources require.	Limited resources may dictate open wardlike environment but need to control spread of infection still exists.
Monitor visitors/caregivers for infectious diseases.	Prevents exposure of client to further infection and may reveal additional cases.
Review individual nutritional needs, appropriate exercise program, and need for rest.	Essential for well-being and recovery.
Instruct client/SO(s) in techniques to prevent spread of infection, protect the integrity of skin, and care for wound/lesions.	Self-care activities that may provide protection for client/others.
Emphasize necessity of taking antibiotics as directed (e.g., dosage and length of therapy).	Premature discontinuation of treatment when client begins to feel well may result in return of infection. On the one hand, unnecessary use of antibiotics may result in development of secondary infections or resistant organisms.
Involve community in education programs geared to increasing awareness of spread/prevention of communicable diseases.	Helps to reduce incidence of disease in the community, and manage the dissemination of information.
Collaborative	
Obtain appropriate specimens for observation and culture/sensitivities testing (e.g., nose/throat swabs, sputum, blood, urine, and feces).	Provides information to diagnose infection, determine appropriate therapeutic interventions.
Assist with medical procedures (e.g., incision and drainage of abscess, bronchoscopy, wound care) as indicated.	Helps determine causative factors for appropriate treatment and facilitates recovery.
Administer/monitor medication regimen (e.g., antimircrobials, topical antibiotics) and note client's response.	Determines effectiveness of therapy/presence of side effects.
Provide passive protection (e.g., immune globulin), active protection (e.g., vaccination), or chemoprophylaxis as appropriate.	May prevent development of infection following exposure or reduce the likelihood of acquiring disease in the future. (Refer to Chart 15–2 at end of plan of care.)
Alert proper authorities to presence of specific infectious agent and number of cases.	Diseases that could be caused by biologic releases or that spread rapidly through populations have reporting requirements to local, state, and national agencies, such as the state health department or the Centers for Disease Control and Prevention (CDC). These agencies in turn have responsibilities for the public safety and welfare.

NURSING DIAGNOSIS: Anxiety (severe/panic)/Fear

May be related to

Situational crisis, exposure to toxins
Real or perceived threat to physical well-being, threat of death
Interpersonal transmission of concerns/fears
Unconscious conflict about essential values (beliefs)
Unmet needs

Possibly evidenced by

Persistent feelings of apprehension and uneasiness, sense of impending doom
Scanning and vigilance, or lack of awareness of surroundings
Sympathetic stimulation, extraneous movements (restlessness, foot shuffling, hand/arm fidgeting, rocking movements)
Focus on self, overexcited
Impaired functioning; verbal expressions of having no control or influence over situation, outcome, or self-care

DESIRED OUTCOMES/EVALUATION CRITERIA—CLIENT WILL:

Anxiety [or] Fear Self-Control (NOC)

Acknowledge and discuss feelings.
Verbalize accurate knowledge of current situation and potential outcomes.
Identify healthy ways to successfully deal with stress.
Report anxiety is reduced to a manageable level.
Demonstrate problem-solving skills appropriate for individual situation.
Use resources/support systems effectively.

ACTIONS/INTERVENTIONS	RATIONALE
Crisis Intervention (NIC)	
Independent	
Determine degree of anxiety/fear present, associated behaviors (e.g., laughter, crying, calm or agitation, excited/hysterical behavior, expressions of disbelief and/or self-blame), and reality of perceived threat.	Clearly understanding client's perception is pivotal to providing appropriate assistance in overcoming the fear. Individual may be agitated or totally overwhelmed. Severe anxiety increases risk for client's own safety as well as the safety of others in the environment.
Note degree of disorganization.	Client may be unable to handle ADLs or work requirements and need more intensive evaluation/intervention.
Maintain and respect client's personal space boundaries (approximately 4-foot circle around client).	Entering client's personal space without permission/invitation could result in an overwhelming anxiety response, and possibly an overt act of violence.
Create quiet area as able. Maintain a calm, confident manner. Speak in even tone using short simple sentences.	Decreases sense of confusion/overstimulation, enhances sense of safety. Helps client focus on what is said and reduces transmission of anxiety.
Develop trusting relationship with client.	Trust is the basis of a therapeutic nurse/client relationship and enables them to work together effectively.
Identify whether incident has reactivated preexisting or coexisting situations (physical/psychologic).	Concerns/psychologic issues will be recycled every time trauma is re-experienced and affect how the client views the current situation.
Determine presence of physical symptoms, (e.g., numbness, headache, tightness in chest, nausea, and pounding heart).	Physical problems need to be differentiated from anxiety symptoms so that appropriate treatment can be given.

ACTIONS/INTERVENTIONS	RATIONALE
Identify psychologic responses (e.g., anger, shock, acute anxiety, panic, confusion, denial). Record emotional changes.	Although these are normal responses at the time of the trauma, they will recycle again and again until they are dealt with adequately.
Discuss with client perception of what is causing anxiety/panic.	Increases ability to connect symptoms to subjective feeling of anxiety, providing opportunity to gain insight/control and make desired changes.
Assist client to correct any distortions being experienced. Share perceptions with client.	Perceptions based on reality will help to decrease fearfulness. How the nurse views the situation may help client to see it differently.
Explore with client/SO the manner in which the client has coped with anxiety-producing events before the trauma.	May help client regain sense of control and recognize significance of trauma.
Engage client in learning new coping behaviors (e.g., progressive muscle relaxation, thought-stopping).	Replacing maladaptive behaviors can enhance ability to manage and deal with stress. Interrupting obsessive thinking allows client to use energy to address underlying anxiety, while continued rumination about the incident can actually retard recovery.
Demonstrate/encourage use of techniques to reduce/manage stress and vent emotions such as anger, hostility.	Reduces likelihood of eruptions that can result in abusive behavior.
Give positive feedback when client demonstrates better ways to manage anxiety and is able to calmly and/or realistically appraise own situation.	Provides acknowledgement and reinforcement, encouraging use of new coping strategies. Enhances ability to deal with fearful feelings and gain control over situation, promoting future successes.

Collaborative

Administer medications as indicated; e.g.,	
Antianxiety: diazepam (Valium), buspirone (BuSpar), alprazolam (Xanax), oxazepam (Serax);	Provides temporary relief of anxiety symptoms enhancing client's ability to cope with situation. Also useful for alleviating feelings of panic, intrusive nightmares.
Antidepressants: fluoxetine (Prozac), paroxetine (Paxil), bupropion (Wellbutrin).	Used to decrease anxiety, lift mood, aid in management of behavior, and ensure rest until client regains control of own self. Helpful in suppressing intrusive thoughts and explosive anger.
Refer for additional therapies; e.g., hypnosis, eye movement desensitization/reprocessing (EMD/R), or thought reprocessing therapy as appropriate.	When used by trained therapist, these short-term therapies are particularly effective with individuals who have been traumatized or who have problems with anxiety and depression. Systematic desensitization, reframing, and reinterpretation of memories may be achieved through hypnosis.
Coordinate release/discharge to family, friend, or emergency services as indicated.	Triaging and maximum use of resources may limit time allotted for care and client may not be ready to meet own needs/assume full responsibility for self.
Educate victims and public about risks and steps being taken to deal with problem. Include other members of healthcare teams, stressing risks to themselves. Refer to resources such as CDC, Web sites.	Nurses have a role in community education because they are close to the individuals affected. Providing accurate information and credible resources helps limit level of concern and transmission of anxiety. Current, timely information regarding biologic concerns and healthcare needs can be accessed through Web sites such as *www.cdc.gov/*, *www.hhs.gov/* and *www.fbi.gov/*.

NURSING DIAGNOSIS: Spiritual Distress

May be related to

Physical/psychologic stress, energy-consuming anxiety
Situation, loss(es)/intense suffering
Separation from religious/cultural ties
Challenged belief and value system

Possibly evidenced by

Expressions of concern about disaster, the meaning of life/death and/or belief systems
Inner conflict about current loss of normality and effects of the disaster, anger directed at deity, engaging in self-blame
Seeking spiritual assistance, or chooses not to participate
Reports of somatic symptoms

DESIRED OUTCOMES/EVALUATION CRITERIA—CLIENT WILL:

Spiritual Health (NOC)

Verbalize increased sense of self-concept and hope for future.
Discuss beliefs/values about spiritual issues.
Verbalize acceptance of self as being worthy.

ACTIONS/INTERVENTIONS	RATIONALE
Spiritual Support (NIC)	
Independent	
Determine client's religious/spiritual orientation, current involvement, and presence of conflicts.	Provides baseline for planning care and accessing appropriate resources.
Establish environment that promotes free expression of feelings and concerns. Provide calm, peaceful setting when possible.	Promotes awareness and identification of feelings so they can be dealt with.
Listen to client/SO's reports/expressions of anger, concern, alienation from God, belief that situation is a punishment for wrongdoing, and so forth.	Helpful to understand client's/SO's point of view and how they are questioning their faith in the face of tragedy.
Note sense of futility, feelings of hopelessness and helplessness, lack of motivation to help self.	These thoughts and feelings can result in the client feeling paralyzed and unable to move forward to resolve the situation.
Listen to expressions of inability to find meaning in life, reason for living. Evaluate for suicidal ideation.	May indicate need for further intervention to prevent suicide attempt.
Determine support systems available to client/SO(s).	Presence or lack of support systems can affect client's recovery.
Ask how you can be most helpful. Convey acceptance of client's spiritual beliefs/concerns.	Promotes trust and comfort, encouraging client to be open about sensitive matters.
Make time for nonjudgmental discussion of philosophic issues/questions about spiritual impact of current events/situation.	Helps client to begin to look at basis for spiritual confusion. *Note:* There is a potential for care provider's belief system to interfere with client finding own way. Therefore it is most beneficial to remain neutral and not espouse own beliefs.
Discuss difference between grief and guilt and help client to identify and deal with each, assuming responsibility for own actions, expressing awareness of the consequences of acting out of false guilt.	Blaming self for what has happened impedes dealing with the grief process and needs to be discussed and dealt with.
Use therapeutic communication skills of reflection and Active-Listening.	Helps client find own solutions to concerns.
Discuss use of/provide opportunities for client/SO to experience meditation, prayer, and forgiveness. Provide information that anger with God is a normal part of the grieving process.	Can help to heal past and present pain.

ACTIONS/INTERVENTIONS	RATIONALE
Assist client to develop goals for dealing with life situation.	Enhances commitment to goal, optimizing outcomes and promoting sense of hope.

Collaborative

ACTIONS/INTERVENTIONS	RATIONALE
Identify and refer to resources that can be helpful (e.g., pastoral/parish nurse or religious counselor, crisis counselor, psychotherapy, Alcoholics/Narcotics Anonymous).	Specific assistance may be helpful to recovery, (e.g., relationship problems, substance abuse, suicidal ideation).
Encourage participation in support groups.	Discussing concerns and questions with others can help client resolve feelings.

NURSING DIAGNOSIS: risk for Post-Trauma Syndrome

Risk factors may include

Events outside the range of usual human experience
Serious threat or injury to self/loved ones, witnessing horrors/tragic events (e.g., police, fire, rescue, corrections, healthcare providers, and their family members)
Exaggerated sense of responsibility/survivor's role in the event
Inadequate social support; nonsupportive environment, displacement from home

Possibly evidenced by

[Not applicable; presence of signs and symptoms establishes an *actual* diagnosis.]

DESIRED OUTCOMES/EVALUATION CRITERIA—CLIENT/CAREGIVERS WILL:

Anxiety [or] Fear Self-Control (NOC)

Express own feelings/reactions, avoiding projection.
Demonstrate ability to deal with emotional reactions in an individually appropriate manner.
Report absence of physical manifestations (e.g., pain, nightmares/flashbacks, fatigue) associated with the event.

ACTIONS/INTERVENTIONS — RATIONALE

Crisis Intervention (NIC)

Independent

ACTIONS/INTERVENTIONS	RATIONALE
Determine involvement in event (e.g., survivor, SO, rescue/aid worker, healthcare provider, family member).	All those concerned with a traumatic event are at risk for emotional trauma and have needs related to their situation/involvement in the event. *Note:* Close involvement with victims affects individual responses and may prolong emotional suffering.
Evaluate life factors/stressors currently or recently occurring, such as displacement from home due to catastrophic event (e.g., illness/injury, natural disaster, terrorist attack). Identify how client's past experiences may affect current situation.	Affects client's reaction to current event and is basis for planning care and identifying appropriate supports/resources.
Listen for comments of taking on responsibility (e.g., "I should have been more careful/gone back to get her").	Indicators of "survivor's guilt" and blaming self for actions.
Identify client's current coping mechanisms.	Noting positive or negative skills provides direction for care.

ACTIONS/INTERVENTIONS	RATIONALE
Determine availability/usefulness of client's support systems, (e.g., family, social, community, and so forth).	Family and others close to the client may also be at risk and require assistance to cope with the trauma.
Provide information about signs/symptoms of post-trauma response, especially if individual is involved in a high-risk occupation.	Awareness of these factors helps individual identify need for assistance when they occur.
Identify and discuss client's strengths as well as vulnerabilities.	Provides information to build on for coping with traumatic experience.
Evaluate individual's perceptions of events and personal significance (e.g., rescue worker trained to provide lifesaving assistance but recovering only dead bodies).	Events that trigger feelings of despair and hopelessness may be more difficult to deal with, and require long-term interventions.
Provide emotional and physical presence by sitting with client/SO and offering solace.	Strengthens coping abilities.
Encourage expression of feelings. Note whether feelings expressed appear congruent with events experienced.	It is important to talk about the incident repeatedly. Incongruencies may indicate deeper conflict and can impede resolution.
Note presence of nightmares, reliving the incident, loss of appetite, irritability, numbness and crying, family/relationship disruption.	These responses are normal in the early post-incident time frame. If prolonged and persistent, they may indicate need for more intensive therapy.
Provide a calm, safe environment.	Helps client deal with the disruption in personal life.
Encourage and assist client in learning stress-management techniques.	Promotes relaxation and helps individual exercise control over self and what has happened.

Collaborative

Recommend participation in debriefing sessions that may be provided following major disaster events.	Dealing with the stresses promptly may facilitate recovery from event/prevent exacerbation.
Identify employment, community resource groups.	Provides opportunity for ongoing support to deal with recurrent feelings related to the trauma.
Administer medications as indicated; e.g.,	
Antipsychotics; e.g., phenothiazines such as chlorpromazine (Thorazine), haloperidol (Haldol);	Low doses may be used for reduction of psychotic symptoms when loss of contact with reality occurs, usually for client's with especially disturbing flashbacks.
Carbamazepine (Tegretol).	Used to alleviate intrusive recollections/flashbacks, impulsivity, and violent behavior.

NURSING DIAGNOSIS: ineffective community Coping

May be related to

Natural or man-made disasters (earthquakes, floods, reemerging infectious agents, terrorist activity)
Deficits in social support services and resources
Ineffective or nonexistent community systems (e.g., lack of/inadequate emergency medical system, transportation system, or disaster planning systems)

Possibly evidenced by

Deficits of community participation, community does not meet its own expectations
Expressed vulnerability, community powerlessness
Stressors perceived as excessive
Excessive community conflicts
High illness rates

DESIRED OUTCOMES/EVALUATION CRITERIA—COMMUNITY WILL:

Community Competence (NOC)

Recognize negative and positive factors affecting community's ability to meet its own demands or needs.
Identify alternatives to inappropriate activities for adaptation/problem-solving.
Report a measurable increase in necessary/desired activities to improve community functioning.

ACTIONS/INTERVENTIONS	RATIONALE
Community Disaster Preparedness (NIC)	
Independent	
Evaluate community activities as related to meeting collective needs within the community itself and between the community and the larger society. Note immediate needs (e.g., healthcare, food, shelter, funds).	Provides a baseline to determine community needs in relation to current concerns/threats.
Note community reports of functioning, including areas of weakness or conflict.	Provides a view of how the community itself sees these areas.
Identify effects of related factors on community activities.	In the face of a current threat, local or national, community resources need to be evaluated, updated, and given priority to meet the identified need.
Determine availability and use of resources. Identify unmet demands or needs of the community.	Information necessary to identify what else is needed to meet the current situation.
Determine community strengths.	Promotes understanding of the ways in which the community is already meeting the identified needs.
Encourage community members/groups to engage in problem-solving activities.	Promotes a sense of working together to meet the needs.
Develop a plan jointly with the members of the community to address immediate needs.	Deals with deficits in support of identified goals.
Create plans managing interactions within the community itself and between the community and the larger society.	Meets collective needs when the concerns/ threats are shared beyond a local community.
Make information accessable to the public. Provide channels for dissemination of information to the community as a whole (e.g., print media, radio/television, reports and community bulletin boards, Internet sites, speaker's bureau, reports to committees/councils, advisory boards).	Readily available accurate information can help citizens deal with the situation.
Make information available in different modalities and geared to differing educational levels/cultures of the community.	Using languages other than English and making written materials accessible to all members of the community will promote understanding.
Seek out and evaluate needs of underserved populations.	The homeless and those residing in lower income areas may have special needs requiring additional resources.

NURSING DIAGNOSIS: Potential for enhanced community Coping

May be related to

Social support available
Resources available for problem-solving
Community has a sense of power to manage stressors

Possibly evidenced by

Agreement that community is responsible for stress management
Active planning by community for predicted stressors
Active problem solving by community when faced with issues
Positive communication among community members and between community/aggregates and larger community
Resources sufficient for managing stressors

DESIRED OUTCOMES/EVALUATION CRITERIA—COMMUNITY WILL:

Community Competence (NOC)

Identify positive and negative factors affecting management of current and future problems/stressors.
Have an established plan in place to deal with various contingencies.
Report a measurable increase in ability to deal with potential events.

ACTIONS/INTERVENTIONS	RATIONALE
Program Development (NIC)	
Independent	
Review community plans to monitor for and deal with untoward events.	Provides a baseline for comparison of preparedness with other communities and developing plan to address concerns.
Assess effects of related factors on management of problems/stressors.	Identifies areas that need to be addressed to enhance community coping.
Determine community strengths and weaknesses. Identify limitations in current pattern of community activities that can be improved through adaptation and problem-solving.	Plan can be built on strengths, and areas of weakness can be addressed.
Evaluate community activities as related to management of problems/stressors within the community itself and between the community and the larger society.	Disasters occurring in the community or the country affect the local community and need to be recognized and addressed.
Define and discuss current needs and anticipated or projected concerns.	Agreement on scope/parameters of needs is essential for effective planning.
Identify and prioritize community goals.	Helps to bring the community together to meet a common concern/threat. Helps maintain focus and facilitates accomplishment.
Promote community awareness about the problems of design of buildings, equipment, transportation systems, and workplace practices that may compound disaster/impact disaster response.	Provides opportunity for making changes that promote safety.
Identify available resources (e.g., persons, groups, financial, governmental, as well as other communities).	Important to work together to meet goals. Major catastrophes affect more than local community, and communities need to work together to deal with and accomplish growth.
Seek out and involve underserved/at-risk groups within the community.	Supports communication and commitment of community as a whole.
Assist the community to form partnerships within the community and between the community and the larger society.	Promotes long-term developmental growth of the community.
Establish mechanism for self-monitoring of community needs and evaluation of efforts.	Facilitates proactive rather than reactive responses by the community.
Participate in exercises/activities to test preparedness.	Provides opportunities to verify appropriateness of plans and problem-solve deficiencies.
Use multiple formats, e.g., TV, radio, print media, billboards, computer bulletin boards, speaker's bureau, reports to community leaders/groups on file and accessible to the public.	Keeps the community informed and involved regarding plans, needs, outcomes of tests of the plans.

Chart 15–1: Clinical Characteristics of Critical Biological Agents - 7/1/00

Disease	Signs & symptoms	Physical Exam	Clinical tests	Key differential diagnosis	Incubation period	Duration of illness	Case fatality	U.S. Epidemiology
Inhalational Anthrax	Fever, malaise, cough, mild chest discomfort, possible short recovery phase then onset of dyspnea, diaphoresis, stridor, cyanosis, shock. Death 24–36 hours after onset of severe symptoms. Hemorrhagic meningitis in up to 50%.	Nonspecific physical findings.	Serology, gram stain, culture, polymerase chain reaction (PCR); CXR—widened mediastinum. Rarely pneumonia.	Hantavirus pulmonary syndrome (HPS), dissecting aortic aneurysm (no fever)	1–6 days (up to 45 days)	3–5days	~100% if untreated	None
Pneumonic plague	High fever, chills, headache, hemoptysis and toxemia, rapid progression to dyspnea, stridor, and cyanosis. Death from respiratory failure, shock, and bleeding.	Rales, hemoptysis, purpura	Gram stain, culture, serum immunoassay for capsular antigen, PCR, immunohistochemical stains (IHC)	HPS, TB, community acquired pneumonia (CAP), meningoccoccemia, rickettsioses	2–3 days	1–6 days	Usually fatal unless treated in 12–24 hour	2–3 cases/yr mainly in SW U.S.
Tularemia	Typhoidal–aerosol, gastrointestinal, & intradermal challenge. Fever, headache, malaise, chest discomfort, anorexia, nonproductive cough. Pneumonia in 30–80%. Oculoglandular from inoculation of conjunctiva with periorbital edema.	No adenopathy with typhoidal illness	Serology, culture, PCR, IHC; CXR—pneumonia, mediastinal lymphadenopathy, or pleural effusion.	Atypical CAP, Q fever, brucellosis	1–10 days (average 3–5 days)	>2 wks	10–35% untreated	150 case/yr, transmitted by ticks/deer flies or contact with infected animals
Smallpox	Fever, back pain, vomiting, malaise, headache, rigors. Papules 2–3 days later, progressing to pustular vesicles. Abundant on face and extremities initially.	Papules, pustules, or scabs of similar stage, many on face/extremities, palms/soles	Guamierl bodies on Glemsa or modified silver stain, virions on electron microscopy, PCR, viral isolation, IHC	Varicella, vaccinia, monkeypox, cowpox, disseminated herpes zoster	7–17days (average 12 days)	4 wks	up to 30% higher in flat-type or hemorrhagic disease	None

Botulism	Ptosis, blurred vision, diplopia, generalized weakness, dizziness, dysarthria, dysphonia, dysphagia, followed by symmetrical descending flaccid paralysis and respiratory failure.	No fever, client alert, postural hypotension, pupils unreactive, normal sensation, variable muscle weaknesss	Serology, toxin assays/anaerobic cultures of blood/stool; electromyography studies	Guillain Barré, myasthenia gravis, tick paralysis, Mg^{++} intoxication, organophosphate poisoning, polio	1–5 days	Death 24–72 hour or respiratory support for months	High mortality without respiratory support	30 cases/yr; food intoxication, wound infections, or honey ingestion (infants)
Filoviruses (Maburg, Ebola)	Fever, severe headache, malaise, myalgia, maculopapular rash day 5; progression to pharyngitis, hematemasis, melena, uncontrolled bleeding; shock/death 6–9 days.	Petechia, ecehymoses, conjunctivitis, uncontrolled bleeding	Serology, PCR, IHC, electron microscopy (EM); elevated liver enzymes, thrombocytopenia	Meningococcemia, malaria, typhus, leptospirosis, borreliosis, thrombotic thrombocytopenic purpura (TTP), rickettsiosis, hemolytic uremic syndrome (HUS), arenaviruses	2–19 days (average 4–10 days)	Days to weeks	>80%	None
Arenaviruses (Lassa, Junin, Sabia, Machupo, Guanarito)	Fever, malaise, headache, N/V, pharyngitis, cough, retro-intestinal pain, bleeding, tremors of tongue and hands (Junin), shock, aspetic meningitis, coma, hearing loss in some.	Conjunctivitis, petechia, ecchymoses, flushing over head and upper torso	Serology, viral isolation, PCR, IHC; leukopenia, thrombocytopenia, proteinuria	Leptospirosis, meningococcemia, malaria, typhus, borreliosis, rickettsiosis, TTP, HUS, filoviruses	5–21 days Lassa; 7–16 days Sabia, Junin, Machapo, Guanarito	7–15 days	15–30%	None

Biological Warfare and Terrorism: Medical Issues and Response—Student Material Booklet.
U.S. Army Medical Research Institute of Infectious Diseases, September, 2000.

Chart 15–2: BW Agents: Vaccine, Therapeutics, and Prophylaxis

Disease	Vaccine	Chemotherapy	Chemoprophylaxis (PX)	Comments
Anthrax	Bioport vaccine (licensed) 0.5 mL SC @ 0, 2, 4 wk, 6, 12, 18 mo then annual	Ciprofloxacin 400mg IV q 8–12 h Doxycycline 200 mg IV, then 100 mg IV q 8–12 h Penicillin 2 million units IV q 2 h	Ciprofloxacin 500 mg PO bid × 4 wk if unvaccinated, begin initial doses of vaccine Doxycycline 100 mg PO bid × 4 wk plus vaccination	Potential alternates for Rx: gentamicin, erythromycin, and chloramphenicol PCN for sensitive organisms only
Cholera	Wyeth–Ayerst Vaccine 2 doses 0.5 mL IM or SC @ 0, 7–30 days, then boosters q 6 months	Oral rehydration therapy during period or high fluid loss Tetracycline 500 mg q 6 h × 3 d Doxycycline 300 mg once, or 100 mg q 12 h × 3 d Ciprofloxacin 500 mg q 12 h × 3 d		Vaccine not recommended for routine protection in endemic areas (50% efficacy, short term) Alternates for Rx: erythromycin, trimethoprim and sulfamethoxazole, and furazolidone Quinolones for tetra/doxy resistant strains
Q Fever	IND 610—inactivated whole cell vaccine given as single 0.5 mL s.c. injection	Tetracycline 500 mg PO q 6 × 5–7 d Doxycycline 100 mg PO q 12 h × 5–7 d	Tetracycline start 8–12 d post-exposure × 5 d Doxycycline start 8–12 d post-exposure × 5 d	Currently testing vaccine to determine the necessity of skin testing prior to use.
Glanders	No vaccine available	Antibiotic regimens vary depending on localization and severity of disease—refer to text	Post-exposure prophyaxsis may be tried with TMP-SMX	No large therapeutic human trials have been conducted owing to the rarity of naturally occurring disease.
Plague	Greer inactivated vaccine (FDA licensed) is no longer available: 1.0 mL, IM; 0.2 mL, IM 1–3 mo later; 6.2 mL 5–6 mo after dose 2; 0.2 ml boosters @ 6, 12, 18 mo after dose 3 then q 1–2 years	Streptomycin 30 mg/kg/d IM in 2 divided doses × 10 d (or gentamicin) Doxycycline 200 mg IV then 100 mg IV bid × 10–14 d Chloramphenicol 1 gm IV qid × 10–14 d	Doxycycline 100 mg PO bid × 7 or duration of exposure Ciprofloxacin 500 mg PO bid × 7 d Doxycycline 100 mg PO bid × 7 d Tetracycline 500 mg PO qid × 7 d	Plague vaccine not protective against aerosol challenge in animal studies Alternate Rx: trimethoprim-sulfamethoxazole Chloramphenicol for plague meningitis
Tularemia	IND—Live attenuated vaccine: one dose by scarification	Streptomycin 30 mg/kg IM divided bid × 10–14 d Gentamicin 3–5 mg/kg/d IV × 10–14 d	Doxycycline 100 mg PO bid × 14 d Tetracycline 500 mg PO qid × 14 d	
Brucellosis	No human vaccine available	Doxycycline 200 mg/d PO plus rifampin 600–900 mg/d PO × wk Ofloxacin 400/rifampin 600 mg/d PO × 6 wks	Doxycycline and rifampin × 3 wk	Trimethoprim-sulfamethoxazole may be substituted for rifampin; however, relapse may reach 30%
Viral encephalitides	VEE DOD TC-3 live attenuated vaccine (IND): 0.5 mL SC × 1 dose VEE DOD C-84 (formalin inactivated TC-83) (IND): 0.5 mL SC for up to 3 h EEE inactivated (IND): 0.5 mL SC at 0 & 28 d WEE inactivated (IND): 0.5 mL SC at 0, 7, and 28 d	Supportive therapy: analgesics and anticonvulsants prn	NA	TC-83 rectogenic in 20% No seroconversion in 20% Only effective against subtypes IA, IB, and IC C-84 vaccine used for non-responders to TC-83 EEE and WEE inactivated vaccines are poorly immunogenic; multiple immunizations are required

(Continued on the following page)

Disease	Vaccine	Chemotherapy	Chemoprophylaxis (PX)	Comments
Viral hemorrhagic fevers	AHF Candid #1 vaccine (x-protective for BHF) (IND) RVF inactivated vaccine (IND)	Ribavarin (CCHF/arenaviruses) 30 mg/kg IV initial dose 15 mg/kg IV q 6 h × 4 d 7.5 mg/kg IV q 8 h × 6 d Passive antibody for AHF, BHF, Lassa fever, and CCHF	NA	Aggressive supportive care and management of hypotension very important
Smallpox	Wyeth calf lymph vaccinia vaccine (licensed): 1 dose by scarification	Cidofovir (effective in vitro); animal studies ongoing	Vaccinia immune globulin 0.6 mL/kg IM (within 3 d of exposure, best within 24 h)	Pre- and postexposure vaccination recommended if > 3 years since last vaccine
Botulism	DOD pentavaient toxoid for serotypes A-E (IND): 0.5 ml deep SC @ 0, 2 &12 wk, then yearly boosters	DOD heptavalent equine despeciated antitoxin for serotypes A-G (IND): 1 vial (10 mL) IV CDC trivaient equine antitoxin for serotypes A, B, E (licensed)		Skin test for hypersensitivity before equine antitoxin administration
Straphylococcus enterotoxin B	No vaccine available	Ventilatory support for inhalation exposure		
Ricin	No vaccine available	Inhalation: supportive therapy G-1: gastric lavage, superactivated charcoal, cathartics		
T-2 Mycotoxins	No vaccine available		Decontamination of clothing and skin	

Biological Warfare and Terrorism: Medical Issues and Response—Student Material Booklet.
U.S. Army Medical Research Institute of Infectious Diseases, September, 2000.

PEDIATRIC CONSIDERATIONS

Encompasses problems related to childhood through adolescence.

CARE SETTING

Any setting in which nursing contact with children occurs/care is provided.

Client Assessment Database

Data depend on the specific pathology necessitating therapeutic interventions.

ASSESSMENT FACTORS (IN ADDITION TO ROUTINE ASSESSMENTS)

Age and gender
Developmental level
Patterns of communication with SOs
Perception of body and its functions: in health and illness
Behavior when anxious, afraid, withdrawn, angry, tearful

SIGNIFICANT OTHERS

Nuclear family, extended family
Family developmental cycle
Child's role in family tasks and functions
Peer group, friends

SOCIOECONOMIC

Social class, value system
Social acceptability of current situation

CULTURAL

Ethnic background, heritage, and residence

DISEASE (ILLNESS)

Condition requiring treatment and response of child/family to situation
Nature of condition—acute, chronic, recurrent
Emotional response to current treatments
Past experience with illness, hospitalization, and healthcare providers
If illness is terminal, what do child and family expect?
Availability/use of resources

NURSING PRIORITIES

1. Enhance level of comfort/minimize pain.
2. Reduce anxiety/fear.
3. Provide growth-promoting environment for child and parent(s).
4. Prevent/minimize complications.

DISCHARGE GOALS

1. Reports/indicates pain relieved.
2. Child/family dealing appropriately with current situation.
3. Safe environment maintained.
4. Plan in place to meet needs after discharge.

NURSING DIAGNOSIS: acute Pain

May be related to

Injuring agents (biologic, chemical, physical, psychologic)

Possibly evidenced by

Verbal cues
Changes in appetite and eating, sleep pattern
Guarded/protective behavior; restlessness, moaning, crying, irritability
Autonomic responses

DESIRED OUTCOMES/EVALUATION CRITERIA—CHILD WILL:

Pain Level (NOC)

Report/indicate pain is relieved/controlled.
Manifest decreased restlessness/irritability.
Demonstrate age-appropriate blood pressure, pulse, and respiratory rates.

ACTIONS/INTERVENTIONS	RATIONALE
Pain Management (NIC)	
Independent	
Perform routine comprehensive pain assessment, including location, characteristics, onset/duration, frequency, quality, severity (using 0–10 scale, facial expressions, or color scale).	Assessment of children involves observational skills and may require enlisting the aid of parent/caregiver to clarify cues and verbalizations.
Accept child's description of pain.	Pain is subjective and cannot be experienced by others.

ACTIONS/INTERVENTIONS	RATIONALE
Investigate changes in frequency or description of pain.	May signal worsening of condition or development of complications.
Observe for guarding, rigidity, and restlessness.	Nonverbal expressions may signal pain or changes in pain severity.
Monitor heart rate, blood pressure (BP) (using correctly sized cuff), and respiratory rate, noting age-appropriate normals/variations.	Changes in autonomic responses may indicate increased pain before child verbalizes. *Note*: Autonomic responses change with acute pain, not chronic pain. Blood pressure may be lower than normal, or higher than normal if child has experienced fluid loss (vasoconstriction).
Note location/type of surgical incisions, injuries/trauma.	Influences degree/severity of pain manifestations.
Provide comfort measures; e.g., repositioning, back rub, use of heat/cold.	Nonpharmacologic pain management promotes relaxation, may reduce level of pain and enhance coping.
Encourage diversional activities; e.g., TV, music, reading, playing quiet games.	Helps distract child's attention from pain and reduces tension.
Review procedures/expectations and tell child when it will hurt.	Reduces concern of the unknown and helps child deal with the reality of the anticipated pain.

Collaborative

Encourage rest periods.	Helps reduce fatigue and enhances coping ability.
Administer medications as indicated.	A regular schedule may be required to manage pain effectively. As condition resolves, advancing to a prn schedule may be sufficient.

NURSING DIAGNOSIS; Anxiety/Fear; ineffective Coping

May be related to

Situational/maturational crisis, interpersonal transmission/contagion
Threat to/change in health/role status
Natural/innate origin (e.g., pain, loss of physical support)
Separation from support system in potentially stressful situation (e.g., hospitalization, hospital procedures)
Learned response (e.g., conditioning, modeling from or identification with others)

Possibly evidenced by

Excessive psychomotor activity, restlessness, crying, lack of eye contact, withdrawal, sleep disturbances/nightmares
Avoidance or attack behaviors, reports of being scared, expressed concerns about changes
Social inhibition, shy, withdrawn demeanor

DESIRED OUTCOMES/EVALUATION CRITERIA—CHILD WILL:

Anxiety Level (NOC)

Appear relaxed and report/demonstrate relief from somatic manifestations of anxiety.
Demonstrate a decrease in somatic complaints and physical symptoms when faced with stressful situations (e.g., impending separation from SO).

Anxiety Self-Control (NOC)

Engage in age-appropriate activities in absence of parent/primary caregiver without fear or distress noted.

ACTIONS/INTERVENTIONS	RATIONALE
Anxiety Reduction (NIC)	
Independent	
Establish an atmosphere of calmness, trust, and genuine positive regard.	Trust and unconditional acceptance are necessary for satisfactory nurse/child/family relationship. Calmness is important because anxiety is easily transmitted from one person to another and children are often adept at sensing changes in the moods of adults around them.
Provide explanations in language appropriate for age. Use terms familiar to child (e.g., care activities—"walk" instead of "ambulate"; procedures—"take a picture" instead of "fluoroscope").	Accurate communication promotes trust and creates an atmosphere where child feels free to ask questions. Promotes understanding/accurate expectations. *Note*: Children may become frightened of things they cannot articulate.
Ensure child of his or her safety and security (e.g., listen to child, identify needs, and be available for support).	Strange surroundings, changes in routine, and loss of control in situation create anxiety and can be very frightening. Children may believe that situation is punishment for some wrongdoing (imagined or real) on their part. Providing information, being available can be reassuring.
Be honest with child and parents; e.g., saying "Yes, this will hurt and I will help you manage it."	Promotes trust and enhances relationship with nurse/caregiver.
Refrain from conversations unrelated to child in his or her presence, or failing to include child in conversations regarding him or her.	Ignoring the child/talking about (not to) them or allowing child to overhear partial or unrelated conversations may be very stressful and result in child imagining things that are incorrect.
Maintain home routines whenever possible. Encourage child/parents to bring transitional object from home (e.g., familiar toys, special pillow/blanket, pictures/posters, music) if hospitalized.	Use of age-appropriate object enhances sense of security when child or adolescent is hospitalized or in treatment setting.
Provide consistency of caregivers.	Becoming acquainted with caregiver enhances sense of security, facilitates communication, and lessens anxiety.
Promote family interaction; i.e., child and family contact. Encourage parents to participate in care planning and care provision.	Family involvement in activities promotes continuity of family unit, provides opportunity to learn/practice new skills, and enhances coping skills.
Emphasize importance of staff/family giving verbal prompts in anticipation of absences. Provide honest information about leaving and returning.	Avoidance of these issues increases the likelihood of anxiety responses when separation occurs.
Help family support child emotionally by being available, active-listening.	Conveys acceptance of child and confidence in ability to cope with situation.
Provide child with choices when possible.	Promotes sense of control, demonstrates regard for individual.
Schedule ample time for play and age-appropriate diversions. Use play materials (e.g., puppets, doll house, doctor/nurse kits, fairy tale stories, clay, sand tray).	Promotes normalcy and helps divert attention from situation. Play therapy enables child to explore conflicts, express fears, and release tension.
Engage in exercise program as appropriate to situation.	Provides physical outlet for energy, releasing tension. May stimulate release of endorphins, decreasing anxiety and enhancing child's ability to deal with illness/situation.
Collaborative	
Administer medications as indicated.	Mild sedation can be effective in ameliorating symptoms of anxiety and enhancing child's receptiveness to therapeutic regimen.

NURSING DIAGNOSIS: Activity Intolerance [specify level]/Fatigue

May be related to

Generalized weakness, bed rest or immobility
Imbalance between oxygen supply and demand
Pain, extreme stress

Possibly evidenced by

Report of fatigue or weakness, lack of energy, exertional discomfort or dyspnea, abnormal heart rate or blood pressure response to activity, inability to maintain usual routine; listless, lethargic

DESIRED OUTCOMES/EVALUATION CRITERIA—CHILD WILL:

Endurance (NOC)

Participate in customary activities at desired level.
Report absence of fatigue.

ACTIONS/INTERVENTIONS	RATIONALE
Activity Therapy (NIC)	
Independent	
Ascertain child's usual level of activity, taking into account age and developmental level.	Establishes baseline, in order to determine needed interventions and to assess progress of recovery.
Note how present situation is affecting level of activity: immobilization, use of restraints, casts or traction, presence of heart or respiratory impairment, cancer, and treatments.	Presence of certain disease processes/trauma, treatment modalities have potential for interfering with child's usual/desired level of activity.
Determine usual sleep/rest routine and bedtime rituals/security objects. Plan care with adequate rest periods.	Attempting to maintain usual sleep routines promotes rest and maximizes energy and endurance.
Adjust activities, reduce intensity level or discontinue activities as needed. Assist with activities of daily living (ADLs) and promote exercise as indicated.	Protects child from injury and enhances ability to participate in activity to improve strength.
Promote participation in individually appropriate recreational and diversional activities.	Enhances sense of well-being and expectation of return to usual activities.
Monitor response to activity including BP, pulse, respiratory rate, skin color, and behavior.	Helps identify/monitor degree of fatigue and potential for complications. *Note*: Charts list different respiratory rates for different ages. However, a quick method to use as a guide is—if you feel out of breath watching a child breathe, the rate is abnormally fast; if you feel the need to help a child breathe, the rate is probably too slow.
Collaborative	
Provide/monitor response to oxygen administration via appropriate route and effects of medication.	Oxygen may be needed to improve tolerance to activity, treat underlying cause for fatigue. High-flow oxygen via non-rebreather mask is ideal if child can tolerate it. Blow-by oxygen can provide some benefit if child refuses to wear mask.
Refer to physical/occupational and family therapists.	Helpful to develop activity and exercise programs to meet individual needs.

NURSING DIAGNOSIS: risk for delayed Growth and Development

Risk factors may include

Separation from parents and family, peer group
Environmental and stimulation deficiencies, effects of physical disability/confinement
Inadequate care, multiple caretakers, prolonged, painful treatments

Possibly evidenced by

[Not applicable, presence of signs and symptoms establishes an *actual* diagnosis.]

DESIRED OUTCOMES/EVALUATION CRITERIA—CHILD WILL:

CHILD DEVELOPMENT: [specify age group] (NOC)

Perform motor, social, and/or expressive skills typical of age group within scope of present capabilities.
Demonstrate weight/growth-stabilization or progress toward age-appropriate size.

ACTIONS/INTERVENTIONS	RATIONALE
DEVELOPMENT ENHANCEMENT: Child [or] Adolescent (NIC)	
Independent	
Determine existing factors/condition(s) that could contribute to growth deviation, including familial history of pituitary tumors, Marfan's syndrome, genetic anomalies.	Plan of care will be based on individual factors present, immediacy of threat, and potential long-term complications.
Determine child's birth weight and length and compare present growth. Measure developmental level using age-appropriate tests such as the Denver Developmental Screening Test. Note reported losses/alterations in functional level.	Identifies the child's status compared with other children of the same age. Provides comparative baseline and basis for choosing developmentally appropriate interventions.
Note chronologic age, familial factors (body build/stature). Review expectations for current height/weight percentiles and degree of deviation.	Aids in determining growth expectations.
Note severity/pervasiveness of situation (e.g., individual showing effects of long-term physical/emotional abuse or neglect versus individual experiencing recent onset situational disruption or inadequate resources during period of crisis or transition).	Problems existing over a long period may have more severe effects and require longer course of treatment to reverse.
Determine child's cognitive/perceptual level; e.g., grade level in school, infant ability to roll over or sit unsupported. Note behavioral (e.g., withdrawal/aggression) reaction to environment and stimuli.	Illness/injury can lead to a temporary increase in level of dependency/decline in functional level. Although this may not be of major concern for the short term, chronic/recurrent conditions may delay acquisition of important developmental milestones.
Determine occurrence/frequency of significant stressful events, losses, separation, and environmental changes (e.g., abandonment, divorce, death of parent/sibling, relocation).	Lack of resolution or repetition of stressor can have a cumulative effect over time and result in regression in, or deterioration of, functional level.
Provide information regarding normal growth/development as appropriate, including pertinent reference materials.	Helps parents understand potential changes in relation to current illness/problem.
Identify realistic goals with child/parents. Discuss actions to take to avoid/minimize preventable complications.	Provides anticipatory guidance. Increases probability of reaching goals, managing situation more effectively. Can enhance sense of control/independence.

ACTIONS/INTERVENTIONS	RATIONALE
Identify nature and effectiveness of parenting/caregiving activities (e.g., inadequate, inconsistent, unrealistic/insufficient expectations; lack of stimulation, limit setting, responsiveness).	Assessment of parenting and potential for conflict and negative interaction between parent/caregiver and child identifies interventions needed to maximize care.
Encourage self-care activities as appropriate; e.g., feeding, grooming, play.	Promotes independence and maintenance of self-esteem.

Collaborative

Assist with therapy to treat/correct underlying conditions (e.g., Crohn's disease, cardiac problems, or renal disease), endocrine problems (e.g., hypothyroidism, type 1 diabetes mellitus, growth hormone abnormalities), genetic/intrauterine growth retardation, infant feeding problems, nutritional deficits. (Refer to ND, Nutrition, imbalanced [specify].)	Illness, hospitalization, treatments, and separation from parents/family have a negative effect on physical/psychologic growth and development.
Include family, nutritionist and other specialists (e.g., physical/occupational therapist) in developing plan of care.	Use of multidisciplinary team increases likelihood of developing a well-rounded plan of care that meets child's special and varied needs.
Refer to available community resources as appropriate (e.g., public health programs such as WIC, medical equipment supplies, nutritionist, substance abuse program, specialist in endocrine conditions/genetics.	Although acute situations may be readily resolved with limited support and few ill effects, chronic/recurrent conditions require many resources to maximize growth potential of child and family.

NURSING DIAGNOSIS: risk for imbalanced Nutrition: less than body requirements

Risk factors may include

Inability to ingest or digest food or absorb nutrients because of biologic, psychologic, or economic factors
Increased metabolic demands

Possibly evidenced by

[Not applicable, presence of signs and symptoms establishes an *actual* diagnosis.]

DESIRED OUTCOMES/EVALUATION CRITERIA—CHILD WILL:

Nutritional Status (NOC)

Ingest nutritionally adequate diet for age, activity level, and metabolic demands.
Demonstrate stable weight/progressive weight gain toward goal.

Nutrition Management (NIC)

Independent

ACTIONS/INTERVENTIONS	RATIONALE
Identify children at risk for malnutrition (e.g., intestinal surgery, hypermetabolic states, restricted intake, prior nutritional deficiencies).	Provides opportunity for timely intervention.
Determine ability to chew, swallow, taste; presence of mechanical barriers; or conditions such as lactose intolerance, cystic fibrosis, diabetes, inflammatory bowel diseases, eating disorder.	These factors can affect ingestion/desire to eat and/or digestion of nutrients, and specific dietary choices.

ACTIONS/INTERVENTIONS	RATIONALE
Determine child's current nutritional status using age-appropriate measurements, including weight and body build, strength, activity level, sleep/rest cycles.	Identifies individual nutritional needs and provides comparative baseline.
Elicit information from child/parent of younger child regarding typical daily food intake, determining foods and beverages normally consumed. Note types of snacks. Discuss eating habits and food preferences (likes and dislikes).	Baseline information to determine adequacy of intake. Knowledge of child's specific likes/dislikes may be helpful in meeting child's nutritional needs during a time when appetite is suppressed or child has no interest in food.
Determine psychologic factors, cultural or religious desires/influences on dietary choices.	Dietary beliefs, such as vegetarianism, can affect nutritional intake. Usual ethnic food choices can improve a child's intake when appetite is poor.
Determine whether infant is breast-fed or formula-fed and typical pattern of feedings during a 24-hr period. Note type and amounts of solid foods an infant/young toddler eats.	Providing usual and typical feedings is important to infant well-being and early growth.
Auscultate bowel sounds. Note characteristics of stool (e.g., color, amount, frequency).	Provides information about digestion/bowel function and may affect choice/timing of feeding.
Discuss with parent what types of candy, other sweets, snacks, and sodas child eats/drinks.	Identifies what child eats in a typical day. Provides opportunity for identifying teaching needs and providing healthy snacks.
Emphasize importance of well-balanced, nutritious intake. Provide information regarding individual nutritional needs and ways to meet these needs within financial constraints. Avoid arguing over food intake. Provide food without comment.	Although nutritious intake is important, arguing over food is counterproductive. Providing age-appropriate guidelines to children as well as to parents/care provider may help them in making healthy choices.
Review drug regimen, side effects, and potential interactions with other medications/OTC drugs/herbs.	Timing of medication doses, interaction with certain foods can alter effect of medication or digestion/absorption of nutrients.
Clarify family/caregiver access to/use of resources such as food stamps, budget counseling, WIC, community food bank, and/or other appropriate assistance programs.	May be necessary to improve child's intake and/or availability of food to meet nutritional needs.

Collaborative

Establish a nutritional plan that meets individual needs incorporating specific food restrictions, special dietary needs.	Corrects/controls underlying causative factors (e.g., diabetes, cancer, malabsorption syndrome, and anorexia).
Consult dietitian/nutritional team as indicated.	Useful in determining individual nutritional needs and therapeutic diet/feedings.
Review laboratory studies (e.g., serum albumin/prealbumin, transferring, amino acid profile, iron, blood urea nitrogen [BUN], nitrogen balance studies, glucose, liver function, electrolytes, total lymphocyte count, indirect calorimetry).	Indicators of nutritional health and effects of nutrients in organ function.
Refer for dental hygiene/professional care, counseling/psychiatric/family therapy as indicated.	May be needed to provide assistance, support, and direction for meeting nutritional needs not only in the present but for achieving long-term goals as well.
Refer to home care resources when indicated by specific condition/illness.	To assist with initiation/supervision of home nutrition therapy when used.

NURSING DIAGNOSIS: risk for Injury, (specify: trauma, suffocation, poisoning)

Risk factors may include

Developmental age, cognitive or emotional difficulties
Disease or injury process, use of restraining device

Use of pharmaceutical agents, narrow therapeutic margin of safety of some drugs, exposure to substances (e.g., tobacco, alcohol, street drugs)
Lack of safety or drug education/precautions
Immune/autoimmune dysfunction, malnutrition, exposure to nosocomial agents

Possibly evidenced by

[Not applicable, presence of signs and symptoms establishes an *actual* diagnosis.]

DESIRED OUTCOMES/EVALUATION CRITERIA—CHILD WILL:

Risk Control (NOC)

Be free of injury.

CAREGIVER/PARENT—WILL:

Verbalize understanding of individual risk factors that contribute to possibility of injury.
Take steps to correct identified risks and protect child from hazards.

ACTIONS/INTERVENTIONS	RATIONALE
Risk Surveillance (NIC)	
Independent	
Identify individual risk factors; e.g., airway patency, therapeutic use of potentially toxic medications, invasive lines/procedures, exposure to latex products, impaired neurologic status, seizure activity, exposure to safety hazards, immobility/use of restraints, presence of fractures, malnutrition, fluid deficit/excess.	Provides opportunity to modify environment/eliminate factors that place child at risk.
Handle infant/child gently. Limit use/release restraints periodically per protocol.	Skin/tissues are more fragile and at greater risk for damage.
Provide appropriate level of supervision.	Permits monitoring of child's well-being, allows for timely intervention.
Initiate safety precautions as individually appropriate; e.g., bed in low position, padded side rails, infection precautions, medications in childproof containers.	Preventing injuries and complications is a prime responsibility of parents and caregivers.
Have age-appropriate equipment available; e.g., properly sized BP cuffs, IV catheters, airway adjuncts, and oxygen mask/hood; suction equipment, ventilator bag, low-flow IV pump, warming devices.	Prevents treatment-related injuries and ensures availability of age/size appropriate life-saving equipment.
Monitor medication administration closely, especially dosage measurements and conversions. Use pediatric concentrations of medications when available.	Provides for effective therapeutic management, prevents overdose, and reduces risk for toxic reactions.
Ascertain recurrent exposure to latex gloves, catheters/tubing, etc. Note history of allergies, eczema.	Repeat exposure increases risk of developing sensitivity/adverse reaction to latex products.
Review home situation for safety hazards. Ascertain parent/caregiver knowledge of safety needs, injury prevention in home setting.	Promotes a safe environment.
Provide bibliotherapy/written resources for parent/caregiver and child, including information about smoking, substance use, and safer sex practices.	Provides information for later review and self-paced learning.

ACTIONS/INTERVENTIONS	RATIONALE
Encourage parent/caregiver to learn cardiopulmonary resuscitation (CPR) and individually appropriate procedures or emergency interventions/responses, such as carrying an EpiPen.	Being prepared for emergencies promotes confidence for adults and children in their own ability to deal with their situation.

Collaborative

Refer to community education programs and resources as indicated.	Can provide additional opportunities for improving parenting skills, obtaining necessary equipment.

NURSING DIAGNOSIS: risk for imbalanced Fluid Volume

Risk factors may include

Lack of adequate intake, increase in fluid needs; e.g., fever
Rapid/sustained loss; e.g., hemorrhage, burns, vomiting, diarrhea, fistulas
Rapid/excessive fluid replacement

Possibly evidenced by

[Not applicable; presence of signs and symptoms establishes an *actual* diagnosis.]

DESIRED OUTCOMES/EVALUATION CRITERIA—CHILD WILL:

Hydration (NOC)

Demonstrate adequate fluid balance as evidenced by stable vital signs, palpable pulses/good quality, normal skin turgor, moist mucous membranes; individual appropriate urinary output; lack of excessive weight fluctuation (loss/gain); absence of edema.

PARENT/CAREGIVER WILL:

Verbalize understanding of child's fluid needs.
Promote adequate age-appropriate fluid intake.

ACTIONS/INTERVENTIONS — RATIONALE

Fluid Management (NIC)

Independent

ACTIONS/INTERVENTIONS	RATIONALE
Note potential sources of fluid loss/intake, presence of conditions such as diabetes, burns, use of total parenteral nutrition (TPN).	Causative/contributing factors for fluid imbalances.
Note child's age, size, weight, and cognitive abilities.	Affects ability to tolerate fluctuations in fluid level and ability to respond to fluid needs.
Monitor vital signs, color of palms, soles of feet, mucous membranes; weight, skin turgor, breath sounds, urinary and gastric output, amount of blood draws, hemodynamic measurements.	Indicators of hydration status. *Note*: Hypotension indicative of developing shock may not be readily observed in child until very late in the clinical course, because of vasoconstriction.
Review child's intake of fluids.	Children often do not take in enough oral fluids to meet hydration needs.
Determine child's normal pattern of elimination and whether child is toilet trained.	Provides information for baseline and comparison. If child is in diapers, output may be determined by weighing diapers.

ACTIONS/INTERVENTIONS	RATIONALE
Determine whether child has problems with urination, such as urine retention, bed-wetting, burning, holding.	Evaluation of these issues is important for determining cause and treatment of underlying problem.
Note uses of drainage devices such as NG tube, wound drain; use of laxatives, enemas, and suppositories.	May increase fluid and electrolyte losses.

Collaborative

ACTIONS/INTERVENTIONS	RATIONALE
Administer IV fluids via control device/pump.	Because smaller volumes are administered, close monitoring and regulation is required to prevent fluid overload while correcting fluid balance.
Replace electrolytes as indicated by oral route whenever possible.	Replacement solutions formulated for children are often safer and better tolerated when given orally if time/condition allows. *Note*: Child with mild dehydration not caused by trauma may respond well to oral rehydration starting with 5–10 mL by mouth every 15–20 minutes and increasing according to tolerance.
Monitor laboratory results; e.g., hemoglobin/hematocrit (Hb/Hct), BUN, urine osmolality/specific gravity.	Indicators of adequacy of hydration/effectiveness of therapeutic interventions.
Arrange with laboratory to combine common tests and draw smallest amount of blood that is necessary to perform required studies.	Excessive/repetitive blood draws may markedly reduce Hb/Hct levels in pediatric client.

NURSING DIAGNOSIS: interrupted Family Processes/impaired Parenting

May be related to

Situational transition and/or crises (illness, trauma, disabling/expensive treatments), shift in health status of a family member
Developmental transition, modification in family finances, family social status
Lack of/ineffective role model, lack of support between or from significant other(s)
Interruption in bonding process, lack of appropriate response of child to parent/parent to child
Lack of knowledge; unrealistic expectation for self, child, partner

Possibly evidenced by

Changes in communication patterns, participation in decision making, expressions of conflict within family
Frequent verbalization of disappointment in child, resentment toward child, inability to care for/discipline child
Lack of parental attachment behaviors
Growth and/or developmental lag in child

DESIRED OUTCOMES/EVALUATION CRITERIA—PARENT/CAREGIVER WILL:

Family Functioning (NOC)

Verbalize positive feelings about parenting abilities.
Be involved in problem-solving solutions for current situation.
Develop skills to deal with present situation.
Strengthen parenting skills.

ACTIONS/INTERVENTIONS	RATIONALE
Family Support (NIC)	
Independent	
Determine existing situation and parental perception of the problems, noting presence of specific factors such as psychiatric/physical illness, disabilities of child or parent.	Identification of the individual factors will aid in focusing interventions and establishing a realistic plan of care.
Identify developmental stage of the family (e.g., first child/new infant, school-age/adolescent children, stepfamily).	These factors affect how family members view current problems and choices of solutions.
Determine cultural/religious influences on parenting expectations of self/child, sense of success/failure.	This information is crucial to helping the family identify and develop a treatment plan that meets its specific needs, enhancing likelihood of success.
Assess parenting skill level, considering intellectual, emotional, and physical strengths and limitations.	Identifies areas of need for further education, skill training, and factors that might interfere with ability to assimilate new information.
Note attachment behaviors between parent and child(ren), recognizing cultural background. Encourage parent(s) to hold and spend time with child, particularly newborn/infant.	Lack of eye contact and touching may indicate bonding problems. Failure to bond effectively is thought to affect subsequent parent-child interaction.
Observe interactions between parent(s) and child(ren).	Identifies relationships, communication skills, and feelings about one another.
Note presence/effectiveness of extended family/support systems.	Provides role models for parent(s) to help them develop own style of parenting. *Note*: Role models may be negative and/or controlling.
Stress the positive aspects of the situation, maintaining a positive attitude toward parent's capabilities and potential for improving.	Helping parent(s) to feel accepting about self and individual capabilities will promote growth.
Involve all members of the family in learning activities.	Learning new skills is enhanced when everyone is participating and interacting.
Encourage parent(s) to identify positive outlets for meeting own needs (e.g., going to a movie or out to dinner). Discuss use of home care/respite services as appropriate.	Parent often believes it is "selfish" to do things for own self, that children are primary. However, parents are important, children are important, and the family is important. As a rule, when parents take care of themselves, their coping abilities are enhanced and they are better parents. *Note*: Siblings also require time with parents to attend to their needs/have positive interactions.
Discuss issues of step-parenting and ways to achieve positive relationships in a blended family.	Blending two families can be a very demanding task, and preconceived ideas can be counterproductive.
Collaborative	
Refer to resources such as books, classes, support groups.	Providing information/role models can help people learn to negotiate and develop skills for parenting and living together.

NURSING DIAGNOSIS: risk for imbalanced Body Temperature

Risk factors may include

Extremes of age/weight, dehydration, exposure to cold/hot environments, illness/trauma affecting temperature regulation

Possibly evidenced by

[Not applicable; presence of signs/symptoms establishes an *actual* diagnosis.]

DESIRED OUTCOMES/EVALUATION CRITERIA—CHILD WILL:

Thermoregulation (NOC)

Regain/maintain appropriate body temperature for age/size.

PARENT/CAREGIVER WILL:

Risk Control (NOC)

Provide proper environmental controls and safeguards.

ACTIONS/INTERVENTIONS	RATIONALE
Temperature Regulation (NIC)	
Independent	
Note conditions promoting fevers.	Infection, inflammation, hot environment, dehydration.
Measure/monitor child's temperature, using properly functioning thermometer.	All children experience fever at some time. Inaccurate measurement can result in inappropriate treatment.
Discuss variables in temperature measurements for age of child and where temperature is measured.	Knowledge of normal ranges for age of child (e.g., newborn through adolescent) is critical to knowing when a fever requires treatment. Temperature may be measured orally, rectally, and at the axillary space, with rectal measurement being on average approximately 1 degree higher than oral, and axillary being 1 degree lower than oral. *Note:* Temperature of 101° F or greater in newborns/infants needs immediate attention. (There is a 50% mortality associated with infection.) For toddlers and older children, higher temperatures (up to 104° F) may be tolerated unless accompanied by other signs, such as poor color, breathing problems, severe lethargy, etc.
Be aware of heat loss related to age/body mass.	Newborn is more vulnerable to heat loss than older child because of body surface area, higher metabolic rate, and sensitivity to environmental conditions.
Observe for seizure activity. Provide safety precautions as indicated.	Higher fevers may trigger febrile seizures in susceptible children.
Adjust bedclothes and linens, environment. Apply cool cloth to head, bathe in lukewarm bath.	Limiting linens, use of room fan, can help lower body temperature. *Note*: Use of alcohol sponge bath is contraindicated as fumes are inhaled by infant.
Collaborative	
Administer antipyretics; e.g. acetaminophen [Tylenol] 10–15mg/kg q 4h or ibuprofen [Motrin] 10–15 mg/kg q 6h as indicated.	Some degree of fever may be useful for fighting infection; however, excessive levels may have adverse effects and require intervention.

NURSING DIAGNOSIS: risk for ineffective Health Maintenance

Risk factors may include

Unachieved developmental tasks
Perceptual or cognitive impairment

Ineffective individual/family coping
Lack of material resources, psychosocial supports

Possibly evidenced by

[Not applicable; presence of signs/symptoms establishes an *actual* diagnosis.]

DESIRED OUTCOMES/EVALUATION CRITERIA—PARENT/CAREGIVER WILL:

Health Seeking Behavior (NOC)

Identify necessary health maintenance activities.
Verbalize understanding of factors contributing to current situation.
Develop plan to meet specific needs.

ACTIONS/INTERVENTIONS	RATIONALE
Health System Guidance (NIC)	
Independent	
Explore with parents how child's health status is maintained; e.g. nutrition, exercise, sleep/rest, immunization status, environmental issues such as childcare setting, homelessness.	Identifies strengths, may reveal problems requiring immediate intervention.
Discuss mother's health status when pregnant with child; e.g., exposure to toxic agents, substance use, and complications of pregnancy/birth.	Helps identify issues that may arise in child's future health status.
Ascertain frequency of routine health exams, including eye and dental care, monitoring by primary care provider, and immunizations.	Identifies areas of child's healthcare that may be lacking, and provides parents with information about areas that need to be monitored/care provided for optimum health.
Note desire/level of ability to meet health maintenance needs, as well as self-care ADLs.	Care providers and children who can provide much of their own care may have areas of need, either because of illness or other stressors.
Develop plan with parent/caregiver for child's care.	Allows for incorporating existing strengths or limitations, assistance in adapting and organizing care as necessary.
Provide time to listen to concerns of parent/caregiver.	Long-term care for chronically ill child or acute care for a child can be very challenging to parent's physical, emotional, and financial resources.
Provide anticipatory guidance for periods of wellness, and identify ways parent can adapt when progressive illness/long-term health problems occur.	Information and support is vital for maintaining and managing effective health practices.
Provide for communication and coordination between the healthcare facility team and community healthcare providers.	Promotes continuity of care and continuation of goals.
Monitor adherence to prescribed medical regimen. Determine causes for deviations.	Additional education or problem-solving may be required for success of therapeutic plan.
Provide information about individual healthcare needs. Identify signs and symptoms requiring further evaluation and follow-up.	Provides for prevention of complications and early intervention in times of illness.
Collaborative	
Make referral as needed for community support services (e.g., homemaker/home attendant, skilled nursing care, well-baby clinic).	Provides for childcare and parental support in home setting.

ACTIONS/INTERVENTIONS	RATIONALE
Refer to social services as indicated.	May need assistance with financial, housing, or legal concerns.
Arrange for hospice services if needed.	May be indicated when illness is terminal.

POTENTIAL CONSIDERATIONS following acute hospitalization (dependent on client's age, physical condition/presence of complications, and family resources)

Refer to primary diagnosis for specific concerns.

ineffective Therapeutic Regimen Management—perceived seriousness, economic difficulties, complexity of regimen/excessive demands made on family, family patterns of healthcare

delayed Growth and Development—effects of physical disability, prescribed dependence, environmental and stimulation deficiencies

FLUID AND ELECTROLYTE IMBALANCES

Body fluid is composed primarily of water and electrolytes. The body is equipped with homeostatic mechanisms to keep the composition and volume of body fluids within narrow limits. Organs involved in this mechanism include the kidneys, lungs, heart, blood vessels, adrenal glands, parathyroid glands, and pituitary gland. Body fluid is divided into two types: intracellular (within the cells) and extracellular (interstitial or tissue fluid, intravascular or plasma, and transcellular, such as cerebrospinal or synovial fluids).

RELATED CONCERNS

All plans of care specific to underlying health condition causing imbalance; e.g., DM, HF, upper GI bleeding, renal failure/dialysis.
Metabolic acidosis, page 492
Metabolic alkalosis, page 495
Respiratory acidosis, page 194
Respiratory alkalosis, page 198

NURSING PRIORITIES

1. Restore homeostasis.
2. Prevent/minimize complications.
3. Provide information about condition/prognosis and treatment needs as appropriate.

DISCHARGE GOALS

1. Homeostasis restored.
2. Free of complications.
3. Condition/prognosis and treatment needs understood.
4. Plan in place to meet needs after discharge.

Note: Because fluid and electrolyte imbalances usually occur in conjunction with other medical conditions, the following information is offered as a reference. The interventions are presented in a general format for inclusion in the primary plan of care.

FLUID BALANCE

Total body water, essential for metabolism, declines with age and also varies with body fat content and gender. It constitutes about 80% of an infant's body weight, 60% of an adult's, and as little as 40% of an older person's weight.

Hypervolemia (Extracellular Fluid Volume Excess)

PREDISPOSING/CONTRIBUTING FACTORS

Excess sodium intake including sodium-containing foods, medications, or fluids (PO/IV)
Excessive, rapid administration of hypertonic (or possibly isotonic) parenteral fluids
Increased release of antidiuretic hormone (ADH), excessive adrenocorticotropic hormone (ACTH) production, hyperaldosteronism
Decreased plasma proteins as may occur with chronic liver disease with ascites, major abdominal surgery, malnutrition/protein depletion
Chronic kidney disease/acute renal failure (ARF)
Heart failure (HF)

Client Assessment Database

ACTIVITY/REST

May report: Fatigue, generalized weakness

CIRCULATION

May exhibit: Hypertension, elevated central venous pressure (CVP)
Pulse full/bounding, tachycardia usually present, bradycardia (late sign of cardiac decompensation)
Extra heart sounds (S_3)
Edema variable from dependent to generalized
Neck and peripheral vein distention

ELIMINATION

May report: Decreased urinary output, polyuria if renal function is normal
Diarrhea

FOOD/FLUID

May report: Anorexia, nausea/vomiting
Thirst (may be absent, especially in elderly)

May exhibit: Abdominal girth increased with visible fluid wave on palpation (ascites)
Sudden weight gain, often in excess of 5% of total body weight
Edema initially dependent, pitting may progress to facial/periorbital, general/anasarca

NEUROSENSORY

May exhibit: Changes in level of consciousness, from lethargy, disorientation, confusion to coma, aphasia
Muscle twitching, tremors, seizure activity
Hyperreflexia, rigid paralysis (severe hypernatremia)

PAIN/DISCOMFORT

May report: Headache
Abdominal cramps

RESPIRATION

May report: Shortness of breath

May exhibit: Tachypnea with/without dyspnea, orthopnea, productive cough
Crackles

SAFETY

May exhibit: Fever
Skin changes in color, temperature, turgor; e.g., taut and cool where edematous

TEACHING/LEARNING

Refer to predisposing/contributing factors.

Discharge plan considerations: May require assistance with changes in therapeutic regimen, dietary management

Refer to plan of care concerning underlying medical/surgical condition for possible postdischarge considerations.

DIAGNOSTIC STUDIES

Hematocrit: Elevated in dehydration, decreased in fluid overload.
Serum sodium: May be high, low, or normal (between 135 and 145 mEq/L).
Serum potassium and BUN: Normal or decreased in fluid overload unless renal damage present.
Total protein: Plasma proteins/albumin may be decreased.
Serum osmolality: Usually unchanged, although hypo-osmolality may occur.
Urine sodium: May be low because of sodium retention.
Urine specific gravity: Decreased.
Chest radiographs: May reveal signs of congestion.

NURSING DIAGNOSIS: excess Fluid Volume

May be related to

Excess fluid or sodium intake
Compromised regulatory mechanism

Possibly evidenced by

Signs/symptoms noted in database

DESIRED OUTCOMES/EVALUATION CRITERIA—CLIENT WILL:

Fluid Overload Severity (NOC)

Demonstrate stabilized fluid volume as evidenced by balanced I&O, vital signs within client's normal range, stable weight, and absence of signs of edema.

KNOWLEDGE: Treatment Regimen (NOC)

Verbalize understanding of individual dietary/fluid restrictions.
Demonstrate behaviors to monitor fluid status and prevent/limit recurrence.

ACTIONS/INTERVENTIONS	RATIONALE
Hypervolemia Management (NIC)	
Independent	
Monitor vital signs, also CVP if available.	Tachycardia and hypertension are common manifestations. Tachypnea usually present with/without dyspnea. Elevated CVP may be noted before dyspnea and adventitious breath sounds occur. Hypertension may be a primary disorder or occur secondary to other associated conditions; e.g., HF.
Auscultate lungs and heart sounds.	Adventitious sounds (crackles) and extra heart sounds (S_3) are indicative of fluid excess. Pulmonary edema may develop rapidly.
Assess for presence/location of edema formation.	Edema can be either a cause or a result of various pathologic conditions reflecting four competing forces—blood hydrostatic and osmotic pressures, and interstitial fluid hydrostatic and osmotic pressures. The dynamic interaction of these four forces allows fluid to shift from one body compartment to another. Edema may be generalized or localized in dependent areas. Elderly clients may develop dependent edema with relatively little excess fluid. *Note:* Clients in a supine position can have an increase of 4–8 L of fluid before edema is readily detected.
Note presence of neck and peripheral vein distention, along with pitting edema, dyspnea.	Signs of cardiac decompensation/HF.
Maintain accurate I&O. Note decreased urinary output, positive fluid balance (intake greater than output) on 24-hr calculations.	Decreased renal perfusion, cardiac insufficiency, and fluid shifts may cause decreased urinary output and edema formation.
Weigh as indicated. Be alert for acute or sudden weight gain.	One liter of fluid retention equals a weight gain of 2.2 lb.
Give oral fluids with caution. If fluids are restricted, set up a 24-hr schedule for fluid intake.	Fluid restrictions, as well as extracellular shifts, can aggravate drying of mucous membranes, and client may desire more fluids than are prudent.
Monitor infusion rate of parenteral fluids closely; administer via control device/pump as necessary.	Sudden fluid bolus/prolonged excessive administration potentiates volume overload/risk of cardiac decompensation.
Encourage coughing/deep-breathing exercises.	Pulmonary fluid shifts potentiate respiratory complications.

ACTIONS/INTERVENTIONS	RATIONALE
Maintain semi-Fowler's position if dyspnea or ascites is present.	Gravity improves lung expansion by lowering diaphragm and shifting fluid to lower abdominal cavity.
Turn, reposition, and provide skin care at regular intervals.	Reduces pressure and friction on edematous tissue, which is more prone to breakdown than normal tissue.
Encourage bedrest. Schedule care to provide frequent rest periods.	Limited cardiac reserves result in fatigue/activity intolerance. In addition, lying down favors diuresis and reduction of edema.
Provide safety precautions as indicated; e.g., use of side rails, where appropriate, bed in low position, frequent observation, soft restraints (if required).	Fluid shifts may cause cerebral edema/changes in mentation, especially in the geriatric population. *Note:* Use of restraints may increase agitation and can pose a safety threat.

Collaborative

Assist with identification/treatment of underlying cause.	Refer to listing of predisposing/contributing factors to determine treatment needs.
Monitor laboratory studies as indicated; e.g., electrolytes, BUN, ABGs.	Extracellular fluid shifts, sodium/water restriction and renal function all affect serum sodium levels. Potassium deficit may occur with diuretic therapy. BUN may be increased as a result of renal dysfunction/failure. ABGs may reflect metabolic acidosis.
Provide balanced protein, low-sodium diet. Restrict fluids as indicated.	In presence of decreased serum proteins (e.g., malnutrition), increasing level of serum proteins can enhance colloidal osmotic gradients and promote return of fluid to the vascular space. Restriction of sodium/water decreases extracellular fluid retention.
Administer diuretics: loop diuretic; e.g., furosemide (Lasix); thiazide diuretic; e.g., hydrochlorothiazide (Esidrix); or potassium-sparing diuretic; e.g., spironolactone (Aldactone).	To achieve excretion of excess fluid, either a single diuretic (e.g., thiazide) or a combination of agents may be selected (e.g., thiazide and spironolactone). The combination can be particularly helpful when two drugs have different sites of action, allowing more effective control of fluid excess.
Replace potassium losses as indicated.	Potassium deficit may occur, especially if client is receiving potassium-wasting diuretic. This can cause lethal cardiac dysrhythmias if untreated.
Prepare for/assist with dialysis or ultrafiltration if indicated.	May be done to rapidly reduce fluid overload, especially in the presence of severe cardiac/renal failure.

Hypovolemia (Extracellular Fluid Volume Deficit)

PREDISPOSING/CONTRIBUTING FACTORS

Excessive fluid losses: Vomiting, gastric suctioning, diarrhea, polyuria, diaphoresis, wounds or burns, intraoperative fluid loss, hemorrhage
Insufficient/decreased fluid intake; e.g., preoperative/postoperative NPO status
Systemic infections, fever
Intestinal obstruction or fistulas
Pancreatitis, peritonitis, cirrhosis/ascites, adrenal insufficiency
Kidney disease, diabetic ketoacidosis, hyperglycemic hyperosmotic nonketotic coma (HHNC), diabetes insipidus, syndrome of inappropriate antidiuretic hormone (SIADH)

Client Assessment Database

ACTIVITY/REST

May report: Fatigue, generalized weakness

CIRCULATION

May exhibit: Hypotension, including postural changes
Pulse weak/thready; tachycardia
Neck veins flattened; CVP decreased

ELIMINATION

May report: Constipation or occasionally diarrhea, abdominal cramps
May exhibit: Urine volume decreased, dark/concentrated color, oliguria (severe fluid depletion)

FOOD/FLUID

May report: Thirst, anorexia, nausea/vomiting
Complete, sudden cessation of intake, or prolonged diminished intake of fluids

May exhibit: Weight loss often exceeding 2%–8% of total body weight
Abdominal distention
Mucous membranes dry, furrows on tongue, decreased tearing and salivation
Skin dry with poor turgor or pale, moist, clammy (shock)

NEUROSENSORY

May report: Tingling of the extremities, vertigo, syncope

May exhibit: Behavior change, apathy, restlessness, confusion

RESPIRATION

May exhibit: Tachypnea, rapid/shallow breathing

SAFETY

May exhibit: Temperature usually subnormal, although fever may occur

TEACHING/LEARNING

Refer to predisposing/contributing factors
Use/misuse of diuretics

Discharge plan considerations: May require assistance with changes in therapeutic regimen, dietary management

Refer to plan of care concerning underlying medical/surgical condition for possible considerations after discharge.

DIAGNOSTIC STUDIES

Serum sodium: May be normal, high, or low.
Urine sodium: Usually decreased (less than 10 mEq/L when losses are from external causes; usually greater than 20 mEq/L if the cause is renal or adrenal).
CBC: Hb/Hct and RBC usually increased (hemoconcentration); decrease suggests hemorrhage.
Serum glucose: Normal or elevated.
Serum protein: Increased.
BUN and Cr: Increased, with BUN out of proportion to Cr level.
Urine specific gravity: Increased.

NURSING DIAGNOSIS: deficient Fluid Volume

May be related to

Active fluid loss; e.g., hemorrhage, vomiting/gastric intubation, diarrhea, burns, wounds, fistulas
Regulatory failure; e.g., adrenal disease, recovery phase of ARF; diabetic ketoacidosis (DKA), HHNC; diabetes insipidus, systemic infections

Possibly evidenced by

Signs/symptoms noted in client database

DESIRED OUTCOMES/EVALUATION CRITERIA—CLIENT WILL:

Fluid Balance (NOC)

Maintain fluid volume at a functional level as evidenced by individually adequate urinary output with normal specific gravity, stable vital signs, moist mucous membranes, good skin turgor, and prompt capillary refill.

KNOWLEDGE: Treatment Regimen (NOC)

Verbalize understanding of causative factors and purpose of therapeutic interventions.
Demonstrate behaviors to monitor and correct deficit as appropriate.

ACTIONS/INTERVENTIONS	RATIONALE
Hypovolemia Management (NIC)	
Independent	
Monitor vital signs and CVP. Note presence/degree of postural BP changes. Observe for temperature elevations/fever.	Tachycardia is present along with a varying degree of hypotension, depending on degree of fluid deficit. CVP measurements are useful in determining degree of fluid deficit and response to replacement therapy. Fever increases metabolism and exacerbates fluid loss.
Palpate peripheral pulses; note capillary refill, skin color/temperature. Assess mentation.	Conditions that contribute to extracellular fluid deficit can result in inadequate organ perfusion to all areas and may cause circulatory collapse/shock.
Monitor urinary output. Measure/estimate fluid losses from all sources; e.g., gastric losses, wound drainage, diaphoresis.	Fluid replacement needs are based on correction of current deficits and ongoing losses. *Note:* A diaphoretic episode requiring a full linen change may represent a fluid loss of as much as 1 L. A decreased urinary output may indicate insufficient renal perfusion/hypovolemia, or polyuria can be present, requiring more aggressive fluid replacement.
Weigh daily and compare with 24-hr fluid balance. Mark/measure edematous areas; e.g., abdomen, limbs.	Although weight gain and fluid intake greater than output may not accurately reflect intravascular volume (e.g., third-space fluid accumulation cannot be used by the body for tissue perfusion), these measurements provide useful data for comparison.
Evaluate client's ability to swallow.	Impaired gag/swallow reflexes, anorexia/nausea, oral discomfort, and changes in level of consciousness/cognition are among the factors that affect client's ability to replace fluids orally.
Ascertain client's beverage preferences, and set up a 24-hr schedule for fluid intake. Encourage foods with high fluid content.	Relieves thirst and discomfort of dry mucous membranes and augments parenteral replacement. *Note*: Sense of thirst is often diminished in the older adult.
Turn frequently, gently massage skin, and protect bony prominences.	Tissues are susceptible to breakdown because of vasoconstriction and increased cellular fragility.
Provide skin and mouth care. Bathe every other day using mild soap. Apply lotion as indicated.	Skin and mucous membranes are dry with decreased elasticity because of vasoconstriction and reduced intracellular water. Daily bathing may increase dryness.
Provide safety precautions as indicated; e.g., use of side rails where appropriate, bed in low position, frequent observation, soft restraints (if required).	Decreased cerebral perfusion frequently results in changes in mentation/altered thought processes, requiring protective measures to prevent client injury. *Note*: The use of restraints may increase agitation and can pose a safety risk.
Investigate reports of sudden/sharp chest pain, dyspnea, cyanosis, increased anxiety, restlessness.	Hemoconcentration (sludging) and increased platelet aggregation may result in systemic emboli formation.
Monitor for sudden/marked elevation of BP, restlessness, moist cough, dyspnea, basilar crackles, frothy sputum.	Too rapid a correction of fluid deficit may compromise the cardiopulmonary system, especially if colloids are used in general fluid replacement (increased osmotic pressure potentiates fluid shifts).
Collaborative	
Assist with identification/treatment of underlying cause.	Refer to listing of predisposing/contributing factors to determine treatment needs. *Note:* Dehydration is the most common fluid and electrolyte imbalance in older adults.
Monitor laboratory studies as indicated; e.g., electrolytes, glucose, pH/P_{CO_2}, coagulation studies.	Depending on the avenue of fluid loss, differing electrolyte/metabolic imbalances may be present/require correction; e.g., use of glucose solutions in clients with underlying glucose intolerance may result in serum glucose elevation and increased urinary water losses.

ACTIONS/INTERVENTIONS	RATIONALE
Administer IV solutions as indicated:	
Isotonic solutions; e.g., 0.9% NaCl (normal saline), 5% dextrose/water;	Crystalloids provide prompt circulatory improvement, although the benefit may be transient (increased renal clearance).
0.45% NaCl (half-normal saline), lactated Ringer's (LR) solution;	As soon as the client is normotensive, a hypotonic solution (0.45% NaCl) may be used to provide both electrolytes and free water for renal excretion of metabolic wastes. *Note:* Buffered crystalloids (LR) are used with caution because they may potentiate the risk of metabolic acidosis.
Colloids; e.g., dextran, Plasmanate/albumin, hetastarch (Hespan);	Corrects plasma protein concentration deficits, thereby increasing intravascular osmotic pressure and facilitating return of fluid into vascular compartment.
Whole blood/packed RBC transfusion, or autologous collection of blood.	Indicated when hypovolemia is related to active blood loss.
Administer sodium bicarbonate if indicated.	May be given to correct severe acidosis while correcting fluid balance.
Provide tube feedings, including free water as appropriate.	Enteral replacement can provide proteins and other needed elements in addition to meeting general fluid requirements when swallowing is impaired.

SODIUM

Sodium is the major cation of extracellular fluid and is primarily responsible for osmotic pressure in that compartment. Sodium enhances neuromuscular conduction/transmission of impulses and is essential for maintaining acid-base balance. Normal serum range is 135–145 mEq/L; intracellular, 10 mEq/L. Chloride is carried by Na and will display the same imbalances. Normal serum chloride range is 95–105 mEq/L.

Hyponatremia (Sodium Deficit)

PREDISPOSING/CONTRIBUTING FACTORS

Primary hyponatremia (loss of sodium): Lack of sufficient dietary sodium, severe malnutrition, infusion of sodium-free solutions, excessive sodium loss through heavy sweating (e.g., heat exhaustion), wounds/trauma (hemorrhage), burns, gastric suctioning, vomiting, diarrhea, small-bowel obstruction, peritonitis, salt-wasting renal dysfunction, adrenal insufficiency (Addison's disease)

Dilutional hyponatremia (water gains): Excessive water intake, electrolyte-free IV infusion, water intoxication (IV therapy, tap-water enemas), gastric irrigations with electrolyte-free solutions, presence of tumors or CNS disorders predisposing to SIADH, HF, renal failure/nephrotic syndrome, hepatic cirrhosis, DM (hyperglycemia), freshwater near-drowning, use of certain drugs; e.g., hypoglycemia medications, barbiturates, antipsychotics, aminophylline, morphine (may stimulate pituitary gland to secrete excessive amounts of ADH), anticonvulsants, some antineoplastic agents, or NSAIDs

Note: A pseudohyponatremia may occur in presence of multiple myeloma, hyperlipidemia, or hypoproteinemia but does not reflect an actual abnormality of water metabolism.

Client Assessment Database

(Client may be asymptomatic until serum sodium level is less than 125 mEq/L, depending on rapidity of onset.)

General

ACTIVITY/REST

May report: Malaise
Generalized weakness, faintness, muscle cramps

EGO INTEGRITY

May report: Anxiety
May exhibit: Restlessness, apprehension

FOOD/FLUID

May report: Nausea, anorexia, thirst
Low-sodium diet
Diuretic use

NEUROSENSORY

May report: Headache, blurred vision, vertigo
May exhibit: Loss of coordination, stupor, personality changes

TEACHING/LEARNING

Refer to predisposing/contributing factors
Use of oral hypoglycemic agent, potent diuretics, NSAIDs, other drugs that impair renal water excretion

Discharge plan considerations: May require assistance with changes in therapeutic regimen, dietary management

Refer to plan of care concerning underlying medical/surgical condition for possible considerations after discharge.

Sodium/Water Deficit

(Na less than 135 mEq/L; urine specific gravity elevated, serum osmolality normal.)

CIRCULATION

May exhibit: Hypotension, tachycardia
Peripheral pulses diminished
Pallid, clammy skin

ELIMINATION

May report: Abdominal cramping, diarrhea
May exhibit: Urinary output decreased

FOOD/FLUID

May report: Anorexia, nausea/vomiting
May exhibit: Poor skin turgor, soft/sunken eyeballs
Mucous membranes dry, decreased saliva/perspiration

NEUROSENSORY

May report: Dizziness
May exhibit: Muscle twitching
Lethargy, restlessness, confusion, stupor

RESPIRATION

May exhibit: Tachypnea

SAFETY

May exhibit: Skin flushed, dry, hot
Fever

Sodium Deficit/Water Excess

(Na less than 135 mEq/L, urine specific gravity low, serum osmolality decreased.)

CIRCULATION

May exhibit: Hypertension
Generalized edema

ELIMINATION

May exhibit: Urinary output increased

NEUROSENSORY

May exhibit: Muscle twitching, restlessness, changes in mentation (more severe when problem is acute/develops rapidly)

PAIN/DISCOMFORT

May report: Headache, abdominal cramps

Severe Sodium Deficit

(Na less than 120 mEq/L.)

CIRCULATION

May exhibit:	Hypotension with vasomotor collapse Rapid, thready pulse Cold/clammy skin, fingerprinting on sternum; cyanosis

NEUROSENSORY

May exhibit:	Hyporeflexia Convulsions/coma

DIAGNOSTIC STUDIES (DEPEND ON ASSOCIATED FLUID LEVEL)

Serum sodium: Decreased, less than 135 mEq/L. However, signs/symptoms may not occur until level is less than 120 mEq/L.

Urine sodium: Less than 15 mEq/L indicates renal conservation of sodium due to sodium loss from a nonrenal source unless sodium-wasting nephropathy is present. Urine sodium greater than 20 mEq/L indicates SIADH.

Serum potassium: May be decreased as the kidneys attempt to conserve sodium at the expense of potassium.

Serum chloride/bicarbonate: Levels are decreased depending on which ion is lost with the sodium.

Serum osmolality: Commonly low, but may be normal (pseudohyponatremia) or high (HHNC).

Urine osmolality: Usually less than 100 mOsm/L unless SIADH present; in which case, it will exceed serum osmolality.

Urine specific gravity: May be decreased (less than 1.010) or increased (greater than 1.020) if SIADH is present.

Hct: Depends on fluid balance; e.g., fluid excess versus dehydration.

DESIRED OUTCOMES/EVALUATION CRITERIA—CLIENT WILL:

Electrolyte and Acid/Base Balance (NOC)

Display heart rate, BP, and laboratory results within normal limits (WNL) for client, absence of muscle weakness, neurologic irritability.

ACTIONS/INTERVENTIONS	RATIONALE
ELECTROLYTE MANAGEMENT: Hyponatremia (NIC)	
Independent	
Identify client at risk for hyponatremia and the specific cause; e.g., sodium loss or fluid excess.	Provides clues for early intervention. Hyponatremia is a common imbalance (especially in the elderly) and may range from mild to severe. Severe hyponatremia can cause neurologic damage or death if not treated promptly.
Monitor I&O. Calculate fluid balance. Weigh daily.	Indicators of fluid balance are important, because either fluid excess or deficit may occur with hyponatremia.
Assess level of consciousness/neuromuscular response.	Sodium deficit may result in decreased mentation (to point of coma), as well as generalized muscle weakness/cramps, convulsions.
Maintain quiet environment; provide safety/seizure precautions.	Reduces CNS stimulation and risk of injury from neurologic complications; e.g., seizures.
Note respiratory rate and depth.	Co-occurring hypochloremia may produce slow/shallow respirations as the body compensates for metabolic alkalosis.
Encourage foods and fluids high in sodium; e.g., milk, meat, eggs, carrots, beets, and celery. Use fruit juices and bouillon instead of plain water.	Unless sodium deficit causes serious symptoms requiring immediate IV replacement, the client may benefit from slower replacement by oral method or removal of previous salt restriction.

ACTIONS/INTERVENTIONS	RATIONALE
Irrigate NG tube (when used) with normal saline instead of water.	Isotonic irrigation will minimize loss of GI electrolytes.
Observe for signs of circulatory overload as indicated.	Administration of sodium-containing IV fluids in presence of HF increases risk.

Collaborative

Assist with identification/treatment of underlying cause.	Refer to listing of predisposing/contributing factors to determine treatment needs.
Monitor serum and urine electrolytes, osmolality.	Evaluates therapy needs/effectiveness.
Provide/restrict fluids depending on fluid volume status.	In presence of hypovolemia, volume losses are replaced with isotonic saline (e.g., normal saline), or, on occasion, hypertonic solution (3% NaCl) when hyponatremia is life-threatening. In the presence of fluid volume excess, or SIADH, fluid restriction is indicated. *Note:* Too rapid/excessive administration of hypertonic solutions can be lethal.
Administer medications as indicated; e.g.:	
Furosemide (Lasix);	Effective in reducing fluid excess to correct sodium/water balance.
Sodium chloride;	Used to replace deficits/prevent recurrence in the presence of chronic/ongoing losses.
Potassium chloride;	Corrects potassium deficit, especially when diuretic is used.
Demeclocycline (Declomycin);	Useful in treating chronic SIADH, or when severe water restriction may not be tolerated; e.g., COPD. *Note:* May be contraindicated in clients with liver disease because nephrotoxicity may occur.
Captopril (Capoten).	May be used in combination with a loop diuretic (e.g., Lasix) to correct fluid volume excess, especially in the presence of HF.
Prepare for/assist with dialysis as indicated.	May be done to restore sodium balance without increasing fluid level when hyponatremia is severe or response to diuretic therapy is inadequate.

Hypernatremia (Sodium Excess)

Predisposing/Contributing Factors

Excessive water losses: Polyuria (as may occur with diabetes insipidus); use of osmotic diuretics (such as mannitol); presence of fever, profuse sweating, vomiting, diarrhea; extracellular fluid volume excesses such as renal disease, HF, primary aldosteronism, excessive steroids/Cushing's disease; excessive ingestion or infusion of sodium; saltwater near-drowning

Insufficient water intake: Administration of tube feedings/high-protein diets with minimal fluid intake, self-medication/"ulcer diets" primarily using half and half/whole milk

Client Assessment Database

Sodium Excess/Water Deficit

(Na greater than 145 mEq/L, elevated urine specific gravity.)

ACTIVITY/REST

May report: Weakness

May exhibit: Muscle rigidity/tremors, generalized weakness

CIRCULATION

May exhibit: Decreased blood pressure, postural hypotension
Tachycardia

ELIMINATION

May exhibit: Decreased urinary output

FOOD/FLUID

May report: Thirst
May exhibit: Mucous membranes dry, sticky; tongue dry, swollen, rough

NEUROSENSORY

May exhibit: Irritability, lethargy/coma (depending on rapidity of onset rather than actual serum sodium level)
Delusions, hallucinations
Muscle irritability, seizure activity

SAFETY

May exhibit: Hot, dry, flushed skin
Fever

Sodium/Water Excess

(Na greater than 145 mEq/L, urine specific gravity decreased.)

CIRCULATION

May exhibit: Elevated BP, hypertension

ELIMINATION

May exhibit: Polyuria

FOOD/FLUID

May report: Thirst
May exhibit: Skin pale, moist, taut with pitting edema
Weight gain

NEUROSENSORY

May exhibit: Confusion, lethargy
Delusions, hallucinations

RESPIRATION

May exhibit: Dyspnea

Sodium Excess/Water Deficit or Excess

TEACHING/LEARNING

Refer to predisposing/contributing factors

Discharge plan considerations: May require assistance with changes in therapeutic regimen, dietary management

Refer to plan of care concerning underlying medical/surgical condition for possible considerations after discharge.

DIAGNOSTIC STUDIES

Serum sodium: Increased, greater than 145 mEq/L. Serum levels greater than 160 mEq/L may be accompanied by severe neurologic signs.
Serum chloride: Increased, greater than 106 mEq/L.
Serum potassium: Decreased.
Serum osmolality: Greater than 295 mOsm/L when dehydrated, lower in presence of extracellular fluid excess, and less than 200 mOsm/L with excessive polyuria.
Hct: May be normal or elevated depending on fluid status.
Urine sodium: Less than 50 mEq/L.
Urine chloride: Less than 50 mEq/L.
Urine osmolality: Greater than 800 mOsm/L.
Urine specific gravity: Increased, greater than 1.015 if water deficit present, or less than 1.010 when hypernatremia is due to polyuria.

DESIRED OUTCOMES/EVALUATION CRITERIA—CLIENT WILL:

Electrolyte and Acid/Base Balance (NOC)

Display BP, heart rate, and laboratory results WNL for client, absence of neuromuscular irritability, cognitive impairment.

ACTIONS/INTERVENTIONS	RATIONALE
ELECTROLYTE MANAGEMENT: Hypernatremia (NIC)	
Independent	
Monitor BP.	Either hypertension or hypotension may be present depending on the fluid status. Presence of postural hypotension may affect activity tolerance.
Identify client at risk for hypernatremia and likely cause; e.g., water deficit, sodium excess.	Early identification and intervention prevents serious complications associated with this problem.
Note respiratory rate, depth.	Deep, labored respirations with air hunger suggest metabolic acidosis (hyperchloremia), which can lead to cardiopulmonary arrest if not corrected.
Monitor I&O, urine specific gravity. Weigh daily. Assess presence/location of edema.	These parameters are variable, depending on fluid status, and are indicators of therapy needs/effectiveness.
Evaluate level of consciousness and muscular strength, tone, movement.	Sodium imbalance may cause changes that vary from confusion and irritability to seizures and coma. In presence of water deficit, rapid rehydration may cause cerebral edema.
Maintain safety/seizure precautions, as indicated; e.g., bed in low position, use of padded side rails.	Sodium excess/cerebral edema increases risk of convulsions.
Assess skin turgor, color, temperature, and mucous membrane moisture.	Water-deficit hyponatremia manifests by signs of dehydration.
Provide/encourage meticulous skin care and frequent repositioning.	Maintains skin integrity.
Provide frequent oral care. Avoid use of mouthwash/rinse that contains alcohol.	Promotes comfort and prevents further drying of mucous membranes.
Offer debilitated client fluids at regular intervals. Give free water to client receiving enteral feedings.	May prevent hypernatremia in client who is unable to perceive or respond to thirst.
Recommend avoidance of foods high in sodium; e.g., canned soups/vegetables, processed foods, snack foods, and condiments.	Reduces risk of sodium-associated complications.
Collaborative	
Assist with identification/treatment of underlying cause.	Refer to listing of predisposing/contributing factors to determine treatment needs.
Monitor serum electrolytes, osmolality, and ABGs as indicated.	Evaluates therapy needs/effectiveness. *Note:* Co-occurring hyperchloremia may cause metabolic acidosis, requiring buffering; e.g., sodium bicarbonate.
Increase PO/IV fluid intake; e.g., 5% dextrose/water in presence of dehydration; 0.90% of NaCl if extracellular deficit is present.	Replacement of total body water deficit will gradually restore sodium/water balance. *Note:* Rapid reduction of serum sodium level with corresponding decrease in serum osmolality can cause cerebral edema/convulsions.
Restrict sodium intake and administer diuretics as indicated.	Restriction of sodium intake while promoting renal clearance lowers serum sodium levels in the presence of extracellular fluid excess.

POTASSIUM

Potassium is the major cation of the intracellular fluid and is responsible for maintaining intracellular osmotic pressure. Potassium also regulates neuromuscular excitability, aids in maintenance of acid-base balance, synthesis of protein, and metabolism of carbohydrates. Normal serum range is 3.5–5.0 mEq/L (body total of 42 mEq/L).

Hypokalemia (Potassium Deficit)

PREDISPOSING/CONTRIBUTING FACTORS

Renal loss: Use of potassium-wasting diuretics; diuretic phase of ATN; healing phase of burns; diabetic acidosis; Cushing's syndrome; nephritis; hypomagnesemia; use of sodium penicillins, amphotericin B, carbenicillin, steroids; licorice abuse
GI loss: Profuse vomiting, excessive diarrhea, laxative abuse, prolonged gastric suction, inflammatory bowel disease, fistulas
Inadequate dietary intake: Anorexia nervosa, starvation, high-sodium diet
Shift into cells: TPN, alkalosis, or excessive secretion or administration of insulin
Other: Sweat losses (heavily perspiring person acclimated to heat); liver disease

Client Assessment Database

ACTIVITY/REST

May report: Generalized weakness, lethargy, fatigue

CIRCULATION

May exhibit: Hypotension
Pulses weak/diminished, irregular
Heart sounds distant
Dysrhythmias; e.g., premature ventricular contractions (PVCs), ventricular tachycardia/fibrillation

ELIMINATION

May exhibit: Nocturia, polyuria if factors contributing to hypokalemia include HF or DM
Bowel sounds diminished, decreased bowel motility, paralytic ileus
Abdominal distention

FOOD/FLUID

May report: Anorexia, nausea/vomiting
Thirst

NEUROSENSORY

May report: Paresthesias
May exhibit: Depressed mental state/confusion, apathy, drowsiness, irritability, coma
Hyporeflexia, tetany, paralysis (flaccid quadriparesis)

PAIN/DISCOMFORT

May report: Muscle pain/cramps

RESPIRATION

May exhibit: Hypoventilation/decreased respiratory depth due to muscle weakness/paralysis of diaphragm, apnea, cyanosis

TEACHING/LEARNING

Refer to predisposing/contributing factors
May use/misuse herbal supplements than can cause/exacerbate hypokalemia (e.g., aloe, caraway, castor oil, dandelion, elder flower, flax seed, glycerol, licorice, peppermint oil, psyllium, yarrow).

Discharge plan considerations: May require assistance with changes in therapeutic regimen, dietary management

Refer to plan of care concerning underlying medical/surgical condition for possible considerations after discharge.

DIAGNOSTIC STUDIES

Serum potassium: Decreased, less than 3.5 mEq/L.
Serum chloride: Often decreased, less than 98 mEq/L.
Serum glucose: May be slightly elevated.
Serum magnesium: Levels often decreased when potassium deficit is present.
Plasma bicarbonate: Increased, greater than 29 mEq/L.
Urine osmolality: Decreased.
ABGs: pH and bicarbonate may be elevated (metabolic alkalosis).
ECG: Low voltage, flat or inverted T wave, appearance of U wave, depressed ST segment, peaked P waves, prolonged QT interval, ventricular dysrhythmias.

DESIRED OUTCOMES/EVALUATION CRITERIA—CLIENT WILL:

Electrolyte & Acid/Base Balance (NOC)

Display heart rhythm and laboratory results WNL for client, absence of muscle weakness, paresthesias, cognitive impairment.

ACTIONS/INTERVENTIONS	RATIONALE
ELECTROLYTE MANAGEMENT: Hypokalemia (NIC)	
Independent	
Monitor heart rate/rhythm.	Changes associated with hypokalemia include abnormalities in both conduction and contractility. Tachycardia may develop, and potentially life-threatening atrial and ventricular dysrhythmias; e.g., PVCs, sinus bradycardia, atrioventricular (AV) blocks, AV dissociation, ventricular tachycardia.
Monitor respiratory rate, depth, effort. Encourage cough/deep-breathing exercises; reposition frequently.	Respiratory muscle weakness may proceed to paralysis and eventual respiratory arrest.
Assess level of consciousness and neuromuscular function; e.g., strength, sensation, movement.	Apathy, drowsiness, irritability, tetany, paresthesias, and coma may occur.
Auscultate bowel sounds, noting decrease/absence or change.	Paralytic ileus commonly follows gastric losses through vomiting/gastric suction, protracted diarrhea.
Maintain accurate record of urinary, gastric, and wound losses.	Guide for calculating fluid/potassium replacement needs.
Monitor rate of IV potassium administration using microdrop or pump infusion devices. Check for side effects. Provide ice pack as indicated.	Ensures controlled delivery of medication to prevent bolus effect and reduce associated discomfort; e.g., burning sensation at IV site. When solution cannot be administered via central vein and slowing rate is not possible/effective, ice pack to infusion site may help relieve discomfort.
Encourage intake of foods and fluids high in potassium; e.g., bananas, oranges, dried fruits, red meat, turkey, salmon, leafy vegetables, peas, baked potatoes, tomatoes, winter squash, coffee, colas, tea. Discuss use of potassium chloride salt substitutes for client receiving long-term diuretics.	Potassium may be replaced/level maintained through the diet when the client is allowed oral food and fluids. Dietary replacement of 40–60 mEq/L/day is typically sufficient if no abnormal losses are occurring.
Review drug regimen for potassium-wasting drugs; e.g., furosemide (Lasix), hydrochlorothiazide (Diamox), IV catecholamines, gentamicin (Garamycin), carbenicillin (Geocillin), amphotericin B (Fungizone).	If alternate agents (e.g., potassium-sparing diuretics such as spirinolactone [Aldactone], triamterene [Dyrenium], amiloride [Midamor]) cannot be administered or when high-dose sodium drugs are administered (e.g., carbenicillin), close monitoring and replacement of potassium are necessary.

ACTIONS/INTERVENTIONS	RATIONALE
Discuss preventable causes of condition; e.g., nutritional choices, proper use of laxatives.	Provides opportunity for client to prevent recurrence. Also, dietary control is more palatable than oral replacement medications.
Dilute liquid and effervescent K supplements (K-Tab, K-Lyte/Cl) with 4 oz water/juice and give after meals.	May prevent/reduce GI irritation and saline laxative effect.
Watch for signs of digitalis intoxication when used (e.g., reports of nausea/vomiting, blurred vision, increasing atrial dysrhythmias, and heart block).	Low potassium enhances effect of digitalis, slowing cardiac conduction. *Note:* Combined effects of digitalis, diuretics, and hypokalemia may produce lethal dysrhythmias.
Observe for signs of metabolic alkalosis; e.g., hypoventilation, tachycardia, dysrhythmias, tetany, changes in mentation.	Frequently associated with hypokalemia.

Collaborative

ACTIONS/INTERVENTIONS	RATIONALE
Assist with identification/treatment of underlying cause.	Refer to listing of predisposing/contributing factors to determine treatment needs. *Note:* Hypokalemia is life-threatening, early detection is crucial.
Monitor laboratory studies; e.g.:	
Serum potassium;	Levels should be checked frequently during replacement therapy, especially in the presence of insufficient renal function. Sudden excess/elevation may cause cardiac dysrhythmias.
ABGs;	Correction of metabolic alkalosis raises serum potassium level and reduces replacement needs. Correction of acidosis drives potassium back into cells, resulting in decreased serum levels and increased replacement needs.
Serum magnesium;	Hypomagnesemia occurs with and exacerbates potassium loss and sodium retention, altering cell membrane excitability (affects cardiac and neuromuscular function).
Serum chloride.	Use of diuretics; e.g., furosemide (Lasix), hydrochlorothiazide (HydroDiuril), may cause chloride and potassium depletion.
Administer oral and/or IV potassium.	May be required to correct deficiencies when changes in medication, therapy and/or dietary intake are insufficient. *Note:* Even in severe deficit, parenteral replacement should not exceed 40 mEq/2 hr. Dietary supplementation may also be used to produce a gradual equilibration if client is able to take oral food and fluids.

Hyperkalemia (Potassium Excess)

PREDISPOSING/CONTRIBUTING FACTORS

Potassium retention: Decreased renal excretion (e.g., renal disease/acute failure, hypoaldosteronism, Addison's disease), hypovolemia, use of potassium-conserving diuretics, especially when associated with potassium supplements, use of NSAIDs
Excessive potassium intake: Salt substitutes, drugs containing potassium (e.g., penicillin), improper use of oral potassium supplements, too-rapid IV administration of potassium, massive transfusion of banked blood
Shift or release of potassium out of cells: Severe catabolism, burns, crush injuries, myocardial infarction (MI), severe hemolysis, rhabdomyolysis, chemotherapy with cytotoxic drugs, respiratory or metabolic acidosis, anoxia, hyperglycemia with insulin deficiency, use of some β-adrenergic blockers, profound digitalis toxicity
Other: Use of certain medications such as captopril, heparin, cyclosporine

Client Assessment Database

Data depends on degree of elevation and length of time condition has existed.

ACTIVITY/REST

May report: Vague muscular weakness
May exhibit: Restlessness, irritability

CIRCULATION

May exhibit: Irregular pulse, bradycardia, heart block, asystole

EGO INTEGRITY

May report: Apprehension

ELIMINATION

May report: Intermittent abdominal cramps, diarrhea
May exhibit: Urine volume decreased
Hyperactive bowel sounds

FOOD/FLUID

May report: Nausea/vomiting

NEUROSENSORY

May report: Paresthesias (often of face, tongue, hands, feet)
Slurred speech
May exhibit: Decreased deep-tendon reflexes; progressive, ascending flaccid paralysis, twitching, seizure activity
Apathy, confusion

PAIN/DISCOMFORT

May report: Muscle cramps/pain

TEACHING/LEARNING

Refer to predisposing/contributing factors
Discharge plan considerations: May require assistance with changes in therapeutic regimen, dietary management

Refer to plan of care concerning underlying medical/surgical condition for possible considerations after discharge.

DIAGNOSTIC STUDIES

Serum potassium: Increased, greater than 5.1 mEq/L.
Serum magnesium: Levels may be elevated if renal failure is present.
Renal function studies: May be altered, indicating failure.
Leukocyte or thrombocyte count: Elevation may cause a pseudohyperkalemia, affecting choice of interventions.
ECG changes: T waves tall and peaked/tented, prolonged PR interval, loss of P waves, widening of QRS complex, shortened QT interval, and ST segment depression; atrial/ventricular dysrhythmias; e.g., bradycardia, atrial arrest, complete heart block, ventricular fibrillation, cardiac arrest.

DESIRED OUTCOMES/EVALUATION CRITERIA—CLIENT WILL:

Electrolyte & Acid/Base Balance (NOC)

Display heart rate/rhythm and laboratory results WNL for client, absence of muscle weakness, paresthesias, cognitive impairment.

ACTIONS/INTERVENTIONS	RATIONALE
ELECTROLYTE MANAGEMENT: Hyperkalemia (NIC)	
Independent	
Identify client at risk or the cause of the hyperkalemia; e.g., excessive intake of potassium or decreased excretion.	Influences choice of interventions. Early identification and treatment can prevent complication. *Note:* A major cause of hypokalemia is decreased renal excretion.

ACTIONS/INTERVENTIONS	RATIONALE
Instruct client in use of potassium-containing salts (salt substitutes), taking potassium supplements safely.	The client is often able to prevent hyperkalemia through management of supplements, diet, and other medications.
Monitor respiratory rate and depth. Elevate head of bed. Encourage cough/deep-breathing exercises.	Clients may hypoventilate and retain CO_2, leading to respiratory acidosis. Muscular weakness can affect respiratory muscles and lead to complications of respiratory infection/failure.
Monitor heart rate/rhythm. Be aware that cardiac arrest can occur.	Excess potassium depresses myocardial conduction. Bradycardia can progress to cardiac fibrillation/arrest.
Monitor urinary output.	In kidney failure, potassium is retained because of improper excretion. Potassium should not be given if oliguria or anuria is present.
Assess level of consciousness, neuromuscular function; e.g., movement, strength, sensation.	Client is usually awake and alert; however, muscular paresthesia, weakness, and flaccid paralysis may occur.
Encourage/assist with ROM exercises as tolerated.	Improves muscular tone and reduces muscle cramps and pain.
Encourage frequent rest periods; assist with care activities, as indicated.	General muscle weakness decreases activity tolerance.
Review drug regimen for medications containing potassium/affecting potassium excretion; e.g., penicillin G, spironolactone (Aldactone), amiloride (Midamor), hydrochlorothiazide (Dyazide, Maxzide).	Requires regular monitoring of potassium levels, and may require alternate drug choices or changes in dosage/frequency.
Identify/discontinue dietary sources of potassium; e.g., tomatoes, broccoli, orange juice, bananas, bran, chocolate, coffee, tea, eggs, dairy products, dried fruits.	Facilitates reduction of potassium level and may prevent recurrence of hyperkalemia.
Recommend an increase in carbohydrates/fats and foods low in potassium; e.g., canned fruits, refined cereals, apple/cranberry juice.	Reduces exogenous sources of potassium and prevents catabolic tissue breakdown with release of cellular potassium.
Stress importance of client's notifying future caregivers when chronic condition potentiates development of hyperkalemia; e.g., oliguric renal failure.	May help prevent recurrence.

Collaborative

Assist with identification/treatment of underlying cause.	Refer to listing of predisposing/contributing factors to determine treatment needs.
Monitor laboratory results; e.g., serum potassium, ABGs, BUN/Cr, glucose as indicated.	Evaluates therapy needs/effectiveness. *Note:* Hypoventilation may result in respiratory acidosis, thereby increasing serum potassium levels.
Administer medications as indicated; e.g.:	
Diuretics; e.g., furosemide (Lasix);	Loop or thiazide diuretics promote renal clearance and excretion of potassium.
IV glucose with insulin, sodium bicarbonate;	Short-term emergency measure to move potassium into the cell, thus reducing toxic serum level. *Note:* Use with caution in presence of HF or hypernatremia. Use of glucose is contraindicated in clients who are hyperkalemic.
Calcium gluconate;	Temporary stopgap measure that antagonizes toxic potassium depressant effects on heart and stimulates cardiac contractility. *Note:* Calcium is contraindicated in clients on digitalis because it increases the cardiotonic effects of the drug and may cause dysrhythmias.
Sodium polystyrene sulfonate (Kayexalate, SPS suspension), orally, per NG tube, or rectally;	Resin removes potassium by exchanging potassium for sodium or calcium in the GI tract. Sorbitol enhances evacuation. *Note:* Use cautiously in clients with HF, edema, and in the elderly because it increases sodium level. In addition, Kayexalate may cause hyperchloremia.
β-Adrenergic agonist; e.g., albuterol (Proventil).	Nebulizer administration has been effective in clients receiving hemodialysis, and may also attenuate the hypoglycemic effect of insulin administration.

ACTIONS/INTERVENTIONS	RATIONALE
Infuse potassium-based medication/solutions slowly.	Prevents administration of concentrated bolus, allows time for kidneys to clear excess free potassium.
Provide fresh blood or washed RBCs (when possible) if transfusions required.	Fresh blood has less potassium than banked blood because breakdown of older RBCs releases potassium.
Prepare for/assist with dialysis (peritoneal or hemodialysis).	May be required when more conservative methods fail or are contraindicated; e.g., severe HF.

CALCIUM

Calcium is involved in bone formation/reabsorption, neural transmission/muscle contraction, regulation of enzyme systems, and is a coenzyme in blood coagulation. Normal serum levels are 4.5–5.3 mEq/L, 8.5–10.5 mg/dL (total), or 2.1–2.6 mEq/L (ionized). The ionized calcium is physiologically active and clinically important, especially in critically ill clients. The total serum calcium is directly related to the serum albumin, follows it, and must be considered if only total serum readings are available. Some factors that alter the percentage of ionized calcium are changes in pH (affects how much calcium is bound to protein) or increased serum levels of fatty acids, lactate, and bicarbonate.

Hypocalcemia (Calcium Deficit)

PREDISPOSING/CONTRIBUTING FACTORS

Primary or surgical hypoparathyroidism, transient hypocalcemia following thyroidectomy; hyperphosphatemia, hypomagnesemia
Massive subcutaneous tissue infections, acute pancreatitis, burns, peritonitis, malignancies
Excessive GI losses: Draining fistula, diarrhea, fat malabsorption syndromes, chronic laxative use (particularly phosphate-containing laxatives/enemas)
Extreme stress situations with mobilization and excretion of calcium
Diuretic and terminal phase of renal failure
Inadequate dietary intake, lack of milk/vitamin D, excessive protein diet
Alcoholism: Primary effect of ethanol, plus intestinal malabsorption, hypomagnesemia, hypoalbuminemia, and pancreatitis
Use of anticonvulsants, antibiotics, corticosteroids; loop diuretics, drugs that lower serum magnesium (e.g., cisplatin, gentamycin)
Infusion of citrated blood, calcium-free infusions; rapid infusion of Plasmanate
Malignant neoplasms with bone metastases
Alkalotic states
Decreased ultraviolet exposure

Client Assessment Database

Data depend on duration, severity, and rate of onset of hypocalcemia.

CIRCULATION

May exhibit: Hypotension
Pulses weak/decreased, irregular (weak cardiac contraction/premature dysrhythmias)

ELIMINATION

May report: Diarrhea, abdominal pain
May exhibit: Abdominal distention (paralytic ileus)

FOOD/FLUID

May report: Nausea/vomiting
May exhibit: Difficulty swallowing

HYGIENE

May exhibit: Coarse, dry skin; alopecia (chronic)

NEUROSENSORY

May report: Circumoral paresthesia, numbness and tingling of fingers and toes, muscle cramps

May exhibit: Anxiety, confusion, irritability, alteration in mood, impaired memory, depression, hallucinations, psychoses
Muscle spasms (carpopedal and laryngeal), increased deep-tendon reflexes, tetany, tonic/clonic seizure activity, positive Trousseau's and Chvostek's signs

RESPIRATION

May exhibit: Labored shallow breathing, stridor (spasm of laryngeal muscles)

SAFETY

May exhibit: Bleeding with no or minimal trauma

TEACHING/LEARNING

Refer to predisposing/contributing factors

Discharge plan considerations: May require assistance with changes in therapeutic regimen, dietary management

Refer to plan of care concerning underlying medical/surgical condition for possible considerations after discharge.

DIAGNOSTIC STUDIES

Serum calcium: Decreased, less than 4.5 mEq/L or 8.5 mg/dL (total), 2.1 mEq/L (ionized)
Urine Sulkowitch test: Shows light or no precipitate.
ECG: Prolonged QT interval (characteristic but not necessarily diagnostic). In severe deficiency, T waves may flatten or invert, giving appearance of hypokalemia or myocardial ischemia; ventricular tachycardia may develop.

DESIRED OUTCOMES/EVALUATION CRITERIA—CLIENT WILL:

Electrolyte & Acid-Base Balance (NOC)

Display heart rhythm and laboratory results WNL for client, absence of neuromuscular irritability, respiratory impairment.

ACTIONS/INTERVENTIONS	RATIONALE
ELECTROLYTE MANAGEMENT: Hypocalcemia (NIC)	
Independent	
Monitor heart rate/rhythm.	Calcium deficit along with associated hypomagnesemia weakens cardiac muscle contractility.
Assess respiratory rate, rhythm, effort. Have tracheostomy equipment available.	Laryngeal stridor may develop and result in respiratory emergency/arrest.
Observe for neuromuscular irritability; e.g., tetany, seizure activity. Assess for presence of Chvostek's/Trousseau's signs.	Calcium deficit causes repetitive and uncontrolled nerve transmission, leading to muscle spasms and hyperirritability.
Provide quiet environment and seizure precautions as appropriate.	Reduces CNS stimulation and protects client from potential injury.
Encourage relaxation/stress reduction techniques; e.g., deep-breathing exercises, guided imagery, visualization.	Tetany can be potentiated by hyperventilation and stress. *Note:* Direct pressure on the nerves (e.g., tightening BP cuff) may also trigger tetany.
Check for bleeding from any source (mucous membranes, puncture sites, wounds/incisions, and so on). Note presence of ecchymosis, petechiae.	Alterations in coagulation can occur as a result of calcium deficiency.

ACTIONS/INTERVENTIONS	RATIONALE
Review client's drug regimen; e.g., use of insulin, mithramycin (Mithracin), parathyroid injection, digitalis.	Some drugs can lower magnesium levels, affecting calcium level. The effect of digitalis is enhanced by calcium, and, in clients receiving calcium, digitalis intoxication may develop.
Discuss use of laxatives/antacids.	Those containing phosphate may negatively affect calcium metabolism.
Review dietary intake of vitamins and fat.	Insufficient ingestion of vitamin D and fat impairs absorption of calcium.
Identify sources to increase calcium and vitamin D in diet; e.g., dairy products, beans, cauliflower, eggs, oranges, pineapples, sardines, shellfish. Restrict intake of phosphorus; e.g., barley, bran, whole wheat, rye, liver, nuts, chocolate.	Vitamin D aids in absorption of calcium from intestinal tract. Phosphorus competes with calcium for intestinal absorption.
Encourage use of calcium-containing antacids if needed (e.g., Titralac, Dicarbosil, Tums).	Possible sources for oral replacement to help maintain calcium levels, especially in clients at risk for osteoporosis.
Stress importance of meeting calcium needs.	Adverse effects of long-term deficiency include tooth decay, eczema, cataracts, and osteoporosis.

Collaborative

Assist with identification/treatment of underlying cause.	Refer to listing of predisposing/contributing factors to determine treatment needs.
Monitor laboratory studies; e.g.:	
Serum calcium and magnesium; serum albumin, ABGs;	Evaluates therapy needs/effectiveness. *Note:* Low serum albumin levels or serum pH affects calcium levels; e.g., a low albumin level causes a deceptively low calcium level; alkalosis causes surplus bicarbonate to bind with free calcium, impairing function; acidosis frees calcium, potentiating hypercalcemia.
PT, platelets.	Calcium is an essential part of the clotting mechanism and deficit may lead to excessive bleeding.
Administer the following:	
Calcium gluconate/gluceptate/chloride IV;	Provides rapid treatment in acute calcium deficit (especially in presence of tetany/convulsions). *Note:* Calcium chloride is not used as often because it is irritating to the vein and can cause tissue sloughing if it leaks into tissues.
Oral preparations; e.g., calcium lactate/carbonate;	Oral preparations are useful in correcting subacute deficiencies.
Magnesium sulfate IV/PO if indicated;	Hypomagnesemia is a precipitating factor in calcium deficit.
Vitamin D supplement (e.g., calcitriol).	May be used in combination with calcium therapy to enhance calcium absorption once concomitant phosphate deficiency is corrected.

Hypercalcemia (Calcium Excess)

PREDISPOSING/CONTRIBUTING FACTORS

Hyperparathyroidism, hyperthyroidism, multiple myeloma/other malignancies (e.g., cancer of breast, lung), renal disease, skeletal muscle paralysis, parathyroid tumor, sarcoidosis, adrenal insufficiency, TB

Excessive/prolonged use of vitamins A and D and calcium-containing antacids, prolonged use of thiazide diuretics, theophylline, lithium

Multiple fractures, bone tumors, osteoporosis, osteomalacia, prolonged immobilization causing imbalance between the rate of bone formation and resorption

Milk-alkali syndrome as a side effect of prolonged milk/antacid self-medication for gastric pain/ulcer

Hypophosphatasia, hyperproteinemia
Anticancer drugs; e.g., tamoxifen, androgens/estrogens

Client Assessment Database

ACTIVITY/REST

May report: General malaise, fatigue/weakness
Lethargy

May exhibit: Incoordination, ataxia

CIRCULATION

May exhibit: Hypertension
Irregular pulse, dysrhythmias, bradycardia

ELIMINATION

May report: Constipation or diarrhea

May exhibit: Polyuria, nocturia
Kidney stones/calculi

FOOD/FLUID

May report: Anorexia, nausea/vomiting
Thirst

ABDOMINAL PAIN

May exhibit: Poor skin turgor, dry mucous membranes

NEUROSENSORY

May report: Headache

May exhibit: Hypotonicity/muscular relaxation, flaccid paralysis, depressed/absent deep-tendon reflexes
Drowsiness, apathy, paranoia, personality changes, decreased attention span, memory loss, depression, inappropriate/bizarre behaviors, psychosis, confusion, stupor/coma
Slurred speech

PAIN/DISCOMFORT

May report: Epigastric, abdominal, deep flank pain, or bone/joint pain

TEACHING/LEARNING

Refer to predisposing/contributing factors.

Discharge plan considerations: May require assistance with changes in therapeutic regimen, dietary management

Refer to plan of care concerning underlying medical/surgical condition for possible considerations after discharge.

DIAGNOSTIC STUDIES

Serum calcium: Increased, greater than 2.6 mEq/L (ionized) or 10.5 mg/dL (total).
BUN: Increased (calculi can damage kidney).
Serum phosphorus: Decreased levels may be noted.
Urine Sulkowitch test:: Shows heavy precipitate.
Urine calcium: Increased.
Urine osmolality: Decreased.
Urine specific gravity: Decreased.
Radiography: May reveal evidence of bone cavitation, pathologic fracture, osteoporosis, urinary calculi.
ECG changes: Shortened QT interval, inverted T waves. In severe deficit, QRS may widen, PR interval lengthens, and ventricular prematurities develop.

DESIRED OUTCOMES/EVALUATION CRITERIA—CLIENT WILL:

Electrolyte & Acid-Base Balance (NOC)

Display heart rhythm, muscle strength, cognitive status, and laboratory results WNL for client.

ACTIONS/INTERVENTIONS	RATIONALE
ELECTROLYTE MANAGEMENT: Hypercalcemia (NIC)	
Independent	
Monitor cardiac rate/rhythm. Be aware that cardiac arrest can occur in hypercalcemic crisis.	Overstimulation of cardiac muscle occurs with resultant dysrhythmias and ineffective cardiac contraction. Sinus bradycardia, sinus dysrhythmias, wandering pacemaker, and AV block may be noted. Hypercalcemia creates a predisposition to cardiac arrest.
Assess level of consciousness and neuromuscular status; e.g., muscle movement, strength, tone.	Nerve and muscle activity is depressed. Lethargy and fatigue can progress to convulsion/coma.
Monitor I&O, calculate fluid balance.	Efforts to correct original condition may result in secondary imbalances/complications.
Encourage fluid intake of 3–4 L/day, including sodium-containing fluids (within cardiac tolerance) and use of acid-ash juices; e.g., cranberry and prune if kidney stones present or suspected.	Reduces dehydration, encourages urinary flow and clearance of calcium, reduces risk of stone formation. *Note:* Sodium favors calcium excretion and can be used if not contraindicated by other conditions.
Strain urine if flank pain occurs.	Large amount of calcium present in kidney parenchyma may lead to stone formation.
Auscultate bowel sounds.	Hypotonicity leads to constipation when the smooth muscle tone is inadequate to produce peristalsis.
Maintain bulk in diet.	Constipation may be a problem because of decreased GI tone.
Encourage frequent repositioning and ROM and/or muscle-setting exercises with caution. Promote ambulation if client is able.	Muscle activity may reduce calcium shifting from the bones that occurs during immobilization. *Note:* Increased risk for pathologic fractures exists because of calcium shifts out of the bones.
Provide safety measures; e.g., gentle handling when moving/transferring client.	Reduces risk of injury/pathologic fractures.
Review drug regimen, noting use of calcium-elevating drugs; e.g., heparin, tetracyclines, methicillin, phenytoin.	May affect drug choice or require reduction in oral sources of calcium.
Identify/restrict sources of calcium intake; e.g., dairy products, eggs, and spinach; calcium-containing antacids (Titralac, Dicarbosil, Tums).	Foods or drugs containing calcium may need to be limited in chronic conditions causing hypercalcemia.
Collaborative	
Assist with identification/treatment of underlying cause.	Refer to listing of predisposing/contributing factors to determine treatment needs.
Monitor laboratory studies; e.g., calcium, magnesium, phosphate.	Monitors therapy needs/effectiveness. *Note:* Phosphate levels may be low when parathyroid hormone inversely promotes calcium uptake and calcium competes with phosphate for absorption/transport with vitamin D.
Administer isotonic saline and sodium sulfate IV/orally.	Emergency measures in severe hypercalcemia used to dilute extracellular calcium concentration and inhibit tubular reabsorption of calcium, thereby increasing urinary excretion.

ACTIONS/INTERVENTIONS	RATIONALE
Administer medications as indicated:	
Diuretics; e.g., furosemide (Lasix);	Diuresis promotes renal excretion of calcium and reduces risks of fluid excess from isotonic saline infusion.
Sodium bicarbonate;	Induces alkalosis, thereby reducing the ionized calcium fraction.
Phosphate;	Rapid-acting agent that induces calcium excretion and inhibits resorption of bone.
Glucocorticoid therapy;	Inhibits intestinal absorption of calcium and reduces inflammation and associated stress response that mobilizes calcium from the bone.
Mithramycin (Mithracin);	Cytotoxic antibiotic that lowers serum calcium by inhibiting inappropriate bone resorption, typically seen in malignancies or hyperparathyroidism.
Disodium edetate (EDTA);	Chelating action lowers serum calcium level.
Calcitonin;	Promotes movement of serum calcium into bones, temporarily reducing serum calcium levels, especially in the presence of increased parathyroid hormone.
Neutra-Phos, Fleet Phospho-Soda.	These drugs bind calcium in the GI tract, promoting excretion.
Prepare for/assist with hemodialysis.	Rapid reduction of serum calcium may be necessary to correct life-threatening situation.

MAGNESIUM

Magnesium influences carbohydrate metabolism, secretion of parathyroid hormone, sodium/potassium transport across the cell membrane, and synthesis of protein and nucleic acid. Magnesium activates adenosine triphosphate (ATP) and mediates neural transmission within the CNS. Magnesium deficit is often associated with hypokalemia and promotes intracellular potassium loss and sodium accumulation, altering and exacerbating membrane excitability. Normal serum range is 1.5–2.5 mEq/L or 1.8–3.0 mg/dL.

Hypomagnesemia (Magnesium Deficit)

PREDISPOSING/CONTRIBUTING FACTORS

GI losses: Biliary/intestinal fistula; surgery (bowel resection, small-bowel bypass); severe, protracted diarrhea; laxative abuse; impaired GI absorption/malabsorption syndrome; gastric/colon cancer; prolonged gastric suction
Protein/calorie malnutrition, feeding (enteral or parenteral) without adequate magnesium replacement
Prolonged IV infusion of magnesium-free solutions, multiple transfusions with citrated blood products
Chronic alcoholism, alcohol withdrawal, pancreatitis
Hyperaldosteronism: Primary or secondary (e.g., cirrhosis or HF)
Toxemia of pregnancy
Renal losses: Severe renal disease/diuretic phase of ARF, vigorous and/or prolonged diuresis with mercurial thiazides or loop diuretics, SIADH
Drugs that affect magnesium balance: Aminoglycosides (gentamicin, tobramycin), antifungals (amphotericin B), chemotherapy agents (cisplatin), antirejection agents (cyclosporine), and excessive doses of calcium or vitamin D supplements
Diabetic ketoacidosis, malignancies causing hypercalcemic states, severe burns, sepsis, hypothermia, hypoparathyroidism, hypercalcemia, hyperthyroidism

Client Assessment Database

ACTIVITY/REST

May report: Generalized weakness, insomnia
Ataxia, vertigo

CIRCULATION

May exhibit: Tachycardia, dysrhythmias
Hypotension (vasodilation), occasional hypertension

FOOD/FLUID

May report: Anorexia, nausea/vomiting, diarrhea

NEUROSENSORY

May report: Paresthesia (legs, feet)
Vertigo

May exhibit: Nystagmus
Musculoskeletal fasciculations/tremors, neuromuscular irritability/spasticity, spontaneous carpopedal spasms, hyperactive deep tendon reflexes, clonus
Tetany, convulsions; positive Babinski's, Chvostek's, and Trousseau's signs
Disorientation, apathy, depression, irritability, agitation, hallucinations/psychoses, coma

TEACHING/LEARNING

Refer to predisposing/contributing factors.

Discharge plan considerations: May require assistance with changes in therapeutic regimen, dietary management

Refer to plan of care concerning underlying medical/surgical condition for possible postdischarge considerations.

DIAGNOSTIC STUDIES

Serum magnesium: Decreased, less than 1.5 mEq/L or 1.8 mg/dL. (Usually symptoms do not appear until level is less than 1 mEq/L.)
Calcium: May be decreased unless there is a hypercalcemic condition causing the magnesium deficit.
Potassium: Decrease associated with severe hypomagnesemia.
ECG: Prolonged PR and QT intervals, widened QRS complex, ST segment depression, T wave inversion.

DESIRED OUTCOMES/EVALUATION CRITERIA—CLIENT WILL:

Electrolyte & Acid/Base Balance (NOC)

Display heart rate/rhythm, muscle strength, cognitive status, and laboratory results WNL for client, absence of neuromuscular irritability.

ACTIONS/INTERVENTIONS	RATIONALE
ELECTROLYTE MANAGEMENT: Hypomagnesemia (NIC)	
Independent	
Monitor cardiac rate/rhythm, noting tachydysrhythmias and characteristic ECG changes.	Magnesium influences sodium/potassium transport across the cell membrane and affects excitability of cardiac tissue.
Monitor for signs of digitalis intoxication when used (e.g., reports of nausea/vomiting, blurred vision; increasing atrial dysrhythmias and heart block).	Magnesium deficit may precipitate digitalis toxicity.
Assess level of consciousness and neuromuscular status; e.g., movement, strength, reflexes/tone; note presence of Chvostek's/Trousseau's signs.	Confusion, irritability, and psychosis may occur. However, more common manifestations are muscular; e.g., hyperactive deep tendon reflexes, muscle tremors, spasticity, generalized tetany.
Monitor status of airway and swallowing.	Laryngeal stridor and dysphagia can occur when depletion is moderate to severe.
Take seizure/safety precautions; e.g., padded side rails, bed in low position, frequent observation as indicated.	Changes in mentation or the development of seizure activity in severe hypomagnesemia increases the risk of client injury.
Provide quiet environment and subdued lighting.	Reduces extraneous stimuli; promotes rest.

ACTIONS/INTERVENTIONS	RATIONALE
Encourage ROM exercises as tolerated.	Reduces deleterious effects of muscle weakness/spasticity.
Place footboard/cradle on bed.	Elevation of linens may reduce spasms.
Auscultate bowel sounds.	Muscle weakness/spasticity may reduce peristalsis and bowel function.
Encourage intake of dairy products, whole grains, green leafy vegetables, meat, and fish.	Provides oral replacement for mild magnesium deficits; may prevent recurrence.
Instruct client in proper use of laxatives and diuretics.	Deficit may be the result of abuse of these drugs.
Observe for signs of magnesium toxicity during replacement therapy; e.g., thirst, feeling hot and flushed, diaphoresis, anxiety, drowsiness, hypotension, increased muscular and nervous system irritability, loss of patellar reflex.	Rapid, excessive IV replacement may lead to toxicity and life-threatening complications.

Collaborative

Assist with identification/treatment of underlying cause.	Refer to listing of predisposing/contributing factors. *Note:* Studies have shown that chronic alcoholism with malnutrition is the most common cause of hypomagnesemia in the United States.
Monitor laboratory studies; e.g., serum magnesium, calcium, and potassium levels.	Evaluates therapy needs/effectiveness. *Note:* These electrolytes are interrelated, symptoms may be similar, and deficits of more than one may be present.
Administer medications as indicated:	
Magnesium sulfate or magnesium chloride IV, monitoring administration closely;	IV replacement is preferred in severe deficit because absorption of magnesium from intestinal tract varies inversely with calcium absorption. However, potential for drug interaction with digitalis preparations may lead to increased cardiac dysrhythmias/heart block. *Note:* Calcium gluconate is the antidote should hypermagnesemia be evidenced by depressed deep tendon reflexes or respiratory depression and hypotension (late sign).
Magnesium sulfate IM, or magnesium hydroxide PO (Amphojel, Milk of Magnesia);	May be given for mild deficit or in nonemergent situations. Injections should be deep IM to decrease local tissue reaction.
Magnesium-based antacids; e.g., Mylanta, Maalox, Gelusil, Riopan.	Can supplement dietary replacement. *Note:* Use of these products may cause diarrhea, which can be alleviated by concurrent use of aluminum-containing products; e.g., Amphojel, Basaljel.

Hypermagnesemia (Magnesium Excess)

PREDISPOSING/CONTRIBUTING FACTORS

Reduced renal function (e.g., acute processes or age), chronic renal disease/failure, or dialysis with hard water
Excessive intake/absorption: e.g., too-rapid replacement of magnesium (as in pregnancy-induced hypertension or premature labor), excessive use of magnesium-containing drugs/products; e.g., Maalox, Milk of Magnesia, Epsom salts
Untreated diabetic ketoacidosis
Hyperparathyroidism, aldosterone deficiency, adrenal insufficiency
Extracellular fluid volume depletion (e.g., after diuretic abuse)
Saltwater near-drowning, hypothermia, shock
Chronic diarrhea; diseases that interfere with gastric absorption

Client Assessment Database

ACTIVITY/REST

May report: Generalized weakness, fatigue
May exhibit: Drowsiness, lethargy, stupor

CIRCULATION

May exhibit: Hypotension (mild to severe)
Pulses weak/irregular, bradycardia (12–15 mEq/L), cardiac arrest (greater than 25 mEq/L)

FOOD/FLUID

May report: Nausea/vomiting

NEUROSENSORY

May exhibit: Depressed deep tendon reflexes (7–10 mEq/L) progressing to flaccid paralysis
Decreased level of consciousness, lethargy progressing to coma
Slurred speech

RESPIRATION

May exhibit: Hypoventilation progressing to apnea (12–15 mEq/L)

SAFETY

May exhibit: Skin flushing, sweating

TEACHING/LEARNING

Discharge plan considerations: Refer to predisposing/contributing factors.
May require assistance with changes in therapeutic regimen, dietary management

Refer to plan of care concerning underlying medical/surgical condition for possible considerations after discharge.

DIAGNOSTIC STUDIES

Serum magnesium: Symptomatic levels greater than 3 mEq/L (increase to 10–20 mEq/L results in respiratory depression, coma, and cardiac arrest).
ECG: Prolonged PR and QT intervals, wide QRS, elevated T waves, development of heart block, cardiac arrest.

DESIRED OUTCOMES/EVALUATION CRITERIA—CLIENT WILL:

Electrolyte & Acid/Base Balance (NOC)

Display heart rhythm, muscular strength, cognitive status and laboratory results WNL for client, absence of respiratory impairment.

ACTIONS/INTERVENTIONS	RATIONALE
ELECTROLYTE MANAGEMENT: Hypermagnesemia (NIC)	
Independent	
Monitor cardiac rate/rhythm.	Bradycardia and heart block may develop, progressing to cardiac arrest as a direct result of hypermagnesemia on cardiac muscle.
Monitor BP.	Hypotension unexplained by other causes is an early sign of toxicity.
Assess level of consciousness and neuromuscular status; e.g., reflexes/tone, movement, strength.	CNS and neuromuscular depression can cause decreasing level of alertness, progressing to coma, and depressed muscular responses, progressing to flaccid paralysis.
Monitor respiratory rate/depth/rhythm. Encourage cough/deep-breathing exercises. Elevate head of bed as indicated.	Neuromuscular transmissions are blocked by magnesium excess, resulting in respiratory muscular weakness and hypoventilation, which may progress to apnea.

ACTIONS/INTERVENTIONS	RATIONALE
Check patellar reflexes periodically.	Absence of these reflexes suggests magnesium levels about 7 mEq/L or greater. If untreated, cardiac/respiratory arrest can occur.
Encourage increased fluid intake if appropriate.	Increased hydration enhances magnesium excretion, but fluid intake must be cautious in event of renal/cardiac failure.
Monitor urinary output and 24-hr fluid balance	Renal failure is the primary contributing factor in hypermagnesmia; and, if it is present, fluid excess can easily occur.
Promote bedrest; assist with personal care activities as needed.	Flaccid paralysis, lethargy, and decreased mentation; reduced activity tolerance/ability.
Recommend avoidance of magnesium-containing antacids; e.g., Maalox, Mylanta, Gelusil, Riopan, in client with renal disease. Caution clients with renal disease to avoid OTC drug use without discussing with healthcare provider.	Limits oral intake to help prevent hypermagnesemia.

Collaborative

Assist with identification/treatment of underlying cause.	Refer to listing of predisposing/contributing factors to determine treatment needs. *Note:* Most frequently occurs in clients with advanced renal failure.
Monitor laboratory studies as indicated, e.g; serum magnesium and calcium levels.	Evaluates therapy needs/effectiveness.
Administer IV fluids and thiazide diuretics as indicated.	Promotes renal clearance of magnesium (if renal function is normal).
Administer 10% calcium chloride or gluconate IV.	Antagonizes action/reverses symptoms of magnesium toxicity to improve neuromuscular function.
Assist with dialysis as needed.	In the presence of renal disease/failure, dialysis may be needed to lower serum levels.

DEMENTIA OF THE ALZHEIMER'S TYPE/VASCULAR DEMENTIA

Dementia of the Alzheimer's type (DAT) is a specific degenerative process occurring primarily in the cells located at the base of the forebrain that send information to the cerebral cortex and hippocampus. It is the most common form of dementia and is characterized by a steady and global decline. In comparison, *vascular dementia* reflects a pattern of intermittent deterioration related to multiple infarcts to various areas of the brain. Although the etiologies differ, these two forms of dementia share a common symptom presentation and therapeutic intervention.

In vascular dementia symptoms fluctuate and are determined by the area of the brain that is affected. Deterioration is thought to occur in response to repeated infarcts of the brain. Predisposing factors include various diseases and conditions that interfere with blood circulation, including cerebral and systemic vascular disease, hypertension, cerebral hypoxia, hypoglycemia, cerebral embolism, and severe head injury.

These dementias are characterized by progressive cognitive losses caused by damage to various areas of the brain and depending on underlying pathology. Personality change is common and may be manifested by either an alteration or accentuation of premorbid characteristics with primary deficits in memory and planning and a predisposition to confusion.

Several studies have shown that antibodies are produced in the brains of individuals with Alzheimer's disease. Although the triggering mechanism is not known, the reactions are actually autoantibody production, suggesting a possible alteration in the body's immune system. Although the exact cause of Alzheimer's disease is unknown, several hypotheses have been supported by varying amounts and quality of research data. The exception is research on environmental causes, such as the ingestion of aluminum, which to date have not been supported by research findings. Research has revealed that, in DAT, the enzyme required to produce acetylcholine is dramatically reduced, especially in the areas of the brain where the senile plaques and neurofibrillary tangles occur in the greatest numbers. This decrease in acetylcholine production reduces the amount of neurotransmitter that is released to cells in the cortex, hippocampus, and nucleus basalis, resulting in a disruption of memory processes. Additionally, the neuritic plaques that accumulate are composed of β-amyloid, an insoluble protein that is an abnormal breakdown product of the cell membrane constituent amyloid precursor protein (APP). Furthermore, the formation of the customary plaques and tangles appears to be related to the cholesterol-transporting protein, apolipoprotein-E (ApoE), which has been associated with an earlier-than-average age of onset for the common form of Alzheimer's disease for individuals who carry the $ApoE_4$ genetic variant.

Thus, genetics appears to play a role. Studies suggest a familial pattern of transmission that is four times greater than in the general population. Familial, or early-onset Alzheimer's, has been linked to defects of genes on chromosome 1, 14, or 21, with some families exhibiting a pattern of inheritance that suggests possible autosomal dominant gene transmission. Furthermore, Down's syndrome (extra chromosome 21) may have some relationship to Alzheimer's disease. At autopsy, both disorders have many of the same pathophysiologic changes, and a high percentage of individuals with Down's syndrome who survive to adulthood develop Alzheimer's lesions by age 50. (Incidentally, these individuals carry two copies of the gene for APP.)

Current research suggests that Alzheimer's disease may actually be a lifelong process, with changes in the brain developing decades before the onset of dementia. Other researchers theorize that a rich education may increase a person's reserve of brain cells or connections between nerve cells, either of which could reduce the risk of dementia.

CARE SETTING

Primarily home or assisted living/extended care; however, inpatient care may be required for treatment of other health problems

RELATED CONCERNS

End of life/hospice care, page 880
Extended care, page 810
Pneumonia, page 128
Psychosocial aspects of care, page 770
Sepsis/septicemia, page 701
Total nutritional support; parenteral/enteral feeding, page 478

Client Assessment Database

ACTIVITY/REST:

May Report: Feeling tired; fatigue may increase severity of symptoms, especially as evening approaches
Decreased interest in usual activities, hobbies; inability to recall what is read/follow plot of television program; possibly forced to retire from work

May exhibit: Day/night reversal, wakefulness/aimless wandering, disturbance of sleep rhythms
Lethargy, impaired motor skills, inability to carry out familiar, purposeful movements
Content sitting and watching others
Main activity may be hoarding inanimate objects, repetitive motions (e.g., fold-unfold-refold linen), hiding articles, wandering

CIRCULATION

May report: History of systemic/cerebral vascular disease, hypertension, embolic episodes (predisposing factors)

EGO INTEGRITY

May report: Anxiety and depression related to the knowledge that cognitive abilities are deteriorating (early stages), progressing to apathy
Multiple losses; changes in body image and self-esteem

May exhibit: Behavior often inconsistent, verbal/nonverbal behavior may be incongruent
Suspicious or fearful of imaginary people/situations; clinging to significant other(s)
Misperception of environment, misidentification of objects/people, hoarding objects, belief that misplaced objects are stolen
Emotional lability (cries easily, laughs inappropriately), variable mood changes (apathy, lethargy, restlessness, short attention span, irritability), sudden angry outbursts (catastrophic reactions)
May deny significance of early changes/symptoms, especially cognitive changes, and/or describe vague, hypochondriacal reports (e.g., fatigue, diarrhea, dizziness, occasional headaches)
May conceal limitations (e.g., make excuses for not being able to perform tasks, redirect conversation/avoid direct answers to questions)
Feelings of helplessness, strong, depressive overlay, delusions, paranoia

ELIMINATION

May report/exhibit: Urgency (may indicate loss of muscle tone)
Incontinence of urine/feces
Prone to constipation/impaction, with diarrhea

FOOD/FLUID

May report: Changes in taste, appetite; denial of hunger/refusal to eat (may be trying to conceal lost skills)

May exhibit: Hypoglycemic episodes (predisposing factor)
Lack of interest in/forgetting of mealtimes, dependence on others for food cooking and preparation at table, feeding, using utensils
Loss of ability to chew (silent aspiration)
Weight loss; decreased muscle mass; emaciation (advanced stage)

HYGIENE

May report: Dependence on SO to meet basic hygiene needs

May exhibit: Appearance disheveled, unkempt; body odor present; poor personal habits
Clothing may be inappropriate for situation/weather conditions
Misinterpretation of, or ignoring, internal cues, forgetting steps involved in toileting self, or inability to find the bathroom

NEUROSENSORY

May report: Family members may report a gradual decrease in cognitive abilities, impaired judgment/inappropriate decisions, impaired recent memory but good remote memory, behavioral changes/individual personality traits altered or exaggerated

May exhibit: Concealing inabilities (may make excuses not to perform task, may thumb through a book without reading it)
Loss of proprioception sense (location of body/body parts in space)
Primitive reflexes (e.g., positive snout, suck, palmar) may be present
Facial signs/symptoms dependent on degree of vascular insults
Seizure activity (secondary to the associated brain damage)
Mental status examination:
- Disoriented to time initially, then place; usually oriented to person until late in disease process
- Impaired recent memory, progressive loss of remote memory
- May change answers during the interview
- Difficulty in comprehension, abstract thinking
- Unable to do simple calculations or repeat the names of three objects, short attention span
- Hallucinations, delusions, severe depression, mania (advanced stage)
- May have impaired communication: difficulty with finding correct words (especially nouns); conversation repetitive or scattered with substituted meaningless words; speech may become inaudible; gradually loses ability to write (fine motor skills) or read

SAFETY

May report: History of recent viral illness or serious head trauma, drug toxicity, stress, nutritional deficits (may be predisposing/accelerating factors)
Incidental trauma (e.g., falls, burns)

May exhibit: Forgets how to negotiate places away from home, ignores safety issues
Presence of ecchymosis, lacerations
Disturbance of gait
Striking out/violence toward others

SOCIAL INTERACTIONS

May exhibit: Fragmented speech, aphasia, and dysphasia
Ignore rules of social conduct/inappropriate behavior
Prior psychosocial factors (individuality and personality influence present altered behavioral patterns)
Family roles possibly altered/reversed as individual becomes more dependent

TEACHING/LEARNING

Family history of DAT (four times greater than general population), incidence of primary degenerative dementia is more common in women (who live longer) than in men, vascular dementia occurs more often in men than in women
May present a total healthy picture except for memory/behavioral changes
Use/misuse of medications, OTC drugs, including alcohol
Difficulty managing medications

Discharge plan considerations: May require support and legal services, financial assistance, caregiver support groups, respite and home health care

DIAGNOSTIC STUDIES

Although no diagnostic studies are specific for Alzheimer's disease, these studies are used to rule out reversible problems that may be confused with these types of dementia.

Antibodies: Abnormally high levels may be found (leading to a theory of an immunologic defect).

$ApoE_4$: Screens for the presence of a genetic defect associated with the common form of DAT.

CBC, RPR, electrolytes, thyroid studies: May determine or eliminate treatable/reversible dysfunctions (e.g., metabolic disease processes, fluid/electrolyte imbalance, neurosyphilis).

Vitamin B_{12}: May disclose a nutritional deficit if low.

Folate levels: Low level can affect memory function.

Dexamethasone suppression test (DST): Rules out treatable depression.

ECG: Rules out cardiac insufficiency.

EEG: May be normal or show some slowing (aids in establishing treatable brain dysfunctions), may also reveal focal lesions (vascular).

Skull radiographs: Usually normal but may reveal signs of head trauma.

Vision/Hearing tests: Rule out deficits that may be the cause of or contribute to disorientation, mood swings, altered sensory perceptions (rather than cognitive impairment).

Positron-emission tomography (PET) scan, brain electrical activity mapping (BEAM), magnetic resonance imaging (MRI): May show areas of decreased brain metabolism characteristic of DAT. (In the future, scans may become a screening tool to reveal early changes, such as plaque formation or development of neurofibrillary tangles, for those at risk of developing dementia.)

CT scan: May show widening of ventricles or cortical atrophy.

CSF: Presence of abnormal protein from the brain cells is 90% indicative of DAT.

Tropicamide (Mydriacyl) pupil response test: Hypersensitive to drugs that block the action of acetylcholine. Pupil dilation response to the eyedrops seems equal in clients with mild or early-stage DAT as in severe stage; therefore, this test may provide an early screening tool but is still being researched.

Alzheimer's disease–associated protein (ADAP): Postmortem studies have yielded positive results in more than 80% of DAT clients. Adaptation of ADAP for live testing is being investigated.

Neurologic mental status examination: The client is asked to perform maneuvers or answer questions that are designed to elicit information about the condition of specific parts of the brain or peripheral nerves. Testing will assess mental status and alertness, muscle strength, reflexes, sensory-perception, language skills, and coordination.

NURSING PRIORITIES

1. Provide safe environment, prevent injury.
2. Promote socially acceptable responses, limit inappropriate behavior.
3. Maintain reality orientation/prevent sensory deprivation/overload.
4. Encourage participation in self-care within individual abilities.
5. Promote coping mechanisms of client/significant other(s).
6. Support client/family in grieving process.
7. Provide information about disease process, prognosis, and resources available for assistance.

DISCHARGE GOALS

Not indicated in home/community setting. Following inpatient care, based on underlying condition requiring admission.

NURSING DIAGNOSIS: risk for Injury/Trauma

Risk factors may include

Inability to recognize/identify danger in environment, impaired judgment
Disorientation, confusion, agitation, irritability, excitability
Weakness, muscular incoordination, balancing difficulties, disturbed perception (e.g. missing chairs, steps)
Seizure activity

Possibly evidenced by:

[Not applicable; presence of signs and symptoms establishes an *actual* diagnosis.]

DESIRED OUTCOMES/EVALUATION CRITERIA—FAMILY/CAREGIVER(S) WILL:

Safe Home Environment (NOC)

Recognize potential risks in the environment
Identify and implement steps to correct/compensate for individual factors.

CLIENT WILL: Physical Injury Severity (NOC)

Be free of injury.

ACTIONS/INTERVENTIONS	RATIONALE
ENVIRONMENTAL MANAGEMENT: Safety (NIC)	
Independent	
Assess degree of impairment in ability/competence, presence of impulsive behavior.	Identifies potential risks in the environment and heightens awareness of risks so caregivers are more alert to dangers. Clients demonstrating impulsive behavior are at increased risk of injury because they are less able to control their own behavior/actions.
Assist SO to identify any risks/potential hazards and visual-perceptual deficits that may be present.	Visual-perceptual deficits increase the risk of falls.
Eliminate/minimize identified hazards in the environment.	A person with cognitive impairment and perceptual disturbances is prone to accidental injury because of the inability to take responsibility for basic safety needs or to evaluate the unforeseen consequences (e.g., may light a stove/cigarette and forget about it, mistake plastic fruit for the real thing and eat it, misjudge distance involving chairs and stairs). Preventive measures can contain client without constant supervision. Activities promote involvement and keep client occupied.
Lock outside doors as appropriate, especially in evening/night. Do not allow access to stairwell or exit. Provide supervision and activities for client who is regularly awake during night. Recommend use of "child-proof locks," secure such items as medications, cleaning products, poisonous substances, tools, sharp objects. Remove stove knobs, burners.	As the disease worsens, the client may fidget with objects/locks (hypermetamorphosis) or put small items in mouth (hyperorality), which potentiates possibility of accidental injury/death.
Dementia Management (NIC)	
Monitor behavior routinely, note timing of behavioral changes, increasing confusion, hyperactivity. Initiate least restrictive interventions before behavior escalates.	Early identification of negative behaviors with appropriate action can prevent need for more stringent measures. *Note:* "Sundowner syndrome" (increased restlessness, wandering, aggression) may develop in late afternoon/early evening, requiring programmed interventions and closer monitoring at this time to redirect and protect client.
Distract/redirect client's attention when behavior is agitated or dangerous (e.g., climbing out of bed). Place bed in low position/mattress on floor as indicated.	Maintains safety while avoiding a confrontation that could escalate behavior/increase risk of injury.
Obtain/have client wear identification jewelry (bracelet/necklace) showing name, phone number, and diagnosis.	Facilitates safe return of client if lost. Because of poor verbal ability and confusion, these persons may be unable to state name, address, phone number. Client may wander, exhibit poor judgment, and be detained by police, appearing confused, irritable, or having violent outbursts.
Dress according to physical environment/individual need.	The general slowing of metabolic processes results in lowered body heat. The hypothalamic gland may be affected by the disease process or by aging, causing person to feel cold. Client

ACTIONS/INTERVENTIONS	RATIONALE
	may have seasonal disorientation and may wander out in the cold. *Note:* Leading causes of death in these clients are pneumonia and accidents.
Be attentive to nonverbal physiologic symptoms.	Because of sensory loss and language dysfunction, may express needs nonverbally (e.g., thirst by panting; pain by sweating, doubling over). *Note:* Wandering may be a coping mechanism as client seeks a change in environment (too hot/cold, bored/overstimulated), searches for food/bathroom, or relief from discomfort (pain/adverse drug reaction).
Be alert to underlying meaning of verbal statements.	May direct a question to another, such as, "Are you cold/tired?" meaning client is cold/tired.
Monitor for medication side effects, signs of overmedication (e.g., extrapyramidal signs, orthostatic hypotension, visual disturbances, GI upsets).	Client may not be able to report signs/symptoms, and drugs can easily build up to toxic levels in the elderly. Dosages/drug choice may need to be altered.
Provide quiet room/activity.	Overstimulation increases irritability/agitation, which can escalate to violent outbursts.
Avoid use of restraints. Have SO/others stay with client during periods of acute agitation.	Endangers the individual who succeeds in partial removal of restraints. May increase agitation and potentiate fall-risk and fractures in the elderly.

Collaborative

Administer medications as appropriate; e.g., risperidone (Risperdal), olanzapine (Zyprexa), quetiapine (Seroquel), ziprasidone (Geodon).	Some of the newer antipsychotics are favored to control agitation, aggression, halluncinations, thought disturbances, and wandering because of their lessened propensity to cause anticholinergic and extrapyramidal side effects. May help moderate "sundowning" behaviors. *Note:* Condition may be related to deterioration of the suprachiasmatic nucleus of the hypothalamus (controls the sleep-wake cycle) with disturbance of circadian rhythms.

NURSING DIAGNOSIS: chronic Confusion

May be related to

Irreversible neuronal degeneration

Possibly evidenced by

Disturbed interpretation/response to stimuli
Progressive/long-standing cognitive impairment, impaired short-term memory
Disturbed personality; impaired socialization
Clinical evidence of organic impairment

DESIRED OUTCOMES/EVALUATION CRITERIA— CLIENT WILL:

Personal Well-Being (NOC)

Experience a decrease in level of frustration, especially when participating in daily activities.

FAMILY/CAREGIVER WILL:

CAREGIVER PERFORMANCE: Direct Care (NOC)

Verbalize understanding of disease process and client's needs.
Identify/participate in interventions to deal effectively with situation.
Provide for maximal independence while meeting safety need of clients.
Initiate behaviors/lifestyle changes to maximize client's cognitive functioning.

ACTIONS/INTERVENTIONS	RATIONALE
Dementia Management (NIC)	
Independent	
Assess degree of cognitive impairment (e.g., changes in orientation to person, place, time; attention span; thinking ability). Talk with SO about changes from usual behavior/length of time problem has existed.	Provides baseline for future evaluation/ comparison, and influences choice of interventions. *Note*: Repeated evaluation of orientation may actually heighten negative responses/client's level of frustration.
Maintain a pleasant, quiet environment.	Reduces distorted input, whereas crowds, clutter, and noise generate sensory overload that stresses the impaired neurons.
Approach in a slow, calm manner.	This nonverbal gesture lessens the chance of misinterpretation and potential agitation. Hurried approaches can startle and threaten the confused client who misinterprets or feels threatened by imaginary people and/or situations.
Face the individual when conversing.	Maintains reality, expresses interest, and arouses attention, particularly in persons with perceptual disturbances.
Address client by name.	Names form our self-identity and establish reality and individual recognition. Client may respond to own name long after failing to recognize SO.
Use lower voice register and speak slowly to client.	Increases the chance for comprehension. High-pitched, loud tones convey stress and anger, which may trigger memory of previous confrontations and provoke an angry response.
Give simple directions, one at a time, or step-by-step instructions, using short words and simple sentences.	As the disease progresses, the communication centers in the brain become impaired, hindering the individual's ability to process and comprehend complex messages. Simplicity is the key to communicating (both verbally and nonverbally) with the cognitively impaired person.
Pause between phrases or questions.	Invites a verbal response and may increase comprehension.
Give hints and use open-ended phrases when possible.	Hints stimulate communication and give the person a chance for a positive experience.
Listen with regard despite content of client's speech.	Conveys interest and worth to the individual.
Interpret statements, meanings, and words. If possible, supply the correct word.	Assisting the client with word processing aids in decreasing frustration.
Reduce provocative stimuli: negative criticism, arguments, confrontations.	Any provocation decreases self-esteem and may be interpreted as a threat, which may trigger agitation or increase inappropriate behavior.
Use distraction. Talk about real people and real events when client begins ruminating about false ideas, unless talking realistically increases anxiety/agitation.	Rumination promotes disorientation. Reality orientation increases client's sense of reality, self-worth, and personal dignity.
Refrain from forcing activities and communications.	Force decreases cooperation and may increase suspiciousness, delusions.
Change activity if client loses interest in present activity.	Changing activity maintains interest and reduces restlessness and possibility of confrontation.
Use humor with interactions.	Laughter can assist in communication.
Focus on appropriate behavior. Give verbal feedback, positive reinforcement (e.g., a pat on the back, applause). Use touch judiciously and respect individual's personal space/response.	Reinforces correctness, appropriate behavior. A focus on inappropriate behavior can encourage repetition. Although touch frequently transcends verbal interchange (conveying warmth, acceptance, and reality), the individual may misinterpret the meaning of touch, and intrusion into personal space may be interpreted as threatening because of the client's distorted perceptions.
Respect individuality and evaluate individual needs.	Persons experiencing a cognitive decline deserve respect, dignity, and recognition of worth as an individual. Client's past and background are important in maintaining self-concept, planning activities, communication, etc.

ACTIONS/INTERVENTIONS	RATIONALE
Allow personal belongings.	Familiarity enhances security, sense of self, and decreases feelings of loss/deprivation.
Permit hoarding of safe objects.	This activity may preserve security and counter-balances irrevocable losses.
Create simple, noncompetitive activities paced to the individual's abilities. Provide entertaining, memory-stimulating music, videos, TV programs. Engage in old hobbies, preferred activities (e.g., arts/crafts, music, supervised cooking, gardening, spiritual programs).	Motivates client in ways that will reinforce usefulness and self-worth and stimulate reality.
Make useful activities (jobs) out of hoarding and repetitive motions (e.g., collecting junk mail, creating scrapbook, folding/unfolding linen, bouncing balls, dusting, sweeping floors).	May decrease restlessness and provide option for pleasurable activity. Having a "job" helps client feel useful.
Provide several drawers/baskets that are acceptable to rummage through. Fill with safe items that would be of interest to client; e.g., yarn balls, quilt blocks, fabrics with different texture and colors; baby clothes, pictures, costume jewelry (without pins), small tools, sports magazines.	Availability of this kind of assortment provides stimulation that enhances the sense and promotes memories of past life experiences.
Help client find misplaced items, label drawers/ belongings. Do not challenge client.	May decrease defensiveness when client believes he or she is being accused of stealing a misplaced, hoarded, or hidden item. To refute the accusation will not change the belief and may invite anger.
Monitor phone use closely. Post significant phone numbers in prominent place, secure long-distance numbers.	Can be used as reality orientation. However, client may forget time of day when making calls, try to call dead relative. Impaired judgment does not allow for distinguishing long-distance numbers and makes client easy prey for phone sales pitches.
Evaluate sleep/rest pattern and adequacy. Note lethargy, increasing irritability/confusion, frequent yawning, dark circles under eyes.	Lack of sleep can impair cognitive function and coping abilities. (Refer to ND: disturbed Sleep Pattern.)
Monitor for medication side effects, signs of overmedication.	Drugs can easily build up to toxic levels in the elderly, aggravating confusion. Dosages/drug choice may need to be altered.

Collaborative

Administer medications as individually indicated:	
Acetylcholinesterase inhibitors: e.g., Tacrine (Cognex), donepezil (Aricept), rivastigmine (Exelon), galantamine (Reminyl);	These medications are being used for the treatment of mild to moderate cognitive impairment in Alzheimer's disease. They act by elevating acetylcholine concentrations in the cerebral cortex by slowing the degradation of acetylcholine released by still intact cholinergic neurons. Because their action relies on functionally intact cholinergic neurons, the effects of these medications may lessen as the disease advances. There is no evidence that cholinesterase inhibitors alter the course of the underlying dementia process.
Antipsychotic agents: e.g., haloperidol (Haldol), risperidone (Risperdal), quetiapine (Seroquel), olanzapine (Zyprexa);	Psychotic symptoms (typically paranoid delusions and formed visual hallucinations) respond to neuroleptic management in most clients in dementia. *Note*: Phenothiazines may cause oversedation, excitation, or bizarre reactions. Presence of postural hypotension increases the risk of falls and development of constipation, requiring inclusion of a bowel program.
N-methyl-D-aspartate antagonist: memantine (Namenda, Axura);	This medication was recently approved by the FDA for treatment of moderate to severe Alzheimer's disease. It slows the progression of the disease and has been shown to improve cognitive and physical abilities in the later stages of the disease.

ACTIONS/INTERVENTIONS	RATIONALE
Anxiolytic agents: busipirone (Buspar), diazepam (Valium), trazadone (Desyrel); lorazepam (Ativan), chlordiazepoxide (Librium), oxazepam (Serax);	More useful in early/mild stages for relief of anxiety. It can increase confusion/paranoia in the elderly. *Note*: Serax may be preferred because it is shorter action.
thiamine;	Studies are currently underway to verify the usefulness of high doses of thiamine during the early phase of the disease to slow progression of impairment/slightly improve cognition.
Investigational drugs approved for other uses; e.g.: NSAIDs, such as ibuprofen (Motrin), estrogen, *Ginkgo biloba*, vitamin E, selegiline (Eldepryl), prednisone.	These drugs are being studied for possible benefit of treatment or for delaying the onset/progression of DAT.

NURSING DIAGNOSIS: disturbed Sensory Perception (specify)

May be related to

Altered sensory reception, transmission, and/or integration (neurologic disease/deficit)
Socially restricted environment (homebound/ institutionalized)
Sleep deprivation

Possibly evidenced by

Changes in usual response to stimuli (e.g., spatial disorientation, confusion, rapid mood swings)
Change in problem-solving abilities, altered abstraction/conceptualization
Exaggerated emotional responses (e.g., anxiety, paranoia, and hallucinations)
Inability to tell position of body parts
Diminished/altered sense of taste

DESIRED OUTCOMES/EVALUATION CRITERIA— CLIENT WILL:

Sensory Function Status (NOC)

Demonstrate improved/appropriate response to stimuli.

CAREGIVER(S) WILL:

Risk Control (NOC)

Identify/control external factors that contribute to alterations in sensory/perceptual abilities.

ACTIONS/INTERVENTIONS	RATIONALE
Reality Orientation (NIC)	
Independent	
Assess degree of impairment and how it affects the individual, including hearing/visual deficits.	Although brain involvement is usually global, a small percentage of clients may exhibit asymmetrical involvement, which may cause the client to neglect one side of the body (unilateral neglect). Client may not be able to locate internal cues, recognize hunger/thirst, perceive external pain, or locate body within the environment.

ACTIONS/INTERVENTIONS	RATIONALE
Encourage use of corrective lenses and hearing aids as appropriate.	May enhance sensory input, limit/reduce misinterpretation of stimuli.
Maintain a reality-oriented relationship and environment.	Reduces confusion and promotes coping with the frustrating struggles of misperception and being disoriented/confused.
Provide clues for 24-hr reality orientation with calendars, clocks, notes, cards, signs, music, seasonal hues, scenic pictures; color-code rooms.	Dysfunction in visual-spatial perception interferes with the ability to recognize directions and patterns, and the client may become lost even in familiar surroundings. Clues are tangible reminders that aid recognition and may permeate memory gaps, increasing independence.
Provide quiet, nondistracting environment when indicated (e.g., soft music, plain but colorful wallpaper/paint).	Helps to avoid visual/auditory overload, by emphasizing qualities of calmness, consistency. *Note*: Patterned wallpaper may be disturbing to the client.
Provide touch in a caring way.	May enhance perception to self/body boundaries.
Engage client in individually meaningful activities, supporting remaining abilities and minimizing failures (e.g., daily living skills including meal preparation, setup/cleaning activities, making bed, gardening/watering plants).	Supports client's dignity, familiarizes individual with home/community events, and enables him or her to experience satisfaction and pleasure.
Use sensory games to stimulate reality (e.g., smell mentholated ointment and tell of the time mother used it on client; use of spring/fall nature boxes).	Communicates reality through multiple channels.
Indulge in periodic reminiscence (old music, historical events, photos/mementoes, videos).	Stimulates recollections, awakens memories, aids in the preservation of self/individuality via past accomplishments; increases feelings of security. Helpful in easing adaptation to a changed environment.
Provide intellectual activities (e.g., word games, review of current events, storytime, travel discussions).	Stimulates remaining cognitive abilities and provides a sense of normalcy.
Include in Bible study group, church activities, TV services for shut-ins; or arrange for visitation by clergy/spiritual advisor as appropriate.	Provides opportunity to meet spiritual needs and to maintain connection with religious beliefs; may help reduce sense of isolation from humanity.
Encourage simple outings, short walks. Monitor activity.	Outings refresh reality and provide pleasurable sensory stimuli, which may reduce suspiciousness/hallucinations caused by feelings of imprisonment. Motor functioning may be decreased, because nerve degeneration results in weakness, decreasing stamina.
Promote balanced physiologic functions using colorful Nerfballs/beachballs or beanbags for tossing, target games, marching, dancing, or arm dancing with music.	Preserves mobility (reducing the potential for bone loss and muscle atrophy), provides diversional activity and opportunity for interaction with others.
Involve in activities with others as dictated by individual situation (e.g., one-to-one visitors, animal visitation, socialization groups at an Alzheimer center, occupational therapy including crafts, paintings/finger paints, modeling clay).	Provides opportunity for the stimulation of participation with others and may maintain some level of social interaction.

NURSING DIAGNOSIS: Fear

May be related to

Decreases in functional abilities
Public disclosure of disabilities
Further mental/physical deterioration

Possibly evidenced by

Social isolation
Apprehension, irritability, defensiveness, suspiciousness
Aggressive behavior

DESIRED OUTCOMES/EVALUATION CRITERIA— CLIENT WILL:

Fear Level (NOC)

Demonstrate more appropriate range of feelings and lessened fear.

ACTIONS/INTERVENTIONS	RATIONALE
Anxiety Reduction (NIC)	
Independent	
Note change of behavior, suspiciousness, irritability, defensiveness.	Change in moods may be one of the first signs of cognitive decline, and the client, fearing helplessness, tries to hide the increasing inability to remember and engage in normal activities.
Identify strengths the individual had previously.	Facilitates assistance with communication and management of current deficits.
Deal with aggressive behavior by imposing calm, firm limits.	Acceptance can reduce fear and lessen progression of aggressive behavior.
Provide clear, honest information about actions/events.	Assists in maintaining trust and orientation as long as possible. When the client knows the truth about what is happening, coping is often enhanced, and guilt over what is imagined is decreased.
Discuss feelings of SO/caregivers. Acknowledge normalcy of feelings/concerns and provide information as needed.	Client senses but may not understand reaction of others. This may heighten client's sense of anxiety/fear.

NURSING DIAGNOSIS: anticipatory Grieving

May be related to

Client awareness of something "being wrong" with changes in memory/family reaction, physiopsychosocial well-being
Family perception of potential loss of loved one

Possibly evidenced by

Expressions of distress/anger at potential loss
Choked feelings, crying
Alteration in activity level, communication patterns, eating habits, and sleep patterns

DESIRED OUTCOMES/EVALUATION CRITERIA— CLIENT/FAMILY WILL:

PSYCHOSOCIAL ADJUSTMENT: Life Change (NOC)

Express concerns openly.
Discuss loss and participate in planning for the future.

ACTIONS/INTERVENTIONS	RATIONALE
Grief Work Facilitation (NIC)	
Independent	
Assess degree of deterioration/level of coping.	Information is helpful to understand how much the client is capable of doing to maintain highest level of independence and to provide encouragement to help individuals deal with losses.
Provide open environment for discussion. Use therapeutic communication skills of active-listening, acknowledgment.	Encourages client/SOs to discuss feelings and concerns realistically.
Note statements of despair, hopelessness, "nothing to live for," expressions of anger.	May be indicative of suicidal ideation. Angry behavior may be client's way of dealing with feelings of despair.
Respect desire not to talk.	May not be ready to deal with or share grief.
Be honest; do not give false reassurances or dire predictions about the future.	Honesty promotes a trusting relationship. Expressions of gloom, such as, "You'll spend the rest of your life in a nursing home," are not helpful. (No one knows what the future holds.)
Discuss with client/SOs ways they can plan together for the future.	Having a part in problem solving/planning can provide a sense of control over anticipated events.
Assist client/SO to identify positive aspects of the situation.	Ongoing research, possibility of slow progression may offer some hope for the future.
Identify strengths client and SO see in self/situation and support systems available.	Recognizing these resources provides opportunity to work through feelings of grief.
Collaborative	
Refer to other resources (e.g., support groups, counseling, spiritual advisor).	May need additional support/assistance to resolve feelings.

NURSING DIAGNOSIS: disturbed Sleep Pattern

May be related to

Sensory impairments
Psychologic stress (neurologic impairment)
Changes in activity pattern

Possibly evidenced by

Changes in behavior and performance, irritability
Disorientation (day/night reversal)
Wakefulness/interrupted sleep, increased aimless wandering, inability to identify need/time for sleeping
Lethargy, dark circles under eyes, frequent yawning

DESIRED OUTCOMES/EVALUATION CRITERIA— CLIENT WILL:

Sleep (NOC)

Establish adequate sleep pattern, with wandering reduced.
Report/appear rested.

ACTIONS/INTERVENTIONS	RATIONALE
Sleep Enhancement (NIC)	
Independent	
Provide for adequate rest. Restrict daytime sleep as appropriate; increase interaction time between client and family/staff during day, then reduce mental activity late in the day.	Although prolonged physical and mental activity results in fatigue, which can increase confusion, programmed activity without overstimulation promotes sleep.
Avoid use of continuous restraints.	Restraints may potentiate sensory deprivation, agitation, and restrict rest. *Note*: HCFA guidelines require that clients be free from chemical or mechanical restraint unless warranted by a medical diagnosis and that the least restrictive means of control be used.
Evaluate level of stress/orientation as day progresses.	Increasing confusion, disorientation, and uncooperative behaviors ("sundowner's syndrome") may interfere with attaining restful sleep pattern.
Adhere to regular bedtime schedule and rituals. Tell client that it is time to sleep.	Reinforces that it is bedtime and maintains stability of environment. *Note*: Later-than-normal bedtime may be indicated to allow client to dissipate excess energy and facilitate falling asleep.
Provide evening snack, warm milk, bath, back rub/general massage with lotion.	Promotes relaxation and drowsiness and helps to address skin-care needs.
Reduce fluid intake in the evening. Toilet before retiring.	Decreases need to get up to go to the bathroom/incontinence during the night.
Provide soft music or "white noise."	Reduces sensory stimulation by blocking out other environmental sounds that could interfere with restful sleep.
Allow to sleep in shoes/clothing if client demands.	Provided no harm is done, altering the "normal" lessens the rebellion and allows rest.
Collaborative	
Administer medications as indicated for sleep: antidepressants: e.g., doxepin (Sinequan), sertraline (Zoloft), and paroxetine (Paxil); trazodone (Desyrel);	May be effective in treating pseudodementia or depression, improving ability to sleep. However, tricyclic antidepressants are avoided because the anticholinergic properties can induce side effects, which are not tolerated well.
Sedative-hypnotics; e.g., oxazepam (Serax), triazolam (Halcion), zolpidiem (Ambien).	Used sparingly, low-dose, short-acting, rapid-onset hypotics may be effective in treating insomnia or sundowner syndrome.
Avoid use of diphenhydramine (Benadryl).	Once used for sleep, this drug is now contraindicated because it interferes with the production of acetylcholine, which is already inhibited in the brains of clients with DAT.

NURSING DIAGNOSIS: Self-Care Deficit (specify type/level)

May be related to

Cognitive decline, physical limitations
Frustration over loss of independence, depression

Possibly evidenced by

Impaired ability to perform ADLs (e.g., frustration, forgetfulness, misuse/misidentification of objects, inability to bring food from receptacle to mouth, inability to wash body part(s), regulate water temperature, impaired ability to put on/take off clothing, difficulty completing toileting tasks)

DESIRED OUTCOMES/EVALUATION CRITERIA— CLIENT WILL:

Self-Care Status (NOC)

Perform self-care activities within level of own ability.

CAREGIVER WILL:

Caregiver Home Care Readiness (NIC)

Identify and use personal/community resources that can provide assistance; support client's independence.

ACTIONS/INTERVENTIONS	RATIONALE
SELF-CARE ASSISTANCE: [specify] (NIC)	
Independent	
Identify reason for difficulty in self-care; e.g., physical limitations in motion, apathy/depression, cognitive decline (such as apraxia), or room temperature ("too cold to get dressed").	Underlying cause affects choice of interventions/ strategies. Problem may be minimized by, e.g., changes in environment or adaptation of clothing, or may be more complex, requiring consultation from other specialists. Important to distinguish between partial and total dependence to avoid creating excess disability. *Note:* Clients reported to be unable to perform specific ADLs are often able to do so given the right circumstances (e.g., adequate/knowledgeable caregiver support).
Determine hygienic needs and provide assistance as needed with activities, including care of hair/nails/ skin, brushing teeth, cleaning glasses.	As the disease progresses, basic hygienic needs may be forgotten. Infection, gum disease, disheveled appearance, or harm may occur when client/caregivers become frustrated, irritated, or intimidated by degree of care required.
Inspect skin regularly.	Presence of such lesions as ecchymoses, lacerations, rashes may require treatment, as well as signal the need for closer monitoring/protective interventions.
Incorporate usual routine into activity schedule as possible. Wait or change the time to initiate dressing/hygiene if a problem arises.	Maintaining routine may prevent worsening of confusion and enhance cooperation. Because anger is quickly forgotten, another time or approach maybe successful.
Be attentive to nonverbal physiologic symptoms.	Sensory loss and language dysfunction may cause client to express self-care needs in nonverbal manner (e.g., thirst by panting, need to void by holding self/fidgeting, pain by facial grimacing).
Be alert to underlying meaning of verbal statements.	May direct a question to another, such as "Are you cold?" meaning "I am cold and need additional clothing."
Supervise but allow as much autonomy as possible.	Eases the frustration over lost independence.
Allot plenty of time to perform tasks.	Tasks that were once easy (e.g., dressing, bathing) are now complicated by decreased motor skills or cognitive and physical changes. Time and patience can reduce chaos resulting from trying to hasten this process.
Assist with neat dressing/provide colorful clothes.	Enhances esteem; may diminish sense of sensory loss and convey aliveness.
Offer one item of clothing at a time in sequential order. Talk through each step of the task one at a time. Allow the wearing of extra clothing if client demands.	Simplicity reduces frustration and the potential for rage and despair. Guidance reduces confusion and allows autonomy. Altering the "normal" may lessen rebellion.
Provide reminders for elimination needs. Involve in bowel/bladder program as appropriate.	Loss of control/independence in this self-care activity can have a great impact on self-esteem and may limit socialization. (Refer to ND: Constipation)
Assist with and provide reminders for pericare after toileting/incontinence.	Good hygiene promotes cleanliness and reduces risks of skin irritation and infection.

NURSING DIAGNOSIS: risk for imbalanced Nutrition: less/more than body requirements

Risk factors may include

Sensory changes
Impaired judgment and coordination
Agitation, forgetfulness, regressed habits, and concealment

Possibly evidenced by:

[Not applicable; presence of signs and symptoms establishes an *actual* diagnosis.]

DESIRED OUTCOMES/EVALUATION CRITERIA— CLIENT WILL:

Nutritional Status (NOC)

Ingest nutritionally balanced diet.
Maintain/regain appropriate weight.

ACTIONS/INTERVENTIONS	RATIONALE
Nutrition Management (NIC)	
Independent	
Assess SO/client's knowledge of nutritional needs.	Identifies needs to assist in formulating individual teaching plan. A role-reversal situation can occur (e.g., child now cooking for parent, husband taking over "duties" of wife), increasing the need for information.
Determine amount of exercise/pacing client does.	Nutritional intake may need to be adjusted to meet needs related to individual energy expenditure.
Offer/provide assistance in menu selection.	Poor judgment may lead to poor choices; client may be indecisive/overwhelmed by choices and/or unaware of the need to maintain elemental nutrition. *Note:* In general, metabolic rate decreases with age, requiring caloric adjustment that must be balanced with activity.
Provide privacy when eating habits become an insoluble problem. Accept eating with hands, spills, and whimsical mixtures (e.g., salad dressing in milk, salt and pepper on ice cream). Avoid solo dining or separating client from other people too early in the disease process.	Socially unacceptable and embarrassing eating habits develop as the disease progresses. Acceptance preserves esteem; decreases irritability or refusal to eat as a result of anger, frustration. Early separation can result in client feeling upset and rejected and can actually result in decreased food intake.
Offer small feelings and/or snacks of one or two foods around the clock as indicated.	Large feedings may overwhelm the client, resulting either in complete abstinence or gorging. Small feedings may enhance appropriate intake. Limiting number of foods offered at a single time reduces confusion regarding which food to choose.
Simplify steps of eating (e.g., serve food in courses).	Promotes autonomy and independence; decreases potential frustration/anger over lost abilities.
Anticipate needs, cut foods, provide soft/finger foods.	Coordination decreases as the disease progresses, which impairs the client's ability to chew and handle utensils.
Provide ample time for eating.	A leisurely approach aids digestion and decreases the chance of anger precipitated by rushing.
Place food items in pita bread/paper sack for the client who paces.	Carrying food may encourage client to eat.
Avoid baby food and excessively hot foods.	Baby foods lack adequate nutritional content, fiber, and taste for adults, and can add to client's humiliation. Hot foods may result in mouth burns and/or refusal to eat.

ACTIONS/INTERVENTIONS	RATIONALE
Observe swallowing ability; monitor oral cavity.	Diminished abilities may result in client/caregiver repeatedly placing food in client's mouth, which is not swallowed, increasing risk of aspiration.
Stimulate oral-suck reflex by gentle stroking of the cheeks or stimulating the mouth with a spoon.	As the disease progresses, the client may clench teeth and refuse to eat. Stimulating the reflex may increase cooperation/intake.

Collaborative

Refer to dietitian.	Assistance may be needed to develop nutritionally balanced diet individualized to meet client needs/food preferences.

NURSING DIAGNOSIS: Constipation (specify)/Bowel Incontinence/impaired Urinary Elimination

May be related to

Disorientation, inability to locate the bathroom/recognize need
Lost neurologic functioning/muscle tone
Changes in dietary/fluid intake

Possibly evidenced by

Urgency/inappropriate toileting behaviors
Incontinence/constipation

DESIRED OUTCOMES/EVALUATION CRITERIA— CLIENT/CAREGIVER WILL:

Bowel [or] Urinary Elimination (NOC)

Establish adequate/appropriate pattern of elimination.

ACTIONS/INTERVENTIONS | RATIONALE

Urinary Elimination [or] Bowel Management (NIC)

Independent

ACTIONS/INTERVENTIONS	RATIONALE
Assess prior pattern and compare with current situation.	Provides information about changes that may require further assessment/intervention.
Locate bed near a bathroom when possible; make signs for/color code door. Provide adequate lighting, particularly at night.	Promotes orientation/finding bathroom. Incontinence may be attributed to inability to find a toilet.
Take client to the toilet at regular intervals. Dictate each step one at a time and use positive reinforcement.	Adherence to a daily and regular schedule may prevent accidents. Frequently the problem is forgetting how to toilet (e.g., pushing pants down, positioning).
Establish bowel/bladder training program. Promote client participation to level of ability.	Stimulates awareness, enhances regulation of body function, and helps to avoid accidents.
Encourage adequate fluid intake during the day (at least 2 L as appropriate), diet high in fiber and fruit juices. Limit intake during the late evening and at bedtime.	Essential for bodily functions and prevents potential dehydration/constipation. Restricting intake in evening may reduce frequency/incontinence during the night.
Avoid a sense of hurrying/being rushed.	Hurrying may be perceived as intrusion, which leads to anger and lack of cooperation with activity.

ACTIONS/INTERVENTIONS	RATIONALE
Be alert to nonverbal cues (e.g., restlessness, holding self, or picking at clothes).	May signal urgency/inattention to cues and/or inability to locate bathroom.
Be discreet and respect person's privacy.	Although the client is confused, a sense of modesty is often retained.
Convey acceptance when incontinence occurs. Change promptly; provide good skin care.	Acceptance is important to decrease the embarrassment and feelings of helplessness that may occur during the changing process. Prompt changing reduces risk of skin irritation/breakdown.
Record frequency of voidings/bowel movements.	Provides visual reminder of elimination and may indicate need for intervention.
Monitor appearance/color of urine, note consistency of stool.	Detection of changes provides opportunity to alter interventions to prevent complications or acquire treatment as indicated (e.g., constipation/urinary infection). *Note*: Although it is difficult, the caregiver must try to monitor frequency of bowel movements during the stage of the illness when the client is still toileting self. It is not enough to ask client, "Did you have a bowel movement today?" Client cannot remember. Monitoring is essential to prevent constipation and potential for impaction.

Collaborative

Administer stool softeners, bulk expanders (e.g., Metamucil), or glycerin suppository as indicated.	May be necessary to facilitate/stimulate regular bowel movement.

NURSING DIAGNOSIS: risk for Sexual Dysfunction

Risk factors may include

Altered body function/progression of disease: decrease in habit/control of behavior, confusion, forgetfulness, and disorientation to place or person
Lack of intimacy/sexual rejection by SO
Lack of privacy

Possibly evidenced by:

[Not applicable; presence of signs and symptoms establishes an *actual* diagnosis.]

DESIRED OUTCOMES/ EVALUATION CRITERIA— CLIENT WILL:

Sexual Functioning (NOC)

Meet sexuality needs in an acceptable manner.
Experience fewer/no episodes of inappropriate behavior.

ACTIONS/INTERVENTIONS | RATIONALE

Sexual Counseling (NIC)

Independent

Assess individual needs/desires/abilities of client and partner.	Alternative methods need to be designed for the individual situation to fulfill the need for intimacy and closeness.
Encourage partner to show affection/acceptance.	The cognitively impaired person retains the basic needs for affection, love, acceptance, and sexual expression.

ACTIONS/INTERVENTIONS	RATIONALE
Ensure privacy or encourage home visitation for residential client as appropriate.	Sexual expression or behaviors may differ. The individual may masturbate, expose self. Privacy allows sexual expression without embarrassment and the objections of others.
Use distraction as indicated. Remind client that, when in a public area, sexual behavior is unacceptable.	This tool is useful when there is inappropriate/objectionable behavior (e.g., self-exposure).
Provide time to listen/discuss concerns of SO.	SO may need information and/or counseling about alternatives for sexual activity/aggression.

NURSING DIAGNOSIS: compromised/ disabled family Coping

May be related to

Disruptive behavior of client
Family grief about their helplessness watching loved one deteriorate
Prolonged disease/disability progression that exhausts the supportive capacity of SO
Highly ambivalent family relationships

Possibly evidenced by

Family becoming embarrassed and socially immobilized
Home maintenance becoming extremely difficult, leading to difficult decisions with legal/financial considerations

DESIRED OUTCOMES/EVALUATION CRITERIA— FAMILY WILL:

Family Coping (NOC)

Identify/verbalize resources within themselves to deal with the situation.
Acknowledge client's condition and demonstrate positive coping behaviors in dealing with situation.
Use outside support systems effectively.

ACTIONS/INTERVENTIONS	RATIONALE
Family Support (NIC)	
Independent	
Include family in teaching and planning for home care.	Can ease the burden of home management and increase adaptation. A comfortable and familiar lifestyle at home helps preserve the client's need for belonging.
Review past life experiences, role changes, and coping skills.	Identifies skills that may help individuals cope with grief of current situation more effectively.
Focus on specific problems as they occur, the "here and now."	Disease progression follows no set pattern. A premature focus on the possibility of long-term care or possible incontinence; e.g., impairs the ability to cope with present issues.
Establish priorities.	Helps to create a sense of order and facilitates problem solving.
Be realistic and honest in all matters.	Decreases stress that surrounds false hopes (e.g., that client may regain past level of functioning from advertised or unproven medication).
Reassess family's ability to care for client at home on an ongoing basis.	Behaviors like hoarding, clinging, unjust accusations, angry outbursts, can precipitate family burnout and interfere with ability to provide effective care.

ACTIONS/INTERVENTIONS	RATIONALE
Provide time to listen with regard to concerns/anxieties.	SO/caregiver requires constant support with the multifaceted problems that arise during the course of this illness to ease the process of adaptation and grieving.
Help caregiver/family understand the importance of maintaining psychosocial functioning.	Embarrassing behavior, the demands of care may cause withdrawal from social contact.
Discuss possibility of isolation. Reinforce need for support systems.	The belief that a single individual can meet all the needs of the client increases the potential for physical/mental illness (caregiver role strain). *Note*: Mortality rate for primary caregivers is actually higher than for the client with DAT.
Provide positive feedback for efforts.	Reassures individuals that they are doing their best and provides reinforcement to continue efforts.
Acknowledge concerns generated by consideration/decision to place client in long-term care facility. Answer questions honestly, explore options as appropriate.	Constant care requirements may be more than can be managed by the SO and support systems. Support is needed for this difficult guilt-producing which may create a financial burden as well as family disruption/dissension.
Encourage visitation by extended family/friends as tolerated by client.	Contact with/and familiarity forms a base of reality and can provide a reassuring freedom from loneliness. Recurrent contact helps family members realize and accept situation. *Note* Family members may require ongoing support in dealing with visitation and issues of client's deterioration and their own personal needs.

Collaborative

Involve SO/family members in planning care/problem-solving. Verify presence of Advance Directives/Durable Medical Power of Attorney.	Consensus may be more readily achieved when family participates in decision making. It is important, however, to keep client's wishes in mind when making choices and to be aware of who actually has the power to make decisions for the cognitively impaired client.
Refer to local resources; e.g., adult day care, respite care, homemaker services, or a local chapter of Alzheimer's Disease and Related Disorders Association (ADRDA), National Family Caregivers Association (NFCA).	Coping with these clients is a full-time, frustrating task. Respite/day care may lighten the burden, reduce potential social isolation, and prevent family burnout/caregiver role strain. ADRDA provides group support and family teaching and promotes research. Local groups provide a social outlet for sharing grief and promote problem-solving with such matters as financial/legal advice and home care. NFCA also provides programs for educating caregivers/healthcare providers and a quarterly publication.
Refer for family counseling or to appropriate ethical committee as indicated.	Differing opinions regarding client care/placement can result in conflict requiring professional mediation.

NURSING DIAGNOSIS: impaired Home Maintenance/ineffective Health Maintenance

May be related to

Progressively impaired cognitive functioning
Complete or partial lack of gross and/or fine motor skills
Significant alteration in communication skills
Ineffective individual/family coping
Insufficient family organization or planning
Unfamiliarity with resources, inadequate support systems

Possibly evidenced by

Overtaxed family members (e.g., exhausted, anxious)
Household members express difficulty and request help in maintaining home safely and comfortably
Home surroundings appear disorderly/unsafe
Reported or observed inability to take responsibility for meeting basic health practices
Reported or observed lack of equipment, financial, or other resources, impairment of personal support system

DESIRED OUTCOMES/EVALUATION CRITERIA— FAMILY/CAREGIVER(S) WILL:

Family Resiliency (NOC)

Verbalize ability to cope adequately with existing situation.
Identify factors related to difficulty in maintaining a safe environment for the client.
Assume responsibility for and initiate changes supporting client safety and healthcare goals.
Demonstrate appropriate, effective use of resources (e.g., respite/day care, homemakers, support groups).

ACTIONS/INTERVENTIONS	RATIONALE
Home Maintenance Assistance (NIC)	
Independent	
Evaluate level of cognitive/emotional/ physical functioning (level of independence).	Identifies strengths, areas of need, and how much responsibility the client may be expected to assume. (Refer to ND: Self-Care Deficit.
Assess environment, noting unsafe factors and ability of client to care for self.	Determines what changes need to be made to accommodate disabilities. (Refer to ND: risk for Injury/Trauma).
Identify senior services/community resources for homemaking/cleaning and handyman tasks.	As client's condition worsens, caregiver will require additional support to maintain client in home, especially if family support is limited/not available.
Health System Guidance (NIC)	
Assist client to develop plan for keeping track of/dealing with health needs.	Schedule can be helpful to maintain system for managing routine healthcare services.
Identify support systems available to client/SO (e.g., other family members, friends).	Planning and constant care is necessary to maintain this client at home. If family system is unavailable/unaware, client needs (e.g., nutrition, dental care, eye exams) can be neglected. Primary caregiver can benefit from sharing responsibilities/constant care with others. (Refer to ND: risk for Caregiver Role Strain.)
Evaluate coping abilities, effectiveness, commitment of caregiver(s)/support persons.	Progressive debilitation taxes caregiver(s) and may alter ability to meet client/own needs. (Refer to ND: compromised/disabled family Coping).
Collaborative	
Refer to supportive services as needed.	Medical and social services consultant may be needed to develop ongoing plan/identify resources as needs change.

ACTIONS/INTERVENTIONS	RATIONALE
Identify in home healthcare options; e.g., medical, dental, diagnostic services.	Delivery of health care needs "on site" may prevent exacerbation of confusion, increase cooperation, and provide more accurate picture of client's status.

NURSING DIAGNOSIS: risk for Caregiver Role Strain

Risk factors may include

Illness severity of the care receiver, duration of caregiving required, complexity/amount of caregiving tasks
Caregiver is female, spouse
Care receiver exhibits deviant, bizarre behavior
Family/caregiver isolation, lack of respite and recreation

Possibly evidenced by

[Not applicable; presence of signs/symptoms establishes an *actual* diagnosis.]

DESIRED OUTCOMES/EVALUATION CRITERIA— CAREGIVER WILL:

CAREGIVER PERFORMANCE: Direct Care (NOC)

Identify individual risk factors and appropriate interventions.
Demonstrate/initiate behaviors or lifestyle changes to prevent development of impaired function.

CAREGIVER PERFORMANCE: Indirect Care (NOC)

Use available resources appropriately.
Report satisfaction with plan and support available.

ACTIONS/INTERVENTIONS — RATIONALE

Caregiver Support (NIC)

Independent

ACTIONS/INTERVENTIONS	RATIONALE
Determine family/caregiver's understanding of condition and expectations for the future.	Identifies teaching needs. Provides opportunity to update information and clarify misconceptions.
Provide bibliotherapy.	Materials that can be reviewed as time permits/questions arise can be very helpful in expanding knowledge and providing on-going support.
Identify strengths of caregiver and care receiver.	Helps to use positive aspects of each individual to the best of abilities in daily activities.
Facilitate family conference to share responsibilities as indicated and to stress importance of self-nurturing for caregiver (e.g., pursuing self-development interests, personal needs, hobbies, and social activities).	Helps family to focus on needs of caregiver as well as care receiver. When others are involved in care, the risk of one person becoming overwhelmed is lessened.
Determine available supports and resources currently used.	Organizations (e.g., Alzheimer's Disease and Related Disorders Association [ADRDA], National Family Caregivers Association [NFCA], local support groups) can provide information regarding adequacy of supports, identify needs/possible options, and provide role-models.

ACTIONS/INTERVENTIONS	RATIONALE
Identify alternate-care sources (e.g., sitter/day-care facility), senior care services (e.g., Meals on Wheels/respite care), Alzheimer's programs, home-care agency.	As client's condition worsens, SO may need additional help from several sources to maintain client at home, even on a part-time basis.

Refer to CP: Multiple Sclerosis, ND: risk for Caregiver Role Strain for additional interventions.

NURSING DIAGNOSIS: risk for Relocations Stress Syndrome

Risk factors May include

Little or no preparation for transfer to hospital/extended care setting
Changes in daily routine
Sensory impairment, physical deterioration
Separation from support systems

Possibly evidenced by:

[Not applicable; presence of signs/symptoms establishes an *actual* diagnosis.]

DESIRED OUTCOMES/EVALUATION CRITERIA— CLIENT WILL:

Stress Level (NOC)

Experience minimal disruption of usual activities.
Display limited increase in agitation.

FAMILY/CAREGIVER WILL:

Family Participation in Professional Care (NOC)

Be aware of potential impact of changes on client.
Plan for/coordinate move as situation permits.
Recognize need to provide stability for client during adaptation period.

ACTIONS/INTERVENTIONS	RATIONALE
Relocation Stress Reduction (NIC)	
Independent	
Discuss ramifications of move to new surroundings	Discussing pros and cons of this decision helps those involved to reach an informed decision and feel better about/plan for the future.
Encourage visitation to facility prior to planned move.	Familiarizes family and client with new options to enable them to make informed decision.
Provide clear, honest information about actions/ events.	Decreases "surprises." Assists in maintaining trust and orientation. When the client knows the truth about what is happening, coping may be enhanced.

Refer to CP: Extended Care, ND: risk for Relocation Stress Syndrome for additional interventions.

Bibliography

GENERAL

Books

Deglin, J.H., and Vallerand, AH. (2005). *Davis's Drug Guide for Nurses*, ed 9. Philadelphia: FA Davis.

Doenges, M.E., Moorhouse, M.F., and Geissler-Murr, A.C. (2004). *Nurse's Pocket Guide: Diagnoses, Interventions, and Rationales*, ed. 9. Philadelphia: FA Davis.

Duke, J.A. (2000). *The Green Pharmacy Herbal Handbook.* Kutztown, PA:Rodale.

Ellsworth, A.J., et al. (2004). *Mosby's Medical Drug Reference 2005.* St. Louis: Mosby.

Fetrow, C.W., and Avila, J.R. (2000). *The Complete Guide to Herbal Medicines.* Springhouse, PA: Springhouse.

Gordon, T. (2000). *Parent Effectiveness Training.* New York: Three Rivers Press.

Jaffe, M.S., and McVan, B.F. (1997). *Davis's Laboratory and Diagnostic Test Handbook.* Philadelphia: FA Davis.

Kuhn, M.A. (1998). *Pharmacotherapeutics: A Nursing Approach*, ed 4. Philadelphia: F.A. Davis.

Lewis, S.M., Heitkemper, M.M., and Dirksen, S.R. (2004). *Medical-Surgical Nursing: Assessment and Management of Clinical Problems*, ed 6. St. Louis: Mosby.

Lubkin, I.M., and Larsen, P.D. (2002). *Chronic Illness—Impact and Interventions*, ed. 5. Sudbury, MA: Jones and Bartlett.

McCloskey-Dochterman, J.C., and Bulechek, G.M. (2004). *Nursing Interventions Classification (NIC)*, ed. 4. St. Louis: Mosby.

McNeal, G.J. (2000). *AACN Guide to Acute Care Procedures in the Home.* Philadelphia: Lippincott.

Moorehead, S., Johnson, M., and Maas, M.L. (2004). *Nursing Outcomes Classification (NOC)*, ed. 3. St. Louis: Mosby.

NANDA (2005). *Nursing Diagnoses: Definitions & Classification 2005–2006.* Philadelphia: North American Nursing Diagnosis Association.

Purnell, L.D., and Paulanka, B.J. (2003). *Transcultural Health Care: A Culturally Competent Approach*, ed. 2. Philadelphia: FA Davis.

Rantz, M.J., and Lemone, P. (1999). *Classification of Nursing Diagnosis: Proceedings of the Thirteenth Conference, North American Nursing Diagnosis Association.* Glendale, CA: CINAHL Information Systems.

Sommers, M.S., and Johnson, S.A. (2002). *Diseases and Disorders: A Nursing Therapeutics Manual*, ed. 2. Philadelphia: FA Davis.

Sparks, S.M., and Taylor, C.M. (2005). *Nursing Diagnosis Reference Manual*, ed. 6. Springhouse, PA: Springhouse.

Springhouse (2002). *Diagnostic Tests Made Incredibly Easy!* Springhouse, PA.

Springhouse (2004). *Handbook of Diseases*, ed 3. Springhouse, PA.

Springhouse (2005). *Pathophysiology Made Incredibly Easy!* ed. 3. Springhouse, PA.

Taber's Cyclopedic Medical Dictionary, ed. 20 (2005). Philadelphia: FA Davis.

White, L.B., Foster, S., and the Staff of Herbs for Health. (2003). *The Herbal Drugstore: The Best Natural Alternatives to Over-the Counter and Prescription Medicines!* Kutztown, PA: Rodale.

Wilkinson, J.M. (2005). *Prentice Hall Nursing Diagnosis Handbook: With NIC Interventions and NOC Outcomes*, ed. 8. Upper Saddle River, NJ: Prentice Hall Health.

Articles

Brown, M., and Whalen, P.K. (2000). Red blood cell transfusion in critically ill patients: Emerging risks and alternatives. *Crit Care Nurse/Supplement*, December:1–14.

Dimartino, C. (1999). Herbal therapies: Are there rehab applications? *Rehab Rep*, 10(8):26–29.

Hatcher, T. (2001). The proverbial herb. *AJN*, 101(2):36–43.

Henker, R. (1999). Evidence-based practice: Fever-related interventions. *Am J Crit Care*, 8(1):481–487.

Hussar, D.A. (2000). New drugs 2000. *Nursing2000*, 30(1):55–62.

Mayer, D.M., et al (2001). Speaking the language of pain. *AJN*, 101(2):44–49.

Pasero, C., Gordon, D.B., and McCaffery, M (1999). Pain control: JCAHO on assessing and managing pain. *AJN*, 99(7):22.

Schmidt, L.M. (2004). Herbal remedies: The other drugs your patients take. *Home Healthcare Nurse*, 22(3):169–175.

Journals

Addiction
Advance for Health Information Executives
Advance for Nurses
American Family Physician
American Journal of Critical Care
American Journal of Continuing Care

American Journal of Kidney Disease
American Journal of Nursing
Annals of Internal Medicine
Annals of Neurology
AORN Journal
Archives of General Psychiatry
ARN Network
Burns
Cancer Nursing
Case Manager
CIN: Computers, Informatics, Nursing
Clinical Journal of Oncology Nursing
Critical Care Nurse
Dermatology Nursing
Dimensions of Critical Care Nursing
Electronic Resources
Gastroenterology Nursing
Holistic Nursing Practice
Homecare Provider
Home Healthcare Nurse
Heart and Lung
Image: Journal of Nursing Scholarship
Imprint: The Professional Magazine for Nursing Students
Inside MS
Internal Medicine
Journal of the American Medical Association (JAMA)
Journal of the American Medical Informatics Association
Journal of the Association of Nurses in AIDS Care (JANAC)
Journal of Association of Operating Room Nurses
Journal of Cardiovascular Nursing
Journal of Clinical Investigation
Journal of Legal Nurse Consulting
Journal of Marital and Family Therapy
Journal of Neurology
Journal of Parenteral and Enteral Nutrition
Journal for Prevention and Healing
Journal of Psychosocial Nursing
Journal of School Nursing
Journal of Trauma, Infection and Critical Care
MCN: The American Journal of Maternal/Child Nursing
MD Comput
Neurology
The Nurse Practitioner
Nursing98–Nursing2005
Nursing Diagnosis: The International Journal of Nursing Language and Classification
Nursing Made Incredibly Easy!
Nursing Management
Nursing Times
Nutrition Today
Oncology Nursing Forum
Orthopaedic Nursing
Physical Therapy
Rehabilitation Nursing
Rehab Management
Rehab Report
RN
Seminars in Oncology Nursing
Sexuality and Disability
Team Rehab
Urology Nursing

CHAPTER 1

Articles

Alspach, G. (1998). Patient advocacy: Have we ascended to new heights or fallen to new depths? *Crit Care Nurse,* 18(4):17–19.

Amatayakul, M. (2000). Governmental strategies: The race to standardize medical record information. *MD Comput,* 17(6):22–24.

Aquilino, M.L., and Keenan, G. (2000). Having our say: Nursing's standardized nomenclature. *AJN,* 100(7):33–38.

Blegen, M.A., Goode, C.J, and Reed, L. (1998). Nursing staffing and patient outcomes. *Nurs Res,* 47(1):43–50..

Buerhaus, P.J. (1998). Is a nursing shortage on the way? *Nursing98,* 28(8):34, August.

Harvey, M.A. (1999). Point-of-care laboratory testing in critical care. *Am J Crit Care,* 8(2):72–83.

Haughton, J. (2000). A paradigm shift in healthcare: From disease management to patient-centered systems. *MD Comput,* 17(4):34–38.

Leape, L.L., and Berwick, D.M. (2005). Five years after to err is human: What have we learned? *JAMA,* 293(19):2384–2390.

MacNeil, V. (1999). 2000 and beyond: What's ahead for rehab? *Rehab Rep,* 10(11):12–17.

McFaddin, G.M. (2000). Health care consumers in the internet age. *Advance for Health Information Executives,* 4(6):43–44.

Menninger, B. (2000). The bleeding of healthcare. *Cerner Rep,* 1:4–7.

Millenson, M.L. (2000). The battle for better healthcare. *Cerner Rep,* 1:15–16.

Prescott, P.A. (1993*). Nursing: An important component of hospital survival under a reformed healthcare system. Nurs Econ,* 11(4):192–199.

Spackman, K (2000). SNOMED RT and SNOMED CT: The promise of an international clinical terminology. *MD Comput,* 17(6):29.

Topel, K (2000). Technologies that change patient expectations. *Advance for Health Information Executives,* 4(8)59–66.

Woody, T. (1999). How the net could save your life. *Industry Standard,* 2(6):28–30.

Yang, K.P. (2003). Relationships between nurse staffing and client outcomes. *J Nurs Res, 11*(3):149–58.

No author listed. (2000). Certified nurses report fewer adverse events. *ARN Network,* June/July:8.

Electronic Resources

Abt Associates, Inc. (2003). "Phase II Evaluation of CNO Demonstration, final report to Congress, January 6, 2003. Retrieved May 26, 2004. http://*www.cms.hhs.gov/researchers/reports/2003/CNOPfinalreport.pdf*

State Health Access Data Assistance Center (2002). Characteristics of the uninsured: A view from the states. Prepared by University of Minnesota. Retrieved February 2005 from *http://www.rwjf.org/files/research/BRFFS%20final 3.pdf*

CHAPTER 2

Books

American Nurses Association (1965). *Nursing's Social Policy Statement*. Washington, DC.

American Nurses Association (1991). *Standards of Clinical Nursing Practice*. Kansas City, MO.

Pesut, D.J., and Herman, J. (1999). *Clinical Reasoning, The Art and Science of Critical and Creative Thinking*. Albany, NY: Delmar.

Shore, L.S. (1988). *Nursing Diagnosis: What It Is and How To Do It, A Programmed Text*. Redmond, VA: Medical College of Virginia Hospitals.

Articles

Aquilino, M.L., and Keenan, G. (2000). Having our say: Nursing's standardized nomenclature. *AJN*, 100(7):33–38.

Delaney, C., and Maas, M. (2000). Reliability of nursing diagnoses documented in a computerized nursing information system. *Nurs Diagn*, 11(3):121–134.

CHAPTER 3

Book

Pesut, D.J., and Herman, J. (1999). *Clinical Reasoning, The Art and Science of Critical and Creative Thinking*. Albany, NY: Delmar.

Article

Mueller, A., Johnson, M., and Bligh, D. (2002). Joining mind mapping and care planning to enhance student critical thinking and achieve holistic nursing care. *Nur Diagn*, 13(1):24–27.

CHAPTER 4

Books

Bezruchka, S. (1998 revision). *Altitude Illness Prevention & Treatment*. Seattle, WA: The Mountaineers.

Articles

Aaronson, K. (2000). Exercise for heart failure? *Health News*, 6(8):3.

Abraham, W.T. (2004). The expanding role of natruiretic peptide treatment in management of heart failure. CME Offering. University of Minnesota.

Adams, J.E., and Miracle, V.A. (1998). Cardiac biomarkers: Past, present, and future. *Am J Crit Care*, 7(6):418–423.

Albert, N. (1999). Heart failure: The physiologic basis for current therapeutic concepts. *Crit Care Nurse Suppl*, June:2–13.

American College of Cardiology/American Heart Association Task Force (1999). *Practice Guidelines for the management of patients with AMI*. New York: Elsevier Science.

Artinian, M.T. (2003). The psychosocial aspects of heart failure. *AJN*, 103(12):32–42.

Artinian, M.T. (2004). Innovations in blood presssure monitoring. *AJN*, 104(8):53–60.

Balser, J.R. (2000). Managing arrhythmias after cardiac surgery. *AACN News*, 17(2):10–11.

Bond, E.A., et al. (2003). The left ventricular assist device. *AJN*, 103(1):33–41.

Braun, L.T., and Davidson, M.H. (2003). Cholesterol-lowering drugs bring benefits to high-risk populations even when LDL is normal. *J Cardiovas Nurs*, 18(1):44–49.

Bridges, E.J., and Woods, S.L. (1998). Cardiovascular chronobiology: Implications for critical care nursing. *Crit Care Nurse*, 18(4):49–64.

Cheek, D., and Cesan, A. (2003). What's different about heart disease in women? *Nursing2003* 33(8):36–42.

Chobanian, A.V. et. al. (2003). Seventh report of Joint National Committee (JNC) on detection, evaluation, and treatment of high blood pressure. *Hypertension*, 42(6):1206–1252.

Church, V (2000). Staying on guard for DVT and PE. *Nursing2000*, 30(2):34.

Church, V. (2001). Managing the risk of DVT and PE. *Nursing2001*, 31(12):1–10.

Coviello, J.S., and Nystrom, K.V. (2003). Obesity and heart failure. *J. Cardiovasc Nurs*, 18(5):360–368.

Crowther, M., and McCourt, K. (2004). Get the edge on deep vein thrombosis. *Nurs Manage*, 35(1):21–29.

Crumlish, C.M., et al. (2000). When time is muscle. *AJN*, 100(1):26.

Cucinelli, C. (2000). Minimally invasive coronary artery bypass surgery. *Crit Care Nurse* 23(1): 54.

Curtis, A. (2004). Prophylactic defibrillators for the prevention of sudden cardiac death: The SCD-HeFT trial. American College of Cardiology Presentation March 7–10, New Orleans.

D'Arcy, Y. (1999). Controlling pain: Managing postoperative CABG pain. *Nursing99*, 29(9):17.

Daly, J., et al. (2000). Health status, perceptions of coping and social support immediately after discharge of survivors of acute myocardial infarct. *Am J Crit Care*, 9(1):62–69.

Day, M.W. (2003). Recognizing and managing deep vein thrombosis. *Nursing2003*, 33(5):36–41.

De Jong, M.J., and Morton, P.G. (2000). Predictors of atrial dysrhythmias for patients undergoing coronary artery bypass grafting. *Am J Crit Care*, 9(6):388–396.

Dracup, K.A., and Cannon, C. (1999). Combination treatment strategies for management of acute myocardial infarction: New directions with current therapies. *Crit Care Nurse Suppl*, April:3–15.

Edgar, W.F., Ebersole, N., and Mayfield, M.G. (1999). MIDCAB. *AJN*, 99(7):40.

Fort, C.W. (2003). Can you solve this mystery? The patient might have DVT … or is it FES? *Nursing Made Incredibly Easy*! 1(2):10.

Freeman, J.J., and Hedges, C. (2003). Cardiac arrest: The effect on the brain. *AJN*, 103(6): 51–55.

Futterman, L.G., and Lemberg, L. (1998). Encephalopathies following cardiac surgery. *Am J Crit Care*, 7(6):450–453.

Futterman, L.G., and Lemberg, L. (1999). Low-molecular-weight heparin: Antithrombotic agent whose time has come. *Am J Crit Care*, 8(1):520–523.

Futterman, L.G., and Lemberg, L. (2000). Update on management of acute myocardial infarction: Facilitated percutaneous coronary intervention. *Am J Crit Care*, 9(1):70–76.

Gibbon-Clements, T., et al. (2000). The challenge of warfarin therapy. *AJN*, 100(3):38.

Goldsborough, M.A., et al. (1999). Prevalence of leg wound complications after coronary artery bypass grafting: Determination of risk factors. *Am J Crit Care*, 8(3):149–153.

Gylys, K., and Gold, M. (2000). Acute coronary syndromes—New developments in pharmacological treatment strategies. *Crit Care Nurse Suppl*, April:3–14.

Heidenreich, P.A., et al. (2004). Cost effectiveness of screening with B-type natriuretic peptide to identify patients with reduced left ventricular ejection fraction. *J Am Coll Cardiol* 17; 43(6):1019–1026.

Heller, G.A. (1999). Atrial fibrillation: Soothing the savage beat. *Nursing99*, 29(2):26.

Hill, M.N., Han. H., Dennison C.R., et al. (2003). Hypertension care and control in underserved urban African American men: Behavioral and physiologic outcomes at 36 months. *Am J Hypertens*, 16:906–913.

Hussar, D.A. (1999). New drugs99, part II. *Nursing99*, 29(2):45.

Kearney, K. (2000). Digitalis toxicity. *AJN*, 100(6):51–52.

Khan, N.A., et al, (2004). The Canadian Recommendations for Management of Hypertension. *Can J Cardiol*, 20(1):41–54.

Kline-Rogers, E., Marlin, J.S., and Smith, D.D. (1999). New era of reperfusion in acute myocardial infarction. *Crit Care Nurse*, 19(1):21–31.

Kozuk, J.L. (2000). NSAIDs and anti-hypertensives: An unhappy union. *AJN*, 100(6):40.

Kuncl, N., and Nelson, K.M. (2000). Getting the skinny on lipid-lowering drugs. *Nursing2000*, 30(7):52.

Lewis, A.M. (1999). Cardiovascular emergency. *Nursing99*, 29(6):51.

Livorsi-Moore, J., Gulanick, M., and Rosko, P.H. (1999). Port access: Another advance in cardiovascular surgery. *AJN*, 99(7):52.

Logan P., and Moore, J. (2004). Hypertension: Getting back to the basics. *Nursing2004*, May suppl.

MacCallum, E.M., Hanlon S.J., and Byrne, K.H. (1999). Beyond aspirin: How glycoprotein inhibitors ease acute coronary syndromes. *Nursing99*, 29(12):34.

McKinney, B.C. (1999). Solving the puzzle of heart failure. *Nursing99*, 29(5):33.

Mair, M. (2003). Monophasic and biphasic defibrillators. *AJN*, 103(8):58–60.

Metules, T.J. (1999). Cardiac tamponade. *RN*, 62(12):26.

Mosca, L., et al. (2004). Evidence-based guidelines for cardiovascular disease prevention in women. *J Am Coll Cardiol*, 43(5):900–921.

Murphy, M.J., and Berding, C.B. (1999). Use of measurements of myoglobin and cardiac troponins in acute myocardial infarction. *Crit Care Nurse*, 19(1):58–65

Owens, S.G. (2000). Nursing management of arrhythmias after cardiac surgery. *AACN News*, 17(2):11–12.

Platek, U.N., and Atzori, M. (1999). PTMR. *AJN*, 99(7):64.

Rochett, J.L. (1999). Endothelial dysfunction and the promise of ACE inhibitors. *AJN*, 99(10):44.

Sakallaris, B.R., et al. (2000). Same-day transfer of patients to the cardiac telemetry unit after surgery: The rapid after bypass back into telemetry (RABBIT) program. *Crit Care Nurse*, 20(2):50–68.

Savage, L.S., and Grap, M.J. (1999). Telephone monitoring after early discharge for cardiac surgery patients. *Am J Crit Care*, 8(3):154–159.

Sieck, S. (2000). Acute coronary syndrome: Getting patients on the right treatment track. *RN* March suppl.

Sims, J.M., and Miracle, V.A. (1999). Easy ECG series, part II: Using the ECG to detect myocardial infarction. *Nursing99*, 29(8):41..

Siomko, A.X. (2000). Demystifying cardiac markers. *AJN*, 100(1):36.

Steinke, EE. (2000). Sexual counseling after myocardial infarction. *AJN*, 100(12):38–43.

Tasota, F.J., and Tate, J. (2000). Eye on diagnostics: Assessing digoxin levels. *Nursing2000*, 30(3):24.

Whitman. G.R. (2004). Nursing-sensitive outcomes in cardiac surgery patients. *J Cardiovasc Nurs*, 19(5):293–298.

Woods, A.D. (1999). Managing hypertension: Help your patient keep the lid on high BP. *Nursing99*, 29(3):41.

Yutsis, P. (2000). High blood pressure: Prescription drugs causing more problems than they solve? *J Longev*, 6(1):21.

Zevola, D.R., and Maier, B. (1999). Improving the care of cardiothoracic surgery patients through advanced nursing skills. *Crit Care Nurse*, 19(1):34–44.

No author listed. (1999). Angioplasty vs clot busters. *Harvard Health Lett*, 24(11):7.

No author listed. (2000). Chest pain in women—in the head or in the heart? *Harvard Heart Lett*, 10(12):2.

No author listed. (2000). Heart attacks without chest pain: The danger is greater. *Harvard Heart Lett*, 11(1):5.

No author listed. (2000). New techniques for preventing strokes. *Focus on Healthy Aging*, 3(8):1.

No author listed. (2000). Triglycerides and heart disease. *Harvard Heart Lett*, 11(1):5.

Electronic Resources

Ablation. Article for HeartCenterOnline website. Retrieved November 2004. *http://www.heartcenteronline.com*

American Heart Association (AHA). Cholesterol levels. Article for AHA website. Retrieved November 2004. *http://americanheart.org*

Advances for Patients: Drug-Eluting Stents. Presentation of the 2004 Transcatheter Cardiovasular Therapeutics Symposium. Washington, D.C. Retrieved November 2004. *http://www.pcta.org*

Coronary artery bypass surgery. Article for HeartCenter-Online website. Retrieved November 2004. *http://www.heartcenteronline.com*

Electrophysiology Study. Article for HeartCenterOnline website. Retrieved November 2004. *http://www.heartcenteronline.com*

Ensuring Patient Access to New Medical Technology. Remarks by Art Collins, Chairman and CEO, Medtronic. For Cleveland Clinic Medical Innovation Summit, October 2003, Cleveland OH. Retrieved May 2004. Medtronic website. *http://www.medtronic.com*

Griffin, R.M. (2003). Heart-failure treatment by device. Article for My WebMD website. Retrieved November 2004. *http://www.mywebmd.com*

Maze procedure. Article for HeartCenterOnline website. Retrieved November 2004. *http://www.heartcenteronline.com*

Minimally invasive bypass surgery. Article for HeartCenter-Online website. Retrieved November 2004. *http://heart centeronline.com*

OPCRES. Article for HeartCenterOnline website. Retrieved November 2004. *http://heartcenteronline.com*

NHLBI Issues New High Blood Pressure Clinical Practice Guidelines. Article for U.S. Department of Health and Human Services National Institues of Health (NIH) News website. Accessed November 2004. *http://wwwl.nih.gov/news/pr/may2003/nhlbi-14.htm*

Pacemaker. Article for HeartCenterOnline website. Retrieved November 2004. *http://www.heartcenteronline.com*

Warner, J., and Nazario, B. (2003). New heart failure drug approved by FDA: Inspra reduces risk of death after heart attack. Article for WebMD with AOL website. Accessed November 2004. *http://aolsvc.health.webmd*

CHAPTER 5

Books

Blair, K.A. (2005). The aging pulmonary system. In Stanley, M., Blair, K.A., and Beare, P.G. *Gerontological Nursing: Promoting Successful Aging with Older Adults,* ed 3. Philadelphia: F.A. Davis.

DeConti, R.C. (2003). Carcinomas of the head & neck. In Skeel, R.T., ed. *Handbook of Cancer Chemotherapy,* ed. 6. Philadelphia: Lippincott Williams & Wilkins.

Fink, J.G., and Hess, D.R. (2002). Secretion clearance techniques, In Hess, D.R. et. al., eds. *Respiratory Care: Principles and Practices*. Philadelphia: Saunders.

Ginsberg, R.J., Vokes, E.E., and Rosenzweig, K. (2001). Non–small cell lung cancer. In DeVita, V.T., Hellman, S., and Rosenberg, S.A., eds.. *Cancer Principles and Practice of Oncology,* ed 6. Philadelphia: Lippincott-Raven.

Hoang, T., and Schiller, J. (2003). *Carcinoma of the lung*. In Skee. R., ed. *Handbook of Cancer Chemotherapy,* ed. 6. Philadelphia: Lippincott Williams & Wilkins.

Springhouse (1997). When acids and bases tip the balance. In *Fluids & Electolytes Made Incredibly Easy!* Springhouse, PA.

Articles

Anderson, K.L. (1999). Change in quality of life after lung volume reduction surgery. *Am J Crit Care,* 8(6):389–396.

Boutotte, J.M. (1999). Keeping TB in check. *Nursing99,* 29(3):34.

Burns, S.M. (1999). Pharmacological and ventilatory management of acute asthma exacerbations. *Crit Care Nurse,* 19(4):39–54.

Byers, J.F., and Sole, M.L. (2000). Analysis of factors related to the development of ventilator-associated pneumonia: Use of existing databases. *Am J Crit Care,* 9(5):344–349.

Carroll, P. (1999). Evolutions/revolutions: Respiratory monitoring. *RN,* 62(5):69.

Chrisp, D.R. (2000). Action Stat: Tension pneumothorax. *Nursing2000,* 30(5)33.

Covey, M.L., and Larson, J.L. (2004). Beats and Breaths: Exercise and COPD. *AJN* 104(5):40–43.

DeVito Dabbs, A., Hoffman, L.A., Iacono A.T., et. al. (2003). Pattern and predictors of early rejection after lung transplantation. *Am J Crit Care,*12:497–507.

Endicott, L., et. al. (2003). Operating a sustainable disease management program for chronic obstructive pulmonary disease. *Lippincott's Case Manage,* 8(6):282.

Faul, J.L., et al. (1999). Quality of life and lung volume reduction surgery. *Am J Crit Care,* 8(6):359–360.

Fahlman M.M., Morgan, A.L., McNevin N., et al. (2003). Salivary s-IgA response to training in functionally limited elders. *J Aging Phys Activ,* 11:502–515.

Forastiere, A., Koch, W., Trotti, A., et al. (2001). Head and neck cancer. *N Engl J* 345:1890–1900.

Frakes, M.A., Evans, T. (2004). TB—Your vigilance is vital. *RN,* 67(11):30–35.

Holcomb, S. (2004). Asthma update. *Dimen Crit Care Nurse,* 23(3):101–107

Horne, C., and Derrico, D. (1999). Mastering ABGs. *AJN,* 99(8):26.

Jacavone, J., and Young, J. (1998). Use of pulmonary rehabilitation strategies to wean a difficult-to-wean patient: Case study. *Crit Care Nurse,* 18(6):29–37.

Kinloch, D. (1999). Instillation of normal saline during endotracheal suctioning: Effects on mixed venous oxygen saturation. *Am J Crit Care,* 8(4):231–240.

Kowalski, S.D., and Rayfield, C.A. (1999). A post hoc descriptive study of patients receiving propofol. *Am J Crit Care,* 8(1):507–513.

Kreamer, K.M. (2003). Getting the lowdown on lung cancer. *Nursing2003,* 33(11):36–42.

Legon, K (1999). Teaching incentive spirometry. *Nursing99,* 29(11):60.

Lewis, A.M (1999). Respiratory emergency. *Nursing99,* 29(8):62.

Mason, D.J. (1999). Put this in your pipe and smoke it. *AJN,* 99(11):7.

McEnroe-Ayers, D.M., and Lappin, J.S. (2004). Act fast when your patient has dyspnea. *Nursing2004,* 34(7):36–41.

McGann, E. (1999). Medication compliance in adults with asthma. *AJN,* 99(3):45.

Murphy, K.R., Cecil, B., and Sarver, N.L. (2004). Asthma: Helping patients breathe easier. *Nurs Pract: American J Primary Health Care,* 29(10):38–55.

Owens, C.L. (1999). New directions in asthma management. *AJN,* 99(3):26, 1999.

Pierce, L.N.B. (2000). Protocols for practice: Applying research at the bedside—traditional and nontraditional modes of mechanical ventilation. *Crit Care Nurse,* 20(1):81–86.

Pieterman, R.M., et al. (2000). Preoperative staging of

non–small-cell lung cancer with positron-emission tomography. *N Engl J Med*, 343:254–261.
Powers, J., and Bennett, S.J. (1999). Measurement of dyspnea in patients treated with mechanical ventilation. *Am J Crit Care*, 8(4):254–261.
Rose-Ped, A.M., et al. (2002). Complications of radiation therapy for head and neck cancers: The patient's perspective. *Cancer Nurs*, 25(6):461–467
Ruppert, R.A. (1999). The last smoke. *AJN*, 99(11):26.
Schmelz, J.O., et al. (1999). Effects of position of chest drainage tube on volume drained and pressure. *Am J Crit Care*, 8(5):319–323..
Shortall, S.P., and Perkins, L.A. (1999). Interpreting the ins and outs of pulmonary function tests. *Nursing99*, 29(12):41.
Schultz, T.R. (2003). Community-acquired pneumonia: Hunting the elusive respiratory infection. *Nursing Made Incredibly Easy!*, 1(1):29–34.
Schultz, T.R. (2003). On the trail of community-acquired pneumonia. *Nurs Manage*, 34(2):27–31.
St. John, R.E. (1999). Protocols for practice: Applying research at the bedside—airway management. *Crit Care Nurse*, 19(4):79–83.
Trudeau, M.E., and Solano-McGuire, S.M. (1999). Evaluating the quality of COPD care. *AJN*, 99(3):47.
Wong, F. (1999). A new approach to ABG interpretation. *AJN*, 99(8):34.
Woodruff, D.W. (1999). How to ward off complications of mechanical ventilation. *Nursing99*, 29(11):34.
Yantis, M.A., and Nieman, W. (2000). Resting easy with PAP therapy. *Nursing2000*, 30(4):62.
No author listed. (2002). Bronchial hygiene therapy: From traditional hands-on techniques to modern technological advances. *AJN*, 102(1):37.

Electronic Resources

Lombard, L.E. (2003). Laryngectomy rehabilitation. Article for Emedicine website. Retrieved December 2004. *http://www.emedicine.com*
Payne, K., and Rhoads, C. (2003). Cardiac calcium scoring. Article for WebMDHealth website. Retrieved November 2004. *http://my.webmd.com*
Petrossian, G.A. (2000). Angiojet. Article on HeartCenter Online website. Retrieved November 2004. *http://www.heartcenteronline.com*
Sharma, S. (2004). Pneumonia, bacterial. Article for Emedicine website. Retrieved November 2004. *http://www.emedicine.com*
No author listed. Exercise testing for evaluation of hypoxemia and/or desaturation: 2001 Revision and Update. American Association for Respiratory Care (AARC). Retrieved February 2004 from National Guideline Clearinghouse. *http://www.guideline.gov*
No author listed: Facts about coronary angioplasty (PTCA). Article for North Suburban Cardiology Group, Ltd. Website. Retrieved November 2004. *http://www.nscardiology.com.*
No author listed. Laryngeal & hypopharyngeal cancer. American Cancer Society website. *http://www.cancer.org*

CHAPTER 6

Book

Halper, J., et al. (2000). *Multiple Sclerosis: Best Practices in Nursing Care*. Columbia, MD: Medicallance.

Articles

Abour, R. (1998). Aggressive management of intracranial dynamics. *Crit Care Nurse*, 18(3):30–40.
Black, T., Soltis, T., and Bartlett, C. (1999). Using the functional independence measure instrument to predict stroke rehabilitation outcomes. *Rehab Nur*, 24(3):109–114/121.
Chotikul, L. (2000). Spinal implants. *RN*, 63(5):28–31.
Crimlisk, J.T., and Grande, M.M. (2004). Neurologic assessment for the acute medical surgical nurse. *Orthop Nur*, 23(1):3–9.
Cross, C. (2004). Seizures: Regaining control. *RN*, 67(12): 44–51.
Dryden, T., Baskwill, A., and Preyde, M. (2004). Massage therapy for the orthopaedic patient: A review. *Orthop Nurs*, 23(5):327–332.
Eck, M. (2000). Through the labyrinth: The twists and turns of brain injury. *AJN*, 100(9):25.
Filippini, G., et al. (1994). Sensitivities and predictive values of paraclincal tests for diagnosing MS. *J Neurol*, (3):132–137.
Galvin, T.J. (2001). Dysphagia: Going down and staying down. *AJN*, 101(1):37–42.
Gambrell, M.., and Flynn, N. (2004). Seizures 101. *Nursing 2004*, 34(8):36–41
Gray, M. (2000). Urinary retention: Management in the acute care setting. *AJN*, 100(8):36–43..
Harvey, J. (2004). Countering "brain attacks." *Nurs Manage*, 35(8):27–32.
Hazard, R.G. (2000). Movement brings relief: Using lumbar CPM as a postrehab strategy for patients with recurring low back pain. *Rehab Manage*, 13(7):40–42.
Hilton, L. (2005). We've got your back: Recovery from spinal cord injuries starts with the first hours of critical care. *Nurseweek Mountain West*, January 10, 2005, p. 12.
Kavchak-Keyes, M.A. (2000). Autonomic hyperreflexia. *Rehab Nurs*, 25(1):31–35.
Keating, D.J., et al (2000). Postacute brain injury rehab: Where do we go from here? *Rehab Manage*, 13(7):36–38.
Kennedy, M.S. (2004). News: Growing older, seeing less: Blindness and visual impairment are on the rise in older Americans. *AJN*, 104 (7):21.
Lathbury, K. (2000). The road ahead—Managing a spinal cord injury. *Case Manager*, 11(3):55–57.
Lewis, A.M. (1999). Neurologic emergency! *Nursing99*, 29(10):54.
Manchikanti, L., et al. (2003). Evidence-based practice guidelines for interventional techniques in the management of chronic spinal pain. *Pain Physician*, 6:3—81.
Martin, L. (1996). Computer-assisted management of primary open-angle glaucoma. *CIN: Comput, Inform, Nurs*, 14(5):267.

Modlin, S.J. (2000). Service dogs as interventions: State of the science. *Rehab Nurs*, 25(6):212–219.

Nickolaus, M.J. (1999). Diabetes insipidus: A current perspective. *Crit Care Nurse*, 19(6):18–30.

Offenbacher, H., et al. (1993). Assessment of MRI criteria for a diagnosis of MS. *Neurology*, 43:905–909.

O'Leary, J.M., and Sarkarati, M. (2000). Aging with SCI. *Rehab Manage*, 13(5):66–70,.

Pohl, P.S., and Richards, L.G. (2000). Decreasing stroke deficits. *Rehab Manage*, 13(3):32–35.

Posser, C.M., et al. (1983). New diagnostic criteria for multiple sclerosis: Guidelines for research protocols. *Ann Neurol*, 13:227–231.

Reeves, K., and Barash, S. (1999). Managing intrathecal baclofen pump implantation. *Rehab Rep*, 10(10):28–29.

Rothke, S.E., and Michael, E. (2000). Integrating the head injury team. *Rehab Manage*, 13(2):38–40, 96.

Santoni-Reddy, L.C. (2004). Heads up on cerebral bleeds. *Nursing Made Incredibly Easy!*, 2(3):8–16

Secrest, J.A. (2000). Transformation of the relationship: The experience of primary support persons of stroke survivors. *Rehab Nurs*, 25(3):93–99.

Secrest, J.A., and Thomas, S.P. (1999). Continuity and discontinuity: The quality of life following stroke. *Rehab Nurs*, 24(6):240–246.

Stockert, P.A. (1999). Getting UTI patients back on track. *RN*, 62(3):49–52.

Stuifbergen A.K., and Harrison T.C. (2003). Complementary and alternative therapy use in persons with multiple sclerosis. *Rehab Nurs*, 28:141–147, 158.

Sullivan, M.P., and Sharts-Hopko, N.C. (2000). Preventing the downward spiral: Osteoporosis and MS. *AJN*, 100(8):26–32.

Teasell, R.W., et al. (2000). Cardiovascular consequences of loss of supraspinal control of the sympathetic nervous system after spinal cord injury. *Arch Phys Med Rehab*, April: 81.

Travers, P.L. (1999). Autonomic dysreflexia: A clinical rehabilitation problem. *Rehab Nurs*, 24(1):19–23.

Weeks, S.K., Hubbartt, E., and Michaels, T.K. (2000). Keys to bowel success. *Rehab Nurs*, 25(2):66–69.

Winkelman, C. (2000). Effect of backrest position on intracranial and cerebral perfusion pressure in traumatically brain-injured adults. *Am J Crit Care*, 9(6):373–380.

Wong, F.W. (2000). Prevention of secondary brain injury. *Crit Care Nurse*, 20(5):18–27.

Electronic Resources

Acute seizures and seizure disorder. Guideline from bibliographic source: Texas Tech University Managed Health care Network Pharmacy and Therapeutics. Committee. Retrieved December 2004 from National Guideline Clearinghouse. *htpp://www.guideline.gov*

American Academy of Orthopaedic Surgeons (AAOS). Clinical Guideline on low back pain/sciatica (acute) (phases I and II) (2002). Retrieved January 2005. National Guideline Clearinghouse website. *http://www.guide line.gov*

Bilkovski, R.N. (2003). Transient ischemic attack (mini-stroke). Article for Emedicine website. Retrieved January 2005. *http://www.emedicinehealth.com*

Charite, S.B. (no date listed). Get ADR, Artificial disc replacement surgery at Stenum Hospital. Public information materials from Get ADR.com website. Retrieved January 2005. *http://www.getadr.com*

de Menezes, M.S. (2004). Status epilepticus. Article for Emedicine website. Retrieved December 2004. *http://www.emedicine.com*

Dr. Schiffer.com: Procedures: Spine and Neck Surgical Procedures. Retrieved January 2005. *http://www.spinesearch.com/procedures.html*

Herniated disc. In North American Spine Society phase III clinical guidelines for multidisciplinary spine care specialists. Retrieved January 2005 from National Guideline Clearinghouse. *http://guideline.gov*

Huff, J.S., Huff, M., and Plantz, S.H. (2003). Epilepsy. Article for Emedicine website. Retrieved December 2004. *http://www.emedicine.com*

Medline Plus: Medical Encyclopedia: Herniated nucleus pulposus (slipped disk) Public information materials from National Library of Medicine (NLM) from National Institutes of Health (NIH). Retrieved January 2005. *http://www.nlm.nih.gov*

Pascotto, A., and Soreca, E. (2004). Glaucoma, complications and management of glaucoma filtering. Article for Emedicine website. Retrieved January 2005. *http://www.emedicine.com*

Public Information articles (including Diagnostic tests, and What Is Glaucoma?). Published by the Glaucoma Research Foundation website. Retrieved January 2005. *http://www.glaucoma.org*

Schwanke, J. (2001). Gene putty helps body grow new bone. Article for WebMD Medical News. *http://webmdpractice.health.*

Silver, B. (2004). Medical treatment of stroke. Article for Emedicine website. Retrieved January 2005. *http://www.emedicine.com*

Scott, D.D., and Williamson, S.F. (2004). Multiple sclerosis. Article for Emedicine website. Retrieved January 2005. *http://www.emedicine.com*

CHAPTER 7

Books

American Dietetic Association (2000). *American Dietetic Association Manual of Clinical Dietetics*, ed. 6. pp. 425–426, 395–399, Chicago.

Escott-Stump, S. (2002). *Nutrition and Diagnosis-Related Care*. Philadelphia: Lippincott Williams & Wilkins, pp. 289–290, 291–292.

Mohaned, I., and Skeel, R.T. (2003). Carcinoma of the breast. In Skeel, R.T., ed. *Handbook for Cancer Chemotherapy*, ed. 6. Philadelphia: Lippincott Williams & Wilkins.

Springhouse (1999). Living with irritable bowel syndrome. In *Patient Teaching Made Incredibly Easy!* Springhouse, PA.

Sussman, C., and Bates-Jensen, B. (1998). *Wound Care, A Collaborative Practice Manual for Physical Therapists and Nurses*. Gaithersberg, MD: Aspen.

VanGuilder, T, et al. (2003). *Gastroenterology Nursing: A Core Curriculum.* Chicago: Society of Gastroenterology Nurses and Associates.

Winer, E.P., Morrow M., Osborne, C.K., et al. (2001). Malignant tumors of the breast. In DeVita, V.T, Hellman, S., Rosenberg, S.A., eds. *Cancer: Principles and Practice of Oncology.* Philadelphia: Lippincott Willliams & Wilkins.

Articles

Breitfeller, J.M. (1999). Peritonitis. *AJN*, 99(4):33.

Bryant, D., and Fleischer, I. (2000). Changing an ostomy appliance. *Nursing2000*, 11(30):51.

Farrar, J.A., and Kearney, K. (2001). Acute cholecystitis. *AJN*, 101(1):35–36.

Fries, C.F. (1999). Managing an ostomy. *Nursing99*, 29(8): 26.

Klonowski, E.I., and Masoodi, J.E. (1999). The patient with Crohn's disease. *RN*, 62(3):32.

Neal, L.J. (2000). Rehab's role in incontinence treatment and ostomy care. *Rehab Manage*, 13(5):28–30, 100.

Cancer Facts and Figures 2004. Atlanta: American Cancer Society.

No author listed. (1999). Advice prn: Gastric lavage: Tapping the source. *Nursing99*, 29(10):17

No author listed. (2000). Coping with heartburn. *Focus on Healthy Aging*, 3(12):1.

No author listed. (2000). Infectious disease: *H. pylori* ulcer disease transmission. *AJN*, 100(4):17.

No author listed. (2001). *Helicobacter pylori:* The most common cause of ulcers is easily treated. *Focus on Healthy Aging*, 4(1):7.

O'Brien, B.K. (1999). Coming of age with an ostomy. *AJN*, 99(8):71.

Rayhorn, N. (1999). Understanding inflammatory bowel disease. *Nursing99*, 29(12):57.

Electronic Resources

Barkin, A., Bardou, M., and Marshall, J.K. (2003). Consensus recommendations for managing patients with nonvariceal upper gastrointestinal bleeding. *Ann Intern Med*, 139 (10):843–857. Retrieved January 2005 from National Guideline Clearinghouse. *http://guideline.gov*

Cerulli, M.A. (2004). Upper gastrointestinal bleeding. Article for Emedicine website. Retrieved January 2005. *http://www.emedicine.com*

Craig, S. (2005). Appendicitis, acute. Article for Emedicine website. Retrieved January 2005. *http://www.emedicine.com*

Dandan, I.S., Soweid, A.M., and Abiad, F. (2004). Article for Emedicine website. Retrieved January 2005. *http://www.emedicine.com*

Santen, S. (2004). Cholecystitis and biliary colic. Article for Emedicine website. Retrieved January 2005. *http://www.emedicine.com*

Varma, M.K, and Allen, A.W. (2204). Gastrointestinal bleeding, upper article for Emedicine website. Retrieved January 2005. *http://www.emedicine.com*

CHAPTER 8

Books

Bernal-Mizrachi, E., and Bernal-Mizrachi, C. (2004). Diabetes mellitus and related disorders. In Green, G.B., Harris, I.S., Lin, G.A., et al. eds. *The Washington Manual of Medical Therapeutics*, ed. 31. Washington University in St. Louis School of Medicine. Lippincott Williams & Wilkins.

Clutter, W.E. (2004). Endocrine diseases: Hyperthyroidism. In Green, G.B., Harris, I.S., Lin, G.A., et al. eds. *The Washington Manual of Medical Therapeutics*, ed. 31. Washington University in St. Louis School of Medicine. Lippincott Williams & Wilkins.

Klein, S. (2004). Nutrition support. In Green, G.B., Harris, I.S., Lin, G.A., et al. eds. *The Washington Manual of Medical Therapeutics*, ed. 31. Washington University in St. Louis School of Medicine. Lippincott Williams & Wilkins.

Springhouse (1997). *Fluids & Electrolytes Made Incredibly Easy*! Springhouse, PA.

Articles

Apfell, S.C., et al. (1999). New option for diabetic neuropathy. *AJN*, 99(2):20.

Birn, C.S. (2005). CE 355: Endoscopic ultrasound reveals GI tract secrets. *NurseWeek Mountain West*, January 17, 2005.

Blackwood, H.S. (2004). Obesity: A rapidly expanding challenge. *Nurs Manage*, 35(5):27–35.

Bockhold, K.M. (2000). Who's afraid of hepatitis C? *AJN*, 100(5):26.

Booker, K.J., et al. (2000). Comparison of 2 methods of managing gastric residual volumes from feeding tubes. *Am J Crit Care*, 9(5):318–324.

Bowers, S. (1999). All about tubes: Your guide to enteral feeding devices. *Nursing2000*, 30(12):41.

Cammon, S.A., and Hackshaw, H.S. (2000). Are we starving our patients? *AJN*, 100(5):43–46.

Cheever, K.H. (1999). Early enteral feeding of patients with multiple trauma. *Crit Care Nurse*, 19(6):40–51

Cole, L. (2002). Unraveling the mystery of acute pancreatitis. *Dimen Crit Care Nurs*, 21(3): 86–89.

Corbell, C.F., and Cook, D. (2004). Diabetes ABCs: Do you know them, get them, improve them? *Home Healthcare Nurse*, 22(7):452–459

Davidson, J.E., et al. (2003). Critical care of the morbidly obese. *Crit Care Nurse Quarterly*, 26(2):105–116

Dudek, S.G. (2000). Malnutrition in hospitals: Who's assessing what patients eat? *AJN*, 100(4):36.

Durston, S. (2004). The ABCs—and more—of hepatitis. *Nursing Made Incredibly Easy!*, 2(4):22–32.

Fleming, D.R. (1999). Challenging traditional insulin injection practices. *AJN*, 99(2):72

Funnell, M.M., and Barlage, D.L. (2000). Saying a mouthful about oral diabetes drugs. *Nursing2000*, 30(11):34.

Funnell, M.M., and Kruger, D.F. (2004). Type 2 diabetes: Treat to target. *Nurs Pract*, 29(1):11–13.

Gallagher, S. (1999). Tailoring care for obese patients. *RN*, 62(5):43.

Gallagher, S. (2004). Taking the weight off with bariatric surgery. *Nursing2004*, 34(3):58–64.

Halmi, KA, et al. (1991). Comorbidity of psychiatric diagnosis in anorexia. *Arch Gen Psychiatry*, 48:712–718 .

Halpin-Landry, J.E., and Goldsmith, S. (1999). Feet first: Diabetes care. *AJN*, 99(2):26.

Holleman, C.B. (2000). Monitoring CSII therapy. *AJN*, 100(3):86.

Hussar, D.A. (2003). New Drugs 2003, part III. *Nursing2003*, 33(8), 55–61.

Jorgensen, R.A. (2003). Nonalcoholic fatty liver disease. *Gastroenterol Nurs*, 26(4):150–154.

Klainberg, M. (1999). Primary biliary cirrhosis. *AJN*, 99(12):38.

Kohn-Keeth, C. (2000). How to keep feeding tubes flowing freely. *Nursing2000*, 30(3):58.

Konick-McMahan, J. (1999). Riding out a diabetic emergency. *Nursing99*, 29(9):34.

Lambright, J.A. (1999). Preventing hepatitis. *Nursing99*, 29(8):66.

McConnel, E.A. (1999). Clincal do's and don'ts: Administering an insulin injection. *Nursing99*, 29(12):18.

McInnis, K.J. (2003). Diet, exercise, and the challenge of combating obesity in primary care. *J Cardiovasc Nurs*, 18(2):93–100.

Metheny, N.A., Aud, M.A., and Wunderlich, R.J. (1999). A survey of bedside methods used to detect pulmonary aspiration of enteral formula in intubated tube-fed patients. *Am J Crit Care*, 8(3):160–167.

Noble, K.A. (2003). Name that tube. *Nursing2003*, 33(3):56–62.

O'Brien, B., Davis, S., and Erwin-Toth, P. (1999). G-tube site care: A practical guide. *RN*, 62(2):52.

Olohan, K., and Zappitelli, D. (2003). The insulin pump. *AJN*, 103(4):48–56.

Olson, R.S. (2000). An update in diabetes management. *Rehab Nurs*, 25(5):177–184.

O'Neil, K.M. (1999). Thyrotoxic hypokalemic paralysis: A case study. *Crit Care Nurse*, 19(6):31–34.

Orbanic, S. (2001). Understanding bulimia, signs, symptoms and the human experience. *AJN*, 101(3):35.

Padula, C.A., et al. (2004). Enteral feedings: What the evidence says. *AJN*, 104(7):62–69.

Parini, S. (2003). Hepatitis C: Update your knowledge of this silent stalker. *Nursing2003*, 22(4): 57–63.

Perkins, H.K. (1999). Where is bariatric rehab on the safety scale? *Rehab Rep*, 10(6):19–23, 1999.

Powers, J., et al. (2003). Beside placement of small-bowel feeding tubes in the intensive care unit. *Crit Care Nurse*, 23(1):1624.

Racette, S.B., Deusinger, S.S., and Deusinger, R.H. (2003). Obesity: Overview of prevalence, etiology and treatment. *Phys Ther*, 83:276–288.

Scherer, M.J. (1999). Breaking barriers—Important factors to consider when advising bariatric clients on home modification and assistive technology. *Rehab Manage*, 12(6):74–77.

Shovein, J.T, Damozo, R.J., and Hyams, I. (2000). Hepatitis A: How benign is it? *AJN*, 100(3):43.

Simmons-Holcomb, S. (2002). An update on hepatitis. *Dimen Crit Care Nurs*, 21(5):170–177.

Trujillo, E.B., Robinson, M.K., and Jacobs, D.O. (1999). Nutritional assessment in the critically ill. *Crit Care Nurse*, 19(1):67–78.

Winfield, M. (1999). Bariatric rehab: What you should know about the new drug therapies. *Rehab Rep*, 10(10):13–17.

Young, J. (1999). Action stat! Myxedema coma. *Nursing99*, 29(1):64.

Young, J. (1999). Action stat! Thyroid storm. *Nursing99*, 29(8):33.

Vink, T. et al. (2001). Association between an agouti-related protein gene polymorphism and anorexia nervosa. *Mol Psychiatry*, 6(3)325–328.

No author listed. (2001). Comparing psychotherapies for bulimia. *Harvard Mental Health Lett*, 17(99):8.

No author listed. (2004). Clinical Practice Recommendations by the American Diabetes Association. *Diabetes Care*, 27–S3.

Electronic Resources

American Association of Clinical Endocrinologists Medical guidelines for clinical practice for evaluation of hyperthyroidism and hypothyroidism (2003). Retrieved January 2005 from National Guideline Clearinghouse. *http://www.guideline.gov*

Cirrhosis. Article retrieved from *www.nlm.nih.gov/medlineplus/cirrhosis.*

DA Liburd, J. (2004). Eating disorder: Anorexia. Article for Emedicine website. Retrieved January 2005. *http://www.emdicine.com*

Diseases of the pancreas: *FAQ* Retrieved from Pancreas Foundation web*site, http://www.pancreasfoundation.org*

Foster, R., and Smith-Coggins, R. (2004). Bulimia. Article for Emedicine website. Retrieved January 2005. *http://www.emedicine.com*

Hepatitis Foundation International: Herbs and Nutritional Supplements. Information retrieved from *www.hepatitisresources-calif.org*

Hepatitis, A, B, and C: learn the differences. Retrieved from website. *http://www.immunize.org*

Hepatitis B and C fact sheet and Hepatitis and Liver Disease in the United States. .Retrieved from website. *http://www.liverfoundation.org*

Hepatitis-Central: Some herbs should not be taken. Retrieved from *www.hepatitis-central.com/hcv/herbs/donotuse.html*

Kaye, W.H. (2004). Atypicals in the treatment of anorexia nervosa. In Broadening the Horizon of Atypical Antipsychotic Applications, pp 65–67. CME Article for MedScape from WebMD website. Retrieved January 2005. *http://www.medscape.com http://www.immunize.org*

Patient Information Sheet: Thyroid and Parathyroid Surgery. Department of Surgery, Division of Endocrine Surgery, University of Michigan Health System Website. Retrieved January 2005, *http://www.um-edocrine-surgery.org*

Pancreatic diseases. Retrieved from *http://www.nlm.nih.gov/medlineplus/pancreaticdiseases*

Pancreatitis. Article for Emedicine website. Retrieved from *http://www.emedicinehealth.com*

Patient Information Sheet: Thyroid and Parathyroid Surgery. Department of Surgery, Division of Endocrine Surgery,

University of Michigan Health System Website. Retrieved January 2005, *http://www.um-edocrine-surgery.org*

Payne, K. (2004). Thyroid hormone tests and hyperthyroidism treatment overview. (2) Articles for WebMD with AOL website. Retrieved January 2005. *http://aolsvc.health.webmd.aol.com*

Priestley, M.A., and Lieh-Lai, M. (2004). Alkalosis, metabolic. Article for Emedicine website. Retrieved January 2005. *http://www.emedicine.com*

Ross, D.S. (2004). Patient information: Antithyroid drugs. Retrieved January 2005 from UpToDate website. *http://patients.uptodate.com*

Spengler, R. Thyroid scan and radioactive iodine uptake test. Article for WebMD with AOL Health website. Retrieved January 2005. *http://aolsvc.health.webmd.aol.com*

Thomas, C., and Hamawi, K. (2003). Metabolic acidosis. Article for Emedicine website. Retrieved November 2004. *http://emedicine.com*

T3, T4, TSH: Public resource on clinical lab testing. Lab Tests Online website. Retrieved January 2005. *http://www.labtestsonline.org*

Yakshe, Paul. (2005). Pancreatitis, acute. Article for Emedicine website. Retrieved January 2005, *http://www.emedicine.com*

Youngerman-Cole, S. (2004). Thyroidectomy: Surgery overview. Article for WebMD. Retrieved January 2005. *http://aolsvc.health.webmd.aol.com*

CHAPTER 9

Books

Evens, A., and Tallman, M. (2003). Acute leukemias. In Skeel, R.T., ed. *Handbook of Cancer Chemotherapy*, ed. 6. Philadelphia: Lippincott Williams & Wilkins.

National Institutes of Health (2002). *The Management of Sickle Cell Disease*, ed. 4. Bethesda, MD: NIH Pub #02–2117.

Stein, R., Morgan, D., and Greer, J. (2003). Hodgkin's disease and non-Hodgkin's lymphoma. In Skeel, R.T., ed. *Handbook of Cancer Chemotherapy*, ed. 6. Philadelphia: Lippincott Williams & Wilkins.

Articles

Cerrato, P.L. (2000). Complementary therapies: Diet and herbs for BPH? *RN*, 63(2):63–64.

Day, S.W., and Wynn, L.W. (2000). Sickle cell pain and hydroxyurea. *AJN*, 100(11):34–38.

Gorman, K. (1999). Sickle cell disease: Do you doubt your patient's pain. *AJN*, 99(3):38–43..

Gutaj, D.A. (2000). Oncology today: Lymphoma. *RN*, 63(8):32–37.

Hays, K., and McCartney, S. (1998). Nursing care of the patient with chronic lymphocytic leukemia. *Semin Oncol Nurs*, 25(1):75.

Kanarek, R. (1998). Facing the challenge of childhood leukemia. *AJN*, 98(7):42.

Kosits, C., and Callaghan, M. (2000). Rituximab: A new monoclonal antibody therapy for non-Hodgkin's lymphoma. *Oncol Nurs Forum*, 27(1):51.

Mackey, H., and Klemm, P. (2000). Leukemia: Aggressive therapies predispose patients to a host of side effects. *AJN*, April Suppl:27–31.

Medoff, E., (2000). Oncology today: Leukemia. *RN*, 63(9):42–49.

Mitchell, R. (1999). Sickle cell anemia. *AJN*, 99(5):36–37.

Stremick, K., and Gallagher, E. (2000). Malignant lymphomas. *AJN*, April Suppl:18–22.

Thompson, K.A. (1999). Detecting Hodgkin's disease. *AJN*, 99(5):61–64.

Electronic Resources

The Leukemia and Lymphoma Society website. http://www.leukemia.org

National Cancer Institute website http://www.nci.nih.gov

Pui C.H., Heslop H.E., and Hoelzer. D. (2002). Advances in pediatric and adult acute lymphoblastic leukemia. In Oncology 2002: the American Society of Clinical Oncology 2002 Education Book. Alexandria, VA: American Society of Clinical Oncology, 2002:32–57. Available at http://www.asco.org.

CHAPTER 10

Articles

Arkouche, W., Traeger, J., Delawari, E., et al. (1999). Twenty-five years of experience with out-center hemodialysis. *Kidney Int*, 56(6):2269–2275.

Burrows-Hudson, S. (2005). Chronic kidney disease: An overview. *AJN*, 105(2):40–49.

Calabrese, D.A. (2004). Prostate cancer in older men. *Urol Nurs*, 24(4):258–264.

Cambell, D. (2003). How acute renal failure puts the brakes on kidney function. *Nursing2003*, 33(1):59–63.

Chan, C.T., Floras, J.S., Miller, J.A., Richardson, R. M., and Pierratos, A. (2002). Regression of left ventricular hypertrophy after conversion to nocturnal hemodialysis. *Kidney Int*, 61(6):2235–2239.

Chertow G.M., Ling J., Lew, N.L., et al. (1994). The association of intradialytic parenteral nutrition with survival in hemodialysis patients. *Am J Kidney Dis*, 24:921.

Cook, L. (1999). The value of lab values. *AJN*, 99(5):66–75.

Davison, B.J., et al. (2004). Client evaluation of a discharge program following a radical prostatectomy. *Urol Nurs*, 24(6):483–489.

Gilchrist, K. (2004). Benign prostatic hyperplasia: Is it a precursor to prostatic cancer? *Nurse Practitioner*, 29(6): 30–37.

Gray, M. (2000). Urinary retention: Management in the acute care setting, part 1. *AJN*, 100(7):40–47.

Greifzu, S.P. (2000). Oncology today: Prostate cancer. *RN*, 63(6):26–31.

Held-Warmkessel, J. (1999). How to care for men with prostate cancer. *Nursing99*, 29(11):51–53.

Holcolm. S.S. (2004). Keeping kidney function flowing. *Nursing Made Incredibly Easy!*, 2(5):30–40.

Kaplow, R., and Barry, R. (2002). Continuous renal replacement therapies. *AJN*, 102(11):26–33.

Kearney, K. (2000). Dialysis disequilibrium syndrome. *AJN*, 100(2):53–54.

King, B. (2000). Meds and the dialysis patient. *RN*, 63(7):54–59.

Little, C. (2000). Renovascular hypertension. *AJN*, 100(2):46–51.

McGlynn, B., et al. (2004). Management of urinary incontinence following radical prostatectomy. *Urol Nurs*, 24(6):475–482.

Osborne, D. (2000). Managing patients with a distended bladder. *Clin J Oncol Nurs*, 4(2):103.

Pupim L.B., Flakoll P.J., and Brouillette J.R. (2002). Intradialytic parenteral nutrition improves protein and energy homeostasis in chronic hemodialysis patients. *J Clin Invest*, 110(4):483–492.

Research News Item. (2004). Don't give your kidneys a jolt! *Nutr Today*, 39(5):213.

Sienty, M.K., and Dawson, N. (1999). Preventing urosepsis from indewelling urinary catheters. *AJN*, 99(1):24C–24H.

Young, J. (2000). Kidney stone. *Nursing2000*, 30(7):33.

Zellner, K.M. (1999). Acute tubular necrosis. *RN*, 62(10): 42–45.

Electronic Resources

Argraharkar, M., and Gupta, R. (2004). Acute renal failure. Article for Emedicine website. Retrieved February 2005. *http://www.emedicine.com*

Continent urinary diversion. Public information fact sheet. Retrieved February 2005. from UrologyHealth website. *http://www.urologyhealth.org*

Costa, J.A., and Kreder, K. (2004). Urinary diversions and neobladders. Article for Emedicine website. Retrieved February 2005. *http://www.emedicine.com*

Kidney (renal) failure. Public information fact sheets. Retrieved February 2005 from UrologyHealth website. *http://www.urologyhealth.org*

Leveillee, R.J., and Patel, V. (2004). Prostate hyperplasia, benign. Article for Emedicine website. Retrieved February 2005. *http://emedicine.com*

Mayo Clinic Staff (2004). Bladder cancer. Article for MayoClinic.com website. Retrieved February 2005. *http://mayoclinic.com*

National Institutes of Health. Hemodialysis dose and adequacy. Patient information fact sheet. National Institute of Diabetes and Digestive and Kidney Diseases. NIH Pub No. 03–4556. Available at *http://www.kidneyniddk.nih.gov*

National Institutes of Health (2003). Eat right to feel right on hemodialysis. NIH Pub No. 03–4274. Retrieved February 2005 from the National Kidney and Urologic Diseases Information Clearinghouse. Available at *http://www.kidney.niddk.nih.gov*

National Institutes of Health (2003). Kidney failure: Choosing a treatment that's right for you. NIH Pub No. 03–2412. Retrieved February 2005 from the National Kidney and Urologic Diseases Information Clearinghouse. Available at *http://www.kidney.niddk.nih.gov*

National Institutes of Health (2004). Kidney stones in adults. NIH Public information fact sheet Pub No. 05–2495. Retrieved February 2005 from the National Kidney and Urologic Diseases Information Clearinghouse. *http://www.kidney.niddk.nih.gov*

National Kidney Foundation. (2000). Clinical practice guidelines. Retrieved February 2005 from *http://www.kidney.org/professionals/kdoqi/guidelines.cfm*

Poit, C.A. (2003). The ins and outs of continent urinary diversions. Nursing Spectrum Education/CE Self-Modules. Available at *http://nsweb.nursingspectrum.com*

Rubenstein, J., and McVary, K.T. (2004). Transurethral microwave thermotherapy of the prostate (TUMT). Article for Emedicine website. Retrieved February 2005. *http://www.emedicine.com*

Wolf, J.S. (2004). Nephrolithiasis. Article for Emedicine website. *http://www.emedicine.com*

CHAPTER 11

Books

American Cancer Society (2004). *Cancer Facts and Figures 2004*. Atlanta, GA.

Mohamed, I., and Skeel, R.T. (2003). Carcinoma of the breast. In Skeel R.T., ed. *Handbook for Cancer Chemotherapy*, ed. 6. Philadelphia: Lippincott Williams & Wilkins.

Winer E.P., Morrow, M., Osborne C.K., et al. (2001). Malignant tumors of the breast. In DeVita, V.T., Hellman, S., and Rosenberg, S.A., eds. *Cancer: Principles and Practice of Oncology*. Philadelphia: Lippincott Williams & Wilkins.

Articles

Buren, J.M., and Linton, C. (2000). The role of exercise in treating lymphedema. *Rehab Manage*, 13(6):26–31.

Curry H. (2002). Menorrhagia and Hysterectomy. *AJN*, 102(1):14–19.

DiPalma, A.M., and DiPalma, J.A. (2002). Women's colonic digestive health. *Gastroenterol Nurs*, 25(1):3–8.

Klingman, L. (1999). Assessing the female reproductive system. *AJN*, 99(8):37–43.

Mazmanian, C.M. (1999). Hysterectomy: Holistic care is key. *RN*, 62(6):32–35.

Oetker-Black, S.L. (2003). Preoperative teaching and hysterectomy outcomes. *AORN J*, 77(6):1215–1218, 1221–1231.

Risser, N., and Murphy, M. (2004). Literature review: Women's health care: Sexual function after hysterectomy. *Nurs Pract*, 29(2):49.

Ruth-Sahd, L.A., and Zulkosky, K.D. (1999). Cervical cancer: Caring for patients undergoing total pelvic exenteration. *Crit Care Nurse*, 19(1):46–57.

Sharts-Hopko, N.C. (2001). Hysterectomy for nonmalignant conditions. *AJN*, 101(9):32–36

Thomas, S., and Greifzu, S.P. (2000). Oncology today: Breast cancer. *RN*, 63(4):40–45.

Thomas, S., and Greifzu, S.P. (2000). Oncology today: Breast reconstruction. *RN*, 63(4):45–47.

Electronic Resources

Bachmann, G., and Patel, S. (2004). Hysterectomy. Article for Emedicine website. Retrieved February 2005. *http://www.emedicine.com*

Forchuk, C., Baruth, P., Pendergast, M., et al. (2004). Postoperative arm massage: A support for women with lymph node dissection. *Cancer Nurs,* 27(1):25–32. Retrieved February 2005 from *http://www. medscape.com*

Institute for Clinical Systems Improvement (ICSI) (2003). Cervical cancer screening. Retrieved February 2005 from National Guideline Clearinghouse. *http://www.guideline.gov*

Institute for Clinical Systems Improvement (ICSI) (2004). Menopause and hormone therapy (HT): Collaborative decision-making and management. Retrieved February 2005 from National Guideline Clearinghouse. *http://www.guideline.gov*

National Guideline Clearinghouse (2000). Surgical alternatives to hysterectomy in the management of leiomyomas. American College of Obstetricians and Gynecologists (ACOG). Available at *http://www.guideline.gov*

Walling, A.D. (2004). Laparoscopic vs. abdominal hysterectomy: a comparison. Article for American Family Physician, October 2004. Available at HighBeam Research website *http://www.highbeam.com*

CHAPTER 12

Articles

Bailey, J. (2003). Getting a fix on orthopedic care. *Nursing 2003,* 33(6):58–63.

Bryant, G (2001). Stump care. *AJN,* 101(2):67–71.

Fort, C.W. (2003). How to combat 3 deadly trauma complications. *Nursing2003,* 33(5):58–63.

Frakes, M., and Evans, T. (2004). Major pelvic fractures. *Crit Care Nurse,* 24(2):24–30.

Pasero, C. (1999). Using superficial cooling for pain control. *AJN,* 99(3):24.

Prehoden, M.E. (1999). Crush injury: Compromised circulation can threaten limb survival. *AJN,* 99(3):35.

Wilson, T. (2004). Advanced prosthetic devices aid amputees. *Disabled American Veterans (DAV) Magazine,* November/December, 2004.

Electronic Resources

Clontz, A.S., Annonio, D., and Walker, L. (2004). Trauma nursing: Amputation. Article for RNWeb. Retrieved February 2005. *http://rnweb.com*

Ertl, J.P., and Ertl, W. (2005). Amputations of the lower extremity. Article for Emedicine website. Retrieved February 2005. *http://www.emedicine.com*

NLLIC Staff (2004). Wound care: Preventing infection. Public Information Fact Sheet by Partners against Pain and the National Limb Loss Information Center (NLLIC). Available at *http://amputee-coalition.org*

Pain management and the amputee (2003). Public Information Fact Sheet by Partners Against Pain and the National Limb Loss Information Center (NLLIC). Available at *http://amputee-coalition.org*

Rasul, A.T., and Wright, J. (2004). Total joint replacement rehabilitation. Article for Emedicine website. Retrieved February 2005 *http://www.emedicine.com*

Richeimer, S. (July, 2000). Phantom limb pain. The Richeimer Pain Report. Retrieved February, 2005 *http://www.helpforpain.com/arch2000jul.htm*

Rhodes, L.A. Phantom limb pain. In Malawer, M.M., and Sugarbaker. P.H., eds. (2001). *Musculoskeletal Cancer Surgery.* New York: Springer. Retrieved February, 2005. *http://www.sarcoma.org/publications/mcs/ch24.pdf*

Schuch, C.M. (1998, update 2004). Consumer guide for amputees: A guide to lower limb prosthetics: Part 1—Prosthetic designs: Basic concepts. Article for inMotion: a Publication of the Amputee Coalition of America 8(2). Available at *http://amputee-coalition. org*

Shonski, C. (1998). Pain management: A discussion of the various techniques and types of drugs currently available for pain control with medicines. Article for inMotion: a publication of the Amputee Coalition of America 8(5). Available at *http://www.amputee-coalition.org*

Swain, R., and Ross, D. (1999). Lower extremity compartment syndrome: When to suspect acute or chronic pressure buildup. Article for Postgraduate Medicine Online. Available at *http://www.postgradmed.com*

CHAPTER 13

Articles

Clinical News (1999). Complementary therapy—Massage therapy and burn debridement. *AJN,* 99(1):15.

Demling, R.H., and DeSanti, L. (1999). Management of partial thickness facial burns (comparison of topical antibiotics and bio-engineered skin substitutes). *Burns,* 25: 256–261.

Johnson, R.M., and Richard, R. (2003). Partial-thickness burns: Identification and management. *Adv Skin Wound Care,* 16(4):178–186.

Morgan, E.D, Bledsoe, S,C, Barker, J. (2000). Ambulatory management of burns. *Am Fam Physician,* 62(9):2015–2026.

Sheridan, R.L. (2000). Evaluating and managing burn wounds. *Dermatol Nurs,* 12(1):17–18, 21–28.

Wiebelhaus, P., and Hansen, S.L. (1999). Burns: Handle with care. *RN,* 62(11):52–57.

Wiebelhaus, P., and Hansen, S.L. (2001). What you should know about managing burn emergencies. *Nursing2001,* 31(1):36–41.

Electronic Resources

EAST Practice Management Guidelines Work Group. Practice management guidelines for nutritional support of the trauma patient. Eastern Association for the Surgery of Trauma (EAST). Available at National Guideline Clearinghouse *http:www.guidelines.gov*

Edlich, R.F., and Farinholt, H.M.A. (2004). Burns, thermal. Article for Emedicine website. Retrieved February 2005. *http://www.emedicine.com*

CHAPTER 14

Articles

AIDS file: Achieving medication adherence. *AJN*, 99(1):17, 1999.

AIDS file: Return to unsafe sexual behaviors. *AJN*, 99(9):17, 1999.

Carroll, P. (1999). Monitoring the gut to prevent MODS. *RN*, 62(10):34–37.

Cavanaugh, J.C. (2001). A qualitative study of stress and coping strategies used by well spouses of lung transplant candidates. *Families Systems Health/J Cardiovasc Nurs*, 10(2):58–70.

Coe, P.F. (2000). Managing pulmonary hypertension in heart transplantation: Meeting the challenge. *Crit Care Nurse*, 20(2):22–28

Cook, L. (1999). The value of lab values. *AJN*, 99(5):66–75.

Crone, C.C., and Wise, T.N. (1999). Psychiatric aspects of transplantation, III: Postoperative issues. *Crit Care Nurse*, 19(4):28–38.

Crone, C.C., and Wise, T.N. (1999). Psychiatric aspects of transplantation, II: Preoperative issues. *Crit Care Nurse*, 19(3):51–63.

Good, E.W. (2000). Caring for patients with donor organs. *Nursing2000*, 30(6):34.

Grady, K.L. (1996). When to transplant: Recipient selection for heart transplantation. *J Cardiovasc Nurs, 10*(2):58–70.

Hoffman, R.L., and Reeder, S.J. (1998). Mycophenolate mofetil (CellCept): The newest immunosuppressant. *Crit Care Nurse*, 18(3):50–57.

Kurz, J.M., and Cavanaugh, J.C. (2001). A qualitative study of stress and coping strategies used by well spouses of lung transplant candidates. *Families Systems Health*, 10(2).

Martin, S.A. (1998). Posttransplant lymphoproliferative disease in a pediatric multivisceral transplant recipient. *Crit Care Nurse*, 18(3):74–80.

Moons, P. (1998). Post-transplant immunosuppression. *Heart Lung*, 27:34.

Pressly, K.B., and Quattlebaum, L.S. (2000). Infection control: Vibrio vulnificus sepsis. *Crit Care Nurse*, 20(5):78–83.

Ramsburg, K.L. (2000). Rheumatoid arthritis. *AJN*, 100(11):40–43.

Rayl, J. (2000). Home care of the cancer patient. *Adv Nurses*, 2(14):23–33.

Rayl, J. (2000). Home health care of the post-transplant patient. *Adv Nurses*, 2(12):25–35,

Ress, B. (2001). AIDS/HIV—Caring for patients with HIV disease in the millennium. *Crit Care Nurse*, 21(1):69–76.

Schmelzer, M., and Stam, M.A. (2000). A hidden menace: Hemolytic uremic syndrome. *AJN*, 100(11):26–32.

Sears, J.R., and Ganger, P.M. (2000). Antibiotics to treat RA. *RN*, 63(1):41–42.

Sheff, B. (1999). Reining in a runaway infection. *Nursing99*, 29(10):60–61.

Tahan, H.A. (1998). Patients waiting for heart transplantion: An analysis of vulnerability. *Crit Care Nurse*, 18(4):40–48.

Veitz, A. (2000). Managing the side effects of chemotherapy. *Adv Nurses*, 2(14):11–13.

Webb, A., and Norton, M. (2004). Clinical assessment of symptom-focused health related quality of life in HIV/AIDS. *JANAC*, 15(2):67–81.

Electronic Resource

AIDSinfo Web site: *http://aidsinfo.nih.gov/guidelines*

CHAPTER 15

Books

American Psychiatric Association (2000). *DSM-IV-TR, Diagnostic and Statistical Manual of Mental Disorders*, ed. 4. Text Revision. Washington, DC, pp. 583–595.

Hartung, J., and Galvin, M. (2003). *Energy Psychology and EMDR: Combining Forces to Optimize Treatment*. New York: Norton.

Kowalak, J., Hughes, A., et al. (2002). *Handbook of Signs and Symptoms*. ed. 2. Springhouse, PA: Lippincott Williams & Wilkins.

Schaffer Library of Drug Policy Alcohol Handbook. Updated June 19, 2003.

Skeel R., ed. (2003). *Handbook of Cancer Chemotherapy*. ed. 6. Philadelphia: Lippincott Williams & Wilkins.

Theander, S. Outcome and prognosis in anorexia nervosa and bulimia. In Szmukler, G.I, Slade, P.D., Harris, P., et al., eds. (1985). *Anorexia Nervosa and Bulimic Disorders*. London: Pergamon.

University of Missouri. *Handbook of Disabilitites, Substance Abuse*, Product of RECP7 and Curators of the University of Missouri.

Young, B., Flamm, J.A., and Graham R.M. (2004). Improved options for better care: The role of new HIV-1 protease inhibitors. A continuing education monograph, 3/2004.

Articles

American Cancer Society (2000). Cancer facts & figures 2000. Atlanta, GA.

Amella, E.J. (2004). Presentation of illness in older adults. *AJN*, 104(10):40–51.

Barry, M. (2000). How growth factors help chronic wounds heal. *Nursing2000*, 30(5):52–53.

Bayard, M., et al. (2004). Alcohol withdrawal syndrome. *Am Fam Physician*, 69(6):1443–1450.

Brenner, Z.R. (1999). Preventing postoperative complications: What's old, what's new, what's tried-and-true. *Nursing99*, 29(10):34–39.

Bridges, K.J., Trujillo, E.B., and Jacobs, D.O. (1999). Nutrition: Alcohol-related thiamine deficiency and malnutrition. *Crit Care Nurse*, 19(6):80–85.

Brown, M.K., and Worobec, F. (2000). Hypodermoclysis: Another way to replace fluids. *Nursing2000*, 30(5):58–59.

Chau Patel, CT, et al. (2000). Vacuum-assisted wound closure. *AJN*, 100(12):45–48.

Clinical Rounds: Wound closure. *Nursing2000*, 30(5):62.

Cowley, C. (2003). Pain and chronic illness. *Business briefing: Long-term healthcare strategies*.

Creechan, T. (2000). Combining mechanical ventilation with hospice care in the home: Death with dignity. *Crit Care Nurse*, 20(3):49.

Daus, C. (1999). Maintaining mobility: Assistive equipment helps the geriatric population stay active and independent. *Rehab Manage*, 12(5):58–61.

Deering, C.G., and Jennings, D. (2002). Communicating with children and adolescents. *AJN*, 102 (3):34.

Derby, S.A. (1999). Opioid conversion guidelines for managing adult cancer pain. *AJN*, 99(10):62–65.

Dest, V.M. (2000). Oncology today: New horizons—Colorectal cancer. *RN*, 63(3):54–59.

DiMaria-Ghalili, R.A., and Amella, E. (2005). Nutrition in older adults. *AJN*, 105(3):50.

Egan, K.A., and Arnold, R.L. (2003). Grief and bereavement care. *AJN*, 103(9):42–52.

Ewing, J.A. (1984). Detecting alcoholism: The CAGE questionnaire. *JAMA*, 252:1905–1907.

Ferrell, B., Coyne, P., and Uman, G. (2000). End-of-life care: Nurses speak out. *Nursing2000*, 30(7):54–57.

Furman, J. (2000). Taking a holistic approach to the dying time. *Nursing2000*, 30(6):46.

Gaguski, M.E. (1999). A private place: Consolation for grieving families. *AJN*, 99(4):18.

Giarelli, E., Pisano, R., and McCorkle, R. (2000). Stable and able. *AJN*, 100(12):26.

Ginther, G. (1999). Schuckit Address State of the Art Addiction Treatments. *Psychiatric Times*, April, Vol XVI. Issue 4.

Granholm, E., et al. (2003). Tropicamide effects on pupil size and pupillary light reflexes in Alzheimer's and Parkinson's disease. *Int J Psychophysiol*, 47:95–115.

Gray-Vickery, P. (2000). Combating abuse, Part 1: Protecting the older adult. *Nursing2000*, 30(7):34–38.

Grogan, T.A. (1999). Bringing bloodless surgery into the mainstream. *Nursing99*, 29(11):58–61.

Halmi, K.A., Eckert, E. Marchi, P, et al. (1991). Comorbidity of psychiatric diagnoses in anorexia nervosa. *Arch Gen Psychiatry*, 48:712–718.

Henderson-Martin, B. (2000). No more surprises: Screening patients for alcohol abuse. *AJN*, 100(9):26–32.

Hess, C.T. (1999). Wound care: When to use hydrocolloid dressings. *Nursing99*, 29(11):20.

Hess, C.T. (2000). Wound care: When to use composite dressings. *Nursing2000*, 30(5):26.

Horn L.B. (2000). Reducing the risk of falls in the elderly. *Rehab Manage*, 13(5):36–38/96.

Kearney, K. (2000). Hyperkalemia. *AJN*, 100(1):55–56.

Kirckhoff, K.T., et al. (2000). Intensive care nurses' experiences with end-of-life care. *Am J Crit Care*, 9(1):36.

Kleinbeck, S (1999). Development of the perioperative nursing data set. *AORN* J, 70(1):15–28.

Komurcu, S., et al. (2000). Common symptoms in advanced cancer. *Semin Oncol*, 27(1):24–33.

Mazanec, P., and Tyler, M.K. (2003). Cultural considerations in end-of-life care. *AJN*, 103(3):50–57.

McKee, R.J. (1999). Clarifying advance directives. *Nursing99*, 29(5):52.

Nelson, K., et al. (2000). Common complications of advanced cancer. *Semin Oncol*, 27(1):34–44.

Ott, B.B. (1999). Advance directives: The emerging body of research. *Am J Crit Care*, 8(1):514–519.

Panke, J.T. (2002). Difficulties in managing pain at the end of life. *AJN*, 102(7):26–33.

Pasero, C, and McCaffery, M. (1999). Pain control: Using agonist-antagonist opioids and antagonist drugs. *AJN*, 99(1):20–23.

Pitorak, E.F. (2003). Care at the time of death. *AJN*, 103(7):42–52.

Sachse, D.S. (2000). Emergency: Delirium tremens. *AJN*, 100(5):41–42.

Salati, D.S. (2004). Caring for a sick child in a nonpediatric setting. *Nursing2004*, 34(4):54–61.

Scanlon, C. (2003). Ethical concerns in end-of-life care. *AJN*, 103(1):48–53.

Schiffman, R.F. (2004). Drug and substance use in adolescents. *MCN Am J Matern Child Nurs*, 29(1):21–27.

Schmidt, T.C. (2000). New eye on diagnostics: Assessing a sodium and fluid imbalance. *Nursing2000*, 30(1):18.

Schutzius, P. (1999). Update on wound care. *Rehab Manage*, 12(6):30–34.

Sheehan, D.K., and Schirm, V. (2003). End-of-life care of older adults. *AJN*, 103 (11):48–57.

Skokal, W. (1999). How to spot this catheter complication. *RN*, 62(10):26–28.

Smith, R. (1999). Increasing independence: Advancements in rolling walkers get clients back into the outside world. *Rehab Manage*, 12(5):62.

Snow, D. (1999). Addiction: Working with relapse. *AJN*, 99(7):69.

Sprigle, S. (2000). Prescribing pressure ulcer treatment. *Rehab Manage*, 13(5):72–77.

Star, J.H. (2000). Radiation is lonely. *RN*, 63(8):40–42.

Stewart, K.B., and Richards, A.B. (2000). Recognizing and managing your patient's alcohol abuse. *Nursing2000*, 30(2):56–59.

Stuppaeck, C.H., et al. (1994). Assessment of the alcohol withdrawal syndrome: Validity and reliability for the translated and modified Clinical Institute Withdrawal Assessment for Alcohol scale (CIWA-A). *Addiction*, 89(10):1287–1202

Tesselaar, H. (1999). Joe wanted to die alone … or so he said. *Nursing99*, 29(5):54.

Thompson, J. (2000). A practical guide to wound care. *RN*, 63(1):48–52.

Tilden, V.P. (2000). Advance directives. *AJN*, 100(12):48,.

Vassallo, B.M. (2001). The spiritual aspects of dying at home. *Holistic Nursing Practice*, 15(2):19–29.

Virani, R., and Sofer, D. (2003). Improving the quality of end-of-life care. *AJN*, 103 (5):52–60.

Wolfe, S. (2000). Are you ready for bloodless medicine? *RN*, 63(5):42–46.

Zambroski, C.H. (2004). Hospice as an alternative model of care for older patients with end-stage heart failure. *J Cardiovasc Nurs*, 19(1):76–85.

No author listed (2000). Treatment of alcoholism—Part II. *Harvard Mental Health Lett*, 16(12):1.

No author listed (2002). Disaster and trauma. *Harvard Mental Health Lett*, 18(7):1–5.

Electronic Resources

Association of periOperative Registered Nurses (AORN), Correct site surgery tool Kit..building a safer tomorrow. Available from *www.patientsafetyfirst.org*

Burns, M., and Price, J.B (2004). Delirium tremens. Article for Emedicine website. Available at *http://www.emedicine. com*

Caselli, R.J. (2005). Dementia: Overview of pharmacotherapy. Article for Emedicine website. Available at *http://www.emedicine.com*

Joint Commission on Accreditation of Healthcare Organizations. (2003). Universal protocol for preventing wrong site, wrong procedure, wrong person surgery™. Retrieved January 2005 from *http://www.jcaho.org/index.htm*

Kresevic, D.M., and Mezey. M. (2003). Asssessment of function of critical importance in acute care of older adults. Geriatric guideline. Available at National Guideline Clearinghouse *http://www.guideline.gov*

Kuljis, R.O. (2004). Alzheimer disease. Article for Emedicine website. Available at *http://www.emedicine.com*

Lyons, S.S. (2004). Fall prevention for older adults. University of Iowa Gerontological Interventions Research Center. Available at National Guideline Clearinghouse. *http://www.guideline.gov*

Munetz, M.R., and Benjamin, S. (1988). How to examine patients using the Abnormal Involuntary Movement Scale. *Hosp Commun Psychiatry*, 39(11):1172–1177. Reference Courtesy of the Virtual En-psychlopedia by Dr. Bob *http://www.dr-bob.org*

University of Iowa Gerontological Interventions Research Center (2002). Oral hygiene care for functionally dependent and cognitively impaired older adults. Available at National Guideline Clearinghouse *http://www.guideline.gov*

University of Texas at Austin, School of Nursing, Family Nurse Practitioner Program. (2004). Initiating exercise in adults with chronic illness. Available at National Guideline Clearinghouse *http://www.guideline.gov*

INDEX OF NURSING DIAGNOSES

R

S

T

U

V

W

GORDON'S FUNCTIONAL HEALTH PATTERNS*

HEALTH PERCEPTION—HEALTH MANAGEMENT PATTERN

Health-seeking behaviors (specify)
Ineffective health maintenance Ineffective therapeutic regimen management
Effective therapeutic regimen management
Ineffective family therapeutic regimen management
Ineffective community therapeutic regimen management
Readiness for enhanced therapeutic regimen management
Noncompliance (specify)
Risk for infection Risk for injury (trauma) [this refers to 2 NDs]
Risk for falls
Risk for perioperative positioning injury
Risk for poisoning Risk for suffocation Ineffective protection
Disturbed energy field
Sudden infant death syndrome

NUTRITIONAL-METABOLIC PATTERN

Imbalanced nutrition: more than body requirements
Risk for imbalanced nutrition: more than body requirements
Imbalanced nutrition: less than body requirements
Readiness for enhanced nutrition
Adult failure to thrive
Ineffective breastfeeding
Interrupted breastfeeding
Effective breastfeeding Ineffective infant feeding pattern
Impaired swallowing
Nausea
Risk for aspiration
Impaired oral mucous membrane
Impaired dentition
Deficient fluid volume
Risk for deficient fluid volume
Excess fluid volume
Risk for imbalanced fluid volume
Readiness for enhanced fluid balance
Impaired skin integrity
Risk for impaired skin integrity
Impaired tissue integrity (specify type)
Latex allergy response
Risk for latex allergy response
Ineffective thermoregulation
Hyperthermia Hypothermia Risk for imbalanced body temperature

ELIMINATION PATTERN

Constipation
Perceived constipation Risk for constipation Diarrhea
Bowel incontinence
Impaired urinary elimination Readiness for enhanced urinary elimination
Functional urinary incontinence Reflex urinary incontinence
Stress urinary incontinence
Urge urinary incontinence Risk for urge urinary incontinence
Total incontinence
Urinary retention

ACTIVITY-EXERCISE PATTERN

Activity intolerance Risk for activity intolerance Fatigue
Deficient diversonal activity Impaired physical mobility Impaired bed mobility
Impaired transfer ability
Impaired wheelchair mobility
Impaired walking Wandering
Risk for disuse syndrome
Self-care deficit (specify: bathing/hygiene, dressing/grooming, feeding, toileting)
Delayed surgical recovery Delayed growth and development
Risk for delayed development
Risk for disproportionate growth
Impaired home maintenance
Dysfunctional ventilatory weaning response
Impaired spontaneous ventilation
Ineffective airway clearance
Ineffective breathing pattern
Impaired gas exchange
Decreased cardiac output
Ineffective tissue perfusion (specify)
Autonomic dysreflexia
Risk for autonomic dysreflexia
Disorganized infant behavior
Risk for disorganized infant behavior
Readiness for enhanced organized infant behavior
Risk for peripheral neurovascular dysfunction
Decreased intracranial adaptive capacity
Sedentary lifestyle

SLEEP-REST PATTERN

Disturbed sleep pattern Sleep deprivation
Readiness for enhanced sleep

COGNITIVE-PERCEPTUAL PATTERN

Acute pain
Chronic pain
Disturbed sensory perception (specify) Unilateral neglect
Deficient knowledge (specify)
Readiness for enhanced knowledge (specify)
Disturbed thought processes
Acute confusion
Chronic confusion
Impaired environmental interpretation syndrome
Impaired memory Decisional conflict (specify)

SELF-PERCEPTION-SELF-CONCEPT PATTERN

Fear
Anxiety
Death anxiety Risk for loneliness
Hopelessness
Powerlessness
Risk for powerlessness
Readiness for enhanced self-concept
Situational low self-esteem Risk for situational low self-esteem
Chronic low self-esteem
Body image disturbed
Disturbed personal identity
Risk for violence, self-directed

ROLE-RELATIONSHIP PATTERN

Anticipatory grieving
Dysfunctional grieving
Risk for dysfunctional grieving Chronic sorrow
Ineffective role performance
Social isolation
Impaired social interaction
Relocation stress syndrome Risk for relocation stress syndrome
Interrupted family processes
Dysfunctional family processes: alcoholism
Readiness for enhanced family processes
Impaired parenting
Risk for impaired parenting Readiness for enhanced parenting
Parental role conflict Risk for impaired parent/infant/child attachment
Caregiver role strain
Risk for caregiver role strain Impaired verbal communication
Readiness for enhanced communication
Risk for violence directed at others

SEXUALITY-REPRODUCTIVE

Ineffective sexuality patterns
Sexual dysfunction
Rape-trauma syndrome
Rape-trauma syndrome: compound reaction Rape-trauma syndrome: silent reaction

COPING-STRESS TOLERANCE PATTERN

Ineffective coping
Readiness for enhanced coping
Defensive coping Compromised family coping Disabled family coping
Readiness for enhanced family coping
Ineffective community coping Readiness for enhanced community coping
Ineffective denial
Impaired adjustment Post-trauma syndrome Risk for post-trauma syndrome Risk for suicide
Self-mutilation Risk for self-mutilation

VALUE-BELIEF PATTERN

Impaired religiosity Risk for impaired religiosity
Readiness for enhanced religiosity Spiritual distress
Risk for spiritual distress Readiness for enhanced spiritual well-being